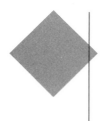

Critical Care
of Infants and Children

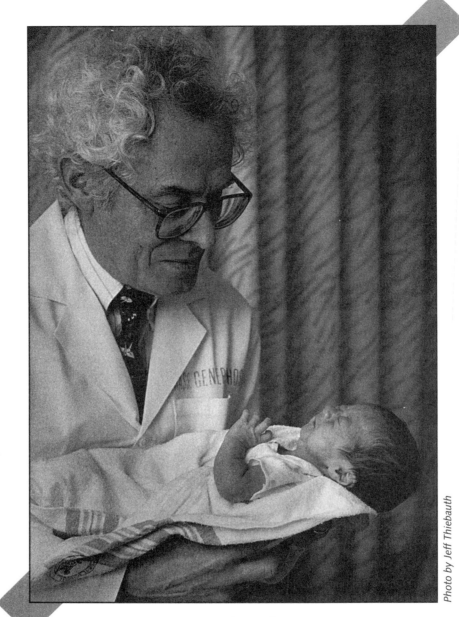

I. David Todres

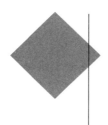

Critical Care
of Infants and Children

Edited by

I. David Todres, M.D.
Associate Professor of Anaesthesia and Pediatrics
Harvard Medical School
Director, Pediatric Critical Care Medicine
Massachusetts General Hospital
Boston

and

John H. Fugate, M.D.
Medical Director, Pediatric Intensive Care
Children's Health Care—Minneapolis

Foreword by
Donald N. Medearis, Jr., M.D.
Professor Emeritus of Pediatrics
Harvard Medical School
Former Chief, Pediatric Service,
Massachusetts General Hospital
Boston

Little, Brown and Company
Boston New York Toronto London

Notice

The indications and dosages of all drugs in this book have been recommended in the medical literature and conform to the practices of the general medical community. The medications described do not necessarily have specific approval by the Food and Drug Administration for use in the diseases and dosages for which they are recommended. The package insert for each drug should be consulted for use and dosage as approved by the FDA. Because standards for usage change, it is advisable to keep abreast of revised recommendations, particularly those concerning new drugs.

Library of Congress Cataloging-in-Publication Data

Critical care of infants and children / I. David Todres, John H. Fugate [editors].
   p. cm.
  Includes bibliographical references and index.
  ISBN 0-316-85020-9
  1. Pediatric intensive care.   2. Pediatric emergencies.
I. Todres, I. David. II. Fugate, John H.
  [DNLM: 1. Critical Care—in infancy & childhood. WS 366 C932 1996]
RJ370.C73 1996
618.92′0028—dc20
DNLM/DLC
for Library of Congress   95-46923
                                                      CIP

Printed in the United States of America
MV-NY

Editorial: Nancy E. Chorpenning
Production Supervisor: Mike Burggren
Cover Designer: Mike Burggren
Cover Illustration: Stephanie Schilling

To our wives and children
Judith and Hillel
and
Carolyn, Jason, and Jonathan

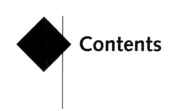

Contents

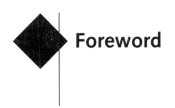 # Foreword

It was almost 30 years ago when Dr. Peter Safar, then Professor and Chairman of the Department of Anesthesiology at the University of Pittsburgh, and I discussed creating a critical care unit at the Children's Hospital of Pittsburgh (at the time I was Chairman of Pediatrics and Medical Director there). Peter had been responsible for significant advances in resuscitation when he was at Baltimore City Hospital and Johns Hopkins.[1] Moreover, in 1958 at Baltimore City Hospital, he had established what was probably the first multidisciplinary intensive care unit in the world, according to Dr. John J. Downes.[2] Dr. Downes also noted, of course, that such events are preceded by other important developments, such as postanesthesia recovery rooms, which appeared in the 1950s. In 1961, Drs. Henning Pontoppidan, Hendrick Bendixen, and Myron Laver established a respiratory intensive care unit at the Massachusetts General Hospital. When Dr. Safar moved to Pittsburgh, he first established an intensive care unit for the care of adult patients at Presbyterian University Hospital. Our discussion occurred about 1968. Beginning then, we upgraded a postoperative surgical unit that provided special nursing care by having critical care medicine fellows from Dr. Safar's program at Presbyterian University Hospital rotate through our pediatric ICU. In 1969, we established a 10-bed ICU and appointed Dr. Stephan Kampschulte its full-time director. According to Dr. Downes, this was only the second pediatric intensive care unit in the United States, the first being the one that Dr. Downes had established at the Children's Hospital of Philadelphia in 1967. Dr. Downes further noted that, insofar as he could determine, the world's first pediatric intensive care unit that was multidisciplinary and physician directed was established at the Children's Hospital of Göteborg, Sweden in 1955. Drs. Daniel Shannon and David Todres established the PICU at the Massachusetts General Hospital in 1971. I am greatly indebted to Dr. Safar for his leadership, his refreshing my memory about these events, and very significantly enlarging my information base about the development of critical care in pediatrics. I want to acknowledge the superb leadership that Dr. Kampschulte provided in this field in Pittsburgh and subsequently in Europe. In this foreword I felt it was entirely appropriate and just to pay great tribute to the pioneers in this important field.

An immense amount of new information, and thus new ways to support, comfort, and cure, has accumulated in the quarter-century since those first units were established. A lot of this information is shared with readers of this book through the expertise of the outstanding group of individuals whom Dr. Todres has recruited to write this text. Dr. Todres is outstandingly well-qualified to editorially orchestrate such an effort. Boarded in Pediatrics and Anesthesiology, he has also earned sub-Board certification in Neonatology and in Critical Care, and he was recently honored by the American Academy of Pediatrics Subspecialty of Critical Care Medicine as

the first recipient of its Distinguished Career Award. Thus, I feel both highly pleased and privileged to have been asked by David to write this foreword.

This opportunity has given me the chance to express my admiration and appreciation to those who have developed the field of pediatric intensive care and its near relative, those who provide intensive care for the newborn, and especially those who have done it here. In our institution, the two units (NICU and PICU) are geographically contiguous, and this has provided for a remarkably productive interchange. That relationship was fostered by those who created it: Doctors Shannon, Talbot, Todres, and Kitz. Whether that relationship can continue as these fields continue to develop is a challenge, as it is in the other linkages I will outline. So with my tribute I also offer a challenge.

Because of the remarkable advances in pharmacology, physiology, and pathophysiology, as well as the support systems that have been developed to sustain the life-threatened child, we have a great need to develop better ways for cardiologists, gastroenterologists, nephrologists, pulmonologists, and others not only to bring their expertise to the bedside of the patient, but to integrate, focus, and prioritize that knowledge to the end of providing better care. I believe that this is the most significant challenge ahead for all pediatricians. That challenge is not unique to those who provide the wonderful services of intensivists that have enabled so many infants and children to survive and subsequently to live productive lives. It applies equally to all aspects of care, primary to quaternary, emergency to rehabilitational. We must link the various system-oriented subspecialists to the intensivist, the intensivist to the emergency transport (as is emphasized in this text), and both of these to rehabilitational services (which ideally should begin much earlier than is our current practice). All must work to achieve an integration of the vast amount of information needed to provide curative and restorative care to the critically ill child. After the next quarter-century, someone may tell that tale. I hope it will be one of success.

In closing, I again extend my admiration and appreciation to those who contributed to this outstanding text, and I wish to those who read it success in their efforts to learn in order to help infants and children.

Donald N. Medearis, Jr., MD

References

1. Safar, P: Initiation of closed-chest cardiopulmonary resuscitation basic life support. A personal history, *Resuscitation 18* (1989) 7-20.
2. Downes, JJ: The historical evolution, current status, and prospective development of pediatric critical care. *Critical Care Clinics 8:1* (1992) 1-22.

 # Preface

Intensivists caring for infants and children with a critical illness must acquire the knowledge and management skills required to support the child and the family through the crisis. These objectives are met through our understanding of the pathophysiology of disease, the application of the principles of applied physiology and pharmacology, and the psychosocial dynamics of critical illness. *Critical Care of Infants and Children* has been edited with this focus in mind. With the assistance of an outstanding group of contributors, we have selected material that will assist the physician's understanding of the specific diseased organ system pathology, the appropriate therapeutic management, and the ethical and psychosocial impact of critical illness.

Although the text is primarily directed at the pediatric patient beyond the newborn stage, we have emphasized aspects of neonatal medicine where it is particularly relevant to the practice of pediatric critical care.

An important aspect of care of the critically ill infant and child is the ability to perform selected technical procedures that assist in providing sophisticated monitoring, diagnosis, and therapy. Hence, the procedures section has received detailed attention with text and illustrations to guide the physician in performing these procedures. We have approached procedures from the viewpoint of not only "what to do" but also "what to avoid," as the latter is critical in ensuring that the procedure is performed safely. Diseases of the cardiac, respiratory, neurological, and renal systems are major components of the problems relating to critical illness; these sections, therefore, have been given additional emphasis. Psychosocial and ethical aspects are dealt with in depth because the successful support of a critically ill child requires healing of the child not only physiologically but also emotionally. In addition, family dynamics are stressed, as they are an integral part of the child's care. We have repeated selected material to provide the reader with the opportunity for a more integrated analysis of the problem without the need for multiple references to other chapters.

We trust *Critical Care of Infants and Children* will not only prove helpful to intensivists in training but that seasoned intensivists might find the text helpful in teaching students and residents. We trust, too, that pediatricians, emergency room physicians, anesthesiologists, and surgeons will find sections of the text of assistance to them as it relates to specific areas of their concern.

We are grateful to the contributors for their commitment to this effort. We appreciate the support and encouragement of Nancy Chorpenning and Rob Stuart of Little, Brown. Eva Panzera provided valuable assistance by "gently" coaxing the contributors and helping to organize the material.

I.D.T.
J.H.F.

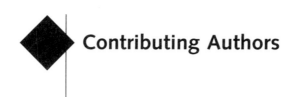

Contributing Authors

Olugbenga A. Akingbola, M.D.
Faculty, Department of Pediatrics, Louisiana State University
School of Medicine in New Orleans

Angela Anderson, M.D.
Assistant Professor of Pediatrics, Brown University School of
Medicine; Attending Physician, Pediatric Emergency Medicine,
Hasbro Children's Hospital and Rhode Island Hospital,
Providence, Rhode Island

Lisa Arguin, B.S.B.M.E.
Clinical Engineering Manager, Department of Respiratory Care,
Massachusetts General Hospital, Boston

John H. Arnold, M.D.
Assistant Professor of Anaesthesia and Pediatrics, Harvard Medical
School; Medical Director, Respiratory Care, Department of
Anesthesia, The Children's Hospital, Boston

Charles B. Berde, M.D.
Professor of Anaesthesia, Harvard Medical School; Director, Pain
Treatment Center, The Children's Hospital, Boston

Susan E. Briggs, M.D.
Assistant Professor of Surgery, Harvard Medical School; Associate
Visiting Surgeon, Massachusetts General Hospital, Boston

Thomas V. Brogan, M.D.
Fellow, Pediatric Intensive Care Unit, Department of
Anesthesiology and Critical Care Medicine, University of
Washington School of Medicine and Children's Hospital and
Medical Center, Seattle

Dorothy I. Bulas, M.D.
Associate Professor of Diagnostic Imaging and Radiology, George
Washington University School of Medicine and Health Sciences;
Staff Radiologist, Children's Hospital National Medical Center,
Washington, D.C.

Joan Burg, M.D.
Assistant Professor of Surgery and Pediatrics, Stanford University
School of Medicine; Associate Director, Pediatric Emergency
Medicine, Stanford University Hospital, Stanford, California

Leticia Castillo, M.D.
Assistant Professor of Pediatrics, Harvard Medical School; Associate
Director, Pediatric Intensive Care Unit, Massachusetts General
Hospital, Boston

Elizabeth A. Catlin, M.D.
Assistant Professor of Pediatrics, Harvard Medical School; Chief
of Neonatology, Massachusetts General Hospital, Boston

Paul H. Chapman, M.D.
Associate Professor of Surgery, Harvard Medical School; Chief of
Pediatric Neurosurgery, Massachusetts General Hospital, Boston

Grace T. Clancy, R.N., M.S.
Clinical Nurse Specialist, Neonatal Intensive Care Unit,
Massachusetts General Hospital, Boston

Charles J. Coté, M.D.
Professor of Anesthesia and Pediatrics, Northwestern University
Medical School; Vice Chairman and Director of Research,
Department of Pediatric Anesthesia, The Children's Memorial
Hospital, Chicago

Michael J. Cunningham, M.D.
Assistant Professor of Otology and Laryngology, Harvard Medical
School; Associate Surgeon, Department of Otolaryngology,
Massachusetts Eye and Ear Infirmary, Boston

Alice A. Curnin, L.I.C.S.W.
Clinical Social Worker, Pediatrics, Massachusetts General
Hospital, Boston

Joseph R. Custer, M.D.
Associate Professor of Pediatrics, University of Michigan Medical
School; Director, Critical Care Medicine, The University of
Michigan Hospitals, Ann Arbor, Michigan

Marco Danon, M.D.
Associate Professor of Pediatrics, State University of New York
Health Science Center at Brooklyn College of Medicine; Director,
Pediatric Endocrinology, Maimonides Medical Center, Brooklyn,
New York

Daniel Doody, M.D.
Assistant Professor of Surgery, Harvard Medical School; Associate
Surgeon, Pediatric Surgery, Massachusetts General Hospital,
Boston

Elizabeth C. Dooling, M.D.
Associate Professor of Neurology, Harvard Medical School;
Neurologist and Associate Pediatrician, Massachusetts General
Hospital, Boston

Morris Earle, Jr., M.D., M.P.H.
Instructor of Pediatrics, Harvard Medical School; Attending
Physician, Pediatric Critical Care Division, Massachusetts General
Hospital, Boston

Roland D. Eavey, M.D.
Associate Professor of Otology and Laryngology, Harvard Medical
School; Director, Pediatric Otolaryngology, Massachusetts Eye and
Ear Infirmary, Boston

E. Marsha Elixson, R.N.C., M.S.
Pediatric Cardiovascular Clinical Nurse Specialist, Massachusetts
General Hospital, Boston

Robert Englander, M.D.
Assistant Professor of Pediatrics, University of Maryland School of
Medicine, Baltimore

Patricia English, M.S., R.R.T.
Respiratory Therapist, Massachusetts General Hospital, Boston

Lars C. Erickson, M.D.
Instructor of Pediatrics, Harvard Medical School; Assistant Pediatrician, Pediatric Cardiology Unit, Massachusetts General Hospital, Boston

Ellen R. Feldman, L.I.C.S.W.
Clinical Social Worker, Massachusetts General Hospital, Boston

William S. Ferguson, M.D.
Instructor of Pediatrics, Harvard Medical School; Chief of Pediatric Hematology-Oncology Unit, Massachusetts General Hospital, Boston

Joseph J. Frassica, M.D.
Associate Professor of Pediatrics and Anesthesia, University of Massachusetts Medical School, Director, Pediatric Critical Care, UMASS Medical Center, Worcester

John H. Fugate, M.D.
Medical Director, Pediatric Critical Care, Children's Health Care—Minneapolis

Jeremy M. Geiduschek, M.D.
Assistant Professor of Anesthesiology, University of Washington School of Medicine; Attending Physician, Anesthesiology and Intensive Care, Children's Hospital and Medical Center, Seattle

Brahm Goldstein, M.D.
Associate Professor of Pediatrics, Oregon Health Sciences University School of Medicine; Chief of Critical Care, Department of Pediatrics, Doernbecher Memorial Hospital for Children, Portland, Oregon

Nishan Goudsouzian, M.D.
Associate Professor of Anaesthesia, Harvard Medical School; Director, Pediatric Anesthesia, Massachusetts General Hospital, Boston

Kristy M. Hendricks, R.D., Sc.D.
Ruby Winslow Linn Professor of Nutrition, Simmons College; Nutrition Support Service, The Children's Hospital, Boston

John T. Herrin, M.B.B.S., F.R.A.C.P.
Associate Clinical Professor of Pediatrics, Harvard Medical School; Director, Clinical Services, Division of Nephrology, The Children's Hospital, Boston

David Herzog, M.D.
Associate Professor of Psychiatry, Harvard Medical School; Chief, Child Psychiatry Consultation Liaison Service, Massachusetts General Hospital, Boston

Dean Hess, R.R.T., Ph.D.
Instructor of Anaesthesia, Harvard Medical School; Research Coordinator, Respiratory Care, Massachusetts General Hospital, Boston

Sarah J. Ilstrup, M.D.
Assistant Professor of Laboratory Medicine and Pathology, University of Minnesota Medical School—Minneapolis; Medical Director, Blood Bank Donor Center, University of Minnesota Hospital and Clinic of the University of Minnesota Health Science Center, Minneapolis

Michael S. Jellinek, M.D.
Associate Professor of Psychiatry (Pediatrics), Harvard Medical School; Chief, Child Psychiatry Service, Massachusetts General Hospital, Boston

Robert Kacmarek, Ph.D.
Assistant Professor of Anaesthesia, Harvard Medical School; Director, Respiratory Care Services, Massachusetts General Hospital, Boston

Harry J. Kallas, M.D.
Assistant Professor of Clinical Pediatrics, University of California, Davis, School of Medicine, Davis, California; Associate Director, Pediatric Critical Care Medicine, University of California, Davis, Medical Center, Sacramento, California

William M. Kauffman, M.D.
Assistant Professor of Diagnostic Imaging, University of Tennessee, Memphis, College of Medicine; Diagnostic Imaging, Saint Jude Children's Research Hospital, Memphis, Tennessee

Mary Etta E. King, M.D.
Assistant Professor of Pediatrics, Harvard Medical School; Director, Pediatric Echocardiography, Massachusetts General Hospital, Boston

Monica Kleinman, M.D.
Assistant Professor of Pediatrics, Brown University School of Medicine; Director, Pediatric Transport Services, Department of Pediatric Critical Care, Rhode Island Hospital, Providence, Rhode Island

Ronald E. Kleinman, M.D.
Associate Professor of Pediatrics, Harvard Medical School; Chief of Pediatric GI and Nutrition, Massachusetts General Hospital, Boston

Elliot J. Krane, M.D.
Professor of Anesthesiology, Stanford University, Stanford, California; Chief of Anesthesiology, Packard Children's Hospital at Stanford, Palo Alto, California

Kalpathy S. Krishnamoorthy, M.D.
Assistant Professor of Neurology and Pediatrics, Harvard Medical School; Associate Neurologist and Associate Pediatrician, Massachusetts General Hospital, Boston

Steve Kurachek, M.D.
Medical Director, Pediatric Intensive Care Unit, Children's Health Care—Minneapolis

David C. Kushner, M.D.
Professor of Radiology and Pediatrics, George Washington University School of Medicine and Health Sciences; Chairman, Department of Diagnostic Imaging and Radiology, Children's Hospital National Medical Center, Washington, D.C.

Peter Lang, M.D.
Associate Professor of Pediatrics, Harvard Medical School; Chief, Department of Pediatric Cardiology, Massachusetts General Hospital, Boston

Richard R. Liberthson, M.D.
Associate Professor of Pediatrics, Harvard Medical School; Pediatrician and Associate Physician, Massachusetts General Hospital, Boston

David Link, M.D.
Assistant Professor of Pediatrics, Harvard Medical School, Boston; Chief of Pediatrics, The Cambridge Hospital and Mount Auburn Hospital, Cambridge, Massachusetts

Alejandro López, M.D.
Clinical Fellow, Pediatric Cardiology, Massachusetts General Hospital, Boston

Denise Lozowski, R.N.
Clinical Pediatric Nurse Specialist, Massachusetts General Hospital, Boston

Ruth Lynfield, M.D.
Instructor of Pediatrics, Harvard Medical School; Assistant, Department of Pediatrics, Massachusetts General Hospital, Boston

M. Claire McManus, Pharm.D.
Clinical Assistant Professor of Pharmacy Practice, Bouvé College of Pharmacy and Health Sciences, Northeastern University; Clinical Pharmacy Specialist in Pediatrics, St. Elizabeth's Hospital, Boston

Tracie L. Miller, M.D.
Assistant Professor of Pediatrics, Harvard Medical School; Assistant in Gastroenterology, The Children's Hospital, Boston

Melinda Morin, M.D.
Clinical Instructor of Pediatrics, Harvard Medical School; Fellow, Department of Pediatric Critical Care, Massachusetts General Hospital, Boston

Natan Noviski, M.D.
Director, Pediatric Intensive Care Unit, The Edith Wolfson Hospital, Holon, Israel

Patricia O'Malley, M.D.
Assistant Professor of Pediatrics, Harvard Medical School; Director, Pediatric Emergency Services, Massachusetts General Hospital, Boston

Kristen Outwater, M.D.
Department of Pediatrics, Michigan State College of Human Medicine, Lansing, Michigan; Attending Physician, Pediatric Intensive Care Unit, St. Luke's Hospital, Saginaw, Michigan

Mark Pasternack, M.D.
Associate Professor of Pediatrics, Harvard Medical School; Chief, Pediatric Infectious Disease, Massachusetts General Hospital, Boston

James M. Perrin, M.D.
Associate Professor of Pediatrics, Harvard Medical School; Director, Ambulatory Care Programs and General Pediatrics, Massachusetts General Hospital, Boston

Elizabeth H. Perry, M.D.
Assistant Professor of Laboratory Medicine and Pathology, University of Minnesota Medical School—Minneapolis; Assistant Director, Memorial Blood Centers of Minnesota, Minneapolis

Myron B. Peterson, M.D., Ph.D.
Associate Professor of Pediatrics, Tufts University School of Medicine; Director, Pediatric Critical Care, New England Medical Center, Boston

Ruth Purtilo, Ph.D.
Interim Director and Professor, Center for Health Policy and Ethics, Creighton University School of Medicine, Omaha, Nebraska

Karen F. Rothman, M.D.
Assistant Professor of Medicine and Pediatrics, University of Massachusetts Medical School, Worcester, Massachusetts

Gary J. Russell, M.D.
Assistant Professor of Pediatrics, Harvard Medical School; Assistant in Pediatrics, Massachusetts General Hospital, Boston

William E. Russell, M.D.
Associate Professor of Pediatrics and Cell Biology, Vanderbilt University School of Medicine; Attending Physician, Children's Hospital of Vanderbilt University Medical Center, Nashville, Tennessee

Daniel P. Ryan, M.D.
Assistant Professor of Surgery, Harvard Medical School; Associate Surgeon, Department of Pediatric Surgery, Massachusetts General Hospital, Boston

John Ryan, M.D.
Associate Professor of Anaesthesia, Harvard Medical School; Anesthetist, Massachusetts General Hospital, Boston

Andrew L. Salzman, M.D.
Assistant Professor, University of Cincinnati College of Medicine; Director, Division of Critical Care Medicine, Children's Hospital Medical Center, Cincinnati

Kenneth R. Scheublin, M.S.W.
Unit Manager, Pediatrics and Obstetrics, Social Service Department, Massachusetts General Hospital, Boston

Daniel C. Shannon, M.D.
Professor of Pediatrics, Harvard Medical School, Boston; Professor of Health Science, Massachusetts Institute of Technology, Cambridge, Massachusetts; Chief, Department of Pediatric Pulmonology, Massachusetts General Hospital, Boston

Michael Shannon, M.D., M.P.H.
Associate Professor of Pediatrics, Harvard Medical School; Associate, Department of Medicine, The Children's Hospital, Boston

Carlos J. Sivit, M.D.
Associate Professor of Radiology, Case Western Reserve University School of Medicine; Director, Division of Pediatric Radiology, University Hospitals of Cleveland, Cleveland

Brenda Stewart, R.N., C.C.R.N.
Organ and Tissue Donation Coordinator, Intensive Care Nursing Service/Transplant, Massachusetts General Hospital, Boston

Brooke Swearingen, M.D.
Assistant Professor of Neurosurgery, Harvard Medical School; Assistant Visiting Professor, Neurosurgical Service, Massachusetts General Hospital, Boston

I. David Todres, M.D.
Associate Professor of Anaesthesia and Pediatrics, Harvard Medical School; Director, Pediatric Critical Care Medicine, Massachusetts General Hospital, Boston

Timothy P. Trompeter, M.D.
Chairman, Department of Pediatrics, Sequoia Hospital, Redwood City, California

John T. Truman, M.D., M.P.H.
Professor of Clinical Pediatrics, Columbia University College of Physicians and Surgeons, New York; Chairman, Department of Pediatrics, Morristown Memorial Hospital, Morristown, New Jersey

Thomas L. Truman, M.D.
Clinical Instructor of Pediatrics, Harvard Medical School; Fellow, Pediatric Critical Care, Massachusetts General Hospital, Boston

Gus J. Vlahakes, M.D.
Associate Professor of Surgery, Harvard Medical School; Associate Visiting Surgeon, Massachusetts General Hospital, Boston

Edward P. Walsh, M.D.
Assistant Professor of Pediatrics, Harvard Medical School; Director, Electrophysiology Service, The Children's Hospital, Boston

H. Shaw Warren, M.D.
Associate Professor of Pediatrics, Harvard Medical School; Associate Pediatrician, Infectious Disease Unit, Massachusetts General Hospital, Boston

Robert H. Wharton, M.D.
Instructor of Pediatrics, Harvard Medical School; Chief of Pediatric Rehabilitation, Massachusetts General Hospital and Spaulding Rehabilitation Hospital, Boston

William Wheeler, M.D.
Medical Director, Pulmonary Diagnostic Program, Children's Health Care—Minneapolis, Minneapolis

James W. Ziegler, M.D.
Assistant Professor of Pediatrics, Brown University School of Medicine; Hasbro Children's Hospital, Pediatric Cardiology, Providence, Rhode Island

Critical Care
of Infants and Children

I ◆ Emergent Evaluation, Management, and Procedures

I. David Todres
Patricia O'Malley
Monica Kleinman

1 Cardiopulmonary Resuscitation

Cardiopulmonary arrest results in the total cessation of oxygen delivery and perfusion to the vital organs of the body. To be successful, cardiopulmonary resuscitation (CPR), or the temporary support of heart and lung function, must be accomplished within minutes while treatment is directed toward restoration of spontaneous circulation. Of necessity, guidelines for pediatric resuscitation have been often derived from adult and animal experience, sometimes without appreciation of the special circumstances imposed by cardiopulmonary arrest in the infant or child. Our best efforts in the apneic and pulseless child may result in resumption of heart and lung function too late or too ineffectively to ensure resuscitation of a normal child. The primary goals of CPR are to maintain myocardial and cerebral perfusion; thus, CPR should be viewed in the context of cardiopulmonary-cerebral resuscitation.

Historical Background

The history of cardiopulmonary resuscitation until the present century makes scant reference to pediatric patients. There is, however, a biblical reference (2 Kings 4:34–35) that suggests the first documented successful mouth-to-mouth resuscitation when Elisha the prophet resuscitated a child: "And he went up, and lay upon the child, and put his mouth upon his mouth, and his eyes upon his eyes, and his hands upon his hands; and he stretched himself upon the child; and the flesh of the child waxed warm."

Successful mouth-to-mouth resuscitation is reported in the treatment of newborn infants in the early part of the nineteenth century. However, physicians abandoned this method because of fear of contracting a contagious disease from a technique that was also perceived as aesthetically vulgar. In addition, it was thought that the carbon dioxide in expired air would have harmful effects on the victim. Thus, except for continued use by midwives, mouth-to-mouth resuscitation was abandoned until its recommendation in 1958 by the National Academy of Sciences as the optimal choice for emergency resuscitation.

Early resuscitation techniques emphasized mechanical means to stimulate breathing. Resuscitation of the depressed infant involved exposure to cold air and stimulation of the infant's skin. The infant was immersed in cold water and vigorously handled to stimulate afferent nerves and initiate respiratory efforts. Not infrequently the rough handling resulted in lethal organ injury. Tobacco fumes were pumped into the rectum in the belief that chemical stimulation would initiate respiratory efforts. In the early part of the twentieth century it was the practice to stimulate the drowned victim to breathe by inserting a corn cob into the rectum!

In the 1920s, Henderson attempted to apply physiological reasoning to methods for resuscitation. He advocated combining oxygen with 5% carbon dioxide because it was known at that time that carbon dioxide was a potent stimulant of the respiratory center in the brain. Henderson described a positive pressure device that provided ventilation for the depressed infant.[1] Tracheal intubation for the depressed infant was advocated by Flagg in 1928 and Blaikley and Gibberd in 1935.[2,3] Oxygen and carbon dioxide were then administered. Blaikley and Gibberd also described a procedure of forced inspiration through a face piece in an effort to cause air to enter the lungs under positive pressure.[3] However, this aggressive approach fell into disfavor and it was some years before resuscitation of the depressed infant and child became once again an active process involving positive pressure via a face mask and ventilatory apparatus (self-inflating bag) and tracheal intubation.

Support of the cardiovascular system in the form of direct cardiac massage and external cardiac massage was experimentally carried out over a hundred years ago. External cardiac massage was carried out successfully in two children (8 years and 13 years) following circulatory arrest precipitated by chloroform anesthesia.[4] In 1906, Crile described the effectiveness of external cardiac compressions in maintaining the circulation in dogs.[5] In 1960, the landmark paper by Kouwenhoven et al. reported successful external cardiac massage in 20 patients (including pediatric patients) with a 70% survival rate.[6] Their paper stated, "Anyone, anywhere can now initiate cardiac resuscitative procedures. All that is needed are two hands." In 1947, Beck successfully employed internal defibrillation of a human heart.[7] In 1956, Zoll performed the first successful external defibrillation of a human patient.[8]

Standards for CPR for infants and children are a relatively recent (1980) development, pioneered by the American Heart Association, and follow the adoption of standards for adult resuscitation.[9] These pediatric standards were revised in 1986 and 1992.[10,11] A well-defined separate pediatric advanced life support (PALS) teaching course, supported both by the American Heart Association (AHA) and the American Academy of Pediatrics, was developed in 1988.[12]

Epidemiology and Outcome of Cardiopulmonary Arrest

Although it has been noted that childhood beyond the first month of age is the healthiest period of life, 40,000 infants under 1 year of age and 16,000 children between 1 and 14 years die annually in the United States. Several studies of pediatric arrest concur with the observation that cardiopulmonary arrest is most common in the child under 2 years of life, the majority of those arrests occurring in infants under 5 months of life.[12–18] It is important to note the multitude of causes of cardiopulmonary arrest in the pediatric patient as compared with the adult. In out-of-hospital arrest, sudden infant death syndrome (SIDS), trauma from motor vehicle accidents and abuse, near-drowning, and upper airway obstruction are leading causes. In the hospital setting, respiratory infections and disorders, congenital diseases, sepsis, and dehydration are the most common. In the pediatric intensive care unit (PICU) itself, leading causes of death include hypoxic-ischemic encephalopathy, postoperative complications, mechanical misadventures, and overwhelming infection.

The most common pathophysiologic pathway leading to arrest in the infant or child involves a primary respiratory dysfunction leading to bradyarrhythmias secondary to hypoxemia, hypercarbia, and acidosis, followed by asystolic arrest. In some patients with sepsis, trauma, or dehydration, respiratory dysfunction may be accompanied or precipitated by circulatory failure. It is rare for the pediatric patient to suffer cardiac arrest from a primary cardiac problem without underlying primary cardiac disease (congenital, surgical, or infectious) or a metabolic/toxicologic problem that precipitates a dysrhythmia. Ischemic heart disease secondary to atherosclerosis, the dominant cause of cardiopulmonary arrest in the adult, is an uncommon cause of death in the pediatric population but has been described in children with Kawasaki's arteritis and anomalous coronary artery.

Published rates of mortality from cardiopulmonary arrest in the pediatric age group have varied from 60% to 95%, although definition of cardiopulmonary arrest (respiratory alone or cardio-respiratory), survival (short- or long-term), location (in- or out-of-hospital), as well as methods of resuscitation have not been comparable among studies.[12–18] Outcome is probably most dependent on underlying condition, location of arrest, and the level of support and duration of CPR required to achieve hemodynamic stability.

In a study of 47 patients, 44% of patients resuscitated in the PICU were long-term survivors as compared with 23% of patients resuscitated outside the PICU.[15] Ninety-two percent of patients requiring only airway support had good long-term outcomes. CPR lasting longer than 15 minutes produced only four out of 25 survivors. Although there are scattered reports of survivors of prolonged CPR efforts, most commonly in hypothermic arrest, it is unusual to have a good outcome following CPR for longer than 45 minutes. Of note is that neither pupillary response nor flaccidity at time of resuscitation was predictive of outcome in this study. A study of 119 out-of-hospital cardiac arrests in children revealed that sudden infant death was the most common cause (32%), with drowning the second most common (22%).[13] Seven percent of patients treated with emergency medical technician and paramedic care survived. A study of 34 patients brought to the emergency room apneic and pulseless revealed that only 21% (N = 7) survived until hospital discharge; of the seven, five remained in a vegetative state.[16] A prospective study of 105 resuscitations concluded that outcomes for respiratory arrest without cardiac arrest were reasonably good (25% mortality). However, prognosis with cardiopulmonary arrest was poor (89% mortality or severe morbidity).[14] A retrospective study of 42 cardiopulmonary arrests in a general ward of a pediatric hospital showed that respiratory arrest had a significantly better outcome than cardiopulmonary arrest, with only 9% of the cardiac arrest patients surviving. Predictors of non-survival were a duration of arrest longer than 15 minutes and administration of more than one intravenous bolus of epinephrine.[17] A study of 113 cardiac arrests in 93 children in a tertiary care children's hospital showed that cardiac arrest had a mortality rate of 90.6% compared with 32.5% for respiratory arrest.[18] The majority of the patients were less than 1 year of age and had at least one underlying chronic disease. None of the 31 cardiac arrest victims receiving more than two doses of epinephrine survived to discharge.

In a study of 38 victims of submersion found in cardiopulmonary arrest, 32% survived, with two thirds of the survivors unimpaired or mildly impaired.[19] Two risk factors noted to be associated with death or severe impairment were submersion longer than 9 minutes and cardiopulmonary resuscitation longer than 25 minutes. These outcomes are better than previously reported for the near-drowning victim and are ascribed to the prompt pre-hospital advanced cardiac life support provided for the victims. A recent review of near-drowning from the same area confirms the earlier findings; namely, that duration of submersion and resuscitation are the two most important indicators of responsiveness to resuscitation efforts.[20] The authors of this study proposed that when the duration of submersion exceeds 10 minutes or resuscitative efforts are required beyond 25 minutes, the victim should be declared dead. The dismal prognosis in victims brought to emergency depart-

ments while still undergoing CPR reflects the prolonged resuscitation times in these patients.

There are important lessons to take away from the differences between adult and pediatric arrests. First of all, pediatric arrest can frequently be anticipated in the patient with progressive respiratory insufficiency, inadequate perfusion, or severe metabolic derangement. When anticipated, cardiopulmonary collapse can potentially be prevented by early and aggressive airway support, intravascular volume support, and correction of metabolic abnormalities.

Management Overview

Although during cardiopulmonary resuscitation many tasks must be accomplished simultaneously, it is important to develop a standard approach that prioritizes tasks to be performed and ensures that important items will not be overlooked. This is particularly true in pediatric resuscitation because any single practitioner will not compile a great number of experiences with pediatric arrest, even in the setting of the PICU. This approach should be practiced on a regular basis to ensure that skills do not deteriorate and that system readiness is checked.

Recognition of cardiopulmonary arrest involves confirmation of unconsciousness by verbal and physical stimulation, absence of respirations by observation and listening, and absence of a major pulse by palpation. The orderly sequence of management then proceeds along the following lines.

Airway

A clear airway is a fundamental requirement for effective CPR. Many apparent arrests in the pediatric population are respiratory emergencies without loss of cardiac function; in these cases, simply positioning and securing the airway to provide oxygenation and ventilation may be all that is necessary to save the child's life. Head extension is the most effective maneuver in opening the airway, according to studies performed on anesthetized adults. Anterior displacement or thrust of the mandible will enhance this effect.[21] Traditional teaching about the unconscious patient has been that the tongue is displaced toward the posterior pharyngeal wall and is primarily responsible for airway obstruction. However, studies on anesthetized (i.e., unconscious) adult patients demonstrated that airway occlusion was most commonly due to displacement of the soft palate toward the posterior pharyngeal wall.[22–24] In the child undergoing CPR, displacement of the tongue, epiglottis, and soft palate toward the posterior pharyngeal wall may all contribute in various degrees to upper airway obstruction. Precisely what contributes to airway obstruction and what is most effective for its relief in children undergoing CPR require further study.

Airway control in the trauma victim with possible cervical vertebrae or spinal cord injury demands specific measures. Positioning the child on a standard backboard to stabilize the neck may be dangerous because the young child's large head places the neck in a relatively flexed position when the child is supine. Thus, during emergency transport and for radiographic examination, the child should be supported on a modified backboard that has a recess for the occiput to lower the head, or on a double mattress pad to raise the chest and shoulders, to provide correct alignment of the cervical spine. This position corresponds approximately to an alignment of the external auditory meatus with the shoulders.[25]

Although endotracheal intubation is the most secure way of providing airway control, the pediatric patient can often be managed for a period of time with bag and mask ventilation alone, particularly if care is taken to vent the stomach of air. Bag and mask ventilation with 100% oxygen via a clear airway should precede any attempt to intubate the trachea.

Future developments in controlling the airway and providing effective ventilation include the use of the laryngeal mask. This device is generally employed by anesthesiologists in the operating room setting. Studies have demonstrated that nurses trained in the use of this device achieved more effective tidal volumes using a Laerdal self-inflating system than with the conventional face mask technique.[26–28]

Ventilation

Great emphasis must be placed on assessment of effective ventilation. **If there is no chest movement, there is no ventilation.** One must **always** exclude upper airway obstruction as a possible underlying cause of inadequate ventilation.

Mouth-to-Mouth and Mouth-to-Mask Ventilation

Mouth-to-mouth and mouth-to-mask resuscitation are effective basic life support methods to achieve adequate ventilation.[29] Mouth-to-mask is becoming more acceptable because of its aesthetic appeal, as well as increasing concerns about the spread of infectious diseases. This technique has an additional advantage if the mask allows for the provision of supplemental oxygen.

Bag-Valve-Mask Devices

Bag-valve-mask (BVM) devices can be employed to ventilate the child. The self-inflating bag is the most commonly utilized and is available in sizes ranging from 240 ml to 2 liters. Small-volume self-inflating bag devices, however, may deliver inadequate tidal volumes to the infant with poorly compliant lungs or high airway resistance. Thus, the child-sized and adult-sized self-inflating bags are appropriate for the entire age range of infants and children. The self-inflating devices may have attached a device to entrain oxygen (oxygen reservoir) to maximize the oxygen concentration delivered. A flow of oxygen at 15 liters/min needs to be delivered to achieve maximum oxygen concentration, which even then may not exceed 90%. Another device for ventilation of pediatric patients is the anesthesia bag; although very effective, it should only be employed by individuals skilled in its use.[30,31] Self-inflating bags have the advantage of being independent of gas flow and thus, should the oxygen tank run out, ventilation may still be effective. In comparison, the anesthesia bag device is gas flow–dependent for its filling and thus, in the absence of gas flow, would be ineffective in ventilating the child.

Some BVM devices are fitted with pop-off valves set at 30 to 35 cm H_2O pressure, which are intended to prevent overinflation of the patient's lungs and the attendant risks of barotrauma, air leaks, and life-threatening tension pneumothorax. The rationale for this preset pop-off pressure level is based on an experimental study of excised newborn lungs. This in vitro observation should not be extrapolated to the clinical situation when increased airway resistance and decreased lung compliance may necessitate ventilation at pressures greater than 30 cm H_2O to achieve effective ventilation.[32] Activation of the pop-off valve may lead to inadequate delivery of the required tidal volume, especially if the lung compliance is reduced or airway resistance increased.[33] In addition, activation of the pop-off valve leads to a reduced delivery of oxygen and thus limits reliability of the device to deliver maximal oxygen concentrations. Thus, when inspiratory pressures are required that would exceed the pop-off pressure, the operator should employ a bag-mask device without a pop-off valve or occlude the pop-off operating valve during ventilation.

Standard adult and pediatric-size BVM devices have been shown to provide equally effective ventilation of an infant mannequin lung model, and the larger resuscitation bags do not cause excessive ventilation. Mask fit on the patient is much more important to ensure adequate ventilation than is the resuscitation bag size, since air leak under the mask will lead to underventilation, particularly in situations of low lung compliance or high airway resistance. Generally, a single operator can effectively ventilate the child with a BVM device. However, when it is difficult to secure an air-tight mask fit to the face, the operator should employ both hands to secure a mask fit and have a second individual provide ventilation by squeezing the bag.[34,35] A recent study has confirmed the superior effectiveness of two-operator ventilation with a bag-mask device, and has also demonstrated that the single operator may have difficulty compressing the bag effectively. In this case, more effective ventilation is provided by using the open-palm method of squeezing the bag against one's body to effectively deliver an adequate tidal volume.[36] When ventilating the patient with a BVM, one should position oneself behind the patient's head to maintain optimal airway control (i.e., head extension and chin lift) while operating the BVM device. Cricoid pressure (Sellick maneuver) can be performed by a second person during BVM ventilations to reduce the risk of gastric distension and regurgitation with its potential for pulmonary aspiration during resuscitation. However, if the patient begins to vomit, cricoid pressure should be released to avoid gastric or esophageal rupture.

The airway in the infant and young child is less structurally stable than in the adult. An obstruction in the infant's or young child's upper airway leads to markedly increased negative pressure on inspiration, which readily produces dynamic collapse of the airway because of relative instability of the child's airway structures. Positive pressure ventilation with a BVM device helps counteract the dynamic airway obstruction by "stenting" the airway open and thus providing effective ventilation to the patient.

Previously published CPR guidelines have noted that "ideally a manometer should be attached to monitor airway pressure." However, it is emphasized that **the primary concern is to focus on visualizing adequate bilateral chest excursions, rather than achieving a preset pressure, to guide adequacy of ventilation.** In the apneic child without cardiac arrest, the recommended rate of artificial ventilations is 20 per minute. In certain clinical situations, such as increased intracranial pressure, hyperventilation at a faster rate may be appropriate.

Tracheal Intubation

Tracheal intubation provides optimal management of the airway for effective ventilation ("Tracheal Intubation," by Todres and Frassica, this volume). Tracheal intubation provides an effective route for ventilating the patient when BVM ventilation is inadequate. Although tracheal intubation provides definitive control of the airway, one should not overlook the fact that BVM ventilation is generally effective, making tracheal intubation an elective procedure. Multiple efforts at intubation by an inexperienced operator may further compromise the child's ability to recover. Ventilation via a tracheal tube ensures that all the gas is directed into the lungs, avoiding distension of the stomach, which may occur with BVM ventilation. Tracheal intubation ensures airway protection from aspiration of gastric contents and provides a route for suctioning secretions and possibly blood from the airway, which may be contributing to airway obstruction. Appreciation of the differences in anatomical structure of the upper airway between children and adults is important in approaching tracheal intubation. These include the following:

1. In the infant, the tongue is relatively larger in proportion to the rest of the oral cavity and thus more readily obstructs one's view in performing tracheal intubation. The large tongue also makes it more difficult to manipulate the laryngoscope blade.

2. The infant larynx is higher in the neck (C_{3-4}) compared with the adult (C_{4-5}). This superior position of the larynx creates a more acute angle between the base of the tongue and the glottis, making it more difficult to visualize the laryngeal structures. For this reason, optimal visualization is best obtained with a straight laryngoscope blade.

3. The infant epiglottis is angled away from the long axis of the trachea and may be "floppy," making it more difficult to lift the tip of the epiglottis with the laryngoscope blade.

4. Infant vocal folds are attached anteriorly at a lower level than posteriorly, and as a result the endotracheal tube may be more difficult to pass as it tends to be "caught" at the anterior commissures.

5. The subglottic area, i.e., the space within the cricoid ring, is the most narrow portion of the infant larynx and may limit the passage of an endotracheal tube once it has passed through the vocal cords. This area is subject to swelling and edema from trauma or infection, resulting in a marked increase in airway resistance.

Tracheal intubation must be carried out expeditiously and skillfully. Proper positioning of the child is essential. Appropriate equipment (laryngoscopes, tubes, suction) must be at hand. Tube size selection is usually estimated by standard formulas using the child's age. More recently, a multicenter study has shown that length-based estimations more reliably predict the proper tube size.[37]

Once the patient is intubated, it is essential to fix and stabilize the tube with the child's head in the neutral position. Flexion and extension of the head may displace the tube either into a mainstem bronchus or up into the pharynx with potential catastrophic consequences.[38,39] Should tracheal intubation be followed by a deterioration in the child's condition, immediate attention must be given to the position and patency of the endotracheal tube. The tube may have been passed accidentally into the esophagus or down a mainstem bronchus, or it may be plugged with mucus, blood, or vomitus.

If available, the simple technique of pulse oximetry (oxygen saturation) will provide valuable information regarding the child's oxygenation status and response to resuscitative measures. It should be noted, however, that in the child who is poorly perfused, the device may not accurately measure oxygen saturations due to peripheral vasoconstriction.

Where available, the measurement of end-tidal carbon dioxide ($ETCO_2$) is a valuable method to determine correct position of the endotracheal tube. Recently, a disposable, colorimetric $ETCO_2$ detector was found reliable in verifying endotracheal tube placement in infants and children.[40] It was noted that during CPR, a positive test correctly indicated the presence of the endotracheal tube in the airway. However, a negative result suggesting esophageal placement may not be a true assessment and needs further investigation for correct placement of the tube.

Transtracheal catheter ventilation may be an effective life-saving maneuver when all other standard attempts to secure an airway and oxygenate the patient have failed. Transtracheal catheter venti-

lation is performed rarely in the child and is particularly difficult to perform on the younger child due to the relatively small and not easily identifiable cricothyroid membrane. Experimental work on animals (dogs weighing 21–30 pounds) has demonstrated that this maneuver effectively oxygenated the animal while resulting in tolerable hypercarbia.[41] In fact, marked hypercarbia (>150 mm Hg) is well tolerated, provided oxygenation is adequate.[42]

Foreign Body Obstruction of the Airway

Foreign body dislodgment and removal has been performed successfully using abdominal thrusts (the Heimlich maneuver).[43] Children over the age of 1 year who have complete airway obstruction due to a foreign body should receive a series of five abdominal thrusts. Once loss of consciousness has occurred, attempts to ventilate should be interposed with abdominal thrust sets, because it may be possible to bypass the obstruction with positive pressure. For infants less than 1 year of age, the AHA does not recommend the use of abdominal thrusts due to concerns for injury to the abdominal organs, especially the liver. Instead, a series of five back blows and five chest thrusts are used in an effort to dislodge the foreign body. Although this is an area of much debate and controversy, there is no scientific evidence to support the use of the Heimlich maneuver in infants.

It is recommended that the victim who undergoes a Heimlich maneuver be medically examined as soon as possible in order to rule out complications such as ruptured stomach, ruptured jejunum, or esophageal rupture.[44-46]

Circulation (Perfusion)

Although positive-pressure artificial respiration is manifestly different from negative-pressure spontaneous breathing, for the most part it is not difficult to take over the function of the respiratory muscles and provide satisfactory gas exchange during a cardiac arrest. It is a much more difficult project to take over the function of the heart in providing adequate perfusion and oxygen delivery. Indeed, it seems clear that the most sophisticated markers of perfusion we have available during experimental cardiac arrest situations, such as coronary and cerebral blood flows and pressures, oxygen and glucose consumption, or $ETCO_2$ measurements, are only the grossest of parameters for what is happening at the cellular level. This is all the more a concern during a pediatric resuscitation where frequently the only indicators that are followed are heart rate, rhythm, and blood pressure. We do not yet understand what constitutes adequate perfusion during a cardiopulmonary resuscitation nor what should be the optimal characteristics of reperfusion in a patient who has suffered cardiac arrest.

In the 1950s, cardiac compressions were performed in the hospital via open-chest cardiac massage. When the technique of closed-chest cardiac massage was described by Kouwenhoven and colleagues in 1960, the benefit of a technique that could be initiated anywhere by anyone was obvious.[6] Closed-chest cardiac compressions continue to be the standard of care recommended by the AHA for cardiac arrest both outside of and within the hospital. The mechanism of forward blood flow during external cardiac compressions continues to be an area of debate. Observations from studies carried out in experimental animals cannot necessarily be extrapolated directly to the child. The cardiac pump theory of CPR states that forward blood flow results from compression of the heart "sandwiched" between the sternum and the vertebral column. In the cardiac pump theory, forward flow occurs during the compression phase (systole). For this to be effective, the mitral valve must close and the aortic valve open. During release of compressions (diastole), left ventricle filling occurs.

In the alternate thoracic pump theory, external cardiac compressions cause an increase in intrathoracic pressure, which is transmitted to all cardiac chambers and major blood vessels within the thorax.[6,47–50] Forward flow occurs because of an arteriovenous pressure differential created by venous valves at the thoracic inlet that prevent the transmission of the increased intrathoracic pressure to the venous circulation. The left side of the heart then acts as a passive conduit for blood ejected into the systemic circulation. The mitral valve remains open during compression. Studies supporting this concept demonstrated forward flow of blood with little change in left ventricular dimensions. It was also noted that simultaneous chest compressions and lung inflation increased blood flow (measured in the carotid artery). Transthoracic echocardiography in adult humans demonstrated that the mitral valve remained open during the entire compression and release phases and that the aortic valve opened only during compression systole. Cardiac filling occurred passively between compressions. In 1990, the thoracic pump concept was challenged with studies using transthoracic and transesophageal echocardiography, showing direct cardiac compression to be the major determinant of stroke volume.[50]

It is likely that multiple factors interact to produce forward blood flow during CPR, including compression technique and thoracic structure. Chest compressions can be characterized by their rate, depth, and duty cycle; location and hand position are related to the patient's anatomy. The recommended rates of compressions for neonates, infants, and children are at least 120, at least 100, and 100 per minute, respectively. In order to preserve forward flow, the appropriate compression rate should be maintained during CPR, although the optimal rate for compressions has not been determined scientifically. A study of pediatric patients receiving CPR showed improved coronary perfusion pressures at an average compression rate of 136 per minute as compared with 96 per minute.[51] Previous recommendations for the depth of compressions consisted of specific depths which might be inadequate.[52] Recently, the AHA provided guidelines based on the patient's size, with a recommendation that the chest be compressed to one third to one half the depth of the thorax. In a study of pediatric CPR, these compression depths have been shown to produce a greater coronary perfusion pressure than the previously recommended techniques.[53]

Duty cycle refers to the percent of a compression/relaxation set spent in the compression phase. In physiologic terms, it represents a balance between cardiac filling and ejection. A short duty time will favor myocardial filling and coronary perfusion, while a longer duty cycle will improve stroke volume and forward flow. The optimal duty time may vary between clinical situations, and is affected by the compression rate and use of vasopressor therapy. The AHA recommends a duty cycle of 50%, although human and animal studies have favored both shorter and longer duty cycles.[54,55]

The thoracic structure influences both the efficacy and mechanism of forward blood flow during CPR. In infants and children, the highly compliant chest wall readily transmits forces to the heart, which is compressed between the sternum and the vertebral column. The AHA recommends that chest compressions in infants and children be performed over the lower one third of the sternum, based on the radiologic location of the heart.[56] In children less than 8 years of age, CPR is performed using direct sternal compression with the heel of one hand. For infants less than 1 year of age, two fingers are used over the sternum, placed one finger-breadth below an imaginary line drawn between the nipples. For neonates and small infants, the chest-encircling or circumferential method may also be utilized. There are several reports of infants receiving CPR that show that this method improves arterial pressure in comparison with the two-finger technique.[52,57] An animal study of pediatric CPR has also demonstrated improved arterial and coronary perfusion pressures while using circumferential compressions.[58]

In adult patients, open-chest CPR has been shown to produce higher cardiac output and improved resuscitation efficacy, as compared with closed-chest massage.[59–61] One advantage of open-chest CPR is avoidance of the elevation in central venous pressure, which accompanies closed-chest compressions. Increased central venous pressure may limit stroke volume by decreasing the arteriovenous pressure difference that contributes to forward flow. An animal study of pediatric CPR demonstrated the superiority of open-chest massage in terms of myocardial and cerebral blood flow.[62] Open and closed-chest CPR have been compared in pediatric patients with traumatic cardiac arrest; there was no difference in the rate of return of spontaneous circulation or in survival.[63] There have been anecdotal reports of successful resuscitation in children who underwent open-chest CPR following a period of closed-chest massage.[64] To date, there has not been a clinical study to compare open- and closed-chest CPR in nontraumatic pediatric cardiac arrest. Open-chest cardiac massage should be considered for a potentially salvageable child who fails to respond to conventional closed-chest CPR and in special situations, such as in the operating room.

Age-related rates of compression during CPR and compression-ventilation ratios are presented in Table 1-1. For adult basic life support, the AHA CPR guidelines include a recommendation to pause between sets of compressions in order to deliver a ventilation. If the patient is intubated, however, compressions and ventilations can be done asynchronously.[11] Pediatric basic life support recommendations also include a pause after each set of five compressions for a ventilation given over 1 to 1.5 seconds. There are no specific recommendations regarding the coordination of compressions and ventilations in the intubated pediatric patient. There is no evidence that simultaneous compressions and ventilations is advantageous. When the airway is secured with an endotracheal tube, the pause for ventilation may not be essential for the following reasons: (1) all ventilation is now directed down the trachea, avoiding gastric distension; (2) positive end-expiratory pressures may be applied; and (3) diffusion oxygenation enhances the ability to oxygenate the child. In a study by Berkowitz et al., simultaneous compressions and ventilations in intubated piglets did not enhance myocardial or cerebral blood flow.[65] The explanation for this observation is

Table 1-1. Guidelines for chest compression and ventilatory rates during cardiopulmonary resuscitation

Age	Chest compression rate (per min)	Ventilatory rate (per min)	Ratio
Neonate	120	40	3:1
Infant (<1 yr)	100	20	5:1
Child (1–8 yr)	100	20	5:1
Older child and adolescent (>8 yr)	80–100	16–20	5:1

that CPR already produces high intrathoracic pressures due to the compliance of the infant animal's chest wall.

CPR investigators have developed several new techniques in an effort to improve the effectiveness of basic life support. These include active compression-decompression (ACD), vest CPR, and interposed abdominal compressions. In animal studies, ACD CPR has been shown to increase myocardial and cerebral blood flow. Adult human studies have demonstrated increased mean arterial pressures during ACD CPR. The technique has not been studied in children and is less likely to have considerable benefit over standard CPR because chest wall compliance is significantly greater in children, as compared with adults.[66] Vest CPR produces blood flow without significant displacement of the chest wall, thus reducing chest deformity during prolonged resuscitation, which could interfere with venous return. Vest CPR has been used in adult humans and resulted in improved blood pressure and initial resuscitation rates.[67] A recent study investigated the use of vest CPR during resuscitation of infant pigs.[68] This technique produced cerebral and myocardial blood flow rates that were comparable to standard CPR. Clinical studies of vest CPR in children are needed to determine its utility during resuscitation. Interposed abdominal compressions have been shown to improve blood flow during CPR in adults. Due to concern for organ injury, it is unlikely that this will be recommended for children.

Drugs and Fluids

Access to the Circulation

Drugs and fluids may be administered through peripheral or central intravenous lines or by the intraosseous or endotracheal route.[69–72] Peripheral intravenous lines may be inserted in the median basilic, antecubital, or cephalic veins of the upper extremity, although these may be difficult to cannulate in children with cardiovascular collapse. The femoral vein provides a reliable alternative to access the circulation. The external jugular vein is an unstable and elusive vein for peripheral line placement. It should especially be avoided when the patient has sustained possible cervical spinal cord injury, as manipulation of the neck to place the line may be seriously detrimental to the patient. The intraosseous route is a method for immediate vascular access in infants and children under the age of 6. It allows for volume expansion as well as drug administration while intravenous routes are being sought. Saphenous vein cutdown as a technique for emergency vascular access, while appropriate in certain cases, is frequently time consuming and unreliable, even in the hands of trained individuals. For infants and children less than 6 years of age, the intraosseous route is preferred.

The endotracheal tube provides an alternative route of drug administration. Epinephrine, atropine, and lidocaine are recommended for administration via the endotracheal tube. It is essential that these drugs be diluted to a volume of 3 to 5 ml with sterile saline (depending on the size of the child) to achieve a volume sufficient to assure adequate absorption through the tracheobronchial tree. Alternatively, these drugs may be given in a smaller volume (1–2 ml) through a catheter that extends past the distal tip of the endotracheal tube, followed by a flush of 3 to 5 ml of saline. The absorption of drugs from the tracheobronchial tree may be unreliable, and higher doses may be required to achieve effective plasma levels. Whenever possible, medications should be administered intravenously rather than endotracheally.[73] Intracardiac administration of drugs is not recommended during external cardiac compressions because intracardiac injections are associated with the risks of pneumothorax, intramyocardial injection, or coronary vessel laceration, and interrupt the cardiac compressions.

Intravascular Volume Expansion

Hypovolemia must be corrected immediately in children who undergo cardiopulmonary resuscitation. Causes of intravascular volume depletion include trauma (blood loss), burns, sepsis, prolonged vomiting or diarrhea, or diabetic ketoacidosis. However, children with a major deficiency of circulating red blood cell mass will require red blood cell transfusions as well as either crystalloid or colloid (e.g., 5% albumin) to restore adequate oxygen carrying capacity and intravascular volume. In most situations, a balanced salt solution, such as lactated Ringer's or normal saline, or a colloid (e.g., 5% albumin) will suffice.

Advantages of **crystalloid** are that it is readily available, inexpensive, and does not put the patient at risk for allergic reactions, hepatitis, or HIV. The major disadvantage of crystalloid resuscitation is that the fluid remains within the vascular space for a relatively short period; therefore, the volume of crystalloid required to replace a given volume of blood loss is 3 ml lactated Ringer's or normal saline for each milliliter of blood. This volume of crystalloid is well tolerated in the healthy child; in the patient with severe cardiac or renal disease, however, pulmonary edema may be precipitated. In patients with severe closed-head injury, excessive crystalloid administration may aggravate cerebral edema and increase intracranial pressure. During the resuscitation of a head-injured patient, however, restoration of adequate intravascular volume status is essential to maintain cerebral perfusion pressure.

Colloid (5% albumin or synthetic colloids; e.g., hydroxethyl starch) is relatively well confined to the vascular space and results in rapid volume expansion. Disadvantages include its potential for adverse reactions and its high cost. Plasma protein fraction and albumin are heat-treated, and thus there is no risk of disease transmission; some of these products, however, contain vasoactive substances, which may cause hypotension. Fresh frozen plasma (FFP) should never be used for volume expansion; its only indication is to replenish clotting factor deficiencies. Rapid transfusion of FFP (>1.0 ml/kg/min) may result in serious hypocalcemia and hypotension or electrical mechanical dissociation (EMD) (pulseless electrical activity [PEA]). Dextran 70, although an effective volume expander, may interfere with normal coagulation and is associated with a high incidence of allergic reactions. Dextran is therefore rarely administered for volume expansion.

The initial management of the patient in hypovolemic shock is the rapid infusion of 20 ml/kg of a crystalloid solution. Either lactated Ringer's or 0.9% sodium chloride is a reasonable initial choice.[74] However, large amounts of sodium chloride may result in hypernatremia and hyperchloremic acidosis. Dextrose-containing solutions are avoided in resuscitation unless there is documented hypoglycemia. The stress of the illness or injury leads to increased output of catecholamines, which tend to produce hyperglycemia. Hyperglycemia may cause an osmotic diuresis, and, in some cases, excessively high levels of glucose in the blood may lead to hypertonic non-ketotic coma. In addition, blood glucose levels above 200 mg/dl have been associated with increased neurologic deficit in the presence of hypoxemia and ischemia.[75,76]

After the initial fluid bolus, the child's circulatory status should be reassessed. Important clinical signs include skin temperature and color, capillary refill time, heart rate, blood pressure, urine output, and mental status. Blood pressure is frequently maintained, even in the presence of other overt signs of hypovolemia, due to the child's ability to compensate with profound peripheral vasoconstriction. If perfusion is still inadequate after the initial fluid bolus, a further 20 ml/kg of crystalloid is administered. A common error in the volume resuscitation of the child in hypovolemic shock is inadequate replacement of intravascular volume. The child with hypovolemic or septic shock will frequently require 40 to 80 ml/kg of crystalloid in the first hour of resuscitation.

In the pediatric trauma patient with significant hemorrhage, transfusion of blood should be considered if signs of shock persist following administration of two boluses (20 ml/kg each) of isotonic crystalloid solution. Typed and cross-matched **blood** should be administered as soon as it is available. If, however, the urgency of the situation does not allow for the complete cross-matching of blood, then type-specific, partially cross-matched or type-specific, non-crossmatched, or type O Rh-negative non-crossmatched blood may be administered in the order of preference listed. Early consultation with a pediatric surgeon is indicated to obtain appropriate diagnostic studies and operative intervention.

Studies on adult patients and experimental models have shown advantages and disadvantages to the use of hypertonic saline in the resuscitation of hypovolemic shock, septic shock, and burn injury.[77,78] Improvement in cardiac output, oxygen transport, oxygen consumption, and less tendency to produce a rise in intracranial pressure compared with isotonic resuscitation, must be weighed against the effects of sodium overload and marked potassium loss with the potential for arrhythmias. There are few studies evaluating the role of hypertonic saline in the resuscitation of pediatric patients, and further research in this area is necessary before it can be generally recommended in clinical practice.

Drug Administration

Epinephrine

In the cardiac arrest setting, epinephrine produces primarily an alpha-adrenergic response that results in vasoconstriction, with increased systemic and coronary perfusion pressures leading to improved myocardial oxygen delivery.[79] It is indicated for asystole, bradyarrhythmias, pulseless electrical activity, and ventricular fibrillation (VF). Epinephrine's beta-adrenergic-receptor action produces an increase in myocardial contractility and heart rate, but the alpha-adrenergic action is the predominant effect.

The effective dose of epinephrine to be employed in CPR has recently undergone re-evaluation. Studies have shown that high-dose epinephrine (up to 200 $\mu g/kg$) improves blood flow in the coronary and cerebral circulation during resuscitation, with a higher rate of return of spontaneous circulation.[80-82] Coronary perfusion pressure is correlated with myocardial blood flow and is a significant predictor of recovery from cardiac arrest in animal models and humans. However, recent studies in adults have demonstrated no advantage of high-dose epinephrine over standard-dose intravenous epinephrine in terms of survival from pre-hospital cardiac arrest.[83,84] In contrast, a study of in-hospital pediatric cardiac arrest demonstrated that high-dose epinephrine (0.1 mg/kg) provided a higher return of spontaneous circulation and improved long-term outcome as compared with standard-dose epinephrine.[85] High-dose epinephrine should be considered at an early stage during resuscitation from cardiac arrest to increase the likelihood that spontaneous circulation is restored and irreversible brain damage is prevented. For pediatric patients in cardiac arrest, the 1992 AHA guidelines recommend a first dose of epinephrine via IV or IO at a dose of 0.01 mg/kg of 1:10,000 solution. Second and

subsequent doses are then given at 0.1 mg/kg every 3 to 5 minutes, with consideration of doses up to 0.2 mg/kg. The recommended dose for endotracheal epinephrine is 0.1 mg/kg of 1:1,000 solution for all doses administered via the endotracheal tube. The actions of epinephrine may be depressed by acidosis, although animal studies have demonstrated no difference in coronary perfusion pressures between animals treated with and without sodium bicarbonate prior to intravenous epinephrine administration.[86,87] Therefore, it is necessary to correct acidosis by ensuring adequate oxygenation, ventilation (even hyperventilation), and perfusion. The administration of sodium bicarbonate to correct metabolic acidosis is controversial (discussed later).

Atropine

Atropine is a parasympatholytic drug that decreases vagal tone in the heart, thereby accelerating sinus node and atrial pacemakers as well as conduction through the AV node. It may be effective in the temporary treatment of symptomatic bradycardia accompanied by hypotension or poor perfusion, and may also enhance conduction in atrioventricular block. It can also be used to prevent the bradycardia associated with intubation that may be provoked by vagal stimulation. Although it has been used routinely in pediatric cardiac arrest with asystole or bradyarrhythmia, these conditions are usually precipitated by hypoxemia and treatment should therefore be directed first to improving ventilation and oxygenation.

Atropine should be given in doses sufficient to be vagolytic, usually at 0.02 mg/kg, with a minimum dose of 0.1 mg to ensure that paradoxical bradycardia does not develop. A maximum dose of 0.5 mg in children and 1 mg in adolescents is recommended and may be repeated. If atropine is administered by endotracheal tube, the dose should be increased by 2 to 3 times to account for reduced absorption. When used prior to intubation, atropine may prevent the bradycardia induced by hypoxemia; scrupulous attention should therefore be paid to pre-oxygenation and to monitoring of oxygen saturations by pulse oximetry during intubation attempts.

Sodium Bicarbonate

Bicarbonate provides the most important buffer system in the body for producing rapid adjustments in pH via the unique system of generating the volatile carbonic acid (H_2CO_3). When combined with an acid, the bicarbonate anion will release carbon dioxide, which can be completely removed from the system if ventilation is intact. Conversely, if ventilation is not functional, sodium bicarbonate administration will have no effect on serum pH, producing parallel increases in serum bicarbonate and pCO_2.

Sodium bicarbonate is indicated when there is documented metabolic acidosis during a prolonged cardiopulmonary arrest or for the treatment of life-threatening hyperkalemia. Circulatory collapse leads to profound tissue hypoxia. Adequate oxygen delivery to the heart and brain is achieved at the expense of skeletal muscle, liver, and the gastrointestinal tract. In hypoxic states, the heart has less oxygen reserve than any other organ or tissue. As hypoxemia progresses, intracellular acidosis and organ failure result.

There is evidence that the administration of sodium bicarbonate may have adverse effects.[88-92] Sodium bicarbonate produces an intracellular acidosis due to the rapid diffusion of carbon dioxide into the cells. The exit of H^+ from the cell is slower, resulting in a lower intracellular pH and cerebrospinal fluid acidosis. The administration of sodium bicarbonate may also have significant effects on the oxygen dissociation curve by causing a leftward shift and reducing oxygen delivery to the tissues at a critical time. Sodium bicarbonate administration may also cause hypernatremia and increased serum osmolality. If serum osmolality is excessive, there is a potential for producing central nervous system dysfunction.

In cardiac arrest, lactic acid production is due to reduction in oxygen delivery to tissue. Administration of sodium bicarbonate does not affect the underlying tissue hypoxia or improve the clinical status of the patient. It is therefore prudent that treatment of lactic acidosis should be aimed at identifying and correcting the underlying cause.[93] The routine administration of sodium bicarbonate is controversial because it has not resulted in significant improvement in success of defibrillation or survival in laboratory animals. It is essential that adequate ventilation be established before sodium bicarbonate is administered to ensure that carbon dioxide produced by the buffer system can be eliminated to avoid a paradoxical respiratory acidosis.

Calcium

The process of myocardial excitation-contraction coupling involves the action of calcium ions. Following cardiac arrest, severe ischemia affects the cell's calcium homeostasis; accumulation of calcium precipitates cardiac arrhythmias and cell death in ischemic tissues. There is no scientific evidence that calcium has a beneficial hemodynamic effect in most patients during CPR.[94–96] On the contrary, calcium may have deleterious effects in ischemic areas of the brain and heart. In fact, calcium-channel blocking agents have been shown to raise the threshold of the ischemic heart to VF.[97]

A randomized, prospective, blind study in a pre-hospital setting suggested a subset of patients who might benefit from calcium administration, namely those with EMD(PEA) and a wide QRS complex.[98] However, there was no demonstrated benefit in the majority of patients who received calcium compared with those who did not receive calcium as part of their CPR management for all other causes of cardiac arrest (VF or asystole). Calcium is thus indicated in (1) proven hypocalcemic cardiac arrest,[96] (2) hyperkalemia and severe cardiac arrhythmias (the calcium may reverse the arrhythmias due to hyperkalemia but does not decrease the serum concentration of potassium), and (3) rhythm disturbances associated with overdose of calcium antagonists. Calcium administration may have a role in EMD(PEA) with a wide QRS complex.[98–100]

Glucose

The role of glucose administration during CPR is controversial because of the observation that there is increased cerebral ischemic damage when hyperglycemia (≥ 200 mg/dl) is present.[75,76,101] This is probably due to conversion of excess glucose to lactic acid in the brain during anaerobic metabolism, which aggravates any neuronal injury that may have been sustained from the cardiac arrest followed by reperfusion with a low cerebral blood flow. In animal studies, glucose administered during CPR results in a higher mortality and worse neurologic outcome.[102,103] However, endogenous release of glucose following **prolonged** resuscitation may explain the association of poor neurologic outcome following cardiac arrest and high blood glucose levels on admission.[104,105] It would seem prudent, therefore, to avoid administration of supplemental glucose during CPR unless there is documented evidence of significant hypoglycemia. In the neonate, hypoglycemia is a relatively common metabolic disorder, particularly in the low-birth-weight infant or the infant of a diabetic mother. Thus, should cardiopulmonary arrest occur in such an infant, one must consider the possibility of hypoglycemia. Measurement of blood glucose

levels is indicated in these circumstance and treatment should be guided accordingly.

Vasopressors

Vasopressor agents (e.g., dopamine and dobutamine for circulatory support), following initial resuscitative efforts, are discussed in Pharmacologic Support of the Circulation by Ziegler, Englander and Fugate, in this volume.

Electrical Defibrillation

Bradyarrhythmias leading to asystole are the most common cause of cardiac arrest in children. In contrast, VF is uncommon in the pediatric patient and may be associated with metabolic disturbances, surgical repair of congenital heart disease, and accidental electric shock. In particular, the presence of VF in a child should prompt a search for hypoxemia, acidosis, hyperkalemia, hypothermia, hypoglycemia, and hypocalcemia. VF has been reported in children with toxicologic exposures, including glue-sniffing and cocaine. The incidence of VF in children may be underestimated if recognition is delayed. A retrospective study of 213 pediatric cardiac arrests found an incidence of VF of 14.5%.[106] Of children who presented with VF, 52% had a witnessed event as compared with only 18% of patients with asystole or EMD(PEA). Furthermore, children with VF had an improved rate of survival to hospital discharge (26% vs. 2%).

When performing defibrillation, it is important to use the appropriate size of electrode paddles. The current delivered to the myocardium is directly proportional to the energy generated by the defibrillator and inversely proportional to the transthoracic impedance. Because impedance is reduced by the use of a larger electrode, defibrillation should be performed using the largest paddle size that provides good chest wall contact and adequate separation. In general, for infants less than 1 year of age (~ 10 kg), the 4.5-cm electrodes, or "pediatric paddles," are appropriate. For children over the age of 1 (>10 kg) the standard 8-cm electrodes (adult paddles) are suitable.[107] When VF is recognized, defibrillation should be performed as quickly as possible at an energy level of 2 joules/kg (2 watt-sec/kg). If VF persists, the energy dose should be doubled to 4 joules/kg, and defibrillation repeated twice as needed. Further attempts at defibrillation following the administration of medications should be done at 4 joules/kg. Proper resuscitation of infants and children requires the availability of a defibrillator that can be adjusted to very low levels of energy (e.g., 5 joules).

Environmental Control

Because the pediatric patient maintains a higher basal metabolic rate and has a greater surface area–to-mass ratio than the adult, critical illness and cardiac arrest can rapidly lead to debilitating degrees of hypothermia, particularly in the unclothed infant or child in an air-conditioned emergency room or intensive care unit. Temperature should always be taken on every child in cardiac arrest, because it may provide clues to etiology and to duration of arrest, and because an alteration in body temperature will require therapy in and of itself. Furthermore, the need to expose the patient during cardiac resuscitation will frequently lead to hypothermia unless proper attention is paid to maintaining thermal control. Measures to control heat loss to the environment include increasing the ambient temperature in the patient's room, decreasing evaporative losses by making sure the patient is not wet, providing heat lamps, heating blankets, warmed intravenous fluids, and warmed nebulized oxygen. The presence of hypothermia may interfere with resuscitative efforts and render therapies such as defibrillation and medications ineffective. On the other hand, hypothermia may also provide a protective effect to the brain and other vital organs by reducing oxygen consumption; therefore, resuscitative efforts in a hypothermic patient should continue until rewarming has been accomplished. Additional measures for warming the child include gastric, rectal, intraperitoneal, and intrathoracic instillation of warmed fluids, and extracorporeal membrane oxygenation with a heat exchanger. A rectal probe thermometer must always be available to confirm rectal temperature below the range of a standard glass thermometer; ear probe thermometers are not accurate enough in pediatric patients to use in the setting of critical hypothermia.

Gastric Dilatation

Stress, critical illness, and BVM ventilation can all produce degrees of gastric dilatation in the pediatric patient, which can cause life-threatening airway compromise by limiting diaphragmatic excursion and increasing the risk of emesis and aspiration. During a cardiac arrest in a pediatric patient, a nasogastric or orogastric tube should be passed to minimize these potential complications.

Postresuscitation Stabilization

Postresuscitation stabilization focuses on (1) preventing secondary organ injury and (2) frequent reassessment of the child's condition. The hypoxic-ischemic insult to major organs may result in varying degrees of tissue injury, resulting in organ failure. A high index of suspicion is necessary to recognize and thus control at the earliest possible time any significant organ injury. For example, should there be signs of cerebral injury, namely seizures, then injury to other target organs, namely, heart, lung, kidney, liver, and GI tract, is a strong possibility. In addition, metabolic dysfunction such as hypoglycemia or hypocalcemia may occur. Effects on the hemopoietic system may lead to the development of disseminated intravascular coagulation. Frequent reassessment of the child's condition is essential, as decompensation may readily occur after an initial stabilizing period. (Management of individual organ failure is discussed in the chapters dealing with the specific organ system.)

Termination of Resuscitation Efforts

The outcome of a pediatric cardiac arrest is related to the nature of the underlying disease process as well as to the time to initiation and duration of resuscitative efforts. Despite appropriate treatment, many patients cannot be resuscitated. The physician directing the resuscitation is responsible for determining at what point to terminate the resuscitative efforts. This involves consideration of history, physical examination, and laboratory findings, which may suggest that the patient has suffered an irreversible cardiac arrest. In addition, failure to respond to appropriate resuscitative efforts within a reasonable period is commonly taken as evidence for nonviability, provided that there are no extenuating circumstances, such as hypothermia or drug overdose. What constitutes a reasonable period of resuscitation depends on the clinical circumstances, including the location of the patient at the time of the cardiac arrest (out-of-hospital vs. in-hospital). There is no established consensus among practicing physicians to guide this decision-making process. Several studies have attempted to determine the time beyond

which no patient can be expected to survive; while none is definitive, predictors of nonsurvival include CPR for longer than 15 to 25 minutes and lack of response to intravenous epinephrine.[15,17–20] During a resuscitation, the potential for intact survival must be assessed and reassessed and consideration given to termination of resuscitation if there is minimal likelihood for success.

The decision to terminate resuscitation of a pediatric patient carries significant emotional and psychological burdens. It is common for members of a resuscitation team to experience physical and psychological symptoms following the death of an infant or child. The use of a debriefing team to discuss the feelings and reactions associated with pediatric resuscitation is a useful process to avoid cumulative stress and burnout among emergency and intensive care personnel. In addition, medical review of the resuscitation efforts is a valuable educational tool that should include all members of the team whenever possible.

The potential for organ donation should be considered as a component of any pediatric resuscitation. Medicolegal issues may require notification of the medical examiner to obtain permission and to determine jurisdiction. Although respectful of the family's psychological and spiritual needs, the physician should discuss postmortem examination at the earliest opportunity.

Teaching Techniques
The Mock Code

Given the infrequency with which the practitioner is presented with a cardiac arrest situation in pediatrics, the practice resuscitation drill or "mock code" is an invaluable tool for teaching the skills necessary for successful resuscitation, as well as for testing the readiness of a system expected to deal with critical pediatric illness. The pediatric intensivist is often looked to as the leader in this sort of endeavor, and may well be called on in the hospital or teaching program to provide direction for a program of training staff to participate effectively in a true cardiac arrest situation. Although emergency departments that see both pediatric and adult patients are much more commonly called on to resuscitate adults, and may therefore be much more at home with the "recipe" for a successful resuscitation, they are far less frequently confident of their skills when applied to the pediatric arrest situation.

Adult educational theory tells us that the adult learner finds the kinetic exercise of theory to be a very useful means of imprinting information, and, obviously, technical skills, into a permanent repertoire. Participants in a mock code can be at any level of training, and may include respiratory therapy, nursing, paramedic, and physician staff. It is most meaningful if a mock code exercise begins with an opportunity to see a well-run pediatric code. This can be followed by a discussion of the principles of pediatric arrest management, then offer the opportunity to practice, in a hands-on fashion, the skills and principles that have been demonstrated. A critique after the exercise can be used. Scenarios might include respiratory arrest from airway obstruction, SIDS, overwhelming infection, traumatic arrest from abuse, drowning, falls, burns or MVA, or the "arrest about to happen"—a child presenting with advanced respiratory or circulatory failure not yet in accomplished cardiac arrest. The principles stressed should include airway control, ventilation, and circulatory support. Use of a critique sheet is helpful not only to evaluate progress over time, but also to make explicit the tasks expected of the leader and participants.

To be effective, a resuscitation scenario should employ equipment and educational aids in an effort to simulate reality as closely as possible. Use of dysrhythmia simulators and mannikins for intubation and intraosseous infusion allows the participant to obtain information and perform skills in the context of the scenario. Despite improved technology, the use of mannikins is inherently limited. In order to become proficient at life-saving skills, the provider must obtain experience with actual patients. To this end, some educators have favored the use of recently deceased patients to teach resuscitation procedures. Such a practice may provide valuable experience in order to benefit other patients. A recently published discussion of this issue proposes a policy for the use of newly deceased patients for training in resuscitation techniques.[108] In particular, it addresses the importance of obtaining informed consent from families. It is recommended that each institution considering the use of recently deceased patients develop a policy for this practice in conjunction with administrators, legal advisors, nursing personnel, and members of the hospital's ethics committee.

References

1. Henderson Y. The prevention and treatment of asphyxia in the newborn. *JAMA* 90:583–586, 1928.
2. Flagg P. The treatment of asphyxia in the newborn. *JAMA* 91:788–791, 1928.
3. Blaikley JB, Gibberd GF. Asphyxia neonatorum. *Lancet* 1:736–739, 1935.
4. Pearson JW. *Historical and Experimental Approaches to Modern Resuscitation.* Springfield, IL: Thomas, 1965. Pp 1–93.
5. Crile GW. The resuscitation of the apparently dead and a demonstration of the pneumatic rubber suit as a means of controlling the blood pressure. *Trans South Surg Gynecol Assoc* 16:362, 1904.
6. Kouwenhoven WB, Jude JR, Knickerbocker GG. Closed-chest cardiac massage. *JAMA* 173:1064–1067, 1960.
7. Beck CS, Pritchard WH, Feil HS. Ventricular fibrillation of long duration abolished by electric shock. *JAMA* 135:985–986, 1947.
8. Zoll PM et al. Treatment of unexpected cardiac arrest by external electric stimulation of the heart. *N Engl J Med* 154:541–546, 1956.
9. Standards and guidelines for cardiopulmonary resuscitation (CPR) and emergency cardiac care (ECC). *JAMA* 244:453–509, 1980.
10. Standards and guidelines for cardiopulmonary resuscitation (CPR) and emergency cardiac care (ECC). *JAMA* 255:2905–2992, 1986.
11. Guidelines for cardiopulmonary resuscitation and emergency cardiac care: Recommendations of the 1992 National Conference. *JAMA* 268:2172–2295, 1992.
12. Chameides L (ed). *Textbook of Pediatric Advanced Life Support.* Dallas-American Heart Association, 1988.
13. Eisenberg M, Bergner L, Hallstrom A. Epidemiology of cardiac arrest and resuscitation in children. *Ann Emerg Med* 12:672–674, 1983.
14. Lewis JK et al. Outcome of pediatric resuscitation. *Ann Emerg Med* 12:297–299, 1983.
15. Nichols DG et al. Factors influencing outcome of cardiopulmonary arrest in children (abstract). *Crit Care Med* 12:287, 1984.
16. O'Rourke PP. Outcome of children who are apneic and pulseless in the emergency room. *Crit Care Med* 14:466–468, 1986.
17. Gillis J et al. Results of inpatient pediatric resuscitation. *Crit Care Med* 14:469–471, 1986.
18. Zaritsky A et al. CPR in children. *Ann Emerg Med* 16:1107–1111, 1987.
19. Quan L et al. Outcome and predictors of outcome in pediatric submersion victims receiving pre-hospital care in King County, Washington. *Pediatrics* 86:586–593, 1990.
20. Quan L, Kinder D. Pediatric submersions: Prehospital predictors of outcome. *Pediatrics* 90:909–913, 1992.
21. Morikawa S, Safar P, DeCarlo J. Influence of the head-jaw position upon airway patency. *Anesthesiology* 22:265–270, 1961.
22. Bordin MP. Airway patency in the unconscious patient. *Br J Anaesth* 57:306–310, 1985.
23. Nandi PR et al. Effect of general anesthesia on the pharynx. *Br J Anaesth* 66:157–162, 1991.
24. Rodenstein DO, Stanescu DC. The soft palate and breathing. *Am Rev Respir Dis* 134:311–325, 1986.
25. Herzenberg JE et al. Emergency transport and positioning of young children who have an injury of the cervical spine: The standard backboard may be hazardous. *J Bone Joint Surg [Am]* 71:15–22, 1989.
26. Brain AIJ. The laryngeal mask airway—A new concept in airway management. *Br J Anaesth* 55:801–805, 1983.
27. Brain AIJ. The laryngeal mask airway—A possible new solution to airway problems in the emergency situation. *Arch Emerg Med* 1:229–232, 1984.
28. Martin PD et al. Training nursing staff in airway management for resuscitation. A clinical comparison of the facemask and laryngeal mask. *Anaesthesia* 48:33–37, 1993.
29. Nickalls RWD, Thomson CW. Mouth to mask respiration. *Br Med J* 292:1350, 1986.
30. Terndrup TE, Kanter RK, Cherry RA. A comparison of infant ventilation methods performed by prehospital personnel. *Ann Emerg Med* 18:607–611, 1989.
31. Kanter RK. Evaluation of mask-bag ventilation in resuscitation of infants. *Am J Dis Child* 61:300–302, 1986.
32. Rosen M, Laurence KM. Expansion pressure and rupture pressures in the newborn lung. *Lancet* 2:721–722, 1965.
33. Hirschman AM, Kravath RE. Venting vs ventilating: A danger of manual resuscitation bags. *Chest* 82:369–370, 1982.
34. Jesudian MCS et al. Bag-valve-mask ventilation: Two rescuers are better than one: Preliminary report. *Crit Care Med* 13:122, 1985.
35. Hess D, Goff G. The effects of two-hand versus one-hand ventilation on volumes delivered during bag-valve ventilation at various resistances and compliances. *Respir Care* 32:1025, 1987.
36. Thomas AN et al. A new technique for two-hand bag valve mask ventilation. *Br J Anaesth* 69:397, 1992.
37. Luten RC et al. Length based endotracheal tube selection in pediatrics (abstract). *Ann Emerg Med* 21:900–904, 1992.
38. Todres ID et al. Endotracheal tube displacement in the newborn infant. *J Pediatr* 57:126–127, 1976.
39. Donn SM, Kuhn LR. Mechanism of endotracheal tube movement with change of head position in the neonate. *Pediatr Radiol* 9:39–40, 1980.
40. Bhende MAS et al. Validity of a disposable end-tidal CO_2 detector in verifying endotracheal tube placement in infants and children. *Ann Emerg Med* 21:142–145, 1992.
41. Coté CJ et al. Cricothyroid membrane puncture: Oxygenation and ventilation in a dog model using an intravenous catheter. *Crit Care Med* 16:615–619, 1988.
42. Goldstein B, Shannon DC, Todres ID. Supercarbia in children: Clinical course and outcome. *Crit Care Med* 18:166–168, 1990.
43. Heimlich HJ, Patrick EA. The Heimlich maneuver: Best technique for saving any choking victim's life. *Postgrad Med* 87:38–53, 1990.
44. Haynes DE, Haynes BE, Yong YV. Esophageal rupture complicating Heimlich maneuver. *Am J Emerg Med* 2:507–509, 1984.
45. Razaboni RM, Brathwaite CE, Dwyer WA Jr. Ruptured jejunum following Heimlich maneuver. *Am J Emerg Med* 4:95–98, 1986.
46. van der Ham AC, Lange IE. Traumatic rupture of the stomach after Heimlich maneuver. *Am J Emerg Med* 8:713–715, 1990.
47. Rudikoff MT et al. Mechanics of blood flow during cardiopulmonary resuscitation. *Circulation* 61:345–352, 1980.
48. Chandra N, Rudikoff M, Weisfeldt ML. Simultaneous chest compression and ventilation at high airway pressure during cardiopulmonary resuscitation. *Lancet* 1:175–178, 1980.
49. Maier GW et al. The physiology of external cardiac massage: High-impulse cardiopulmonary resuscitation. *Circulation* 70:86–101, 1984.
50. Higano ST et al. The mechanism of blood flow during closed chest cardiac massage in humans: Transesophageal echocardiographic observations. *Mayo Clin Proc* 65:1432–1440, 1990.
51. Goetting MG. Higher chest compression rates improve the coronary

perfusion pressure in pediatric cardiopulmonary resuscitation. *Ann Emerg Med* 1:A20, 1994.

52. David R. Closed-chest cardiac massage in the newborn infant. *Pediatrics* 81:552, 1988.

53. Schuster M, Goetting MG. Age-independent chest compression depths: A better method of CPR. *Acad Emerg Med* 1:A89, 1994.

54. Taylor GJ, Tucker WM, Greane HL. Importance of prolonged compression during CPR in man. *N Engl J Med* 296:1515, 1977.

55. Dean JM et al. Improved blood flow during cardiopulmonary resuscitation using a 30 percent duty cycle in infant pigs. *Circulation* 84:896, 1991.

56. Finholt DA et al. The heart is under the lower third of the sternum; Implications for external massage. *Am J Dis Child* 140:646, 1986.

57. Todres ID, Rogers MC. Methods of external cardiac massage in the newborn infant. *J Pediatr* 57:126, 1976.

58. Menegazzi JJ et al. Two-thumb versus two-finger chest compressions during CPR in a swine infant model of cardiac arrest. *Ann Emerg Med* 22:240, 1993.

59. Del Guercio LRM et al. Comparison of blood flow during external and internal cardiac massage in man. *Circulation* 31(Suppl): 1171–1180, 1965.

60. Sanders AB et al. Improved resuscitation from cardiac arrest with open-chest massage. *Ann Emerg Med* 13:672–675, 1984.

61. Schleien CL et al. Controversial issues in cardiopulmonary resuscitation. *Anesthesiology* 71:133–149, 1989.

62. Fleisher G et al. Open- versus closed-chest cardiac compressions in a canine model of pediatric cardiopulmonary arrest. *Am J Emerg Med* 3:305, 1985.

63. Sheikh A, Brogan T. Outcome and cost of open- and closed-chest cardiopulmonary resuscitation in pediatric cardiac arrests. *Pediatrics* 93:392, 1994.

64. Goetting MG. Mastering pediatric cardiopulmonary resuscitation. *Pediatr Clin North Am* 41:1147, 1994.

65. Berkowitz ID et al. Blood flow during cardiopulmonary resuscitation with simultaneous compression and ventilation in infant pigs. *Pediatr Res* 26:558–564, 1989.

66. Lindner KH et al. Effects of active compression-decompression resuscitation on myocardial and cerebral blood flow in pigs. *Circulation* 88:1254–1263, 1993.

67. Halperin HR et al. A preliminary study of cardiopulmonary resuscitation by circumferential compression of the chest with use of a pneumatic vest. *N Engl J Med* 329:762–768, 1993.

68. Shaffner DH et al. Effect of vest cardiopulmonary resuscitation on cerebral and coronary perfusion in an infant porcine model. *Crit Care Med* 22:1817–1826, 1994.

69. Berg RA. Emergency infusion of catecholamines into bone marrow. *Am J Dis Child* 138:810–811, 1984.

70. Seigler RS, Tecklenburg FW, Shealy R. Prehospital intraosseous infusion by emergency medical services personnel: A prospective study. *Pediatrics* 84:173–177, 1989.

71. Fiser DH. Intraosseous infusion. *N Engl J Med* 32:1579–1581, 1990.

72. Ward JT Jr. Endotracheal drug therapy. *Am J Emerg Med* 1:71–82, 1983.

73. Crespo SG et al. Comparison of two doses of endotracheal epinephrine in a cardiac arrest model. *Ann Emerg Med* 20:230–234, 1991.

74. Vincent JL. Fluids for resuscitation. *Br J Anaesth* 67:185–193, 1991.

75. Combs DJ et al. Glycolytic inhibition of 2-deoxyglucose reduces hyperglycemia associated mortality and morbidity in the ischemic rat. *Stroke* 17:989–994, 1986.

76. Lanier WL et al. The effects of dextrose infusion and head position on neurologic outcome after complete cerebral ischemia in primates: Examination of a model. *Anesthesiology* 66:39–48, 1987.

77. Maningas PA et al. Hypertonic saline-dextran solutions for the prehospital management of traumatic hypotension. *Am J Surg* 157:528–533, 1989.

78. Kien ND, Kramer GC, White DC. Acute hypotension caused by rapid hypertonic saline infusion in anesthetized dogs. *Anesth Analg* 73:597–602, 1991.

79. Otto CW, Yakaitis RW, Blith CD. Mechanism of action of epinephrine in resuscitation from asphyxial arrest. *Crit Care Med* 9:364–365, 1981.

80. Brown CG et al. The effect of graded doses of epinephrine on regional blood flow during cardiopulmonary resuscitation in swine. *Circulation* 75:491–497, 1987.

81. Brunette DD, Jameson SJ. Comparison of standard versus high-dose epinephrine in the resuscitation of cardiac arrest in dogs. *Ann Emerg Med* 19:8–11, 1990.

82. Paradis NA et al. The effect of standard and high-dose epinephrine on coronary perfusion pressure during prolonged cardiopulmonary resuscitation. *JAMA* 265:1139–1144, 1991.

83. Stiell IG et al. High-dose epinephrine in adult cardiac arrest. *N Engl J Med* 327:1045–1050, 1992.

84. Brown CG et al. A comparison of standard-dose and high-dose epinephrine in cardiac arrest outside the hospital. *N Engl J Med* 327:1051–1055, 1992.

85. Goetting MG, Paradis NA. High-dose epinephrine improves outcome from pediatric arrest. *Ann Emerg Med* 20:22–26, 1991.

86. Zaritsky A, Chernow B. Use of catecholamines in pediatrics. *J Pediatr* 105:341–350, 1984.

87. Bleske BE et al. The effect of sodium bicarbonate on the vasopressor effect of high-dose epinephrine during cardiopulmonary resuscitation. *Am J Emerg Med* 11:439–443, 1993.

88. Graf H, Leach W, Arieff AI. Evidence for a detrimental effect of bicarbonate therapy in hypoxic lactic acidosis. *Science* 227:754–756, 1985.

89. Stacpoole PW. Lactic acidosis: The case against bicarbonate therapy. *Ann Intern Med* 105:276–279, 1986.

90. Guerci AD et al. Failure of sodium bicarbonate to improve resuscitation from ventricular fibrillation in dogs. *Circulation* 74(Suppl IV):75–79, 1986.

91. Cooper DJ, Worthley LI. Adverse hemodynamic effects of sodium bicarbonate in metabolic acidosis. *Intensive Care Med* 13:425–427, 1987.

92. Berenyi KJ, Wolk M, Killip T. Cerebrospinal fluid acidosis complicating therapy of experimental cardiopulmonary arrest. *Circulation* 52:319–324, 1975.

93. Arieff AI. The indications for use of bicarbonate in patients with metabolic acidosis. *Br J Anaesth* 67:165–177, 1991.

94. Harrison EE, Avery BD. The use of calcium in cardiac resuscitation. *Am J Emerg Med* 3:267–273, 1983.

95. Thompson BM et al. Calcium: Limited indications, some danger. *Circulation* 74(Suppl IV):90–93, 1990.

96. Erdmann E, Reuschel-Janetschek E. Calcium for resuscitation? *Br J Anaesth* 67:178–184, 1991.

97. Resnekov L. Calcium antagonist drugs—Myocardial preservation and reduced vulnerability to ventricular fibrillation during CPR. *Crit Care Med* 9:360–361, 1981.

98. Steuven HA et al. The effectiveness of calcium chloride in refractory electromechanical dissociation. *Ann Emerg Med* 14:626–629, 1985.

99. Salerno DM et al. Post-resuscitation electrolyte changes: Role of arrhythmia and resuscitation efforts in their genesis. *Crit Care Med* 17:1181–1186, 1989.

100. Oszko MA, Klutman NE. Use of calcium salts during cardiopulmonary resuscitation for reversing verapamil-associated hypotension. *Clin Pharm* 6:448–449, 1987.

101. Kraig RP et al. Hydrogen ions kill brain at concentrations reached in ischemia. *J Cereb Blood Flow Metab* 7:379–386, 1987.

102. Lundy EF et al. Infusion of 5 percent dextrose increases mortality and morbidity following six minutes of cardiac arrest in resuscitated dogs. *J Crit Care* 2:4–14, 1987.

103. D'Alecy LG et al. Dextrose containing intravenous fluid impairs outcome and increases death after eight minutes of cardiac arrest and resuscitation in dogs. *Surgery* 100:505–511, 1986.

104. Longstreth WT Jr, Inui TS. High blood glucose level on hospital admission and poor neurologic recovery after cardiac arrest. *Ann Neurol* 15:59–63, 1984.

105. Longstreth WT Jr et al. Neurologic outcome and blood glucose levels during out-of-hospital cardiopulmonary resuscitation. *Neurology* 36:1186–1191.

106. Coffing CR et al. Etiologies and outcomes of the pulseless, nonbreathing pediatric patient presenting with ventricular fibrillation. *Ann Emerg Med* 21:1046, 1992.

107. Atkins DL et al. Pediatric defibrillation: Importance of paddle size in determining transthoracic impedance. *Pediatrics* 82:914–918, 1988.

108. Burns JP, Reardon FE, Truog RD. Using newly deceased patients to teach resuscitation procedures. *N Engl J Med* 331:1652, 1994.

Joan Burg

Melinda Morin

Daniel Doody

2 Care of the Injured Child

Injuries are the leading cause of death in children ages 1 to 14 years, resulting in four times the mortality of any other cause. Each year nearly one in four U.S. children will be sufficiently injured to seek medical attention, resulting in 10 million emergency department visits and 360,000 hospitalizations.[1-3] Approximately 10,000 children between 0 to 14 years and 22,000 youths 0 to 19 years die annually from injuries, resulting in an annual lifetime cost of $165 billion.[4-6]

The two leading causes of injury-related death in children are motor vehicle crashes and firearms. Since the late 1980s, the death rate from motor vehicle crashes has been decreasing and that from firearms increasing; in 1994 the death rate from firearm injuries surpassed that from motor vehicle crashes for the first time.[7] Other common causes of childhood injury include drowning, house fire, struck pedestrians, and bicycle-related injuries. Homicide is the leading cause of traumatic death in infants under 1 year of age, while homicide and suicide are the leading causes of death in adolescents. Falls are the leading cause of nonfatal injuries in the United States.[5,8]

In addition to the tragic loss of life, more than three times this number of children suffer disability at an estimated cost of $7.5 billion each year. The subsequent loss of productive years of life is greater than that resulting from any other etiology, including heart disease, stroke, and cancer.[5,6,8] To decrease the frequency of childhood injuries, a system-wide approach must be applied which incorporates all aspects of care, including prevention, access to care, pre-hospital care, in-hospital care and rehabilitative services.

Anatomy and Physiology

Traumatic injury in a child can be markedly different from that in an adult patient due to the significant anatomic and physiologic differences in this population (Table 2-1).[9-12] Vital signs vary by age, and knowledge of the normal values for age will assist in the recognition of respiratory or hemodynamic compromise (Table 2-2). Due to a greater percent body surface area, the child can rapidly lose body heat and become hypothermic. As children have a proportionately larger head relative to body mass, head injuries are more common and result in significant morbidity and mortality. The child's neck is shorter and the musculature less developed,

Table 2-1. Anatomic and physiologic features unique in children

Variable vital signs with age

Compensatory and reactive arterial tone

Greater body surface area

Proportionately large head

Short, poorly developed neck musculature

Cephalad larynx with narrow subglottic region

Pliable thoracic cage with a mobile mediastinum

Poorly protected abdominal contents

Intraperitoneal bladder

Presence of growth plates in long bones

Table 2-2. Pediatric vital signs

Age	Heart rate (beats/min)	Blood pressure (systolic mm Hg)	Respiratory rate (breaths/min)
Newborn	110–170	>60	30–50
1 year	100–160	>80	<40
5 years	80–130	>90	<30
Adolescent	<90	>90	<20

making determination of tracheal deviation or neck vein distension more difficult. In infants and young children, a more cephalad larynx and a smaller oropharynx make for a more difficult intubation, and short trachea may lead to mainstem bronchial placement. The thoracic cage in a child is more pliable, with less overlying musculature, allowing blunt trauma to cause significant internal chest injuries without fracturing ribs. The mediastinum is less firmly fixed than in the adult, which allows tension pneumothorax to develop more rapidly. The abdominal contents are protected by less rib and muscle, allowing for injuries to the spleen and liver. The bladder is an intraperitoneal organ and can be more readily injured than in the adult. The ligamentous structures in a child are stronger than the growth plates of the bones, making epiphyseal injuries more common than sprains.

Management

Considerable progress has occurred in the pre-hospital care of the acutely injured patient, but pediatric components of trauma systems have been slow to evolve (Table 2-3). The injury-related death rate in children is two times that of the adult patient.[13,14] Attempts at advanced life support (ALS) intervention in the pre-hospital setting in pediatric patients have a higher failure rate than in the adult population. Unlike in adult patients, where endotracheal intubation has a high success rate (86%–97%), the success rate in children, particularly those under 1 year, is as low as 50%. In addition, intravenous line placement and intubation can prolong field time. Ongoing training of pre-hospital and hospital personnel, in addition to a well-organized systematic approach, will assure that optimal care is provided to the pediatric trauma victim.

Being prepared necessitates having a designated trauma team with clearly assigned roles. All children with severe trauma should

Table 2-3. Management of traumatic injuries

The most common error is underestimating the severity of the injury.

Airway management must be aggressive and precise.

Fluid resuscitation must be aggressive and precise.

Progressive organ damage is frequent.

Consequences of hypoxemia and acidosis are often worse than the primary injury.

be transported to a pediatric trauma center, when available, for stabilization and management. This allows for involvement of appropriate pediatric and surgical specialties and has been shown to result in lower morbidity and mortality.[15,16]

The initial approach to the multiple trauma patient has been clearly defined in the Advanced Trauma Life Support course of the American College of Surgeons.[17] This two-tiered approach includes a primary survey, resuscitation phase, secondary survey, and definitive care. The sequential methodology helps to organize resuscitative efforts and avoid missing life-threatening injuries.

Primary Survey

The search for any life-threatening conditions and resuscitation proceed simultaneously. As with adults, the goals of resuscitation of the pediatric trauma patient include gaining control of external blood loss, establishing and maintaining a stable airway, assuring adequate ventilation, supporting the circulation, and assessing global neurologic status.

Airway and Cervical Spine Control

In any child who has significant trauma, the presence of a cervical spine injury must be assumed, and immobilization of the head and neck is mandatory.[18] Cervical spine injuries are less common in children than in adults, but when they occur, they often involve the upper cervical spine (Table 2-4).[19–21] This is due to the increased laxity of the cervical ligaments, a more horizontal alignment of the facets, and larger head size. Spinal cord injury without radiographic abnormality (SCIWORA) is a recognized cause of pediatric neurologic injury and accounts for a large number of pre-hospital deaths previously thought to be due to severe closed-head injury.[22]

The goal of airway management in the pediatric trauma patient is to assure adequate oxygen delivery and ventilation while protecting the cervical spine. Any child who has sustained significant injury should receive high-flow oxygen by face mask. Airway obstruction is common, and causes include anatomy (tongue or head position), an altered level of consciousness, a foreign body (blood or vomitus), trauma (maxillofacial fractures), and inflammation and edema (burns). A child with normal phonation or a strong cry is not likely to immediately obstruct his airway. Simple airway maneuvers include repositioning, airway opening with the jaw thrust technique, and suctioning, which will often return airway patency. Oral and nasal airways are useful alternatives.

Children involved in fires require a detailed airway evaluation. Patients with burns of the face or lips, a history of enclosed-space fire, and soot in the nares or mouth are at high risk for airway compromise. Thermal injury most commonly involves supraglottic tissues, and early intubation is recommended before edema progresses to obstruction.[23]

Any child who cannot be adequately ventilated with a bag and mask device or who is unable to protect her own airway (lacks an active gag and cough reflex) requires endotracheal intubation. Indications for elective intubation should be more liberal in the pediatric population given their tendency for upper airway obstruction. Indications for endotracheal intubation are listed in Table 2-5.

The key to a successful intubation is adequate preparation, and efforts must be well planned and communicated. Adhering to a protocol, such as the SOAP mnemonic (suction, oxygen, airway, pharmacology), can prevent mistakes from happening in the fray of resuscitation. Generally, oral intubation is easier and more successful while immobilizing the cervical spine. The Sellick maneuver, applying pressure to the cricoid cartilage and occluding the esophagus, can aid in preventing reflux and aspiration.

Nasotracheal intubation is rarely indicated and is contraindicated in the patient with maxillofacial injuries. Laryngeal fractures and severe maxillofacial trauma may require a surgical airway. Currently, needle cricothyroidotomy rather than emergent tracheostomy is the emergency procedure advocated in children who cannot be intubated or effectively bag-mask ventilated.[17]

Breathing

Airway and pulmonary injuries may be subtle, and high-flow oxygen by face mask should be provided to all major trauma patients, even in the absence of respiratory distress. As gastric distension can easily compromise ventilation in children, all pediatric patients with significant trauma benefit from gastric decompression.

In the spontaneously breathing child, the adequacy of ventilation must be assessed with attention to the depth and work of breathing. If ventilation is inadequate, bag-mask ventilation should be performed. Intubation with artificial ventilation is indicated if there is difficulty maintaining a stable airway with a face mask and bagging or if prolonged assisted ventilation is expected. The chest should be inspected for evidence of external trauma, asymmetry of chest wall movement with respirations, or flail segments. If breath sounds are absent on one side, assessment should be interrupted to initiate treatment (i.e., needle decompression of a pneumothorax or repositioning of the endotracheal tube). Pneumothorax and hemothorax should always be considered in the child with blunt chest trauma with hemodynamic instability.[22] Direct needle aspiration with an intravenous catheter introduced

Table 2-4. Indications for cervical spine immobilization

High-speed motor vehicle accident

Fall from significant height

Significant trauma above the level of the clavicles

Complaints of neck pain

Altered mental status or history of loss of consciousness

Neurologic deficit or paresthesias

Diving injury

Table 2-5. Indications for tracheal intubation

Cardiopulmonary arrest

Airway obstruction

Respiratory failure

Absent gag reflex

Glasgow coma score ≤ 8

Controlled hyperventilation

Prolonged airway control

Severe maxillofacial injury

Flail chest

into the second intercostal space in the midclavicular line can be life-saving. Chest tube placement should be performed once initial stabilization is complete.

Circulation

Adequate tissue perfusion must be maintained in all trauma patients. Signs of shock are subtle in children and often not apparent until approximately 25% of blood volume has been lost. Rapid assessment of rate and quality of pulse, capillary refill time, and mental status give valuable information about the adequacy of perfusion. Hypotension is a late finding in the hypovolemic child.

Vascular access should be obtained during the circulatory assessment of all children who have sustained major trauma. Unfortunately, rapid vascular access can be a challenge. If attempts at rapid percutaneous peripheral vascular access are unsuccessful, another form must be obtained. Alternatives include percutaneous central venous placement, intraosseous insertion, and surgical cutdown. Femoral vein cannulation is a convenient method in the patient undergoing intubation or CPR. The intraosseous route provides rapid and easy access for infusion of resuscitation medications.

Prior to fluid resuscitation, blood samples for type and crossmatch should be sent. Previous practice has dictated the immediate institution of fluid resuscitation in any child who has evidence of shock.[17] Administration of a rapid initial bolus of 20 ml/kg of isotonic crystalloid solution (lactated Ringer's or normal saline) is recommended. If vital signs fail to improve after the initial bolus, another 20 ml/kg bolus should be given. Vital signs and clinical parameters need to be followed carefully. If the child still fails to respond, 20 ml/kg of blood should be infused. If possible, crossmatched blood should be given if available; however, type-specific or O negative blood may be substituted.

Ongoing hidden blood loss usually involves the lungs (hemothorax), abdomen (intraperitoneal, retroperitoneal, or pelvic hemorrhage), or extremities (femur fracture). To provide adequate fluid replacement, 3 ml of crystalloid must be replaced for every 1 ml of blood lost.

In the persistently unstable patient, unresponsive to fluid and blood product resuscitation, the use of military antishock trousers (MAST) or pneumatic antishock garments (PSAG) may be beneficial. The PSAG have been used as an adjunct to the treatment of shock in adult trauma victims. Their effectiveness, previously thought to be largely a result of "autotransfusion" due to an increase in the total peripheral resistance, is probably limited to only 5% to 10% of the blood volume. There are limited data on their effectiveness for children, although they may afford temporary pelvic stability until definitive treatment can be obtained.

Recent evidence suggests that aggressive preoperative fluid resuscitation may be detrimental in adult trauma victims.[24] The delay of fluid resuscitation until operative intervention in children needs further investigation before this approach is applied to childhood injury victims.

Disability

A rapid neurologic assessment is essential in every trauma patient. A pupillary response should be evaluated early in the primary survey before any medications are given. Initial assessment will identify any severe head or spine injury. Appropriate response to questions such as "what happened" or "what is your name" indicates that the child is alert. The mnemonic AVPU can be used to assess mental status rapidly:

A. Alert

V. Responds to verbal stimuli

P. Responds to painful stimuli

U. Unresponsive

An improving neurologic status generally follows appropriate resuscitation with increased cerebral blood flow. Deterioration argues for significant, global neurologic injury or expanding intracranial mass lesion.[25]

Exposure

The pediatric trauma patient must be completely undressed to avoid missing major injuries. The larger body surface area of the child, however, renders her susceptible to hypothermia, so heating lamps should be available.

Secondary Survey

Continued focus on the airway, breathing, and circulation occurs during the secondary survey, but a more thorough evaluation of other systems begins. Details of the patient's past medical history, including allergies, medications, and surgical history, should be obtained. Diagnostic procedures, consultation, or operative intervention takes place. Serial examinations of the trauma patient help to determine the need for operative intervention. Any child with persistent hemodynamic instability without another obvious source of bleeding is likely to need surgical exploration. Monitoring of urine output is essential as a reflection of cardiac output and peripheral perfusion.

A rectal examination should be performed, specifically noting rectal tone as well as the location and consistency of the prostate. If there is evidence of trauma to the urethra (inability to void, external bleeding at the urethral meatus, or perineal bruising), a bladder catheter should not be passed. A retrograde urethrogram is the diagnostic procedure of choice. It is essential that a urinalysis be obtained on all multiply injured patients. If gross hematuria is present or greater than 50 RBC/HPF is found on urinalysis, additional radiographic studies are indicated.

The past decade has seen a less invasive approach to children with abdominal injuries, both in diagnosis and management. Occult abdominal injury is common in the pediatric trauma victim. In general, the initial evaluation of abdominal or suspected renal injuries should be contrast-enhanced CT scan. For blunt trauma to the kidney, liver, and spleen, close monitoring in the pediatric intensive care unit (PICU) is the preferred management.[26,27]

Diagnostic peritoneal lavage (DPL), although used extensively in the adult population, is not often utilized in children. As many solid organ injuries are now being successfully managed nonoperatively in the intensive care unit, the diagnosis of hemoperitoneum no longer mandates surgical exploration. DPL can be helpful if other surgical procedures need to be performed immediately on the multiply injured victim and in the patient with penetrating injury between the areola and the costal margin, given the potential for injury to the diaphragm. In the lower chest injuries, a peritoneal lavage, which yields greater than 10^4 RBC/ml is highly predictive of a diaphragmatic injury.

Intensive Care Unit Management

The transition to the ICU requires accurate transfer of information, including known events at the scene, presentation in the emergency ward, resuscitation details, and ongoing concerns.[28] As with other patients requiring intensive care management, anticipation of potential problems is the key to effective management. The trauma patient can be challenging due to the involvement of multiple surgical and medical specialists. Most ICU controversy involves the diagnosis and management of the more subtle injuries. The role of the intensivist, however, in concert with the pediatric trauma surgeon, is to organize coordinated care, keeping a "big picture" view of the patient.

Indications for ICU admission include evidence of hemodynamic instability on presentation, an unstable airway or the potential for respiratory deterioration, ongoing bleeding or potential for significant hemorrhage, a Glasgow coma score (GCS) less than or equal to 8, or an unstable spine. Approximately 30% of trauma deaths occur in the first hours following an injury. An additional 20% occur within days to weeks following the injury.[29] In the ICU there is the potential to decrease this mortality through organized and meticulous care (Fig. 2-1).

Cardiovascular Dysfunction

All multiple trauma patients should have ongoing cardiac monitoring and an ECG. Any evidence of ST or T wave changes require thorough investigation; however, ECGs are unreliable indicators of cardiac contusion in children.[30] Cardiac arrhythmias more commonly are warning signs of hypoxemia and hypoperfusion. Other methods of monitoring, such as temperature probe, pulse oximetry, and noninvasive blood pressure, should be utilized. Arterial line placement for monitoring blood pressure and blood gas evaluation is indicated in the patient with respiratory or hemodynamic instability. Central venous pressure (CVP) monitoring is an important adjunct in the trauma patient, with risks of significant fluid shifts seen in traumatic shock or significant burn injuries. Any patient who has undergone aggressive fluid resuscitation or a significant hypoxic injury with resultant capillary leak, or who will undergo fluid restriction (head injury patient), is a likely candidate for CVP monitoring.

Pulmonary artery catheters, although utilized less in the pediatric population than in the adult population, can be useful in the patient with significant cardiac dysfunction, adult respiratory distress syndrome (ARDS), or multiple organ failure syndrome. Burn patients often manifest evidence of cardiac dysfunction secondary to direct asphyxial damage as well as the depressant effect of the burn injury.[23,31] Pulmonary artery catheters may also be useful in the patient with left ventricular dysfunction following severe hypovolemic shock or cardiac arrest. With the hemodynamic information provided by a pulmonary artery catheter, a trial of inotropic or vasopressor therapy can be helpful in the patient not responding to fluid resuscitation. In addition, this information can assist in titrating fluid administration to avoid fluid overload with subsequent increase in capillary leak.

Respiratory Dysfunction

Progressive respiratory compromise following severe traumatic injury must be anticipated in the ICU. The pediatric trauma patient has multiple factors leading to respiratory embarrassment, includ-

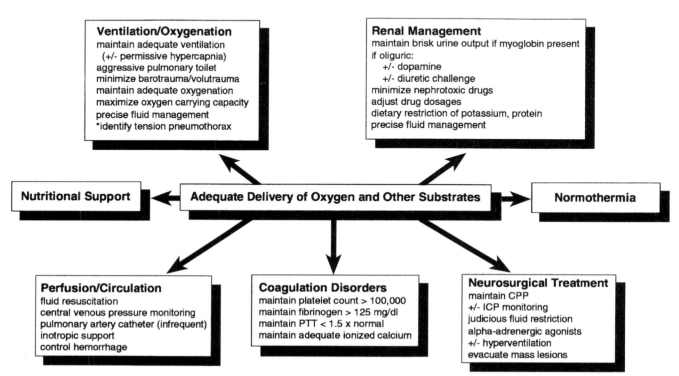

Figure 2-1. Priorities in the ICU management of the injured child. The primary goal is the adequate delivery of oxygen and other necessary substrates. Adequate ventilation, oxygenation, and perfusion are required to ensure this goal. Maintaining normothermia, renal function, neurologic stability, and correcting coagulation dysfunction are integral parts of the overall prioritization of care.

ing a baseline high oxygen consumption, potential for chest wall edema and disrupted capillary membranes, and the use of sedation and pain medications.

After the initial stabilization of the airway in the emergency setting, respiratory failure may occur secondary to progression of primary lung injury. Pulmonary contusion from blunt chest trauma is common and results in focal disruption of capillary membrane integrity and discrete areas of atelectasis. Patients exhibit progressive respiratory distress with hypoxemia due to intrapulmonary shunting. Careful titration of fluid is essential to minimize intraparenchymal shunting. Positive end-expiratory pressures (PEEP) at high levels may be helpful in providing internal stenting of alveoli in contused areas.

Other causes of delayed respiratory dysfunction include aspiration and pulmonary embolism. As aspiration often occurs before initial evaluation, aspiration pneumonitis frequently is an overlooked cause of respiratory deterioration with focal radiographic findings. Recent data suggest that children with trauma are at risk for developing deep vein thrombosis and pulmonary embolism.[32] Attention to this possibility should be given to the injured child with the sudden onset or unexpected worsening of respiratory distress, particularly if there are additional risk factors (i.e., the presence of a central venous catheter).

Another common cause of respiratory failure in the trauma patient is ARDS (see Respiratory Failure, by Fugate, Truman, and Todres, this volume), which frequently develops in the first 24 hours following extensive trauma. While often associated with pulmonary contusion, ARDS is seen as a final common pathway in patients with no known parenchymal damage (i.e., shock, long-bone trauma). ARDS is defined by the presence of noncardiogenic pulmonary edema from injury to the parenchymal microvasculature. Management remains largely supportive, and there is no known prophylaxis to its development. In established ARDS, the treatment goals of mechanical ventilation are to minimize barotrauma (including permissive hypercapnia), maintain distending pressures with PEEP, promote adequate tissue oxygen delivery and intravascular volume, maximize oxygen carrying capacity with packed RBC transfusion, identify other septic foci, and treat other organ dysfunction.[33]

All multiple trauma patients need aggressive pulmonary toilet. Atelectasis is a frequent complication in the heavily sedated patient (because of underventilation) and in those patients with untreated pain due to muscle splinting. The risk of aspiration with the use of uncuffed endotracheal tubes and frequent associated ileus is increased. Although less frequent, aspiration can occur around a cuffed endotracheal tube, so appropriate preventive measures should be taken.

Neurologic Dysfunction

Head injuries are the leading cause of morbidity and mortality in childhood trauma and occur in approximately 75% of children sustaining multiple traumas. The overall mortality from head injury is approximately 6%.[2,34] A number of these patients will die before arrival at an emergency department (ED), but efforts in the ED and in the ICU must be made to prevent further potential damage from secondary injury. The most common injury in children is diffuse brain edema and increased intracranial pressure (ICP).[17] Specific injuries and their management are described in Head Trauma by Swearingen, this volume.

The goal of effective management of neurologic injury is prevention of hypotension with subsequent cerebral hypoxia and isch-

emia. Fluid restriction in the initial resuscitation is inappropriate and can severely compromise cardiopulmonary function. Traditionally, fluid restriction has been advocated. However, this approach has recently been questioned with a current management that recommends normovolemia so that cardiovascular stability and adequate cerebral perfusion are not sacrificed.

Current management strategies advocate the early consultation of neurosurgery. Endotracheal intubation is advised for any trauma patient with a GCS less than or equal to 8. Although controversial, many trauma services recommend placement of ICP monitoring devices in this population and in all cases where surgical intervention is required prior to transfer to an ICU. Intraventricular drain placement, although associated with higher rates of infection and bleeding, offers the benefit of the ability to lower ICP by withdrawing cerebrospinal fluid (CSF). Even small changes in CSF volume can result in a significant reduction in ICP.

Traditionally, the management of intracranial hypertension centered around the reduction of ICP. Fluid restriction, hyperventilation, and the aggressive use of osmotic diuretics formed the basis of therapy. An alternative treatment strategy attempts not to minimize ICP, but to increase the mean arterial pressure (MAP) to maintain an adequate cerebral perfusion pressure (CPP):

$$CPP = MAP - ICP$$

It is hoped that this management scheme will lead to improved outcome in the pediatric population. At present, a minimum CPP of 50 mm Hg in the adult and 40 mm Hg in the child is suggested.[25] Current techniques in use are judicious fluid restriction, maintenance of a CPP greater than 40 mm Hg using vasopressors (dopaminergic or alpha-adrenergic agents, e.g., neosynephrine), maintenance of oxygen delivery with an adequate hemoglobin, avoidance of hyperthermia, and intermittent administration of mannitol for acute deterioration in the neurological examination.

Renal Dysfunction

The risk of renal dysfunction remains high in the severely injured PICU patient. Significant muscle injury, hemodynamic instability, third space losses with resulting intravascular depletion, and nephrotoxic drug use and sepsis threaten the health of the kidney. The onset of renal failure greatly reduces survival. Ischemic injury can occur from decreased blood flow secondary to fall in perfusion pressure, or due to splanchnic vasoconstriction. Duration of renal ischemia only loosely correlates with degree of renal injury.[35] In the trauma patient, hemoglobinuria complicating burn injuries and myoglobinuria from rhabdomyolysis may worsen any renal insult and need to be treated with alkalinization of the urine and induction of a brisk urine output with mannitol and diuretics.

Urine output remains the gold standard for monitoring perfusion and is a reflection of cardiac performance in most pediatric patients. A urine output of 1 ml/kg/hour or more indicates adequate volume status and cardiac function. When urine output falls, initial focus should be on the general hemodynamic status of the patient. The child with prerenal failure characteristically excretes a concentrated urine with high urine-plasma ratio of solutes including creatinine and urea. If renal damage worsens, the reabsorptive properties of the kidney are impaired and sodium appears in the urine. As renal function deteriorates, progressive metabolic acidosis, fluid overload, hyperkalemia, and toxin accumulation occur. Patients respond with increased levels of catecholamines and cortisol, initiating increased catabolism and protein breakdown.

Traditionally, prophylaxis for renal failure has included diuretic therapy and low-dose dopamine. Both mannitol and loop diuretics have a vasodilatory effect; a proven beneficial effect, however, has not been consistently documented. Dopamine at 3 to 5 μg/kg/min has also been used at doses felt to decrease renal vascular resistance. Although no clear benefit has been documented, dopamine administration remains a commonly held practice in the ICU. In the oliguric patient, diuretics are utilized frequently to reverse early renal failure by inducing urine flow. Diuretics may not reverse severe dysfunction, but conversion of oliguric to nonoliguric renal failure makes fluid and electrolyte management easier.

Although renal failure in the trauma patient has traditionally been treated with hemodialysis or peritoneal dialysis, new methods of fluid and toxin removal are available that may lead to improved outcome when utilized early in the disease course.[35] Before severe uremia and hyperkalemia develop, continuous hemofiltration can help to reduce fluid overload. Continuous venous hemofiltration provides effective control of fluid balance with fewer fluid restrictions and less hemodynamic instability. It does require access to large central veins, however. Concomitant use of a dialysate provides excellent elimination of solutes. In the absence of significant abdominal trauma, peritoneal dialysis provides a viable alternative for the treatment of acute renal failure.

Once renal insufficiency is diagnosed, careful fluid and electrolyte management is essential. Potassium and free water must be carefully restricted. Nutritional adjustments should include minimizing protein intake to less than 1 g/kg/day. Drug dosages should be adjusted and sepsis should be aggressively treated.

Disorders of Hemostasis and Coagulation

Coagulation dysfunction in the immediate postinjury period is generally secondary to iatrogenic causes. The severely traumatized patient is aggressively fluid resuscitated, at times receiving greater than 80 ml/kg in crystalloid solutions. The patient with persistent hemodynamic instability or evidence of active bleeding receives multiple packed RBC transfusions, often without adequate replacement of platelets and clotting factors. Dilution of these blood components can result in a coagulopathy. After one blood volume exchange with packed RBC alone, the platelet and coagulation factors are approximately one fourth of the original level.[36]

Hemostasis or the prevention of excessive blood loss involves three stages: (1) constriction of injured blood vessels, (2) primary hemostasis involving formation of a platelet plug, and (3) coagulation where fibrin is added to the platelet plug forming the definitive clot. Thrombocytopenia, the primary effect of which in hemostasis occurs early in the clotting cascade, is therefore a greater threat to the patient than diminished coagulation factors.

Hematologic dysfunction not related to dilution can be due to an abnormal rate of blood component consumption. At the site of injury, this consumption is not a pathologic process, but when disseminated intravascular coagulation (DIC) occurs systemically, the response is no longer appropriate. In DIC, two separate processes are initiated. Tissue damage and release of endogenous tissue factors lead to thrombi formation throughout the arterial and venous system, resulting in decreased peripheral blood flow and organ ischemia. Also occurring is the consumption of platelets and clotting factors, including fibrinogen, factor V, factor VIII, and prothrombin. When coagulation and fibrinolysis continues, the body's synthetic abilities are overwhelmed and the levels of platelets and factors decrease below that necessary for normal hemostasis. This is manifested by widespread bleeding.

Management of DIC generally involves treatment of the under-

lying cause; therapy in the trauma patient, however, must include attention to hemodynamic stability, normothermia, and treatment with blood products. A platelet count of greater than 10⁵, a fibrinogen greater than 125 mg/dl, and treatment of coagulopathy with fresh frozen plasma to decrease partial thromboplastin time (PTT) to less than 1.3 times normal is desirable. Cryoprecipitate is indicated only in cases of hypofibrinogenemia because the blood product is expensive and carries an increased risk of infectious disease transmission through exposure to multiple donors. Anticipated response to transfusion with packed RBC or platelets is represented in Table 2-6.

Blood product transfusions are associated with a number of known complications. Platelet transfusions can be complicated by symptoms of hypotension and rash, felt to be a systemic response to leukocytes present in the sample. The trauma patient with poor myocardial function is at risk for the negative inotropy associated with the drop in calcium secondary to chelation by the citrate contained in banked blood. Patients with hyperkalemia are at significant risk when receiving packed RBC transfusions, particularly older aliquots of banked blood, which have a higher content of hemolyzed cells. Although blood products are often valued for their colloid effect, the patient with severe injury and vascular leak will allow a highly osmolar substance in the extravascular space. This results in increased interstitial edema with slow mobilization back into the intravascular space.

Nutritional Support

Provision of adequate nutrition following trauma is a high priority because nutritional status has been shown to correlate with survival.[37] Starvation and malnutrition are associated with loss of lean body mass and subsequent organ dysfunction. In the multiply traumatized patient, caloric and energy needs can often double. In the pediatric patient with high baseline requirements, this can prove overwhelming. Major injury induces a catabolic state. Although nutritional support can decrease the degree of catabolism, it rarely converts the patient to an anabolic state.[38] If severe catabolism is allowed to persist, the effects on the immune system, pulmonary and hepatic function, wound healing, as well as growth of the child are significantly compromised. Providing adequate nutrition may help to minimize the stress-induced immune depression witnessed in the trauma patient.

The rationale for early nutritional support focuses on the gut as an active immunologic organ. Gut atrophy favors bacterial translocation, which has been seen to occur during the first few hours following a critical injury.[37] Enteral feeds maintain the gut wall integrity by providing luminal cells with nutrients and preventing bacterial overgrowth.

Some trauma and burn units initiate enteral feeds within the first 12 hours following injury, although similar studies in the pediatric population have yet to demonstrate an improved outcome. Although it may be desirable to begin nutrition early in the ICU course, enteral feedings may be problematic due to paralytic ileus from direct injury, response to indirect injury, or medica-

Table 2-6. Principles of transfusion

Packed RBC transfusion: 3 ml/kg will raise the hemoglobin by 1 g/dl

Platelet transfusion: 1 unit platelet/10 kg will raise platelet count by 10⁵

tion effect. The stomach and colon are areas of the gut most frequently and severely affected in the postinjury or postoperative patient.[38] Gastric atony can be bypassed with the use of duodenal or jejunal feeding tubes, the passage of which can be expedited with the use of intravenous metoclopramide. Carefully monitored continuous feedings can be started at rates of 1 ml/kg/hr with gradual increases. Enteral feedings in this manner can provide potential protection against bacterial translocation, even if adequate caloric needs cannot be met. Frequent side effects include abdominal distension and diarrhea.

In those patients unable to tolerate enteral feeds or when the gut cannot be used, parenteral nutrition should be used. In the immediate postinjury period, third space losses and hemodynamic instability often preclude the use of nutritional support. Peripheral formulations are limited by the minimal concentration of glucose (osmolarity) tolerated by peripheral veins, the primary use of fat as a calorie source, and the dependence on large volumes of fluid for delivery. Central venous formulations require central venous access with the associated risks, but provide glucose at higher concentrations than can be provided peripherally.

Protein catabolism is the hallmark of metabolism in the trauma patient, with protein providing approximately 15% to 20% of energy needs via gluconeogenesis.[39] The initial metabolic response to injury is a stress response with release of catecholamines, growth hormone, and glucagon. The result is antagonism of insulin action, with a concomitant rise in blood sugar. Any continued or new stress, such as sepsis, can result in prolonged catabolism with significant lean body mass loss.

The goal of total parenteral nutrition is to provide adequate nonprotein calories via fat and glucose to minimize the amount of protein used for energy and to encourage anabolism. Although the composition of parenteral nutrition varies with each patient, it is recommended that the ratio of nonprotein calories to nitrogen be 150 to 200:1. Glucose infusions should be limited to less than 4 mg/kg/min because higher rates can result in inadequate glucose clearance from the liver, resulting in conversion to fat with deposition in the liver. The other risk of glucose loading is the concern over increased carbon dioxide production. As excess glucose is converted to fat, greater carbon dioxide production occurs, adding potential stress to a patient with a tenuous respiratory status and perhaps complicating weaning the patient from a ventilator.

Pain and Anxiety

The ICU management of the pediatric trauma patient must include treatment of pain and anxiety. The PICU patient suffers pain from injuries of trauma, undergoes painful procedures, is separated from family or caregivers, frequently has an altered level of consciousness, and is surrounded by constant activity, light, and stimulation. Careful attention must be paid to the pain and sedation needs of the acutely injured child.

Pediatric patients often are very sensitive to the respiratory depressive effects of agents used for analgesia and sedation. These should be used with particular caution in non-intubated infants under 3 to 6 months of age, patients with hemodynamic or airway instability, patients with evolving neurologic conditions, or patients with altered ventilatory control. Opioids, when coupled with benzodiazepines, often induce hypoventilation because the effects on the central respiratory drive are synergistic. This problem may be exacerbated in the hypovolemic patient. Analgesia and sedation at continuous, low-dose infusions are more efficacious than bolus dosing.

Many of the commonly used analgesic agents are also useful for their sedating effect. In the patient with pain, however, in whom sedation is contraindicated, regional anesthesia and newer agents (e.g., ketorolac) offer analgesia without the concern of masking an evolving neurological examination. Epidural analgesia can provide pain relief with fewer side effects associated with systemic narcotic use. An epidural catheter can deliver local anesthetics (lidocaine or bupivacaine) or opioids (morphine or fentanyl). Ketorolac, a prostaglandin inhibitor, does not produce respiratory depression or sedation; in adult studies, however, this drug has been associated with an increased risk of gastrointestinal bleeding and renal dysfunction, particularly in the hypovolemic patient. Its use in children requires further evaluation.

In the ICU patient, agitation equals hypoxemia and/or underventilation until proven otherwise. The progressively anxious patient should be examined closely for evidence of airway compromise, ventilatory disturbances, and alterations in blood gas. Short-acting sedation agents (e.g., midazolam) are helpful, particularly in the head-injured patient with agitation, who requires close observation for potential deterioration of neurologic function. The decision to administer opioids or benzodiazepines should be made in consultation with the pediatric trauma surgeon or neurosurgeon to ensure that the effects of the drug will not compromise the patient's clinical evaluation.

The severely injured child can become chemically dependent when receiving continuous infusions of opioids or benzodiazepines. Withdrawal from these agents must be anticipated and appropriately treated. The stress response associated with withdrawal can have adverse effects, including increased catabolism and poor wound healing (see Sedation and Pain Control by Arnold and Berde, this volume).

References

1. Christoffel KK. Violent death and injury in US children and adolescents. *Am J Dis Child* 144:88, 1982.
2. Division of Injury Control, Center for Health and Injury Control, Centers for Disease Control. Childhood injuries in the United States. *Am J Dis Child* 144:627, 1990.
3. National Safety Council Tabulations of National Center for Health Statistics and Mortality Data. *Accident Facts*, 1994 edition.
4. Guyer B, Gallagher S. An approach to the epidemiology of childhood injuries. *Pediatr Clin North Am* 32:5, 1985.
5. Rice DP et al. Cost of injury in the United States; a report to Congress 1989. San Francisco: Institute for Health and Aging, University of California and Injury Prevention Center, The Johns Hopkins University, 1989.
6. Runge JW. The cost of injury. *Emerg Med Clin North Am* 11:187, 1993.
7. Fingerhut L, Jones C, Makue D. Firearm and motor vehicle injury mortality variations by state, race and ethnicity: United States 1990–91. Advance data from vital and health statistics; no. 242. Hyattsville, Maryland: National Center for Health Statistics. 1994.
8. Waller AE, Baker SP, Szocka A. Childhood injury deaths: National analysis and geographic variations. *Am J Public Health* 79:310, 1989.
9. Anderson PA et al. The epidemiology of seatbelt-associated injuries. *J Trauma* 31:60, 1991.
10. Burdi AR, Huelke DF. Infants and children in the adult world of automobile safety design: Pediatric and anatomical considerations for design of child restraints. *Biomechanics* 2:267, 1969.
11. Eichelberger MR et al. Comparative outcomes of children and adults suffering blunt trauma. *J Trauma* 28:430, 1988.
12. Inaba AS, Seward PN. An approach to pediatric trauma. Unique anatomic and pathophysiologic aspects of the pediatric patient. *Pediatr Emerg* 9:523, 1991.

13. Holmes MJ, Reyes HM. A critical review of urban pediatric trauma. *J Trauma* 24:253, 1984.

14. McKoy C, Bell MJ. Preventable traumatic deaths in children. *J Pediatr Surg* 4:505, 1983.

15. Durch JS, Lohr KN (eds). *Emergency Medical Services for Children.* Washington, DC: National Academy Press. 1993.

16. Lowe DK et al. Patterns of death, complication and error in the management of motor vehicle accident victims: Implications for a regional system of trauma care. *J Trauma* 23:503, 1983.

17. American College of Surgeons Committee on Trauma. *Advanced Trauma Life Support Program Instructors Manual.* 1989.

18. Holley J, Jorden R. Airway management in patients with unstable cervical spine fractures. *Ann Emerg Med* 18:1237, 1989.

19. Hadley AJ et al. Pediatric spinal trauma. Review of 122 cases of spinal cord and vertebral column injuries. *J Neurosurg* 68:18, 1988.

20. Pang D, Wilberger JE. Spinal cord injury without radiographic abnormalities in children. *J Neurosurg* 57:114, 1982.

21. Ruge JR et al. Pediatric spinal injury: The very young. *J Neurosurg* 68:25, 1988.

22. Trauma resuscitation. In Chameides L (ed): *Textbook of Pediatric Advanced Life Support.* Dallas: American Heart Association, 1994.

23. Spear RM, Munster AM. Burns, inhalational injury and electrical injury. In Rogers MC (ed): *Textbook of Pediatric Intensive Care.* Baltimore: Williams & Wilkins, 1987. Pp 1506–1512.

24. Bickell WH et al. Immediate versus delayed fluid resuscitation for hypotensive patients with penetrating torso injuries. *N Engl J Med* 331:1105, 1994.

25. Fink M. Emergency management of the head injured patient. *Emerg Med Clin North Am* 5:783, 1987.

26. Meredith JW, Young JS, Bowling J. Nonoperative management of blunt hepatic trauma: The exception or the rule? *J Trauma* 36:529, 1994.

27. Morse MA, Garcia VF. Selective nonoperative management of pediatric blunt splenic trauma: Risk for missed associated injuries. *J Pediatr Surg* 29:23, 1994.

28. Moront ML et al. The injured child: An approach to care. *Pediatr Clin North Am* 41:1201, 1994.

29. Trunkey D. Initial treatment of patients with extensive trauma. *N Engl J Med* 324:1259, 1991.

30. Ildstad S et al. Cardiac contusion in pediatric patients with blunt thoracic trauma. *J Pediatr Surg* 25:287, 1990.

31. Reynolds EM et al. Left ventricular failure complicating severe pediatric burn injuries. *J Pediatr Surg* 30:264, 1995.

32. Andrew M et al. Venous thromboembolic complications (VTE) in children: First analyses of the Canadian Registry of VTE. *Blood* 83:1251, 1994.

33. Kacmarek RM, Hickling KG. Permissive hypercapnia. *Respir Care* 38:373, 1993.

34. Tepas JJ et al. Mortality and head injury: The pediatric perspective. *J Pediatr Surg* 25:92, 1990.

35. Pascual JF, Lopez JD, Molina M. Hemofiltration in children with renal failure. *Pediatr Clin North Am* 34:803, 1987.

36. Dawson RB. Acute coagulation disorders after trauma. In Siegel JH (ed): *Trauma. Emergency Surgery and Critical Care.* New York: Churchill Livingstone, 1987. Pp 737–745.

37. Zaloga GP. *Nutrition in Critical Care.* St. Louis: Mosby, 1994. Pp 59–62.

38. Ott L, Young B. Metabolic and nutritional management. In Andrews BT (ed): *Neurosurgical Intensive Care.* New York: McGraw-Hill, 1992. Pp 163–171.

39. Askanazi J et al (eds). Nutritional support. *Crit Care Clin* 3:1, 1987.

Brahm Goldstein

John H. Fugate

I. David Todres

3 ▸ Transport of Critically Ill and Injured Children

The Emergency Medical Services (EMS) Systems Act of 1973 was designed to improve the pre-hospital and in-hospital care of the acutely ill or injured patient. Adults have a higher prevalence of diseases requiring EMS (those resulting from trauma, poisoning, ischemic heart disease, and acute treatable diseases) than do children. As a result, pediatric EMS systems initially suffered because of lack of interest, education, money, and resources.[1] As regionalized trauma and neonatal centers and their associated transport systems developed, those centers with pediatric intensive care facilities began transporting acutely ill children from outlying hospitals to tertiary care facilities.

Improvements have been made in EMS systems for children (EMS-C), and many states are now served by regionalized pediatric critical care transport systems. Despite these advances, pre-hospital care of the critically ill child still lags behind that for the adult, neonate, or trauma victim. Holbrook stated that the "pre-hospital phase is the most underdeveloped area in the care of critically ill children."[2] He reported that in 1976 approximately 60% of deaths in children between the ages of 1 to 14 years were caused by diseases that usually require EMS. Seidel et al. concluded that needs of children are often not met in the pre-hospital setting.[3] Furthermore, EMS programs "often fail to recognize the special needs of the critically ill child." In a follow-up report, Seidel reported that 40% of paramedic and emergency medical technician (EMT) training programs offered less than 10 hours of didactic and clinical experience in caring for children and many lacked proper equipment used in the care of pediatric patients.[4]

Viewing pre-hospital care of children from a different perspective, Applebaum concluded that priority should be given to adult emergencies, as children were less likely to benefit from advanced levels of pre-hospital care.[5] This appears to be relevant to children who suffer out-of-hospital cardiac arrest.[6–8] However, a large number of acutely ill and injured children would likely benefit from advanced pre-hospital treatment and transport to a regional pediatric intensive care unit (PICU). Survival of critically ill and injured children is increased when they are hospitalized at pediatric critical care centers rather than local hospitals.[9]

Unlike neonatal and trauma EMS systems, pediatric transport systems and PICUs lack formal regionalization in many parts of the United States. Bushore calls for macroregions of pediatric emergency care.[10] The American Academy of Pediatrics, Committee on Hospital Care states that in order to "achieve maximum cost effectiveness and optimal patient care, the [pediatric] transport system should be regional in scope and used by multiple facilities."[11] The Society of Critical Care Medicine joint task force has issued guidelines for the safe transportation of critically ill patients.[12]

Patient Population

Table 3-1 lists the results from published reports of pediatric transport. Of the studies listed, the most common diagnostic categories are respiratory, neurologic, and trauma (including head trauma). These are also the most common diagnostic categories of children admitted to a multidisciplinary PICU. There is a seasonal variation in the number of pediatric critical care team transports, with an increase during the fall and winter months when the most likely cause is an increased incidence of respiratory pathogens.[13,14]

The age range for pediatric critical care transport varies from the newborn through late adolescence or early adulthood. The large array of diseases prevalent at different ages, combined with developmental differences in physiologic features, necessitate that pediatric critical care transport personnel be well versed in cardiology, pulmonology, neurology, infectious disease, pharmacology, and trauma management as well as have formal training in pediatric surface and air transport.

Table 3-1 Pediatric critical care transport studies

Study	No. of transports	Air/ground	Most common diagnostic category	Age range	No. of intratransport deaths	In-hospital mortality
Harris et al. 1975[13]	22	22/—	Surgical trauma	—	0	—
Dobrin et al. 1980[14]	125	54/71	Resp, neuro	1 mo–18 yr	0	11.2
Duncan et al. 1981[41]	46	—	Resp	—	0	10.9
Black et al. 1982[30]	752	713/39	Neuro, resp	3 wk–16 yr	1	—
Smith and Hackel 1983[17]	115	—	Neuro, resp	2 wk–18 yr	0	—
Owen and Duncan 1983[18]	158	73/85	Resp	—	0	—
Mayer and Walker 1984[19]	636	604/32	Neuro, resp	3 wk–16 yr	0	7.0
Colombani et al. 1985[31]	267	73/194	Trauma	<15yr	—	6.7
Kisson et al. 1988[34]	72	—	Neuro, resp	—	—	16.7
Kanter and Tompkins 1989[47]	117	—/117	Trauma, resp	—	0	16.2
Kanter et al. 1992[15]	177	—/177	Trauma, resp	—	—	—

Modified with permission from Goldstein B. Pediatric critical care transport. In Chernow B, Todres ID (eds): *Problems in Anesthesia*. Philadelphia: Lippincott, 1989.

Components of a Pediatric Critical Care Transport System

Personnel

Expert, well-trained personnel are essential for a successful pediatric transport system. Kanter et al. showed in 1992 that there was increased morbidity in patients transferred with a nonspecialized team as opposed to patients in a PICU during their first 2 hours of admission.[15] Edge et al. demonstrated significantly increased intensive care adverse events in patients transported with a nonspecialized team when compared with a specialized team.[16] However, the optimal makeup of the "transport team" remains controversial. Various centers use combinations of pediatric, anesthesia, and pediatric surgery house officers, PICU fellows, nurses, respiratory therapists, and EMTs in the composition of their pediatric transport teams.[17–21] Beyer et al. showed that intubated pediatric patients could be transported safely without a physician as long as the transport team was well trained in pediatric transport and was well supervised.[22]

The American Academy of Pediatrics, Committee on Hospital Care proposed guidelines for air and ground transportation of pediatric patients.[11] They concluded that the composition of the pediatric transport team should vary, depending "on the patient's diagnosis and clinical condition and with the availability of different types of medical personnel in a given system." Furthermore, the selection of the transport team should be made from a pool of trained personnel, including physicians (beyond intern level), nurses, respiratory therapists, and EMTs. A pediatric intensivist should also be available. McCloskey et al. have demonstrated in separate articles that physician need for transport can be predicted and that physicians are not always needed on pediatric transports.[23,24] Rubenstein et al. noted that need for a physician could not always be predicted according to their criteria for physician intervention.[25] The National Leadership Conference could not reach a consensus on this issue.[26]

Whatever criteria are used to select the pediatric critical care transport team, two important factors deserve mention. (1) The key to any successful pediatric transport system is intensive training and experience of all medical personnel in the rapid diagnosis and acute management of the critically ill or injured child, especially under transport conditions. (2) A pediatric intensivist or pediatric emergency medicine physician must be available at all times to make critical decisions regarding triage of patients, transport team composition, and mode of transport, and to provide continuous communication between the referring physician, transport team, and receiving hospital throughout the transport process. The National Leadership Conference on Pediatric Interhospital Critical Care Transport reached the following consensus.[26]

1. Pediatric patients should be transported by staff with the cognitive and technical skills required for pediatric patients and sufficient experience to maintain those skills.
2. Each critical care transport should be supervised by an attending physician who is expert in pediatric critical care or emergency medicine.
3. Possession of appropriate skills by team members is a more critical issue than the presence of a physician.
4. For some programs, a stratified team with a flexible response tailored to the anticipated needs of the patient may be optimal.
5. The ideal system for classifying patient status is as yet unidentified. A multicenter study using a common data base would be useful for validating such a system

Equipment

Basic lists of equipment and medications required for pediatric transport are shown in Tables 3-2 and 3-3, respectively. Previous reports have detailed similar lists.[11,14,27] One principle that must be observed at all times is that the transport team should bring **all** equipment and drugs necessary for stabilization and return transport. Although the list of medications on Table 3-3 will apply to most transport situations, the individual case must be assessed as to its specific needs (e.g., prostaglandin E-1 for transport of the infant with a congenital cardiac defect). The referring hospital should be presumed to have limited pediatric equipment and resources.

The transport equipment and medications should be organized by the transport coordinator. (We have found a nurse to be very effective in this position.) A centralized storage area holds the necessary monitors, medical equipment, and medications. Routine maintenance and restocking of all transport equipment and medications is done after all transports and on a weekly basis in conjunction with the biomedical engineering and pharmacy departments. Prior to departure, the transport nurse goes through a rapid checklist of equipment and medications. An emergency medication dosage schedule is also prepared for each patient based on the patient's weight in kilograms (Fig. 3-1).

Table 3-2. Pediatric transport equipment

Monitoring equipment
    ECG monitor and electrodes
    Blood pressure—cuff and invasive
    Thermometer—regular, low grade
    Pulse oximeter

Respiratory equipment
    Oxygen tank (full)
    Oxygen facemask and tubing
    Airways—oral, nasopharyngeal
    Bag-valve-mask systems
    PEEP valves and manometer
    Endotracheal tubes
    Magill forceps
    Laryngoscopes

Suction equipment
    Suction catheters
    Portable suction device

Procedure equipment
    Intravenous catheters
    Intraosseous needles
    Central venous catheters
    Chest tubes
    Heimlich valve
    Syringes

Fluids and intravenous infusion equipment
    D_5W, dextrose 5% in water
    Normal saline
    Ringer's lactate solution
    5% albumin
    Infusion pumps and appropriate tubing

Miscellaneous
    NG tube
    Tape
    Flashlight

MASSACHUSETTS GENERAL HOSPITAL
PEDIATRIC INTENSIVE CARE UNIT

PEDIATRIC EMERGENCY DRUG THERAPY

NAME:_____ DATE:_____ MD_____

RN:_____

weight (max 40 kg)_____ ETT size_____ Landmark:_____

DRUG	DOSE	CALCULATION	
EPINEPHRINE (1:10,000)	0.1 ML/KG (MAX 5 ML)	____ KG X 0.1 ML/KG	_____ML
ATROPINE (0.4 MG/ML)	0.02 MG/KG (MAX 0.5 MG)	____ KG X 0.05 ML/KG	_____ML MIN = 0.25 ML MAX = 1.25 ML
SODIUM BICARB. (0.5 mEQ/ML	PREEMIES: 1Meq/KG	____ KG X 2 ML/KG	_____ML
(1 mEQ/ML)	1 - 2 mEQ/KG	____ KG X 1-2 ML/KG	_____ML
DEXTROSE 10% (.10 GM/ML) for neonatal hypoglycemia	.5 GM/KG	____ KG X 4 - 5 ML/KG	_____ML
DEXTROSE (.25 GM/ML) FOR PEDIATRIC EMERGENCY GLUCOSE REPLACEMENT	0.5 GM/KG TO 1 GM/KG	____ KG X 2 ML/KG ____ KG X 4 ML/KG	_____ML _____ML
CALCIUM CHLORIDE 10%	3 MG EL. CA/KG (STARTING DOSE)	____ KG X 0.1 ML/KG	_____ML
GLUCONATE 10%		____ KG X 0.3 ML/KG	_____ML
LIDOCAINE (20 MG/ML)	1 MG/KG	____ KG X 0.05 ML/KG	_____ML
DEFIBRILLATION	EXTERNAL: 2 J/KG	____ KG X 2 J/KG	_____J
	INTERNAL: 0.02 J/KG (double dose if ineffective)	____ KG X 0.2 J/KG	_____J
CARDIOVERSION	0.5 JOULES/KG (double dose if ineffective)	____ KG X 0.5 J/KG	_____J
BREVITAL (10 MG/ML)	1 MG/KG	____ KG X 0.1 ML/KG	_____ML
SUCCINYLCHOLINE	< 1 YEAR: 2 MG/KG > 1 YEAR: 1 MG/KG	____ KG X 0.1 ML/KG ____ KG X 0.05 ML/KG	_____ML _____ML
PANCURONIUM (2 MG/ML)	0.1 MG/KG	____ KG X 0.05 ML/KG	_____ML

Figure 3-1. Emergency drug therapy form.

DRUG	DOSE	CALCULATION
EPINEPHRINE ISOPROTERENOL NOREPINEPHRINE PHENYLEPHRINE	MIX: 0.06 MG X WT IN 100 ML D5W I ML/HR = 0.1 MCG/KG/MIN	_____KG X 0.6 = _____MG IN 100 ML
START AT 1 ML/HR TITRATE FOR EFFECT TO 10 ML/HR		
DOPAMINE DOBUTAMINE	MIX: 6 MG X WT IN 100 ML D5W 1 ML/HR = 1 MCG/KG/MIN	_____KG X 6 = _____MG IN 100 ML
START AT 5 ML/HR TITRATE FOR EFFECT TO 20 ML/HR		
NITROPRUSSIDE NITROGLYCERIN	MIX: 6 MG X WT IN 100 ML D5W 1 ML/HR = 1 MCG/KG/MIN	_____KG X 6 = _____MG IN 100 ML
MAXIMUM CONCENTRATION FOR NIPRIDE SHOUD NOT EXCEED 100 MG IN 100 ML. START AT 1 ML/HR. TITRATE FOR EFFECT TO 8 ML/HR.		
AMRINONE	MIX: 6 MG X WT IN 100 ML NS 1 ML/HR = 1 MCG/KG/MIN	_____KG X 6 = _____MG IN 100 ML
GIVE AT 0.75 MG/KG TO START. MAY REPEAT LOADING DOSE X 3 TOTAL EVERY FIVE MINUTES IF NO RESPONSE.		
PROSTAGLANDIN E1	MIX: 0.6 MG X WT IN 100 ML D5W 1 ML/HR = 0.1 MCG/KG/MIN	_____KG X 0.6 = _____MG IN 100 ML
START AT 1 ML/HR. TITRATE FOR EFFECT TO 2 ML/HR.		
LIDOCAINE	MIX: 6 MG X WT IN 100 ML D5W 1 ML/HR= 1 MCG/KG/MIN	_____KG X 6 = _____MG IN 100 ML
START AT 30 - 40 MCG/KG/MIN. IF BREAK THRU ARRHYTHMIAS REBOLUS AND TITRATE TO 50 MCG/KG/MIN.		

Figure 3-1. (cont.)

Table 3-3.   Pediatric transport medications

Resuscitation
  Epinephrine 1:10,000 and 1:1000
  Bicarbonate (sodium)
  Atropine
  10% calcium chloride
  25% dextrose
  Narcan
  Dopamine
  Dobutamine

Antiarrhythmics
  Lidocaine
  Adenosine

Airway/pulmonary
  Racemic epinephrine
  Methylprednisolone
  Aminophylline
  Albuterol nebulizers

Muscle relaxants/sedatives
  Midazolam
  Morphine sulfate
  Ketamine
  Methohexital
  Succinylcholine
  Pancuronium
  Vecuronium

Neurologic/anticonvulsants
  Phenobarbital
  Diphenylhydantoin
  Diazepam
  Lorazepam
  Mannitol

Antihypertensives
  Labetalol
  Nifedipine

Antibiotics
  Ampicillin
  Aminoglycoside
  Cephalosporin

Diuretic
  Furosemide

Communication

Communication between the transport team and referring hospital is essential for safe and successful transport. Beginning with the initial telephone call from the referring physician, optimally via a well-publicized "Hot Line" number, a concise and accurate description of the patient and the patient's condition must be communicated. A transport data form used by the transporting team is shown in Fig. 3-2.

The triage physician is trained to obtain the information required to initiate a transport. Recommendations are made to the referring physician to help stabilize the patient until the transport team arrives. Often, follow-up phone calls to check on the patient's progress are made while the transport team is enroute. The transport team should contact the referring hospital on successful completion of the transport and continue to notify them of the child's progress.

The referring hospital has an important role in facilitating communications between the transport team and the family of the critically ill child. In addition, the referring hospital should be advised to have prepared copies of all relevant medical notes, x-rays, and laboratory values.

Various severity of illness scores may be used as a triage device by the receiving institution in making decisions concerning transport mode, personnel, and equipment. The Therapeutic Intervention Scoring System (TISS),[19,20,27-29] Glasgow Coma Scale (GCS),[30-32] Modified Injury Severity Scale (MISS),[31,33] Physiological Stability Index (PSI) Scoring System,[34,35] Pediatric Risk of Mortality Index (PRISM),[15,36] and the Denver Patient Status Category (DPSC) system[14,34] have been used in assessing pretransport severity of illness. The Pediatric Trauma Score may also prove to be a useful tool for triage of pediatric trauma patients.[37-39] Other reasons for obtaining an objective measure of patient illness are for quality assurance, utilization review, cost analysis, and clinical studies of pediatric critical care patients and transport systems

Mode of Transport

Modern ground ambulances, helicopters, and fixed-wing aircraft are equipped to function as mobile ICUs, capable of monitoring various physiologic functions almost as well as in the PICU. Ground ambulance is the most common form of critical care transport. Due to geographic conditions in the Boston area, ground transport accounts for the majority of all pediatric transports. This varies considerably between centers. Pediatric transport programs in large rural geographic areas, such as Colorado and Utah, have reported using mostly air transport.[14,19,30]

There are a number of advantages to ground ambulance transportation. Ambulances can carry almost any type of equipment necessary to provide intensive care during transport, such as mechanical ventilators, defibrillators, and monitoring devices. If the patient suddenly deteriorates during transport, the ambulance may stop along the roadside until the transport team can restabilize the patient. Ambulances are also relatively fast and inexpensive over short distances (<50 miles) compared with air transport. The disadvantages of ground transport include noise, vibrations, and sudden, unexpected movements. We have found the incidence of motion sickness experienced by transport team members to be increased in ground ambulance transport. This can be ameliorated or even prevented by the use of scopolamine dermal patches placed prior to transport.

Modern air transport of critically ill patients involves both helicopter and fixed-wing aircraft. The advantages of using helicopters over ground ambulance or fixed-wing aircraft include ease of access to either the accident scene or referring hospital, rapid departure time, and overall speed. Many hospitals use a hospital-based helicopter with helipad. Disadvantages of helicopter transport include noise; difficulty in access to the patient; hypothermia in cold weather; inability to fly if inclement, unsafe weather conditions exist; and a limited range, usually 200 to 350 miles.

Fixed-wing aircraft are used for long-range transports of greater than 300 to 400 miles. These aircraft can be modified to resemble an ICU environment. There is minimal noise and vibration, and access to the patient is relatively easy. Disadvantages include the necessity of using a second ground ambulance transport, both from the referring hospital to the airport and from the airport to the receiving hospital. The effects of high altitude on patients have been well documented.[11] Expanding gas secondary to a decrease in the ambient pressure can result in pneumothorax, ruptured viscus, pressure on a vital organ, and sinus or middle ear pain. The reduction in the partial pressure of oxygen results in a lowered

MASSACHUSETTS GENERAL HOSPITAL

NEONATAL AND PEDIATRIC
INTENSIVE CARE UNITS

TRANSPORT DATA
FOR ADMISSION

DATE _____ TIME OF CALL _____ CHILD'S NAME _____

BIRTH DATE _____ BIRTH TIME _____ GEST AGE _____ WEIGHT _____

SEX M ___ F ___ REFERRING HOSPITAL _____ TEL # _____

REFERRING PHYSICIAN _____ TEL # _____

PRIMARY PEDIATRICIAN _____ TEL # _____

PATIENT LOCATED IN: EW _____ PEDI FLOOR _____ NEWBORN UNIT _____ L&D _____

SIGNIFICANT INFORMATION (DIAGNOSIS, BIRTH HX, P.M. HX, APGARS)

CULTURES DONE: YES ____ NO ____ TYPE OF FLUID LINE IN _____
ANTIBIOTICS: YES ____ NO ____ TYPE _____

CURRENT STATUS OF CHILD

TEMP _____ HEART RATE _____ RESP RATE _____ B.P. _____

D-STICK _____ HCT _____ CURRENT BLOOD GAS: ART _____ CAP _____

OTHER SIGNIFICANT BLOOD WORK: _____ X-RAYS _____

RESPIRATORY STATUS: INTUBATED _____ FiO2 _____ HOOD _____ FACE MASK _____
TRACH _____ OTHER _____ O2 SAT _____

VENT MODE: BAGGING _____ RESPIRATOR _____ INSP PRESSURE _____
PEEP _____ RATE _____

RECOMMENDATIONS FROM MGH TO THE REFERRING PHYSICIAN

CALL TAKEN BY: _____

Figure 3-2. Massachusetts General Hospital Pediatric and Neonatal Intensive Care Units' transport data form. (Reprinted with permission from Goldstein B. Pediatric critical care transport. In Chernow B, Todres ID (eds): *Problems in Anesthesia*. Philadelphia: Lippincott, 1989.)

alveolar PO_2 and subsequent hypoxemia, even in pressurized cabins. Changes in barometric pressure can alter flow rates of intravenous solutions. Therefore, infusion pumps should be used to provide accurate IV flow rates during all air transports.

The mode of transportation for pediatric critical care transport is determined by the following factors: (1) the nature and severity of the patient's illness, (2) the capabilities and resources of the referring hospital, (3) the type of transport vehicles and personnel available, (4) geography, (5) weather, (6) traffic patterns, and (7) cost (Fig. 3-3).

The patient's condition and need for rapid and expert stabilization and treatment are of primary importance. In cases in which the patient is unstable or the referring hospital lacks the proper personnel or expertise to correctly stabilize and treat the patient,

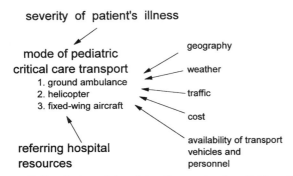

Figure 3-3. Factors determining the mode of pediatric critical care transport. (Reprinted with permission from Goldstein B. Pediatric critical care transport. In Chernow B, Todres ID (eds): *Problems in Anesthesia.* Philadelphia: Lippincott, 1989.)

rapid transport may be life-saving. Baxt et al. compared ground versus air transport in adult trauma patients transported from the scene of injury.[40] By the use of helicopter versus ground ambulance, they reported a significant decrease in predicted mortality for adult patients suffering from blunt trauma.

Geography plays an important role in determining transport mode. The most common reason for choosing air transport is the shorter time needed for air transport when the referring hospital is isolated a great distance away from the receiving medical center. Reviewing Table 3-1, a marked geographic influence on the primary mode of transport is evident. Areas such as Utah, Colorado, and Australia rely heavily on air transport because of the greater distances involved.[14–19,30,41] For example, Mayer and Walker reported that in Denver the mean distance of pediatric transport was 207 miles.[19] In contrast, Colombani et al., reporting results from a major pediatric trauma center in Maryland,[31] and the authors' experience at the Massachusetts General Hospital in Boston, found that these facilities serve geographically smaller and more densely populated areas.

Another reason for using air transport involves topographical obstacles such as mountains or ocean. For instance, emergency transports from Nantucket Island, located off the coast of Cape Cod, to the Massachusetts General Hospital may only be accomplished by helicopter.

Traffic patterns likewise can determine the mode of transport in large urban areas. In Boston, a 45-minute transit time by ambulance late at night without any traffic congestion can turn into a 2-hour transit time during rush hour; for the latter, emergency transport by helicopter is necessary.

Weather conditions should be an absolute determination of the feasibility of air transport by either helicopter or fixed-wing aircraft. In order to ensure optimal safety, the aircraft pilot should make this determination without any knowledge of the prospective patient's status. Weather conditions should also determine safe ground ambulance speed during transport. In winter, when snow and icy road conditions often exist, good judgment and caution must be exercised.

Cost may be a factor in determining the mode of transportation. Black et al. reported a cost analysis of the pediatric air transport program in Salt Lake City, Utah.[30] They determined that the charge per mile of air transport was similar (within 1%) to ground transport for distances between 25 and 200 miles and substantially less for transports of greater distances.

Preparation for Transport

Initially, a "scoop-and-run" approach toward transportation of critically ill patients was believed to be optimal. The concept was to transport patients after minimal stabilization, regardless of their underlying illness or condition, as rapidly as possible to a regional medical center for further stabilization and treatment. This approach has worked well in selected adults, trauma victims, and the subset of patients in whom restorative measures can be instituted only at the medical center.[42] In pediatric patients, the scoop-and-run policy—especially with inadequately trained personnel—has been shown to be detrimental. Sharples et al. noted that 32% of children dying from head injury had potentially avoidable factors, including inadequate management of the airway.[43] Edge et al. reported that adverse clinical events occurred in only 2% of children when a specialized transport team was employed, as opposed to 20% of children with adverse effects when nonspecialized staff was used.[16,44] Stabilization may take some hours, especially if the patient is hemodynamically unstable and requires inotropes in addition to assisted ventilation.[45] However, this is time well spent in the interests of the child. It is useful to have a checklist prior to departure from the referring hospital for the PICU (Table 3-4).[46] The list ensures that optimal stabilization has

Table 3-4. Checklist prior to transport of the critically ill child

Airway
- Is the airway clear?
- If obstructed or potentially obstructed, perform tracheal intubation.
- Is the tube adequately fixed and correctly positioned, i.e., mid-trachea? (Chest x-ray may be needed to confirm.)
- Suction airway prior to departure.

Ventilation
- Is the chest moving adequately and equally on both sides?
- Are the ventilation settings appropriate?
- Check ETCO$_2$/blood gases when available.

Oxygenation
- Is the patient's color satisfactory?
- Are the O$_2$ saturations adequate?
- Is there an adequate supply of O$_2$ for transport?

Perfusion (circulation)
- Is perfusion adequate?
- Check extremity warmth, capillary refill, pulses (distal compared with central), blood pressure, urine output.
- Appropriate IV catheters in place and well secured.
- Appropriate IV fluid infused (preferably with pumps).

Drugs
- Is the patient adequately sedated and pain controlled?
- Are there adequate supplies of necessary drugs required for transport?

Monitors/devices
- Are monitors functioning and alarms appropriately set?
- Are all drains and catheters secure and protected?

Records, x-rays
- Are all necessary records and x-rays available?

Miscellaneous
- Are parents informed of the management plans and the destination for their child's care; provided telephone numbers and names of responsible physician staff?
- Is the PICU notified of the needs of the child for ICU care and the approximate time of arrival to the unit?
- Is the transport environment temperature appropriate?

been achieved and is likely to remain so in transport. The list has general application; specific disease states, however, will warrant special considerations.

Because of differences in development, anatomy, and disease states, critically ill or injured children often need expert and sometimes definitive treatment by the transport team prior to departure from the referring hospital. For example, to ensure safe transport, the 2-year-old child with life-threatening acute airway obstruction needs establishment of a patent airway through endotracheal intubation or surgical tracheostomy while at the referring hospital.

The goal of pediatric critical care transport should be delivery of care that approximates that received in the PICU, within the limits of the transport process. While the focus of this chapter is on the foundations of safe transport from one hospital or scene of trauma to a tertiary ICU, the same principles apply to the "short transport" for the patient **within** the hospital (e.g., from radiological examinations, operating room, etc.).

Outcome

Mortality data are shown in Table 3-1. Only one intratransport death was reported.[30] The patient had suffered a cardiac arrest prior to air transport and died while in flight.

The low frequency of transport deaths implies that most programs stress stabilization and initiation of corrective treatment measures prior to departure from the referring hospital. It may be advisable to perform prophylactic procedures before the return transport to ensure patient safety. For example, in a child with a deteriorating respiratory or neurologic status, endotracheal intubation to ensure airway patency and assisted ventilation performed electively at the referring hospital under controlled circumstances are preferable to a possible sudden respiratory arrest and the need for emergency intubation in an ambulance or helicopter.

Overall mortality rate subsequent to transport to the PICU ranges from 6.7% to 16.7%. Black et al. reported a higher mortality rate in trauma versus non-trauma patients (9% vs. 5.2%).[30] This higher rate seemed most likely related to the presence of head injury in many trauma patients. Mayer and Walker and Colombani et al. concluded that unlike adult trauma victims, the pediatric trauma victim mortality does not correlate with multiple organ injury but directly correlates with the presence of head injury.[19,31] Furthermore, they suggested that with aggressive management, including airway control, ventilation, and maintenance of stable heart rate and blood pressure, mortality and morbidity can be minimized. The use of mannitol, furosemide, head positioning, and hyperventilation to control increased intracranial pressure is recommended when appropriate.

Morbidity following pediatric critical care transport has been assessed in two studies. Black et al. reported an 8% disability (2% severe and 6% moderate) as assessed by the GCS in their report of 752 pediatric air transport patients.[30] Using the same scale,[31] Colombani et al. reported a 9.4% incidence of mild-to-severe neurologic deficits in 160 head injury patients.

References

1. Goldstein B. Pediatric critical care transport. In Chernow B, Todres ID (eds): *Problems in Anesthesia*. Philadelphia: Lippincott, 1989.
2. Holbrook PR. Prehospital care of critically ill children. *Crit Care Med* 8:537, 1980.
3. Seidel JS et al. Emergency medical services and the pediatric patient: Are the needs being met? *Pediatrics* 73:769, 1984.
4. Seidel JS. Emergency medical services and the pediatric patient: Are the needs being met? II. Training and equipping emergency medical services providers for pediatric emergencies. *Pediatrics* 78:808, 1986.
5. Applebaum D. Advanced prehospital care for pediatric emergencies. *Ann Emerg Med* 14:656, 1985.
6. Eisenberg M, Bergner L, Hallstrom A. Epidemiology of cardiac arrest in children. *Ann Emerg Med* 12:672, 1983.
7. Friesen RM et al. Appraisal of pediatric cardiopulmonary resuscitation. *Can Med Assoc J* 126:1055, 1982.
8. O'Rourke PP. Outcome of children who are apneic and pulseless in the emergency room. *Crit Care Med* 14:466, 1986.
9. Pollack MM et al. Comparison of tertiary and nontertiary intensive care: A statewide comparison (abstract). *Pediatr Res* 23:234, 1988.
10. Bushore M. Emergency care of the child. *Pediatrics* 79:572, 1987.
11. American Academy of Pediatrics, Committee on Hospital Care. Guidelines for air and ground transportation of pediatric patients. *Pediatrics* 78:943, 1986.
12. Society of Critical Care Medicine joint task force. Guidelines for the safe transfer of critically ill patients. *Crit Care Med* 21:931, 1993.
13. Harris BH, Orr BE, Boles ET. Aeromedical transportation of infants and children. *J Pediatr Surg* 10:719, 1985.
14. Dobrin RS et al. The development of a pediatric emergency transport system. *Pediatr Clin North Am* 27:633, 1980.
15. Kanter RK et al. Morbidity associated with interhospital transport. *Pediatrics* 90:893, 1992.
16. Edge WE et al. Reduction of morbidity in interhospital transport by specialized pediatric staff. *Crit Care Med* 22:486, 1994.
17. Smith DF, Hackel A. Selection criteria for pediatric critical care transport teams. *Crit Care Med* 11:10, 1983.
18. Owen H, Duncan AW. Towards safer transport of sick and injured children. *Anaesth Intens Care* 11:113, 1983.
19. Mayer TA, Walker ML. Severity of illness and injury in pediatric air transport. *Ann Emerg Med* 13:108, 1987.
20. McCloskey KA, King WD, Bryan L. Pediatric critical care transport: Is a physician always needed on the team? *Ann Emerg Med* 18:247, 1989.
21. Orr RA et al. Transportation of critically ill children. In Rogers MC (ed): *Textbook of Pediatric Intensive Care* (2nd ed). Baltimore: Williams & Wilkins, 1992.
22. Beyer AJ, Land G, Zaritsky A. Nonphysician transport of intubated pediatric patients: A system evaluation. *Crit Care Med* 20:961, 1992.
23. McCloskey KA, Johnston C. Critical care interhospital transports: Predictability of the need for a pediatrician. *Pediatr Emerg Care* 6:89, 1990.
24. McCloskey KA, King WD, Byron L. Pediatric critical care transport: Is a physician always needed on the team? *Ann Emerg Med* 18:247, 1989.
25. Rubenstein JS et al. Can the need for a physician as part of the pediatric transport team be predicted? A prospective study. *Crit Care Med* 21:1657, 1993.
26. Day S et al. Pediatric interhospital critical care transport: Consensus of a national leadership conference. *Pediatrics* 88:696–704, 1991.
27. Cullen DJ et al. Therapeutic intervention scoring system: A method for a quantitative comparison of patient care. *Crit Care Med* 2:57, 1974.
28. Yeh TS et al. Assessment of pediatric intensive care application of the therapeutic intervention scoring system. *Crit Care Med* 10:497, 1982.
29. Rothstein P, Johnson P. Pediatric intensive care: Factors that influence outcome. *Crit Care Med* 10:34, 1982.
30. Black NE et al. Air transport of pediatric emergency cases. *N Engl J Med* 307:1465, 1982.
31. Colombani PM et al. One-year experience in a regional pediatric trauma center. *J Pediatr Surg* 20:8, 1985.
32. Jennett B et al. Severe head injuries in three countries. *J Neurol Neurosurg Psychiatry* 40:291, 1977.
33. Mayer T et al. Causes of morbidity and mortality in severe pediatric trauma. *JAMA* 245:719, 1981.

34. Kisson N et al. The child requiring transport: Lessons and implications for the pediatric emergency physician. *Pediatr Emerg Care* 4:1, 1988.

35. Yeh TS et al. Validation of physiologic stability index for use in critically ill infants and children. *Pediatr Res* 18:445, 1984.

36. Pollack MM, Ruttiman UE, Getson PR. Pediatric risk of mortality (PRISM) score. *Crit Care Med* 16:1110, 1988.

37. Ramenofsky ML et al. The predictive value of the Pediatric Trauma Score. *J Trauma* 28:1038, 1988.

38. Tepas JJ et al. The Pediatric Trauma Score as a predictor of injury severity in the injured child. *J Pediatr Surg* 22:14, 1987.

39. Tepas JJ et al. The Pediatric Trauma Score as a predictor of injury severity: An objective assessment. *J Trauma* 28:425, 1988.

40. Baxt WG et al. Hospital-based rotocraft aeromedical emergency care services and trauma mortality: A multicenter study. *Ann Emerg Med* 14:859, 1985.

41. Duncan AW et al. A pediatric emergency transport service. *Med J Aust* 2:673, 1981.

42. Brill JC, Geideman JM. A rationale for scoop-and-run: Identifying a subset of time-critical patients. *Topics Emerg Med* July: 37, 1981.

43. Sharples PM et al. Avoidable factors contributing to death of children with head injury. *Br Med J* 300:87, 1991.

44. Edge WE et al. Reduction of morbidity in interhospital transport by specialized pediatric staff. *Crit Care Med* 20:S38, 1992.

45. Whitfield JM, Buser NNP. Transport stabilisation times for neonatal and pediatric patients prior to interfacility transfer. *Pediatr Emerg Care* 9:69, 1993.

46. Macrae DJ. Paediatric intensive care transport. *Arch Dis Child* 75:175, 1994.

47. Kanter RK, Tompkins JM. Adverse events during interhospital transport: Physiological deterioration associated with pretransport severity of illness. *Pediatrics* 84:43, 1989.

4 Airway Procedures

I. David Todres

Joseph J. Frassica

4.1 Tracheal Intubation

Tracheal intubation is a vital procedure required in selected critically ill children. The physician in the intensive care unit therefore must be skilled in carrying out the procedure, both in the patient with a normal airway and in those with a "difficult airway." In appropriate situations (i.e., a conscious patient and one who is developmentally able to comprehend), the child should be apprised of the procedure and its effects. This involves explaining that a tube will be coming through the mouth or nose, which will temporarily make them unable to talk and may be uncomfortable. Reassurance and appropriate medication should be provided.

Anatomic Considerations

Tongue

The infant tongue is relatively large with respect to the oral cavity, making it more likely to obstruct the upper airway during bag-mask ventilation. The tongue may also present an obstruction to the passage of the endotracheal tube if not properly controlled during insertion of the laryngoscope blade.

Larynx

The infant's larynx is located high in the oropharynx at the level of cervical vertebrae 3-4. With advancing age, the laryngeal opening descends to the level of C4-5. The relatively cephalad position of the infant larynx may make exposure of the laryngeal inlet more difficult than in the older child.

Airway Shape

The infant and child upper airway is shaped differently than in the adult. The adult upper airway has a relatively constant cross-sectional diameter below the glottic opening. In the infant, the upper airway takes the shape of an inverted cone with the narrowest point at the cricoid ring. Therefore, the glottic opening of the infant and child larynx may appear larger than the airway's smallest dimension, which is hidden just below the vocal cords.

Epiglottis

The infant epiglottis is firm and omega-shaped, making it potentially difficult to lift directly to expose the glottic opening, in which case the laryngoscope blade placed in the vallecula will displace the epiglottis indirectly. However, direct lifting of the epiglottis may be necessary to achieve full visualization of the glottic opening.

Preparation for Intubation

Identification of the Difficult Airway

The majority of airways are normal and relatively easily managed. It is prudent, however, to approach all patients as having a potentially difficult airway so that one is well prepared to deal with the difficult situation when it arises. The approach to the potentially difficult airway includes a careful physical examination and radiologic examination, if necessary.[1,2] Tracheal intubation is potentially difficult in the presence of a pathology of the maxillofacial area, neck, pharynx, and larynx. With a congenital anomaly, the defect may be associated with anomalies of other organ systems (e.g., cardiac), and this must be taken into account in the selection of drugs with which to intubate the child.

Limitation of extension of the head at the atlanto-occipital joint is an important cause of difficult intubation.[3] With extension limited by the approximation of the occiput and the posterior tubercle of the atlas, attempts at extension lead to forward or anterior displacement of the larynx and difficulty in visualizing the glottic opening.[4] Forward displacement of the upper teeth and backward displacement of the tongue also contribute to difficulties with intubation. The shape of the mandible and the size and position of the tongue and its mobility are important factors in determining the ease of laryngeal visualization. A receding mandible, (e.g., Pierré Robin, Treacher Collins syndromes) is associated with difficult intubation.

To assess the potential for difficult intubation, one should perform the following three evaluations of the patient's anatomy prior to intubation attempts. First, one should assess, preferably in the sitting patient, the visibility of the uvula and soft palate. When these are obstructed by the base of the tongue, laryngoscopy and visualization of the glottis may be extremely difficult.[5] Second, an assessment should be made of the patient's ability to extend the atlanto-occipital joint by having the patient extend the neck actively (this test should not be performed in the patient with suspected cervical injury). Finally, the length of the thyromental space should be evaluated (i.e., the distance from the thyroid cartilage to the inside of the mental portion of the mandible) with the head fully extended.[6] An abnormally shortened space (in the adolescent, the average is a distance of 5–6 cm or 3 finger breadths; in the infant one finger breadth is normal) may be a predictor of a difficult intubation.[7] Thus, adequate mouth opening with observation of the uvula, base of tongue, and soft palate; extension of the atlanto-occipital joint; and thyromental space are important factors in predicting the ease of laryngeal visualization. Utilizing these three assessments probably provides the most accurate indication of a potentially difficult intubation. It should be kept in mind, however, that these tests may fail to predict difficult intubations in a number of patients, who subsequently prove to be difficult to intubate, and conversely may predict difficult intubations in some normals.[8,9]

Based on the pre-intubation evaluation, a plan must be formulated to ensure that skilled personnel are available to assist with the management of the difficult airway prior to undertaking intubation. In some cases, it may be indicated to have personnel standing by who can perform emergent bronchoscopy or tracheostomy should this be necessary.

Special techniques have been introduced to assist in carrying out tracheal intubation in a child with a difficult airway. The use of a modified laryngoscope blade (Oxyscope) provides supplemental oxygenation during laryngoscopy and minimizes the potential for hypoxemia. The fiberoptic bronchoscope may allow one to pass an endotracheal tube under direct vision and be able to circumvent "obstructions" to standard laryngoscopic examination. The laryngeal mask airway may provide a means to ventilate the patient who proves to be difficult to intubate and ventilate with bag-mask while attempts are being made to establish a secure airway either through fiberoptic intubation or tracheostomy.[10]

Equipment

Endotracheal Tube Size Selection

Selection of an appropriate endotracheal tube (ETT) size is an important part of preparation for intubation. A simple formula based on the child's age is a helpful guide (Table 4.1-1), although recent studies indicate that the height of the child correlates more accurately with appropriate tube size selection.[11,12] Another simple method for determining ETT size requires examining the child's little finger and comparing the middle phalanx to the potential tube selections; the closest match should be the appropriate size. Regardless of the calculated size, one should have available one size smaller and one size larger than the calculated sized tube to allow for individual variation. Generally, uncuffed tubes are selected for children under 9 years of age because the cricoid ring is the narrowest point in the upper airway and usually provides an adequate seal for the tube. Some situations, however, may call for a cuffed ETT in patients younger than 9 years. These situations include intubation for bowel obstruction surgery and severe respiratory failure requiring peak inspiratory pressures greater than 20 cm H_2O. It should be kept in mind that a cuffed ETT has an external diameter 1 mm larger than the same internal diameter size uncuffed ETT. This may be of significance in the smaller airway where 1 mm may make a significant difference in airway resistance. Cuffed ETT may be used at any age if care is taken to maintain cuff pressure within a range that allows adequate perfusion of tracheal tissues. ETT cuff pressures should not exceed 20 mm Hg. For a child beyond approximately 9 years of age, cuffed tubes are necessary. The appropriate size tube should allow an air leak around the tube at 20 to 30 cm H_2O peak inflation pressure.

Laryngoscope Blade

A straight blade (e.g., Miller) is more suitable in infants and young children than a curved blade (e.g., Macintosh) because the larynx is higher in the neck and the angle between the base of the tongue to the glottis is more acute in the young child.

Suction

An operating suction with an appropriately sized suction tip should be positioned within reach of the right hand of the operator. A firm suction tip, such as the pediatric Yankauer, is preferable to a suction catheter for clearing the airway of all but the smallest children during intubation.

Bag-Valve Mask with Oxygen Supply

A means to provide positive pressure ventilation and appropriately sized mask (Mapleson, or self-inflating bag-mask) should be available prior to initiating endotracheal intubation.

Oral/Nasal Airways

Appropriate sized oral and nasal airways should be available to facilitate establishment of an adequate mask airway.

Technique

Oral Intubation

After preparation and airway assessment are complete, laryngoscopy and tracheal intubation are performed with the child sedated (breathing spontaneously) or sedated and muscle relaxed (paralyzed). Proper equipment is needed (Table 4.1-2). The appropriate choice of drugs will depend on the child's clinical status. The operator performing the procedure must give **clear** instructions to assistants regarding positioning of the patient, applying cricoid pressure (Sellick maneuver) whenever regurgitation and pulmonary aspiration are significant possibilities, and directions for appropriate administration of drugs to facilitate laryngoscopy and tracheal intubation.

Position of the child's head and neck is critical in providing optimal conditions for intubating the trachea. The position corresponds to an alignment of the axes of the structures of the mouth, oropharynx, and trachea, thus permitting direct visualization of the glottic opening with the laryngoscope in proper position. Figure 4.1-1 demonstrates the maneuvers necessary for alignment of the oral, pharyngeal, and tracheal axes. To achieve this, a folded blanket or pillow approximately 2 inches high is placed beneath the child's occiput, providing flexion of the cervical spine. Extension of the head at the atlanto-occipital joint now aligns the axes; the patient is now in the classic "sniffing" position.

In children younger than 2 years of age, because the head is relatively large in proportion to the trunk, it is usually unnecessary to elevate the occiput; head extension at the atlanto-occipital joint

Table 4.1-1. Endotracheal tube size for children

Age	Size (mm ID)
Neonate–6 mo	3.0–3.5
6 mo–1 yr	3.5–4.0
1 yr–2 yr	4.0–5.0
Over 2 yr	$\dfrac{Age\ (yr)\ +\ 16}{4}$

ID = internal diameter

Table 4.1-2. Tracheal intubation equipment

Suction (functional, immediately available)
Endotracheal tubes
Laryngoscope (bright light)
Bag-mask device with O_2
Oral airways
Assistant for cricoid pressure
Drugs

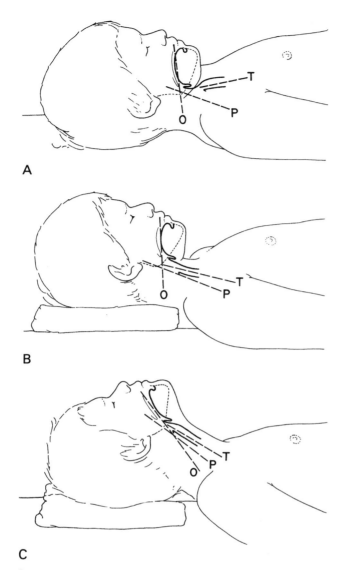

A

B

C

Figure 4.1-1. Correct positioning for ventilation and tracheal intubation. With a patient flat on the bed **(A)** the oral (O), pharyngeal (P), and tracheal (T) axis passes through three divergent planes. **(B)** A folded sheet or towel placed under the occiput of the head aligns the pharyngeal (P) and tracheal (T) axis. **(C)** Extension of the atlanto-occipital joint results in alignment of the oral (O), pharyngeal (P), and tracheal (T) axes. From: Coté CJ and Todres ID. The pediatric airway. In Coté CJ, Ryan JF, Todres ID, and Goudsouzian N (eds): *A Practice of Anesthesia for Infants and Children*. Philadelphia: Saunders, 1992. With permission.

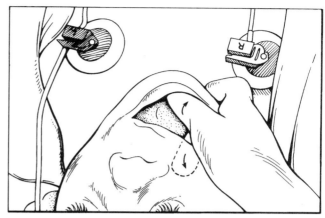

Figure 4.1-2. A method for opening the mouth to introduce the laryngoscope blade.

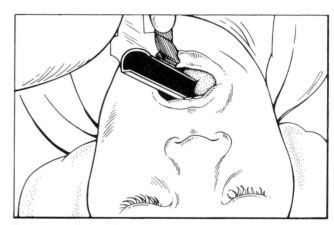

Figure 4.1-3. In placing the laryngoscope blade correctly, the tongue should be swept over to the left side of the mouth. Improper control of the laryngoscope blade and tongue leads to a "spill over" of the tongue, as depicted, and obscures an adequate view of the glottic opening.

will align the airway axes. In addition, because the larynx has a relatively high position in the neck, flexion does not aid visualization. However, external pressure on the larynx may increase the intubation angle and facilitate visualization of the glottis.[13] An assistant can be helpful in maintaining the patient's head in the mid-line.

Any loose teeth should be noted and care taken to avoid trauma to them. Suction equipment must be at hand to ensure clear visibility as one introduces the laryngoscope blade. The laryngoscope blade is introduced **gently** after opening the child's mouth

(Fig. 4.1-2). The blade is introduced along the dorsum of the tongue from the right corner of the mouth, gently sweeping the tongue toward the left. Care should be taken to avoid the tongue's "spilling" over the laryngoscope blade and obscuring visibility (Fig. 4.1-3). The blade is then gently directed down the mid-line and the landmarks are identified—first the uvula and then the epiglottis (Fig. 4.1-4). In many situations, introduction of the tip of the laryngoscope blade into the vallecula and then the gentle lifting of the base of the tongue provides a direct view of the glottic opening (Fig. 4.1-5). In some cases, this maneuver is inadequate for viewing the glottic opening, in which case the tip of the laryngoscope blade is introduced behind the epiglottis and then lifts the epiglottis with the base of the tongue to expose the glottic opening. The operator should then pass the appropriate ETT through the glottis, noting the depth to which the tube has been passed (Fig. 4.1-6). In the normal airway, direct visualization of the passage of the tube is possible. The use of a stylet within the tube may be helpful in shaping the curve of the tube and thus facilitating

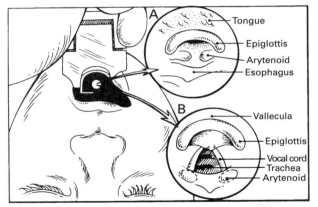

Figure 4.1-4. As the laryngoscope blade is advanced, anatomical landmarks are identified. **(A)** The epiglottis is noted, but a complete view of the glottic opening is not yet achieved because the blade needs to be further introduced into the vallecula or beyond the tip of the epiglottis.

tracheal intubation. The stylet should **not** protrude beyond the tip of the tube.

ETT insertion distance is determined by the length of the trachea as measured from glottic opening to carina. In children up to 1 year of age, this varies between 5 and 7 cm. In our experience, when the 10-cm mark on the ETT is at the alveolar ridge of the child between 3 and 12 months of age, the tip of the tube rests in a proper position above the carina. At age 2 years, the 12-cm mark on the tube is a useful guide. For a child beyond 2 years of age, the correct length for oral intubation corresponds to

$$\frac{age\ (years)}{2} + 12 \quad or \quad \frac{weight\ (kg)}{5} + 12$$

Markings on the distal end of the ETT may be used as a guide to the depth of tube placement. The ETT should be positioned initially with the double-line marks at the level of the vocal cords. Correct positioning is confirmed by chest inspection and auscultation for equal bilateral chest excursion and breath sounds. Placement within the trachea is confirmed with end-tidal carbon dioxide

detection. The ETT tip moves relative to the carina with motion of the head. The ETT tip moves away from the carina with neck extension and toward the carina with flexion. A simple way to remember this is to recall that the ETT tip "follows the nose" with movement of the head. Following clinical assessment of ETT position, it is secured with adhesive tape. A chest x-ray may then be taken to confirm the correct tube position.

Nasotracheal Intubation

We generally recommend initial placement of an orotracheal tube. Should nasotracheal tube placement be indicated, switching to this position is done with the patient optimally oxygenated, employing 100% oxygen, and ventilated via the orotracheal tube. The ETT chosen for nasal intubation is generally one half size smaller than the appropriately sized oral tube. The nasal mucus membranes should first be sprayed with neosynephrine or a similar vasoconstrictor to allow for easier, less traumatic passage. The tube should be softened in warm saline prior to introduction into the naris. The appropriate size of nasotracheal tube is then passed along the floor of the nose via the naris, which allows the easiest passage. This procedure should be carried out gently because adenoidal hypertrophy is common in children and trauma may lead to significant bleeding and obstruction of the airway. The tip of the nasotracheal tube is advanced into the oropharynx; the tip is then grasped with a Magill forceps and directed toward the glottic opening (occupied by the orotracheal tube). An assistant removes the orotracheal tube on instruction from the operator, who passes the nasotracheal tube to the proper depth. The nasotracheal tube is then fixed with tape at the nose. The patient's head is steadied in the neutral position to avoid flexion and extension with movements of the head, which could lead to accidental right mainstem intubation or extubation, respectively.

Management of the Difficult Airway

In patients with a predicted difficult airway, spontaneous ventilation should be maintained if at all possible. The use of neuromuscular blocking agents to facilitate intubation, prior to establishment of an adequate mask or laryngeal mask airway, may have disastrous consequences because of loss of muscle tone in the tongue and

Figure 4.1-5. Lateral views of the upper airway demonstrating the position of the tip of the laryngoscope blade. **(A)** The Macintosh laryngoscope blade is placed deep into the vallecula. **(B)** A straight blade laryngoscope lifts the epiglottis to expose the glottic opening.

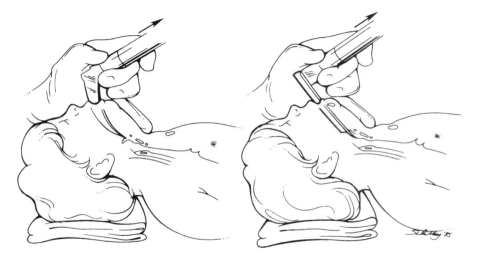

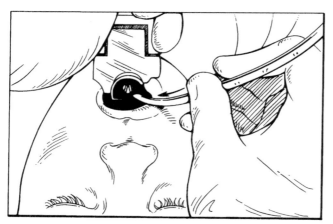

Figure 4.1-6. With the glottic opening in full view, the ETT is introduced from the right corner of the mouth, and its passage through the glottis is visually followed until the tube is properly positioned.

larynx, leading to total airway obstruction and inability to ventilate the patient manually.

Airway Management Situations

All patients who need emergency intubation should be evaluated for the potential for aspiration of stomach contents during the procedure. In general, patients who require emergency intubation should be treated as if they have a "full stomach" with its attendant risk for aspiration. In this situation, rapid-sequence intubation (RSI) should be followed (Table 4.1-3). The choice of specific sedatives and muscle relaxants depends on the clinical situation and indications for intubation. Commonly encountered clinical scenarios in the ICU will be discussed in greater detail, but generally, atropine (0.02 mg/kg) may be administered preceding the sedative and muscle relaxant in order to block vagal reflexes leading to bradycardia. If the patient is tachycardic, however, atropine may be withheld but should be readily available. The dose of succinylcholine for RSI is 2 mg/kg in children less than two years and 1 mg/kg in older children.

Respiratory Failure

The patient with respiratory failure who is able to cooperate may be intubated with sedation via the blind nasal route. In the patient who is younger or unable to cooperate, induction may be accom-

Table 4.1-3. Rapid-sequence intubation technique

Prepare equipment

Evaulate airway

Preoxygenate

Sedation + muscle relaxant

Cricoid pressure

Intubate

If unsuccessful and O_2 saturation drops, mask ventilate with continued cricoid pressure

plished with ketamine or sodium thiopental. Muscle relaxation may be achieved with succinylcholine for RSI or with vecuronium. Care must be taken to oxygenate the patient well prior to intubation attempts because respiratory failure from all causes is often accompanied by a marked reduction in functional residual capacity and thus a tendency toward rapid arterial desaturation during intubation (Fig. 4.1-7).

The asthmatic patient may be intubated, if able to cooperate, with sedation via the blind nasal route. For the younger asthmatic or the patient who is unable to cooperate with intubation under sedation, intubation may be carried out with anesthesia induced with ketamine and muscle relaxation with succinylcholine. Ketamine is recommended because of its properties as an anesthetic coupled with its potent bronchodilator effects. Atropine should be administered with ketamine to minimize secretions.

Head Injury/Cervical Spine Injury

The head injury patient should be intubated with care with attention directed toward the potential for accompanying cervical injury, shock, and a "full stomach."

It is important to immobilize the cervical spine with either suspected or actual injury prior to laryngoscopy. This requires manual in-line immobilization of the head and neck. Precisely how this is done has not always been clear from reports—whether it is manual restraint of the head in the neutral position or application of axial traction. One paper evaluating this problem states that "the oral route for tracheal intubation clearly has a good clinical trial record and the objections to its use in cervical spine injury remain unproved."[14]

In the absence of accompanying shock, induction should be accomplished with sodium thiopental and muscle relaxation with succinylcholine. Patients with accompanying shock or hypovo-

Figure 4.1-7. Algorithm for airway management during respiratory failure.

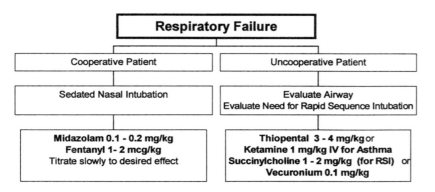

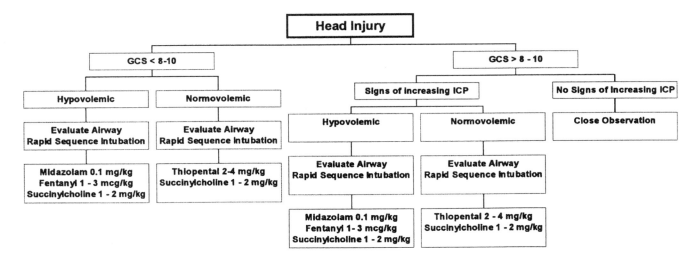

GCS = Glasgow Coma Scale

Figure 4.1-8. Algorithm for airway management following a head injury. GCS, Glasgow Coma Score; ICP, intracanial pressure.

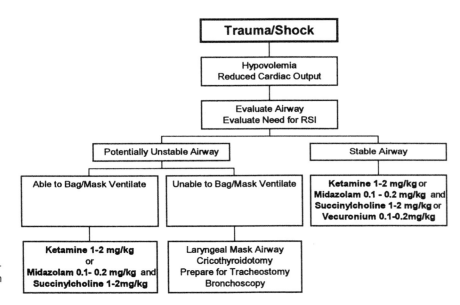

Figure 4.1-9. Algorithm for airway management following trauma or for the child in shock. RSI, rapid sequence intubation.

lemia should be treated with fentanyl and midazolam for sedation and succinylcholine for muscle relaxation. Ketamine, however, is the preferred agent in the patient with severe shock, although there is concern that this drug may transiently increase intracranial pressure and lower seizure threshold. Thus one needs to balance the risks and benefits in each situation (Fig. 4.1-8).

Trauma/Shock

If there is upper airway trauma or injuries that may complicate airway management and the patient needs emergent intubation due to hypoxemia, intubation may be accomplished with the modified rapid-sequence technique establishing an airway with mask or laryngeal mask airway **prior** to muscle relaxation. Keep in mind that patients who have airway trauma may present some of the most difficult airway management problems, and as such, a plan

for alternative methods of ventilation (laryngeal mask airway, transtracheal jet ventilation, tracheostomy) should be formulated as the initial assessment of the airway is made. In some cases of facial or airway injury, if the patient is not hypoxemic, it may be prudent to plan to establish a secure airway emergently in the operating room, with personnel and preparations for emergency tracheostomy in place, rather than attempt to intubate in the emergency department. The management of children who present with shock requires careful attention to the selection of drugs to facilitate intubation. As these patients are hemodynamically compromised, agents selected should be those that have the least depressant effect on the cardiovascular system. Hence, ketamine is a preferred agent to provide sedation and analgesia, followed by succinylcholine for muscle relaxation, during intubation (Fig 4.1-9). If the mechanism of injury suggests the possibility of cervical or head injury, the patient should be managed as described for head injury patients (Fig. 4.1-8).

Burns

The patient with burns presents unique problems from the perspective of airway management (Fig. 4.1-10). All burns of the face and airway should be considered airway emergencies and triaged for immediate airway management. All burn patients should be evaluated carefully for signs of airway involvement. Signs of airway burn usually requiring immediate airway management include white, swollen, or erythematous mucosa; stridor; hypoxia; or history suggestive of superheated gas inhalation. Signs of airway burn that could potentially require intervention include singed nasal hairs, soot around the mouth and pharynx, and minor facial burns. In general, emergent intubation for airway burns should be instituted for all except the most minor of injuries. Intubation should be accomplished with a modified rapid-sequence technique. Induction with ketamine should be followed by muscle relaxation with vecuronium. Succinylcholine is contraindicated in the burn patient because of its potential to produce extremely high serum potassium levels in this population.

Seizures

Seizures are frequently encountered in the pediatric population. In selected cases, emergent tracheal intubation is required for control of the airway and ventilation. These patients may have airway obstruction, loss of reflexes, hypoventilation, hypoxemia, and risk for pulmonary aspiration. Also, patients who need CNS imaging may need to be intubated.

Rapid-sequence intubation is usually indicated, as most patients should be considered to have a full stomach. Midazolam or thiopental is usually used for sedation because of its added benefit as an anticonvulsant. Succinylcholine is generally used for muscle relaxation unless contraindicated, as seen in patients with muscle dystrophies, paralysis, or spasticity. In this situation vecuronium would be a satisfactory choice (Fig. 4.1-11).

Open Eye Injury

Patients with open eye injury often have other traumatic injuries that may take priority over treatment of the ocular injury. In patients with open eye injury who require emergent intubation in the absence of signs of hypovolemia, induction may be carried

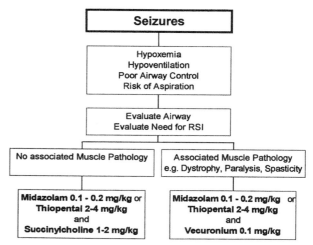

Figure 4.1-11. Algorithm for airway management in the patient with seizures.

out with sodium thiopental or fentanyl and midazolam and muscle relaxation with vecuronium. Succinylcholine is usually avoided in patients with open eye injuries because its use has been associated with transient rises in intraocular pressure during intubation. This, theoretically, may be associated with an increased risk of extrusion of intraocular contents during the intubation procedure.

Complications of Tracheal Intubation

While tracheal intubation may be a necessary and life-saving procedure in the child, one must be aware of the possible complications associated with the procedure and how to avoid them. Some of the complications are minor; others, however, may be life-threatening.

Complications during the Procedure of Laryngoscopy and Intubation

Cardiovascular

Tachycardia and hypertension often are associated with laryngoscopy and intubation. Arrhythmias may occur. Should bradycardia occur, however, one must immediately rule out hypoxemia as the cause. Bradycardia may also represent a profound vagal response to the procedure.

Respiratory

Bronchospasm may result in susceptible subjects from the irritation of the tracheal tube on the respiratory mucus membrane. Laryngospasm occurs when the patient is inadequately sedated or receives an inadequate dose of muscle relaxant.

During the procedure, regurgitation and pulmonary aspiration may occur. This is a particular risk in patients with gastrointestinal reflux, obese patients, and those who have recently eaten.

Central Nervous System

Increased intracranial pressure may occur. Thus, one must be especially cautious in patients with existing intracranial hypertension. This includes adequate sedation and muscle relaxation and expeditious and skilled intubation techniques.

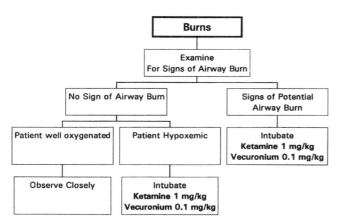

Figure 4.1-10. Algorithm for airway management in the patient with burns.

Trauma

Trauma to lips, teeth, upper airway, and trachea may occur. Tracheal perforation has occurred particularly when a stylet has been employed, thus, the importance of ensuring that the stylet does not protrude beyond the distal end of the ETT. Trauma to teeth is avoided by making sure that in carrying out the laryngoscopy, the operator does not use the patient's teeth as a fulcrum for elevating the tongue.

Complications with the Tracheal Tube Positioned

Misplacement of the Tube

The tube may be inadvertently misplaced into a mainstem bronchus, particularly the right. Also, movements of the patient's head and neck may displace the tube such that extension leads to accidental extubation and flexion to mainstem bronchial intubation. The tube may obstruct due to secretions, blood, kinking, or the patient's biting down on the tube.

Complications Following Extubation

Early

Laryngospasm—usually subsides with positive pressure ventilation and 100% oxygen.

Laryngeal edema—may follow intubation and is more likely to occur with children who have upper respiratory infections or when the ETT fit has been "tight." Hence, the importance of choosing the appropriate size tube, one which enables one to provide effective ventilation with a minimal leak around the tube; that is, a leak is detected at peak inspiratory pressures of 20 to 25 cm H_2O. These children present with stridor (inspiratory), chest wall retractions, and distress.

Sore throat and hoarseness—may occur and usually subsides in a few days.

Delayed

Subglottic stenosis—may occur, especially with prolonged intubation; appropriate size ETTs lessen this risk.

Tracheomalacia—occurs especially with cuffed ETT as a result of pressure necrosis of the trachea and destruction of the cartilaginous support.

Vocal tube injury—and granulomas are occasionally seen.

Infection—from nasotracheal intubation and may be associated with possibly serious infections of the maxillary sinus and middle ear.

References

1. Samsoon GLT, Young JRB. Difficult tracheal intubation: A retrospective study. *Anesthesia* 42:487–490, 1987.
2. Wilson ME et al. Predicting difficult intubation. *Br J Anaesth* 61: 211–216, 1988.
3. Nichol HC, Zuck D. Difficult laryngoscopy—The "anterior" larynx and the atlanto-occipital gap. *Br J Anaesth* 153:141–143, 1983.
4. Mallampati SR et al. A clinical sign to predict difficult intubation: A prospective study. *Can Anesth Soc J* 32:429–434, 1985.
5. Benumof JL. Management of the difficult adult airway. *Anesthesiology* 75:1087–1110, 1991.
6. Lewis M et al. What is the best way to determine oropharyngeal classification and mandibular space length to predict difficult laryngoscopy? *Anesthesiology* 81:69–75, 1994.
7. Pennant JH, White PF. The laryngeal mask airway: Its uses in anesthesiology. Anesthesiology 79:144–163; 1993.
8. Hinkle AJ. A rapid and reliable method of selecting endotracheal tube size in children. *Anaesth Analg* 67:S-592, 1988.
9. Luten RC et al. Length-based endotracheal tube and emergency equipment selection in pediatrics. *Ann Emerg Med* 21:900–904, 1992.
10. Wood PR, Lawler PGP. Managing the airway in cervical spine injury. *Anaesthesia* 47:792–797, 1992.
11. Westhorpe RN. The position of the larynx in children and its relationship to the ease of intubation. *Anaesth Intensive Care* 15:384–388, 1987.
12. Belhouse CO, Doré C. Criteria for estimating likelihood of difficulty of endotracheal intubation with the Macintosh laryngoscope. *Anaesth Intensive Care* 16:329–337, 1988.
13. Matthew M, Hanna LS, Aldrete JA. Pre-operative indices to anticipate difficult tracheal intubation. *Anaesth Analg* 68:187, 1989.
14. Practice Guidelines. Practice guidelines for management of the difficult airway: A report by the American Society of Anesthesiologists Task Force on Management of the Difficult Airway. *Anesthesiology* 78:597–602, 1993.

Daniel P. Ryan

Natan Noviski

I. David Todres

4.2   Bronchoscopy

Endoscopic evaluation of the upper and lower airways has both diagnostic and therapeutic applications in the critical care unit.[1–3] Recent developments with fiberoptic instrumentation have expanded their diagnostic uses to very small infants without the need for general anesthesia, but the rigid systems remain unsurpassed in their clarity and optical definition.[4,5]

Bronchoscopy alone visualizes the lower airway but should always be accompanied by an inspection of the larynx, pharynx, and, when indicated, the nasal passages for a complete evaluation of the airway. Direct laryngoscopy under anesthesia or sedation using the rigid telescope for a close inspection of the larynx with magnification gives the best view of the anatomy. Fiberoptic instruments, however, offer a view of the awake and phonating larynx for a better dynamic evaluation, but with less clarity.

Rigid Bronchoscopy

Rigid bronchoscopes are sized similar to endotracheal tubes, that is, by their internal diameter. One must remember that the Hopkins telescope system occupies a significant proportion of the overall internal diameter of the smaller bronchoscopes and may produce difficulty with ventilation. The telescope provides a superb view, but one cannot examine the airway past the second or third order of bronchi. An advantage of the rigid tube is complete control of the airway once the bronchoscope is passed between the vocal cords. The indications for both rigid and flexible bronchoscopy are seen in Table 4.2-1. Rigid bronchoscopy is especially reserved for foreign body removal, hemoptysis evaluation, and the need for biopsy. There may be situations in which flexible bronchoscopy is impossible (i.e., uncooperativeness, small size, or poor airway control), thus making rigid bronchoscopy the preferred choice.

The rigid bronchoscope can be quite traumatic, so a very controlled situation is required (usually meaning the use of general anesthesia). The large opening of the rigid tube allows visualization and treatment of foreign bodies, thick secretions, massive hemoptysis, and cryotherapy or laser resection of lesions with complete airway control. The choice of anesthesia depends on the indication for the endoscopy, but usually spontaneous ventilation can be maintained in cases of possible airway obstruction to avoid complete loss of control of the airway. Essential monitors include ECG, blood pressure, precordial stethoscope, pulse oximetry, and optional use of an end-tidal carbon dioxide capnograph or a transcutaneous carbon dioxide monitor.

After induction of anesthesia, the child is placed in a "sniffing position," which straightens the upper airway. This may require support behind the child's shoulders, due to the relatively large size of the head, in order to prevent trauma to the teeth and gums. Direct laryngoscopy is done first, and the appropriate rigid bronchoscope with telescope is passed under vision between the vocal cords. Once the bronchoscope is inside the larynx, the anesthesia team can maintain oxygenation and ventilation through it. When using the 3.5-mm scope (or smaller), ventilation may be difficult with the telescope in place, and the scope may need to be intermittently removed while ventilation is maintained through the bronchoscope tube to prevent hypercapnia.

Table 4.2-1. Indications for bronchoscopy

	Flexible	*Rigid*
Stridor	+	+
Acute airway obstruction	+ *	+
Sleep-associated airway obstruction	+	−
Persistent cough or wheezing	+	+/−
Suspected congenital anomalies	+	+/−
Foreign body	−	+
Hemoptysis	−	+
Tracheal stenosis	+	+
Laryngeal trauma	+	+
Smoke inhalation	+	−
Lobar atelectasis	+/−	+
Pulmonary infection	+	+/−
Lung abscess	−	+
Suspected airway compression	+	+/−
Bronchial toilet—diagnosis/therapy	+	+
Evaluation of tracheostomy stoma	+	+
Aid in difficult intubations	+	−
Biopsy	−	+

*To assist with intubation.

When dealing with foreign bodies in the airway, rigid bronchoscopy is preferable to maintain control of the airway during manipulations. The optical foreign body forceps give superb visualization and control when working through the rigid tube. Small, distal foreign bodies can sometimes be dislodged by using a Fogarty balloon catheter passed beyond the object and inflating the balloon to allow the object to be manipulated within the bronchoscope, or to move it within the reach of forceps. One must always inspect all of the airway after the last piece of foreign body is removed to be certain of complete clearance.

Bronchoscopy in skilled hands is usually a very safe technique. During manipulation within the airway, injury can occur, and even diagnostic evaluations can lead to acute, serious problems. Induction of laryngospasm with resultant hypoxia and hypercapnia can be avoided with adequate depth of anesthesia and proper selection of patients and technique. Hypoxia and hypercapnia during the procedure must be avoided, and for this, the technology of pulse oximetry, transcutaneous carbon dioxide monitor, and capnography can be invaluable. Pneumothorax, pneumomediastinum, and tension pneumothorax can easily occur,[6] and a chest x-ray should be obtained following any manipulation or at the slightest hint of a problem. When working to remove an impacted foreign body, bleeding may occur but is rarely massive. Loss of airway control can occur if a foreign body is broken or displaced into both mainstem bronchi or impacted onto the carina. Biopsy of lesions should be done carefully; avoid lymphangiomas and hemangiomas because of the risk of bleeding. Care must be taken to avoid contamination of clean areas of the lung when encountering an infectious process like a lung abscess, and if massive bleeding is found or produced, the uninvolved lung must be protected. Finally, injury to the nasal passages, pharynx, larynx, trachea and distal airways, teeth, lips, and gums should be avoided.

Wiseman et al. showed that 30% of a series of 277 pediatric patients who had rigid bronchoscopies had evidence of upper airway obstruction. These patients usually present with stridor, and the differential diagnosis is quite long, as seen in Table 4.2-2. Wiseman's group found that about half of the patients with upper airway obstruction had congenital lesions on bronchoscopy, while the rest had acquired lesions. In 85% of this series, a specific diagnosis was reached for both upper and lower airway problems.[7]

Flexible Fiberoptic Endoscopy

Equipment

A flexible fiberoptic bronchoscope of appropriate size, with a light source, is required. Flexible fiberoptic equipment is sized according to the outer diameter (e.g., 3.5 mm) and should therefore allow room for the patient to breathe around it. The distal 2 to 2.5 cm of the device is flexible and controlled through a range of approximately 160 degrees in one direction and 60 degrees in the opposite direction. A suction channel is used to suction, irrigate the airway, and perform bronchial lavage. Smaller diameter bronchoscopes (i.e., 1.8 mm and 2.2 mm) have no suction channel. The "suction" channel may also be used to insufflate oxygen.

Monitoring (Equipment and Personnel)

The bronchoscopist should be assisted by one person who is dedicated to monitoring the patient's condition while he or she is undergoing bronchoscopy. This includes direct visualization of the patient and the monitoring of vital signs, especially heart

Table 4.2-2. Differential diagnosis of stridor

Laryngomalacia

Congenital laryngeal stenosis and webs

Cleft larynx

Papilloma

Laryngeal cyst

Epiglottitis (supraglottitis)

Diphtheria

Acute croup

Recurrent nerve paralysis

Foreign body of airway

Vascular ring

Tracheal esophageal fistula

Tracheomalacia

Congenital goiter

Cystic hygroma

Thymic abscess or cyst

Mediastinal adenitis

Congenital/acquired tracheal stenosis

Esophageal foreign body impinging on trachea

Subglottic hemangioma or lymphangioma

Laryngeal trauma

Bronchogenic cysts

rate, with appropriate monitors; oxygen saturation monitoring with pulse oximetry is essential throughout the procedure. In addition to monitoring equipment, provision must be made for resuscitation equipment should this be necessary. This includes the means to deliver oxygen with bag and mask devices and appropriate medications.

Indications and Contraindications

The indications for flexible fiberoptic bronchoscopy are summarized in Table 4.2-1. The procedure should be performed only when the benefits outweigh the risks. A factor in the risk equation is inexperience on the part of the operator, and thus the procedure should be performed only by experienced personnel or trainees who are closely supervised. Situations that pose serious risks for the child undergoing bronchoscopy include (1) bleeding diathesis, (2) massive hemoptyses, (3) severe airway obstruction, (4) severe refractory hypoxemia, and (5) unstable hemodynamics including dysrhythmias.[8]

Procedure

The patient should be adequately sedated and the airway anesthetized with topical agents.[9]

1. *Sedation.* This is most effectively accomplished via the intravenous route. Morphine or meperidine may be used. Benzodiazepines (diazepam and midazolam) are favored by some but should be used cautiously, as they may precipitate respiratory depression. The key to successful sedation is titration of the drug for the individual patient's needs, recognizing that the critically ill patient may not tolerate "normal" doses of the drug.

2. *Topical anesthesia.* Lidocaine is an effective topical anesthetic agent. One should carefully titrate the dose administered up to 5 mg/kg, as systemic absorption of "large" doses may produce toxic effects. To achieve optimal anesthesia of the larynx and tracheal tree, it is necessary not to rush the procedure and to allow 2 to 3 minutes for the local anesthesia to take effect.

The fiberoptic bronchoscope is best passed through the nose in the nonintubated patient.[10] In the intubated patient, passage via the endotracheal tube through a modified adaptor at the tube allows one to have the patient continually ventilated during the examination. In children with a tracheostomy, examination may take place through the tube or the stoma.

Flexible fiberoptic bronchoscopy provides optimal conditions for visualizing dynamic movements of the larynx (vocal cords, etc.) and the trachea (tracheomalacia). Examination of the airway takes place on both insertion and removal of the bronchoscope. During the procedure, supplemental oxygen is administered. This may be carried out via a cannula in the open nostril or through a clear oxygen mask in which a central hole has been cut to allow the bronchoscope to pass through. This allows the patient to receive supplemental oxygen throughout the procedure. Oxygen saturations are continually checked with a pulse oximeter.

Flexible fiberoptic devices may be extremely useful in facilitating tracheal intubation in the difficult airway (oropharyngeal and cervical spine abnormalities) when conventional laryngoscopy has failed to identify the glottic opening. The 3.5-mm bronchoscope fits a 4.5-mm (internal diameter) endotracheal tube, while the smaller ultrathin bronchoscope (2.2 mm) fits a 3.0- and 3.5-mm tube. Once intubated, bronchoscopy also helps to identify the distal end of the tube in relationship to the carina.

Complications

Possible complications arising out of the procedure of flexible fiberoptic bronchoscopy are

1. adverse effects of the drugs used to sedate and locally anesthetize the patient
2. complications related to the bronchoscopic examination

Hypoxemia occurring during the procedure is a potential major concern. This may be due to excessive sedation, leading to depressed ventilation with resultant disturbance of ventilation and perfusion in the lung; in addition, the increased airway resistance afforded by the bronchoscope may contribute to hypoxemia. Close monitoring of the patient with pulse oximetry (oxygen saturations) and the use of supplemental oxygen during the procedure should limit the occurrence of significant hypoxemia during the bronchoscopy procedure.

Bradycardia occurring during the procedure should immediately signal the possibility of hypoxemia. Bradycardia, however, may also reflect a vagal mediated reflex when the procedure is performed on a patient who has received inadequate amounts of local anesthesia. Should bradycardia occur during the procedure, the bronchoscope should be withdrawn and adequate oxygenation and ventilation ensured.

Transient elevations of carbon dioxide have been reported. We generally do not monitor carbon dioxide levels, as the usual rapidity of the procedure does not lead to serious elevations of the $PaCO_2$.

Infections due to the procedure are rare. Nonetheless, adequate cleaning and sterilization of the equipment is necessary following each use. Pneumothorax occurs very rarely. One paper cited an incidence of two cases in 1095 bronchoscopic procedures.[11] Trauma to the nasal passages and larynx may occur but is generally preventable with good technique. Epistaxis and hemoptysis have been documented; generally, the bleeding subsides spontaneously. Occasionally, the child experiences postbronchoscopic glottic and subglottic edema presenting with stridor. Racemic epinephrine inhalations may be necessary in more severe cases.

References

1. Wood RE, Postma D. Endoscopic endoscopy of the airway in infants and children. *J Pediatr* 112:1, 1988.
2. Puhakka H et al. Pediatric bronchoscopy; a report of methodology and results. *Clin Pediatr* 28:253, 1989.
3. Fan LL, Sparks LM, Fix EJ. Flexible fiberoptic endoscopy for airway problems in a pediatric intensive care unit. *Chest* 93:556, 1988.
4. Fan LL, Sparks LM, Dulinski JP. Applications of an ultrathin flexible bronchoscope for neonatal and pediatric airway problems. *Chest* 89:673, 1986.
5. Vigneswaran R, Whitfield JM. The use of a new ultra-thin fiberoptic broncho-scope to determine endotracheal tube position in the sick newborn infant. *Chest* 80:174, 1981.
6. Gallagher MJ, Muller BJ. Tension pneumothorax during pediatric bronchoscopy. *Anesthesiology* 55:685, 1981.
7. Wiseman NE, Sanchez I, Powell RE. Rigid bronchoscopy in the pediatric age group: Diagnostic effectiveness. *J Pediatr Surg* 27:1294, 1992.
8. Official statement of the American Thoracic Society. Flexible endoscopy of the pediatric airway. *Am Rev Respir Dis* 145:233, 1992.
9. Godfrey S. Bronchoscopy in childhood. *Br J Dis Chest* 81:225, 1987.
10. Noviski N, Todres ID. Fiberoptic bronchoscopy in the pediatric patient. *Anesthesiol Clin North Am* 9:163, 1991.
11. Wood RE. Spelunking in the pediatric airways: Explorations with the flexible fiberoptic bronchoscope. *Pediatr Clin North Am* 31:785, 1984.

Michael J. Cunningham **4.3** **Tracheostomy**
Roland D. Eavey

Historical Perspective

Of all procedures performed in the pediatric intensive care unit, tracheotomy most probably lays claim to the longest history.[1,2] The procedure was discussed as far back as the second century A.D. in the medical writings of Galen, Aretaeus, and Asclepiades. The first successful adult tracheotomy was reported by the Italian physician Barsovala in the sixteenth century. In 1620 Nicholas Habicot described four tracheotomies, one on a 14-year-old boy who had swallowed a bag of gold coins. The bag had become lodged in the boy's esophagus, compressing and obstructing his trachea. Habicot performed the first pediatric tracheotomy in order to manipulate the bag further down the esophagus with its eventual recovery from the rectum! In 1766 Caron subsequently performed a tracheotomy on a 7-year-old boy in order to remove a bean from the airway itself. Andree, in 1782, and Chevalier, in 1814, also recorded successful tracheotomies in pediatric patients.

In the year 1825 Bretonneau published an additional surgical indication for tracheotomy which would significantly facilitate its use; he defined the clinical entity of diphtheria, distinguished it from other inflammatory processes of the airway, and successfully performed a tracheotomy in a 5-year-old girl with this disease.[3] By 1833, Trousseau reported having salvaged 50 of 200 children with diphtheria by use of the procedure. Further refinements came from Chevalier Jackson who, in 1921, demonstrated that the morbidity was low when the procedure was performed properly through the tracheal rings and when meticulous postoperative care was provided.[4]

Galloway[5] further enlarged the scope of the procedure when he reported in 1943 its usefulness for the respiratory care of patients with poliomyelitis. Up to this time, the procedure had been mainly performed for the acute relief of airway obstruction. This change in the application of tracheotomy to patients with chronic as well as acute airway problems paralleled the era of intensivist care, and served to establish this operation as the airway procedure of choice in both adult and pediatric respiratory care units.

Indications

Although *tracheostomy* and *tracheotomy* are commonly used interchangeably, *tracheotomy* is derived from the Greek word *tome* (to cut) whereas *tracheostomy* is derived from the word *stomoun* (to furnish with an opening or mouth).[6] *Tracheotomy* more properly describes the performance of the procedure itself whereas *tracheostomy* better describes the permanent tracheal stoma so-created.

The specific indications for tracheotomy remain in evolution (Table 4.3-1). Epiglottitis and laryngotracheobronchitis replaced diphtheria as the principal infectious diseases causing acute airway obstruction necessitating tracheotomy in the latter half of the twentieth century.[7,8] Such acute inflammatory airway conditions still remain the primary indication for tracheotomy in the underdeveloped world today.[9] In modern intensive care settings, the successful employment of orotracheal and nasotracheal intubation has drastically reduced this particular need for surgical intervention. Instead, noninfectious congenital and acquired airway lesions constitute the principal obstruction bypass indication for tracheotomy.[7,8,10–13] Acquired subglottic stenosis heads this list, reflecting the greater likelihood of survival of long-term intubated infants in neonatal intensive care settings.

Prolonged mechanical ventilation due to poliomyelitis is likewise a rare indication for tracheotomy today. Myeloneuropathies such as Guillain-Barré's syndrome remain an important problem,[10,11] but prolonged respiratory support is more often a need in the overall ICU care of head trauma patients or children with other debilitating central nervous system lesions.[7,8,10–13] Short-term airway support via tracheotomy may also be part of the planned management of children undergoing craniofacial or extensive cardiovascular surgery.[7,8,10–13] Tracheotomy may additionally play a role as an adjunct to laryngeal closure or laryngotracheal separation in the prevention of chronic aspiration in selected children.[14,15]

The actual decision to perform a tracheotomy as opposed to alternative means of airway support frequently requires the consideration of multiple factors, most important of which is the antici-

Table 4.3-1. Clinical indications for tracheotomy

Allergy	Metabolic	Prophylactic	Degenerative; Idiopathic	Sleep disorders
Angioneurotic edema Anaphylaxis		Head and neck surgery Craniofacial surgery Prolonged endotracheal tube placement	Vocal cord paralysis	Pharyngeal musculature collapse Adenotonsillar hypertrophy
Asthma	Cystic fibrosis Coma secondary to diabetes, Reye syndrome uremia, etc. Respiratory distress syndrome Bronchopulmonary dysplasia	Neurosurgery Cardiothoracic surgery	CNS or neuromuscular failure as in Guillain- Barré syndrome, polymyositis, myasthenia gravis, botulism, cardiac arrest, respiratory arrest	Central hypoventilation syndrome

Congenital	Trauma	Toxic	Infection	Neoplastic
Choanal atresia Macroglossia Pierre-Robin anomaly Laryngomalacia Laryngeal stenosis Vocal cord paralysis Laryngeal webs, cysts Subglottic stenosis Vascular ring Tracheal hypoplasia Tracheomalacia	Facial injury Oral injury Foreign body Burns Laryngeal edema Recurrent laryngeal nerve injury Laryngeal fracture	Corrosive aspiration	Epiglottitis Laryngotracheobronchitis Bacterial tracheitis Diphtheria Retropharyngeal abscess Ludwig's angina Faciitis/cellulitis Tetanus Rabies Plague	Laryngeal tumors Tracheal tumors Obstructive tumors of the oral cavity and pharynx
Congenital heart disease Congenital heart failure Esophageal atresia secondary to tracheoesophageal fistula Hypoplastic lung secondary to diaphragmatic hernia Bilateral phrenic nerve paralysis	Head trauma Crushed chest Shock lung Intrapulmonary hemorrhage Pneumothorax Post-bypass lung	Coma secondary to toxins such as phenobarbital Hydrocarbon lung Aspiration syndromes such as from meconium	Meningitis Encephalitis Brain abscess Pneumonia Bronchiolitis Poliomyelitis Recurrent pulmonary aspiration with/without laryngeal closure	Brain tumors Spinal cord tumors

Adapted from Stool SE, Eavey RD. Tracheotomy. In *Pediatric Otolaryngology*. CD Bluestone and SE Stool (eds), 2nd edition. WB Saunders Co., Philadelphia, 1990.

pated course of the patient's illness. A condition with no likelihood of a quick recovery, such as a severe neurological injury, is much more suitable for tracheotomy than one with an anticipated rapid recovery like epiglottitis. Patient-specific factors of significance include the child's overall degree of medical health and suitability for operation. In neonates, the age and size (weight) of the infant also influence the morbidity of the procedure.[16,17] Care-specific factors involve the experience and comfort of hospital personnel with tracheotomy patients, as well as the ability of the parents or alternative caretakers to potentially provide homecare if a long-dwelling tracheostomy proves necessary. At times, the decision making can be sufficiently complicated, and a medical ethicist must be brought into the picture.

Tracheostomy Tubes

Tracheostomy tubes have evolved over the centuries in concert with the varying indications for tracheotomy. The principal tracheostomy tubes of the infectious era were of the Jackson and Hollinger variety made of metal and silver, respectively. They were designed with inner sleeves or cannulas to allow for easy cleaning of thick secretions and maintenance of lumen patency (Fig. 4.3-1). Mechanized respiratory support was limited so adaptation to ventilator equipment was not necessary.

The tracheostomy tubes of the modern era needed to be more suitable for longer term use and to be amenable to the associated demands of a variety of ventilator support systems. Tubes made from synthetic materials (polyvinyl chloride, silicone) were developed with the goals of pliability, nonreactivity, sterility, easy disposability, and affordable cost. Universal hubs became standard for the attachment of ventilation equipment. Variations in size and length were maintained and expanded on to increase the suitability of tubes to different clinical situations. This became particularly important as tracheotomy was more frequently performed in the infant and neonatal populations.[18]

The most critical characteristics of a tracheostomy tube are its length and internal/external diameters. Unfortunately, the numbers used to categorize tracheostomy tubes are not part of a standardized system but rather vary among manufacturers. Table 4.3-2 lists several types of tubes and compares their sizes according to each manufacturer's numbering system.

The selection of a particular tube depends on the indication

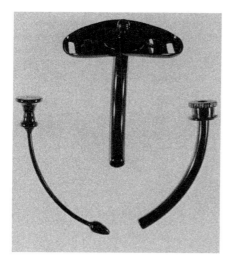

Figure 4.3-1. Silver Hollinger tracheostomy tubes with inner cannulas and insertion obturators. Two sizes—0 and 1—are shown.

for the procedure and the size of the child. For example, if an obstruction bypass tracheotomy is being performed solely to provide an alternative airway, the tube usually does not need to fill the entire tracheal lumen. However, should the tracheotomy be performed for mechanical ventilation, the external diameter of the tube should be sufficiently large relative to the size of the airway in order to prevent excessive air leakage. This works particularly well in young children in whom it has been a common

experience not to require a cuffed tube. In older children and adolescents, a cuff may be required in order to achieve adequate ventilation parameters.

The more critical diameter in most clinical situations is actually the inner lumen size. Individualization to the clinical situation at hand is obviously necessary. Endotracheal tube size can be of help in previously intubated patients. Bronchoscopic evaluation and calibration may be of major assistance in difficult airway cases.

At times, the length of the tube is an even more pertinent dimension than its diameter. In the preterm infant, for example, the length of a standard tube may be such that it contacts the carina repeatedly or inserts itself into one of the mainstem bronchi on movement of the child. Two manufacturers (Shiley, Bivona) have a neonatal series of reduced-length tracheostomy tubes to minimize this complication (Fig. 4.3-2). Alternatively, it may be necessary to design a custom-made, shorter tracheostomy tube to solve this problem.

As mentioned previously, metal and silver tubes do not adapt well to ventilatory equipment, requiring special inner cannulas to do so. The majority of synthetic material tubes, in contrast, are designed with a universal hub for immediate connection to anesthesia and/or respiratory equipment. The tracheostomy tubes manufactured by the Shiley and Bivona companies, for example, have direct coupling capability due to a built-in 15-mm connector (see Fig. 4.3-2). Portex tubes are also available with a 15-mm connector or can be adapted to a low-profile swivel connector with additional securement features (Fig. 4.3-3). The Tracoe tracheostomy tube features multiple inner cannulas, one of which has a universal hub for respiratory equipment attachment (Fig. 4.3-4).

Unique circumstances occasionally require the use of special

Table 4.3-2. Approximate gauge equivalents of frequently used endotracheal and tracheostomy tubes* (based on nearest inner diameter measurement)

Endotracheal[1]			Shiley[2]				Portex[3]				Tracoe[4]				Bivona[5]			
ID	OD	FR#	ID	OD	Lg	Size	ID	OD	Lg	Size (Jackson)	D	OD	Lg	Size	ID	OD	Lg	Size (Jackson)
2.5	3.5	10													2.5	4.0	38 (30)	000
3.0	4.2	12	3.1	4.5	39 (30)	00	3.0	5.0	36	0								
3.5	4.9	15	3.4	5.0	40 (32)	0	3.5	5.5	40	1	3.5	4.6	46	3	3.0	4.7	39 (32)	00
4.0	5.5	16	3.7	5.5	41 (34)	1	4.0	6.0	44	2	4.0	5.3	55	4	3.5	5.3	40 (34)	0, 1
4.5	6.1	18	4.1	6.0	42	2	4.5	6.5	48	—					4.0	6.0	41 (36)	2
5.0	6.8	20	4.8	7.0	44	3	5.0	7.0	48.5	3	5.0	6.3	57 •	5				
5.5	7.4	22	5.5	8.0	46	4									4.5	6.7	42	3 –
6.0	8.0	24					6.0	8.1	55	4	6.0	6.0	76	6	5.0	7.3	44	3 +
															5.5	8.0	46	4

*All measurements except French number and sizes are expressed in millimeters
[1]The French number (FR#) is arrived at by multiplying the outside diameter by 3.
[2]The Shiley tube is made by Shiley Laboratories, Irvine, CA. This tube is stamped with the size and inner and outer diameters. The length measurements in parentheses refer to the Neonatal series; all other measurements refer to the Pediatric series and/or are shared in common by both series for size 00, 0, and 1 tubes.
[3]The Portex tube is made by Portex Inc., Wilmington, MA. The Portex company uses Jackson-size measurements as well as an internal system in which the last two series numbers denote the internal diameter of the tube (e.g., 500030, 500035, etc.).
[4]The Tracoe tube is made in West Germany and is distributed by Boston Medical Products, Waltham, MA. The Tracoe series employs both an outer cannula and inner cannula tube. The size number refers to the inner diameter of the outer cannula tube.
[5]The Bivona tube is made by Bivona Medical Technologies, Gary IN. This tube is stamped with the inner and outer diameters as well as the PED (Pediatrics) or NEO (Neonatal) line designation. The length measurements in parentheses refer to the Neonatal series; all other measurements refer to the Pediatric series and/or are shared in common by both series for ID (mm) size 2.5, 3.0, 3.5, and 4.0 tubes.
Adapted from Stool SE, Eavey RD. Tracheotomy. In *Pediatric Otolaryngology*. CD Bluestone and SE Stool (eds), 2nd edition. WB Saunders Co., Philadelphia, 1990, p. 1231.

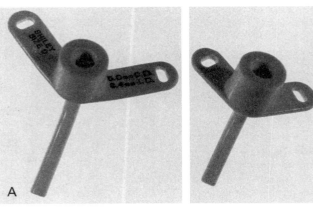

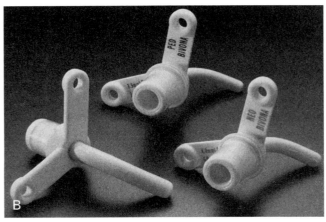

Figure 4.3-2. **(A)** The Shiley polyvinyl chloride and **(B)** Bivona silicone single cannula tracheostomy tubes are each available in two lines of various lengths and diameters for specific use in the pediatric and neonatal age group. Pediatric and neonatal size 0 tubes are demonstrated for comparison purposes. Note the built-in 15-mm connector for respiratory equipment. (**A**: Courtesy of Mallaninckrodt Medical/TPI, St. Louis, MO; **B**: Courtesy of Bivona Medical Technologies, Gary, IN.)

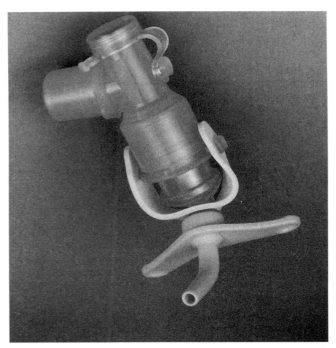

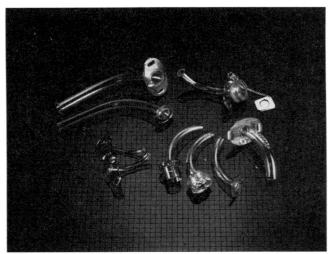

Figure 4.3-4. The Tracoe tracheostomy tube series features a standard outer tube of different lengths and diameters with a corresponding array of different inner cannulas including a ventilation equipment adapter and two speaking valves. An extra long (Hautant) tube is also shown. (Courtesy of Boston Medical Products, Waltham, MA.)

Figure 4.3-3. The Portex tracheostomy tube with low-profile swivel adapter designed for attachment of respiratory equipment. (Courtesy of Concord/Portex, Keene, NH.)

tubes. The Bivona company manufactures a Hyperflex wire-reinforced silicone tube which conforms well to the deformed airways of children with skeletal anomalies such as kyphoscoliosis or achondroplasia (Fig. 4.3-5). Children with extensive tracheomalacia may require stenting either with tracheostomy tubes custom made to a specific length or with an adjustable neck flange (see Fig. 4.3-5). A special group of patients are those with chronic hypoventilation syndrome or specific lower respiratory tract problems who require mechanical ventilation only at night. They can benefit from a solid stoma obturator or plug during the day (Fig.

4.3-6)[19]; alternatively, the Bivona TTS (tight to the shaft) cuffed tracheostomy tube offers the benefits of a cuff when inflated but the profile of a cuffless tube when deflated during the day (Fig. 4.3-7).

There are multiple ways to enhance the speech of tracheotomized children who do not require constant ventilator support. The Passy-Muir and Montgomery valves are silicone and plastic (respectively) one-way valve adaptors that attach externally to the universal hub of most tracheostomy tubes.[20] The Tracoe tube system has two different inner cannulas with silver speaking valves for enhanced communi-

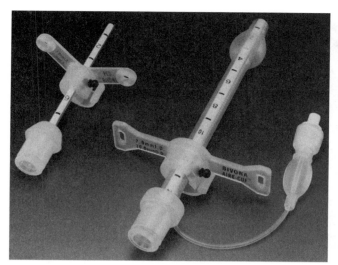

Figure 4.3-5. The Bivona Hyperflex wire-reinforced silicone tracheostomy tube with adjustable neck flange allows for bedside customization in children with anatomical deformation and other special airway needs. (Courtesy of Bivona Medical Technologies, Gary, IN.)

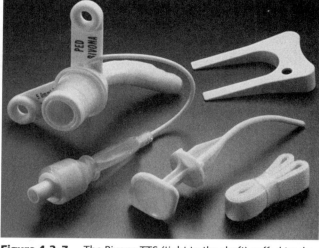

Figure 4.3-7. The Bivona TTS (tight to the shaft) cuffed tracheostomy tube has the profile of a cuffless tube when the cuff is deflated as shown. (Courtesy of Bivona Medical Technologies, Gary, IN.)

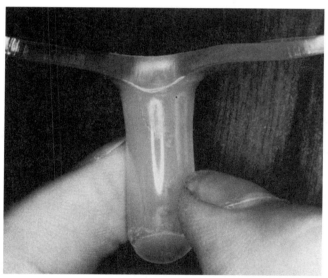

Figure 4.3-6. A custom-shortened, silicone-filled Aberdeen design Franklin tube can function as a stoma plug or obturator. (Courtesy of J.G. Franklin & Sons, Ltd., High Wycombe England.)

cation. Polyvinyl chloride tracheostomy tubes are also manufactured with fenestrations created on the tubes' superior surface; occlusion of the lumen of these tubes on expiration will force air to pass through superiorly, allowing vocalization. Many children with uncuffed tracheostomy tubes demonstrate the ability to cry or vocalize surprisingly well without the need for such speaking valves or fenestrations; this requires a sufficiently large tracheal lumen relative to the external diameter of the tube.

A final concern from the standpoint of tracheostomy tube adaptations is the need for humidification. Mechanized systems provide adequate humidification at bedside. Tiny portable humidifiers known by several names (heat and moisture exchanger, regenerative humidifier, artificial nose) can be placed on the universal adaptor at the end of most synthetic tracheostomy tubes. Such devices have been shown to provide quite adequate moisture levels for transient periods of time.[21]

Technique

Tracheotomy is preferably performed as an elective procedure under general anesthesia in children. If an endotracheal tube is not already in position, it is placed prior to surgery. If intubation cannot be readily performed, a bronchoscope should be passed and left in position until the tracheotomy is completed. The light of the bronchoscope can provide an unmistakable target in a particularly difficult procedure.

The child is positioned at the head of the table with ready access to both the anesthesia and surgical teams. The shoulders are elevated on a roll so that the neck can be hyperextended (Fig. 4.3-8). An attempt is made to clearly identify both the thyroid and cricoid cartilages. The cricoid cartilage is the key tracheotomy landmark; in the neonatal age group, however, it is typically less prominent than the surrounding hyoid and thyroid structures. The tracheal rings are palpated down to the sternal notch. Placement of the neck incision one finger breadth above the sternal notch is recommended. Either a horizontal or vertical skin incision can be utilized. Dissection should be confined strictly to the midline thereafter, transecting the fascial layers and separating the strap muscles down to the level of the trachea. Palpation is as important as visualization during this portion of the operation. If the thyroid gland is encountered, it can be mobilized superiorly or inferiorly, or the isthmus divided to provide access to the airway.

Various incisions in the trachea can be utilized. The options include a vertical incision, horizontal incision, or the inferiorly based tracheal flap.[22,23] Excision of the anterior tracheal wall is not recommended as it results in tracheal stenosis in the pediatric age group.[24] We prefer a vertical incision with stay sutures placed on each side of the incision. These silk sutures are later taped to the neck. They can be lifted laterally to pull the trachea to the

Figure 4.3-8. The ideal positioning of the child for tracheotomy requires elevation of the shoulders and hyperextension of the neck. The anesthetist may be utilized to pull the chin up and cephalad if necessary. (From SE Stool, RD Eavey. Tracheotomy. In CD Bluestone, SE Stool (eds): *Pediatric Otolaryngology.* Vol. 2. Philadelphia: Saunders, 1990. P. 1231. With permission.)

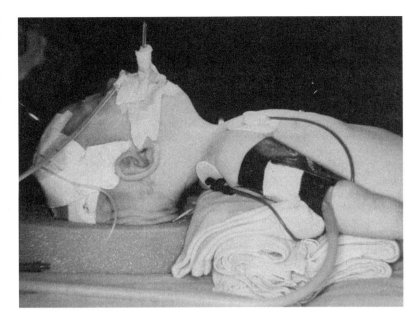

Figure 4.3-9. Stay sutures are intraoperatively placed through the trachea bilaterally in vertical fashion parallel to the midline tracheotomy incision. They are individually tied and secured to the child's chest with tape. In the event of accidental decannulation, they can be lifted laterally, opening the stoma and bringing the trachea closer to the skin surface, facilitating replacement of the tracheostomy tube. (From SE Stool, RD Eavey. Tracheotomy. In CD Bluestone, SE Stool (eds): *Pediatric Otoloaryngology.* Vol. 2. Philadelphia: Saunders, 1990. P. 1231. With permission.)

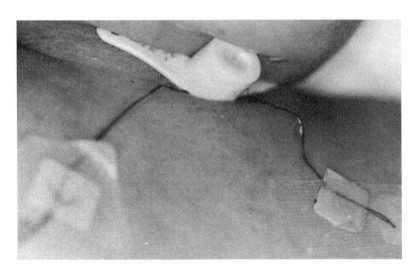

stoma surface, allowing for emergency replacement of the tracheostomy tube, should the patient be accidentally decannulated before a stomal tract becomes permanently established (Fig. 4.3-9). Intraoperative placement of the tube is carefully performed in order to avoid creation of a false passage. The incision is typically left open around the tube. If the incision is very wide, loose sutures or packing can be used to partially close the gap. A tight closure is contraindicated as it predisposes to the accumulation of subcutaneous emphysema. The tube is secured with tracheotomy tape. Stitching of the tracheostomy tube flange to the skin of the neck is additionally used in some centers. Approximately two fingers should be able to be inserted between the neck and the tape to avoid strangulation effect.

Over the first several postoperative days the tracheostomy tube tape will become blood-stained and unsightly. If an experienced team is present that can reestablish the tracheostomy tube should it be accidentally expelled, then the tape can be restrung. If there is any uncertainty about losing the tube, however, the tape should not be changed until the date of the first tracheostomy tube change

by the surgical team. The timing of this first tube change will vary depending on the surgeon. Our preference is approximately 5 to 7 days postoperatively. We find that by this time the stoma generally has a patent lumen that does not collapse when the tube is removed.

Emergency Tracheotomy

Emergency tracheotomy should be avoided if possible. In an acute respiratory distress situation, positive pressure ventilation or intubation is a much preferred initial maneuver. In the infant or very young child, emergent tracheotomy or cricothyroidotomy can be quite difficult due to the small airway and absence of clearly palpable landmarks. An alternate method of establishing oxygenation in a desperate situation is to insert a needle into the cricothyroid membrane. Coté et al have demonstrated the following needle technique to be effective in maintaining a supranormal pO_2 in an animal model.[25] A large bore, preferably Medicut, needle is attached to a syringe and inserted through the cricothyroid membrane angling toward the carina. Aspiration will ensure placement in the airway. An endotracheal tube adaptor can be inserted into the distal end of the syringe (plunger removed) to provide the hook-up for ventilation equipment.

Problematic Operative Consequences

As with any procedure, troublesome consequences can occur despite optimal anesthesia and surgical technique.

Hemorrhage

Preoperative coagulation studies may detect a bleeding tendency secondary to the child's medical condition. Unanticipated hemorrhage may occur due to transection of an aberrant midline anterior jugular vein or superiorly located innominate artery. The inferior thyroid veins also lie anterior to the trachea. Ligatures rather than electrocautery are advocated to control venous bleeding. Fortunately most surgical bleeding is capillary oozing, which is readily controlled by electrocautery and/or pressure, and is likely to stop spontaneously. Persistent oozing may necessitate a return to the operating room, because probing around a freshly placed tracheostomy tube can be difficult from both a surgeon-visualization and patient-comfort standpoint.

Air Entry

Air dissection can occur during tracheotomy between the fascia layers of the neck and extend into the mediastinum.[26] Puncture of the pleural dome can also produce pneumothorax. The former is usually clinically insignificant, but the latter may result in respiratory compromise. A postoperative radiograph of the chest is routinely recommended.

Anatomic Damage

A tracheotomy incision is routinely recommended at the level of the second through fourth tracheal rings so as to avoid trauma to the cricoid cartilage. Should the cricoid be incised, subglottic stenosis could occur. The membranous posterior tracheal wall or esophagus potentially can be lacerated from a tracheotomy incision that is too deep.[27] The placement of an endotracheal tube or bronchoscope preoperatively prevents this injury. The recurrent laryngeal nerves and great vessels of the neck are also at potential risk during tracheotomy.

Tracheostomy Tube Difficulties

A false passage may inadvertently be created on forceful placement of the tracheostomy tube. Good operative visualization and proper selection of tracheostomy tube size will prevent this problem. Difficulty ventilating the patient immediately after placement of the tracheostomy tube can also be caused by an inadequate internal tube diameter, luminal blockage, or tube dislodgement. Tube changes intraoperatively should be made until adequate ventilation is assured.

Respiratory Arrest

Patients undergoing tracheotomy for relief of upper airway obstruction are at risk for postoperative respiratory arrest. This has been attributed to the rapid washout effect of retained carbon dioxide,

with resultant loss of ventilatory drive, hypotension, and cardiac arrythmia.[28]

Pulmonary Edema

The acute development of pulmonary edema status posttracheotomy has been attributed to the extravasation of fluids through the alveolar wall secondary to rapid changes in airway pressures. Children with hypoxia and hypercapnia secondary to airway obstruction are particularly at risk. The use of continuous positive airway pressure postoperatively can prevent this problem.[29]

Problematic Postoperative Consequences

Hemorrhage

Common etiologies of postoperative tracheostomy tube hemorrhage include inflammation of the tracheal mucosa and intraluminal granulation tissue. Humidification and antibiotics are the recommended treatment if tracheitis is the cause.

Tracheal granulomas typically occur at the superior edge of the internal stoma along the anterior tracheal wall; granulation tissue can also occur in the trachea distal to the stoma secondary to either suctioning or movement of the tip of the tracheostomy tube. Modifications in suctioning technique or changes in tracheostomy tube size can often result in a disappearance of distal granulation tissue. Suprastomal granulomas require bronchoscopic removal.[30] The role of interval endoscopic examination in preventing excessive granulation tissue formation in tracheotomized children is controversial.[31]

Massive postoperative hemorrhage is a rare but quite dramatic event. The most common mechanism is arterial erosion, usually of the innominate artery.[32] The innominate artery often indents the anterior portion of the lower trachea. The tip of the tracheostomy tube may lie against this pulsatile indentation, predisposing the anterior tracheal wall to erosion, fistula formation, and arterial hemorrhage. The problem may be heralded by pulsating tracheostomy tube motion or by brief "sentinal" bleeds. This complication can usually be avoided by proper selection of tracheostomy tube size. Should a massive bleed occur, emergent treatment consists of pressure tamponade produced either by inflating the cuff of an inserted endotracheal tube or by compressing with a bronchoscope the tracheal wall against the posterior sternum. Median sternotomy is required for definitive treatment.

Air Entry

In addition to the difficulties that can be encountered at the time of surgery, high inflation pressures can result in alveolar rupture. This leaking of alveolar air dissects along the perivascular and perilymphatic channels back to the hilum with resultant pneumomediastinum and pneumothorax. This problem has even been reported after decannulation.[33]

Tracheal Lesions

Subglottic stenosis secondary to cricoid disruption has been mentioned previously. Both tracheal stenosis and tracheomalacia may occur at the tracheotomy site; suprastomal depression of the anterior tracheal wall is particularly prevalent.[34] These problems become an issue at decannulation, at which time they can potentially cause significant airway obstruction. A pre-decannulation endoscopic evaluation is strongly recommended.

Tracheostomy Tube Difficulties

Tracheostomy tube obstruction by thick secretions or dry crusts can be avoided or minimized by constant humidification and frequent suctioning. Ventilation difficulties can often be solved by changing the tracheostomy tube size or occasionally changing the brand of tube.

Erythema and skin excoriation at the stoma site can usually be diminished with the use of antibiotic ointments and/or Telfa to act as a water barrier. Should the flange of the tube impinge on the skin of the neck in an uncomfortable fashion, surgical sponges can be inserted in between to cushion the tube. Additionally, the tube can be modified to conform better to the anterior neck.[35]

Infection

Due to the trachea's communication with the external environment, a mild degree of inflammation and infection in the peristomal region is expected. Organisms such as pseudomonas or staphylococcus are frequently recovered from the tracheostomy site. Burn patients are especially prone to bacterial colonization.[36,37] Purulent secretions occur periodically; chest radiographs should be obtained to rule out pneumonia and, if negative, humidification and oral antibiotics should suffice.

Swallowing Difficulties

A tracheotomy can cause both dysphagia and aspiration. Pain on attempted swallowing over the initial postoperative days is not uncommon. More long-standing tracheostomy tube effects include impairment of laryngeal elevation due to tethering of the strap muscles and decompression of normally sustained subglottic pressure, both of which may contribute to aspiration during swallowing.[38]

Impaired Phonation

The initial postoperative inability to communicate can be very distressing to the neurologically intact child. Once the proper size of tube that is adequate enough for ventilation is determined, many children with uncuffed tubes do demonstrate the ability to vocalize and communicate, albeit with a dysphonic vocal quality. The speaking valves mentioned previously may be of additional use. Early routine involvement of speech-language therapy is recommended in neurologically intact children.[39]

Tracheocutaneous Fistula

With time, epithelium from the skin of the neck will migrate internally through the stoma and connect with the mucosa of the trachea. This maturing of the tracheostoma produces a fistula that may persist after the patient is decannulated. The tracheocutaneous fistula and surrounding scar can be excised in such cases to produce a water- and air-tight seal as well as an improved cosmetic result.[40]

Postoperative Care

A tracheostomy tube provides a life-saving alternate airway. In doing so, it bypasses normal physiologic processes that must then be replicated artificially.

Inhaled air must be warmed, filtered, and humidified to prevent tracheobronchial mucosa drying and discomfort and to diminish the incidence of obstruction and infection. Because the ability to cough is greatly diminished, tracheal secretions must be artificially suctioned. Frequent changes of equipment and the use of aseptic technique can minimize the risk of infection. Suctioning should be gentle and done as frequently as is necessary to maintain airway patency.

Cardiorespiratory and oxygen saturation monitoring in the intensive care setting is an absolute necessity in the immediate postoperative care period. Children of all ages require constant reassurance and urgent attention to airway needs. Older children should be provided with means of gaining staff attention, such as a bell, buzzer and writing equipment. Family instruction in tracheotomy care, proficiency in tube changes, and CPR is essential. Individual nursing practices and care arrangements vary greatly between institutions. An instructional booklet written by a multispecialty group is provided to all families of tracheotomized children in our institution.

Decannulation

Decannulation is a time of both excitement and anxiety. The decannulation trial should occur in at least an intermediate care intensive setting. Not all decannulations are successful. Some guidelines are suggested to help facilitate this process.

The timing should obviously be appropriate for the underlying condition. Epiglottitis, for example, resolves quickly, and decannulation can be attempted in a very few days. Long-term tracheotomies, in contrast, are much more prone to the consequences previously discussed and typically prove more difficult to remove. A pre-decannulation laryngoscopy/bronchoscopy is strongly recommended in such cases for removal of granulation tissue and general airway assessment.[41]

The medical personnel should have established a very comfortable rapport with the child so that there will be a minimum of anxiety at the time of decannulation. It is very helpful to have a parent present so that if the child is anxious when medical personnel manipulate the tube, the parent can actually perform the removal.

Airway resistance increases markedly following tube removal. To lessen the suddeness of such a change, the patient may be prepared by prompting laryngeal breathing prior to attempted decannulation. Such maneuvers include periodic occluding of the tube with a finger and changing the tracheostomy tubes in sequence, utilizing progressively smaller diameter tubes.

Occasionally, even despite such measures, a patient will not tolerate the initial decannulation attempt. In infants, this has been attributed to their small airway size; a miniscule diminution in the cross-sectional lumen may be quite significant to the free flow of air.[42] Young children also have more pliable cartilage; the increased force of respiration postdecannulation may cause tracheal collapse, especially in the anterosuperior stomal region.[43] Although consideration has been given to the psychological factors involved in decannulation, present opinion is that the majority of difficulties with decannulation are anatomic/mechanical and not psychological.[44,45] In long-term tracheotomized patients, in the absence of a correctable cause of failure, a repeat trial in 4 to 8 months, simply anticipating further airway growth, is recommended.

References

1. Eavey R. The evolution of tracheotomy. In Myers E, Stool S, Johnson J (eds): *Tracheotomy*. New York: Churchill Livingstone, 1985. Pp 1–11.
2. Stool S, Eavey R. Tracheotomy. In Bluestone C, Stool S (eds): *Pediatric Otolarynogology*. Philadelphia: Saunders, 1983. Pp 1226–1243.
3. Goodall EW. The story of tracheotomy. *Br J Child Dis* 31:167–273, 1934.
4. Jackson C. High tracheotomy and other errors—The chief causes of chronic laryngeal stenosis. *Surg Gynecol Obstet* 32:392, 1923.
5. Galloway TC. Tracheotomy in bulbar poliomyelitis. *JAMA* 123:1096, 1943.
6. *Dorland's Illustrated Medical Dictionary* (25th ed). Philadelphia: Saunders, 1974. P. 1626.
7. Line WS et al. Tracheotomy in infants and young children: The changing perspective 1970–1985. *Laryngoscope* 96:510–575, 1986.
8. Arcand P, Granger J. Pediatric tracheotomies: Changing trends. *J Otolaryngol* 17:121–124, 1988.
9. Prescott CAJ, Vanlierde MJRR. Tracheostomy in children—The Red Cross War Memorial Children's Hospital Experience 1980–1985. *Int J Pediatr Otorhinolaryngol* 17:97–107, 1989.
10. Freezer NJ, Beasley SW, Robertson CE. Tracheostomy. *Arch Dis Child* 65:123–126, 1990.
11. Crater P, Benjamin B. Ten-year review of pediatric tracheotomy. *Ann Otol Rhinol Laryngol* 92:398–400, 1983.
12. Crysdale WS, Feldman RI, Naito K. Tracheotomies: A 10 year experience in 319 children. *Ann Otol Rhinol Laryngol* 97:439–443, 1988.
13. Wetmore RF, Handler SD, Postic WP. Pediatric tracheotomy. Experience during the past decade. *Ann Otol Rhinol Laryngol* 91:628–632, 1982.
14. Eavey RD. Airway interruption in encephalopathic children: A clinical and histological analysis. *Laryngoscope* 95:1455–1460, 1985.
15. Cohen SR, Thompson JW. Varients of Möbius' syndrome and central neurologic impairment. Lindeman procedure in children. *Ann Otol Rhinol Laryngol* 96:93–100, 1987.
16. Kenna MA, Reilly JS, Stool SE. Tracheotomy in the preterm infant. *Ann Otol Rhinol Laryngol* 96:68–71, 1987.
17. Gianoli GJ, Miller RH, Gurrisco JL. Tracheotomy in the first year of life. *Ann Otol Rhinol Laryngol* 99:896–901, 1990.
18. Mullins JB et al. Airway resistance and work of breathing in tracheostomy tubes. *Laryngoscope* 103:1367–1372, 1993.
19. Eavey R, Shannon D, Montgomery S. Customizing tracheotomy tubes. *Laryngoscope* 95:1407–1408, 1985.
20. Passy V. Passy-Muir tracheostomy speaking valve. *Otolaryngol Head Neck Surg* 95:247–248, 1986.
21. Myer CM III. The heat and moisture exchanger in post-tracheotomy care. *Otolaryngol Head Neck Surg* 96:209–210, 1987.
22. Fry TL et al. Comparisons of tracheotomy incisions in a pediatric model. *Laryngol* 94:450–453, 1985.
23. Waki EY et al. An analysis of the inferior based tracheal flap for pediatric tracheotomy. *Int J Pediatr Otorhinolaryngol* 27:47–54, 1993.
24. Kirchner JA. Avoiding problems in tracheotomy. *Laryngoscope* 96:55–57, 1986.
25. Coté C et al. Cricothyroid membrane puncture: Oxygenation and ventilation in a dog model using an intravenous catheter. *Crit Care Med* 16:615–619, 1988.
26. Forbes GB, Salmon G, Herweg JC. Further observations on post-tracheotomy mediastinal emphysema and pneumothorax. *Pediatrics* 31:172–194, 1947.
27. Crysdale WS, Forte V. Posterior tracheal wall disruption: A rare complication of pediatric tracheotomy and bronchoscopy. *Laryngoscope* 96:1279, 1986.
28. Greene NM. Fatal cardiovascular and respiratory failure associated with tracheotomy. *N Engl J Med* 261:846–848, 1959.
29. Galvis AG, Stool SE, Bluestone CD. Pulmonary edema following relief of acute upper airway obstruction. *Ann Otol Rhinol Laryngol* 89:124, 1980.
30. Tom LWC et al. Endoscopic assessment in children with tracheotomies. *Arch Otolaryngol Head Neck Surg* 119:321–324, 1993.
31. Rosenfeld RM, Stool SE. Should granulomas be excised in children with long-term tracheotomy? *Arch Otolaryngol Head Neck Surg* 118:1323–1327, 1992.
32. Hafez A et al. Late cataclysmic hemorrhage from the innominate artery after tracheostomy. *Thorac Cardiovasc Surg* 32:315–319, 1984.
33. Lehmann WB. Bilateral pneumothorax five days after tracheotomy decannulation. *Ann Otol Rhinol Laryngol* 83:128, 1974.
34. Prescott CAJ. Peristomal complications of pediatric tracheostomy. *Int J Pediatr Otorhinolaryngol* 23:141–149, 1992.
35. Rothfield RE, Petruzzelli GJ, Stool SE. Neonatal tracheotomy tube modification. *Otolaryngol Head and Neck Surg* 103:133–134, 1990.
36. Eckhauser FE et al. Tracheostomy complicating massive burn injury: A plea for conservatism. *Am J Surg* 127:423, 1974.
37. Calhoun KH et al. Long-term airway sequelae in a pediatric burn population. *Laryngoscope* 98:721–725, 1988.
38. Gilbert RW et al. Management of patients with long-term tracheotomies and aspiration. *Ann Otol Rhinol Laryngol* 96:561–564, 1987.
39. Arvedson JC, Brodsky L. Pediatric tracheotomy referrals to speech-language pathology in a children's hospital. *Int J Pediatr Otorhinolaryngol* 23:237–243, 1992.
40. White AK, Smitheringale AJ. Treatment of tracheocutaneous fistulae in children. *J Otolaryngol* 18:49–52, 1989.
41. Friedberg J. Tracheotomy revision in infants: To facilitate extubation and restore phonation. *Int J Pediatr Otorhinolaryngol* 13:61–68, 1987.
42. Mallory GB Jr et al. Tidal flow measurement in the decision to decannulate the pediatric patient. *Ann Otol Rhinol Laryngol* 94:454–457, 1985.
43. Benjamin B, Curley JWA. Infant tracheotomy—Endoscopy and decannulation. *Int J Pediatr Otorhinolaryngol* 20:113–121, 1990.
44. Black RJ, Baldwin DL, Johns AN. Tracheostomy 'decannulation panic' in children: Fact or fiction? *J Laryngol Otol* 98:297–304, 1984.
45. Kearns DB et al. Functional assessment of the paediatric laryngeal airway. *Clin Otolaryngol* 15:53–58, 1988.

I. David Todres

John H. Fugate

4.4   Percutaneous Cricothyroidotomy

Percutaneous cricothyroidotomy is reserved for emergency situations when life-threatening hypoxemia cannot be controlled by either mask-bag device with 100% oxygen or tracheal intubation.[1-4] For those experienced with the use of a laryngeal mask airway, this device may provide access to the airway and ability to ventilate the patient and thus obviate the need for percutaneous cricothyroidotomy. When percutaneous cricothyroidotomy is performed, it should be appreciated that the cricothyroid membrane through which the needle is passed is extremely small in infants and small children and not easily identified. Attempts at cricothyroidotomy may damage cricoid and thyroid cartilages.

A minimal amount of equipment is required:

Figure 4.4-1. **(A–D)** Schematic depictions of the procedure of percutaneous cricothyroidotomy. (From Cote CJ, Eavey RD, Todres ID et al. Cricothyroid membrane puncture: Oxygenation and ventilation in a dog model using an intravenous catheter. *Crit Care Med* 16:615–619, 1988. With permission.)

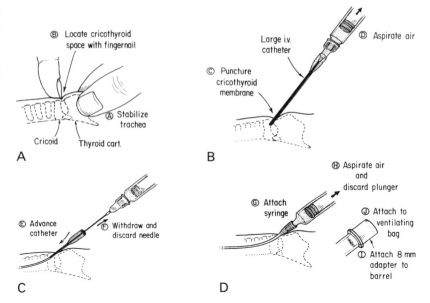

1. Intravenous catheter and syringe
2. Adapter 12–16 (e.g., adapter of 3-mm ID endotracheal tube)
3. Oxygen source and bag-valve device

Technique

What to Do

1. The patient is positioned supine with the head extended in the midline (a rolled towel under the shoulders).

2. The trachea is located and the cricothyroid membrane identified. The cricothyroid membrane extends from the thyroid to the cricoid cartilage (Fig. 4.4-1A).

3. An intravenous catheter (12–16 gauge) is inserted through the cricothyroid membrane and air aspirated (Fig. 4.4-1B).

4. The catheter is advanced into the trachea and the needle withdrawn. Correct intratracheal positioning is confirmed by attaching a 3-ml syringe to the catheter and aspirating air (Fig. 4.4-1C).

5. A 3-mm ET tube adapter is attached to the catheter and a self-inflating bag (with pop-off valve action eliminated) is attached and oxygen insufflated (Fig. 4.4-1D).

What to Avoid

1. rushing to perform the procedure without adequate efforts at face mask-and-bag ventilation and tracheal intubation

2. failure to call for experienced personnel (e.g., anesthesia, ENT surgeons, etc.) to assist in a timely manner

3. relying on this procedure to provide extended relief of the life-threatening hypoxemia

General Considerations

Although the resistance to inflation with percutaneous cricothyroidotomy is extremely high, leading to elevated $PaCO_2$, adequate diffusion of oxygen has been demonstrated and may be life-saving.[3,4] Markedly elevated $PaCO_2$ may be well tolerated in children without sequelae.[5]

Jet ventilation is a method of ventilation via a high-resistance catheter that provides more effective ventilation (i.e., elimination of carbon dioxide). However, significant morbidity may result from the development of massive subcutaneous emphysema or tension pneumothorax. This technique should be used with great caution in children.[6]

References

1. Smith RB, Schaer WB, Pfaeffle H. Percutaneous transtracheal ventilation for anaesthesia and resuscitation: A review and report of complication. *Can Anaesth Soc J* 22:607–612, 1975.
2. Stinson TW. A simple connector for transtracheal ventilation. *Anesthesiology* 47:232, 1977.
3. Frumin MJ, Epstein RM, Cohen G. Apneic oxygenation in man. *Anesthesiology* 20:789–798, 1959.
4. Coté CJ et al. Cricothyroid membrane puncture: Oxygenation and ventilation in a dog model using an intravenous catheter. *Crit Care Med* 16:615–619, 1988.
5. Goldstein B, Shannon DC, Todres ID. Supercarbia in children: Clinical course and outcome. *Crit Care Med* 18:166–169, 1990.
6. Steward DJ. Percutaneous transtracheal ventilation for laser endoscopic procedures in infants and small children. *Can J Anaesth* 34:429–430, 1987.

5 ◆ Vascular Procedures

John H. Fugate
I. David Todres

5.1   Central Venous Cannulation

Indications

For each child, the benefits versus the risks of central venous cannulation must be evaluated to justify the use of this procedure. For example, if adequate fluid resuscitation can be given through a peripheral vein, then this should be used. The indications for central venous cannulation include the following:

1. A way to provide a secure and guaranteed means for administration of fluid, blood, and medications, especially when major shifts of intravascular volume have occurred or are anticipated
2. Unattainable access to the peripheral circulation
3. Access for drugs and fluids that require central administration (e.g., vasopressors, hyperalimentation fluids, contrast medications)
4. Need to monitor central venous pressure
5. Access for performing hemodialysis, plasmapheresis, CAVH, and CAVHD
6. Emergency transvenous pacemakers
7. Access in neurosurgical patients undergoing posterior fossa craniectomy or cervical laminectomy for aspiration of potential air embolus to the right ventricle

Procedure

The equipment need for central venous cannulation is shown in Table 5.1-1.

Technique

What to Do

There are general principles to all central venous catheter procedures that are independent of site. These include

1. Use of the Seldinger technique. This technique is illustrated in Fig. 5.1-1. The advantage of this technique is that a small-gauge needle with a guidewire minimizes trauma and hematoma

Table 5.1-1.

Preparation	Insertion
Prep solution	Appropriate kit for different ages and different-sized patients
Adequate sedation	Monitoring tubing, transducer, and equipment
Xylocaine 1–2%	Patient monitoring devices, i.e., ECG, pulse oximeter

formation and enhances successful cannulation. The procedure is carried out with proper aseptic technique.

2. Adequate sedation to minimize movement. If the patient is on the ventilator, consideration should be given to use of muscle relaxants to provide optimal conditions for cannulation and avoidance of possible complications (e.g., diminishing the risk of pneumothorax with subclavian vein cannulation).

3. Proper catheter tip location that avoids placement in the areas where serious complication may result (e.g., low right atrium or ventricle) and free of vessel or myocardial wall contact. It is important to verify catheter position with regular chest x-rays.

4. Proper caution should be employed when the patient suffers from a bleeding diathesis; for example, subclavian puncture may be hazardous because of inability to control serious hemorrhage.

5. Constant monitoring of the patient's condition (i.e., vital signs and oxygen saturations).

External Jugular Vein Cannulation

The external jugular vein is usually identified easily. It can be cannulated in the presence of a coagulopathy. It avoids the risk of a pneumothorax. The main disadvantage of this approach is the difficulty that may be encountered in trying to thread the catheter past the clavicle centrally.

1. The anatomy of the external jugular vein is shown in Fig. 5.1-2.
2. A pillow or rolled towel is placed under both shoulder blades to extend the head and allow access to the neck.
3. The patient is placed in Trendelenburg position and the head is turned 45 degrees away from the side of cannulation.
4. The patient is then prepared using aseptic conditions. The distal end of the vein (at the clavicle) is compressed to distend it. This also helps to stabilize the vein. The vein is entered with the needle at 15 to 20 degrees. A J-wire is generally used to help in circumventing the plexus of veins at the clavicle. The catheter is passed to a depth that approximates the midsubclavian vein.
5. The line is sutured in place, an antibiotic ointment covers the venipuncture site, and a nonocclusive dressing is placed.
6. It is not uncommon that a catheter will not pass beyond the clavicle into the subclavian vein. The right external jugular vein has been shown to be more successful than the left in threading a catheter centrally.[1,2] Placing the head in a neutral position or pushing down on the ipsilateral shoulder may enhance the passage of the guidewire or catheter.

Complications of External Vein Cannulation

Complications are minimal because of the superficial position of the cannulation vein and the ability to compress the vein to prevent hemorrhage.

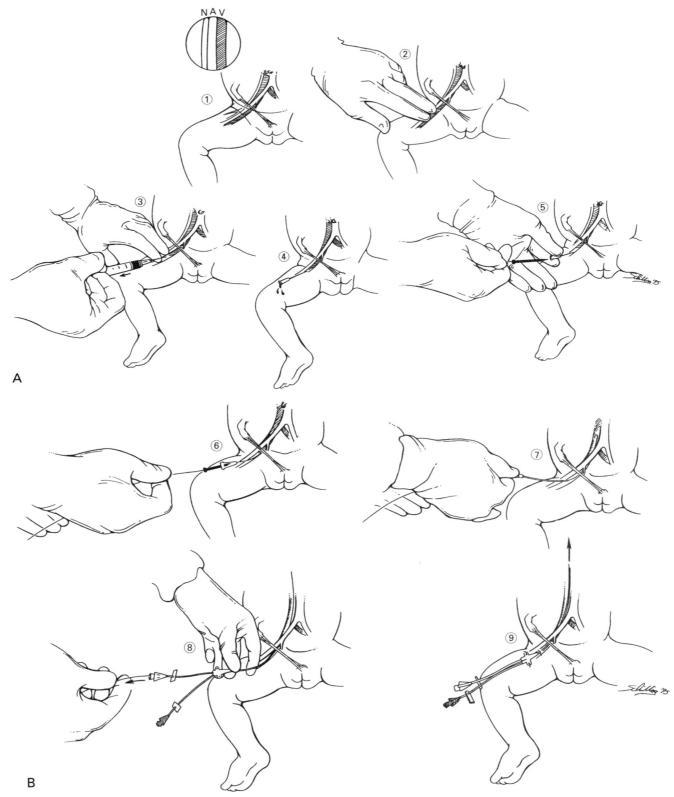

Figure 5.1-1. The Seldinger technique for insertion of a catheter is schematically illustrated. In **(1)** and **(2),** the anatomy of the vessel to be cannulated is identified. A needle and syringe are then directed at the vessel, and blood is aspirated **(3)** and **(4).** A guidewire with introducer is passed through the needle into the vessel **(5)** and **(6).** A dilator is passed over the guidewire **(7).** After the dilator has been removed, the catheter is threaded over the guidewire to the appropriate distance and secured in place **(9).**

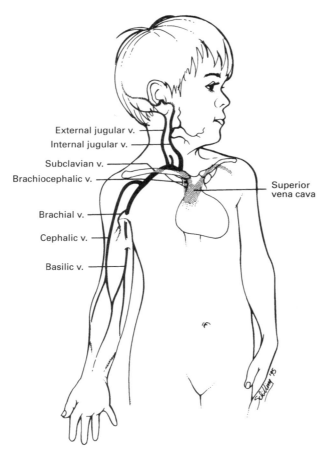

Figure 5.1-2. Venous anatomy of the neck and upper extremity.

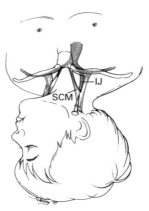

Figure 5.1-3. Internal jugular **(IJ)** vein cannulation (high approach). Note the triangle formed by the clavicle and sternomastoid muscle **(SCM).** The needle is inserted at the apex of the triangle at 30 degrees and directed at the ipsilateral nipple.

needle should be removed simultaneously with the wire to avoid shearing of the wire.

5. The catheter is sutured in place, and the puncture site is covered with antibiotic ointment and protected with a nonocclusive dressing.

6. A posterior approach is preferred by some operators and may be employed if the anterior approach fails (Fig. 5.1-4). The sternomastoid is identified and the point of entry of the needle is midway between the mastoid process and the suprasternal notch. The needle is directed under the belly of the sternomastoid toward the suprasternal notch. Successful entry of the internal jugular vein usually occurs on withdrawal of the needle after transfixing the vein.

Internal Jugular Vein Cannulation

Internal jugular vein cannulation provides an excellent approach to the central circulation with a high success rate and minimal complications.

1. The patient is positioned as in external jugular vein cannulation. There are numerous approaches and techniques, but we have had the most success with the high approach.[3–6] The high approach is used because the most common complications—arterial puncture and pneumothorax or hemothorax—are more easily avoided.

2. The apex of the triangle formed by the two bellies of the sternocleidomastoid muscle and the clavicle is located. The apex is usually where the external jugular vein crosses the sternocleidomastoid, or is midpoint between the mastoid process and the sternal notch (Fig. 5.1-3).

3. The carotid artery is palpated and the needle is introduced at the apex of the triangle at a 30-degree angle just lateral to the carotid artery. The needle is advanced while continually aspirating. The needle is aimed at the ipsilateral nipple. If no blood is freely obtained, having transfixed the vein, the needle is then slowly withdrawn while maintaining aspiration. Frequently, blood is aspirated on withdrawal.

4. Once there is free aspiration of blood, the syringe is carefully removed and the end of the needle occluded to prevent air embolism, especially if the patient is spontaneously breathing. A flexible guidewire is inserted, the needle is removed, and the catheter is advanced over the guidewire. If the wire cannot be advanced, the

Complications of Internal Jugular Vein Cannulation

1. Carotid artery puncture is the most common complication. Usually the amount of bleeding is inconsequential and only requires compression to stop. With bleeding diathesis, however, the hematoma may become quite large and compress central neck structures. An uncorrected coagulopathy is a relative contraindication in children with a bleeding diathesis.

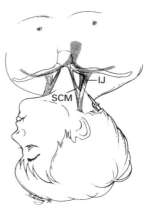

Figure 5.1-4. Internal jugular **(IJ)** vein cannulation (posterior approach). With extension of the neck, the needle is inserted at the midpoint of the lateral border of the sternomastoid muscle **(SCM)** and directed toward the suprasternal notch.

2. Pneumothorax may occur, though the incidence is quite low, usually when needle puncture is just superior to the clavicle.[7]

3. With left-sided cannulation there is potential for injury to the thoracic duct, and there is a higher risk for pneumothorax because the apex of the left lung is higher than on the right. There is also potential for the tip of the catheter to rest against the wall of the superior vena cava (SVC), causing possible erosion.

4. Worsening of increased intracranial pressure may occur because of venous obstruction from the catheter or because of use of the Trendelenburg position during insertion.

Subclavian Vein Cannulation

The subclavian vein is the preferred site in patients with long-term catheter requirements because of its relatively high level of patient comfort and ease of catheter maintenance. In patients with hypovolemia, the subclavian vein does not collapse as readily as some of the other major vessels because of its fibrous attachments directly below the clavicle. It is the site generally used for acute hemodialysis, and in patients with increased intracranial pressure, the subclavian or femoral vein is the preferred site. Because of a higher complication rate, only experienced personnel should use this site.[8,9] Two techniques have been described (infraclavicular and supraclavicular) with equal success and complication rates with experienced operators.[10–12] Following is a description of the more commonly used infraclavicular technique.

Technique: What to Do

1. The anatomy of the subclavian vein is seen in Fig. 5.1-2. The vein is a continuation of the axillary vein and has a set of valves just distal to the junction of the external jugular vein.

2. The patient is prepared as previously described for external jugular vein puncture. A small roll or towel is placed between the shoulder blades; the patient is in a 15- to 30-degree Trendelenburg position, and the head is turned to the contralateral side.

3. The needle is inserted as shown in Fig. 5.1-5. It is inserted immediately below the clavicle at a point one half to two thirds of its length from the sternoclavicular junction and "walked down" the clavicle until it clears the inferior body of the clavicle. The needle is then advanced while it is hugging the under surface of the clavicle and is directed at the suprasternal notch while continuously aspirating.

4. The needle should be inserted bevel up into the subclavian vein, and once blood is freely aspirated, the level should be turned 90 degrees in the direction of the heart, so that when the guidewire is advanced, it goes toward the heart rather than up the internal jugular.

5. As soon as free blood is obtained, the guidewire is advanced as previously described in the Seldinger technique (see Fig. 5.1-1). If free blood is not obtained on insertion or withdrawal of the needle, then the needle should be directed slightly cephalad on the next attempt.

6. Once the catheter is inserted, the site is covered with antibiotic ointment and sutured in place, and a nonocclusive dressing is applied.

Complications of Subclavian Vein Cannulation

1. The major complication of the subclavian vein cannulation is pneumothorax or occasionally hemothorax, especially in patients

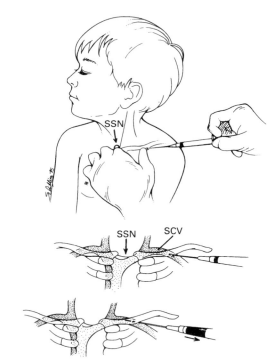

Figure 5.1-5. Subclavian vein **(SCV)** cannulation. The needle is inserted at a point one half to two thirds of its length from the sternoclavicular junction and directed to a point slightly above the suprasternal notch **(SSN)**.

who have a bleeding diathesis, which is a relative contraindication.[13,14] X-rays should be done after placement to verify correct position of the catheter and rule out possible pneumothorax. One fourth to one half of pneumothoraces may be managed without a chest tube.[15–17]

2. The second most common complication is subclavian artery puncture. Usually this is handled by applying pressure above and below the clavicle. In patients with a coagulopathy, such a puncture may be catastrophic. AV fistula is a rare complication of arterial puncture.

3. Other rare complications include thoracic duct injury (from left-sided puncture), central venous thrombosis, and erosion of the catheter, especially if the tip of the catheter abuts the vessel wall.

Femoral Vein Cannulation

In many institutions, femoral vein cannulation is the most common site for central vein cannulation. It is easily accessible and avoids possible pleura and lung complications. The Trendelenburg position is not needed and serious complications are rare. All of these reasons make it popular in the pediatric patient, especially in the patient needing airway management or cardiopulmonary resuscitation.

Technique: What to Do

1. The anatomy of the femoral vein and artery is seen in Fig. 5.1-6. At the inguinal ligament the vein lies in the femoral sheath

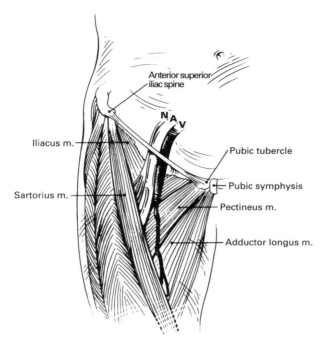

Figure 5.1-6. The anatomy of the neurovascular structures at the groin. Note the relationship of the femoral nerve, artery, and vein **(NAV)**. The femoral artery is midway between the anterior superior iliac spine and the pubic symphysis.

just below the skin line. It lies just medial to the femoral artery, which is just medial to the femoral branch of the genitofemoral nerve.

2. The patient is placed in the supine position with the leg extended and slightly abducted at the hip. Some operators recommend placing a small towel under the hips. Either side may be used. The groin is prepped with betadine, and the skin is infiltrated with xylocaine.

3. The femoral artery is palpated at a point midway between the pubic tubercle and the anterior superior iliac spine.

4. The vein is entered just medial to the femoral artery and 1 cm below the inguinal ligament. The catheter is inserted using the Seldinger technique (see Fig. 5.1-1). If central access is indicated, a long catheter will be needed. The catheter generally does not need to be placed centrally unless accurate cardiac filling pressure measurements are needed. Central pressure trending may be done by measuring the pressures of the inferior vena cava.

5. Once the catheter is inserted, it should be sutured in place, an antibiotic ointment applied, and an occlusive dressing used to prevent any urine or stool from contaminating the insertion site.

Complications of Femoral Vein Cannulation

1. Arterial puncture occurs in a small percentage of pediatric patients.[18] Only a very small percentage (1%) develops a major hematoma, and even in coagulopathy hematomas are of no serious consequence.[19,20]

2. Infectious complications appear to be less than 5% in adults and children and are similar to rates at other sites even though cannulations are in the pubic area.[18-22]

3. A major complication is deep vein thrombosis. This is more common with long-dwelling catheters, but it is still uncommon.

Antecubital Vein Cannulation

In pediatric patients, antecubital vein cannulation for central access with a thin silastic catheter is employed primarily for long-term use. These catheters may be used for antibiotic therapy or for hyperalimentation. With thin silastic catheters, advanced centrally, there is a low incidence of complications, and this makes them ideal for prolonged use. A typical catheter is the PerCuCath catheter, which uses a break-away needle that is placed into the vein; the catheter is then advanced through the needle.

Technique: What to Do

1. The anatomy of the antecubital vein is seen in Fig. 5.5-2. The basilic vein is the easiest to cannulate centrally as it is a direct path to the axillary and subclavian veins. A catheter placed in the cephalic vein, which is the other frequently palpable vein, is usually more difficult to advance centrally.

2. The arm is prepared and aseptic technique used. The basilic vein, if found, is usually tried first. The needle is inserted after local infiltration with xylocaine, and the small silastic catheter is advanced to a central location. This usually requires preplacement measuring. After the catheter is inserted, the needle is removed, split apart, and discarded.

3. If the catheter cannot be advanced past the shoulder, cephalad positioning of the arm and anterior displacement of the shoulder may help in advancing the catheter. X-ray is needed to confirm proper location.

4. In older patients with large antecubital veins, the Seldinger technique may be used occasionally to place large catheters into the central veins. These should be left in only a short time (48–72 hours) because of the high frequency of thrombophlebitis.

Complications of Antecubital Vein Cannulation

There are few complications from use of this technique other than local trauma, but there is a high incidence of inability to pass a catheter centrally.[23-25] With movement of the arm, there may be significant catheter migration. Infection and thrombophlebitis of the arm are the two most common complications.

Summary of What to Avoid
1. Placing lines in an uncooperative, moving patient
2. Lack of patient monitoring
3. Multiple sticks at the same site
4. Placing subclavian or internal jugular catheters in a patient with an uncorrected coagulopathy (unless no other site is available)
5. Air embolism—more common in a spontaneously breathing patient
6. Improper site location (There are numerous sites for central lines, and general guidelines are noted in Table 5.1-2.)

Central Venous Catheter Maintenance and Long-Term Complications

There are three long-term complications common to all central venous catheters and to all sites: (1) vascular erosions, (2) vein thrombosis, and (3) infection. Proper catheter maintenance may prevent these complications.

Table 5.1-2. Preferred choices for central line placement according to medical indication

Indication	First choice	Second choice	Third choice
Emergency airway management or CPR	FV	SV	AV
Brain-injured or increased intracranial pressure	FV	SV	—
Long-term parenteral nutrition	AV* or SV	IJV	—
Acute hemodialysis or plasmapheresis	SV	FV	—
Coagulopathy	FV	EJV	IJV
General access (i.e., for surgery, medicine)	IJV	FV or SV	EJV
Emergency transvenous pacemaker	RIJV	SV	LIJV or FV

*Using small silastic catheter.
AV, antecubital vein; FV, femoral vein; SV, subclavian vein; IJV, internal jugular vein; EJV, external jugular vein; R, right; L, left.

Vascular Erosions

Vascular erosions usually occur several days after line placement and are associated with catheter stiffness, hyperosmolar solutions, position of the tip of the catheter within the vessel lumen, and insertion site. The most common sites associated with vessel erosion are the left internal and left external jugular vein cannulations because the tips of the catheters are frequently positioned against the SVC wall.[26–30] Patients with catheters that have migrated into the thoracic cavity usually present with acute dyspnea and pleural effusion. Occasionally, patients may have catheters that erode through the SVC or right atrium and allow fluid to fill the pericardial space. Acute pericardial tamponade can be a serious complication and presents with symptoms of severely compromised cardiac output. It is important to note that aspiration of blood from the catheter does not preclude the erosion of the vessel by the catheter.

Thrombosis

All catheter placement in patients is potentially thrombogenic to some extent. Catheter materials, size of catheter in relation to the vessel, and duration of cannulation appear to be the major causes of thrombi development. The best catheters are soft and pliable within the vessels and have a smooth surface. Silastic and polyurethane catheters appear to be the least thrombogenic. Hydromer coating of polyurethane catheters and heparin bonding also help decrease thrombogenicity.[31–34]

There is a spectrum of thrombosis, ranging from fibrin sleeve formation around the catheter (very common) to mural thrombi (10%–30%) to total venous occlusion (rare). The insertion site does not appear related to thrombi development, and only a small percentage (<3%) have clinical symptoms.[35–37]

Infection

Infectious complications from central venous catheters most commonly occur from colonized bacteria at the skin site invading the catheter tract to the tip and developing a foci for infection.[38–41] Other less common causes include infection entering at the catheter hub (thus multilumen catheters have a higher infection rate), hematogenous seeding from catheters, and, rarely, contamination of the infusate.

Central line infections range from local cellulitis or abscess formation to systemic complications including bacteremia, septic shock, and occasionally metastatic infection. Rates of bacteremia and sepsis are 2% to 8%, although some studies have shown less than 2% infection rate with newer technologies. The most common organisms are Gram-positive, especially *Staphylococcus* species, although Gram-negative organisms are not uncommon. *Candida* infections also occur, especially in immunocompromised patients.

Catheter maintenance, catheter material, and catheter duration have an impact on the incidence of infection. Insertion site does not appear to affect infection rate. Catheter maintenance includes proper sterile insertion technique and the use of standardized protocols for care after insertion. This includes sterile technique in cleaning and dressing the site along with minimizing the number of "piggyback" infusions and catheter site manipulations. Tubing changes are not needed more than every 2 to 3 days.

Silastic catheters have the lowest infection rates. Catheters that have antibiotic bonding and bacteria-resistant cuffs at the skin site have lower infection rates. Increased duration of the catheter indwelling time increases the rate of infection. There is much controversy over the optimal duration of catheter placement, with many institutions recommending changing catheter sites every 3 to 4 days. Also, guidewire exchange of the catheter as an infection control measure does not appear effective.[42,43]

In children, site change every 3 to 4 days is frequently impractical, as the low risks of infection must be balanced against the risks associated with central line placement. We recommend placement of a catheter at a new site every 7 days unless impractical. This usually prevents all the long-term complications of erosion, thrombosis, and infection. To minimize all of these complications, small caliber polyurethane or silastic catheters are used, with a minimal amount of infusion changes and manipulation.

Management of the febrile patient with an indwelling central line is somewhat controversial, and care must be individualized depending on several issues. Obviously, not all febrile patients must have their central lines removed, as the source of infection is frequently unrelated to the line. The following is an example of guidelines for managing the febrile patient with a central line.

Guidelines for Management of the Febrile Patient

1. Does the patient require the catheter? If not, remove it. If the catheter is needed, examine the site. If the site is infected, remove the catheter, start antibiotics, and place the catheter at another site.

2. Does the patient have clinical sepsis? If there is no evidence for clinical sepsis, a source of infection should be investigated. If a source is found, appropriate antibiotics should be instituted.

If there is no alternative source for the fever, the duration of the catheter placement should be considered. Catheters that have been in place for fewer than 3 days are an unlikely source for infection, and only observation of the patient and blood cultures are needed. If the line has been in place 6 days or longer, the catheter should be removed, and an alternative site should be cannulated. If there is high risk for new catheter placement (severe coagulopathy) or technical impossibility, guidewire replacement may be considered. If the catheter has been in place 4 to 5 days, the catheter should be rewired and the tip of the catheter sent for culture. If the catheter tip culture and blood cultures are positive, the wired catheter should be removed and another site chosen, if a central line is needed. Antibiotics should be given appropriately.

Rewiring an existing catheter should be done using sterile technique. The wire should not be placed through the hub of the existing catheter but should be placed through a transected segment of catheter, preferably through a segment that had been within the vessel prior to the wire's being withdrawn. This cannot be done with short catheters in small infants. It should be emphasized that a rewired catheter will quickly become colonized and a source of infection, as the tract was colonized and infected.[44–47]

3. If the patient is septic and there is no other identifiable source of infection, the catheter should be strongly suspected as the culprit! If the catheter has been in longer than 3 to 4 days, a new site and catheter should be considered (unless there is a higher risk or technical problems). Catheters in place for fewer than 3 to 4 days or catheters in high-risk patients should be rewired and the catheters cultured. If the patient is improved and the catheter tip culture is negative, the rewired catheter may be kept in place; otherwise it should be removed.

4. If catheter-related sepsis does develop, appropriate antibiotics should be used for 7 to 14 days, with continued observation for metastatic infection.

References

1. Belani KG et al. Percutaneous cervical central venous line placement: A comparison of the internal and external jugular vein routes. *Anesth Analg* 59:40–44, 1980.
2. Blitt CD et al. J-wire versus straight wire for central venous system cannulation via the external jugular vein. *Anesth Analg* 61:536–537, 1982.
3. Brinkman AJ, Costley DO. Internal jugular venipuncture. *JAMA* 223:182–183, 1973.
4. Jernigan WR et al. Use of the internal jugular vein for placement of central venous catheter. *Surg Gynecol Obstet* 130:520–524, 1970.
5. Mostert JW, Kenny GM, Murphy GP. Safe placement of central venous catheter into internal jugular vein. *Arch Surg* 101:431–432, 1970.
6. Rao TLK, Wong AY, Salem MR. A new approach to percutaneous catheterization of the internal jugular vein. *Anesthesiology* 46:362–364, 1977.
7. Coté CJ et al. Two approaches to cannulation of a child's internal jugular vein. *Anesthesiology* 50:371–373, 1979.
8. Tremper KK. Central venous catheterization: A perspective. *J Intens Care Med* 2:121, 1987.
9. Sznadjer JI et al. Central vein catheterization: Failure and complication rates by three percutaneous approaches. *Arch Intern Med* 146:259, 1986.
10. James PM, Myers R. Central venous pressure monitoring: Complications and a new technique. *Am Surg* 39:75, 1981.
11. Dronen S et al. Subclavian vein catheterization during cardiopulmonary resuscitation: Comparison of supra- and infraclavicular percutaneous approaches. *JAMA* 247:3227, 1982.
12. Sterner S. A comparison of the supraclavicular approach and the infraclavicular approach for subclavian vein catheterization. *Ann Emerg Med* 15:421, 1986.
13. Defalque RJ. Subclavian venipuncture: A review. *Anesth Analg* 47:677–682, 1968.
14. Groff DB, Ahmed N. Subclavian vein catheterization in the infant. *J Pediatr Surg* 9:171–174, 1974.
15. Eerola R, Kaukinen L, Kaukinen S. Analysis of 13,800 subclavian catheterizations. *Acta Anaesthesiol Scand* 29:193, 1985.
16. Simpson ET, Aitchison JM. Percutaneous infraclavicular subclavian vein catheterization in shocked patients: A prospective study in 172 patients. *J Trauma* 22:781, 1982.
17. McCormack T et al. Complications of subclavian vein cannulation. *Ir Med J* 74:373, 1981.
18. Kanter RK et al. Central venous catheter insertion by femoral vein: Safety and effectiveness for the pediatric patient. *Pediatrics* 77:842, 1986.
19. Getzen LC, Pollak EW. Short-term femoral vein catheterization. *Am J Surg* 138:875, 1979.
20. Williams JF et al. The use of femoral venous catheters in critically ill adults: A prospective study. *Crit Care Med* 19:843, 1991.
21. Swanson RS. Emergency intravenous access through the femoral vein. *Ann Emerg Med* 13:244, 1979.
22. Dailey RH. Femoral vein cannulation: A review. *J Emerg Med* 2:367, 1985.
23. Kuramoto T, Sakabe T. Comparison of success in jugular versus basilic vein technics for central venous pressure catheter positioning. *Anesth Analg* 54:696–697, 1975.
24. Webre DR, Arens JF. Use of cephalic and basilic veins for introduction of central venous catheters. *Anesthesiology* 38:389–392, 1973.
25. Burgess GE III, Marino RJ, Peuler MJ. Effect of head position on the location of venous catheters inserted via basilic veins. *Anesthesiology* 46:212–213, 1977.
26. Seneff MG. Central venous catheterization: A comprehensive review, part 1. *J Intens Care Med* 2:163, 1987.
27. Ellis LM, Vogel SB, Copeland EM. Central venous catheter vascular erosions: Diagnosis and clinical course. *Ann Surg* 209:475, 1989.
28. Ghani GA, Berry AJ. An unusual complication following cannulation of an external jugular vein. *Anesthesiology* 58:93, 1983.
29. Iberti TJ et al. Hydrothorax as a late complication of central venous indwelling catheters. *Surgery* 94:842, 1983.
30. Duntley P et al. Vascular erosion by central venous catheters. *Chest* 101:1633, 1992.
31. Nichols PKT, Major E. Central venous cannulation. *Curr Anaesth Crit Care* 1:54, 1989.
32. Hoar PF et al. Heparin bonding reduces thrombogenecity of pulmonary artery catheters. *N Engl J Med* 305:992, 1981.
33. Mangano DT. Heparin bonding and long-term protection against thrombogenesis. *N Engl J Med* 307:894, 1982.
34. Kido DK et al. Thrombogenicity of heparin and non-heparin coated catheters. *Am J Roentgenol* 139:957, 1982.
35. Ahmed N, Payne RF. Thrombosis after central venous cannulation. *Med J Aust* 1:217, 1976.
36. Efsing HO et al. Thromboembolic complications from central venous catheters: A comparison of three catheter materials. *World J Surg* 7:419, 1983.
37. Bagwell CE, Marchildon MB. Mural thrombi in children: Potentially lethal complication of central venous hyperalimentation. *Crit Care Med* 17:295, 1989.
38. Raad II, Bodey GP. Infectious complications of indwelling vascular catheters. *Clin Infect Dis* 15:197, 1992.
39. Passerini L et al. Biofilms on indwelling vascular catheters. *Crit Care Med* 20:665, 1992.
40. Cooper GL, Schiller AL, Hopkins CC. Possible role of capillary action

in pathogenesis of experimental catheter-associated dermal tunnel infections. *J Clin Microbiol* 26:8, 1988.

41. Make DG. Pathogenesis, prevention, and management of infections due to intravascular devices used for infusion therapy. In Bisno A, Waldvogel F (eds): *Infections Associated with Indwelling Medical Devices*. Washington, DC: American Society for Microbiology, 1989. Pp 161–177.

42. Eyer S et al. Catheter-related sepsis: Prospective, randomized study of three methods of long-term catheter maintenance. *Crit Care Med* 18:1073, 1990.

43. Cobb DK et al. A controlled trial of scheduled replacement of central venous and pulmonary artery catheters. *N Engl J Med* 327:1062, 1992.

44. Olson ME et al. Evaluation of strategies for central venous catheter replacement. *Crit Care Med* 20:797, 1992.

45. Mermel LA et al. The pathogenesis and epidemiology of catheter-related infection with pulmonary artery Swan-Ganz catheters: A prospective study utilizing molecular subtyping. *Am J Med* 91(Suppl B): 197S, 1991.

46. Pettigrew RA et al. Catheter-related sepsis in patients on intravenous nutrition: A prospective study of quantitative catheter cultures and guidewire changes for suspected sepsis. *Br J Surg* 72:52, 1985.

47. Graeve AH, Carpenter CM, Schiller WR. Management of central venous catheters using a wire introducer. *Am J Surg* 142:752, 1981.

John H. Fugate

I. David Todres

◆ 5.2   Arterial Catheterization

Indications

Indications for arterial lines include the need (1) to monitor blood pressure continuously and (2) to monitor blood samples frequently, especially arterial blood gases. Intraarterial blood pressure monitoring is especially important in the hemodynamically unstable patient. Automatic oscillometric devices may replace intraarterial blood pressure monitoring in the relatively stable patient. The inaccuracy in the unstable patient, however, necessitates intraarterial monitoring. Arterial cannulation for blood gas sampling purposes is limited because pulse oximetry (O_2 saturations) and end-tidal carbon dioxide provide approximate data for patients on mechanical ventilation when the patient is relatively stable. Once the indications for the placement of the catheter have passed, the catheter should be removed as the burdens (i.e., complications) at this stage will outweigh the benefits. The equipment requirements for arterial line cannulation are shown in Table 5.2-1.

Radial Artery Cannulation

Radial artery cannulation is a primary site of arterial cannulation in infants and children. Right radial artery cannulation is selected when preductal arterial oxygen tensions are important in evaluating and treating infants with congenital heart disease. Percutaneous radial artery cannulation is widely practiced with minimal morbidity. Failure to cannulate the artery percutaneously may be followed successfully by direct arterial cutdown.

Technique

The anatomy of the radial and ulnar arteries is depicted in Fig. 5.2-1. Adequacy of ulnar artery collateral flow is confirmed by the modified Allen test. The radial and ulnar arteries are compressed at the wrist, and the hand is repeatedly clenched. The ulnar artery is then released and flushing (reperfusion) of the blanched hand is noted. If the entire hand is well perfused while the radial artery remains occluded, indicating adequate collateral flow, catheterization of the radial artery is performed.

The hand is secured on an arm board with slight extension of the wrist to avoid excessive median nerve stretching. The fingertips should be left exposed when the hand is taped down so that any peripheral ischemic changes due to spasm, clot, or air can be observed.

The course of the radial artery may be observed in an infant with the aid of a fiberoptic light source. A Doppler device also may be helpful in identifying the course of the radial artery. A 20-gauge needle is used to make a small skin puncture over the maximal pulsation of the radial artery, usually at the second proxi-

Table 5.2-1.   Equipment needed for an arterial line cannulation

Prep solution, (e.g., betadine)

Xylocaine 1–2%

Sterile needles, syringes, and arm or foot boards

Catheter system, intravenous catheters, or an appropriate arterial cannulation kit

T-connector

Noncompliant tubing and stop cocks

Continuous infusion set-up

Monitor

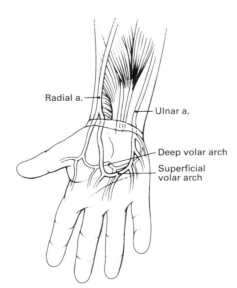

Figure 5.2-1.   Anatomy of the radial artery showing the collateral circulation to the ulnar artery through the deep volar arterial and dorsal arches.

mal wrist crease. This step eases passage of the cannula by reducing resistance offered by the skin. Cannulation is accomplished either on direct entry of the artery at an angle of 15 to 20 degrees or on withdrawing the cannula after transfixion of the artery (Fig. 5.2-2). The catheter is then firmly attached to a T-connector to permit continuous infusion of heparinized isotonic saline (1 U/ ml) at the rate of 1 to 2 ml/hr via a constant-infusion pump. Antibiotic ointment is applied, the surrounding skin is coated with tincture of benzoin, and the catheter is taped securely in place. A pressure transducer is connected to allow continuous arterial pressure monitoring. In order to ensure accurate blood pressure measurement, it is essential that the transducer be calibrated with mercury to the patient's heart level, that all air bubbles be removed from the system, and that no more than 3 feet of tubing be used between the patient and the transducer to minimize artifacts caused by the monitoring tubing.

To facilitate cannulation of the radial artery, the Seldinger technique may be extremely helpful (Fig. 5.2-3). Most difficulties in cannulating the radial artery involve advancing the catheter once blood is aspirated on needle puncture. The guidewire is placed through the needle as blood appears, and the catheter is then threaded over the guidewire.

Blood samples are obtained by clamping off the distal end of the T-connector, cleaning the injection port of the T-connector with povidone-iodine, introducing a 22-gauge needle, and withdrawing a small amount of blood to clear the line. Alternatively, a stopcock attached to the T-connector provides access for sampling. A sample of blood is obtained by use of a heparinized

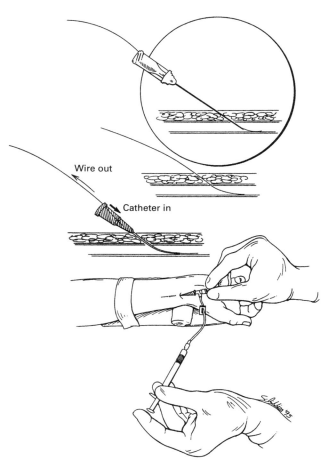

Figure 5.2-3. Placement of the radial artery cannula with the Seldinger technique. The hand is fixed as in Fig. 5.2-2. The artery is entered with a needle and syringe. Blood is aspirated. The wire introducer is then advanced through the needle into the artery. The cannula is then threaded over the wire and advanced while the wire is withdrawn. A T-type connector is attached and blood aspirated to confirm the presence of the cannula in the artery.

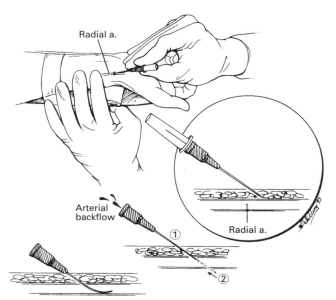

Figure 5.2-2. Cannulation of the radial artery. Note position of hand—extended but avoiding over extension. The hand is immobilized with tape leaving the extremities exposed to assess peripheral circulation. The operator palpates the artery for maximal pulsation and introduces the cannula (20- or 22-gauge angiocath) at an angle of 30 degrees. Making a nick into the skin at the point of entry with a larger needle facilitates introduction of the cannula. The artery is entered as one introduces the cannula or may be transfixed. With the latter method, blood enters the cannula as it is **gently** withdrawn. It is then advanced and fixed in position. Blood is aspirated to confirm the intraarterial position of the cannula.

syringe, with minimal blood loss and minimal manipulation of the system. After sampling, continuous infusion is resumed. Bolus flushes should be avoided because they have been associated with retrograde blood flow to the brain. Disastrous results may occur if an air bubble or blood clot should accompany a bolus flush. Heparinized solutions are infused. All arterial lines must be identified clearly (red tape) to avoid accidental infusion of hypertonic solutions and sclerosing medications.

Complications

1. Disconnection of the catheter from the infusion system. Blood loss may be life-threatening, especially in an infant.

2. Ischemia. The radial artery cannula should be withdrawn if ischemic changes develop.

3. Emboli. A blood clot or air may embolize to the digits or centrally, resulting in arteriolar spasm or more serious ischemic necrosis.

4. Arterial thrombus formation. This is dependent on the size of catheter inserted, the material of which it is constructed, the technique of insertion, and duration of cannulation.

5. Infection at the site of the catheter insertion, with possible septicemia

6. Peripheral neuropathy

Femoral Artery Cannulation

The femoral artery is used more commonly in adults but is being increasingly used in children. If the radial artery cannulation is unsuccessful, the femoral artery provides a good alternative site, especially in patients who have poorly palpable peripheral pulses. Multiple studies in adults have shown that femoral artery cannulation has equally low or lower complication rates than radial artery cannulation.[1-6] There are no published studies concerning children.

Technique

The femoral artery is located by palpation at the groin. Anatomically, it is situated midway between the anterior superior iliac spine and the pubic tubercle.

After sterile preparation of the skin, a catheter of appropriate size is inserted into the femoral artery by use of the Seldinger technique (see Vascular Procedures, Central Venous Cannulation, by Fugate and Todres, this volume). The artery is entered at the point of maximal pulsation, approximately 1 cm below the line joining the anterior superior iliac spine and the pubic tubercle. After cannulation, the catheter is connected to a continuous-flow system and pressure transducer. The catheter is sutured in place, the insertion site is covered with antibiotic ointment, and an occlusive dressing is applied. The likelihood of fecal and urinary contamination makes this last step particularly important.

Complications

1. Infection
2. Emboli of clot and air, leading to ischemic necrosis of the lower limb
3. Retroperitoneal hemorrhage
4. Bowel perforation
5. AV fistula
6. Poor arterial puncture technique, leading to osteoarthritis of the hip joint

Axillary Artery Cannulation

The axillary artery offers an excellent alternative site because of its central location and rich collateral circulation. It is frequently palpable when more peripheral sites cannot be felt. The left axilla artery is usually the preferred site because any air bubbles or clots injected into the right subclavian artery (from the right axillary artery) are more likely to enter the aortic arch.[7] The complication rates have been reported as quite low in adult studies (no studies concerning children).[7-9]

The arm is positioned by placing the patient's hand behind the head. This abducts and externally rotates the arm. The artery is maximally palpated at the inferior border of the pectoralis major muscle and then held against the shaft of the humerus. After prepping and infiltrating, an appropriately sized catheter is introduced and placed by use of the Seldinger technique. It is important to use caution when flushing axillary artery catheters because of their proximity to the central circulation, and it is recommended that only hand flushing with small volumes be employed.[10-12]

Complications

1. Infection
2. Cerebral embolization of air or clot
3. Brachial plexus neuropathy

Brachial Artery Cannulation

The brachial artery is not commonly used in most centers because of its relatively poor collateral circulation and therefore its implied risk of distal ischemia. However, reports of its use do show low complication rates.[6,13,14]

A modified Allen test should be performed on both the ulnar and radial arteries to ensure good peripheral circulation. If there is a question of poor peripheral circulation, the brachial site should not be used. The brachial artery is palpated in the anticubital fossa with the arm extended, just medial to the bicipital tendon (Fig. 5.2-4). The artery is punctured at this point and either an intravenous catheter is directly placed or the Seldinger technique is used as previously described.

Complications

1. Infection
2. Cerebral or peripheral embolization leading to ischemic necrosis
3. Median nerve damage; usually a temporary paresthesias, but median nerve palsy has been reported

Dorsalis Pedis and Posterior Tibial Artery Catheterization

The dorsalis pedis (Fig. 5.2-5) and posterior tibial arteries (Fig. 5.2-6) are additional useful sites for arterial cannulation in children when more desirable locations are inaccessible. Collateral circulation should always be checked. If one cannulates or attempts to cannulate one artery in the foot, the other should always be left uninstrumented to ensure adequate collateral blood flow.

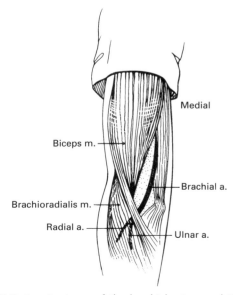

Figure 5.2-4. Anatomy of the brachial artery and its division into radial and ulnar arteries at the elbow.

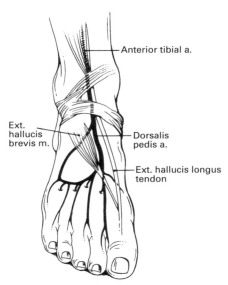

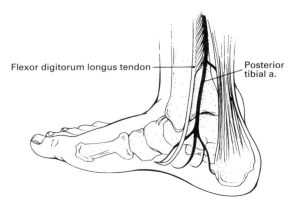

Figure 5.2-6. Anatomy of the posterior tibial artery. Note its relationship to the flexor digitorum longus tendon and the Achilles tendon.

Figure 5.2-5. Anatomy of dorsalis pedis artery. Note its course along a line midway between the medial and laterial malleoli and the juncture of the great and second toes.

Technique

The artery is cannulated in the same manner as the radial artery. The cannulation is attempted at a point of maximal pulsation. One should have a clear picture of the anatomy of the dorsalis pedis and posterior tibial arteries before attempting this procedure. If percutaneous cannulation is impossible, the cutdown technique should be carried out to ensure successful cannulation. Systolic pressures are generally 5 to 15 mm Hg higher in these arteries than in the radial arteries, but mean pressures are usually the same.

Summary of What to Avoid

1. Not checking for adequacy of collateral circulation
2. Improper positioning of patient and extremity
3. Large hematoma, especially in patient with coagulopathy
4. Multiple attempts that may damage the artery
5. Attempting to cannulate both arteries in the same distal extremity, e.g., radial and ulnar
6. Uncooperative, moving child
7. Air or clot embolization
8. Disconnection of tubing
9. Not carrying out ongoing monitoring of adequacy of circulation in the distal extremity

References

1. Soderstom CA et al. Superiority of the femoral artery for monitoring: A prospective study. *Am J Surg* 44:309, 1982.
2. Gurman GM, Kriemerman S. Cannulation of big arteries in critically ill patients. *Crit Care Med* 13:217, 1985.
3. Russell JA et al. Prospective evaluation of radial and femoral artery catheterization sites in critically ill adults. *Crit Care Med* 11:936, 1983.
4. Norwood SH et al. Prospective study of catheter-related infection during prolonged arterial catheterization. *Crit Care Med* 16:836, 1988.
5. Pinilla JC et al. Study of the incidence of intravascular catheter infection and associated septicemia in critically ill patients. *Crit Care Med* 11:21, 1983.
6. Gordon LH et al. Alternative sites for continuous arterial monitoring. *South Med J* 77:1498, 1984.
7. Bryan-Brown CW et al. The axillary artery catheter. *Heart Lung* 12:492, 1983.
8. DeAngelis J. Axillary artery monitoring. *Crit Care Med* 4:205, 1976.
9. Brown M et al. Intravascular monitoring via the axillary artery. *Anaesth Intensive Care* 13:38, 1984.
10. Harman EM. Arterial cannulation. In Mallory DL, Venus B (eds): *Problems in Critical Care*. Philadelphia: Lippincott, 1988.
11. Sladen A. Arterial pressure monitoring. In: *Invasive Monitoring and Its Complications in the Intensive Care Unit*. St. Louis: Mosby, 1990.
12. Lipchik EO, Sugimoto H. Percutaneous brachial artery catheterization. *Radiology* 160:842, 1986.
13. Barnes RW et al. Safety of brachial arterial catheters as monitors in the intensive care unit: A prospective evaluation with the Doppler ultrasonic velocity detector. *Anesthesiology* 44:260, 1976.
14. Mann S et al. The safety of ambulatory intra-arterial pressure monitoring: A clinical audit of 1000 studies. *Int J Cardiol* 5:585, 1984.

John H. Fugate

I. David Todres

 5.3

Pulmonary Artery Cannulation

Pulmonary artery (PA) catheters were introduced in 1970 by Swan, Ganz, and associates. Since then they have found widespread clinical application in adults and children.[1,2] PA catheters provide data to better evaluate cardiopulmonary performance and aid in decision making, especially in patients who are unstable or who have significantly impaired cardiac function. Benefits versus risks must be weighed in every patient when PA catheters are considered.

Indications

1. The need to assess left and right ventricular function
2. The need to evaluate pulmonary artery pressures
3. Assistance in guiding therapy in unstable patients or selected patients for long-term pharmacologic treatment
4. Assistance in providing prognostic data

5. Specialty catheters
   a. The need to measure mixed versus oxygen saturation (SvO_2) continuously
   b. Providing temporary cardiac pacing

Most commonly, PA catheters are used in pediatric patients who have significant lung disease (i.e., ARDS) or to help in the assessment of shock. Occasionally, they are needed to help in fluid management or to evaluate therapy or progress in patients with chronic respiratory failure, chronic heart failure, or primary pulmonary hypertension.

Procedure

Equipment

Pictures of PA catheters are seen in Figs. 5.3-1 and 5.3-2. The catheter is balloon-tipped (Fig. 5.3-2), thus becoming flow-directed when the balloon is inflated and has a thermistor at the tip, multiple lumens, and an electronic connection to measure cardiac output and temperature. Specialty PA catheters may have extra lumens, a pacing port, or an oxygen sensor to measure SvO_2 continuously. Catheters come in various sizes: 3F, 4F, 5F, 7F, and 7.5F, along with various lengths. Other equipment needs are noted in Table 5.3-1.

Technique

What to Do

1. Choose the appropriately sized catheter and appropriate insertion site. Table 5.3-2 gives guidelines for insertion site.

Table 5.3-1. Equipment for pulmonary artery catheters

Prep solution, e.g., betadine

Local anesthetic—1%–2% xylocaine

Introducer sheath kit

Sterile gowns, gloves, masks, drapes, syringes, stopcocks

Flush bags (heparinized saline) and transducers with appropriate tubing and monitor

Suture and dressing materials

Lidocaine or other antidysrhythmic agents

2. The patient is sedated and muscle-relaxed if on a ventilator.

3. The patient is positioned according to the site chosen as seen in central venous cannulation section. Prep solution and sterile drapes are applied, and the appropriate skin site is infiltrated with xylocaine.

4. The PA catheter is prepared by placing stopcocks and syringes of normal saline to all infusion sites. Monitoring tubing with transducer and monitor are put in place. All ports are flushed, and the distal port is readied for continuous monitoring of pressure. The balloon is inflated and deflated to ensure proper functioning; the electronic connection is also evaluated. The PA catheter is kept sterile during preparation.

5. The introducer sheath is placed by use of the Seldinger technique. First, the needle is inserted into the appropriate vein, blood is aspirated, the guidewire is placed, and the needle is removed (see Fig. 5.3-1). The vessel dilator-sheath apparatus is

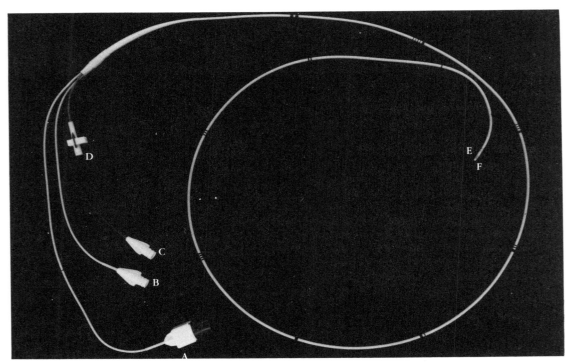

Figure 5.3-1. Pulmonary artery catheter. **(A)** Connection to thermodilution cardiac output computer. **(B)** Connection to distal lumen. **(C)** Connection to proximal lumen. **(D)** Stopcock connected to balloon at the catheter tip for balloon inflation. **(E)** Thermistor. **(F)** Balloon. The catheter is marked in 10-cm increments. (From JM Rippe et al. *Procedures and Techniques in Intensive Care Medicine*, Boston: Little, Brown, 1995. p. 50. With permission.)

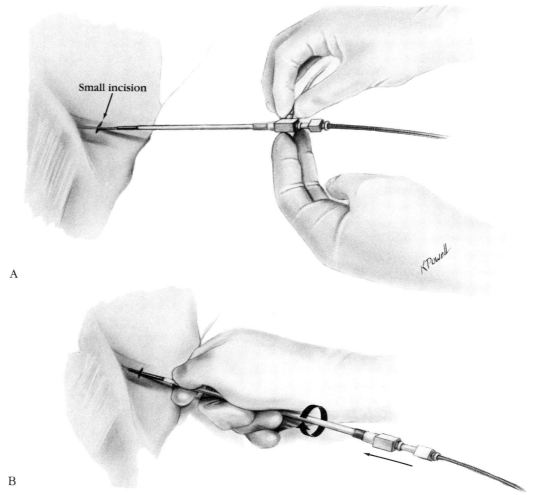

A

B

Figure 5.3-2. **(A)** The vessel dilator-sheath apparatus is threaded over the guidewire and advanced into the vessel. **(B)** A twisting motion is used to thread the apparatus into the vein. (From JM Rippe et al. *Procedures and Techniques in Intensive Care Medicine,* Boston: Little, Brown, 1995. p. 55. With permission.)

Table 5.3-2. Insertion sites for pulmonary artery catheters

Patient condition	Site Selection Choice		
	1st	2nd	3rd
General need	RIJV	LIJV or LSV	FV
Patient with coagulopathy	FV	EJV	RIJV
Patient with high PEEP	RIJV	FV or LIJV	EJV
Patient with increased ICP or acute brain injury	FV	LSV	

FV, femoral vein; EJV, external jugular vein; IJV, internal jugular vein; SV, subclavian vein; R, right; L, left.

then threaded over the guidewire after a small incision in the skin has been made. The apparatus is inserted into the vein with a twisting movement, and then the guidewire and vessel dilator are removed (see Fig. 5.3-2).

6. The PA catheter is then inserted through a sterile sleeve protector, and the sleeve is pulled back to the proximal portion of the catheter and out of the way.

7. The catheter is then advanced through the introducer

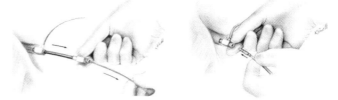

Figure 5.3-3. The pulmonary artery catheter is passed through the introducer sheath into the vein. (From JM Rippe et al. *Procedures and Techniques in Intensive Care Medicine,* Boston: Little, Brown, 1995. p. 55. With permission.)

sheath into the vein (Fig. 5.3-3). Once the catheter is advanced to a point near the right atrium (RA), the balloon is inflated with the appropriate amount of air according to the directions. There should be a slight resistance on inflation; if there is none, it may mean that the balloon has ruptured, or if there is excessive resistance, the balloon may be in a peripheral vein.

8. As the catheter is being advanced, a continuous pressure tracing from the distal port is monitored. A right atrial tracing is identified, and the catheter is advanced until a right ventricular

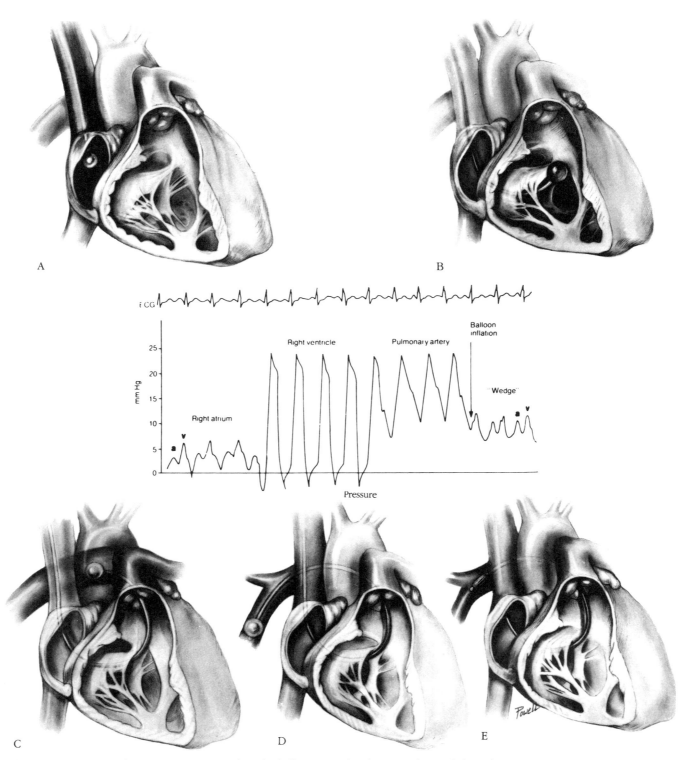

Figure 5.3-4. Waveform tracings generated as the balloon-tipped catheter is advanced through the right heart chambers into the pulmonary artery. **(A)** With the catheter tip in the RA, the balloon is inflated. **(B)** The catheter is advanced into the RV with the balloon inflated, and RV pressure tracings are obtained. **(C)** The catheter is advanced through the pulmonary valve into the PA. A rise in diastolic pressure will be noted. **(D)** The catheter is advanced to the PAWP position. A typical PAWP tracing will be noted with A and V waves. **(E)** The balloon is deflated. Phasic PA pressure should reappear on the monitor. Note that the balloon is inflated to facilitate passage through the heart and minimize damage. (See text for details.) RA, right atrium; RV, right ventricle; PA, pulmonary artery; PAWP, pulmonary artery wedge pressure. (From JM Rippe et al. *Procedures and Techniques in Intensive Care Medicine,* Boston: Little, Brown, 1995. p. 56. With permission.)

(RV) tracing is noted. There is a significant risk for dysrhythmia once the catheter is in the RV. Appropriate antidysrhythmic medication should be nearby, and if there is significant decompensation from ectopy, the catheter should be withdrawn immediately.

9. Not uncommonly, there is difficulty in floating the balloon into the PA from the RV. If the balloon has been advanced 10 to 15 cm in the RV with no PA trace, it most likely is coiling in the RV; the balloon should be deflated and the catheter pulled back into the RA and then tried again. Occasionally, the procedure will need the aid of fluoroscopy in floating the catheter into the PA.

10. The PA pressure tracing usually has the same systolic pressure as the RV, but the higher diastolic tracing indicates the catheter position in the PA. The catheter is further advanced into the wedge position (tracing of lower systolic values) (Fig. 5.3-4).

11. The balloon is deflated, and the PA tracing should return. If the wedge tracing continues, the catheter should be pulled back until PA tracing returns. The pressure tracing should be monitored continuously to ensure that the catheter does not become wedged again (blocking distal flow) or that it doesn't slip back into the RV.

12. The introducer sheath, the protector sleeve, and the catheter are firmly secured in their proper positions and then covered with a sterile dressing. A chest x-ray should be obtained for placement and to observe for complications.

What to Avoid

1. Placing a catheter in any uncooperative, moving patient
2. Lack of patient monitoring
3. Having significant ectopy without appropriate therapy nearby
4. Knotting the catheter. This usually occurs when loops form in the intracardiac chambers, especially when the catheter is repeatedly withdrawn and advanced.[3–5] This can be avoided by not advancing the catheter significantly beyond anticipated entry points for the RV and PA. Knotted catheters usually can be removed with guidewire placement, venotomy, or occasionally, surgery.[6]
5. Balloon rupture. This happens secondary to overinflating the balloon, inflating it too rapidly, or overuse. It may lead to air embolus to the arterial side if right-to-left communication is present, or the balloon remnants may cause distal obstruction of the pulmonary arteries. It is avoided by not overdistending the balloon, inflating it slowly, and not overusing.
6. Pulmonary infarction. There are several mechanisms for the development of pulmonary infarction. The most common is peripheral migration of the catheter tip and wedging in a small arteriole.[7] This is usually asymptomatic. Other causes include leaving the balloon dilated in a more central artery, injecting hypertonic solutions at high pressure, or the development of thrombus in the pulmonary artery. These may lead to large pulmonary infarcts at significant risk to the patient. These complications are rare if the PA waveform is monitored continuously and heparin flush solution is used continuously.[8,9] Also, the wedge pressure measurement should be done only for a maximum of 8 to 15 seconds.[10]
7. Intracardiac damage. Most intracardiac damage occurs during withdrawal of the catheter when the balloon is inflated. This especially injures the cardiac valves and supporting chordae.[1] RV endocardial damage may occur during insertion or manipulation of the catheter.[11–14]
8. Obtaining inaccurate data. All pressures should be measured at the end of expiration to minimize the effects of intrathoracic

pressure swings, including if the patient is breathing spontaneously or receiving positive pressure breaths.[10] Pulmonary artery wedge pressures (PAWP) generally reflect left atrial (LA) pressure as long as there is no distal obstruction (anatomic or functional) from the tip of the PA catheter, through the pulmonary vasculature, to the LA. It is important that the catheter tip is in zone 3 of the lung, below the LA, where capillaries remain open because both pulmonary artery and venous pressures exceed alveolar pressures. This may be ascertained by taking a lateral chest x-ray. Tuman et al[15] have suggested other techniques for confirming zone 3 catheter tip placement:

a. A and V wave forms should be present on a phasic pulmonary capillary wedge pressure (PCWP) tracing when the balloon is inflated; they should disappear when the balloon is deflated.
b. It should be possible to aspirate blood easily through the catheter's distal port; this ensures adequate blood flow.
c. Mean PCWPs should be no greater than the end-diastolic pulmonary artery pressure and less than the mean pulmonary artery pressure.

What is important to remember is that as long as the catheter tip remains below the left atrium, zone 3 conditions will exist, despite even high levels of PEEP. Thus, wedge pressures can still provide reasonably accurate estimates of mean LA atrial pressure; concomitant intrapleural or intraesophageal pressure measurements are unnecessary.[15]

Clinical Application of the Pulmonary Artery Catheter

The primary use of PA catheters is to measure cardiac output and cardiovascular parameters, then to use these measurements to calculate the patient's hemodynamic values. Table 5.3-3 lists the normal ranges for measurements obtained from a PA catheter. Table 5.3-4 lists the normal values for the commonly calculated hemodynamic measurements.

With these measurements, the patient's diagnosis may be more easily ascertained, and selective therapy may be utilized to improve the patient's condition. Table 5.3-5 depicts hemodynamic parameters found in common clinical situations. PA catheters help in providing selective therapy to maximize cardiac output oxygenation with minimal detriment to pulmonary and cardiac function. Specific details of this are provided elsewhere in this book.

Table 5.3-3. Normal ranges of pulmonary artery catheter measurements

Measurement	Range
Central venous pressure	4–8 mm Hg (mean)
Right atrial pressure	4–8 mm Hg (mean)
Right ventricular pressure (systolic)	12–30 mm Hg
Right ventricular pressure (diastolic)	0–8 mm Hg
Pulmonary artery pressure (systolic)	12–30 mm Hg
Pulmonary artery pressure (diastolic)	5–15 mm Hg
Pulmonary artery wedge pressure	6–12 mm Hg (mean)
Cardiac output	age-dependent
PO_2 mixed venous blood	35–45 mm Hg

Table 5.3-4. Calculations and normal ranges for hemodynamic measurements

Values	Calculation	Normal range
Cardiac index (CI)	$\dfrac{\text{CO (l/min)}}{\text{Body surface area (M}^2)}$	2.5–4.0 l/min/M^2
Stroke volume index (SI)	$\dfrac{\text{CO (ml/min)}}{\text{Heart rate (beats/min)} \times \text{BSA (M}^2)}$	30–65 ml/beat/m^2
Systemic vascular resistance index	$\dfrac{\text{MSAP-CVP (mm Hg)} \times 79.8^*}{\text{CI (l/min)}}$	800–1500 dynes $\times$ sec $\times$ cm^{-5}
Pulmonary vascular resistance index	$\dfrac{\text{MPAP-PAWP (mm Hg)} \times 79.8^*}{\text{CI}}$	150–240 dynes $\times$ sec $\times$ cm^{-5}
Left ventricular stroke work index	SI $\times$ (MSAP-PAWP) $\times$ 0.0136	43–61 g-meters/M^2
Right ventricular stroke work index	SI $\times$ (MPAP-CVP) $\times$ 0.00136	7–12 g-meters/M^2
% shunt	$\dfrac{\text{CcO}_2 - \text{CaO}_2}{\text{CcO}_2 - \text{CvO}_2}$	<5%
Oxygen uptake	CO (CaO$_2$ − CvO$_2$)	Age-dependent 3–6 ml O$_2$/kg/min

MSAP, mean systemic arterial pressure; CVP, central venous pressure; MPAP, mean pulmonary arterial pressure; PAWP, pulmonary artery wedge pressure; BSA, body surface area; CO, cardiac output; CaO$_2$, CvO$_2$, CcO$_2$, oxygen content of arterial blood, mixed venous blood, and end capillary blood, respectively.
*79.8 = conversion factor to obtain resistance units in dynes $\times$ sec $\times$ cm^{-5}.

Table 5.3-5. Hemodynamic parameters in common clinical situations

	RA	RV	PA	PAWP	SAP	CI	SVRI	PVRI
Normal	4–8 mean	12–30 sys / 0–8 dias	12–30 sys / 5–15 dias	6–12 mean	80–120 / 40–90	2.5–4.0	800–1500	150–240
Hypovolemic shock	↓	↓	↓	↓	↓	↓	↑	± ↓
Cardiogenic shock	± ↑	↑	↑	↑	↓	↓	↑	± ↓
Septic shock								
Early	± ↓	± ↓	± ↓	± ↓	± ↓	↑	↓	↓
Late	± N	± N	± N	± N	± N	↓	±	↑
Pulmonary embolism	↑	↑	↑	± N	± ↓	↓	↑	↑
Cardiac tamponade	↑	↑ dias	± N	↑	↓	↓	↑	± ↓
Cor pulmonale	↑	↑	↑	± N	± N	± ↓	± ↑	↑
Primary pulmonary hypertension	± N	↑	↑	± N	± N	↓	↑	↑

Measurements are listed in Tables 5.3-3 and 5.3-4.
RA, right atrium; RV, right ventricle; PA, pulmonary artery; PAWP, pulmonary artery wedge pressure; SAP, systemic arterial pressure; CI, cardiac index; SVRI, systemic vascular resistance index; PVRI, pulmonary vascular resistance.

Complications

The major complications of PA catheters include the common complications associated with any central venous catheter and are discussed in the central venous cannulation section of this chapter. Other complications specific to PA catheters include arrhythmias, knotting the catheter, balloon rupture, pulmonary infarction, and intracardiac damage, which has been discussed previously.

One of the most serious complications associated with PA catheters is PA rupture. Rupture of the PA may lead to massive hemorrhage, may be fatal, and may occur on insertion of the catheter or several days later.[16–24] There are several mechanisms by which rupture may occur and they include peripheral catheter migration, eccentric balloon distention, a damaged catheter tip contacting the vessel wall repeatedly, or chronic wedging of the catheter.

PA perforation usually presents with hemoptysis, which is an ominous sign. Management of PA rupture may include bronchoscopy, wedge arteriogram, intubation of the unaffected lung, and possible emergent lobectomy. Catheter balloon tamponade may also be tried to stop bleeding. Infectious complications of PA catheters are of lower incidence than central lines generally, because PA catheters are only used for 3 to 4 days, and the same guidelines for therapy are used in both PA catheters and central lines.

References

1. Swan HJC et al. Catheterization of the heart in man with use of a flow-directed balloon-tipped catheter. *N Engl J Med* 283:447, 1970.

2. Swan HJC, Ganz W. The balloon-tipped flow-directed pulmonary catheter. *Perspect Crit Care* 3:1–18, 1990.
3. Swaroop S. Knotting of two central venous monitoring catheters. *Am J Med* 53:386, 1972.
4. Meister SG et al. Knotting of a flow-directed catheter about a cardiac structure. *Cathet Cardiovasc Diagn* 3:171, 1977.
5. Lipp H, O'Donoghue K, Resnekov L. Intracardiac knotting of a flow directed balloon catheter. *N Engl J Med* 284:220, 1971.
6. Mond HG et al. A technique for unknotting an intracardiac flow-directed balloon catheter. *Chest* 67:731, 1975.
7. Foote GA, Schabel SI, Hodges M. Pulmonary complications of the flow-directed balloon-tipped catheter. *N Engl J Med* 290:927, 1974.
8. Boyd KD et al. A prospective study of complications of pulmonary artery catheterizations in 500 consecutive patients. *Chest* 84:245, 1983.
9. Sise MJ et al. Complications of the flow directed pulmonary artery catheter: A prospective analysis of 219 patients. *Crit Care Med* 9:315, 1981.
10. Devendra KA, Prediman KS, Swan HFC. The Swan-Ganz catheter: Techniques for avoiding common errors. *J Crit Ill* 8:1263, 1993.
11. O'Toole JD et al. Pulmonary valve injury and insufficiency during pulmonary artery catheterization. *N Engl J Med* 301:1167, 1979.
12. Becker RC, Martin RG, Underwood DA. Right sided endocardial lesions and flow directed pulmonary artery catheters. *Cleve Clin J Med* 54:384, 1987.
13. Ford SE, Manley PN. Indwelling cardiac catheters: An autopsy study of associated endocardial lesions. *Arch Pathol Lab Med* 106:314, 1982.
14. Smith WR, Glauser FL, Jenison P. Ruptured chordae of the tricuspid valve: The consequence of flow-directed SwanGanz catheterization. *Chest* 70:790, 1976.
15. Tuman KJ, Carroll GC, Ivankovich AD. Pitfalls in interpretation of pulmonary catheter data. *J Cardiothorac Anesth* 3:625, 1989.
16. Barash PG et al. Catheter-induced pulmonary artery perforation: Mechanisms, management and modifications. *J Thorac Cardiovasc Surg* 82:5, 1981.
17. Pape LA et al. Fatal pulmonary hemorrhage after use of the flow-directed balloon-tipped catheter. *Ann Intern Med* 90:344, 1979.
18. Lapin ES, Murray JA. Hemoptysis with flow-directed cardiac catheterization. *JAMA* 220:1246, 1972.
19. Haapaniemi J et al. Massive hemoptysis secondary to flow-directed thermodilution catheters. *Cathet Cardiovasc Diagn* 5:151, 1979.
20. Golden MS et al. Fatal pulmonary hemorrhage complicating use of a flow-directed balloon-tipped catheter in a patient receiving anticoagulant therapy. *Am J Cardiol* 32:865, 1973.
21. Page DW, Teres D, Hartshorn JW. Fatal hemorrhage from Swan-Ganz catheter. *N Engl J Med* 291:260, 1974.
22. Chun GMH, Ellestad MH. Perforation of the pulmonary artery by a Swan-Ganz catheter. *N Engl J Med* 284:1041, 1971.
23. Fleischer AG et al. Management of massive hemoptysis secondary to catheter-induced perforation of the pulmonary artery during cardiopulmonary bypass. *Chest* 95:1340, 1989.
24. Carlson TA et al. Catheter induced pulmonary artery hemorrhage: Diagnosis and management in cardiac operations. *J Thorac Cardiovasc Surg* 82:1, 1981.

Brahm Goldstein **5.4** ## Intraosseous Infusion

The establishment of intravenous access in critically ill infants and children can be an extremely difficult and time-consuming process. A review of pre-hospital care of pediatric emergencies showed an IV success rate of only 29% in infants 2 to 12 months old, and 66% in children 1 to 6 years old.[1] As many as 24% of pediatric cardiopulmonary arrest victims studied in a pediatric emergency department required more than 10 minutes to obtain IV access, and in 6% IV access was never achieved.[2] These studies and similar clinical experience in the emergent treatment of critically ill children have resulted in the reintroduction of intraosseous (IO) infusion, a technique for intravenous access that was widely used in the 1940s.[3–18] The IO route has been used successfully to provide rapid and safe administration of fluids and drugs in children suffering from cardiopulmonary arrest, shock, multiple trauma, seizures, near drowning, and burns.[5–23] The American Heart Association (AHA) and The American Academy of Pediatrics (AAP) currently recommend IO infusion as a temporary measure in the resuscitation of critically ill infants and children when other vascular sites are not immediately available.[20]

Physiology

Fluids and drugs infused via the IO route into the medullary cavity of long bones are rapidly absorbed into the central venous circulation through the rich vascular network within the bone. The distribution of fluids and drugs administered by the IO route is similar to that after IV injection and may more closely resemble central rather than peripheral kinetics and distribution.[8,22]

Method

The technique of IO infusion is rapid and simple. While there are several specially designed IO needles commercially available, any short needle with a stylet, such as an 18- or 20-gauge 1.5-inch spinal needle or a bone marrow needle, will work well.

The most commonly used sites for IO infusion are the proximal tibia, distal tibia, and distal femur. Due to differences in cortical thickness, the proximal tibia along the flat anteromedial surface of the shaft, 1 to 2 cm below the tibial tuberosity, is the preferred site in infants and young children. The distal tibia at the junction of the medial malleolus and the shaft of the tibia is the preferred site in older children. The distal one third of the femur along the midline and approximately 3 cm above the sternal condyle can also be used (Fig. 5.4-1).

Procedure

The equipment and technique are as follows:

Equipment

1. Disposable IO infusion needle (16, 18, or 20 gauge), 18- or 20-gauge spinal needle with stylet, or bone marrow needle
2. 1% lidocaine
3. 5-ml syringe
4. Heparinized saline flush
5. IV tubing and solution

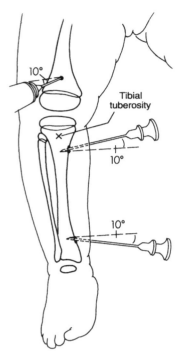

Figure 5.4-1. Insertion sites for IO infusion in the proximal tibia, 1 to 2 cm anteromedial from the tibial tuberosity, the distal tibia at the junction of the medial malleoulus and the shaft of the tibia, and the distal one third of the femur, 3 cm above the external condyle.

Technique

What to Do

1. Using aseptic technique, prepare the site with an iodine solution.

2. Inject the skin with 1% lidocaine for anesthesia in the awake patient.

3. Insert the needle (IO or spinal with stylet in place) at a 10- to 15-degree angle to the vertical away from the joint space (caudad for the proximal tibia, cephalad for the distal tibia and femur). Apply pressure and a to-and-fro rotary motion. As the needle passes into the marrow, a "give" will be felt. The needle should stand without support.

4. Remove the stylet. Proper placement is confirmed by aspiration of bone marrow into a 5-ml syringe or a free flowing of a heparinized saline flush.

5. Connect the needle to the desired IV tubing and solution.

6. Observe for extravasation of fluids into the surrounding soft tissue. This indicates superficial needle placement or that the bone has been pierced posteriorly.

What to Avoid

1. Malpositioning of the needle puncture site
2. Under- or overpenetration of the needle
3. Failure to monitor extremity for fluid extravasation
4. Failure to use the appropriate equipment (needle without trocar)
5. Failure to provide adequate analgesia or sedation in an awake child

Clinical Applications

IO infusion of fluid and medications is a temporary measure used during emergencies when other vascular sites are not readily available. The AHA and AAP recommend administration of medi-

Figure 5.4-2. Severely hypovolemic patient with 80% total body surface area burns. Arrows point to sites of IO needles. Note IO needles are placed bilaterally, and fluids are given under pressure by hand.

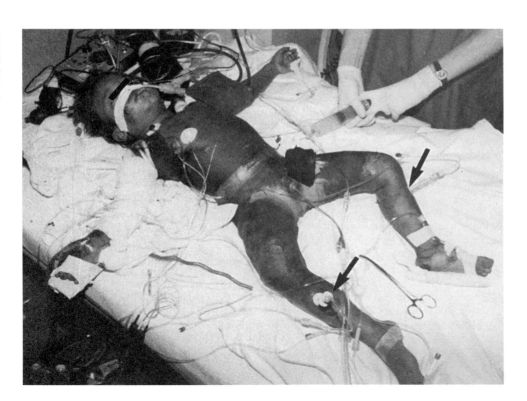

cations via the endotracheal tube initially and then immediate placement of an IO cannula in critically ill children under 3 years of age.[20] Our experience at the Massachusetts General Hospital has been similar to that reported by Kanter et al.[13] We recommend IO infusion in any critically ill patient in which adequate IV access is not obtained within 3 to 5 minutes. While IO infusion is most commonly used in the emergency department, successful employment of this technique has been reported by pre-hospital personnel in the field and is occasionally required in the ICU or operating room.[23–27]

IO infusion may be used to administer a wide variety of fluids and drugs, including saline, glucose, blood and blood products, sodium bicarbonate, atropine, anticonvulsants, antibiotics, succinylcholine, and catecholamines.[3–22,28–34]

Flow rates obtained during IO infusion have been reported from 24 ml/min using a 20-gauge needle to over 50 ml/min using a 13-gauge needle.[33,35,36] In our experience, successful volume resuscitation in severely hypovolemic patients usually requires bilateral IO infusions and pressure infusion of fluids by pump or by hand (Fig. 5.4-2).

Complications and Contraindications

Potential complications include osteomyelitis, subcutaneous abscess, extravasation of fluid into subcutaneous tissue, epiphyseal trauma, and fat embolism.[6–10,34,37] The overall incidence of osteomyelitis is less than 1%, with most cases occurring in patients previously bacteremic with local skin infections, or where the needle was not removed for a prolonged period.[10] At the Massachusetts General Hospital, we have observed no cases of osteomyelitis in patients in which the IO needle was removed within 6 hours of insertion.

IO infusion should be used only in life-threatening situations. Fractured bones, bones with holes in the cortex from unsuccessful attempts at IO infusion, areas of cellulitis, osteogenesis imperfecta, and osteopetrosis may be considered contraindications to IO infusion.

Summary

IO infusion is a rapid, safe, and effective means of providing rapid emergency IV access in critically ill infants and children and should be used as a temporary measure when other vascular sites are not immediately available.

References

1. Tsai A, Kollsen G. Epidemiology of pediatric prehospital care. *Ann Emerg Med* 16:284, 1987.
2. Rossetti V et al. Difficulty and delay in intravascular access in pediatric arrests. *Ann Emerg Med* 13:406, 1984.
3. Tocantins IM, O'Neil JF. Infusion of blood and other fluids into circulation via the bone marrow. *Proc Soc Exp Biol Med* 45:782, 1940.
4. Tocantins IM, O'Neil JF, Jones HW. Infusions of blood and other fluids into the general circulation via the bone marrow. *JAMA* 117:1229, 1941.
5. Tocantins IM, O'Neill JO, Price AH. Infusions of blood and other fluids via the bone marrow in traumatic shock and other forms of peripheral circulatory failure. *Ann Surg* 114:1085, 1941.
6. Heinild S, Sondergaard J, Tudvad F. Bone marrow infusions in childhood: Experiences from a thousand infusions. *J Pediatr* 30:400, 1947.
7. Macht DI. Studies on the intraosseous injections of epinephrine. *Am J Physiol* 38:269, 1943.
8. Spivey WH. Intraosseous infusions. *J Pediatr* 111:639, 1987.
9. Hodge D. Intraosseous infusions: A review. *Pediatr Emerg Care* 1:215, 1985.
10. Rossetti V, Thompson BM, Miller J. Intraosseous infusion: An alternative route of pediatric intravascular access. *Ann Emerg Med* 14:103, 1985.
11. Vlades MM. Intraosseous fluid administration in emergencies. *Lancet* 1:1235, 1977.
12. Mayer TA. Emergency pediatric vascular access. Old solutions to an old problem. *Am J Emerg Med* 4:98, 1986.
13. Kanter RK et al. Pediatric emergency intravenous access. *Am J Dis Child* 140:132, 1986.
14. McNamara RM, Spivey WH, Sussman C. Pediatric resuscitation without an intravenous line. *Am J Emerg Med* 4:31, 1986.
15. Parrish GA, Turkewitz D, Skiendzielewski JJ. Intraosseous infusions in the emergency department. *Am J Emerg Med* 4:59, 1986.
16. Iserson KV, Criss E. Intraosseous infusions: A usable technique. *Am J Emerg Med* 4:540, 1986.
17. Glaeser PW, Losek JD. Emergency intraosseous infusions in children. *Am J Emerg Med* 4:34, 1986.
18. McNamara RM et al. Emergency applications of intraosseous infusions. *Am J Emerg Med* 5:97, 1987.
19. Morris RE, Schonfeld N, Hafter AJ. Treatment of hemorrhagic shock with intraosseous administration of crystalloid fluid in the rabbit model. *Ann Emerg Med* 16:1321, 1987.
20. Chameides L, Hazinski MF (eds). *Textbook of Pediatric Advanced Life Support.* Dallas: American Heart Association, 1994.
21. Goldstein B, Doody D, Briggs S. Emergency intraosseous infusion in severely burned children. *Pediatr Emerg Care* 6:195, 1990.
22. Spivey WH et al. Comparison of intraosseous, central and peripheral routes of sodium bicarbonate administration during CPR in pigs. *Ann Emerg Med* 14:1135, 1985.
23. Smith RJ et al. Intraosseous infusions by prehospital personnel in critically ill pediatric patients. *Ann Emerg Med* 17:491, 1988.
24. Stroup CA. Intraosseous infusion. Prehospital use in the critically ill pediatric patient. *J Emerg Med Surg* 12:38, 1987.
25. Altieri M, Ahrens J, Friery J. The pediatric lifeline. Intraosseous infusion in the field. *J Emerg Med Surg* 12:36, 1987.
26. Zimmerman JA, Coyne M, Logsdon M. Implementation of intraosseous infusion technique by aeromedical transport programs. *J Trauma* 29:687, 1989.
27. Seigler RS, Tecklenberg FW, Shealy R. Prehospital intraosseous infusion by emergency medical services personnel: A prospective study. *Pediatrics* 84:173, 1989.
28. Walsh-Kelly CM et al. Intraosseous infusion of phenytoin. *Am J Emerg Med* 4:523, 1986.
29. Prete MR, Hannan CJ, Burkle FM. Plasma atropine concentrations via the intravenous, endotracheal and intraosseous routes of administration. *Ann Emerg Med* 15:195, 1986.
30. Spivey WH et al. Intraosseous diazepam suppression of pentylenetetrazol-induced epileptogenic activity in pigs. *Ann Emerg Med* 16:156, 1987.
31. Berg RA. Emergency infusion of catecholamines into bone marrow. *Am J Dis Child* 138:810, 1984.
32. Neish SR et al. Intraosseous infusion of hypertonic glucose and dopamine. *Am J Dis Child* 142:878, 1988.
33. Schoffstal JM et al. Intraosseous crystalloid and blood infusion in a swine model. *J Trauma* 29:384, 1989.
34. Spivey WH et al. The effect of intraosseous sodium bicarbonate on bone in swine. *Ann Emerg Med* 16:773, 1987.
35. Shoor PM, Berryhill RE, Benumof JL. Intraosseous infusion: Pressure-flow relationship and pharmacokinetics. *J Trauma* 19:772, 1979.
36. Hodge D, Delgado-Paredes C, Fleisher G. Intraosseous infusion flow rates in hypovolemic "pediatric" dogs. *Ann Emerg Med* 16:305, 1987.
37. Orlowski JP et al. Safety of intraosseous infusions: Risks of fat and bone marrow emboli to the lungs. *Crit Care Med* 16:388, 1988.

I. David Todres

John H. Fugate

6 Pulmonary Procedures

6.1 Thoracentesis

Indications

Thoracentesis is performed to evacuate air or fluid from the patient's pleural space. It is both a diagnostic and a therapeutic procedure. Clinically applicable information was found in greater than 90% of patients requiring thoracentesis in one study.[1] Generally, if the child's condition should require repeated thoracentesis, a chest tube to underwater seal and suction is preferred. Fluid may be in the form of a transudate or exudate (serous, serosanguinous, blood, or pus). When thoracentesis is used for diagnostic purposes, fluid is sent to the laboratory for evaluation of cell count and morphology, protein and glucose, LDH and pH, cultures for organisms (bacterial, fungal, viral), and pathologic smears for possible malignant cells. Thoracentesis is used for therapeutic purposes when large collections of pleural fluid compromise ventilatory function. The procedure is performed only when evidence exists for the presence of fluid in the pleural cavity as determined by clinical and radiologic examination.

Contraindications

1. Uncooperative child
2. Uncorrected coagulopathy
3. Risks outweigh benefits. One of the authors recalls a child who was recovering from pneumonia associated with a relatively small pleural effusion. A thoracentesis was performed. The spleen was lacerated in the procedure, and the patient underwent a splenectomy.
4. Persistent inability to draw fluid would suggest a loculated effusion, and the operator should consider desisting from further attempts until the procedure can be performed under radiographic guidance (i.e., CT scan, ultrasound).

Equipment

The equipment necessary to perform this procedure is listed in Table 6.1-1.

Table 6.1-1. Thoracentesis equipment

Preparation
    Sterile gloves, drugs, needles, syringes
    Xylocaine 1%–2%
    Prep solution, e.g., betadine
Equipment
    Appropriately sized intravenous catheter, 16–20 gauge
    Three-way stopcock and tubing
    Sterile collection tubes for cultures, cell count, and pathology

Technique

What to Do

The first step in thoracentesis is to ensure that fluid is present in the area of thoracentesis. Decubitus films are helpful in demonstrating free fluid that shifts with movement. If there is any question that the fluid is loculated or scant, ultrasound localization is required prior to thoracentesis.[2] Total opacification of a hemithorax frequently causes a diagnostic problem, and CT scan of the chest is considered the most informative procedure to differentiate fluid, atelectasis, tumor, and so on.[3,4] The procedure is then carried out with the patient appropriately sedated and properly positioned. Standard positioning for the alert and mobile patient is shown with the patient positioned upright and leaning forward (Fig. 6.1-1). For patients intubated and ventilated, they should be positioned in the lateral decubitus position with the pleural effusion dependent.[5] The back should be positioned near the edge of the bed;

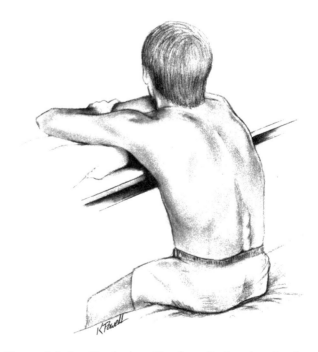

Figure 6.1-1. Standard position for patient undergoing thoracentesis. The patient is comfortably positioned, sitting up and leaning forward over a pillow-draped, height-adjusted bedside table. The arms are crossed in front of the patient to elevate and spread the scapulae. (From JM Rippe et al. *Procedures and Techniques in Intensive Care Medicine,* Boston: Little, Brown, 1995. p. 159. With permission.)

the procedure may be safely performed in this position.[5,6] The procedure is carried out under aseptic precautions. The site of entry is anesthetized with local anesthetic. The landmark for evacuation of the fluid is the angle of the scapula that corresponds approximately to the eighth rib interspace. One should avoid entry below the angle of the scapula, as subdiaphragmatic viscera might be penetrated. An appropriate catheter over needle is used. The needle is introduced immediately above the superior edge of the rib to avoid puncturing the intercostal artery and vein. Once the pleural space is entered and fluid is aspirated, the catheter is advanced as the needle is withdrawn. The catheter is connected to a three-way stopcock and syringe (10–20 ml). It is important to control the aspiration of fluid such that air is not allowed to enter the pleural space from the outside.

While the operator performs the thoracentesis, a designated individual is responsible for monitoring the effects of sedation (possible respiratory depression) and cardiovascular stability. The patient's oxygen saturations are monitored continuously with pulse oximetry. Any signs of hypoxemia must be investigated and treated immediately.

What to Avoid

1. Puncture of lung, heart, or abdominal viscera (i.e., going too far or too low)
2. Hitting the intercostal artery by not aiming at the superior border of the rib
3. Performing the procedure on a patient with coagulopathy
4. Not monitoring a patient's vital signs (i.e., ECG and oxygen saturations) during the procedure
5. Uncooperative and moving patient

Interpretation

Pleural fluid is usually a transudate or exudate. Transudates have a pleural fluid protein to serum protein ratio of less than 0.5 and an LDH of less than 200. Transudates are usually seen with congestive heart failure, cirrhosis, nephrotic syndrome, peritoneal dialysis, central line displacement, or acute atelectasis.

Exudative fluid has greater than 0.5 pleural fluid protein to serum protein ratio and an LDH greater than 200. Exudates are seen in parapneumonic effusions (bacterial, viral, or fungal infections), pulmonary infarctions, malignancies, connective tissue disease, gastrointestinal disease, pancreatitis, chylothorax, and lymphatic abnormalities. The clinical history and examination, together with laboratory studies, will usually provide the correct diagnosis.

Complications

Thoracentesis is relatively safe, but one must always balance the benefits versus the risks.[1,7,8]

1. Respiratory depression or cardiac compromise from excessive sedation
2. Intercostal artery puncture with severe hemorrhage
3. Development of pneumo- or hemothorax
4. Malpositioning of the thoracentesis needle, leading to abdominal viscera or lung parenchymal puncture

References

1. Collins TR, Sahn SA. Thoracentesis: Clinical value, complications, technical problems, and a patient experience. *Chest* 91:817, 1987
2. Light RW. *Pleural Diseases*. Philadelphia: Lea & Febiger, 1983.
3. Light RE et al. Pleural effusions: The diagnostic separation of transudates and exudates. *Ann Intern Med* 77:507–513, 1972.
4. Yu C et al. Ultrasound in unilateral hemothorax opacification. Image comparison with computed tomography. *Am Rev Respir Dis* 147:430–434, 1993.
5. McCartney JP, Adams JW, Hazard PB. Safety of thoracentesis in mechanically ventilated patients. *Chest* 103:1920–1921, 1993.
6. Godwin JE, Sahn SA. Thoracentesis: A safe procedure in mechanically ventilated patients. *Ann Intern Med* 113:800–801, 1990.
7. Seneff MG et al. Complications associated with thoracentesis. *Chest* 89:97, 1986.
8. Qureshi N, Momin ZA, Brandstetter RD. Thoracentesis in clinical practice. *Heart Lung* 23:376–383, 1994.

 6.2   **Thoracentesis: Chest Tube Placement**

Indications

Indications for chest tube placement are evacuation of air or fluid over an extended period because of the mechanical effects that are produced on the affected side, which may lead to collapse of the lung. The situations in which this occurs are mainly pneumothorax, hemothorax, pleural effusion, empyema, and chylothorax.[1–5] Diagnosis of these conditions is determined by the clinical history, physical examination, and radiographic confirmation.

In children, the most common indication for placement of a chest tube is a pneumothorax, especially in patients on positive pressure ventilation. In some cases, children who develop a spontaneous pneumothorax (e.g., severe asthma) require chest tube placement to relieve life-threatening cardiopulmonary decompensation.

Parapneumonic effusions and empyemas may require chest tube

placement for drainage to improve lung mechanics and to promote resolution of the inflammatory processes. Children suffering trauma may develop both pneumothoraces and hemothoraces. This situation may be aggravated by mechanical ventilation. Chylothorax occasionally follows thoracic surgery. This requires chest tube placement for drainage until the situation resolves spontaneously. This may require an extended period (weeks) of drainage. If the chylothorax persists, scleral therapy via the chest tube may be successful in stopping the process.

Contraindications

1. Uncorrected coagulopathy
2. Abdominal contents in the chest following trauma (must be considered)

Equipment

The equipment required for chest tube placement is listed in Table 6.2-1.

Technique

What to Do

Under aseptic conditions, the chest tube is generally placed in either of two sites: (1) midaxillary line, fourth to fifth interspace; or (2) midclavicular line, second interspace to avoid puncturing abdominal structures and pectoral muscles (Fig. 6.1-1). There are generally three techniques that are used.

1. Surgical technique
   a. The patient is placed in a supine position and sedated to optimal comfort, with the involved side slightly elevated. Xylocaine infiltration is performed through tissue to the top of the rib (Fig. 6.2-1).
   b. Thoracentesis may be performed to ensure the presence of air or fluid at the site chosen for tube placement.
   c. The surgical technique involves an incision in the skin and subcutaneous tissues, followed by forceps dissection of the intercostal muscles and penetration into the pleura (Fig. 6.2-2). The chest tube is placed to the appropriate distance, ensuring all holes of the chest tube are within the pleural space. It is important to prove that air and/or fluid is being evacuated at the final positioning.
   d. The chest tube is secured firmly with sutures and taped and connected to an underwater seal system with suction.
2. The Seldinger technique uses the same principles as the surgical technique in regard to positioning, sedation, infiltration, and sterility. The approach involves introducing a needle, followed by a guidewire, into the pleural space at the appropriate site. Over the guidewire, dilators of increasing diameter are passed until the appropriately sized chest tube can be advanced. The advantages of this technique include avoidance of surgical incision and dissection, increased safety (smaller needle compared with the larger trocar), and better control of the puncture of the chest wall.
3. Trocar and cannula. This method uses the same initial principles but has the risk of being less controllable and could therefore inadvertently penetrate major organs. The trocar and catheter are advanced throught the chest wall and into the plural space. To increase safety with this technique, an artery forceps should be clipped to the trocar and cannula at a predetermined point to limit the distance of advancement.

Table 6.2-1. Chest tube insertion equipment

Preparation
    Prep solution, e.g., betadine
    Xylocaine 1%–2%
    Sterile needles, syringes, sponges, towels, and drapes
Insertion
    Chest tube kit
        Surgical kit: Kelly clamp, forceps, scapel, chest tube, sutures
        Seldinger kit: needle, guidewire, dilators, chest tube
        Trocar and chest tube
    Chest tube drainage system

What to Avoid

1. Malposition of tube, especially going subdiaphragmatic
2. Placement of needles or tube at inferior position of rib because of presence of intercostal vessels
3. Leaving side holes of chest tube outside pleural space

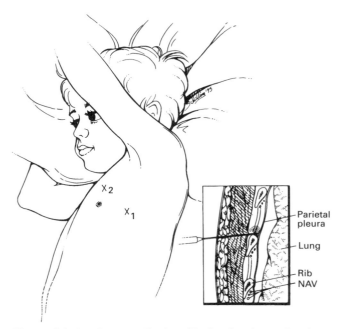

Figure 6.2-1. Proper patient positioning for chest tube placement. Note that the involved side is slightly elevated and the arm is flexed over the head. Preferred sites include (1) midaxillary line, 4th–5th intercostal space (opposite nipple), or (2) midclavicular line, 2nd intercostal space. Inset demonstrates lidocaine infiltration through the tissue to the top of the rib.

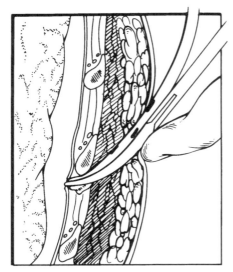

Figure 6.2-2. Surgical technique demonstrating forceps dissection through the muscle and pleura and placement of the chest tube into the pleural space.

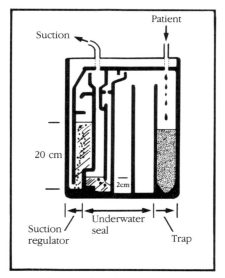
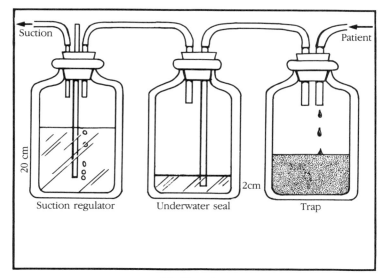

Contained single plastic unit   3 bottle system

Figure 6.2-3.   Chest tube drainage systems: contained, single plastic unit in contrast with three-bottle system. (From JM Rippe et al. *Procedures and Techniques in Intensive Care Medicine.* Boston: Little Brown, 1995. With permission.)

4. Puncturing lung with disection, needles, or tubes
5. Moving, uncooperative child

Chest Tube Management

Once the chest tube is connected to its drainage system, it must be checked constantly to see that it is functioning properly. The drainage system is a three-chambered system: (1) collection trap for fluid; (2) underwater seal, which allows air to escape and prevents air entering the chest via the tube, thus maintaining a negative pleural pressure; and (3) a suction regulator, which is controlled by the height of a water column set at approximately 10 to 20 cm H_2O (Fig. 6.2-3). The chest tubes are stripped intermittantly to ensure their patency. Chest x-rays are assessed to evaluate the resolution of the collection of fluid or air in the pleural space. It is important to ensure that the chest tube remains in position and that the drainage holes in the tube have not migrated outside the pleural cavity. Constant bubbling of air suggests an ongoing air leak. It is worth checking the system by briefly clamping the tube to verify whether the air leak is continuing or the bubbling is related to the suction system. Once the air leak has ceased for 24 to 48 hours, the chest tube is pulled, making sure that the chest wall opening is immediately sealed with petroleum gauze and dressings. Following chest tube removal, a chest x-ray is taken to check for any reaccumulation of air. Another x-ray is performed within 24 hours in case air or fluid has reaccumulated.

Complications

1. Respiratory depression or cardiac compromise from excessive sedation

2. Intercostal artery puncture with severe hemorrhage
3. Development of pneumo- or hemothorax[6,7]
4. Malpositioning of the thoracostomy that has led to abdominal viscera puncture (e.g., liver, spleen, or puncture of the lung parenchyma)[8,9]
5. Secondary infection within the pleura or chest tube insertion site[10]

References

1. Bernard RW, Stahl WM. Subclavian vein catheterization: A prospective study, I. Non-infectious complications. *Ann Surg* 173:184, 1971.
2. Hayes DF, Lucas CE. Bilateral tube thoracostomy to preclude tension pneumothorax in patients with acute respiratory insufficiency. *Am Surg* 42:330, 1976.
3. Staats RA et al. The lipoprotein profile of chylous and unchylous pleural effusions. *Mayo Clin Proc* 55:700, 1980.
4. Hausheer FH, Yarbro JW. Diagnosis and treatment of malignant pleural effusions. *Semin Oncol* 12:54, 1985.
5. Bergh NP et al. Intrapleural steptokinase in the treatment of hemothroax and empyema. *Scand J Thorac Cardiovasc Surg* 11:265, 1977.
6. Daly RC et al. The risk of percutaneous chest tube thoracostomy for blunt thoracic trauma. *Ann Emerg Med* 14:865, 1985.
7. Millikan JS et al. Complications of tube thoracostomy for acute trauma. *Am J Surg* 140:738, 1980.
8. Trapneel DH, Thurston JGB. Unilateral pulmonary edema after pleural aspiration. *Lancet* 1:1367, 1970.
9. Waqaruddin M, Bernstein A. Re-expansion pulmonary oedema. *Thorax* 30:54, 1975.
10. Neugebauer MK, Fosburg RG, Trummer MJ. Routine antibiotic therapy following pleural space intubation: A reappraisal. *J Thorac Cardiovasc Surg* 61:882, 1971.

7 Cardiac Procedures

Lars C. Erickson ◆ 7.1 ◆ **Drainage of Pericardial Effusions**

Any patient with signs of elevated venous pressures (jugular venous distension, hepatomegaly, pulmonary edema), tachycardia, and a prominent pulsus paradoxus must be suspected of having pericardial tamponade. Ideally, confirmation of the diagnosis can be obtained by echocardiography, although in some cases the patient may not tolerate any delay, and immediate intervention may be required.

When practical, pericardiocentesis should be performed in the cardiac catheterization laboratory with electrocardiographic and hemodynamic monitoring and fluoroscopic imaging. If echocardiography is not available in the catheterization laboratory, prior echocardiographic imaging is recommended to localize and size the effusion.

Prepackaged kits are available containing all of the specialized supplies required for pericardiocentesis, including a pericardiocentesis needle, syringe, stopcock, guidewire, and drainage catheter. Equipment specifically designed for pericardiocentesis has certain advantages over generally available supplies such as spinal needles (which are sharper than necessary and increase the risk of myocardial laceration) and catheters designed for intravascular manipulation (which may be less rigid and prone to kink).

The patient is positioned with the head of the table slightly elevated to promote anterior pooling of the effusion. The route of percutaneous entry is guided to some extent by the location of the effusion on echocardiography, although the standard subxiphoid approach is preferred because it avoids the pleural space and presents less risk of laceration of the coronary arteries. For the subxiphoid approach, the thorax is prepped and draped in sterile fashion and the skin is infiltrated with lidocaine. A small stab incision is made with a no. 11 blade just below and to the left of the tip of the xiphoid process. An 18-gauge pericardiocentesis needle is ideal for percutaneous drainage, although other large-bore needles with relatively short bevels have been used. A syringe containing 1% lidocaine without epinephrine is attached to the needle via a three-way stopcock so that local anesthesia may be administered as the needle is advanced. The three-way stopcock is attached to tubing, which may be used to monitor intrapericardial pressure. Although many centers advocate the use of an ECG lead clipped to the pericardiocentesis needle, this feature is not essential, and may pose a small additional risk of compromising the sterile field (unless sterile leads are available) or inducing ventricular arrhythmias (if the ECG machine is not grounded in an equipolar fashion).

The needle is introduced through the stab wound, at an angle of about 45 degrees to the skin, and directed toward the left nipple (Fig. 7.1-1). The needle is advanced slowly but steadily, aspirating and injecting lidocaine at regular intervals until pericardial fluid is aspirated. Once pericardial fluid is obtained, the intrapericardial pressure is recorded. In the setting of pericardial tamponade, the intrapericardial pressure should equal the central venous pressure (if central venous pressure monitoring is available). The stopcock

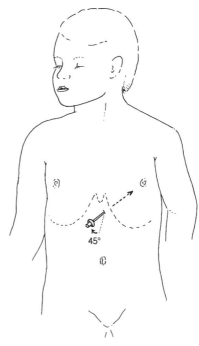

Figure 7.1-1. Note the angle of the needle to the sternum and its direction toward the left nipple of the patient.

is disconnected and a floppy J-tipped guidewire is introduced into the pericardial space. A pigtail or specially designed pericardial catheter is advanced over the guidewire into the pericardial space and the guidewire is removed. At this point, the pericardial effusion may be evacuated and samples sent for appropriate studies. All fluid should be aspirated, and the intrapericardial pressure following the procedure should be less than 3 mm Hg with negative deflections during spontaneous inspiration. The catheter may be withdrawn immediately after the procedure or left in place for up to 24 to 48 hours if there is concern of reaccumulation of fluid. Echocardiography should be performed following the procedure to document evacuation of the fluid, as loculated effusions may not be completely evacuated by pericardiocentesis.

If the cardiac monitor displays ST segment elevation or ventricular premature beats as the needle is initially advanced, it is likely that the tip of the needle has come into contact with the epicardium. In this case, the needle should be withdrawn promptly with continuous aspiration. If fluid is obtained, proceed as outlined previously. Otherwise, the needle is withdrawn completely, and the procedure may be repeated after flushing the needle of any tissue or thrombus that may be lodged in the lumen.

If blood is aspirated as the needle is advanced, contrast may be injected under fluoroscopic visualization: Contrast in the pericardial space will disperse very slowly or not at all. Also, a recording of the pressure will identify intraventricular placement if a ventricular waveform is noted, although this is not a reliable way of ruling out intracardiac placement.

Emergency pericardiocentesis is performed in a similar fashion, except that fluoroscopy and invasive monitoring may not be available. Even in an emergency it is preferable to use a pericardiocentesis needle and catheter, although an 18-gauge angiocatheter may be substituted if necessary. It is quite hazardous to attempt to drain a pericardial effusion with a needle alone because of the possibility of laceration of the myocardium or coronary arteries.

Fluid aspirated at the time of pericardiocentesis should be sent for the laboratory examinations listed in Table 7.1-1. Cultures should be innoculated as soon as possible, preferably by injecting fluid directly into broth and plating onto agar.

Table 7.1-1. Laboratory examination of pericardial fluid

Protein, amylase, glucose, cholesterol

Cell count with differential

Stain for bacteria and mycobacteria

Cytology

Bacterial culture (aerobic and anaerobic)

Fungal culture

Viral culture

Latex agglutination or counterimmuncelectrophoresis for bacterial pathogens

---

Lars C. Erickson
E. Marsha Elixson

 7.2   **Cardiac Pacing**

Cardiac Pacing

Transvenous Temporary Pacing Wires

Usually, transthoracic atrial and/or ventricular pacing wires are placed by the surgeon at the time of surgery. If not, a temporary transvenous pacing catheter may have to be placed, ideally under fluoroscopic guidance. Without the aid of fluoroscopy, it is difficult to place a transvenous pacing catheter in the right ventricle from the femoral vein, and a subclavian or internal jugular vein approach is often necessary.

Temporary transvenous pacing catheters are relatively stiff and, with time, carry a significant risk of erosion through the ventricular wall. Generally, temporary transvenous pacing catheters should be removed within 2 or 3 days.

Transthoracic Temporary Pacing Wires

In children for whom surgical intervention involves tissue near the conduction system (e.g., ventricular septal defect, tetralogy of Fallot, complete atrioventricular canal, truncus arteriosus communis), pacing may be required within the first 10 hours postoperatively as endocardial swelling occurs. Temporary epicardial pacing wires can be attached to the right atrium and right ventricle. By convention, pacing wires exiting the right side of the sternum are atrial wires; those exiting the left side are ventricular.

Permanent Pacing Wires

In children with known heart block or certain other conduction disorders, the cardiac surgeon may choose to place permanent pacing wires at the time of surgery. These wires may be attached to the outside surface of the heart (epicardial leads) or the inside surface via a large vein such as the subclavian vein (transvenous leads). The other end of the wires are routed to an intramuscular pocket within the chest wall or, in infants and small children, over the abdomen, where the pacemaker itself will be implanted.

Modes of Pacing

The Intersociety Commission for Heart Disease Resources (ICHD) and North American Society of Pacing and Electrophysiology (NASPE) have, over the years, developed a standard nomenclature for designation of pacemaker functions.[1] A series of five letters describes the modes of pacing for any permanent or temporary pacemaker (Table 7.2-1).

The first letter designates the chamber that is paced. Atrial, ventricular, and dual pacings (both atrial and ventricular) are abbreviated as A, V, and D, respectively.

The second letter designates the chamber that is sensed for the purpose of inhibiting or triggering pacing (see also next paragraph). Analogous to the first letter, atrial, ventricular, and dual chamber sensings are abbreviated as A, V, and D. Occasionally, it is necessary for a pacemaker to sense no chamber, in which case the second letter is O. It can be very hazardous to pace the ventricle without sensing, because this mode predisposes to dangerous ventricular arrhythmias.

The third letter represents the response to sensed depolarizations. Inhibition (I) takes place when a spontaneous cardiac depolarization sensed by the pacemaker inhibits the next pacemaker-generated beat. Triggering (T) takes place when the pacemaker generates a beat in response to a sensed depolarization. Pacemakers that are both inhibited and triggered by sensed beats are designated dual (D) response.

The fourth letter represents programmability and cardioversion response (see Table 7.2-1).

To manage paced patients in the postoperative setting, it is essential to have a solid understanding of the relationships between at least the first three letters. One common pacing mode, for example, is VVI, which corresponds to ventricular pacing, ventricular sensing, and inhibition of pacing with sensed ventricular beats. It is frequently used in the setting of complete heart block when atrioventricular sequential pacing is not considered important. There is no atrial sensing or pacing, nor will atrial beats trigger ventricular pacing.

Table 7.2-1. Pacemaker modes: The NASPE/BPEG Generic (NBG) Pacemaker Code

Position	I	II	III	IV	V
Category	Chamber(s) paced	Chamber(s) sensed	Response to sensing	Programmability, rate modulation	Antitachyarrhythmia function(s)
	O = None	**O** = None	**O** = None	**O** = None	**O** = None
	A = Atrium	**A** = Atrium	**T** = Triggered	**P** = Simple Programmable	**P** = Pacing (antitachyarrhythmia)
	V = Ventricle	**V** = Ventricle	**I** = Inhibited	**M** = Multiprogrammable	**S** = Shock
	D = Dual (A + V)	**D** = Dual (A + V)	**D** = Dual (T + I)	**C** = Communicating	**D** = Dual (P + S)
				R = Rate modulation	
Manufacturer's designation only	**S** = single (A or V)	**S** = single (A or V)			

Note: Positions I through III are used exclusively for antibradyarrhythmia function.
Source: From Bernstein AD et al. The NASPE/BPEG generic pacemaker code for antibradyarrhythmia and adaptive-rate pacing and antitachycardia devices. *PACE* 10:794–799, 1987. With permission.

Another common pacing mode is used in patients with symptomatic sinus bradycardia or sinus arrest. They require only an atrial wire. The pacemaker would be set to AAI, so that the atrium is sensed and paced, and spontaneous atrial beats would inhibit paced beats.

Because cardiac output can be adversely affected when the atria and ventricles do not beat synchronously, pacing wires may be attached to both the atrium and ventricle and used with a dual-chamber pacemaker. The pacing mode used in this setting is DDD: Both chambers are paced and sensed. The third letter designates dual response. The pacemaker will not pace either chamber if it detects a spontaneous depolarization. In addition, if the pacemaker senses an atrial depolarization, and a ventricular beat does not follow within a fixed period of time (the AV delay), the pacemaker will be triggered to pace the ventricle. Pacemakers in the DDD mode require setting the AV delay separately.

The Temporary Pacemaker

General Considerations

On admission to the pediatric intensive care unit, the staff will attach the temporary pacing wires to the external pacemaker generator. The ventricular or atrial wire is attached to the negative pole of the generator. A skin ground or second pacing wire is attached to the positive pole. When normal atrioventricular conduction exists, atrial wires alone may be used. Atrial wires can also be used to record an atrial electrocardiogram. Ventricular wires are necessary whenever there is concern over the integrity of the atrioventricular conduction system, as is often the case following certain types of surgical procedures, particularly repair of various types of ventricular septal defects. Ventricular wires may be used alone or with atrial wires when atrioventricular sequential pacing is indicated.

During testing of the temporary pacemaker, the external cardiac monitoring leads should be checked to be sure that they do not sense pacing spikes as a QRS complex. Usually, spike sensing can be minimized by changing leads or gain, but occasionally the placement of the monitoring leads must be changed.

It is not recommended that any pacemaker be programmed, tested, or used without the supervision of a person qualified and knowledgeable in their use. The following information is provided for reference only.

Checking the Sensitivity

It is critical that the pacemaker be able to detect spontaneous depolarization of the heart so that pacing does not occur at electrically vulnerable moments in the cardiac cycle when the potential for inducing dangerous arrhythmias is high. The sensitivity of a temporary pacemaker is the electrical voltage generated by the myocardium, which the pacemaker can detect. This voltage is measured in millivolts (mV), or may be represented in arbitrary units on some pacemaker generators.

Because of the differences in the electrical properties of the myocardium, and variations in the quality of contact between the wires and the myocardium, different degrees of sensitivity may be required in different patients to reproducibly sense depolarization of the heart. In addition, a pacemaker generator with the sensitivity set too high may misinterpret extraneous electrical signals as a cardiac contraction, leading to inappropriate suppression of pacing. Also, during the early postoperative period, when a lot of inflammation and healing is taking place at the site of the pacemaker wire insertion into the myocardium, the voltage required to sense depolarization of the heart may change considerably over a short period.

The lowest voltage at which the pacemaker will sense myocardial depolarization is called the "threshold" sensitivity. The lower this threshold voltage, the higher the sensitivity of the pacemaker. Consequently, the numbers on the pacemaker generator SENSITIVITY dial get smaller in the clockwise direction. To determine the threshold sensitivity of a pacemaker for a child with ventricular wires:

1. The patient must be constantly electrocardiographically monitored during any testing of the pacemaker.

2. If there is any underlying ventricular rhythm, the pacemaker cannot operate safely when it is not sensing consistently. Before checking the sensitivity, turn the ventricular OUTPUT current to 0 mA. If there is no underlying ventricular rhythm, the sensitivity may be checked while pacing.

3. Turn the SENSITIVITY all the way down.

4. Watching the ECG, slowly turn up the sensitivity (mA) until the SENSE light begins to flash with every ventricular beat. Some units have a deflection dial rather than a SENSE light. A deflection of the needle to the SENSE side indicates sensing. The sensitivity at which every ventricular beat is sensed is the threshold sensitivity.

It is generally safe to set the pacemaker at about 1.5 to 2 times the threshold sensitivity (half the threshold mV) to guarantee consistent sensing. Because the threshold may change over time, it is optimal to recheck the sensitivity threshold at least daily for the first few days following surgery, and every few days thereafter.

The procedure for setting the sensitivity for atrial and ventricular pacers is the same. In patients with both atrial and ventricular wires, the sensitivities must be set individually.

Setting the Output Current

The output of a temporary pacemaker is the electrical current that is applied to the myocardium via the pacemaker wires. This current is measured in milliamperes (mA). Because of the differences in the electrical properties of the myocardium, and variations in the quality of contact between the wires and the myocardium, different patients require different amounts of current to depolarize the heart. As mentioned earlier, during the early postoperative period when a lot of inflammation and healing is taking place at the site of the pacemaker wire insertion into the myocardium, the current required to depolarize the heart may change considerably over a short period.

The lowest current that will depolarize the myocardium is called the "threshold" current. To determine the threshold current required to capture the ventricle in a child with ventricular wires:

1. The patient must be constantly electrocardiographically monitored during any testing of the pacemaker.
2. Be sure the pacemaker is set to the SYNCHRONOUS mode (not ASYNCH). The SENSE light should flash for every spontaneous beat. If not, check the pacemaker sensitivity.
3. Turn the OUTPUT to 0 mA
4. Turn the RATE up to about 20 bpm greater than the underlying rhythm. The PACE light should begin to flash, signaling paced beats. None of the paced beats should cause contraction in the heart, however, because the current is still set to 0 mA.
5. Watching the ECG, turn up the OUTPUT (mA) until the cardiac rhythm is entrained. Pacing spikes may or may not be apparent on the ECG. The output current at which the ventricle is entrained is the threshold current.

It is generally safe to set the pacemaker at about twice the threshold to guarantee consistent pacing. Because the threshold may change over time, it is optimal to recheck the output threshold at least daily for the first few days following surgery, and every few days thereafter.

The procedure for setting the output for atrial and ventricular pacers is the same. In patients with both atrial and ventricular wires, the outputs must be set individually.

Setting the Rate

Most pacemakers have a dial on which the rate in beats per minute can be set. This represents the minimum rate below which the pacemaker will begin pacing while in the inhibited mode (see earlier discussion). If pacemaker inhibition is turned off (e.g., AOO mode), the pacemaker will pace at the set rate regardless of the underlying rhythm. This mode, sometimes called asynchronous, is a very dangerous pacing mode for the ventricle and should be used only while testing the function of the pacemaker and only with close monitoring.

Most postoperative patients are likely to have an indwelling arterial catheter that allows continuous monitoring of the arterial pressure. The optimal paced heart rate can often be determined by experimenting with the rate until the highest mean BP is achieved.

Pacemaker Emergencies

Because of the complexities of both cardiac rhythm generation and pacemaker function, there is a very wide variation in the types of problems that can occur in the paced heart. These problems may be related to an irregular cardiac rhythm or to a malfunctioning or poorly "tuned" electronic pacemaker.

When the cardiac rhythm of an electronically paced patient becomes slower or faster than the preset pacing rate, or there is concern that the pacemaker is not sensing properly, the best option is to determine the mechanism of the concerning rhythm from analysis of rhythm strips. If the mechanism is still not clear, there are several options:

1. Check the integrity of the circuit. Be sure the pacing wires have not pulled out of the heart or become broken. Check the connections of the pacing wires to the cable adapter and the connector of the adapter to the pacemaker generator itself. The adapter usually attaches to the wire with small tightening screws, which must be tight and in electrical contact with the metal ends of the pacing wires. The adapter has two pins that fit into the tightening rings on the pacemaker generator: The pins must be all the way in, and the tightening rings must be tight. Make sure the batteries in the pacemaker generator are fresh.
2. Turn the pacemaker off. If the arrhythmia is being caused by a pacemaker malfunction, it usually is safer to eliminate the pacemaker and consider replacing it with a different one.
3. Reset the pacemaker to VVI mode: Turn the atrial SENSITIVITY and OUTPUT to off. Many pacemaker malfunctions are related to atrial sensing errors.
4. If the rate is too high and both chambers are being sensed and paced (DDD mode), try lowering the SENSITIVITY of the atrial lead: If the atrial lead is sensing ventricular depolarization, it could be triggering a ventricular beat after each ventricular beat (pacemaker tachycardia). Retrograde conduction up the AV node to the atrium also can trigger inappropriate tachycardia, in which case, resetting the pacemaker to VVI mode may be required to terminate the rhythm.
5. If the rate is too low and the SENSE light is flashing when there is no beat on ECG, try decreasing the SENSITIVITY: The pacemaker may be oversensing.
6. If the rate is too low and the PACE light is flashing but there is no ventricular beat on the ECG, try increasing the OUTPUT: The output threshold may have increased.

Paced Diaphragm

Occasionally, the pacing wires can be sufficiently close to the phrenic nerve or the diaphragm itself so that the pacing pulse causes contraction of the diaphragm. Evidence of this is often a sudden increase in the precordial impulse or an abdominal twitch. A respiratory rate equal to the paced rate is also suggestive. Diaphragmatic pacing is unpleasant for the patient and can hamper attempts at ventilation. Occasionally, diaphragmatic pacing may create a false impression of adequate ventilation, leading to inappropriate withdrawal of respiratory support.

There are four approaches to diaphragmatic pacing, in descending order of desirability:

1. Discontinue electronic pacing if it is no longer strongly indicated.

2. Reduce the OUTPUT of the atrial or ventricular leads. Sometimes the heart can be paced at a lower output than would capture the diaphragm. Unfortunately, sometimes the reverse is true, and the diaphragm can be paced without capturing the heart.

3. If a unipolar system is being used with an ECG lead on the skin for the negative (ground) contact, try moving the ECG lead to another location on the body.

4. If a bipolar system is being used (two wires each in the ventricular or atrial muscle), reverse the polarity of the pacemaker leads. Because patients in the ICU are rarely electrically isolated, the tissue in the region of the positive pacing lead should be exposed to a larger current flow than the negative (ground) lead. If there are two wires embedded in the myocardium, decreasing the current in the vicinity of one or the other lead may reduce the chance of diaphragmatic pacing.

5. Abandon the current pacing wires and resume pacing using new wires placed surgically or via the transvenous or transesophageal routes.

Temporary Pacemaker Applications

In a few circumstances, the control afforded by a temporary pacemaker allows creative interventions for certain rhythm disturbances. A patient with reentrant supraventricular tachycardia may be converted by setting the temporary pacemaker to a rate slightly higher than that of the tachycardia and pacing in short bursts in the AAI mode. The ventricular OUTPUT should be turned to 0.

A patient with junctional ectopic tachycardia may have a more stable rhythm restored by overdriving the AV node at a rate sufficiently faster than the underlying rhythm so that the AV node blocks 2:1, resulting in a ventricular rate of half the atrially paced rate. For example, if a child with junctional ectopic tachycardia at a rate of 200 bpm is atrially paced at a rate of 300 bpm and has 2:1 block at the AV node, his ventricular rate will be 150 bpm. Of course, the ventricular output **must** be off in this situation, otherwise the ventricle will be paced at the same rate as the atrium. This is a measure to be used only in an urgent situation when other methods of controlling junctional ectopic tachycardia have failed and the patient is hemodynamically compromised. Any child in whom this approach is used must be monitored carefully: If the AV node begins to conduct 1:1, the ventricle may be susceptible to dangerous arrhythmias. Pacing may have to be discontinued immediately, or the rate increased until 2:1 block is again achieved. The administration of digoxin may supplement this technique by enhancing block at the AV node.

Finally, the atrial lead may be helpful in the diagnosis of arrhythmias that involve the atrium. A sharp atrial depolarization can be recorded by connecting the atrial wire to one of the V leads on the 12-lead ECG in place of the usual precordial contact. This technique can be very useful in differentiating reentrant supraventricular tachycardia, atrial flutter, atrial fibrillation, and ectopic atrial tachycardia.

Reference

1. Bernstein AD et al. The NASPE/BPEG generic pacemaker code for antibradyarrhythmia and adaptive-rate pacing and antitachycardia devices. *PACE* 10:794–799, 1987.

John H. Fugate
David Link

8.1 ◆ **Hemofiltration and Hemodiafiltration**

Hemofiltration

Continuous arteriovenous hemofiltration (CAVH) or continuous veno-venous hemofiltration (CVVH) and continuous hemodiafiltration (CAVHD or CVVHD) are particularly useful techniques for the control of acute fluid and electrolyte problems arising in the ICU setting.[1-6] These are not new technologies; rather, they are modifications in both theory and application of hemodialysis techniques. In hemofiltration, the principle of convective solute transport is used via an extracorporeal process to generate an ultrafiltrate of blood by hydrostatic pressure exerted across a dialysis membrane more permeable than usual. The purpose of this process is to extract larger amounts of fluid from the patient more rapidly than is possible with conventional hemodialysis. In a sense, hemofiltration mimics the glomerulus by utilizing the patient's blood pressure (or pressure augmented by an in-line blood pump) to generate an ultrafiltrate much as the glomerulus performs its function (Figs. 8.1-1 and 8.1-2). The ultrafiltrate collects below the filtration cartridge, and the fluid is continuously measured and discarded. Whereas the human glomerulus modifies the ultrafiltrate by tubular reabsorption of valuable components and then permits the waste products to proceed out the urinary tract, hemo-

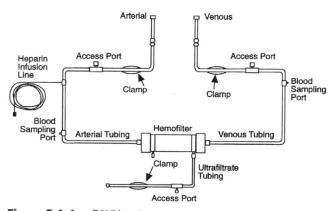

Figure 8.1-1. CAVH system

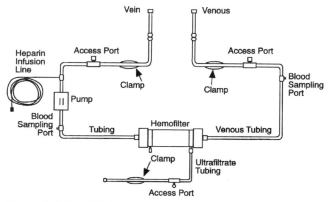

Figure 8.1-2. CVVH system

filtration substitutes fresh "ultrafiltrate replacement" for the discarded liquid. This mode of operation permits (1) substitution of standard fluids, plasma, or albumin for the abnormal ultrafiltrate; (2) downward adjustment of volume in the hypervolemic patient; and (3) bulk removal of toxic substances of the small and middle molecular variety, such as the chemical by-products of tumor lysis.

Hemofiltration is a very attractive procedure for certain circumstances in the ICU. Because the process can be run continuously for many hours (or days), there will be less acute wear and tear on the BP, allowing for more patient comfort. It may obviate the need for vasopressors in an unstable patient or even permit hemofiltration in a patient who cannot tolerate hemodialysis. Moreover, much higher rates of fluid removal can be achieved with hemofiltration than with conventional dialysis and without the need to resort to the high pressures necessary when cranking up dialysis machines for fluid removal. In the situation of tumor lysis, hemofiltration permits bulk removal of the offending chemicals potassium, calcium, phosphate, and uric acid, particularly when used in conjunction with simultaneous dialysis (CAVHD or CVVHD), that is, in serial arrangement. The advantages of continuous renal substitute therapies are listed in Table 8.1-1.

Utilization of these two techniques in the ICU is not aimed at control of chronic renal failure. The appropriate use of hemodialysis or chronic peritoneal dialysis for long-term management of renal failure is reviewed elsewhere in this volume (see Acute Renal Failure by Herrin and Trompeter). However, these methods expand the range of dialysis by including patients whose abdominal complications make them unsuitable for standard peritoneal dialysis and also permit control of severe volume overload by rapid fluid removal and reduction of chemical toxicity from tissue catabolism through bulk removal of potassium, calcium, phosphorous, and uric acid. Table 8.1-2 lists the medical indications for the use of hemofiltration or hemodiafiltration.

Several factors affect the ultrafiltration rate (UFR). The two major factors are hydrostatic pressure and oncotic pressure. Hydrostatic pressure, which is increased with increased BP, blood flow, ultrafiltration column height, and added suction, will augment UFR. Oncotic pressure, as evidenced by higher levels of plasma proteins, will decrease UFR (Fig. 8.1-3). Other factors affecting UFR include (1) shorter and larger caliber catheters (decreased resistance and increased flow), (2) blood viscosity (lower viscosity increases flow), (3)

Table 8.1-1. Advantages of hemofiltration

Control of volume-overloaded states without dramatic fluid shifts

Correction of electrolyte abnormalities

Removal of toxic metabolites

Correction of acid-base status

Ability to increase nutrition

Ease of set-up and may be run by critical care nurse

No complement activation and leukopenia as seen with hemodialysis

Table 8.1-2. Medical indications for hemofiltration or hemodiafiltration

Inability to use peritoneal dialysis secondary to abdominal or thoracic problems

Tumor lysis syndromes

Massive fluid overload

Restricted nutrition because of fluid overload

Respiratory compromise in renal failure

Cardiogenic shock, especially with pulmonary edema

Sepsis

blood pathway patency and venous back pressure (higher resistances decrease flow), and (4) filter surface area and membrane characteristics. Most hemofiltration systems now use hollow-fiber hemofilters, although flat-plate filters may be used. When using CAVH, the UFR is obtained by observing how much fluid is collected in 1 minute. This may be increased by dropping the ultrafiltrate line to the floor (increased gravity) or decreased by partially clamping the line and limiting the amount of filtrate. The blood flow rate may be determined by the following formula:

$$\text{Blood flow rate} = \frac{\text{UFR} \times \text{Hct (venous)}}{\text{Hct (venous)} - \text{Hct (arterial)}}$$

where UFR is ultrafiltration rate and Hct is the hematocrit at the different ports. When hemofiltration is used with two venous cannulations, a pump is used to control the blood flow rate. This is usually set between 30 and 60 ml/min of blood flow for adequate filtration.

The most important consideration in hemofiltration is convective solute removal, which is the movement of molecules in the plasma across the filter into the filtrate. Small- and medium-sized molecules cross into the filtrate and are removed in exact proportion to plasma water. Particles of high molecular weight (albumin, protein, protein-bound drugs) are too large to pass through the filter and are returned to the patient; glucose and ion-bound drugs vary according to blood flow.

When using hemofiltration, it is important to prime the circuit with blood to prevent anemia in the patient and to use anticoagulation to prevent circuit clotting and patient emboli. The most commonly used hemofilters are hollow-fiber capillary hemofilters (e.g., Amicon Diafilter), which may require more heparinization than plate filters. Generally, a bolus dose of heparin (20 units/kg) is given intravenously a few minutes prior to using the circuit. A heparin infusion of 10 units/kg/hr is then started, and the drip is placed into the circuit before the hemofilter. The goal of heparinization is to keep the prothrombin time (PTT) in the circuit at about 90 seconds and in the patient at about 45 seconds. The PTT should be followed every 4 to 6 hours, or more frequently if unstable. It should be noted that the hemofilter does not cause complement activation and the associated drop in leukocytes as occurs in hemodialysis.

In the pediatric population, veno-venous hemofiltration (CVVH) is generally used because there may be very inconsistent blood flow rates with arteriovenous systems due to the small caliber of the blood vessels and variations in patient BP.[7] With an in-line pump, stable blood flows and ultrafiltration may be achieved. Minute blood flows at 30 to 50 ml/min are adequate for normal filtration. Rates for any age may be 5 to 10 ml/kg/min, although at higher rates there may be some tubing collapse. Shorter catheters between 3F and 7F size most commonly are placed in each femoral vein to ensure good blood flow and low resistance, although other areas of central access may be used. Double-lumen single catheters, usually 7F size or greater, may be used in older children. There are data to suggest that, with consistent blood flow and high UFR, urea clearance is dependent on net ultrafiltration regardless of whether hemodiafiltration is employed.[7]

Hemodiafiltration

When hemodiafiltration is used, a dialyzer is primed and placed into the system, which permits the solute transfer between the plasma and the dialysate directly (Fig. 8.1-4). Hemodiafiltration is very efficient in small solute removal and is especially useful in problems of urea management (high BUN secondary to increased catabolism and/or inadequate filtration). It is also efficient in stabilizing electrolyte abnormalities. Peritoneal dialysate fluid is frequently used as the dialysate, and Table 8.1-3 gives the composition of two commonly used dialysates. Dianeal, which represents a standard peritoneal dialysate, has 1.5% dextrose, which may result in a significant dextrose transfer to the patient; this needs to be accounted for in caloric administration. Dianeal also has a sodium concentration of 132 mEq/l, which may induce mild hyponatremia. It is important to note that there is no potassium in standard peritoneal dialysis formulas, and that hypokalemia may develop quickly because of the efficiency of hemodiafiltration. Therefore, it is important to add potassium (0.5–4.0 mEq/l) to the dialysate

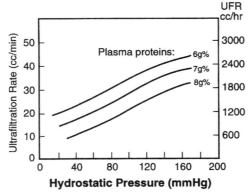

Figure 8.1-3. Effect of plasma proteins (increased oncotic pressure) and hydrostatic pressure on UFR. (Modified with permission from Laver et al. Continuous arterialvenous hemofiltration in critically ill patients. *Ann Intern Med* 99:455–460, 1983.)

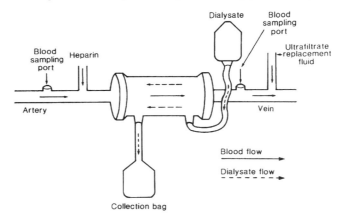

Figure 8.1-4. Hemodiafiltration system. The dialysate runs countercurrent at high volume rates to the blood in the hemodialyzer filter.

Table 8.1-3. Composition of commonly used dialysates for hemodiafiltration

	1.5% Dianeal	*Hospal CAVHD*
Na (mEq/l)	132	140
K (mEq/l)	0	4
Ca (mEq/l)	3.5	3.5
Mg (mEq/l)	1.5	1.5
Cl (mEq/l)	96	96
Lactate (mEq/l)	35	0
Acetate (mEq/l)	0	30
Dextrose (mEq/l)	1.5	0.8

once hyperkalemia has been corrected. Hospal CAVHD formula has been made specifically to account for these issues.[8]

Specialized hemodiafiltration formulas may be made to correct acidosis (adding bicarbonate or acetate for the anion) or to treat any electrolyte disturbance by decreasing, increasing, or omitting the electrolyte of concern; for example, severe hypercalcemia may be treated by omitting calcium. The appropriate dialysate runs countercurrent to the blood flow through the hemodialyzer filter at high volume rates. Usually 300 ml/hr is the minimal rate in infants, and up to 1500 ml/hr may be needed in larger children to meet therapeutic goals. Increasing the dialysate rate and/or the countercurrent blood flow increases the efficiency of the dialysis. Specialized formulas (made in the hospital pharmacy) require significant expense and work time, especially at high volume rates.

There is some controversy about the therapeutic role continuous hemofiltration or hemodiafiltration plays in sepsis.[9-12] There have been several animal and human studies indicating that continuous hemofiltration may improve the clinical state of the septic patient. This may occur because of filtering cytokines or other toxic mediators and possibly by reducing hyperthermia and increased metabolic production, because the blood is cooled going through the circuit. There is very strong evidence that the alternative for renal replacement therapy (hemodialysis) has many important adverse immunologic consequences, making continuous hemofiltration the

preferred therapy because it is much more biocompatible and it does remove cytokines and possibly other toxic mediators. Continuous hemofiltration may also be preferred over hemodiafiltration in septic patients because of the membrane differences; hemodiafiltration should therefore be used only for severe renal failure.

A recent paper by Fleming et al.[13] compared hemofiltration and peritoneal dialysis in children developing renal failure after surgical repair of congenital heart disease. The results showed that hemofiltration as renal replacement therapy offered significant advantages over peritoneal dialysis. This included much greater net negative fluid balance achieved, as well as a marked increase in the ability to provide nutritional support in the form of calorie intake.[13]

Complications of the procedure are both technical and infectious. The filtration cartridge can rupture with consequent blood loss, although this should be less likely with a parallel plate device. To function, the system requires anticoagulation with heparin, and this, too, carries morbidity for ICU patients. Finally, with large-bore catheters in major blood vessels, patients are exposed to the ever-present risk of local or systemic infection. Although this is not a new problem, it simply adds to the burden of risk for a fragile ICU patient already in an environment of increased risk for nosocomial infections. Fortunately, in the typical medical circumstances discussed, hemofiltration or hemodiafiltration will provide a short-term remedy, and the patient will likely recover from the acute insult and then stabilize with more conventional treatment. Thus, the risks associated with the procedure will be short term and quite acceptable in view of the lack of alternative therapies in the most difficult cases. Table 8.1-4 lists common problems and complications.

References

1. Lieberman KV. Continuous arteriovenous hemofiltration in children. *Pediatr Nephrol* 1:330, 1987.
2. Assadi FK. Treatment of acute renal failure in an infant by continuous arteriovenous hemodialysis. *Pediatr Nephrol* 3:320, 1988.
3. Zobel G, Ring E, Zobel V. Continuous arteriovenous renal replacement systems for critically ill children. *Pediatr Nephrol* 3:140, 1989.
4. Golper TA. Continuous arteriovenous hemofiltration in acute renal failure. *Am J Kidney Dis* 6:373, 1985.
5. Stevens PE et al. Continuous arteriovenous haemodialysis in critically ill patients. *Lancet* ii:150, 1988.

Table 8.1-4. Problems and complications with hemofiltration

Problem	Etiology	Therapy or correction of problem
Blood leak (seen as blood-tinged ultrafiltrate)	Ruptured membrane in filter	Replace filter
Clotting of hemofilter (decreased UFR, separation of blood in tubing, darkening of filter, deceased temperature in venous line)	Decreased blood flow Insufficient heparinization Obstruction	Replace filter and tubing Improve blood flow and heparinization
Decreased ultrafiltration rate	Hypotension Clotting Membrane coating	Increase blood flow Check filter clotting Increase intravascular volume
Electrolyte or fluid imbalance	Inadequate monitoring of fluid volume and electrolyte status Inadequate replacement fluids	Accurate records Frequent evaluations Adequate monitoring
Infection	Line or wound infection Circuit contamination Sepsis	Sterile technique Antibiotics Appropriate dressing change protocols Monitor WBC
Exsanguination	Improperly secured circuit Improperly secured vascular access Patient movement	Secure all connections Restrain patient movement if needed Do not cover up system

6. Ronco C et al. Arteriovenous hemodiafiltration associated with continuous hemofiltration: A combined therapy for acute renal failure in the hypercatabolic patient. *Blood Purif* 5:33, 1987.

7. Werner HA, Herbertson MJ, Seear MD. Functional characteristics of pediatric veno-venous hemofiltration. *Crit Care Med* 22:320, 1994.

8. Geroremus R, Schneider N. Continuous arteriovenous hemodialysis. Third International Symposium on Acute Continuous Renal Replacement Therapy, 1987.

9. Gomez A et al. Hemofiltration reverses left ventricular dysfunction during sepsis in dogs. *Anesthesiology* 73:671, 1990.

10. Gootendorst AF et al. High volume hemofiltration improves right ventricular function in endotoxin-induced shock in the pig. *Intensive Care Med* 16:235, 1992.

11. Bellomo R, Tipping P, Boyce N. Continuous veno-venous hemofiltration with dialysis removes cytokines from the circulation of septic patients. *Crit Care Med* 21:522, 1993.

12. Bellomo R, Tipping P, Boyce N. Letter to the editor. *Crit Care Med* 22:719, 1994.

13. Fleming F et al. Renal replacement therapy after repair of congenital heart disease in children. A comparison of hemofiltration and peritoneal dialysis. *J Thorac Cardiovasc Surg* 109:322, 1995.

David Link

John H. Fugate

 8.2   **Peritoneal Dialysis**

Acute Peritoneal Dialysis

Peritoneal dialysis has been available for the management of uremia and manipulation of fluid and solutes in patients since the 1940s. The method retains its attraction because of its simplicity, effectiveness, rapidity of startup, and safety. While hemodialysis is more widely used in pediatrics for dialytic management of chronic renal failure, peritoneal dialysis has many advantages to recommend it in the ICU. Generally, the ICU team cannot manage hemodialysis without consultant help; peritoneal dialysis can be carried out without resort to specialists and technicians. In most pediatric ICUs peritoneal dialysis is quicker to arrange than waiting for the actual start up of hemodialysis. The capital investment for peritoneal dialysis is trivial and equipment is disposable. Factors that influence peritoneal dialysis are listed in Table 8.2-1.

In weighing the advantages and disadvantages of acute peritoneal dialysis vs. hemodialysis, several factors are clinically relevant. Peritoneal dialysis does not result in abrupt change in blood volume. This problem can be of particular concern in patients with compromised circulation or in the infant. No priming transfusion is required. Since peritoneal dialysis typically runs for one to several days, one can adjust the composition of the dialysate to reflect changes in the patient's status and for fine-tuning of the end result. This is more difficult during a 3–4 hour run of hemodialysis since less time is available for correction. Although peritoneal dialysis generally involves heparinization of the dialysate (1 unit/ml), it is rare for generalized anticoagulation to ensue in the patient. This makes peritoneal dialysis particularly attractive in patients with a bleeding tendency or those who are post-surgery with potential for vital organ hemorrhage. On the other hand, there are limitations to peritoneal dialysis. If severe volume overload is the indication for dialysis, rapid fluid removal is better effected by CAVH performed vigorously. Peri-

toneal dialysis can be ineffective in the face of severe abdominal trauma or following extensive surgery. Leakage of peritoneal fluid may occur through wounds or drains, either impairing the efficacy of the procedure or necessitating its termination. A particularly vexing problem with peritoneal dialysis occurs in the patient on maximal-assisted ventilation. The reduction in thoracic volume incurred during instillation of dialysate can bring about respiratory decompensation. Another disadvantage of peritoneal dialysis is the slow, ongoing loss of protein with protracted peritoneal lavage. Also, the ever present problem of bacterial contamination of the peritoneal cavity via the tubing or dialysate is of particular concern in immunocompromised hosts or those patients who are severely catabolic and malnourished. Pain and discomfort may also limit the patient's ability to tolerate the procedure.

While not strictly a disadvantage, the relative impermeability of the peritoneal membrane to certain compounds makes peritoneal dialysis unsuitable for their removal. Particularly in cases of drug ingestion, the use of hemoperfusion through activated charcoal cartridges may be far more effective for drug removal than peritoneal dialysis. Some problems loom larger in theory than in practice. For example, bowel perforation, a constant worry of those inserting peritoneal catheters, seems uncommon and usually self-healing. Bacterial peritonitis often can be cured by the addition of antimicrobials (aminoglycocide or cephalosporin) to the dialysate. Even perforation of a major artery when inserting the trocar for dialysis tends to take care of itself if the patient is not anticoagulated.

In addition to considering peritoneal dialysis for acute renal failure, one can utilize the procedure for removal of other chemicals and toxins. The principal limiting factor for peritoneal dialysis is urgency of removal of the offending substance. Since in general, peritoneal dialysis has a clearance only one-fifth that of hemodialysis, the latter treatment is appropriate when life threatening consequences of chemical imbalance, i.e., malignant hyperkalemia, or toxins (lethal levels of poison) need prompt removal. However, excepting these uncommon circumstances, peritoneal dialysis will successfully control blood levels of low molecular weight chemicals or toxins effectively. For example, hyperuricemia, hypercalcemia (using calcium-free dialysate), and acidosis all respond to peritoneal dialysis by slow removal of the offending ion. Note that peritoneal dialysis can serve as adjunctive therapy for hyperkalemia but kayexalate given orally or by enema (1 g/kg) will be more effective in the acute situation than peritoneal dialysis.

Peritoneal dialysis has a role to play in inherited amino acid disorders, particularly in pediatrics. Thus, infants have been treated with peritoneal dialysis for the severe metabolic acidosis of maple syrup urine disease, lactic acidosis, methylmalonic acidemia, and

Table 8.2-1.   Factors which influence peritoneal dialysis

Anatomic:	Area of peritoneal membrane
	Perfusion of peritoneum
	Permeability of capillary circulation
	Volume of peritoneal cavity available for dialysis
Chemical Factors:	Concentration gradient of ions and molecules
	Solute composition (concentrations, additives)
	Osmotic gradient
Mechanics of Dialysis:	Volume of dialysate
	Dwell time
	Duration of cycle
	Glucose concentration in dialysate

propionic acidemia. The technique should be considered for infants who present with severe acidosis, nonspecific severe neurologic impairment, and suspected inherited metabolic disorder (especially if family history is suggestive). While the putative metabolic product may not be amenable to peritoneal dialysis, little harm can ensue and the acidosis certainly will be improved pending definitive molecular diagnosis.

Technique of Peritoneal Dialysis

A. Equipment

Catheter with trocar—adult size or catheter kit using Seldinger techniques

Dialysis administration set (plumbing)

Dialysis solutions—1.5%, 4.25% (dextrose)

Surgical equipment—antiseptic solutions, sterile sponges, gloves, 4 × 4 gauze, tape, surgical uniform, abdominal paracentesis tray

3½ inch spinal needle—18 or 20 gauge

Drugs—heparin, xylocaine, KCl—concentrated solution in vial (3 mEq/ml)

Warming facility for dialysis solution

Closed drainage urine collector

B. Insertion of Catheter

1. Pre-warm dialysis solution—use 1.5% dextrose solution without K⁺. Prepare and fill dialysis in administration set.
2. Ensure empty bladder by spontaneous voiding or catheterization.
3. Sterile prep and drape of patient's abdomen.
4. Infiltrate puncture site with 1% xylocaine—midline 2–3 cm below umbilicus.
5. Insert #18 gauge spinal needle, or the needle from a Seldinger kit, 3½ inches into peritoneal cavity. Infuse 20ml/ kg of warm dialysate to distend the peritoneal cavity.
6. Using #11 surgical blade, make a puncture wound down to peritoneum. Advance a disposable adult peritoneal catheter into the incision using a drilling motion with a steady pressure until it pops through the peritoneum. Keep the trocar perpendicular to the abdomen. An alternative is using a catheter kit with guidewire. After the needle has been introduced through the peritoneum, a guidewire is advanced. Then the peritoneal catheter is placed into proper position over the guidewire, which is then removed.
7. Withdraw the trocar from the catheter approximately 1 cm; swing the catheter up towards the spleen and advance a bit to clear omentum and then direct down towards the right gutter. Advance the catheter so that all fenestrations are within the peritoneum.
8. Attach dialysis administration tubing to the catheter and allow previously instilled fluid to drain out (watch for blood or fecal matter). Run in and then drain 10 ml/kg warm

dialysis fluid several times (3–5) to ensure that it returns freely from the peritoneal cavity. Cut off excess catheter tubing about 2 cm above the skin and secure the catheter with a single pursestring suture. Use a minimal wound dressing so that fluid leakage will be immediately apparent.

9. Dialysis drainage should enter a closed system that allows accurate measurement of volume. Various devices are available for closed urinary drainage and with suitable modification of their connectors, these can be used for dialysis.

C. Dialysate and Dwell Time

1. Composition of dialysis solutions (See Table 8.2–2)
2. The nature of the underlying problem influences choice of dialysis solution and dwell time. Furthermore, changing patient status will alter dialysis technique.
3. 1.5% dextrose solution is used to initiate dialysis and for routine treatment. Potassium should be added unless hyperkalemia is present. Add 4 mEq/l KCl if renal function is normal and 2 mEq/l for renal failure or for anticipated catabolism or tissue necrosis.
4. Generally, 10 ml/kg of fluid is inserted for each run. Up to 20 ml/kg (or occasionally more) may be used if it does not compromise ventilation or cause significant pain. The larger volumes will augment fluid removal.
5. 4.25% solution augments ultrafiltration and leads to net fluid loss. However, it can produce hypocalcemia, hyperglycemia, and hypernatremia. In cases with pulmonary edema or circulatory overload, 4.25% dialysate permits rapid removal of excess volume.
6. By alternating 4.25% and 1.5% solution or using 4.25% every fourth run, one can remove fluid at a lesser rate.
7. Acetate-containing dialysate should not **be used when** there is lactic acidosis. For hypernatremia use dialysate containing 132 mEq/l of Na⁺.
8. Infuse fluid over 10–15 minutes. For usual dialyses, allow 20–30 minutes for equilibration and then drain over 15–20 minutes.
9. To enhance fluid removal, use rapid dialysis with 4.25% solution. Perform 3–5 exchanges with a dwell time of 5–10 minutes. With good drainage, a cumulative negative balance will ensue. Follow Na⁺, K⁺, glucose, osmolality every 12 hours.

D. Dialysis Technique

1. Add 500 units heparin per liter to each bottle and warm to 37°C. Add potassium as indicated.
2. Maintain desired circulatory volume during dialysis with parenteral fluids.
3. Keep accurate record of inflow and drainage. WEIGH PATIENT TWICE DAILY. Adjust IV rate periodically.
4. Culture dialysate drainage every 12–24 hours.
5. Continue dialysis for as long as required, recognizing that the risk of peritonitis rises substantially with prolonged dial-

Table 8.2-2. Composition of dialysis solutions.

Solution	Dextrose g/l	Na⁺ (mEq/l)	Cl	Ca⁺⁺	Mg⁺⁺	Acetate	Osm
McGaw 1.5%	15	140	101	4	1.5	45	371
4.25%	42.5	140	101	4	1.5	45	521
Travenol 1.5%	15	132	102	3.5	1.5	35	354
4.25%	42.5	132	102	3.5	1.5	35	504
Abbott 1.5%	15	140	101	3.5	1.5	45 lactate	
4.25%	42.5	132	99	3.5	1.5	35 lactate	

ysis. Culture catheter tip when removed.
6. If drainage is poor, reposition patient, catheter or both.
7. Monitor: intake and output
weigh infant every hour; child BID
electrolytes
Ca^{++}
glucose

If performed by an experienced group of physicians and nurses, peritoneal dialysis is generally free of major complications. In the patient who has preexisting abdominal problems (infection, perforated viscus, surgical repair, trauma, etc) the risk of complications increases. If initial insertion of the catheter proceeds smoothly, the most common problem encountered will be peritonitis. Early peritonitis may be treated with systemic antibiotics and antibiotics added to the dialysate fluid. Culturing the dialysis effluent every 12–24 hours will often identify early bacterial contamination. Also, a negative culture in the face of cloudy fluid may suggest either fungal infection or a sterile peritonitis. While white cells will be evident in this circumstance, no bacteria will appear on Gram stain. Occasionally a combination of sterile dialysate with local tenderness or extrusion of pus around the catheter will suggest a tunnel abscess. While antibiotics may help, the presence of this focal infection usually mandates removal of the catheter.

Metabolic disturbances such as hyperglycemia, hypernatremia, or hypokalemia can reflect vigorous peritoneal dialysis and can be corrected with intravenous infusion to offset the effect. If used at proper low doses only at the initiation of dialysis, heparin will not induce systemic anticoagulation. Unfortunately, a common technical difficulty in dialysis is plugging of the catheter pores with fibrin membrane. Both mechanical flushing and heparinization of dialysate can help with this situation. Occasionally, one may need to relocate the catheter in order to clear the problem. A greater difficulty occurs if the omentum wraps itself around the catheter completely occluding the openings. This situation requires manipulation of the catheter to reposition it free of the omentum. Table 8.2-3 lists the common complications seen during peritoneal dialysis treatment and Table 8.2-4 gives the dosages commonly added to the dialysate.

Special Considerations

In the small infant, the dialysis catheter should be inserted in the upper part of the left flank between umbilicus and the hip. If available, a pediatric surgeon can perform the procedure with simple dissection and minimize any possible complication. In patients where one can reasonably predict the need for prolonged peritoneal dialysis, consideration should be given at the outset to utilizing a chronic peritoneal catheter. For patients with severe and prolonged acidosis, sodium bicarbonate can be added to dialysate at 40 mEq/l. However, avoid any calcium in the dialysate since the two may co-precipitate. Unless magnesium is present in dialysate fluid, hypomagnesemia may ensue and should be monitored.

Treatment of acute salt poisoning in infants can readily be carried out by peritoneal dialysis using a hypotonic intravenous solution in place of standard peritoneal dialysis fluid. Fairly rapid exchange will permit efflux of sodium into the dialysate and its physical removal from the body fairly promptly. In management of the tumor lysis syndrome, peritoneal dialysis can be quite effective in controlling the sudden chemical load from tumor cell destruction.

Table 8.2-3   Complications of peritoneal dialysis

1. Perforation of viscus—apparent if catheter returns fecal material or dialysate drains from bladder. Requires surgical correction.
2. Pain—dialysate too cold, use of sorbitol, perforation of viscus, catheter pressure.
3. Poor drainage—obstructed catheter due to clot, omentum, malposition—manipulate catheter and unplug by flushing catheter with dialysate.
4. Hyperosmolarity, hypernatremia—correct with hypotonic IV fluid
5. Hyperglycemia—change from 4.25% to 1.5% dialysate; may require low-dose IV insulin.
6. Dehydration—from excessive use of hypertonic dialysate.
7. Ca^{++} or K^+ derangement—adjust dialysate level to correct.
8. Infection—enteric organisms or staph aureus. Can treat IV and IP. Note: since most drugs cleared by dialysis, need to follow blood levels. Add heparin to avoid plugging of catheter by fibrin.

Table 8.2-4   Drug doses for peritoneal dialysate

Drug	Dose
Heparin	500u/liter
KCl	0–4 mEq/l
Ampicillin	50 mg/l
Cephalothin	250 mg/l
Gentamicin	5-8 mg/l
Vancomycin	25 mg/l
Methicillin	100 mg/l

However, phosphorus may be difficult to remove by this method and requires careful monitoring. In the hemolytic uremic syndrome, early and vigorous peritoneal dialysis will often control hyperkalemia and severe azotemia. Despite the coagulopathy, peritoneal dialysis usually proceeds without added serious risk of bleeding. In the setting of abrupt and severe glomerulonephritis, the main dangers of pulmonary edema from volume overload and hyperkalemia can be well controlled with aggressive peritoneal dialysis. If available, hemodialysis or CAVHD will probably prove more efficient; however, when these modalities are unavailable peritoneal dialysis will generally work well.

Severe hypothermia is a condition seen in children in the northern United States and Canada either because of cold exposure during winter activities or, more commonly, falling through the ice into a pond. Children can arrive at the hospital in asystole and with a core body temperature below 30°C. Rewarming of these children is essential if vital functions are to be restored. Because of accumulating case reports of good neurologic recovery following drowning in very cold water, aggressive efforts are warranted in resuscitation. Peritoneal dialysis can play a major role in rewarming by heat diffusion from warm dialysate into the very large peritoneal cavity and through the extensive abdominal circulation. Dialysis technique is the same as that outlined above; frequently, however, potassium must be added to the dialysate. Dialysate must be prewarmed above room temperature although no precise scheme of rewarming has been proven most effective. Generally, patients have no problem with dialysate warmed to 40°C. As long as the fluid is above body temperature, rapid infusion and short dwell-time peritoneal dialysis will help bring up core temperature to the point where successful restoration of cardiac rhythm can be carried out.

I. David Todres
John H. Fugate

9 ▶ Abdominal Paracentesis

Indications

Abdominal paracentesis is generally used for diagnostic purposes in order to determine the etiology of the peritoneal fluid and to determine whether infiltration is present. It may also be used as a therapeutic tool to remove large volumes of abdominal fluid when these volumes impinge on respiratory function; this is becoming less common, especially with judicious use of chronic diuretics. Occasionally a peritoneal tap is used to remove air when a pneumoperitoneum exists which causes respiratory compromise.

Procedure

Equipment

The equipment required to perform an abdominal paracentesis is listed in Table 9-1.

Technique

What to Do

The patient is placed in a supine position, and the bladder is drained of urine. If there is a coagulopathy, it must be corrected. Sedation is prescribed as needed. If there is a question as to the precise location of the fluid, ultrasound guidance is indicated.

The common sites for paracentesis are shown in Fig. 9-1. These sites are on the anterior abdominal wall. The preferred sites are in the lower abdomen inferior to the umbilicus, through the linea alba midway between the umbilicus and the symphysis pubis. The other sites are just lateral to the rectus abdominous muscle (midclavicular line) and inferior to the umbilicus. These sites are chosen to avoid puncture of underlying vessels or viscera. If punctured, the epigastric artery or vein may cause significant hemorrhage, especially if portal hypertension is present. Usually, the left lower quadrant is preferred to the right in critically ill children because they may have cecal distention. If there has been previous abdominal surgery, the upper abdomen may have to be used, in which case, ultrasound guidance is required.

After the site has been chosen, local infiltration of xylocaine with a small needle is used to produce a skin wheel. The skin is then pulled anteriorly so that further infiltration into the subcutaneous

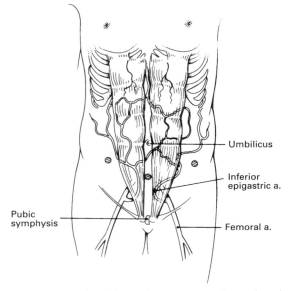

Figure 9-1. Sites for abdominal paracentesis. The preferred sites are the linea alba (midway between the umbilicus and pubic symphysis) and lateral to the rectus abdominous muscle. (Note notched circles.)

tissue is in a different plane (Z tracking). A needle or over-the-needle catheter is then advanced using the Z tracking technique and at an angle perpendicular to the skin. Continued aspiration of the needle is used until peritoneal fluid is aspirated. If an over-the-needle catheter is used, the catheter is advanced as the needle is removed. Approximately 20 ml of fluid is aspirated for studies. Appropriate studies may include cultures and Gram stain, cell count, cytology, amylase, LDH, bilirubin, triglycerides, albumin, and protein.

If the paracentesis is performed for therapeutic purposes to remove large amounts of fluid or occasionally air, a catheter should be placed. Occasionally, the Seldinger technique, as described elsewhere in this volume, may be implemented to place a longer catheter for extended use.

What to Avoid
1. Not emptying the bladder
2. Malpositioning of puncture and hitting a blood vessel or viscera
3. Moving, uncooperative patient

Complications

1. Hemorrhage
2. Persistent fluid leak
3. Intestinal or bladder perforation
4. Hypotension, if large volumes are removed

Table 9-1. Equipment required for abdominal paracentesis

Prep solution, e.g., betadine

Xylocaine 1%–2%

Sedation medication as needed

Sterile needles, syringes

Sterile drapes and towels

Collection containers

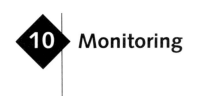

10 | Monitoring

Dean Hess

Patricia English

10.1 | Respiratory Monitoring with Pulse Oximetry and Capnography

Monitoring is the activity of continuously, or nearly continuously, evaluating the physiologic function of a patient in real time to guide management decisions and to assess the impact of treatment.[1] Monitoring differs from measurement in that monitoring is continuous, whereas measurements take place intermittently. There has been increasing interest in noninvasive monitoring of respiratory function over the past 10 years. Two commonly used noninvasive respiratory monitors are the pulse oximeter and the capnograph, and these are discussed in this chapter.

Pulse Oximetry

Pulse oximetry, a technology unavailable until the mid-1980s, is now commonly used in every critical care unit of the modern world. With little scientific evaluation of its impact on outcome, continuous pulse oximetry has become a standard of critical care. A large randomized trial of pulse oximetry in the operating room and postanesthesia care unit failed to show any effect in the overall rate of postoperative complications,[2,3] but similar studies in the critical care environment have not been conducted. Although strong evidence of the benefit of pulse oximetry on patient outcomes is lacking, the reality is that pulse oximetry has become an integral component of critical care monitoring.

The technical and physiologic aspects of pulse oximetry have been reviewed in detail elsewhere.[4-8] Two wavelengths of light (660 nm and 940 nm) are passed through a pulsating vascular bed between two light-emitting diodes (LEDs) and a photodetector. Some of the light emitted from the LEDs is absorbed by each constituent of the tissue, but the only variable absorption is due to arterial pulsations. This is translated into a plethysmographic waveform at each wavelength, the ratio of which is translated into a display of oxygen saturation. A variety of disposable and reusable pulse oximetry probes are available, including digit probes, ear probes, nasal probes, and foot probes. Although most pulse oximeters use transmission oximetry (i.e., the light from the LEDs is transmitted through the tissue, and the photodetector is opposite the LEDs), other designs use reflectance oximetry (i.e., the light from the LEDs is reflected from the tissue, and the photodetector is on the same side of the tissue as the LEDs).

Pulse oximeters use empiric calibration curves developed from studies of healthy adult volunteers. Many clinical evaluations of the accuracy of pulse oximeters have been published, each comparing the pulse oximeter saturation (SpO_2) to the saturation of a simultaneously obtained arterial sample. The accuracy of pulse oximetry is about $\pm 4\%$ to 5% at saturations greater than 80%, but is worse below 80%. To appreciate the implications of the limits of accuracy of pulse oximetry, one must consider the oxyhemoglobin dissociation curve (Fig. 10.1-1). If the pulse oximeter displays an SpO_2 of 95%, the true saturation could be as low as 90% or as high as 100%. If the true saturation is 90%, the PO_2 will be about 60 mm Hg, but one does not know how high the PO_2 might be if the saturation is 100%. Clinically, pulse oximeters should be considered "desaturation meters," with a low SpO_2 considered to reflect hypoxemia until proven other-

wise. However, a SpO_2 greater than 95% does not accurately predict how high the PaO_2 might be.

The pulse oximeter is unique as a respiratory monitor in that it requires no user calibration. However, manufacturer-derived calibration curves programmed into the software vary from manufacturer to manufacturer, and can vary among pulse oximeters of a given manufacturer. The output of LEDs can also vary from probe to probe. The result of these factors is that the accuracy of pulse oximetry varies among devices. For these reasons, the same pulse oximeter and probe should ideally be used for each SpO_2 determination on a given patient.

There are a number of limitations of pulse oximetry that should be appreciated by everyone who uses these devices (Table 10.1-1). Most pulse oximeter errors can be explained as too little signal (e.g., low perfusion, improper probe placement) or too much noise (e.g., motion, ambient light). Although pulse oximetry is generally considered safe, pressure necrosis at the probe site and burns as the result of defective probes may occur. Fetal hemoglobin may affect the accuracy of oxygen saturation measured on blood gas samples (e.g., CO-oximetry), but it does not affect the accuracy of pulse oximetry. Hyperbilirubinemia also does not affect pulse oximetry accuracy.

Although outcome studies are lacking, the use of pulse oximetry should not be withheld when it is indicated. Pulse oximetry is indicated in unstable patients likely to desaturate, in patients receiving a therapeutic intervention that is likely to produce hypoxemia (e.g., bronchoscopy), and in patients having interventions likely to produce changes in arterial oxygenation (e.g., changes in P_IO_2 or PEEP). The pulse oximeter is probably no better at detection of a

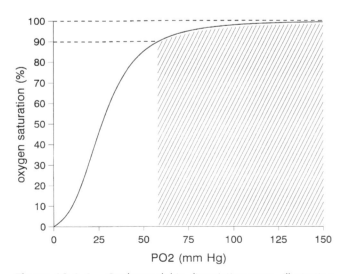

Figure 10.1-1. Oxyhemoglobin dissociation curve, illustrating range of PO_2 due to typical error in pulse oximetry ($\pm 5\%$) when $SpO_2 = 95\%$. Note that SpO_2 of 95% could result in a PaO_2 as low as 60 mm Hg to as high as >150 mm Hg.

Table 10.1-1. Limitations of pulse oximetry

Limitation	Effect
Penumbra effect	With poor probe fit, light can be shunted from the LEDs directly to the photodetector, causing a falsely low SpO_2 at >85% and a falsely elevated SpO_2 at <85%.
Dyshemoglobinemias	Elevations of COHb and metHb result in inaccuracy.
Dyes and pigments	Vascular dyes (e.g., methylene blue) and nail polish affect accuracy.
Skin pigmentation	Accuracy and reliability affected by deeply pigmented skin.
Perfusion	Unreliable results with conditions of low flow (e.g., cardiac arrest or severe peripheral vasoconstriction)
Anemia	Less accurate and reliable with conditions of severe anemia.
Motion	Motion of the probe can produce considerable artifact, causing unreliable and inaccurate readings.
Ambient light	High-intensity ambient light can produce interference.
Abnormal pulses	Venous pulses and a large dicrotic notch may affect accuracy.

disconnect than the alarms already available on the ventilator. There may be a relatively long lag time between disconnect and desaturation (particularly if the PaO_2 is high before the disconnect), although this lag time may be short in neonates with small tidal volumes.

Jubran and Tobin[9] evaluated the use of pulse oximetry to titrate F_IO_2 in 54 critically ill adult ventilator-dependent patients. In White patients, they found that an SpO_2 of 92% was reliable to predict a PaO_2 equal to or greater than 60 mm Hg. In Black patients, however, an SpO_2 of 95% was required. Although pulse oximetry is useful to titrate a level of arterial oxygenation that does not produce hypoxemia, it does not eliminate the need for periodic arterial blood gases. When pulse oximetry is used to titrate F_IO_2, the final F_IO_2 setting should be confirmed by an arterial blood gas. Interestingly, no study similar to that of Jubran and Tobin has been done to evaluate the reliability of pulse oximetry to titrate PEEP, although anecdotal experience has found pulse oximetry useful to adjust PEEP levels.

Despite concern related to the detection of hyperoxemia, pulse oximetry is commonly used in neonatal patients. Blanchette et al.[10] evaluated the ability of pulse oximetry to predict normoxemia in the neonatal intensive care unit (ICU). They evaluated 353 SpO_2-PaO_2 data pairs in 52 infants (mean age 4.6 days with a variety of diagnoses). They found that an SpO_2 between 92% and 96% limited hyperoxemic episodes ($PaO_2 > 90$ mm Hg) to 3% and hypoxemic episodes ($PaO_2 < 45$ mm Hg) to 4%.

Pulse oximetry has been used in neonates to assess cardiac right-to-left shunting. One pulse oximeter probe is placed on the right upper extremity and another is placed on a lower extremity. If there is a large anatomic right-to-left shunt (e.g., patent ductus arteriosus), the preductal SpO_2 may be significantly greater than the postductal SpO_2. For this same reason, it is important to note the probe site when assessing SpO_2 (e.g., preductal versus postductal).

If pulse oximetry is to be clinically useful, it must have a low failure rate. Intraoperative pulse oximeter failure is relatively low, but failures are greater in sicker patients. Pulse oximetry failure in the critical care unit has not been studied, but our suspicion is that failures are more common in the ICU than in the relatively controlled environment of the operating room. Perhaps the most frequent causes of pulse oximetry failure in the ICU are accidental disconnection of the probe from the patient and poor peripheral perfusion.

Capnography

Capnography is measurement of carbon dioxide at the airway during the ventilatory cycle and display of a waveform called the capnogram. Most bedside capnographs measure carbon dioxide by infrared absorption.[11-13] The mainstream capnograph places the measurement chamber at the airway, whereas the sidestream capnograph aspirates gas through fine-bore tubing to the measurement chamber inside the capnograph. There are advantages and disadvantages of each design, and neither is clearly superior. Water is a problem, because it occludes sample lines in the sidestream capnograph and condenses in the cell of mainstream devices. Manufacturers use a number of features to overcome this problem, including water traps, purging of the sample line, construction of the sample line with water-vapor permeable nafion, and heating of the mainstream cell. Generally, capnography is more technically challenging than pulse oximetry.

The normal capnogram is illustrated in Fig. 10.1-2. During inspiration, PCO_2 is 0. At the beginning of exhalation, PCO_2 remains 0 as gas from anatomic dead space leaves the airway (Phase I). The PCO_2 then sharply rises as alveolar gas mixes with dead space gas (Phase II). During most of exhalation, the curve levels and forms a plateau (Phase III). This represents gas from alveoli ("alveolar plateau"). The PCO_2 at the end of the alveolar plateau is end-tidal PCO_2 ($PetCO_2$).

The $PetCO_2$ represents alveolar PCO_2 ($PACO_2$). $PACO_2$ is determined by the rate at which carbon dioxide is added to the alveolus and the rate at which carbon dioxide is cleared from the alveolus. Thus, $PACO_2$ is the result of the ventilation-perfusion ratio ($\dot{V}/\dot{Q}$). With a normal $\dot{V}/\dot{Q}$, the $PACO_2$ will approximate the arterial PCO_2 ($PaCO_2$). If the $\dot{V}/\dot{Q}$ decreases, $PACO_2$ rises toward mixed venous PCO_2 ($P\bar{v}CO_2$). With a high $\dot{V}/\dot{Q}$ (i.e., dead space), $PACO_2$ will approach the inspired PCO_2, which is usually 0. Theoretically, $PetCO_2$ could be as low as the inspired PCO_2 (0) or as high as the $P\bar{v}CO_2$.

An increase or decrease in $PetCO_2$ can be the result of changes in carbon dioxide production (i.e., metabolism), carbon dioxide delivery to the lungs (i.e., circulation), or changes in alveolar ventilation. Due to homeostasis, however, compensatory changes may occur so that $PetCO_2$ remains constant. In practice, $PetCO_2$ is a nonspecific indicator of cardiopulmonary homeostasis and usually does not indicate a specific problem or abnormality.

The gradient between $PaCO_2$ and $PetCO_2$ [$P(a-et)CO_2$] is often calculated. This gradient is usually small (<5 mm Hg). In patients with dead space–producing disease (i.e., high $\dot{V}/\dot{Q}$), however, the $PetCO_2$ may be considerably less than $PaCO_2$ (Table 10.1-2). Although not commonly appreciated, the $PetCO_2$ occasionally may be greater than the $PaCO_2$.

There is considerable intra- and interpatient variability in the relationship between $PaCO_2$ and $PetCO_2$. The $P(a-et)CO_2$ is often too variable to allow precise prediction of $PaCO_2$ from $PetCO_2$.[14-16]

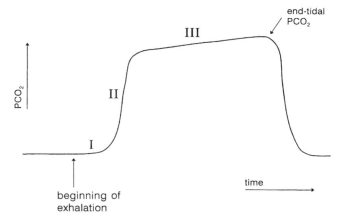

Figure 10.1-2. Typical capnogram. See text for details.

$PetCO_2$ is useful for monitoring iatrogenic hyperventilation in head-injured patients, which is probably because these patients often have relatively normal lung function.

Due to their smaller tidal volumes and more rapid respiratory rates, monitoring of $PetCO_2$ is more difficult in infants and children than adults. This causes difficulty in producing a valid capnogram and identification of the $PetCO_2$. One concern with capnography in children with small tidal volumes is the effect of the mechanical dead space of the airway adapter. However, there are very low dead space airway adapters available for use with both mainstream and sidestream capnographs. There is also a concern related to aspiration of gas from the airway with sidestream capnographs, but this is probably not an issue with continuous flow ventilation systems, in which the total flow through the ventilator circuit far exceeds the sample rate of the capnograph. The usefulness of capnography in critically ill infants and children has not been clearly established. Much work remains to establish the appropriate role of capnography in neonatal and pediatric patients.

Coté et al.[17] conducted a single-blind study of combined pulse oximetry and capnography in 402 pediatric cases in the operating room. They found that the pulse oximeter was superior to the capnograph and clinical judgment in providing an early warning of desaturation. Capnography also provided an early warning of significant morbidity (e.g., esophageal intubations and disconnections), but the incidence of these types of events was not affected by the use of capnography. In these anesthetized children with relatively normal lung function, use of capnography did reduce the incidence of hypercarbia and hypocarbia. Although this study provides useful data related to the use of capnography during anesthesia, one must be cautious about extrapolation of these data to critically ill patients with abnormal pulmonary function.

A useful application of capnography is the detection of esophageal intubation. Because there is normally very little carbon dioxide in the stomach, intubation of the esophagus and ventilation of the stomach result in a very low $PetCO_2$. Of the methods available to

Table 10.1-2. Causes of increased $PaCO_2$-$PetCO_2$

Pulmonary hypoperfusion

Pulmonary embolism

Cardiac arrest

Positive pressure ventilation (especially with PEEP)

High-rate, low-tidal volume ventilation

Table 10.1-3. Recommended applications for pulse oximetry and capnography

Pulse oximetry
  Unstable patients likely to desaturate
  Patients receiving a therapeutic intervention likely to produce hypoxemia (e.g., bronchoscopy)
  Patients in whom FIO_2 or PEEP levels are changed
Capnography
  Verification of proper endotracheal tube position
  Assessment of $PaCO_2$ in patients with normal lung function (e.g., head-injured patients)
  Evaluation of deadspace ($PaCO_2$-$PetCO_2$ gradient)
  Evaluation of pulmonary blood flow during resuscitation

detect esophageal intubation, measurement of $PetCO_2$ is regarded as the most reliable. A potential problem with the use of capnography to confirm endotracheal intubation occurs during cardiac arrest, because of very low $PetCO_2$ values related to decreased pulmonary blood flow. A relatively low-cost disposable device for detecting esophageal intubation is commercially available (Nellcor EasyCap). This device fits between the endotracheal tube and the ventilation device and produces a color change in the presence of exhaled carbon dioxide. It is useful to detect esophageal intubation in adults and children.

Capnography also has been shown to be potentially useful to evaluate pulmonary blood flow during resuscitation. During resuscitation, changes in blood flow are reflected by changes in $PetCO_2$—low pulmonary blood flow results in low $PetCO_2$, and vice versa. It has also been found that patients likely to be resuscitated have a higher $PetCO_2$ (>15 mm Hg) than patients who cannot be resuscitated ($PetCO_2$ <15 mm Hg). The use of $PetCO_2$ as a real-time objective indicator of resuscitation effectiveness is promising, but it is premature to recommend its routine use during resuscitation.

Use of capnography in the operating room has become a standard of care. The use of capnography in the critical care unit, however, has not been as enthusiastically supported. Part of this relates to the fact that capnographs are technically more difficult to use than pulse oximeters. More importantly, $PetCO_2$ is often an imprecise predictor of $PaCO_2$ in patients with lung disease (precisely those in whom its use might be most desirable). Although the use of capnography has been advocated as a back-up ventilator disconnect alarm, there is no evidence that it is any better than the alarms currently available on ventilators.

Summary

Recommendations for appropriate use of pulse oximetry and capnography are listed in Table 10.1-3. Pulse oximetry is useful to evaluate oxygenation in many critically ill infants and children. Unfortunately, $PetCO_2$ is not a very good indicator of $PaCO_2$ in many critically ill patients. Capnography is useful to assess correct endotracheal tube position, but this often can be achieved by using relatively inexpensive qualitative devices.

References

1. Moller JT et al. Randomized evaluation of pulse oximetry in 20,802 patients: I. Design, demography, pulse oximetry failure rate, and overall complication rate. *Anesthesiology* 78:436–444, 1993.

2. Moller JT et al. Randomized evaluation of pulse oximetry in 20,802 patients: II. Perioperative events and postoperative complications. *Anesthesiology* 78:445–453, 1993.

3. Hess D, Kacmarek RM, Stoller JK. Perspectives on monitoring in

respiratory care. In Kacmarek RM, Hess D, Stoller JK (eds): *Monitoring in Respiratory Care.* St. Louis: Mosby, 1993.

4. Hess D, Kacmarek RM. Techniques and devices for monitoring oxygenation. *Respir Care* 38:646–671, 1993.

5. Kelleher JF. Pulse oximetry. *J Clin Monit* 5:37–62, 1989.

6. Welch JP, DeCesare R, Hess D. Pulse oximetry: Instrumentation and clinical applications. *Respir Care* 35:584–901, 1990.

7. Severinghaus JW, Kelleher JF. Recent developments in pulse oximetry. *Anesthesiology* 76:1018–1038, 1992.

8. McCarthy K et al. Pulse oximetry. In Kacmarek RM, Hess D, Stoller JK (eds): *Monitoring in Respiratory Care.* St. Louis: Mosby, 1993. Pp. 309–347.

9. Jubran A, Tobin MJ. Reliability of pulse oximetry in titrating supplemental oxygen therapy in ventilator-dependent patients. *Chest* 97: 1420–1425, 1990.

10. Blanchette T, Dziodzio J, Harris K. Pulse oximetry and normoxemia in neonatal intensive care. *Respir Care* 36:25–32, 1991.

11. Hess D. Capnography: Technical aspects and clinical applications. In Kacmarek RM, Hess D, Stoller JK (eds): *Monitoring in Respiratory Care.* St. Louis: Mosby, 1993. Pp. 375–405.

12. Hess D. Capnometry and capnography: Technical aspects, physiologic aspects, and clinical applications. *Respir Care* 35:557–576, 1990.

13. Gardner RM. Sensors and transducers. In Kacmarek RM, Hess D, Stoller JK (eds): *Monitoring in Respiratory Care.* St. Louis: Mosby, 1993. Pp. 35–70.

14. Hess D et al. An evaluation of the usefulness of end-tidal PCO_2 to aid weaning from mechanical ventilation following cardiac surgery. *Respir Care* 36:837–843, 1991.

15. Hoffman R et al. End-tidal carbon dioxide in critically ill patients during changes in mechanical ventilation. *Am Rev Respir Dis* 140: 1265–1268, 1989.

16. Graybeal JM, Russell GB. Capnometry in the surgical ICU: An analysis of the arterial-to-end-tidal carbon dioxide difference. *Respir Care* 38: 923–928, 1993.

17. Coté CJ et al. A single-blind study of combined pulse oximetry and capnography in children. *Anesthesiology* 74:980–987, 1991.

 10.2

Lisa Arguin

Monitoring in the Intensive Care Unit

The intensive care clinician of today is confronted with far more bedside technology than the clinician of years past. This medical technology is intended to provide information to aid with patient assessment. Unfortunately, this can be confusing and challenging due to the increased level of complexity and availability of advanced monitoring and diagnostic devices. Additionally, technology provides a great deal of information and capability, which has resulted in increased pressure from the nonmedical community. Near perfection has become the expectation, and there is far less tolerance of error. It is for these reasons, as well as unmentioned others, that now more than ever a clinician must understand the basis on which medical instrumentation operates. The intent of this chapter is not to educate a clinician to all of the specifics of medical instrumentation, but rather to make one aware, in the very broadest sense, of some of the capabilities and limitations of bedside monitoring technology and to spur further investigation.

Then and Now

Over the past 30 years there have been many advances that have made the information obtained from medical devices more accurate, consistent, and reliable. However, one cannot lose sight of the fact that these devices are still merely tools and should be regarded as such. Measurements should always be questioned and coupled with sound clinical judgment. Blind acceptance of information can potentially lead to adverse patient care. To question information, a clinician must at least possess a basic understanding of how the measurement is obtained and processed. Without this minimal understanding, a clinician is not capable of examining a situation completely and is therefore not making a fully informed decision.

Technical advances in electronics, materials, power sources, display technology, and manufacturing techniques have enabled devices to become smaller, lighter, more reliable, and more accurate. Gone are the days of vacuum tubes and discrete components. Today's bedside monitors are essentially high-powered computers that are capable of processing very specialized and complex software algorithms. No longer does one require a unique device for each monitored parameter. Several measurements can now be integrated into one housing. For instance, the device shown in

Fig. 10.2-1 was designed approximately 25 years ago and is used to monitor ECG and a pulse. The device in Fig. 10.2-2 was designed within the past few years and is approximately half the size, lighter, and is capable of monitoring ECG, two temperatures, noninvasive BP, two invasive BPs, and oxygen saturation; can provide real-time and on-alarm waveform recordings; and has a 6-hour power source. As these illustrations show, technology has improved greatly.

In addition to the aforementioned parameters, almost all monitoring manufacturers have the capability of monitoring respiration, apnea, multiple invasive pressures, end-tidal CO_2, cardiac output, $TcPO_2$, $TcPCO_2$, F_IO_2, SvO_2, and ECG arrhythmias. With all of these measurements available, which should be utilized? It can be tempting to monitor all parameters on all patients simply because there exists the means to do so. This presents a challenge

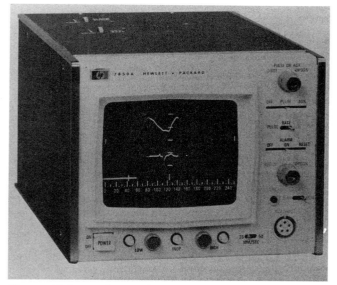

Figure 10.2-1. The Hewlett Packard Patient Monitor Model 7830A. This monitor was designed in the 1960s and is capable of monitoring ECG and a pulse.

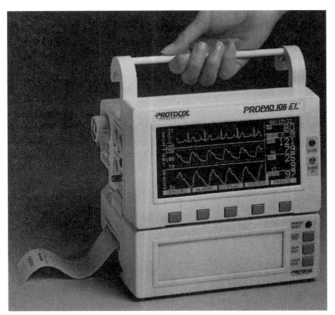

Figure 10.2-2. A Protocol Systems patient monitor: the Propaq 106EL with the expansion module. This monitor was designed in the 1980s and is capable of monitoring ECG, noninvasive BP, two invasive BPs, oxygen saturation, and temperature, and has a printer and a built-in power source.

to manufacturers with regard to the way in which they choose to display this abundance of information. Monitor displays become cluttered quickly when presenting more than a few waveforms and the alphanumerics for five or six parameters. Questions like the following abound: Should alarm limits be displayed? How should color be used? Should pressure scales be displayed and for all pressures being monitored? Should systolic, diastolic, and mean values be displayed at all times? Should one, two, three, or more leads of ECG be displayed simultaneously? These are just a few of the questions that manufacturers have addressed, each in their own particular fashion. Overall, most manufacturers offer the same menu of measurements, and the means used to obtain and process the signals are usually very similar. Bedside monitoring is approaching the point where devices are homogenous, and the only major distinction between them is the way in which the user views and accesses information.

In addition to a multitude of monitored parameters and a display that is congested with information, bedside monitors offer various forms of trended information and calculations. Most monitors can store patient information in memory for at least 24 hours. This trended information can be presented graphically, and with some monitors, in a tabular format. The information can be sent to either a multichannel recorder or a printer and be included in the patient's chart if desired. Trended information can be valuable when looking for changes over time and the effect one parameter may impose on another. It must be remembered, however, that the trended information is taken directly from the monitor, and if there are periods of inaccurate monitoring, this same inaccuracy will be contained in the trended information. Some monitors will allow the user to manually edit information from the history, especially with ECG arrhythmia systems. This is the responsibility of the user. The monitor assumes that the processed information is correct unless otherwise indicated. An example of inaccurate information that would be part of a patient's history is the inaccuracy that respiratory artifact imposes on a pulmonary artery (PA)

pressure (Fig. 10.2-3). This artifact can be seen clearly on a monitor's display and is obvious to a clinician. Unfortunately, most monitors are not capable of completely filtering the respiratory effect. The result is inaccurate information, especially systolic and diastolic values. Given this situation, one method of obtaining accurate information is to read the waveform manually. This can be done either by making a hard copy recording, which has pressure scales on the paper (Fig. 10.2-4), or by freezing the waveform on the display and utilizing on-screen pressure scales or an on-screen cursor. Given this scenario, the PA pressure information stored in trends is erroneous.

Some monitors can perform calculations, such as hemodynamic, respiratory, and cardiac, easily and automatically. Unfortunately, the same problem that exists with trended information is also present with the calculations. Some of the values required to perform the calculations are obtained by the monitor automatically. Depending on the calculation and the required values, the monitor might be gathering data either at the time of the calculation (i.e., real time) or from memory. If erroneous information exists either at the present moment or in the history, the misinformation will be incorporated into the calculations as well. Therefore, it is important that one evaluate the criteria used to derive any calculation and edit as needed.

Along with these sophisticated and complex bedside monitors, companies have developed ways in which to provide continuous

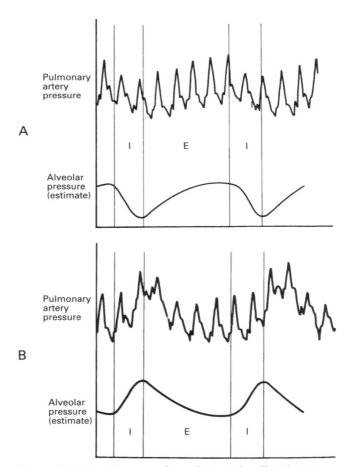

Figure 10.2-3. These waveforms illustrate the effect that airway pressure can have on PA pressure. **(A)** The top tracing is of alveolar pressure during normal, spontaneous respirations. **(B)** The bottom tracing is of alveolar pressure on a mechanically ventilated patient. **(A,B)** The top tracings are of the measured PA pressure.

Figure 10.2-4. A recorder strip taken from the Hewlett Packard M1117A multichannel thermal array recorder. Pressure values can be obtained from a recording such as this when the monitor's digital values are not reliable, such as in the case of PA pressures that are affected by respiratory artifact.

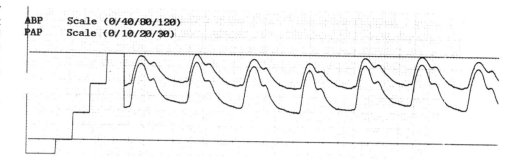

monitoring when transporting patients. Transport monitors have existed for many years; however, it was always necessary to disconnect the patient from the monitor at the bedside, connect to the transport monitor that has a portable power source, and then reconnect to the bedside monitor on returning to the intensive care unit (ICU). Transport systems now exist that utilize the bedside monitor's parameter modules. These modules have built-in power sources that maintain pressure zeroes, alarm limits, and other patient information. The modules attach to a low-power portable display, such as a liquid crystal display (LCD) or an electroluminescent (EL). This transport device (Fig. 10.2-5) enables a patient to be monitored continuously. There are no unmonitored periods during disconnection from or reconnection to the bedside monitor as before. A device of this type greatly simplifies patient transport and minimizes patient risk at a time of potential confusion and stress.

Patient Care Networks

In addition to increased bedside and transport capability, monitoring networks have changed and improved as well. Almost all of the major monitoring manufacturers offer networks as part of their

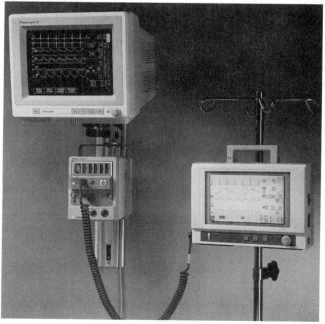

Figure 10.2-5. The Marquette Electronics bedside monitor, Tramscope 12, interfaced to a Tram 600 and a noninvasive BP module. The Tram 600 multiparameter module is also interfaced to the Tram Transport Display. Patients can be monitored continuously throughout the entire transport process with no loss of information.

monitoring systems. The network is simply the communication link that must exist in order to interface devices. It serves as a road, or means of transport, for high-speed transmission of patient data and information. Groupings of bedside monitors, central station displays, central recorders and printers, arrhythmia processing and review terminals, and alarm annunciation systems are just some of the devices that can be connected with networks. Some of the capabilities provided by a network are the linking together of individual monitors so that a patient's information can be accessed and viewed on other monitors, either by demand or on alarm; two-way communication between bedside monitors and central stations; and the remote annunciation, both visually and audibly, of alarm information. Networks have enabled clinicians to access information in many different locations, and they lend a surveillance feature to the system. The exact capabilities and features of each network vary depending on the manufacturer. Regardless of the specific protocols and cabling used, monitoring networks have made patient care more comprehensive and safer.

One of the latest foci of engineering time and corporate resources—an extension of the monitoring network—is that of patient data management, or clinical information systems. Manufacturers realize that there is far more information utilized in patient care than is directly provided by the bedside monitor. The technology that enables the networking of multiple areas—operating rooms, laboratories, diagnostic areas, ICUs, SDUs, clinician's offices, and nonclinical areas—has existed for some time. Patient data can be accessed, viewed, and interacted with from locations that have the appropriate hardware and software. For instance, a computer terminal can be installed in a physician's office and wired to an ICU monitoring network; then data from any patient on that network can be viewed from the office terminal. This capability is costly, yet very powerful.

A piece of the patient data management puzzle, which companies are grappling to master and implement, is bedside charting. It is no secret that in the last few years hospitals have been forced to operate more efficiently, cutting costs and budgets wherever possible. However, the expectation is that patient care will not be adversely affected in any way. These pressures provide a clear indication that it is crucial to simplify the daily tasks required of clinicians. Manufacturers feel that one way to accomplish this is to have a virtually paperless charting system—paperless in the sense that there is no hard copy bedside chart. Instead, all information—vital signs, care plan, medications, lab results, staff notes—is entered into a computer database via a terminal located at or near the patient's bedside (Fig. 10.2-6). Networking enables vital signs to be documented from the monitor and into the chart automatically at intervals determined by the user. It also allows for lab results to be sent back to the appropriate patient location and entered automatically into the computer patient chart. This all appears relatively straightforward; however, patient notes are not quite as simple. The

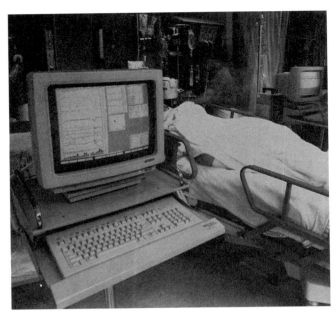

Figure 10.2-6. The Marquette Electronics Clinicomp Clinical Information Systems bedside data terminal. It is an extension of the monitoring network and allows for the consolidation and standardization of patient documentation.

entering of this text requires more than just hardware and software; it requires interaction with the clinicians via a keyboard, mouse, trackball, or other data entry device. This raises the outstanding importance of ease of use. It is not sufficient for a new system to be merely as simple to interact with as the old, which in this case is writing with a pen and is something with which everyone is quite comfortable and familiar. The new method must prove to be easier and quicker to execute, as well as yield a superior result. If this is not the case, individuals may feel that changing to the new system is not worthwhile, and they may oppose the implementation of such a system. A few of the advantages of a clinical information system are complete and legible documentation, increased medical record storage capability, and relatively easy access to past records. Some of the disadvantages include cost and a tremendous learning curve. As with any new concept, the opinions regarding automated patient data management and a paperless medical record vary. Some individuals feel that a paperless bedside chart is a realistic concept that can be achieved. Others believe it to be a somewhat naive goal that stands little chance of complete implementation anytime in the near future.

Another networking concept that has been discussed for the past several years is that of a medical information bus (MIB). The basic idea of the MIB is to design medical devices so that they can interface and communicate with other devices, such as the bedside monitor. Infusion pumps, ventilators, and other peripheral devices send data such as waveforms and alarm and patient information to the monitor for display. One advantage of this is the consolidation of information into one device. Rather than scan multiple instruments for the source of an alarm or a patient's status, all information is housed on one display, thus simplifying the access of information for the clinician. For this concept to succeed, it requires the cooperation and consensus of medical manufacturers, who must agree on and incorporate this communication capability into the design of their devices, and the medical community, to help guide the development. Because this concept has not come to fruition after years of discussion, some manufactur-

ers have developed their own means of interfacing peripheral devices to their bedside monitors.

Monitoring the Neonatal and Pediatric Patient

Thus far, the text has been directed uniformly at all patient populations. However, these generic applications are not always possible. In the past, much of the software and hardware for monitoring was originally designed and perfected for the adult population. Pediatric and neonatal patients were somewhat of an afterthought, and in some instances very few changes were made to the adult technology to accommodate the specific requirements of pediatric patients. An example of this that still exists with some monitors is the ECG. Almost all adult ECG monitors have pacer rejection circuitry that identifies and filters pacer spikes so that they are not considered when determining a patient's heart rate. A neonate's QRS complex is much more narrow and sharp than an adult's and, to a monitor, may resemble a pacer spike. If the same pacer rejection circuit found in adult monitors was also contained in neonatal monitors, there would exist the potential for a false low rate to be determined by the monitor and subsequently displayed. As a result, some manufacturers have eliminated this circuit from their neonatal monitor. The problem that then occurs is with a paced neonate. How does one monitor this patient accurately? Without the rejection circuit, there exists the potential for a false high rate because both the R waves and the pacer spikes may be counted. With these monitors, lead placement, lead selection, and a manual mode for determining the sensing threshold are a few ways of obtaining an accurate rate. An accurate rate on a paced neonate is certainly achievable; but it is unfortunate that not all manufacturers have made obtaining an accurate heart rate as simple and straightforward with neonates as it is with adults.

Another parameter that is monitored routinely in neonatal and pediatric patients is respiration, which is used to determine a rate and detect apnea. The method most often used to monitor respiration is impedance pneumography. Impedance pneumography is a simple, cost-effective, and noninvasive method, but it has definite limitations.[1] The same electrodes used to monitor ECG are used with impedance pneumography. The basic principle is that a harmless electrical signal is input to the patient through one of the chest electrodes. Air in the chest is nonconductive, blood is conductive, and when an individual breathes, the air-blood ratio changes. This change can be measured in terms of impedance, which is then processed by the monitor as a breath.[2] There have been various studies done that indicate that impedance pneumography is not a reliable means of detecting apnea caused by upper airway obstruction where the patient is still making respiratory efforts.[2,3] It has also been shown that it is ineffective in monitoring patients that have very low-level signals. These patients require maximum sensitivity settings, which are to the point where cardiac activity is misinterpreted as a breath. Inappropriately high sensitivity settings can also result in false high rates due to double counting. In addition, vibrations from nearby equipment, patient movement, chest wall fluctuations due to cardiac impulses, and personnel movement may all result in undetected episodes of apnea.[1,3,4] There is little that can be done to improve the device's capability of accurately detecting apnea due to upper airway obstruction, but there are some steps that should be taken to ensure that the best possible respiration signal, and thus information, is obtained. The most basic is lead placement, although this can be somewhat difficult in small patients whose chest surface areas are restricted. It is also crucial that the appropriate sensitivity setting for each individual patient be ascertained.[1,4]

Hemodynamic Monitoring

As the previous examples illustrate, there are limitations with any technology. In the neonatal and pediatric environment, this fact is more profound. The mere physical limitations of the neonatal patient can make the task of accurate monitoring very challenging. Although all patients could benefit from reduced invasive monitoring, the physical limitations of a neonate, coupled with an immature immune system and a low tolerance for stress, make this patient the ideal candidate for noninvasive technology. A noninvasive measurement is obviously not as direct as an invasive one and may not provide the same level of accuracy or precision. An example of this is illustrated with hemodynamic monitoring. The direct and invasive technique, which involves a well-positioned catheter connected to a high-fidelity tubing, transducer, and monitoring system, measures actual pressure, while indirect, noninvasive methods typically measure flow or changes in the volume of a pressure cuff.

Invasive pressure monitoring provides the clinician with direct and continuous hemodynamic information (i.e., systolic, diastolic, and mean pressures) as well as patient access. To achieve this measurement, a catheter is inserted into the patient at the site of choice. Radial arterial, pulmonary arterial, and central venous pressures are all monitored routinely in critical care. In addition, umbilical arterial and venous lines are sometimes placed in neonates, intracranial (IC) catheters are placed in patients whose IC pressure is critical, and left heart catheters are often found in cardiac surgical units. The indwelling catheter provides the input signal to the transducer. This input signal is the patient's pressure signal, which is actually a very complex waveform. Figure 10.2-7 illustrates how various pressure waveforms and an ECG waveform correlate during a cardiac cycle. The catheter is a fluid-filled tube that transmits the pulse signal to another fluid-filled tube outside the patient. These tubes are usually connected via a stopcock. This tubing, which is typically 48 inches in length, is connected to a transducer. The transducer changes the mechanical pressure signal to an electrical signal. This electrical signal is connected via a transducer cable to the monitor where it is filtered and processed. The pressure waveform is displayed along with the systolic, diastolic, and mean pressure values as determined by the monitor's specific software algorithm. Many manufacturers employ a weighted averaging algorithm to compute the pressure values. Varying degrees of value, or weight, are assigned to a certain number of beats. The weight applied to each beat is typically dependent on the variation of the mean pressures from beat to beat.[5,6] A typical adult transducer-tubing system is shown in Fig. 10.2-8. In neonatal and pediatric patients, the pressurized flush bag is usually replaced with a syringe and a pump. This is to eliminate any potential for harmful fast flushes and to more closely and accurately control the infusion of the flush solution.[7] Figure 10.2-9 shows a typical neonatal/pediatric set-up.

The arterial pressure waveform seen on the monitor will depend on the site of the catheter. The further the site (i.e., the catheter tip) is from the heart, the more dramatic the difference will be. Not only will the systolic pressure be greater peripherally, but the entire shape of the waveform will change. These changes include a more severe slope in the upstroke of the wave, a more narrow and peaked curve, and a delay in the rise in pressure after the aortic valve has opened.[8] Figure 10.2-10 illustrates this point.

In addition to changes based on catheter site, hemodynamic

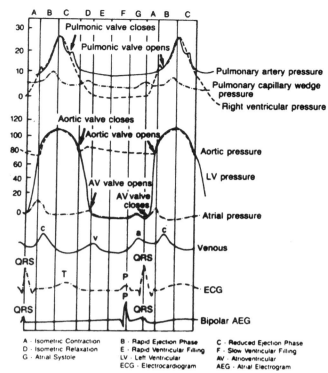

Figure 10.2-7. Various pressure waveforms and an ECG waveform. The graph depicts how pressures and cardiac activity correlate.

waveforms and values are influenced by other factors, such as the patient's condition. One example of this is shock. There are many causes of shock, but in children the most common is hypovolemia.

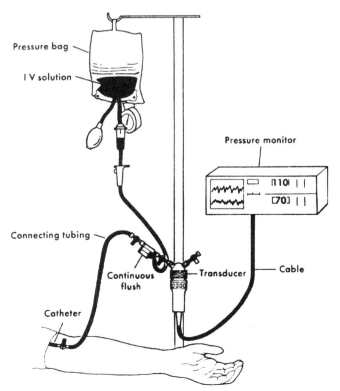

Figure 10.2-8. Typical adult pressure-monitoring set-up.

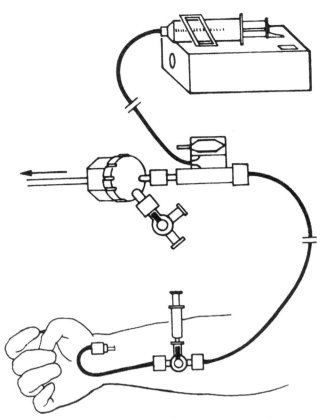

Figure 10.2-9. A neonatal/pediatric pressure-monitoring set-up. Note the absence of a pressurized flush bag, which is replaced by a syringe pump.

Regardless of the cause, shock always results in inadequate tissue perfusion. Although children have less blood than adults, the percent of their weight due to blood volume is greater than in an adult. Therefore, the adverse effects of fluid loss will be realized much quicker in children than in adults. The hemodynamic

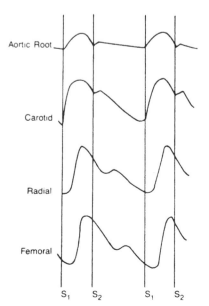

Figure 10.2-10. Different arterial pressure waveforms. S_1 is the aortic valve opening, and S_2 is the valve closing.

changes in patients with shock are that the BP may become variable, the atrial filling pressures (CVP, RA, PAW, and LA) will decrease, and the heart rate will increase. Other factors, such as cardiac output and stroke volume, will also vary depending on the specific type and cause of shock.[7,9]

Many factors, such as various physiologic states, therapies, and treatments, will alter the hemodynamic information as determined by the technology. There are also things, however, that are in no way related to the status of the patient that will also affect the data. Any form of obstruction along the pathway between the tip of the indwelling catheter and the transducer will alter the pressure signal, and thus the waveform and numerical values. Air bubbles and clots located in the tubing-stopcock system are probably the most common causes of damped waveforms. If the catheter tip is resting against the vessel wall, a damped waveform will also result. Leveling of the transducer to heart level (with the exception of an ICP, which is referenced to the middle ear) is critical to hemodynamic accuracy. If the transducer is physically above heart level, a lower than real value will result, and conversely, if the transducer is lower than heart level, a higher value will be obtained. Motion artifact introduced to either the patient or the tubing system will also yield inaccuracies. As mentioned previously, respiratory artifact can have a significant effect on accuracy, and pressure signals that are prone to the effects of respiratory artifact must be measured manually by the clinician to ensure accuracy.

Noninvasive BP can be obtained using different methods, the most common of which are auscultation, palpation, and oscillometry. Palpation and auscultation are two noninvasive methods that can yield varying results with varying users. Auscultation is quite simple. It requires a pressure cuff attached to a sphygmomanometer, a stethoscope, and a listening mechanism, which is usually the observer's ear. The cuff is placed on the upper arm and inflated to a level greater than the patient's typical systolic pressure. The air is gradually bled from the cuff while the stethoscope is used to detect Korotkoff sounds in the brachial artery. The observed pressure at which the first pulsations are detected is the systolic pressure. The observed pressure at the cessation of pulsations is the diastolic pressure. The mean arterial pressure (MAP) can then be calculated by using a simple formula, referred to as the standard triangular estimate.

$$MAP + DP + 1/3 \, (SP - DP)$$

where SP and DP are the systolic and diastolic pressures, respectively.

Palpation is very similar to auscultation. Instead of an observer's ear, it relies on her tactile sense. A pressure cuff is placed as with auscultation (a leg can be substituted for an arm), and a pulse point distal to the cuff is used as the measuring site. The observer inflates the cuff as with auscultation, places one or two fingers on the pulse point, slowly bleeds the air from the cuff, and then notes the pressure at which a pulse is first felt. This is the systolic pressure. Oftentimes a doppler is substituted for an observer's fingers.[6] Obviously, palpation is dependent on the observer's tactile sense, and auscultation is dependent on the observer's ability to hear. Appropriate stethoscope application and the rate of cuff deflation are critical for an accurate reading.[5] Also obvious is that a large degree of inconsistency is likely when using either of these techniques.

Oscillometry, which is dependent on cuff size and cuff placement and is very susceptible to motion artifact, is the most commonly used noninvasive method and is the most consistent and reproducible. Oscillometry is an automated method whereby all of the measurements are determined by a device. The clinician, however, must select the most appropriate cuff size and apply it correctly or the results may be inaccurate. As with the other two techniques, the cuff is inflated to a pressure greater than the patient's systolic, and air is slowly bled from the cuff. The difference is that there is a transducer connected to the cuff via an air hose and this measures the pressure in the cuff. The lowest pressure at which there are maximum oscillations from the pulsations is equal to the mean pressure. Some devices consider systolic pressure to be the value at which two consecutive beats, equal in amplitude, are first detected and diastolic to be the point at which pulsations rapidly diminish in amplitude. Algorithms, however, vary among manufacturers. In addition to motion artifact, oscillometric devices have difficulty obtaining accurate information from patients that are hypotensive or hypertensive.[6]

With all of the described noninvasive techniques, the measured systolic value is for the brachial artery and is typically lower than that measured invasively in the radial artery for various reasons, one of which is that the pulsations that are heard, or the oscillations that are sensed, occur after the artery has begun to reopen. Diastolic pressure is almost always higher with noninvasive methods than with invasive techniques.[10] A reliable device that can provide both an accurate pressure waveform and numerical information would help to eliminate the need for invasive catheters, which, although more accurate, pose the threat of infection and other undesirable complications.

Cardiac Output

Cardiac output (CO) is yet another parameter that is monitored frequently in the critical care setting. Cardiac output is the product of stroke volume (SV) and heart rate.

$$CO \ (liter/min) = SV \ (liter/beat) \times HR \ (beats/min)$$

The SV is the volume of blood that is ejected with each ventricular contraction, or beat. Normal cardiac-output ranges vary from patient to patient. A large patient requires a greater cardiac output than that of a slight patient. A way of normalizing cardiac output to make comparisons between patients is to use the cardiac index (CI), which takes body surface area (BSA) into consideration.

$$CI = CO/BSA$$

During times of increased oxygen demand, such as during exercise in a healthy individual or fever in a sick patient, cardiac output requirements increase. Conversely, when at rest, cardiac output requirements decrease.[8]

Two invasive methods of obtaining CO measurements that are briefly touched on here are the dye indicator dilution method and the thermodilution method. The dye indicator dilution method is not usually used outside of cardiac catheterization areas. A specified amount of dye, usually indocyanine (also known as cardiogreen), is injected intravenously. A densitometer, which is a device that uses spectrophotometry to measure dye concentration over time, is connected to the patient's peripheral artery. As the dye is injected, a steady flow of arterial blood is withdrawn for analysis by the densitometer. The device generates a curve and derives the cardiac output using the Stewart-Hamilton equation.

$$CO = \frac{(l)(60)}{(Cm)(t)} \times \frac{l}{K}$$

where: CO = cardiac output (liter/min)

l = amount of injected dye (mg)

60 = seconds per minute

Cm = mean indicator concentration (mg/liter)

t = mean in seconds of total curve duration

K = calibration factor (mm deflection produced by known concentration of dye)

The most commonly used technique, and the one that is used in all bedside monitors, is thermodilution. This involves injecting a known amount of either iced or room-temperature solution (usually 10 ml in adults and 5 ml in children) into the patient. A flow-directed, balloon-tipped catheter is used for the injectate pathway. The solution is injected into the right atrium, and a thermistor on the catheter tip, located in the PA, monitors the temperature of the blood flowing by. The time of injection is a known, and the time at which the cooler solution passes the thermistor is detected. This period is used in the CO calculation. A modified, somewhat complex, Stewart-Hamilton equation is used to calculate the cardiac output.[7,8]

$$CO = \frac{V(T_B - T_I)}{A} \times \frac{(S_I)(C_I)}{(S_B)(C_B)} \times \frac{(60)(C)(K)}{l}$$

where: CO = cardiac output

V = volume injected

A = area under the thermodilution curve

T_B, T_I = temperature of blood and injectate

S_B, S_I = specific gravity of blood and injectate

C_B, C_I = specific heat of blood and injectate

60 = seconds per minute

C = correction factor

K = calibration constant

Fortunately, the clinician does not need to carry his own calculator for the purpose of performing this calculation. The monitor's software algorithm does this automatically. In addition to performing the calculation, most monitors will create an on-screen array of curves—one per injection. The user can then review the curves and delete those that appear in error, and an average CO value will be calculated based on the acceptable curves.

As with all measurements, CO also has its limitations. Although accurate ($\pm 5\%$), especially with high cardiac outputs, the dye indicator dilution method is somewhat difficult to set up. A pump for withdrawing blood, a densitometer for measuring concentration, and a recorder for curve generation are needed. Delayed injection times, inconsistent blood withdrawal, old dye, and incomplete injection can all cause erroneous readings. Also, the densitometer requires calibration to ensure results. Thermodilution is fast and easy, and multiple measurements can be performed at one time. At least 1 minute should be allowed between injections to ensure adequate remixing and temperature stabilization. As with the dye method, proper injection is critical. Each injection must be smooth and timely. Improper catheter and thermistor placement will also contribute to false readings. The curves should always be critiqued by the clinician before the data are accepted. Judgment on the part of the clinician is crucial when obtaining cardiac output information.

Conclusion

Accurate, noninvasive monitoring should become one of the foci for bedside monitoring in neonatal and pediatric environments. There are many parameters that, if monitored noninvasively, would increase the quality of care for all patients, particularly neonatal and pediatric patients. Without the support from manufacturers, however, these devices may never be designed and implemented. Unfortunately, in the past, many companies have felt that the neonatal and pediatric patient areas are too small a portion of the overall marketplace, and that it is not financially attractive to dedicate extensive resources in these areas. Corporate attitudes among manufacturers have been changing, however, and over the past few years more interest has been expressed for technology specifically designed for these patients.

Bedside monitoring technology has experienced tremendous changes over the past 3 decades. In fact, the monitors used during the 1960s and 1970s in some ways bear no resemblance to those used today. Not only have advances in technology enabled more measurements to be monitored, but also the information obtained is more accurate, consistent, and is presented and used in many more ways. Manufacturers that are involved with new technologies have a tremendous responsibility to design devices that are user friendly, cost-efficient, reliable, physically desirable, and above all, accurate. An equal, if not greater, responsibility also rests with those who apply the technology. An individual who does not understand the limitations of a device, and therefore does not understand the potential inaccuracies, should not be applying the technology nor interpreting the results. It is unfortunate when individuals accept information at face value without asking some questions, the most basic of which is, does this make sense? — a simple question, yet one that often goes without mention. This chapter was not written with the intent of providing answers. The hope was to provoke and encourage the asking of questions. In the future, technology will continue to change and, it is hoped, improve. Coupled with the guidance and sound judgment of knowledgeable clinicians, patient care will continue to change and improve as well.

References

1. ECRI. Infant home apnea monitors. *Health Devices* 16:79–109, 1987.
2. Warburton D, Stark A, Taeusch HW. Apnea monitor failure in infants with upper airway obstruction. *Pediatrics* 60:742–744, 1977.
3. Brouillette RT et al. Comparison of respiratory inductive plethysmography and thoracic impedance for apnea monitoring. *J Pediatr* 111:377–383, 1987.
4. Staewen W. Apnea monitoring basics. *Biomed Instr Technol* 25:322–323, 1991.
5. Geddes LA. *Handbook of Blood Pressure Measurement.* Clifton, NJ: Humana, 1991.
6. Kacmarek RM, Hess D, Stoller JK. *Monitoring in Respiratory Care.* St. Louis: Mosby, 1993.
7. Daily EK, Schroeder JS. *Techniques in Bedside Hemodynamic Monitoring.* St. Louis: Mosby, 1985.
8. Price MS, Fox JD. *Hemodynamic Monitoring in Critical Care.* Rockville, MD: Aspen, 1987.
9. Mayer TA. *Emergency Management of Pediatric Trauma.* Philadelphia: Saunders, 1985.
10. Venus et al. Direct versus indirect blood pressure measurements in critically ill patients. *Heart Lung* May 14:228–231, 1985.

Willam M. Kauffman

Dorothy I. Bulas

Carlos J. Sivit

David C. Kushner

11 ▶ Radiologic Imaging

The purpose of this chapter is to provide an overview of current trends in diagnostic and therapeutic imaging of the severely ill or injured child who requires intensive care. This chapter will interrelate two topics: specific imaging technologies and the clinical situations in which they are essential. The discussion will include standard methods such as film images as well as the newer types of imaging such as doppler ultrasound and magnetic resonance. Examples of clinical situations that require imaging support in the intensive care unit (ICU) will include sepsis, renal failure, trauma, neurologic catastrophe, and acquired immune deficiency syndrome.

Technologies

Standard Film Technology

Despite the advent of sophisticated new technologies, standard film roentgenography remains essential for the evaluation of severely ill children. Film roentgenography requires that ionizing radiation be passed through the patient. The image is formed by variable attenuation of the x-ray beam passing through the patient's body to encounter the x-ray screen (cassette) and film. Compared with other types of imaging, film roentgenography has unique and important strengths. For example, performing the examination is safe and relatively easy. The mobile x-ray device is relatively small and easy to maneuver in the confines of the ICU. Furthermore, the so-called spatial resolution of film roentgenography (the physical terminology for the ability to see small or difficult abnormalities) is superior to any other imaging modality. The disadvantages of standard film roentgenography are those of relatively low-contrast resolution (or the ability to see abnormalities that are not very different from normal tissues), the difficulty of predicting how many photons will be needed to form an image of excellent quality (or how much voltage and amperage to be selected on the machine), and the necessity of exposing the patient to radiation in any instance.

The most frequently ordered standard film roentgenographs that are performed in the pediatric intensive care unit (PICU) are examinations of the chest and abdomen. On these examinations, the physician can determine the position of tubes, catheters, and appliances such as endotracheal tubes, nasogastric tubes, central venous catheters, thoracotomy tubes, parenchymal lung changes, or spontaneous pneumothorax (Figs. 11-1–11-4). It should be cautioned that in making these determinations, the physician must be assured that a full inspiratory film was obtained because a film obtained at expiratory lung volume may imitate parenchymal disease. Bilateral decubitus films (horizontal x-ray beam through a patient who is positioned on his side) may be used to produce an inspiration in one lung while causing the other lung to deflate. In this instance, the dependent lung will be underinflated (a reasonable test for emphysema) and the nondependent lung will demonstrate full volume inspiration. Standard roentgenographs are also useful for the diagnosis of complications of intensive care and respiratory therapy, including pneumothorax, pneumopericardium, pneumomediastinum, pneumoperitoneum, and subcutaneous emphysema (Fig. 11-5). Abdominal roentgenography may be useful in diagnosing pneumoperitoneum (Fig. 11-6) (particularly if a lateral cross-table horizontal beam film is performed). Also, abdominal roentgenography may permit the diagnosis of paralytic ileus or mechanical bowel obstruction by the demonstration of areas of bowel dilatation in the presence in the first instance of gas in the rectum. This specific observation

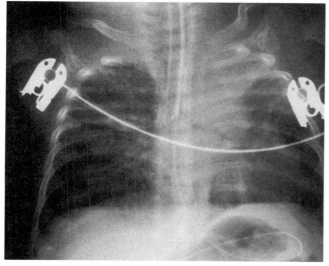

Figure 11-1. An endotracheal tube is seen in the right mainstem bronchus with associated collapse of the left upper lobe.

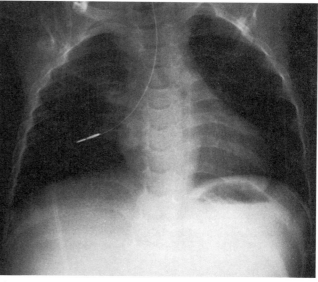

Figure 11-2. A PH probe is seen in the right bronchial system.

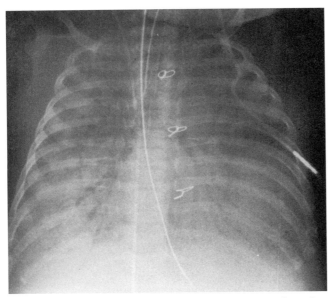

Figure 11-3.   Diffuse opacification of the lungs with air bronchograms in a patient with pulmonary edema.

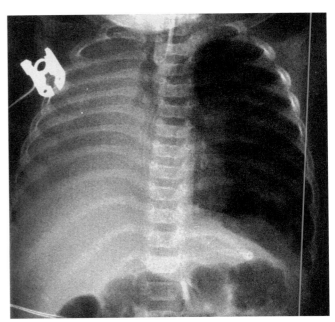

Figure 11-5.   Collapse of the right lung with shift of the mediastinum to the right and hyperinflation of the left lung.

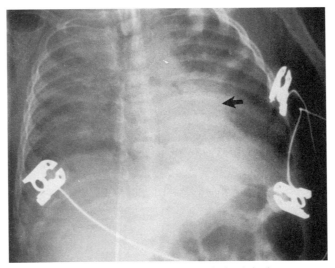

Figure 11-4.   A triangle opacity is seen behind the heart, representing left lower lobe atelectasis or consolidation *(arrow).*

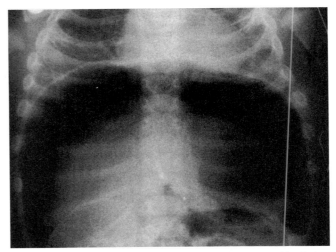

Figure 11-6.   A large pneumoperitoneum is seen with air between the diaphragm and the liver.

may be made more reliably on prone rather than supine examination. Ischemic bowel may contain areas of submucosal hemorrhage that may be recognized as classic **thumb-printing** or localized, rounded, small thickenings of the mucosal outline. Also, the absence of haustral markings that can normally be observed along the outline of the colon may alert one to the presence of inflammation or enteritis. The position of an indwelling tube or catheter can be verified by roentgenography following careful, sterile injection of the tube with an appropriate isotonic, water-soluble contrast agent such as dilute sodium diatrizoate. This technique may be used for locating a central vascular catheter, gastrostomy tube, or enterostomy tube. The technique may be used to evaluate either the patency of the tube itself

or possibility of obstruction or occlusion of the vessel or viscus in which the tube or catheter is located.

Ultrasound

Ultrasound is an imaging modality that uses high-frequency sound waves to produce an image. The sound beam is generated by a single crystal with piezoelectric properties. That is, the crystal is able to convert electrical current to a vibration that is emitted at the frequency of inaudible sound (3 to 10 MHz). This single crystal generates the initial sound beam and then subsequently receives the sound echoes from the part of the body that is under examination. The time that elapses between transmission and reception of the sound waves is used by the ultrasound computer to determine the position of the abnormality being studied, and the strength of the returning echo (amplitude) is used to determine the brightness of the image (shades of gray).

Ultrasound has become an essential, relatively common component of pediatric intensive care imaging, with many clear benefits to the patient. The examination requires no special patient preparation or sedation. **Real-time** ultrasound provides literally instant visualization of anatomic detail, providing the examiner with an infinite combination of views. Also, the motion of the part that is being examined, such as the diaphragm or heart, is shown by real-time ultrasound. There is no ionizing radiation involved and thus no concern about radiation safety. Finally, most modern high-quality ultrasound devices are mobile, easy to move, and relatively small.

One characteristic of ultrasound is that it is **operator-dependent.** This may be viewed as either an advantage or a disadvantage. Specially trained and skilled technologists and physicians are necessary to assure that the patient receives the best possible examination (Fig. 11-7).

The selection of appropriate equipment is an important factor in the performance of a high-quality examination. A variety of transducers may be used to maximize the diagnostic information. Choice of inappropriate transducer frequency may result in inadequate display of superficial or deep structures. In practice, higher frequency transducers are associated with greater detail resolution but less penetrating power. Alternatively, transducers of lower frequency have greater penetration but lower spatial resolution. At any frequency, ultrasound is unable to penetrate gas, including gas-filled bowel and lung, bony structures, and calcification. Therefore, the limitations of ultrasound must be taken into account when chosen as the method to evaluate intensive care patients. For instance, gaseous distention of the abdomen is common in patients who are maintained on mechanical ventilation. This may preclude the use of ultrasound for the evaluation of the pancreas due to overlying gas in the transverse colon and small bowel.

Computerized Tomography

Computerized tomography (CT) requires that ionizing radiation be passed through the patient, where it is partially attenuated in a manner similar to standard roentgenography. The image is formed by the portion of the x-ray beam that passes through the patient. Unlike standard roentgenography, the x-ray beam is received by solid-state electronic detector crystals rather than a cassette containing a screen and sheet of film. The fundamental concept behind CT is that the internal structure of the body can be visualized if multiple beams of x-ray are passed through the patient and detected in circular image.[1] The absorption of the x-ray beam by the patient determines the level of gray scale (brightness) in the image.

CT allows one to see objects that are approximately 1 mm in diameter (spatial resolution). Thus, in comparison, CT is inferior to standard roentgenography that can be used routinely to identify abnormalities that are submillimeter in size. This is exemplified in the clinical situation of attempting to detect small pulmonary nodules or pneumonias. In this instance the **partial volume artifact** may occur as two separate objects that are present in the lung very close together at a separation distance that may be less than the millimeter spatial resolving power of the scanner. When this artifact occurs, the two small objects in question may be displayed as a single object that consists of an **average** of the two original lesions. On the other hand, CT is far superior to other modalities, except magnetic resonance imaging, in the characteristic of **contrast** resolution. This superior contrast resolution has the effect of permitting the detection of abnormalities that may be very similar to normal tissues in absorption of x-rays (density), regardless of the size of the abnormalities.

CT images are cross-sectional in nature, usually oriented in the

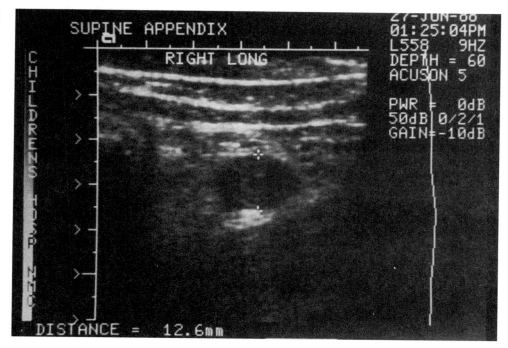

Figure 11-7. The lucent round structure represents a portion of a noncompressible appendix—a sign consistent with an inflamed, diseased appendix—hence appendicitis.

axial plane, particularly in patients that are severely ill. Virtually any part of the body can be imaged (Fig. 11-8). In contrast to ultrasound, high-quality CT images can be performed with little **operator dependency.** The performance of the images is governed primarily by the technology. Nevertheless, specific training and experience are required to be assured that the imaging technique and use of contrast media are appropriate for the clinical problem posed by the patient.

There are some significant disadvantages to CT that should be considered when dealing with the intensive care patient, not the least of which is the requirement for transporting the very ill child out of the intensive care environment to the room that houses the scanner. Also, CT scanning requires that the patient remain relatively motionless for short periods, and thus the administration of sedation for control of involuntary movements must be considered. Artifacts can significantly reduce the diagnostic quality of the image. Motion-induced artifacts can be recognized as **streak** or star-like lines radiating through the image. There may be a **ring** artifact that can occur if the x-ray detectors are not properly calibrated. Degradation of the image may also occur from **beam-hardening** that results from preferential absorption of low-energy x-rays, usually by bony structures such as the occiput or temporal bone. This type of artifact can interfere with visualization of abnormalities in the posterior or middle cranial fossa. The final disadvantage of CT concerns the necessity to expose the patient to ionizing radiation. Although acceptable by all practice guidelines and regulations, the radiation dose from CT is among the highest administered during diagnostic imaging. The actual level of radiation exposure depends on the type of CT scanner used and the number and thickness of the sectional images that are performed.[1]

Nuclear Medicine Modality

Nuclear medicine is a widely used imaging modality that is of significant value in pediatric intensive care. Nuclear medicine techniques can be used to evaluate many abnormalities of body systems, including brain, kidney, liver, heart, lungs, bone, and leukocytes. The examination consists of the administration to the patient of a pharmaceutical agent that has been labeled with a radioactive substance such as Technicium 99m. Each radiopharmaceutical agent is selected specifically for its ability to attach to or reflect the function of a specific organ system, such as the brain or liver. The radiopharmaceutical agents may be injected or administered via any appropriate route. An image is obtained after positioning the patient under a nuclear camera (gamma camera) that consists of detector crystals that are linked to an imaging computer system. Images of the organ can be performed in any projection that is permitted by the condition of the patient. Advantages of this technique include the dual ability to image structure and measure function. In addition, some nuclear equipment is relatively mobile although quite large. Therefore, in selected patients whose condition might be quite fragile, the examination can be performed in the ICU without moving the patient. Disadvantages of the nuclear technique include the requirement for the administration of substances that emit ionizing radiation. Although within the guidelines and regulations for allowable exposure, there must be clear benefit to the patient before any such exposure is made. Also, many examinations take a relatively long time to perform, occasionally necessitating sedation of the patient to control motion.

A comprehensive discussion of all types of nuclear medicine scanning that may be relevant to pediatric intensive care is

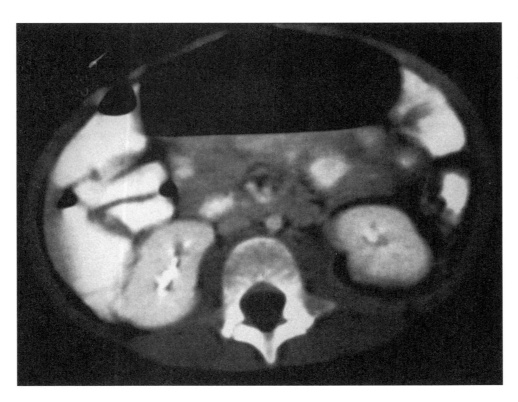

Figure 11-8. CT scan of abdomen—standard view with left kidney on right of image. Air around the left kidney is seen, indicating a perinephric abscess.

beyond the scope of this chapter. Several examples, however, may demonstrate both the relevance and practicality of the techniques. These examples include brain scanning, renal scanning, and scanning for the localization of suspected abdominal abscesses (Fig. 11-9).

Brain scanning can be used in the evaluation of patients who are brain injured and suspected of brain death. For this examination, the most commonly used radiopharmaceutical is sodium pertechnetate labeled with Technicium 99m, although newer agents are being investigated. The radiopharmaceutical is injected intravenously after which it is virtually confined to the vascular compartments within the brain. In the circumstance of brain death, there is no arterial perfusion of the brain, and thus no isotope would be seen in the normal vascular distribution. Patients who fulfill the definition of brain death exhibit virtually no cerebral radioactivity or radioactivity in the superior sagittal sinus.[2] Thus a nuclear medicine study that demonstrates absence of brain perfusion can add credence and support to the appropriate clinical and electroencephalogic evidence of brain death.[3–5]

Renal function can be evaluated with nuclear medicine techniques in the PICU. Common applications of this technique occur in patients who have renal failure or hypertension. Commonly used radiopharmaceutical agents are Technicium 99m–labeled DTPA (diethylenetriamine-pentacetic acid) and Technicium 99m–labeled DMSA (dimercaptosuccinic acid). TcDPTA is excreted rapidly from the bloodstream by glomerular filtration. It can be used, therefore, to evaluate renal perfusion, glomerular function, and the integrity of the renal collecting systems. TcDMSA is initially bound to plasma protein, after which it is absorbed by the renal tubules and subsequently excreted via an active transport mechanism. Therefore, TcDMSA is useful in imaging the structure of the renal cortex as well as the function of the cortical active excretion mechanism.[6] Inflammation and abscesses can be evaluated with the use of several agents, including Gallium 67– and Indium 111–labeled leukocytes.

Gallium 67 citrate is a radiopharmaceutical that emits gamma radiation that is detectable with standard nuclear cameras. Gallium has been shown empirically to localize in inflammatory processes, abscesses, and some tumors. The mechanism of gallium labeling is largely unknown, although possible routes include uptake by leukocytes, extracellular lactoferrin, or directly in the bacteria.[6]

Indium 111–labelled leukocytes have been used infrequently in children, but they have been shown to be effective in the localization of acute inflammatory conditions and abscesses in the adult patient. Indium 111–labeled leukocytes will probably be shown to be as effective for abscess localization in children as it is in adults. However, Indium 111 has the disadvantage of relatively high radiation dose, particularly when compared with gallium.[7]

Interventional Radiology

Interventional procedures that are guided by imaging techniques are not a standard of practice in caring for severely ill children. The development of high-resolution computed tomography, real-time high-resolution ultrasound, and variable projection fluoroscopy (C-arm) has made it possible to image and localize abnormalities with an accuracy and precision that was previously unknown. Also, the development of fine-bore aspiration and biopsy needles, in addition to new catheter materials and design, has encouraged the widespread application of the percutaneous image-guided approach for abscesses and fluid collections that were previously thought to require surgery[8] (Fig. 11-10).

Procedures that require CT or fluoroscopy must be performed in the interventional imaging suite of the radiology department, unless the ICU is specially equipped. Interventional procedures using ultrasound guidance can be performed at the bedside if patient condition dictates and the abnormality is visible and the approach clear and safe. The patient must be supervised and monitored carefully. ECG, pulse oximetry, and BP monitoring devices are frequently used. A specially trained radiology nurse is also important; duties frequently include patient coordination, communication with parents, administration of medications, moni-

Figure 11-9. Gallium scan. Arrow indicates an area of decreased uptake surrounded by increased uptake (doughnut shape) indicating a buttock abscess.

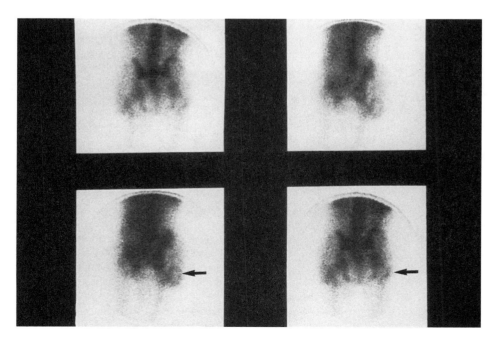

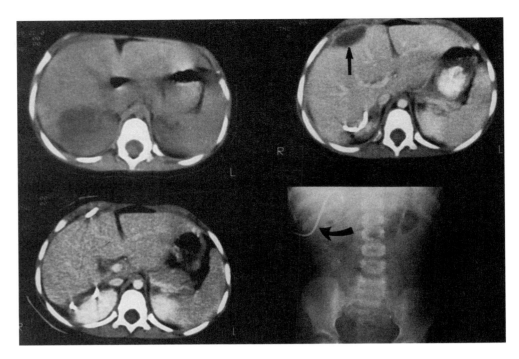

Figure 11-10. Fluid is seen between the liver and diaphragm, representing a subphrenic abscess *(straight arrow)*. Note also the percutaneous catheter in the right upper quadrant for drainage *(curved arrow)*.

toring during the procedure, and assistance with the follow-up care.[9]

In one large study, the results of 104 interventional procedures were reviewed. The procedures included 50 nephrostomies, 11 ureteral or urethral dilations, 8 internal ureteral stent placements, 8 percutaneous transluminal renal angioplasties, 6 drainages of perirenal fluid collections, 4 vascular embolizations for hemorrhage, 4 percutaneous removals of calculi, 3 percutaneous pyeloplasties, 2 placements of circular tubes for drainage of fluid, and 2 renal biopsies of focal lesions. Ninety-five percent of the procedures were concluded to be either curative or beneficial. None of the patients was jeopardized by the procedures.[9]

Contraindications for percutaneous interventional procedures that are performed in the imaging department include inability to adequately visualize the suspected abnormality, lack of a safe route for needle placement, and the presence of an incorrectable coagulopathy.[8] Percutaneous procedures may prevent the necessity for standard surgical procedures that require general anesthesia. When performed with the support of colleagues from the department of surgery, percutaneous interventional imaging procedures can be of benefit to a significant number of children in intensive care situations.

Magnetic Resonance Imaging Modality

Magnetic resonance imaging (MRI) is a new and essential component in the care of severely ill children. The MRI scanner is physically similar to a CT scanner except for the longer length and more tubular shape of the circle in which the patient is positioned. MR images are formed by the use of a large, strong magnet in conjunction with a radiofrequency transmitter. The control of the magnetic fields, the timing and shape of the radiofrequency pulses, and the formation of the images on detection of signals that are emitted from the patient are facilitated by a powerful computer system. The MR image is formed by the interaction of the magnetic fields and radiofrequency pulses with the protons of tissue water. When the patient is positioned in the scanner, tissue protons become aligned with the magnetic moment of the machine. Subsequently, there is activation of radiofrequency pulses that are absorbed by and perturb the protons. On cessation of the radiofrequency pulses, the patient's protons become realigned with the original magnetic moment of the machine as they emit signals that can be detected by the scanner. These signals are then reconstructed by the MRI computer to form an image (Fig. 11-11).

There are many advantages of MRI scanning. MRI does not use ionizing radiation. There are no known harmful biological effects at the energy levels that are used in clinical patient scanning.[10] Unlike CT, the cross-sectional scan planes may be obtained directly in virtually any orientation without varying the position of the patient or sacrificing image quality. The contrast resolution is superior to all other imaging modalities. Finally, MRI can image the position of blood vessels due to the fact that moving blood generates no detectable standard MRI signal, and thus the vessel appears as a void (flow-void phenomenon).

MRI also has three major disadvantages. First, patient motion can be a problem that causes degradation of the image. Patients must remain motionless, except for respiration, for relatively long periods. Many pediatric patients require sedation and careful observation. Second, many metal materials (ferromagnetic) cannot be permitted in the scanner room. These metals would be physically drawn into the scanner by the strong magnetic force. This disadvantage has either precluded the use of MRI in patients who are supported by respiratory, standard monitors, and other life-support equipment or made it very inconvenient by requiring manual ventilatory assistance and monitoring. Recently, prototype nonferromagnetic respiratory and standard monitors have been developed that may make it more convenient and safe for intensive care patients to be evaluated with MRI.[11] The final disadvantage is that

Figure 11-11. A cardiac-gated MRI with measurement of the aortic root in a patient with Marfan's syndrome.

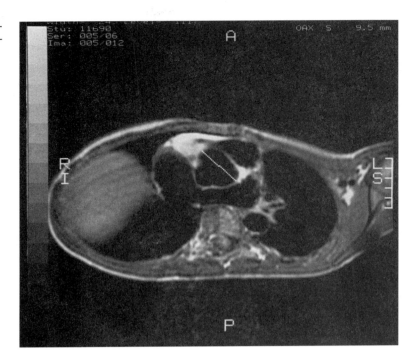

standard MRI proton imaging does not detect signal from cortical bone. Therefore, orthopedic applications are related to evaluation of bone marrow and cartilage rather than the traditional evaluation of bone cortex.

Clinical Situations

It is important to note that imaging in the PICU is a single component of a multifactorial evaluation process that must take place constantly. Indications for the performance of an imaging study must be individualized to each patient's clinical problem and status. History, physical examination, and laboratory values are essential data in making decisions about imaging. Any form of imaging by protocol, algorithm, or daily routine will lead to overutilization of procedures, unnecessary exposure to imaging energy, and a less thoughtful standard of patient care.

Sepsis

Fever of unknown origin is a common problem in the PICU, especially involving the postoperative patient. Imaging modalities that may be appropriate include standard roentgenography, computerized axial tomography, and nuclear medicine.

Standard roentgenography is the most frequently used method for evaluating the septic child. Chest roentgenograph may show a consolidation of the lung parenchyma or loculated fluid in the pleural space (Fig. 11-12). Abdominal roentgenography may show gas-fluid levels or a localized ileus (sentinel ileus), suggesting the presence of localized inflammatory disease such as that associated with pancreatitis or appendicitis. Mechanical bowel obstruction may be shown by dilatation of small bowel without sufficient gas seen in the distal colon.

Ultrasound may be used to supplement information provided

Figure 11-12. Before-and-after treatment images of a pulmonic abscess. Note fluid level in left upper lobe on first examination.

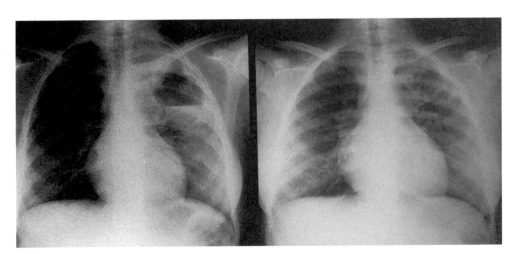

by standard roentgenography, particularly when examining the abdomen. Intraperitoneal and extraperitoneal fluid collections, such as empyema in the basal pleural space or basal lung abscess, subphrenic abscess, the subhepatic abscess, and the pelvic abscess, can be recognized. An abscess has the appearance of a partly cystic (lucent) mass that is surrounded by a thick, echogenic periphery and contains internal **echos,** which suggest that there is more than simple clear fluid present (e.g., exudate).

CT has proven to be somewhat more effective than ultrasound in evaluating the septic patient. This is due largely to the ability of CT to produce diagnostic images in all patients as long as motion is controlled. Certainly, ultrasound is the first line of evaluation because it can be performed easily at the bedside. However, sound waves are attenuated by bowel gas and the presence of large amounts of gas frequently present in children who are maintained on assisted ventilation. This situation can severely limit the effectiveness of ultrasound examination. Therefore, it may be reasonable to elect to transport the patient to the CT scanner, with its attendant risk and inconvenience. Abscesses may have different appearances on CT scan. Usually they are recognized as lucent fluid collections that are surrounded by thick borders that may enhance following the administration of intravenous contrast medium. Gas may be present in the center of the lesion, suggesting an area of necrosis. When an intraabdominal abscess is recognized by any modality, prompt therapy may be instituted by percutaneous drainage. CT can also be used to investigate other areas of the body that may be the source of fever of unknown origin. Examples include the deep compartments of the neck, the paranasal sinuses, and the intracranial area.

Occasionally, the site of infection is not demonstrated by roentgenograph, ultrasound, or CT. In these circumstances, gallium scanning or Indium 111 leukocyte scanning should be considered. Indium 111–labeled leukocytes have been shown to be effective in localizing infections in adult patients. The sensitivity of the labeled leukocyte technique has been reported to vary from 73% to 93%, and the specificity from 91% to 98%.[7] Gallium scanning has been shown to have a higher sensitivity (true positive frequency) but a lower specificity than the leukocyte technique. Considerations of radiation exposure usually lead radiologists to recommend gallium scanning in children in preference to Indium 111–labeled leukocytes. For selected patients, the higher radiation exposure of the leukocyte technique may be indicated.[7]

Renal Insufficiency

Modern methods for the imaging evaluation of renal function include ultrasound and nuclear medicine. The initial evaluation is usually by ultrasound for determination of the structure of the renal parenchyma and to exclude obstructive uropathy as a cause of renal failure. After the kidneys are shown to be structurally normal, nuclear medicine and/or Doppler ultrasound techniques are considered.

Nuclear medicine scanning can be used to evaluate renal structure, perfusion, and function. The most commonly used radiopharmaceutical agent for renal imaging is TcDPTA. Renal function can be determined by quantification of the uptake of TcDPTA in the kidneys relative to uptake of the agent by the liver and soft tissues. Images and quantitative counts of the kidneys are made immediately following injection during the perfusion phase as well as during the later phases that demonstrate renal parenchymal structure and excretion. Children who have renal insufficiency

will show a relatively high **background** activity due to delay in or decreased excretion of the circulating radiopharmaceutical. There is also delayed or decreased excretion of the circulating radiopharmaceutical, as well as delayed or decreased activity in the bladder. TcDTPA can normally be visualized in the renal pelves and ureters as early as 5 minutes after the injection. Children who have decreased renal function from any cause may not begin to excrete the radiopharmaceutical until more than 5 minutes after injection. Severe renal insufficiency may be associated with the delay of excretion for as much as 10 to 15 minutes.

Children who have undergone renal transplantation frequently require intensive care. The evaluation of the child who may have renal transplant rejection includes both nuclear medicine and Doppler ultrasound techniques. The abnormalities that can be shown with nuclear medicine in acute transplant rejection are decreased perfusion, decreased parenchymal uptake, and decreased excretion. These abnormalities are similar to those seen in children who have acute tubular necrosis (ATN). The differential diagnosis between ATN and acute transplant rejection is made by evidence of prolonged decreased function, which is more characteristic of acute transplant rejection than ATN, which usually demonstrates only transient decreased function.[6]

Doppler ultrasound has an increasingly important role in the diagnosis of acute transplant rejection. Standard grey-scale ultrasound is valuable in the evaluation of possible complications of transplantation surgery, such as postoperative urinary obstruction, urinoma, and lymphocele formation. Doppler ultrasound can show changes in the pattern of blood flow in the arcuate arteries of the kidney that may be associated with transplant rejection. Doppler ultrasound studies of acute renal transplant rejection in children can reliably predict the abnormalities found at renal biopsy. Acute transplant rejection may be suggested by Doppler ultrasound evidence of an alteration of the Doppler waveform characterized by an increase in pulsatility accompanied by a decrease in diastolic flow. Unfortunately, this pattern has also been reported in ATN, and therefore the Doppler ultrasound abnormalities may prove to be incompletely distinctive.[12]

Trauma

Trauma is the leading cause of death in the United States in children who are more than 1 year of age. Children who undergo nonfatal trauma are frequently patients in ICU.

Abdominal Trauma

Abdominal trauma in children can result in rupture of a hollow viscus such as the duodenum or injury or rupture of a solid organ such as liver, spleen, or kidney. Such injuries can lead to pneumoperitoneum, hemoperitoneum, or urinoma formation. Children who have undergone significant injury are frequently cared for in the ICU. In these children, significant injuries always raise the consideration of possible surgical exploration, the decision for which requires careful clinical and imaging evaluation.

Ultrasound and nuclear medicine studies can be partially diagnostic in the child who has significant abdominal injury. This may be particularly valuable if the child cannot be moved to the CT scanner. In almost all instances, however, CT is the imaging procedure of choice. CT is the technique that has the highest likelihood of demonstrating the wide range of abnormalities that may occur.

CT has largely replaced diagnostic peritoneal lavage in the evaluation of the stable child who has undergone abdominal trauma. CT reliably and rapidly shows intraperitoneal or retroperitoneal hemorrhages with or without rupture or laceration of the liver, spleen, kidney, or pancreas.[13-21] CT is less reliable in demonstrating injury to bowel or mesentery.[15,18,22,23] The administration of intravenous contrast medium is essential in diagnosing injuries to solid organs. This is because acute intraparenchymal or subcapsular hemorrhage may have the same appearance (isodense) as the normal organ parenchyma or adjacent normal bowel (Fig. 11-13). Careful physiologic monitoring must be performed during the examination. Frequently, sedation must be administered to minimize patient movement. The surgical decision for laparotomy is based on the physiologic condition of the child, supplemented by the extent of anatomic injury that has been shown on CT.[17,20]

Craniocerebral Trauma

After physical examination and laboratory evaluation, CT is the most important step in evaluation of the child who has undergone head trauma. CT has dramatically affected the care of the head-injured child. CT rapidly and reliably demonstrates hemorrhage, particularly subdural, epidural, and intraparenchymal hematomas, and facilitates identification of children who will need surgery.[24-29] Depressed skull fractures can be shown on CT as overriding bony edges or indentation of the skull. High-velocity acceleration and deceleration injuries may cause white matter axons to shear and tear.[30,31] These shearing injuries most commonly occur at the interfaces between grey and white matter, the corpus collosum, basal ganglia, and brain stem. Injury to the axonal system may be accompanied by hemorrhage that can be shown by CT.[32] Nonhemorrhagic axonal disruption, however, is not well demonstrated by CT.[30,33]

MRI has been shown to be very sensitive in detecting most cerebral traumatic injuries.[34-37] MRI offers several imaging advantages in evaluating CNS injury. MRI is superior to CT in detecting intra- and extracranial hemorrhages, except for subarachnoid hemorrhage. This is due to the unique sign of characteristics of blood as well as the multiplanar imaging capability of MRI.[34-36,38,39] Axonal disruption may not be apparent on CT, while areas of high signal intensity are clearly seen on MRI due to the increased water content of the edema.[40] MRI is superior to CT in detecting brain stem injuries, due to the bony artifact caused on CT by the skull base; MRI also surpasses CT in its multiplanar capability.[38] In a similar fashion, MRI is superior to CT in the identification of acute spinal cord injury.[31-44] Epidural hematomas, parenchymal cord injury, and cervical disc herniation can be clearly shown on sagittal MRI images. Although MRI is superior to CT in demonstrating soft tissue and spinal cord injury, CT is superior to MRI in the detection of bony injury to the spine, particularly with three-dimensional reconstruction. In the circumstance of suspected spinal fracture, CT myelography is the only effective method of demonstrating small bony fragments that may lie within the spinal canal.[43]

In a practical sense, the intensive care physician should be aware of the effectiveness of both CT and MRI in the care of the child who has sustained significant trauma. The use of MRI in the acute situation has been limited due to limited availability of MRI instrumentation and the lack of life support and monitoring systems that allowed these patients to be studied in safety. Such systems are presently being developed. In current practice, MRI is important for the follow-up, especially when the patient's status does not correlate with CT findings.

Child Abuse

CT and MRI have become essential tools for the evaluation of the child who is suspected of having undergone abuse[45-52] (Fig. 11-14). Shaking causes injury to the brain by alternating acceleration and deceleration which cause shearing of parenchyma, rupture of bridging veins, and subdural hematoma formation. As in

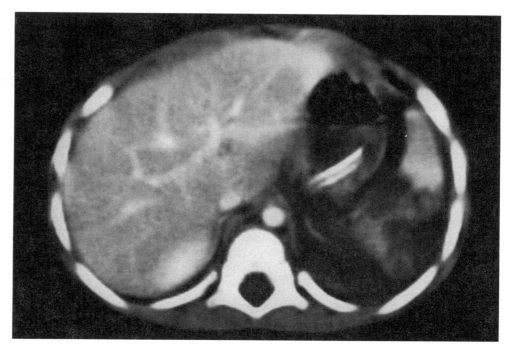

Figure 11-13. CT with intravenous contrast demonstrates a splenic laceration with surrounding hematoma. Note portions of normally homogeneously enhancing spleen on right side of the image. Hematoma is posterior to this area.

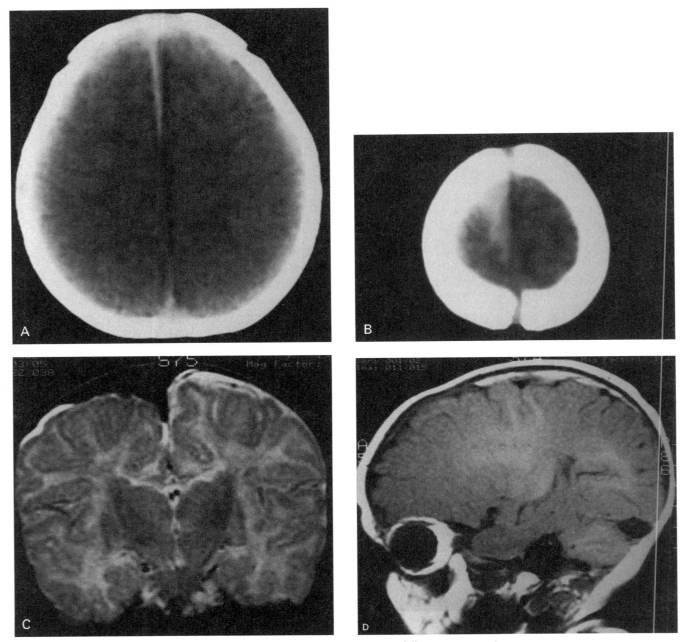

Figure 11-14. Four-month-old infant presented to the emergency room following an apneic episode. **(A, B)** CT demonstrates a small collection of blood over the right convexity and interhemispheric fissure. **(C, D)** MRI more clearly demonstrates fluid along the convexities of both hemispheres. This fluid contains layers of both high and low signal consistent with acute and chronic subdural hematomas. Findings are suggestive of abuse.

other forms of injury, CT is more effective in demonstrating acute subarachnoid hemorrhage and detecting skull fracture. White matter injuries caused by shearing effects of child abuse may be shown only by MRI.[50,51] A unique characteristic of MRI is that there is a change in the characteristics of the MRI signal from blood as it ages and becomes liquified. Therefore, subdural effusions can be estimated as being acute, subacute, or chronic, with injuries of differing ages identified. The existence of lesions of differing ages may suggest that the child has been abused repeatedly.

Thoracic Trauma

Chest injury frequently coexists in the child who has abdominal or craniocerebral injuries.[53–56] Standard chest roentgenography provides useful information on the presence of pleural, parenchymal, mediastinal, or bony injury. CT of the chest may be necessary to distinguish parenchymal injury or consolidation from pleural fluid accumulation. Injury to the tracheobronchial tree and mediastinum can also be evaluated most effectively with CT. Careful evaluation of the lower chest when abdominal CT examination

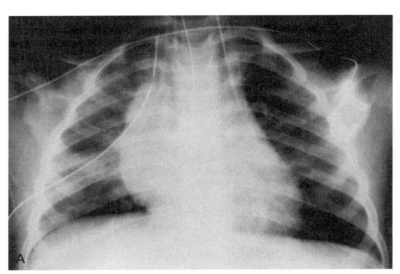
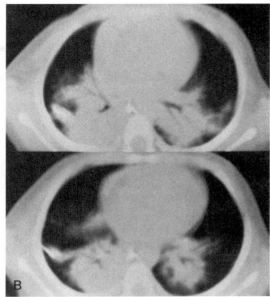

Figure 11-15. **(A)** AP chest radiograph of a 12-year-old injured in a motor vehicle accident demonstrates a small, patchy area of parenchymal density in the right mid-lung field. The left lung appears normal. **(B)** CT of the chest in the same patient demonstrates bilateral pulmonary contusions. The left contusion was not seen on the chest radiograph. Note the ill-defined borders and nonsegmental appearance of the contusions.

is performed may demonstrate occult pneumothorax or injury to the pulmonary parenchyma[57,58] (Fig. 11-15).

Acquired Immunodeficiency Syndrome

The principle complications of the acquired immunodeficiency syndrome (AIDS) that may be encountered in the ICU are respiratory failure, renal failure, and severe gastrointestinal disease. Imaging plays an important role in the evaluation of children who have these abnormalities.

Respiratory Failure

Respiratory failure is the most common cause of death in children who have AIDS.[54,55] These children may have pneumonia caused by *Pneumocystis carinii*, bacteria, viruses, or multisystem failure due to generalized bacterial sepsis. The most common associated organism is pneumocystis.[59-61] Pneumocystis may be found in association with other opportunistic agents, including cytomegalovirus (CMV), mycobacterium avium-intracellular (MAI), and *Candida*.[62] Chest roentgenography may be normal during the early period of clinical disease, followed by rapid evolution of diffuse parenchymal consolidation. The roentgenographic progression frequently begins as subtle, diffuse interstitial opacities that are followed by a coalescent, air-space consolidative process[63,64] (Fig. 11-16). These children usually manifest low (expiratory) lung volumes due to interstitial disease and low pulmonary compliance. It is not possible to differentiate PCP from other opportunistic agents or from lymphocytic interstitial pneumonitis (LIP) without the aid of lung biopsy.[65] High oxygen concentrations and mechanical ventilation may be required. These may lead to complications, including adult respiratory distress syndrome, interstitial emphysema, pneumomediastinum, and pneumothorax.[66,67] Severe bacterial pneumonia may be caused by Gram-negative bacteria,

particularly *Pseudomonas* or *Klebsiella*.[62,68] The chest roentgenography usually shows lobar or segmental consolidation, with or without pleural fluid, that is distinct from the appearance of opportunistic infection.

Severe Gastrointestinal Tract Disease

The gastrointestinal tract is the second most commonly affected site in children who have AIDS.[69] Opportunistic infection may

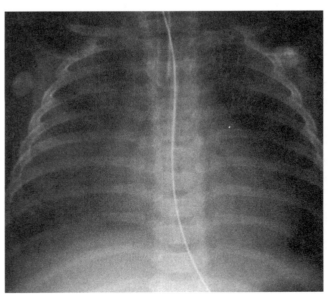

Figure 11-16. AP chest radiograph in child with pneumocystis pneumonia demonstrates coalescent, air-space consolidative densities.

be caused by organisms including *Candida*, CMV, cryptosporidium, and MAI, as well as more common bacterial pathogens such as *Salmonella* and *Shigella*.[60,61,69,70] Most gastrointestinal disorders that are associated with AIDS are not life-threatening. Occasionally, severe complications may occur. These include gastrointestinal hemorrhage, toxic megacolon, and severe inflammatory bowel disease.[60] It is important to recognize the potential for surgical gastrointestinal complication, such as bowel obstruction and perforation, that may arise due to severe widespread bowel inflammation (Fig. 11-17). Standard roentgenographic examination may show thickening of the bowel wall, dilatation of loops of bowel, evidence of obstruction, or free intraperitoneal air. Contrast examination may show erosions, ulcerations, or fistula formation.[71,72]

Renal Failure

Progressive renal failure may result from AIDS-related nephropathy. A variety of glomerular and tubular changes have been identified in this condition.[73–75] In addition, acute renal failure may result from dehydration, hypoxia, or drug toxicity. Renal ultrasound may show increased cortical echogenicity. Duplex or color Doppler ultrasound may show changes in perfusion. Radionuclide scanning may show abnormalities that are associated with renal failure from any cause.

Central Nervous System Infection

Children who have CNS infection frequently require intensive care while posing significant diagnostic problems. CT and MRI are important in the evaluation of the PICU patient in whom

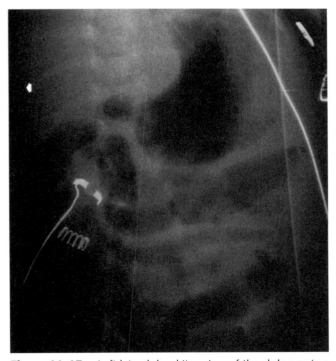

Figure 11-17. Left lateral decubitus view of the abdomen in a 2-month-old infant with AIDS with bowel perforation due to severe enteritis. Separation of bowel loops due to bowel wall edema and free intraperitoneal air *(arrow)* is noted.

intracranial infection is suspected. Uncomplicated meningitis usually does not require imaging of any type.[76–78] Children who develop complications such as seizures, raised intracranial pressure, or poor response to the therapy, however, frequently require imaging to plan appropriate management. CT may demonstrate areas of infarct or edema due to arterial spasm associated with inflammation.[79] Communicating or noncommunicating hydrocephalus may be present due to obstruction of cerebrospinal fluid pathways. Subdural effusions, empyemas, or brain abscesses may be found. CT enhancement by administration of intravenous contrast medium may be useful to demonstrate ventriculitis or abscess.[79–82]

MRI has proven to be more effective than CT in demonstrating cerebritis and regions of infarction.[83] Also, at certain stages of evolutions, subdural effusions and empyemas are demonstrated more effectively on MRI than on CT. MRI is the initial procedure of choice for those children who are suspected of having spinal infections such as disc space infection with or without osteomyelitis, paraspinal abscess, or transverse myelitis.[84,85] CT and administration of intrathecal contrast medium should be reserved for those children in whom meningitis and concomitant epidural abscess are suspected and in whom the MRI is not diagnostic.[86]

Viral infections of the CNS may cause a wide variety of imaging abnormalities, including hemorrhage, edema, necrosis, and vascular congestion.[87] Patients who have herpes simplex encephalitis may benefit from aggressive diagnostic imaging, as early detection and treatment may prevent permanent neurologic damage. CT scan, even with contrast administration, may not show abnormalities in herpes encephalitis until the fifth day, long after the radionuclide scan is abnormal.[88–91] Radionuclide brain scans have been shown to be useful in demonstrating focal uptake of isotope in the temporal lobes early in the course of the infection.[92] More recently, MRI has been shown to be sensitive for the early detection of herpes encephalitis[92–94] (Figs. 11-18 and 11-19).

Hypoxia and Hypotension

Hypoxia and hypotension are associated with many forms of illness or injury that cause a child to be managed in the ICU. Furthermore, these physiologic states may occur during the course of intensive care and require ongoing evaluation. CT is frequently performed to evaluate the results of hypoxia or hypotension. The reaction of brain tissue to hypoxia and ischemia is edema, either focal or diffuse, especially in specific areas such as the basal ganglia or cerebral cortex. CT may show edema and cerebral damage, including loss of differentiation between gray and white matter (Fig. 11-20), effacement of sulci and cisterns by edema, focal areas of edema in the basal ganglia and cortex, and hemorrhagic infarcts in the basal ganglia.[95–100] Unfortunately, there is no reliable method of predicting the patient's neurologic status from the initial CT abnormalities.[101] In some children, the CT scan can be normal despite a poor neurologic outcome. Radionuclide brain scans may be useful in documenting cerebral perfusion. CT scans are more useful as predictors of neurologic outcome when used to follow up the sequelae of the hypoxic or hypotensive episode. Cerebral atrophy may be noted several weeks after the event.[95,101]

Children undergoing intensive care may experience cerebral infarction during initial injury or management. Cerebral infarcts may be caused by embolism, thrombosis, or arteritis[102] (Fig. 11-21). CT scan may show areas of low attenuation within the brain. Unfortunately, regions of infarct may not be apparent early in the course of the abnormality.[103–105] Enhancement by administration of intravenous contrast medium may aid in the diagnosis

Figure 11-18. An 8-year-old boy presented with seizures and behavioral changes. **(A, B)** CT scans, with and without contrast, demonstrate a mild decrease in attenuation of both grey and white matter, suggesting generalized edema. There was no obvious enhancement following contrast administration. **(C)** Brain scan demonstrates a striking increase in tracer uptake throughout the brain. Findings are compatible with encephalitis.

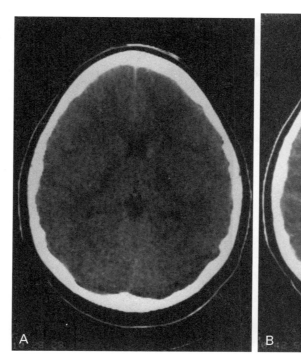

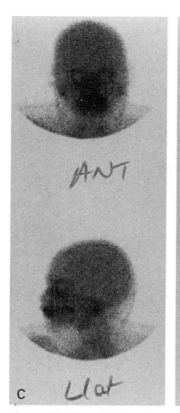

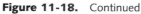

Figure 11-18. Continued

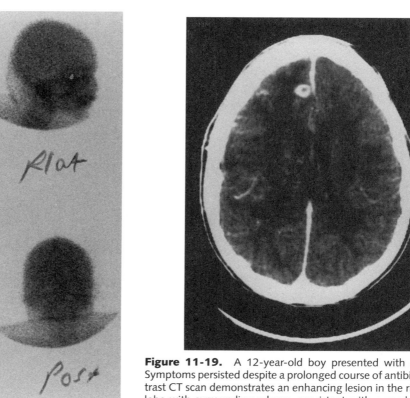

Figure 11-19. A 12-year-old boy presented with meningitis. Symptoms persisted despite a prolonged course of antibiotics. Contrast CT scan demonstrates an enhancing lesion in the right frontal lobe with surrounding edema, consistent with a cerebral abscess (left side of image).

Figure 11-20. An 8-month-old infant was found strangled with her head caught in a slotted fence. **(A, B)** Initial CT was normal. **(C, D)** Five days later, CT demonstrates diffuse low density of both grey and white matter as well as obliteration of the basilar cisterns. Findings were consistent with diffuse cerebral edema secondary to hypoxia.

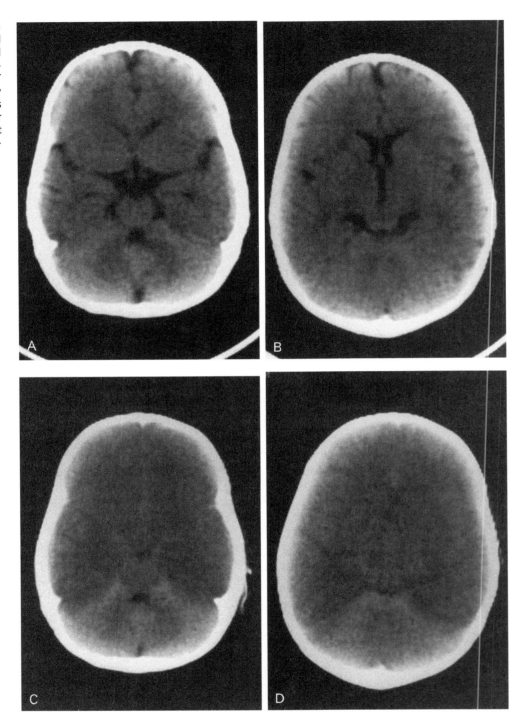

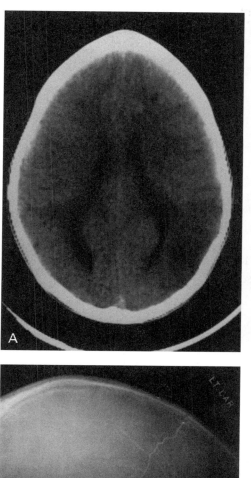

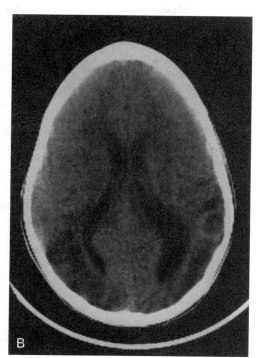

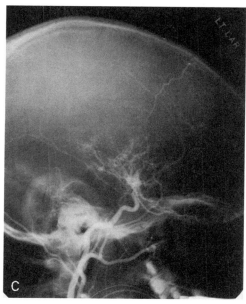

Figure 11-21. A 6-year-old boy presented with a history of headaches and sudden onset of hemiplegia and visual changes. **(A)** The initial CT demonstrates a low-density lesion in the left occipital lobe as well as an old left frontal lobe infarct. **(B)** Two weeks later, the patient developed sudden blindness. CT shows maturation of the left occipital infarct and a new right occipital infarct. **(C)** Angiography demonstrates significant stenosis of both middle, anterior, and posterior cerebral arteries consistent with severe Moya Moya disease.

of an infarct but may be contraindicated due to possible neurotoxicity of contrast agents in regions of acute ischemia.[106-108] MRI has been shown to be more sensitive than CT scanning in demonstrating infarcts, especially in the deep white matter.[109] Visualization of vascular anatomy by MRI may show a cause for the acute ischemic event. Angiography should be reserved for those patients in whom the etiology remains unknown.[110-112]

References

1. Haaga JR, Alfidi RJ. *Computed Tomography of the Whole Body.* St. Louis: Mosby, 1983. Pp 1–16.
2. Treves ST, Crane RK, Lipp A. *Pediatric Nuclear Medicine.* New York: Springer, 1985. Pp 210–213.
3. Mishkin F. Determination of brain death by radionuclide angiography. *Radiology* 115:135–137, 1975.
4. Ashwal S et al. Radionuclide bolus angiography: A technique for verification of brain death in infants and children. *J Pediatr* 91:722, 1977.
5. Wilson K, Gordon L, Selby JB. Diagnosis of brain death with tC-99m HMPAO. *Clin Nucl Med* 18:428, 1993.
6. Walker JM, Margouleff D. *A Clinical Manual of Nuclear Medicine.* Norwalk, CT: Appleton-Century-Crofts, 1984. P 74.
7. Williamson SL et al. Indium III white blood cell scanning in the pediatric population. *Pediatr Radiol* 16:493–497, 1986.
8. Towbin RB, Strife JL. Percutaneous aspiration and biopsies in children. *Radiology* 157:81–85, 1985.
9. Towbin RB, Ball WS. Pediatric interventional radiology. *Radiol Clin North Am* 26:419–429, 1988.

10. Stark D, Bradley WG. *Magnetic Resonance Imaging.* St. Louis: Mosby, 1988. P 3.

11. McArdle CB et al. Monitoring of the neonate undergoing MR imaging: Technical considerations. *Radiology* 159:223–226, 1986.

12. Rigsby CM et al. Doppler signal quantification in renal allografts: Comparison in normal and rejecting transplants with pathologic correlation. *Radiology* 162:39–42, 1987.

13. Baxt WG, Moody P. The impact of rotocraft aero-medical emergency care service on trauma mortality. *JAMA* 249:3047–3051, 1983.

14. Federle MP et al. Evaluation of abdominal trauma by computed tomography. *Radiology* 138:637–644, 1981.

15. Berger PE, Kuhn JP. CT of blunt abdominal trauma in childhood. *AJR* 136:105–110, 1981.

16. Kaufman RA et al. Upper abdominal trauma in children: Imaging evaluation. *AJR* 142:449–460, 1984.

17. Brick SH et al. Hepatic and splenic injury in children: Role of CT in the decision of laparotomy. *Radiology* 165:643–646, 1987.

18. McCort JJ. Caring for the major trauma victim: The role of radiology. *Radiology* 163:1–9, 1987.

19. Kane NM et al. Pediatric abdominal trauma: Evaluation by computed tomography. *Pediatrics* 82:11–15, 1988.

20. Taylor GA et al. The role of computed tomography in blunt abdominal trauma in children. *J Trauma* 28:1660–1664, 1988.

21. Taylor GA, Eichelberger MR. Abdominal CT in children with neurologic impairment following blunt trauma. *Ann Surg* 210:229–233, 1989.

22. Bulas KI, Taylor GA, Eichelberger MR. The value of CT in detecting bowel perforation in children after blunt abdominal trauma. *AJR* 153:561–564, 1989.

23. Sivit CJ et al. Blunt trauma in children: Significance of peritoneal fluid. *Radiology* 178:185–188, 1991.

24. Zimmerman RA, Bilaniuk LT. CT in pediatric head trauma. *J Neuroradiol* 8:257–271, 1981.

25. Zimmerman RA et al. Cranial CT in diagnosis and management of acute head trauma. *AJR* 131:27–34, 1978.

26. Peyster RG, Hoover ED. CT in head trauma. *J Trauma* 22:25–38, 1982.

27. Han BK et al. Reversal sign on CT: Effect of anoxic/ischemic cerebral injury in children. *AJR* 154:361–368, 1990.

28. Dublin AB, French BN, Rennick JM. CT in head trauma. *Radiology* 123:345–350, 1977.

29. de Villansante JM, Taveras JM. CT in acute head trauma. *Radiology* 126:765–768, 1976.

30. Gentry LR, Godersky JC, Thompson BH. MR imaging of head trauma: Review of distribution and radiopathological features of traumatic lesions. *AJNR* 9:101–110, 1988.

31. Adams JF et al. Diffuse axonal injury due to nonmissile head injury in humans: An analysis of 45 cases. *Ann Neurol* 12:557–563, 1982.

32. Zimmerman RA, Bilaniuk LT, Gennarelli. CT of shearing injuries of cerebral white matter. *Radiology* 127:393–396, 1978.

33. Lobato RD et al. Normal CT scans in severe head injury. *J Neurosurg* 65:784–789, 1986.

34. Gentry LR et al. Prospective comparative study of intermediate field MR and CT in the evaluation of closed head trauma. *AJR* 150:673–682, 1988.

35. Mark AS. MRI evaluation of cerebral trauma. *MRI Decisions* 26–33, 1989.

36. Zimmerman RA et al. Head injury: Early results of comparing CT and high field MR. *AJNR* 7:757–764, 1986.

37. Gentry LR, Godersky JC, Thompson B. MR imaging of head trauma: A review of the distribution and radiopathologic features of traumatic lesions. *AJR* 150:663–672, 1988.

38. Gentry LR, Godersky JC, Thompson BH. Traumatic brainstem injury: MR imaging. *Radiology* 171:177–187, 1989.

39. Gomori JM et al. Intracranial hematomas imaging by high field MR. *Radiology* 157:87–93, 1985.

40. Gentry LR, Thompson B, Godersky JC. Trauma to corpus collosum MR features. *AJNR* 9:1129–1138, 1988.

41. Goldberg AL, Daffner RH, Shapiro RL. Imaging of acute spinal trauma: An evolving multi-modality approach. *Clin Imag* 14:11–16, 1990.

42. Hackney DB et al. Hemorrhage and edema in acute spinal cord compression: Demonstration by MR imaging. *Radiology* 161:387–390, 1986.

43. Mirvis SE et al. Acute cervical spine trauma evaluation with 1.5 TMR imaging. *Radiology* 166:807–816, 1988.

44. Zinneich SJ et al. 3-D CT improves accuracy of spinal trauma studies. *Diagn Imag* 102–107, 1990.

45. Tsai FY et al. CT in child abuse head trauma. *CT* 4:277–286, 1980.

46. Cohen RA et al. Cranial CT in the abused child with head injury. *AJR* 146:97–102, 1986.

47. Zimmerman RA et al. CT of craniocerebral injury in the abused child. *Radiology* 130:687–690, 1979.

48. Merten DR et al. Cranio-cerebral trauma in the child abuse syndrome: Radiological observations. *Pediatr Radiol* 14:272–277, 1984.

49. Sinai SH, Ball MR. Head trauma due to child abuse: Serial CT in diagnosis and management. *South Med J* 80:1505–1512, 1987.

50. Alexander RC, Scor DP, Smith WL. Magnetic resonance imaging of intracranial injuries from child abuse. *J Pediatr* 109:975–979, 1986.

51. Sato Y et al. Head injury in child abuse: Evaluation with MR imaging. *Radiology* 173:653–657, 1989.

52. Sivit CJ, Taylor GA, Eichelberger MR. Visceral injury in battered children: A changing perspective. *Radiology* 173:659–662, 1989.

53. Shackford SR. Blunt chest trauma: The intensivist perspective. *J Intens Care Med* 1:125–136, 1986.

54. Eichelberger MR, Anderson KD. Sequelae of thoracic injury in children. In Eichelberger MR, Pratsch GL (eds): *Pediatric Trauma Care.* Rockville, MD: Aspen, 1988. Pp 59–67.

55. Velek FT et al. Traumatic deaths in urban children. *J Pediatr Surg* 12:375–384, 1977.

56. Sivit CJ et al. Efficacy of chest radiography in pediatric intensive care. *AJR* 152:575, 1989.

57. Tocino IM et al. CT detection of occult pneumothorax in head trauma. *AJR* 143:987–990, 1984.

58. Sivit CJ, Taylor Ga, Eichelberger MR. Chest injury in children with blunt abdominal trauma: Evaluation with CT. *Radiology* 171:815–818, 1989.

59. Rubinstein A et al. Pulmonary disease in children with acquired immune deficiency syndrome and AIDS-related complex. *J Pediatr* 108:498–503, 1986.

60. Amodio JB et al. Pediatric AIDS. *Semin Roentgenol* 22:66–76, 1987.

61. Haney PJ et al. Imaging of infants and children with AIDS. *AJR* 152:1033–1041, 1989.

62. Vernon DD et al. Respiratory failure in children with acquired immunodeficiency syndrome and acquired immunodeficiency syndrome-related complex. *Pediatrics* 82:223–228, 1988.

63. Suster B et al. Pulmonary manifestations of AIDS: Review of 106 episodes. *Radiology* 161:87–93, 1986.

64. Nadich DP et al. Radiographic manifestations of pulmonary disease in AIDS. *Semin Roentgenol* 22:14–30, 1987.

65. Zimmerman BL et al. Children with AIDS: Is pathologic diagnosis possible based on chest radiographs? *Pediatr Radiol* 17:303–307, 1987.

66. Goodman PC, Daley C, Minagi H. Spontaneous pneumothorax in AIDS patients with pneumocystis carinii pneumonia. *AJR* 147:29–31, 1986.

67. Sivit CJ et al. Spectrum of chest radiographic abnormalities in children with AIDS and pneumocystis carinii penumonia. *Pediatr Radiol* (in press).

68. Bernstein LJ et al. Bacterial infection in the acquired immunodeficiency syndrome of children. *Pediatr Infect Dis* 4:472–475, 1988.

69. Bradford BF et al. Usual and unusual manifestations of AIDS and HIV infection in children. *Radiol Clin North Am* 26:341–353, 1988.

70. Winters WD, Kirkpatrick JA. Radiology of AIDS in the pediatric patient. *Contemp Diagn Radiol* 11:1–5, 1988.

71. Sivit CJ et al. Bowel obstruction in an infant with AIDS. *AJR* 154:803–804, 1990.

72. Rusin JA et al. AIDS related cholangitis in children: Sonographic findings. *AJR* 159:626, 1992.

73. Rousseau E et al. Renal complications of acquired immunodeficiency syndrome in children. *Am J Kidney Dis* 11:48–50, 1988.

74. Connor E et al. Acquired immunodeficiency syndrome-associated renal disease in children. *J Pediatr* 113:39–44, 1988.

75. Strauss J et al. Renal disease in children with the acquired immunodeficiency syndrome. *N Engl J Med* 321:625–630, 1989.

76. Cabral DA et al. Prospective study of CT in acute bacterial meningitis. *J Pediatr* 111:201–205, 1987.

77. Snyder RD, Stroving J. The follow-up CT scan in childhood meningitis. *Neuroradiology* 16:22–23, 1978.

78. Feigin RD et al. Prospective evaluation of treatment of haemophilus influenzae meningitis. *J Pediatr* 88:542–548, 1976.

79. Synder RD et al. Cerebral infarction in childhood bacterial meningitis. *J Neurol Neurosurg Psychiatry* 44:581–585, 1981.

80. Biliniuk LT et al. CT in meningitis. *Neuroradiology* 16:13–14, 1978.

81. Stroving J, Snyder RD. CT in childhood bacterial meningitis. *J Pediatr* 96:820–823, 1980.

82. Smith HP, Hendrick EB. Subdural empyema and epidural abscess in children. *J Neurosurg* 58:392–397, 1983.

83. Hanigan WC, Wright SM, Wright RM. Clinical utility of magnetic resonance imaging in pediatric neurosurgical patients. *J Pediatr* 108:522–529, 1986.

84. Donovan-Post MJ et al. Spinal infection: Evaluation with MR imaging and intraoperative US. *Radiology* 169:756–771, 1988.

85. Angtuaco EJC et al. MR imaging of spinal epidural abscess. *AJNR* 8:879–883, 1987.

86. Modi MT et al. Vertebral osteomyelitis: Assessment using MR. *Radiology* 151:157–166, 1985.

87. Leestmo JE. Viral infection of the nervous system. In Davis RL, Robertson DM (eds): *Textbook of Neuropathology*. Baltimore: Williams & Wilkins, 1985. Pp 704–787.

88. Davis JM et al. CT of herpes simplex encephalitis with clinicopathological correlation. *Radiology* 129:419–427, 1978.

89. Enzmann DR et al. CT of herpes simplex encephalitis. *Radiology* 129:419–425, 1978.

90. Zimmerman RD et al. CT in the early diagnosis of herpes simplex encephalitis. *AJNR* 134:61–66, 1980.

91. Kim EE, Deland FH, Montebello J. Sensitivity of radionuclide brain scan and CT in early detection of viral meningoencephalitis. *Radiology* 132:425, 1979.

92. Karlin CA et al. Radionuclide imaging in herpes simplex encephalitis. *Radiology* 126:181–184, 1978.

93. Schroth G et al. Early diagnosis of herpes simplex encephalitis by MRI. *Neurology* 37:179–183, 1987.

94. Lester JW, Carter MP, Reynolds TL. Herpes encepahlitis: MR monitoring of response to acyclovir therapy. *Comput Tomogr* 12:941–943, 1988.

95. Neils EW et al. MRI and CT scanning of herpes simplex encepahlitis. *J Neurosurg* 67:529–594, 1987.

96. Fitch SJ et al. CNS hypoxia in children due to near drowning. *Radiology* 156:647–650, 1985.

97. Han BK et al. Reversal sign on CT: Effect of anoxic/eschemic cerebral injury in children. *AJR* 154:361–368, 1990.

98. Toutant SM et al. Absent or compressed basal cisterns on first CT scan: Ominous predictors of outcome in severe head injury. *J Neurosurg* 61:691–694, 1984.

99. Kjos BO, Brandt-Zawodski M, Young RG. Early CT findings of global CNS hypoperfusion. *AJNR* 4:1043–1048, 1983.

100. Murray RR et al. Cerebral CT in drowning victims. *AJNR* 5:177–179, 1984.

101. Bruce DA et al. Diffuse cerebral swelling following head injuries in children: The syndrome of malignant brain edema. *J Neurosurg* 54:170–174, 1981.

102. Taylor SB et al. CNS anoxic-ischemic insult in children due to near drowning. *Radiology* 156:641–646, 1985.

103. Wall SD et al. High frequency CT findings within 24 hours after cerebral infarction. *AJR* 138:307–311, 1982.

104. Inoue Y et al. Sequential CT scans in acute cerebral infarction. *Radiology* 135:655–662, 1980.

105. Ladurner G et al. A correlation of clinical findings and CT in ischemic cerebrovascular disease. *Eur Neurol* 18:281–288, 1979.

106. Valk J. *CT and Cerebral Infarctions with an Introduction into Practice and Principles of CT Reading*. New York: Raven, 1980.

107. Yock DH Jr, Marshal WH Jr. Recent ischemic brain infarcts of CT, appearances pre and post contrast infusion. *Radiology* 117:599–608, 1975.

108. Hayman LA et al. Delayed high dose contrast CT: Identifying patients at risk of massive hemorrhagic infarction. *AJNR* 2:139–147, 1981.

109. Harbedo JE, Nilsson B. Hemodynamic changes in brain caused by local infusion of hyperosmolar solutions in particular relation of blood-brain barrier opening. *Brain Res* 181:45–49, 1980.

110. Brandt-Sawodski M et al. MR imaging and spectroscopy in clinical and experimental cerebral ischemia: A review. *AJNR* 8:39, 1987.

111. Matthews VP et al. Cerebral infarction: Effects of dose and magnetization transfer saturation of gadolinium enhanced MR imaging. *Radiology* 190:547, 1994.

112. Lee C et al. Cerebral infarction: Assessment of patterns using ultrafast MR contrast imaging. *AJNR* 13:277, 1992.

II Respiratory System

Daniel C. Shannon

12 Control of Breathing

In this review there will be a brief discussion of developmental features of the regulation of ventilation and of breathing pattern. With this background there will be a focus on three clinical questions: (1) What provokes hyperventilation (as opposed to hyperpnea)? (2) What provokes hypoventilation? (3) What causes instability in the breathing pattern?

Chemical Regulation of Ventilation

The purpose of chemical regulation of ventilation is to maintain gaseous homeostasis by moment-to-moment changes in ventilation in proportion to changes in the metabolic production of carbon dioxide. This regulation is carried out by a feedback and control system that involves peripheral and central chemoreceptors and their influences on neural outflow from the brainstem to the muscles of respiration.

Peripheral Chemoreceptors

Peripheral chemoreceptors are in the carotid bodies and are perfused by a branch from the aorta. Aortic bodies are of uncertain importance in the regulation of ventilation. The prevailing hypothesis is that glomus cells supported by sustentacular cells are the chemical transducers that release from vesicles preformed transmitters that then alter the firing of sensory nerves. Although many neurotransmitters have been identified, their respective roles are unknown. The carotid body is mainly sensitive to elevated levels of PCO_2 and [H^+] ion concentration. A rise in $PaCO_2$ of only a few torr (mm Hg) elicits a doubling of tidal volume (V_T) within 10 seconds. This chemoreceptor is also sensitive to hypoxemia.

In utero, at the prevailing PaO_2 of 25 to 30 mm Hg, the afferent nerve from the carotid body is silent and becomes active when the umbilical cord is clamped. The carotid sinus nerve contains both baroreceptor and chemoreceptor fibers that change their firing pattern in response to different stimuli. Stimulation of sympathetic fibers that supply carotid body blood vessels increases firing of chemoreceptor cells similar to cord clamping. Progressive reduction in PaO_2 in the animal model is associated with a hyperbolic increase in chemoreceptor firing. However, this pattern is not matched by a parallel change in ventilation. Ventilation increases at a sustained reduction in PaO_2 for about 1 minute and then decreases. The same pattern of ventilation is seen in human infants. The time delay of the increase in ventilation in the infant is 4 seconds and in the adult is about 7 seconds. The magnitude of the subsequent decrease in ventilation in the preterm infant is greater than in the adult (Table 12-1). The neurochemical basis of this decrease in ventilation is unexplained but may arise from the effects of hypoxia on brain stem norepinephrine concentration. The net increase in ventilation in response to moderately severe hypoxia is small, averaging about 35% in older infants and children; this change is generally too small to be observed as an increase in tidal volume or frequency except at extreme altitude when hypoxemia is severe.

Change in sensitivity of the carotid body to hypoxia with age is difficult to measure because the stimulus acts on several organ systems that might alter ventilation. For example, alveolar hypoxia evokes different responses in pulmonary vascular smooth muscle

Table 12-1. The percent change in ventilation during hypoxia in preterm infants compared with adults

	Duration of hypoxia	
Age	*1 min*	*5 min*
35-wk preterm	+ 15%	− 10%
Adult	+ 43%	+ 14%

in infants compared with adults. These effects may confound the ventilatory response by changing the dynamics of gas exchange in the lung. Sensitivity also changes with exposure to chronic hypoxia. The ventilatory response to acute hypoxia is diminished or absent in residents of high altitude and patients with uncorrected cyanotic heart disease.

Central Chemoreceptors

Central chemoreceptors are chemosensitive sites in the brain stem without identified anatomic counterparts. Their response is coupled to changes in local [H^+] ion concentration determined mainly by changes in arterial $PaCO_2$. Because they are physically removed from direct contact with arterial blood, in contrast to peripheral chemoreceptors, the time constant of their response is much longer—about 1 minute. (Note here that the term *time constant* is used in the strict sense of 63% of the maximal response, while the term *time delay*, used previously, refers to the time lapse between presentation of the stimulus and the onset of the response.) Thus, the central chemoreceptors can modulate ventilation in response to sustained increase in metabolic rate, but the long time constant minimizes their contribution to events of brief duration, such as the response to a sigh or to the cycle of respirations that accompanies periodic breathing. These cycles exhibit a cycle duration of 15 to 30 seconds.

These receptors can be activated in utero by evoking arousal and then challenging the fetus with an elevated PCO_2. Immediately following birth, a continuous increase in inspired carbon dioxide concentration evokes a sustained increase in ventilation that is linear over a wide range of $PaCO_2$ values.

Interactions between the ventilatory responses to progressive or sustained hypoxia and hypercapnia have been explored. They have shown that hypoxia depresses the hypercapnic response in infants but has the opposite effect in adults. The response to progressive or sustained hypoxia might be qualitatively different from a transient response. For example, the ventilatory response to transient hypoxia, even if repeated at the cycle duration of periodic breathing (15–30 seconds), may elicit repeated potentiation rather than ventilatory depression because the cycle duration is significantly shorter than the time required to elicit the ventilatory depression during sustained hypoxia. This may explain why in preterm infants oscillations in PaO_2 can occur coincident with oscillations in ventilation during periodic breathing without causing progressive decrease in ventilation.

In summary, the neural basis for chemoreceptor-mediated ventilatory responses is present in the fetus. Qualitatively, the responses to elevated inspired carbon dioxide or reduced inspired oxygen are similar in both newborns and adults. The ventilatory response to hypoxia is mediated by peripheral chemoreceptors, while the response to hypercapnia is mediated by both peripheral (initial response) and central (later response) receptors. Quantitative comparisons will not be possible until both controller and controlled system variables are measured from birth to maturity.

Clinical Questions

1. What factors provoke hyperventilation or hyperpnea?
2. What factors provoke hypoventilation?
3. What factors destabilize breathing pattern?

Hyperventilation versus Hyperpnea

Hyperventilation is a sustained increase in alveolar ventilation (V_A), which by definition results in a disturbance in the balance between carbon dioxide production (VCO_2) and alveolar ventilation so that $PaCO_2$ is reduced. Thus,

$$PaCO_2 = \frac{VCO_2}{V_A} P_B - 47 \qquad (1)$$

where $PaCO_2$ is alveolar partial pressure of carbon dioxide, P_B is barometric pressure, VCO_2 is carbon dioxide production, and V_A is alveolar ventilation.

Hyperpnea is a sustained increase in minute ventilation. It is not necessarily associated with reduced arterial PCO_2. It is worth recalling that frequency is readily estimated by eye, while V_T is not. On average, V_T at rest increases lung volume (FRC) by about 20%. If we simplify the geometry and consider the thorax a cylindrical ellipse, this change in volume requires an average increase in radius and length of 6%. Each incremental increase in dimensions of 6% of the initial values increases volume by an additional 20% of FRC. Thus, the transthoracic diameter at V_T increases by 6 mm in the infant and 12 mm in the adult. A doubling of V_T results from a doubling of these changes in dimensions. It is thus not surprising that changes in dimensions within this range or changes of half those at resting V_T are not apparent to an examiner.

This observation implies that a measurement of V_T is far more reliable than a visual estimate and that the hyperpnea cannot be accurately identified unless it is severe. Given a patient with an evident increase in V_T and/or frequency (f) (i.e., hyperpnea), the most common explanation will be found in disease of the airways or alveoli. The increase in V_T or f indicates that the control system is attempting to restore equilibrium in lung volume or arterial blood gases.

Once hyperpnea has been objectively demonstrated, and there is no evidence of lung disease or physical or radiographic examination and physiologic measurement (note that significant interstitial lung disease can be present without adventitious sounds or radiographic signs), an arterial blood gas measurement is the next best step in evaluating the problem. The acid-base status will reflect one of three conditions: metabolic acidosis, respiratory alkalosis, or normal.

1. Metabolic acidosis causes hyperpnea with alveolar hyperventilation. The stimulus is increased [H^+] ions in arterial blood acting on peripheral chemoreceptors and possibly also acting on medullary chemoreceptors. The classic example is diabetic ketoacidosis.

2. Respiratory alkalosis results from alveolar hyperventilation triggered by anxiety, arterial blood hyperammonemia, or selective increase in CSF [H^+] ions. For completeness, hypoxemia should be included, but this is a rather weak stimulus under most clinical conditions. It is true that severe hypoxemia at high altitude can cause profound alveolar hyperventilation; alveolar PCO_2 levels less than 10 torr have been recorded on top of Mount Everest. In patients with severe lung disease, however, other stimuli from airway and alveolar stretch receptors appear to dominate the increased level of ventilation so that relief of hypoxemia fails to reduce ventilation.

With decreased ammonia detoxification in the liver, the degree of respiratory alkalosis correlates best with brain stem ammonia concentration in experimental subjects and with arterial ammonia concentration in patients. Examples are conditions associated with absence or inactivation of ornithine carbamyl transferase, the rate-limiting enzyme in the urea cycle as a result of congenital deficiency or acquired deficiency with Reye's syndrome or liver failure. In patients with subarachnoid hemorrhage, red blood cells in the CSF metabolize glucose to lactic acid. The increased [H^+] ions stimulate ventilation. This phenomenon has been described in adults but not in children.

3. Normal acid-base balance in a patient with hyperpnea implies either a proportional increase in metabolic rate and alveolar ventilation (see Eq. 1) or an increase in dead space that demands increased total ventilation in order to maintain $PaCO_2$ in the normal range. An example of the first instance is a febrile illness that spares the lung. Recall also that acid-base balance remains normal during all but the most extreme exercise when carbon dioxide production is tenfold that at rest. Examples of increased dead space are congenital absence of a pulmonary artery (most commonly the left) and pulmonary embolus.

In all examples of alveolar hyperventilation, the respiratory control system is a passive victim of disease in either the respiratory system or other organ system. Thus, management is directed at the underlying disease rather than at altering the control system.

Alveolar Hypoventilation

Alveolar hypoventilation is defined by an elevated $PaCO_2$ where $PaCO_2$ depends on the balance between metabolic carbon dioxide production and alveolar ventilation. Alveolar hypoventilation can be associated with a decrease in frequency, VT, or both. As with alveolar hyperventilation, visual assessment is quite misleading, except in extreme cases. Furthermore, most clinical examples are characterized by reduction in VT rather than frequency, making the assessment even more difficult. Recall that approximately one third of every breath is wasted in anatomic dead space and that any reduction in VT reduces alveolar ventilation proportionally. Thus, a one-third reduction in VT of an infant would be accompanied by a reduction in the average change in chest wall radius of about 1 mm. This represents a 50% reduction in alveolar ventilation! Reinspection of the alveolar gas equation shows that a halving of V_A results in a doubling of $PaCO_2$ at the new equilibrium. It is easy to see that visually undetectable reduction in VT can result in profound alveolar hypoventilation. Vigilance and measurement are the only defenses for the clinician.

Alveolar hypoventilation results when respiratory muscles are unable to perform the work required to move the ventilatory pump and maintain the normal ratio of VCO_2/V_A; alveolar ventilation falls because the patient cannot breathe (diseases of the respiratory system) or will not breathe (faulty neuromuscular mechanism).

In those who cannot breathe, the neuromuscular control apparatus is intact, but disease of the respiratory system prevents its adequate performance. Thus, muscular effort is insufficient to accomplish normal alveolar ventilation in the presence of a severe increase in respiratory system resistance or a decrease in compliance. Examples are asthma, adult respiratory disease syndrome, or bronchopulmonary dysplasia (BPD). In BPD, resistance is increased and compliance is decreased.

In those who will not breathe, the respiratory system mechanics are normal but the neuromuscular apparatus is faulty. Examples are pharmacologic effect from narcotics, generalized muscle weakness associated with various dystrophies, phrenic nerve disruption from surgical trauma, and congenital central hypoventilation syndrome (CCHS).

In all cases, the diagnosis is suspected from observation of cyanosis that is unexplained by cardiopulmonary disease and is confirmed by measurement of arterial blood gases and VTs. A word of caution is warranted regarding interpretation of arterial blood gases in patients suspected of having CCHS. Their ventilation is generally normal while awake, so that $PaCO_2$ may be normal. Further, if they are awake more hours than they are asleep, the net flux of bicarbonate over 24 hours through the kidney may be normal, so that plasma bicarbonate may not be above the normal range. Thus, it is crucial to measure $PaCO_2$ and VT while the patient sleeps.

All diseases that result in alveolar hypoventilation may be associated with serious cardiovascular complications. These begin with hypoxic pulmonary vasoconstriction and end with biventricular cardiac failure. The sequence appears to be the following: Global reduction in alveolar PO_2 activates global pulmonary vasoconstriction. This vasoconstriction is sustained for hours, even after restoration of normal $PaCO_2$. Pulmonary blood flow rate is sustained against the increased flow resistance by a higher driving pressure. Prolonged vasoconstriction is followed by anatomic remodeling of pulmonary blood vessels with an increase in all wall components. Thus, a variable reflex increase in flow resistance is followed by a fixed anatomic increase. Right ventricular hypertrophy develops. When resistance is sustained at high levels, the interventricular septum shifts into the left ventricle during systole. The net effect is high afterload on the right ventricle and high preload on the left. This entire sequence can develop in less than 1 month. With appropriate ventilatory support, pulmonary vascular resistance can be expected to return to normal in 1 to 2 months.

A special case is the patient who exhibits so-called hyperoxic ventilatory depression. For decades it has been observed that administration of high concentrations of inspired oxygen can provoke carbon dioxide retention in patients with severe obstructive lung disease, such as asthma or emphysema. The traditional interpretation has been that the patient's carbon dioxide receptors had become desensitized by chronic lung disease, and that the patients were existing on **hypoxic drive**. Removal of that drive by hyperoxia was proposed as the explanation for carbon dioxide retention. This explanation is probably incorrect. It is much more likely that carbon dioxide retention is provoked by inhibition of hypoxic-induced pulmonary vasoconstriction in regions of lung with low V/Q ratios. Pulmonary vasoconstriction in response to alveolar hypoxia in regions of low V/Q ratios is proposed as the mechanism whereby the lung minimizes the decrease in arterial blood oxygen pressures. If Q could be reduced in exact proportion to the reduc-

tion in V, there would be no drop in arterial PO_2. What is generally overlooked is that this same mechanism also minimizes the rise in PCO_2 that would be incurred in the absence of vasoconstriction. Thus, administration of increased inspired oxygen to a patient with airways disease releases the hypoxic-induced pulmonary vasoconstriction without affecting the net ventilation in that region. The result is that arterial oxygenation improves at the expense of worsening carbon dioxide retention.

In the management of alveolar hypoventilation, it may be necessary to supplant the respiratory control system by providing alveolar ventilation as needed to eliminate metabolically produced carbon dioxide. It should be noted, however, that hypoxemia and the accompanying cyanosis can be eliminated in a patient with alveolar hypoventilation simply by increasing the FiO_2. This should be considered a temporary measure.

Unstable Breathing Pattern

The term *unstable* implies excessive variation in either VT or tidal frequency. Those patients with excess variation in VT generally have periods during which breathing movements continue but air flow ceases; they are said to have obstructive apnea. Others have periods during which breathing movements cease; they are said to have central apnea. Some periods and some patients exhibit both characteristics; they are said to have mixed apnea. All healthy subjects have periods of one or the other type of apnea, especially during sleep. The clinician is concerned only with those patients who exhibit prolonged apnea or excessive short apnea that is generally periodic and is called periodic breathing. The operational definition of prolonged apnea is an episode of no gas movement for a period of greater than 20 seconds, or of shorter duration if accompanied by cyanosis or abnormal cardiac slowing. The definition of periodic breathing is three or more consecutive episodes of apnea of 3 seconds or greater, separated by clusters of breaths of 20 seconds or less.

Apnea

Obstructive apnea arises because of an imbalance between the forces that dilate, compared with those that narrow, the upper airway. Dilating forces are dependent on the activity of the alae nasi, tensor palati, genioglossus, and posterior cricoarytenoid muscle. Narrowing forces are neck flexion, pharyngeal constriction, tissue elasticity, surface forces, and Bernoulli effects. When the narrowing forces dominate, the patient is prone to obstructive apnea. When the diaphragm fails to generate the force necessary to move air, central apnea ensues. The duration of apnea depends on the interaction of a number of factors: the intrinsic rhythmic drive of the respiratory controller, potentiation of phrenic nerve activity by developing hypercapnia and hypoxemia, feedback from chest wall muscle spindles, relief of diaphragmatic muscle fatigue, and a shift in the balance of dilating and narrowing forces. Arousal or awakening is often sufficient to terminate apnea.

The sequence of events that leads to prolonged apnea and its consequences can be best illustrated by an example: the child with enlarged adenoids. The intensivist is not likely to see such a patient until prolonged apnea leads to one of its serious consequences, seizures or cardiac failure.

During sleep, especially REM sleep, all skeletal muscles, including those that dilate the upper airway, relax and fail to increase their tone in phase with diaphragmatic contraction. Thus, the stage is set for upper airway obstruction during sleep. If narrowing of the airway is added (e.g., enlargement of adenoids), the resistance to inspired airflow increases. Breathing through the nose doubles the flow resistance found even during normal mouth breathing. The increased resistance is tolerated, perhaps, because the required ventilation is less during sleep, thereby reducing the work of respiratory muscles. As the resistance to flow increases at the site of adenoid enlargement, the pressure difference across the site must be increased to sustain air flow. This is accomplished by a greater than normal reduction in pleural pressure, a reduction that is transmitted up the airway to the site of obstruction. The combination of this reduction in pressure and the acceleration in air flow, which exaggerates the Bernoulli effect, adds dynamic obstruction to the anatomic narrowing. This can be prevented only if the dilating muscles develop opposing forces. Turbulence develops in the nasopharynx where the energy is transmitted to surrounding structures. The soft palate is the most free to vibrate and does so at its resonant frequency, causing snoring. When air flow required to maintain alveolar ventilation is insufficient, alveolar hypoventilation and its consequences develop. In some patients, repeated alveolar hypoxia is associated with seizures. Patients with neuromuscular disorders accompanied by hypotonia of brain stem muscles are prone to critical obstruction at lesser degrees of adenoid enlargement than are those with normal muscles.

Once such a patient is admitted, the airway can be supported in whatever way possible until surgical excision can be arranged. The next critical time in the child's care arrives during induction of anesthesia. Anesthetics have the effect of setting all dilating forces to 0 and promoting total obstruction with no possibility for compensation. Application of positive end-expiratory pressure will counteract the tendency to dynamic obstruction and assist in maintaining an adequate airway.

Periodic Breathing

Periodic breathing is especially prevalent in infants and is a normal phenomenon. It arises from the dynamic interactions between the respiratory controller (brain stem and chemoreceptors) and the controlled system (lung and blood volume) separated by the circulation, which imposes a further dynamic factor. Such a system is prone to oscillate by its very structure. This oscillation is most likely to occur at a critical frequency, which is determined by the summation of all the dynamic elements of the system: the rate of mixing of fresh air with pulmonary capillary blood, the circulation time from pulmonary capillary to chemoreceptors, and the dynamic response time of those receptors in changing phrenic nerve drive to the diaphragm. Because the time constants of the peripheral and central chemoreceptor responses are very different (15 versus 60 seconds) the resulting dynamic changes in phrenic drive occur at very different frequencies as well. From the observation that the cycle duration of periodic breathing averages 15 seconds in infants and 30 seconds in adults, it is clear that peripheral rather than central chemoreceptor activity is primarily involved in periodic breathing. Empirically we find that periodic breathing is associated with increased chemoreceptor sensitivity, reduced lung volume, metabolic alkalosis, and reduced cardiac output. Thus, periodic breathing is made more stable by reversing the previously mentioned factors. Periodic breathing is probably not related to neurologic maturation except to the extent that such maturation is associated with alterations in the parameters just noted. If periodic breathing is found greatly increased in a patient, the first step is to correct abnormalities in any of these parameters if possible (e.g., correction of inadequate fluid intake or elimination of the cause of repeated vomiting). Whether the pattern itself needs to be stabilized has not been demonstrated.

In summary, episodic prolonged apnea and periodic breathing result from instabilities in the interaction between neuromuscular control and the cardiovascular and respiratory systems. This instability is provoked by structural abnormalities in the neuromuscular system, the airways, or the thoracic components of the system.

William Wheeler   **12.1**   ## Clinical Management of the Infant with Apnea

Infants presenting with the symptoms of apnea, bradycardia, or cyanosis are often admitted to the pediatric intensive care unit (PICU) for diagnosis, close monitoring, and specific therapeutic interventions. Most infants have presented with an apparent life-threatening event (ALTE) defined as "an episode that is frightening to the observer and is characterized by some combination of apnea (central or obstructive), color change (cyanotic or pallid but occasionally plethoric), marked change in muscle tone (usually marked limpness), choking, or gagging. In some cases, the observer fears that the infant has died."[1] The pediatric intensivist must recognize the symptoms of ALTE, provide physiologic stability for the infant, and institute an appropriate diagnostic plan and therapeutic intervention.

Clinical Presentation

Most infants present with an ALTE between 2 and 12 weeks of age, which coincides with the peak incidence of sudden infant death syndrome (SIDS).[2] Usually these infants do not represent "aborted or near-miss SIDS" cases, but the pediatric intensivist will encounter some of these infants as well. Infants may appear physiologically stable at the time of medical intervention, or they may appear moribund. The intensivist should quickly evaluate the infant for signs of ongoing cardiopulmonary instability and intervene as necessary to maintain normal gas exchange and tissue oxygenation. The sicker the infant appears, the more likely a specific etiology for the ALTE will be found. Once the infant is admitted to the medical facility, close monitoring of heart rate, respiratory rate, oxygenation, and overall appearance is mandatory. Leaving the infant unattended by medical personnel is strongly discouraged.

After stabilization, a detailed history and physical examination should be performed. Historical factors should focus on environmental circumstances prior to the episode, the physical appearance and character of the infant during the episode, and intervention necessary to terminate the episode. This history is extremely important. Multiple individuals may need to be interviewed to supply the pertinent facts (i.e., mother, baby-sitter, emergency medical responder, emergency room nurse, etc.) (Table 12.1-1). Physician observation of subsequent events and sleeping breathing patterns is mandatory in formulating the correct diagnosis. Diagnostic considerations are myriad and range from diaphragmatic palsy to suffocation by the caregiver. In approximately 60% to 80% of the cases, a diagnosis can be made following a thorough evaluation guided by a detailed history and physical examination (Table 12.1-2). Diagnostic considerations are outlined in Table 12.1-3. It cannot be overemphasized that the presenting examination and history allow one to focus the workup in a productive fashion, rather than perform multiple diagnostic screening studies on every infant; that is, one would not do metabolic testing on the infant with a prior history of URI and RSV-induced apnea but would on the baby with apnea, hypoglycemia, and hepatomegaly.

Management

Once stabilization is achieved, the physician should assess the infant for signs of tissue hypoxia, including laboratory evaluation of arterial blood gases, serum lactate, and plasma bicarbonate measurements. This enables the physician to assess the magnitude of cellular insult from the ALTE. Other diagnostic studies are indicated based on the infant's presenting and historical symptoms. Infants who have suffered a severe near-miss SIDS event show evidence of tissue hypoxia with metabolic acidosis, decreased serum bicarbonate levels, and increased lactate values. These in-

Table 12.1-1. Historical features of event

Awake/asleep

Body position

Respiratory effort/color

Motor tone/eye deviation

Relationship to feeding/vomiting

Environmental circumstances (temperature, cigarette smoke, type of bedding)

Medication use

Pre-event behavior/wellness (recent infection, irritability, breathholding episodes)

Caregiver response to episode

Infant response to caregiver

History of feeding abnormalities

Table 12.1-2. Physical examination

Anthropomorphic measurements (weight, length, head circumference)

Stridor/snoring and relation to behavioral state

Wheezing, crackles, chest wall retractions

Tachycardia, pathologic murmur, asymmetric pulses

Thorough neurologic examination (especially cranial nerve function and motor strength)

Thorough abdominal examination (pyloric tumor, hepatomegaly, paradoxical respirations)

Table 12.1-3. Diagnostic consideration in the infant with severe apnea/ALTE

Infections
  Sepsis (bacterial or viral)
  Respiratory syncytial virus/parainfluenza
  Bordetella pertussis
  Meningoencephalitis

Respiratory
  Bronchiolitis/pneumonia
  Congenital airway malformation with upper or central airway obstruction (i.e., micrognathia, tracheomalacia, laryngomalacia, vascular rings, subglottic hemangioma, etc.)
  Respiratory muscle/neuromuscular disorders (congenital myopathy, diaphragm palsy, spinal muscular atrophy)
  Impaired central controller/abnormal drive (central hypoventilation syndrome)

Neurologic/behavioral
  Breathholding spells
  Seizure disorder
  Intracranial hemorrhage/thrombosis (i.e., subarachnoid hemorrhage, subdural hematoma, sagittal vein thrombosis, etc.)
  Cerebral palsy

Cardiovascular
  Congenital heart disease (coarctation, patent ductus arteriosus, VSD/ASD)
  Supraventricular tachycardia/arrhythmia
  Cardiomyopathy
  Pulmonary hypertension

Metabolic
  Hypoglycemia (non-ketotic, hyperinsulinemia, glycogen storage disease, fatty acid disorders, etc.)
  Hypothyroidism, adrenal insufficiency
  Hypo- or hypernatremia (salt poisoning, water intoxication, inadequate breast feeding)
  Metabolic alkalosis

Digestive
  Gastroesophageal reflux
  Swallowing dysfunction/laryngospasm
  Pyloric stenosis
  Esophagitis

Environmental
  Toxic ingestion (sedatives, narcotics, cocaine, antihistamines)
  Smothering (Munchhausen by proxy, attempted homicide)
  Hyperthermia
  Hypercarbia from CO_2 rebreathing (thick bedding, sheepskin, waterbed)

fants have a benign pre-event history and a nonfocal examination (except for the effects of the event), and diagnostic studies aimed at finding an underlying disorder are negative. This is usually determined retrospectively. These infants are often categorized as having idiopathic apnea of infancy.

In the less critically ill infant with spontaneous respiratory effort and a stable cardiovascular system, multichannel recordings are of value in defining respiratory physiologic perturbations, especially in the evaluation of obstructive or central apnea, episodic bradycardia, and oxygen desaturation. These studies are easily done at the bedside and allow one to quantitate the degree of respiratory dysfunction. These studies are not, however, predictive of future episodes of apnea, bradycardia, or SIDS. The etiology of ALTE cases admitted to the PICU at Minneapolis Children's Medical Center is noted in Table 12.1-4.

Table 12.1-4. Specific diagnoses causing severe ALTE presenting to MCMC PICU 1990–1994

Infectious	
RSV/viral bronchiolitis-associated apnea	25
Sepsis	10
Bordetella pertussis	3
Neurologic	
Seizures	11
Meningoencephalitis	5
Intracranial hemorrhage/thrombosis	5
Werdnig-Hoffman disease	2
Brainstem dysfunction (e.g., Arnold Chiari)	3
Gastrointestinal	
Gastroesophageal reflux/laryngospasm	19
Pyloric stenosis	2
Near-miss SIDS/idiopathic apnea	20
Congenital airway lesions	8
Metabolic	
Severe hypernatremia/hyponatremia	3
Hypoglycemia due to nesidioblastosis	1
MCAD (medium chain acyl dehydrogenase deficiency)	2
Congenital heart disease (coarctation of aorta, VSD, AV canal)	3
Other	
Suffocation (abuse, accidental)	6
Drug-induced (morphine, cocaine)	4
Postanesthesia in ex-premature infant	3

Specific management of these patients depends on the individual diagnosis. However, it is important to focus initially on the most common probabilities in arriving at the definitive diagnosis. Excluding infants with near-miss SIDS or idiopathic apnea (diagnosis made by exclusion), the majority of cases fall into four groups: (1) infectious etiologies, which require a full septic workup to be done, and specific bacterial and viral nasal swabs obtained; (2) neurologic etiologies, which require CNS imaging (CT scan or MRI) be obtained, and lumbar puncture when indicated; (3) gastrointestinal etiologies, which require gastroesophageal reflux workup and therapy and imaging to rule out congenital malformations; and (4) congenital airway lesions, which require bronchoscopy for the definitive diagnosis when indicated. Patients should have routine metabolic blood work and two-dimensional echocardiography when indicated.

Outcomes and Home Monitoring

Infants with severe ALTE have variable outcomes based on the underlying etiology of their events. Large series suggest that the recurrence rate for episodes in all ALTE infants is in the 15% to 40% range, with certain high-risk groups identified.[3,4] These include infants with underlying seizures and recurrent ALTE episodes (mortality 50%), victims of child abuse or Munchhausen syndrome by proxy (mortality 10%), and idiopathic apnea of infancy with two or more episodes requiring CPR (mortality 28%).[4] If the infant survives the event and is normal at age 1 year, he will most likely be normal at 5 years.[5]

Home monitoring with a transthoracic impedance monitor is recommended for idiopathic apnea of infancy, siblings of SIDS experiencing an ALTE, and infants with an underlying condition that is not effectively treated (i.e., upper airway lesions, tracheostomy, recurrent seizures with apnea, severe gastroesophageal reflux that is poorly responsive to medical management, metabolic diseases, etc.). Monitoring should be provided through an apnea home monitoring program wherein the family will receive appropriate education, (i.e., CPR and intervention during monitoring), psychosocial support during the monitoring period, and counseling regarding discontinuation of monitoring. A monitor with computer-chip memory is preferred so that objective criteria can be used to discontinue the monitor, which usually takes place after 4 to 8 weeks of no true events as noted by documented monitoring.[6] More effective monitoring may be utilized in the future by monitoring indices of oxygenation rather than thoracic impedance.[7]

References

1. Apnea (infantile) and home monitoring. Report of a consensus development conference. U.S. Department of Health and Human Services. Publication NIH 87-2905, Bethesda, MD, 1986.
2. Carroll J, Marcus C, Loughlin G. Disordered control of breathing in infants and children. *Pediatr Rev* 14:51–66, 1993.
3. Brooks J. Apparent life threatening events in apnea of infancy. *Clin Perinatol* 19:809–839, 1992.
4. Oren J, Kelly D, Shannon D. Identification of a high risk group for sudden infant death syndrome among infants who were resuscitated from sleep apnea. *Pediatrics* 7:495–499, 1986.
5. Kahn A, Souttiaux M, Appelboom-Fondu I. Long-term development of children monitored as infants for an apparent life threatening event during sleep: A 10 year follow-up study. *Pediatrics* 83:668–673, 1989.
6. Weese-Mayer D et al. Assessing clinical significance of apnea exceeding 15 seconds with event recording. *J Pediatr* 117:568–574, 1990.
7. Poets C et al. Home event recordings of oxygenation breathing movements and heart rate and rhythm in infants with recurrent life threatening events. *J Pediatr* 123:693–701, 1993.

I. David Todres

Charles J. Coté

13 Critical Upper Airway Obstruction in Infants and Children

Acute upper or lower airway obstruction in the infant or child may become life-threatening. The suddenness with which this occurs is often unpredictable; hence, astute recognition and anticipation of the problem is essential to prevent respiratory failure and possible death. Knowledge of the embryologic development, anatomy, and physiology of the upper airway is essential to understanding the pathology and rationally managing airway obstruction.

Developmental Anatomy

The respiratory tract in the embryo develops from the ventral surface of the foregut. The laryngotracheal sulcus is first noted at 3.5 weeks of embryonic life. The tracheobronchial grooves grow medially and unite to separate the laryngotracheal tube from the esophagus. The larynx is formed from the cranial end; caudal growth forms the lung buds. A definable larynx is observed at 6 weeks gestation, and by the tenth to eleventh week, the major structures of the larynx have developed.[1,2] Failure of the true cords to separate results in a complete or partial laryngeal web. By 26 weeks' gestation, the laryngeal epithelium has developed from primitive mesenchyme to cuboidal and stratified squamous cells or epithelium.

Receptors that respond to irritant stimuli causing glottic closure followed by cough develop in the larynx and subglottic space. As the larynx continues to grow and develop, its position changes. It originates in the upper pharynx and moves further into the neck throughout life. In senescent adults, it is often found within the thoracic inlet.

The prime function of the larynx is protection of the lower respiratory tract from aspiration during swallowing. This is achieved by a neurally controlled mechanism for closure of the glottis. The act of swallowing is associated with movement of the closed larynx away from the cervical spine, leading to opening of the relaxed cricopharyngeal sphincter. Peristaltic waves in the esophagus then carry the bolus of food down into the stomach.

Cartilaginous support for the airway extends from the trachea to airways as small as 1 to 2 mm in diameter. Airway patency is maintained despite changes in intrathoracic pressure with the phases of respiration. In some infants this cartilaginous support is ineffective, and collapse of the airway readily takes place with extreme changes in intrathoracic pressure (e.g., coughing). In the subglottic region, the cricoid cartilage, which is in continuity with the trachea, completely encircles the airway and protects the laryngeal structures. The cricoid ring is the only complete ring of cartilage in the entire respiratory tract.

There are significant developmental differences between the infant and adult airways. The infant, for the first few months of life, is primarily an obligate nose breather. This is age-dependent; that is, only 8% of infants at 31 weeks' gestation are able to convert to oral breathing following nasal obstruction, whereas 40% of term infants are able to convert to oral breathing.[3,4] By 5 months of age, nearly all infants are capable of regular oral breathing. The choana (at the junction of the posterior nose and nasopharynx) can readily limit the child's breathing, particularly those who are primarily dependent on nasal breathing. For example, infants born

with choanal atresia or stenosis may present with life-threatening respiratory distress.

The child's tongue is relatively large for the oral cavity and the relatively undeveloped mandible and readily obstructs the airway. An increase in the size of the tongue (e.g., hemangioma, Down syndrome, hypothyroidism) will further increase the potential for airway obstruction.

The infant larynx is higher in the neck (C_{3-4}) than in the adult (C_{5-6}), thereby creating a more acute angle between the oropharynx and trachea, leading to a potentially more difficult laryngoscopy to view the glottic opening. For this reason, straight laryngoscope blades are generally more efficient than curved blades. Infants with a marked hypoplastic mandible (e.g., Pierré Robin, Treacher Collins, Goldenhar's syndromes) are more difficult to intubate because the angle between the oropharynx and the trachea is more acute and the entire larynx is located more posteriorly than normal. Attempts at visualizing the larynx generally provide a view of the esophagus with the laryngeal inlet **anterior** and out of view.

In the infant and child, the attachment of the vocal cords is lower anteriorly than posteriorly. In the adult, the vocal cords are perpendicular to the long axis of the trachea. This occasionally may make endotracheal intubation, particularly nasal intubation, more difficult in the infant as a result of the endotracheal tube being held up at the anterior commissure.

The subglottic region (the cricoid cartilage) is the narrowest part of the child's upper airway; in the adult, it is the rima glottidis (Fig. 13-1). The relatively narrow subglottic area is predisposed to edema from infection (croup) or mechanical trauma (endotracheal intubation or bronchoscopy). This may result in significant respira-

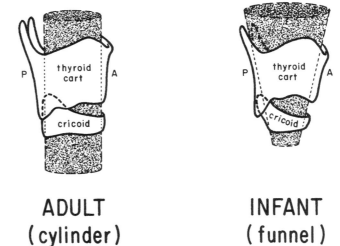

ADULT (cylinder)   INFANT (funnel)

Figure 13-1. Schematic of the larynx of the adult compared with the infant. Note the cylinder shape of the adult larynx and the funnel shape of the infant larynx. (Reproduced from Coté CJ and Todres ID. The pediatric airway. In: *A Practice of Anesthesia for Infants and Children.* Eds. Coté CJ, Ryan JF, Todres ID, Goudsouzian N. Philadelphia: Saunders. 1992. With permission.

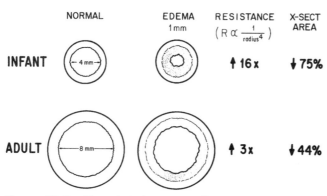

Figure 13-2. The relatively greater effect of airway edema in the infant compared with the adult. For example, in the infant with 1-mm circumferential edema, the cross-sectional area is reduced 75%, and resistance to airflow increases 16-fold. (Reproduced from Coté CJ and Todres ID. The pediatric airway. In: *A Practice of Anesthesia for Infants and Children.* Eds. Coté CJ, Ryan JF, Todres ID, Goudsouzian N. Philadelphia: Saunders. 1992. With permission.

tory distress. An equivalent degree of edema in the adult would have minimal effects due to the much larger airway diameter. Resistance to air flow is inversely proportional to the radius of the lumen of the airway (Fig. 13-2). Laminar flow resistance increases in proportion to the fourth power of the radius of the lumen. This is described by the Hagen-Poiseuille equation:

$$Q = \frac{Pr^4}{8ln}$$

where Q = flow, P = pressure drop across the length of the tube, r = radius, l = length, and n = viscosity of gas. With turbulent flow, this resistance is increased proportionally to the radius of the lumen to the fifth power! For example, the child making vigorous respiratory efforts, (e.g., crying) will have increased resistance to air flow compared with a resting state.

The mucosa of the mouth is continuous with that of the larynx and trachea and is covered with squamous and pseudostratified, ciliated epithelium that is tightly adherent to the vocal cords and tracheal surface of the epiglottis but loosely adherent elsewhere.

Inflammatory changes above the vocal cords are limited by the **barrier** formed by the tightly adherent mucosa at the vocal cords. Thus, supraglottitis (epiglottitis) is usually limited to the supraglottic area. Similarly, in the subglottic region, inflammation (laryngotracheitis) or trauma (by the endotracheal tube, bronchoscopy) leads to subglottic edema in the loosely adherent mucosa below the vocal cords but does not usually spread above the level of the vocal cords.

Physiology

In the neonate, the nasal passages account for 25% of the total resistance to airflow, compared to 60% in the adult. The major resistance to airflow in the infant occurs because of lack of supportive structures.

The larynx, trachea, and bronchi in the infant are considerably more compliant than in the adult, thus making the infant's airway highly susceptible to distending and compressive forces. The **extra**thoracic trachea is subject to different stresses than the **intra**thoracic trachea. With inspiration, negative pressure within the chest is transmitted to the large airways, including the intrathoracic trachea, tending to cause dilation. At the thoracic inlet, however, dynamic collapse results from the differential pressure between the atmosphere and the negative pressure within the **extra**thoracic trachea. With normal inspiration, this collapse is slight, and patency of the airway is not compromised (Fig. 13-3a). Normal expiration is a passive process driven by the elastic recoil of the lung. Transmural pressures are positive along the entire intrathoracic tracheobronchial tree. No clinically significant changes in airway caliber occur (Fig. 13-3b). With obstruction of the extrathoracic airway (e.g., laryngotracheobronchitis, supraglottitis, foreign body), increased inspiratory effort leads to greater negative pressure within the chest and airway. This results in a greater pressure differential between the atmosphere and pressure within the extrathoracic trachea. Thus, significant dynamic inspiratory collapse of the extrathoracic trachea will occur, particularly at the thoracic inlet. This dynamic airway collapse creates airway obstruction adding to that already present. Intrathoracic airway caliber is affected only minimally because inspiratory pressures within the airways and pleural pressure fall to a similar extent (Fig. 13-3c). With lower airway obstruction (e.g., bronchiolitis, asthma, intrathoracic foreign body), forced expiratory

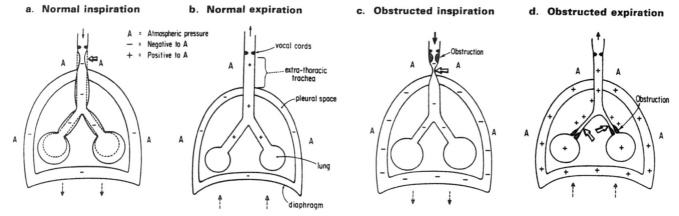

Figure 13-3. Schematic representing the phases of respiration and the dynamic effects on the upper airway with obstruction to inspiration and expiration. (Reproduced from Coté CJ and Todres ID. The pediatric airway. In: *A Practice of Anesthesia for Infants and Children.* Eds. Coté CJ, Ryan JF, Todres ID, Goudsouzian N. Philadelphia: Saunders. 1992. With permission.

effort results in increased intrathoracic pressure, which is transmitted to all intrathoracic airways down to the alveoli, and dynamic expiratory collapse occurs, further limiting expiratory flow (Fig. 13-3d). A good example of this effect is worsening of lower airway obstruction in the crying asthmatic child.

Understanding the phenomenon of dynamic airway collapse is particularly important in treating acute airway obstruction. Agitation and crying lead to marked transmural pressure changes. Efforts to relieve anxiety and crying are crucial in minimizing dynamic airway collapse, which exaggerates the airway obstruction created by the underlying pathologic process. Applying continuous positive airway pressure with a well-sealed face mask and adjustable pop-off valve may counteract dynamic airway collapse and facilitate gas exchange.

History and Physical Examination

In evaluating a child with airway obstruction, a detailed history is important. Progression of the illness may provide a clue to the etiology. Laryngotracheobronchitis is usually insidious in onset, whereas a more sudden and acute onset is usually associated with supraglottitis. The age of the child at the onset of the illness may suggest a congenital abnormality, that is, symptoms starting at birth or shortly after. An infant presenting with **inspiratory stridor** at 1 month of age should not be diagnosed as having **classical** croup. The infant is more likely suffering from a congenital lesion (e.g., subglottic stenosis, subglottic hemangioma, vascular ring). Sudden onset of airway symptoms is suggestive of foreign body aspiration.

The initial physical examination involves observing the child to assess the severity of obstruction and whether immediate therapeutic intervention is necessary. Listening to the child provides clues to the approximate location of the obstruction. Inspiratory stridor is characteristic of upper airway obstruction (e.g., croup, supraglottitis, vocal cord paralysis), while expiratory stridor has its origin in obstruction of the intrathoracic trachea (e.g, intrathoracic foreign body, compression from a vascular ring).[5,6] In severe obstructions, a to-and-fro stridor may exist. Obstruction further down the respiratory tract in the bronchi and bronchioles (e.g., bronchiolitis, asthma) is accompanied by an expiratory wheeze and prolonged expiration. With exhaustion and poor respiratory effort, the intensity of the stridor or wheeze will **diminish**. This may be interpreted incorrectly as an improving situation when in fact the child's condition has seriously deteriorated!

Signs of acute distress are reflected by an increased respiratory rate, nasal flaring, retractions (suprasternal, sternal, intercostal, and subcostal), and desaturation and/or cyanosis while breathing room air. Cyanosis reflects severe hypoxemia. The child may be leaning forward with an open mouth and drooling (e.g., supraglottitis). Drooling of saliva occurs because of an inability to swallow due to pain. Dysphagia occurs with both supraglottitis and some esophageal foreign bodies. The agitated child is often agitated due to hypoxemia.

Direct pharyngeal examination should be performed only by skilled personnel prepared to correct further airway compromise. In suspected cases of supraglottitis, direct examination of the throat is best avoided, as attempts at visualizing the pharynx with a tongue blade may precipitate acute airway obstruction.

Special Investigations

Roentgenograms

Radiologic studies are performed following the history and physical examination. The necessity for these studies must be weighed carefully against the risks of precipitating increased airway obstruction from the procedure. The procedure should be performed with the child in the upright position, as this is usually the least distressing for the patient; for example, placing a child with supraglottitis in the supine position may aggravate the life-threatening airway obstruction. The roentgenogram is examined for secondary signs of airway obstruction. Increased tension in the dilating muscles of the upper airway counterbalances the collapsing negative respiratory pressure force of severe upper airway obstruction causing distention of the hypopharynx. The chest roentgenogram may reveal underaeration because obstruction limits air entry or hyperinflation from air-trapping (e.g., bronchiolitis, asthma, or foreign body). Fluoroscopy helps define the degree of dynamic airway collapse secondary to laryngomalacia or tracheomalacia and may reveal asymmetric lung expansion due to a foreign body. A chest roentgenogram may also reveal the presence of acute pulmonary edema, which is occasionally observed with severe upper airway obstruction. Most commonly, this manifests immediately following relief of airway obstruction (e.g., following tracheal intubation).[7-9] Roentgenographic evaluation should include both anterior-posterior and lateral projections of the upper airway and chest so as to define pathology of the upper airway as well as the chest. In long-standing airway obstruction associated with hypoxemia and pulmonary hypertension, there may be radiologic evidence of cardiac failure. Computerized axial tomography (CAT scan) may be particularly valuable in defining the site and extent of airway obstruction when standard x-rays are equivocal. CAT scans have replaced the need for traditional tomography and xerograms. A barium swallow may be helpful in defining compression of the trachea by a vascular ring (e.g., double aortic arch). All radiologic studies must be carried out under the supervision of personnel equipped to deal with deterioration of the airway obstruction. Furthermore, the child's condition may be so critical that radiologic investigation may have to be postponed.

Endoscopy

Laryngoscopy and bronchoscopy are necessary for the diagnosis of the site, extent, and cause of the airway obstruction.[10] Despite negative radiologic investigation, endoscopic examination should be performed because pathology is frequently found when other tests are negative or equivocal. Flexible fiberoptic bronchoscopy may be a particularly helpful technique. Instruments are available that have an outer diameter as small as 1.8 mm (no suction channel). Fiberoptic bronchoscopy is a safe and effective instrument for examining the pediatric airway.[11-13] It is performed with topical anesthetic and light sedation, thus eliminating the need for rigid bronchoscopy under general anesthesia. It is of particular value in assessing the cause of stridor, as there is less distortion of the child's airway anatomy. Dynamic airway collapse during respiration is often better appreciated than would be the case under general anesthesia because the child's natural airway mechanisms are less affected as spontaneous respiration is maintained while ventilatory effort is not compromised by the light sedation. When rigid bronchoscopy is performed, the procedure must be carried out under appropriate conditions with skilled surgeons and anesthesiologists.

Airway obstruction may be due to a foreign body in the esophagus compressing the trachea. Frequently, the history of a foreign body is not forthcoming. It may be asymptomatic or associated with dysphagia. Thus, evaluation of the child with upper airway

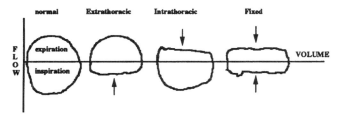

Figure 13–4. Flow volume loops (Courtesy Bernard Kinane, M.D.)

obstruction should include a search for an esophageal foreign body.

Physiologic Studies

Physiologic studies of airway resistance by measuring inspiratory and expiratory airflow produces flow-volume loops. Three types of upper airway obstruction can be identified on flow volume loops. Limitation of flow occurs during inspiration in extrathoracic obstruction (laryngomalacia, croup, post-extubation edema), during expiration in intrathoracic obstruction (tracheomalacia, vascular rings, compression by tumor) and during both inspiration and expiration in fixed airway obstruction (undersized endothracheal tube, tracheal stenosis) (Fig. 13-4).

Diseases of the Upper Airway

Epiglottitis (Supraglottitis)

Epiglottitis (supraglottitis) is a life-threatening infection occurring predominantly in children between the ages of 9 months and 7 years, but it is increasingly noted in adolescents and adults.[14,15] The inflammatory process involves the lingual surface of the epiglottis and aryepiglottic folds. This results in swelling of the epiglottis, which rapidly fills the vallecula. The infection may begin in the aryepiglottic folds and causes partial obstruction before significant involvement of the epiglottis. The organism causing the infection is usually *Hemophilus influenzae* type B.[16] Incidence of this disease appears to be decreasing as the vaccine to prevent *H. influenzae* infection controls the disease.

Clinical Presentation

The child is usually acutely ill with a temperature greater than 101°F. The child sits propped up with the head pushed forward to achieve a less obstructed airway. Inability to swallow (dysphagia) and drooling may be evident. Inspiratory stridor may not be as marked as that heard with laryngotracheobronchitis, probably due to less vigorous respiratory efforts. The stridor is softer and lower pitched. The voice and cry may be muffled. The **unpredictable** and **rapid** progression of symptoms may cause acute total airway obstruction, making this condition one that requires urgent evaluation and treatment.[17]

Differential Diagnosis

Epiglottitis (supraglottitis) should be differentiated from other significant life-threatening causes of upper airway obstruction (e.g., laryngotracheobronchitis [croup], bacterial tracheitis).[18] A retropharyngeal abscess may present with acute upper airway obstruction. Occasionally, acute tonsillitis in severely hypertrophied tonsils may cause acute upper airway obstruction. Diphtheria, a rare but important bacterial infection occurring in the nonimmunized child, may be responsible for acute upper airway obstruction. Other causes include angioneurotic edema, infectious mononucleosis, and laryngeal papillomatosis. A foreign body aspiration should always be considered in **any** acute upper airway obstruction.

Management

A well-defined protocol is necessary for the management of the child with epiglottitis (supraglottitis). Acute and total obstruction may be precipitated by interventions that cause crying and agitation as a result of severe dynamic airway collapse. It is therefore necessary to minimize these responses; that is, throat examination, arterial puncture for blood gas analysis, and placement of an intravenous line should be deferred until control of the airway has been secured by placement of an endotracheal tube or, if necessary, tracheostomy.[19,20] The unpredictable progression and the significant risks for morbidity and mortality make insertion of an artificial airway the safest course. The choice of artificial airway (i.e., endotracheal tube or tracheostomy) will depend on the experience of the physician and the facility where this procedure is performed. Our preference is endotracheal intubation. We have not performed a tracheostomy for supraglottitis for the past 25 years.

X-rays of the upper airway may be helpful in confirming the diagnosis of epiglottitis (supraglottitis) (Fig. 13-5) and in differentiating it from laryngotracheitis (Fig. 13-6) or a radioopaque foreign body. If the child is in acute distress, however, x-ray procedures may delay life-saving intervention; control of the airway should

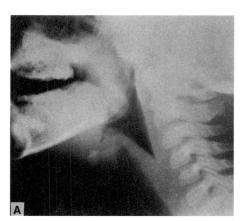

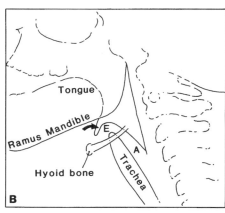

Figure 13-5. (A) Lateral neck roentgenogram of the child with epiglottitis (supraglottitis). Note the marked thickening of the aryepiglottic folds and the swollen epiglottis "hugged" by the hyoid bone. **(B)** Schematic representation of the lateral roentgenogram of the neck. (Reproduced from Todres ID and Berdel B. Pediatric emergencies. In Coté CJ, Ryan JF, Todres ID, Goudsouzian N, eds. *A Practice of Anesthesia for Infants and Children.* Philadelphia: WB. Saunders. 1992. With permission.

Figure 13-6. (A) Roentgenogram (anteroposterior view) of the normal upper airway compared with **(B)** the airway of a child with croup. Note the subglottic area filled in with inflammatory exudate *(arrows).* (Reproduced from Todres ID and Berdel B. Pediatric emergencies. In Coté CJ, Ryan JF, Todres ID, Goudsouzian N, eds. *A Practice of Anesthesia for Infants and Children.* Philadelphia: WB Saunders. 1992. With permission.

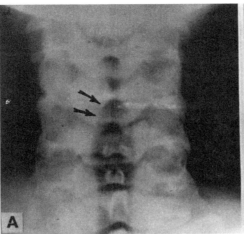 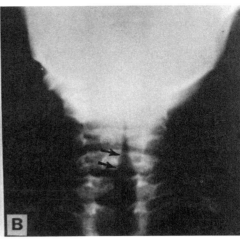

not be compromised in order to obtain radiologic evaluation. X-ray films of the upper airway should be taken only in the relatively stable child. Skilled personnel must accompany the child and be prepared to secure the airway (intubate) should critical obstruction occur.

Our management plan consists of transferring the child from the emergency room to the operating room where, under controlled conditions, general anesthesia is administered for placement of the endotracheal tube. In the procedure of tracheal intubation, prevention of hypoxemia and cardiovascular collapse is critical. Gentle, continuous positive end expiratory pressure (CPAP) may help prevent dynamic airway collapse, ensure adequate oxygenation, and provide an emergency temporary measure until tracheal intubation is achieved. Oxygen insufflation during laryngoscopy, using a modified laryngoscope (Oxyscope), may be helpful.[21] Some centers perform this maneuver in the pediatric intensive care unit (PICU). Generally, oral intubation is easier to perform and should be the first approach. If oral intubation was particularly difficult, the endotracheal tube should **not** be changed to a nasotracheal tube. Cultures of the blood and supraglottic structures are taken once the artificial airway has been secured. Antibiotics (ampicillin and chloramphenicol or third-generation cephalosporins) are administered and given for 10 days once organism sensitivity has been determined. Removal of the endotracheal tube is usually performed in 24 to 36 hours, and this may be signaled by the development of an air leak around the endotracheal tube.

On occasion, it may not be possible to establish an artificial airway with an endotracheal tube. In this desperate situation, percutaneous cricothyroid membrane puncture with an intravenous (IV) catheter and oxygen insufflation may be life-saving prior to a formal tracheostomy.[22,23] This procedure should accomplish oxygenation that will be life-saving; hypercarbia is generally well tolerated in the adequately oxygenated patient. Ventilation (i.e., elimination of carbon dioxide) is exceptionally difficult to achieve with intravenous catheter cricothyrotomy and is not absolutely essential. Any standard IV catheter, preferably 14- to 18-gauge (age-dependent), may be used to puncture the cricothyroid membrane. The patient must be properly positioned to bring the larynx forward; this may be accomplished by placing a rolled towel under the shoulders, allowing the head to fall back. Following aspiration of air, ensuring proper intratracheal position, the adaptor (15 mm of a 3-mm inner diameter endotracheal tube) is attached to the IV catheter. Oxygen is then insufflated with an Ambu bag capable

of an FiO_2 approaching 1.0. Note that in order to attempt ventilation, the pop-off valve must be disabled because the high resistance of the IV catheter necessitates very high inflation pressures. Alternatively, one could interpose a standard IV extension tubing between the oxygen flow metered delivery system and the IV catheter and insufflate oxygen. Caution is advised because excessively high flow rates may result in jet-type ventilation with possible rupture of alveoli, leading to pneumomediastinum and pneumothorax with massive subcutaneous emphysema. Generally, low flows of 20 to 50 cc/kg are preferred. Excess flows will generally decompress through the partially obstructed area. Note that the cricothyroid membrane is extremely small in the infant and child; the procedure is thus more difficult to accomplish in the young child, compared with the adult.

Occasionally, pulmonary edema may be associated with epiglottitis (supraglottitis) and is noted when relief of the airway obstruction is achieved with an endotracheal tube. Metastatic infection, which may lead to pneumonia, meningitis, pericarditis, or periarticular abscess, must be suspected when toxicity and fever do not resolve or when new symptoms appear.[24–28] Steroid therapy has been advocated by some, but there are no properly controlled studies demonstrating its effectiveness. Rifampin prophylaxis is usually administered to intimate contacts and to siblings under 8 years of age (see Antimicrobial Treatment of Sepsis by Lynfield and Warren, this volume).

Laryngotracheobronchitis

Dr. William Buchan, in *Treatise on the Prevention and Care of Diseases* (1803), wrote of the croup:

Children are often seized suddenly with this disease which, if not quickly relieved, proves mortal. It is known by various names. On the east coast of Scotland, it is called the croup. On the west, they call it the chock. In some parts of England, the good women call it the rising of the spirits. The disease generally prevails in cold and wet seasons. Children of a gross and lax habit are most liable to it. It is attended with a frequent pulse, quick and laborious breathing, which is performed with a peculiar kind of croaking noise that may be heard at a considerable distance—a sound compared by some to the crowing of a cock.

Laryngotracheobronchitis (croup) is the most common cause of acute upper airway obstruction in children from 6 months to

5 years of age. The disease is most often caused by a viral infection; the parainfluenza group is responsible for the majority of cases. *Mycoplasma* infection also may be responsible. The subglottic area at the level of the cricoid cartilage is primarily affected. Edema and swelling in this region causes an increase in resistance to breathing and retention of tracheobronchial secretions. The effect of narrowing the child's relatively small airway causes a disproportionate increase in airway resistance, compared with the older child or adult.

Clinical Presentation

The onset of laryngotracheobronchitis is insidious, usually with a few days of upper respiratory tract infection characterized by hoarseness and a "barking cough" followed by the development of inspiratory stridor. The child is tachypneic with chest retractions and becomes cyanotic breathing room air. This indicates severe hypoxemia due to ventilation-perfusion mismatching.[29] Increasing tachypnea, tachycardia, sternal and chest retractions, and deepening cyanosis signal life-threatening airway obstruction. A roentgenogram of the upper airway, particularly the anteroposterior view, demonstrating subglottic narrowing (sharpened pencil or steeple sign) may be helpful when the history and physical examination are atypical (Fig. 13-6). The differential diagnosis must consider other causes of a severe acute upper airway obstruction, for example, supraglottitis, bacterial tracheitis, foreign body, subglottic hemangioma, diphtheria, or esophageal foreign body.

Management

Management of the child with croup will depend on the severity of the disease. In assessing this, a number of croup scoring systems have been used. One such system, known as the Syracuse Croup Scoring System, has recently been validated.[30,31] The scoring system provided an excellent indication of whether the child was at risk of upper airway obstruction and thus required admission to the PICU rather than to the general pediatric unit. The scoring system employs assessment of stridor, presence of cyanosis, sternal retractions, respiratory rate, and heart rate. In the majority of cases, management includes allaying patient and family anxiety and providing oxygen therapy to treat hypoxemia. Sedatives to allay the child's anxiety and distress generally should be avoided and reliance placed more on the parents' calming of the child. Moist air therapy is traditional, but its efficacy in reducing glottic and subglottic edema associated with croup is not supported by scientific data.[32,33] The use of steroids remained controversial until recently. Metaanalyses and further studies on the use of steroids in croup have shown steroid administration to be effective in decreasing the severity of croup symptoms.[34–38] In some cases, tracheal intubation may be averted. Also, it may be possible to extubate intubated patients earlier. How steroids work in croup is uncertain. One factor may be their antiinflammatory action by inhibiting release of mediators such as interleukin-2, tumor necrosis factor, and metabolites of arachidonic acid. Corticosteroids also decrease capillary permeability, and this may be a factor in reducing subglottic edema. The steroids may be administered via the oral and IV routes or by inhalation.[39,40] We have used dexamethasone intravenously (0.3 mg/kg).

Inhalation of racemic epinephrine (0.5 ml in 3.0-ml saline) may benefit the child on a short-term basis by producing mucosal vasoconstriction and decreasing subglottic edema. Racemic epinephrine consists of both dextro- and levo-forms with the levorotatory form the active component. The agent is usually administered by a nebulizer. Previously, it had been administered by intermittent

positive pressure, but there appears to be no significant benefit over the nebulizer method.[41] This form of treatment probably does not affect the duration or ultimate severity of the child's illness. The treatments may need to be repeated every 1 to 3 hours due to the so-called rebound phenomena. It is unclear whether this rebound is progression of the disease or an actual exacerbation of the underlying pathology. Close monitoring of the child's cardiovascular status and airway patency is necessary.[42–44]

Should airway obstruction not respond to the initial epinephrine inhalation or become refractory with worsening symptoms or inability to clear secretions, tracheal intubation is necessary. The procedure is best performed under controlled conditions in the operating room with general anesthesia. The urgency of the situation may, however, dictate tracheal intubation at the bedside. In some circumstances, progressive respiratory distress is due to the presence of inspissated secretions that the child is unable to expectorate. Tracheal intubation provides a means for clearing secretions and maintaining airway patency. The endotracheal tube should be a 0.5- to 1.0-mm internal diameter smaller than would normally be chosen to avoid ischemic necrosis due to pressure in the subglottic region with potential for development of stenosis. Tracheostomy is an alternative procedure, and its practice will depend on the preference of the practitioner and the locale.

Extubation is carried out in the PICU after 3 to 5 days, or earlier, as an air leak develops around the endotracheal tube and the viscosity of secretions has diminished. Because the disease is viral in origin, it is inappropriate to administer antibiotics. However, one must exclude bacterial causes of airway obstruction that would require antibiotic therapy (e.g., epiglottitis and bacterial membranous tracheitis).

In arriving at the diagnosis of the underlying etiology of acute upper airway obstruction with croup-like symptoms, an unusual cause may need to be considered, as illustrated by the following case.[45]

A twelve year old female with a diagnosis of autoimmune neutropenia and rectal abscess developed sudden onset of inspiratory stridor, cyanosis and marked suprasternal retractions. This acute episode was preceded by 3 days of coryza, headache, and sore throat with a temperature of 101°F. X-rays of the upper airway showed extensive subglottic narrowing. The examination of the pharynx was normal and barium swallow and chest x-rays were negative. The child's symptoms improved slightly with oxygen therapy and racemic epinephrine inhalation. Three days following the onset of these symptoms, the child suddenly complained of severe difficulty breathing, became agitated, and developed respiratory arrest. Tracheal intubation was performed. Copious frothy secretions were aspirated from the endotracheal tube and the chest x-ray was suggestive of pulmonary edema. During tracheal toilet, a large plug of necrotic material was suctioned from the trachea. Over the next four days she developed signs of increased intracranial pressure unresponsive to all therapeutic maneuvers. At autopsy a large "membrane" was found in the subglottic area [Fig. 13-7]. Microscopy revealed the hyphae of *Aspergillus* [Fig. 13-8].

This case illustrates a rare cause of acute airway obstruction when the immune response of the body is compromised.

The use of helium-oxygen mixtures in the management of acute upper airway obstruction due to croup was practiced many years ago. There has been renewed interest in this method of treatment.[46,47] Although endotracheal intubation or tracheostomy remains the definitive treatment for life-threatening airway obstruction, this technique may be helpful in reducing the excessive work of breathing and in guiding the child through a crisis so that definitive therapy may be carried out under more optimally

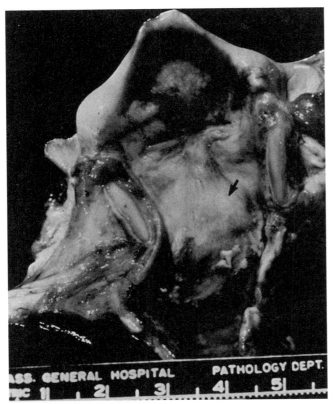

Figure 13-7. The larynx has been opened to show the subglottic membrane causing airway obstruction (*arrow*).

controlled conditions. Note that there is a limit to the inspired oxygen concentration of 40% for an effective amount of helium to reduce gas density. Thus, if the child's condition is complicated by severe hypoxemia requiring FiO_2 greater than 0.4, this technique is not suitable.

Bacterial Tracheitis

A severe form of croup is becoming more prevalent, namely, bacterial tracheitis, also referred to as pseudomembranous croup and membranous croup.[48–50] It is a primary airway infection most commonly due to *Staphylococcus aureus*; occasionally *H. influenzae* and *Streptococcus* are responsible. Severe subglottic edema occurs, followed by tracheal mucosa sloughing. There is inadequate mucociliary clearance, with production of copious mucopurulent secretions; this state may progress rapidly to life-threatening airway obstruction.

Clinical Presentation

The disease affects infants and children until early adolescence. It starts with an upper respiratory infection that progresses rapidly to acute toxicity and severe respiratory distress. Symptoms of stridor, hoarseness, and cough are prominent. Airway obstruction may lead to fatigue, inability to clear the airway, obstruction, and death from hypoxemia. Pulmonary infiltrates may be noted on the chest roentgenogram. With progression of the disease, establishment of an artificial airway by tracheal intubation is necessary to prevent serious hypoxemia. Bronchoscopy may be helpful in clarifying the diagnosis and clearing the airway of sloughing debris. Appropriate IV antibiotics, usually antistaphylococcal, are administered. Bacterial tracheitis should be considered in the differential diagnosis if the child does not respond to conventional therapy for viral croup.

Critical Airway Obstruction Due to Foreign Bodies

Acute life-threatening airway obstruction may follow aspiration of a foreign body.[51–56] On the other hand, the aspiration may be clinically undetected, initially leading to severe lung damage. Children in the first 2 to 3 years of life are particularly prone to aspirate foreign objects. In one study, 81% of cases occurred in children under 3 years of age.[57] The most common offending agents are peanuts, popcorn, hot dogs, plastic objects, and pins.

Most foreign bodies lodge in the trachea or a mainstem bronchus (right > left). Sharp foreign bodies (e.g., plastic, egg

Figure 13-8. Microscopic examination of the subglottic membrane (see Fig. 13-6) revealed hyphae of *Aspergillus*.

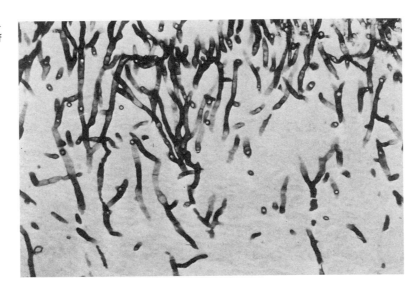

shell pieces, and pins) may impact in the larynx, producing symptoms of acute laryngeal edema. Black et al. reported on 548 children aged 4 months to 18 years, with successful identification and removal of aspirated foreign bodies in 440 children.[58] The foreign bodies were found in the right bronchus in 49%, in the left in 44%, and in the trachea and hypopharynx in 4%. Two thirds of the objects were lodged in the mainstem bronchi, and the remainder in the distal bronchi. When foreign body aspiration is suspected, one must always consider the possibility of multiple foreign bodies. Foreign body aspiration must be considered in all cases of sudden respiratory distress, regardless of age—an older sibling may be responsible for introducing the foreign body! Foreign body aspiration of a balloon has been reported in a 3-month-old infant.[59]

Clinical Presentation

The diagnosis of foreign body aspiration is usually made within the first few days in two thirds of cases; however, the diagnosis is **delayed** in one third of cases. The clinical picture is therefore modified by the interval from aspiration to diagnosis. The clinical presentation is also modified by the location of the foreign body. Thus, an extrathoracic location will present with **inspiratory stridor,** whereas an intrathoracic location will present with **wheezing.** In cases presenting acutely in the first 24 hours, there is usually a history of paroxysms of coughing, choking, gagging, wheezing, and severe respiratory distress from airway obstruction. The classic diagnostic triad (wheezing, coughing, decreased breath sounds on auscultation over the affected side) is more commonly encountered in the late diagnosed cases.[60] In some cases, following acute symptoms, the child may settle down with persistent cough and wheezing without respiratory distress, or there may be an asymptomatic interval followed by symptoms of complications such as obstruction, erosion (hemoptysis), or infection (pneumonia, lung abscess). It must be appreciated that children who wheeze are not necessarily asthmatic; foreign body aspiration may be the underlying cause.

Chest roentgenogram and fluoroscopy are important diagnostic procedures. It should be noted that the majority of aspirated foreign bodies are **not** radioopaque, as plastic foreign bodies are increasingly the objects of aspiration. Obstructive emphysema or atelectasis may be observed on the obstructed side with shift of the mediastinum; initially, hyperinflation is due to a ball-valve effect allowing air to enter the lung but impeding its exit. Once total obstruction occurs, the air distal to the obstructing foreign body is absorbed, resulting in atelectasis of the lung. Hyperinflation may be enhanced by forced expiration. In the study by Black et al., inspiratory and expiratory chest radiographs were positive in 83% of the children.[58] Fluoroscopy findings were positive for 67% of patients. In the Wolach et al. study, fluoroscopy was diagnostic in 92% of patients.[57]

Should the diagnosis of an aspirated foreign body be delayed, pneumonitis may follow. Recurrent, persistent, localized pneumonitis that does not respond to standard medical therapy requires investigation for an underlying foreign body. Bronchial obstruction by a foreign body is probably the most common cause of "recurrent" pneumonia.

Esophageal foreign bodies impacting at sites of anatomical constriction (i.e., the posterior cricoid region and at the level of aortic arch) may produce compression of the trachea and serious airway obstruction. Thus, if bronchoscopy is unable to locate the cause of airway obstruction, esophagoscopy also should be performed.

Management

Debate continues over the emergency measures used to dislodge a foreign body. Back blows have been blamed for causing further distal impaction of the foreign body; abdominal thrusts, (Heimlich maneuver) have been reported to be effective.[61] In infants (<1 year), however, back blows followed by chest thrusts are recommended, as abdominal thrusts are considered potentially traumatic to the infant's abdominal viscera. Abdominal thrusts are recommended for children over 1 year of age. These guidelines continue to be a subject of debate and controversy.

A victim who undergoes a Heimlich maneuver should be medically examined as soon as possible to rule out complications such as ruptured stomach, ruptured jejunum, esophageal rupture, and hepatic or splenic injury.[62,63]

Anesthesia and bronchoscopy for removal of the foreign body should be carried out by skilled personnel with appropriate equipment (i.e., rigid bronchoscope such as the Storz bronchoscope with Hopkins rod-lens system). Removal of the foreign body is usually accomplished with a forceps.[64-68] The tracheobronchial tree is completely inspected because multiple foreign bodies may have been aspirated. A Fogarty embolectomy balloon catheter is often used to dislodge a distally impacted foreign body.[69] The catheter is advanced beyond the foreign body, the balloon inflated, and then pulled back together with the bronchoscope to the pharynx from where the foreign body is removed. Extraction may be difficult with foreign bodies that tend to crumble, such as peanuts and egg shells. Very rarely, the foreign body, if deeply lodged in the bronchus, may have to be removed via a thoracotomy and bronchotomy. Following removal of the foreign body, the child may continue to have symptoms due to the presence of residual foreign bodies. Flexible fiberoptic bronchoscopy is a useful technique to further evaluate distal airways for residual foreign body fragments.[70]

Following a difficult removal of a foreign body, the child may have glottic and airway edema and require steroid therapy and racemic epinephrine inhalations. The use of steroids, while frequently advocated, remains uncertain in this situation, although recent studies have shown its value in infectious croup.[34-40] Early extraction through bronchoscopy will reduce local lung damage and distal parenchymal complications such as bronchiectasis. Esophageal foreign bodies may be removed with the aid of a Fogarty-type catheter in a manner such as that described for airway foreign bodies. The extraction of the esophageal foreign body with this technique, however, without endotracheal intubation, may lead to its movement from the esophagus (as it is extracted into the pharynx) into the airway, causing airway obstruction.

Tracheal Stenosis

Tracheal stenosis in infants and children may be congenital or acquired.[71]

Congenital Tracheal Stenosis

Congenital tracheal stenosis is a rare life-threatening condition.[72] Pathologically, the luminal narrowing is due to the presence of complete tracheal rings. This may present as an isolated lesion or be associated with other anomalies. There is a high association between congenital tracheal stenosis and pulmonary artery sling. In this condition, compression and narrowing of the posterior tracheal wall is due to the anomalous origin of the left pulmonary artery from the right pulmonary artery. Despite surgical correction of the vascular anomaly, some degree of tracheal stenosis remains because of the underlying tracheal defect. Compression of the trachea causing tracheal stenosis may be due to other vascular anomalies (e.g., double aortic arch). Correction of the vascular anomaly generally relieves the airway obstruction, although some infants continue to have respiratory difficulty for prolonged periods. In other cases, the ligamentum arteriosum is responsible for the compression but remains unsuspected because it will not be visualized on an angiogram. Innominate artery compression of the trachea may be severe enough in some children to cause significant narrowing of the airway lumen. In this situation, aortopexy relieves the airway obstruction.

Acquired Tracheal Stenosis

Acquired tracheal stenosis is associated with (1) postintubation (endotracheal tube or tracheostomy), (2) posttrauma, (3) thermal and/or chemical burns, or (4) primary tumors (rare).[73] Tracheal stenosis is relatively uncommon in neonates and occurs more frequently in older children. Tracheal pressure necrosis from an endotracheal or tracheostomy tube causes mucosal injury with the formation of granulation tissue, perichondritis, and scar formation, resulting in stenosis. This is associated with varying degrees of obstruction, which may be life-threatening.

Clinical Presentation

Congenital tracheal stenosis must be considered in any infant who has episodes of stridor cyanosis, wheezing, recurrent pneumonias (inability to clear secretions), or sudden respiratory arrest. With congenital tracheal stenosis, symptoms may appear at birth or shortly thereafter as the stenosed airway becomes inadequate for the growing child's greater ventilatory needs. With upper respiratory infection, mucus plugs and edema secondary to inflammation may acutely narrow the tracheal lumen even further and precipitate respiratory failure. Respiratory distress, stridor, and retractions increase with agitation and crying as a result of dynamic collapse of the airway associated with increased respiratory efforts. Airway obstruction is aggravated by the inability to clear mucus. With distal tracheal obstruction, wheezing may be heard and may be misdiagnosed as allergic asthma. Tracheal stenosis should be suspected when there is a history of recent tracheal intubation or tracheostomy and particularly if a diagnosis of asthma has been made, but it has not responded to standard therapeutic maneuvers.

Examination of the child should include a search for other anatomic anomalies, especially vascular. This includes echocardiography and, in selected cases, angiography. Roentgenograms, MRIs, or CT scans of the anterior-posterior and lateral neck and chest may provide visualization of the location and extent of the tracheal pathology. Airway fluoroscopy demonstrates the dynamic movements of the airway with respiration and any associated degree of tracheomalacia. Tracheobronchography is potentially dangerous because of possible reaction to the contrast material, causing further airway obstruction. Barium swallow may further assist in diagnosing a vascular anomaly (e.g., double arotic arch). Complete radiologic study of the airway may necessitate temporary removal of the endotracheal tube. In this situation, sudden severe obstruction of the airway may occur. A physician skilled in airway control should be in attendance at the x-ray facility to replace the endotracheal tube if necessary.

Management

Bronchoscopy is performed for the definitive diagnosis. At that time, the trachea may then be dilated.[74] The bronchoscopy and dilation may be accompanied by bleeding and edema, which may aggravate the respiratory distress. This problem should be anticipated and postbronchoscopy admission to the PICU planned. Racemic epinephrine inhalation may partly alleviate obstruction due to edema; however, progressively increasing distress from obstruction may require tracheal intubation. Prior to intubation, if this is required, positive end expiratory pressure with a face mask, 100% oxygen, and an adjustable pop-off PEEP valve can force oxygen into the lungs by counteracting the dynamic airway collapse that occurs with increasing respiratory efforts.

The child should remain in an ICU, carefully monitored and treated aggressively should deterioration occur. With significant airway obstruction, narcotics and sedatives should be avoided, as they may cause central respiratory depression and precipitate acute respiratory failure. If the child is relatively stable and able to cope with physical restriction, conservative management is preferred, delaying surgical resection until the child is at an age when tracheal resection would be considered a safer procedure.[75,76]

Different treatments are employed before tracheal resection is performed. These include dilation, steroid injection, diathermy, resection, cryosurgery, and laser surgery. These techniques may be particularly helpful when granulation tissue is present and in the early stages of scar formation. Resection, even in small infants, offers the best chance for success once the scar tissue becomes hard and fibrous.[77,78] As much as 50% of the tracheal length may be resected and a primary anastomosis performed. With extensive tracheal stenosis, however, newer techniques, such as the use of cartilage grafts, pericardial patch, and stents made of a flexible steel spring coated with silicone rubber, have been employed.[79–82] Cardiopulmonary bypass may be required.

Because the presence of an endotracheal tube (foreign body) may predispose to breakdown of the anastomosis, it is generally recommended that the child be extubated, if possible, at the conclusion of surgery. Judicious use of analgesics and sedatives is necessary, especially in the infant. Overzealous use of opioids and benzodiazepines may lead to respiratory arrest and the need for artificial ventilation. Should the child have to remain intubated, endotracheal tube positioning is critical, as the infant's shortened trachea and flexed head position (to prevent stretching of the anastomosis) may predispose to accidental mainstem bronchial intubation or extubation with minimal movement.

Tracheomalacia

Abnormal flaccidity of the tracheal wall leading to tracheal collapse during respiration is referred to as tracheomalacia. Flexible fiberoptic bronchoscopy allows visualization of the airway dynamics and has revealed a more frequent occurrence of tracheomalacia than was previously reported. Malformation of the tracheobronchial cartilages leads to inadequate support, thereby allowing expiratory collapse. The condition may be associated with tracheoesophageal fistula where there is deficiency of tracheal cartilage or secondary to extrinsic compression from vascular anomalies or mediastinal masses. Acquired tracheomalacia may follow tracheostomy or prolonged tracheal intubation, especially with cuffed endotracheal tubes. For this reason, when we employ cuffed endotracheal tubes, high-volume–low-pressure cuffs inflated to the minimum pressure and allowing adequate ventilation are preferred. Tracheomalacia may extend into the mainstem bronchi (bronchomalacia), making this a much more difficult problem for the child, clinically and surgically.

Clinical Presentation

In primary tracheomalacia, the presentation is that of an infant with unexplained respiratory distress manifested by stridor and cyanosis. The symptoms appear after the first few weeks of life, aggravated by infections and agitation. Spontaneous resolution may take as long as 2 years.[83] The clinical history of previous intubation or tracheostomy may suggest this diagnosis in a child who has symptoms of airway obstruction that are aggravated by stress, crying, and agitation.

Airway fluoroscopy defines the dynamic aspects of tracheomalacia, that is, constriction and dilation of the tracheal wall related to phases of respiration. Rigid bronchoscopy at **light** levels of general anesthesia with spontaneous ventilation or fiberoptic bronchoscopy using sedation and local anesthesia provide the best conditions for assessing the airway dynamics. In making the diagnosis of innominate artery compression as the cause of the underlying respiratory distress, care should be taken in interpreting the bronchoscopic findings due to distortion of the airway with a rigid bronchoscope.

Management

The natural history for most children with tracheomalacia is for the tracheal wall to become more stable. This usually occurs by 2 years of age, and thus surgery is rarely indicated. However, underlying causes for secondary tracheomalacia should be identified and treated. Occasionally, a temporary tracheostomy may be required. Those children requiring tracheostomy to maintain a safe, clear airway appear to take longer to stabilize their airways. In selected cases, vascular suspension of the aorta or innominate artery relieves the problem. Long-term (up to 24 months) positive end-expiratory pressure of 8 to 10 cms H_2O via a tracheostomy tube has been effective in stabilizing the upper airway until the tracheal wall has become firm and less compliant.[84,85] Surgical treatment using an implanted synthetic graft has been successfully carried out, apparently without compromising airway growth.[86]

Mediastinal Masses

Mediastinal masses occur in the anterior, middle, and posterior mediastinum. Common mediastinal masses according to location are

1. Anterior mediastinum: lymphoma, teratoma, cystic hygroma, pericardial cyst, diaphragmatic hernia (via foramen of Morgagni)
2. Middle mediastinum: lymphoma, tuberculous lymphadenopathy
3. Posterior mediastinum: neurogenic tumor (neuroblastoma, ganglioneuroma, neurofibroma), esophageal duplication, bronchogenic cyst, diaphragmatic hernia (via foramen of Bochdalek)

The effect of mediastinal masses on the airways, lungs, and cardiovascular system through airway compression is impaired pulmonary ventilation and/or decreased cardiac output. Anesthesia, bronchoscopy, and surgery may be hazardous unless careful investigation and preparation are carried out.[87,88]

Anterior Mediastinum

Anterior mediastinal masses may produce severe respiratory and cardiovascular complications. Obstruction of major airways, cardiac compression producing tamponade, and superior vena caval obstruction may occur (Figs. 13-9 and 13-10). Malignant lymphoma may envelope the heart with infiltration of the pericar-

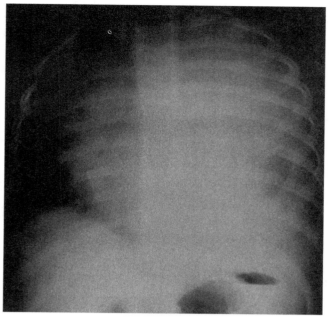

Figure 13-9. Roentgenogram (anteroposterior view) in an 18-month-old presenting with stridor, retractions, cyanosis, and superior vena caval syndrome. The roentgenogram shows a massive lesion (lymphoma) in the chest originating in the anterior mediastinum but growing to involve virtually the entire left chest. The trachea is deviated to the right. (Courtesy of Lynne Ferrari, MD)

dium, producing pericardial tamponade.[89] Most anterior mediastinal masses are lymphomatous in origin (Hodgkin's and non-Hodgkin's lymphoma). It is important to appreciate that cervical masses may also extend into the mediastinum, causing airway compression (e.g., cystic hygroma).

Clinical Presentation

Anterior mediastinal masses may be clinically asymptomatic and detected incidentally on chest x-ray for an unrelated problem. Clinical symptoms and signs associated with the anterior mediastinal mass include cough (especially in the supine position), symptoms of superior vena caval obstruction, stridor, wheezing, retractions, decreased breath sounds, or onset of a new heart murmur related to the pulmonary artery. A night cough is particularly significant as a symptom of airway compression.

Posterior Mediastinum

Posterior mediastinal masses (e.g., esophageal duplication cyst) may cause respiratory distress through pressure on adjacent lung parenchyma. In addition, compression of the esophagus can lead to dysphagia, reflux, and aspiration. On occasion, the symptoms may be incorrectly attributed to other conditions. The authors have seen a child present with "asthma" unresponsive to treatment with bronchodilators, who, on further evaluation, was found to have a large mediastinal mass (neurogenic tumor) obstructing the airway. Surgical removal of the tumor cured the "asthma"!

Preoperative preparation of the child with a mediastinal mass includes evaluation of the degree of airway obstruction and cardiovascular compromise. In addition to clinical evaluation, specific x-rays and laboratory studies are performed. Tomography, fluoroscopy, CT scans, and/or MRI of the airway provide definition of the obstruction. Pulmonary flow-volume loop studies in the upright

Figure 13-10. CT scan of infant referred to in Fig. 13-8, showing the very large lymphoma filling virtually the entire left chest. Note the trachea has been compressed *(arrow).* (Courtesy of Lynne Ferrari, MD)

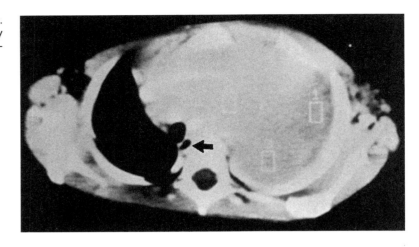

and supine positions provide sensitive indicators of obstructive lesion of the major airways in older children; peak flow rate may show a significant decrease even when the CT scan has revealed no airway obstruction. These can be performed only in the cooperative child. These patients are at general risk for acute life-threatening compromise if sedated for their procedures; thus, it may not be appropriate to pursue these studies in all patients. In evaluating hemodynamic stability, the possibility of cardiac tamponade must be considered; thus, it is important to examine for pulsus paradoxus and perform echocardiography.

In some cases, especially in Hodgkin's disease, where compression of the trachea and bronchi by the mediastinal mass is perceived as life-threatening, irradiation of the tumor prior to anesthesia may ameliorate the degree of airway obstruction and provide a safer anesthetic induction. Preradiation tissue diagnosis may be indicated, however, so that an accurate tissue diagnosis is made. Radiation therapy may affect cellular morphology and preclude an accurate tissue diagnosis and thus lead to suboptimal chemotherapy and/or radiation treatment. General anesthesia, and especially the use of muscle relaxants, in these patients may be extremely hazardous. In the absence of spontaneous respiration, it may be extremely difficult to ventilate the patient, even with an endotracheal tube in place. Sudden airway obstruction or cardiovascular collapse may necessitate turning the patient to one side, or even prone, to relieve mechanical impairment of ventilation or cardiac output. If carefully performed, however, with a full understanding of the patient's cardiorespiratory status, general anesthesia has been successfully carried out prior to radiation therapy.[90] Local anesthesia in preference to general anesthesia may be used for the biopsy procedure, if suitable, although this may be difficult to accomplish in young or uncooperative children. In rare situations, standby cardiopulmonary bypass is necessary. Thoracotomy is usually necessary to make the specific diagnosis. Excision of the entire mediastinal mass is undertaken, if possible. If airway compromise is encountered on induction or maintenance of general anesthesia, the child should remain intubated in the ICU pending tissue-specific radiation or chemotherapy. Following treatment, the airway obstruction will be relieved and the patient safely extubated.

References

1. Tucker JA, O'Rahilly R. Observations on the embryology of the human larynx. *Ann Otol Rhinol Laryngol* 81:520, 1972.

2. Tucker JA, Tucker GF. Some aspects of fetal laryngeal development. *Ann Otol Rhinol Laryngol* 81:49, 1975.

3. Miller MJ et al. Effect of maturation on oral breathing in sleeping premature infants. *J Pediatr* 109:515, 1986.

4. Miller MJ et al. Oral breathing in newborn infants. *J Pediatr* 107:465, 1985.

5. Holinger LD. Etiology of stridor in the neonate, infant and child. *Ann Otol Rhinol Laryngol* 89:397, 1980.

6. Maze A, Bloch E. Stridor in pediatric patients. *Anesthesiology* 50:132, 1979.

7. Travis KW, Todres ID, Shannon DC. Pulmonary edema associated with croup and epiglottitis. *Pediatrics* 59:695, 1977.

8. Oswalt CE, Gates GA, Holmstrom FMG. Pulmonary edema as a complication of acute airway obstruction. *JAMA* 238:1833, 1977.

9. Kanter RK, Watchko JF. Pulmonary edema associated with upper airway obstruction. *Am J Dis Child* 138:356, 1984.

10. Benjamin B. Endoscopy in congenital tracheal anomalies. *J Pediatr Surg* 15:164, 1980.

11. Nussbaum E. Flexible fiberoptic bronchoscopy and laryngoscopy in infants and children. *Laryngoscope* 93:1073, 1983.

12. Wood RE. Spelunking in the pediatric airways: Explorations with the flexible fiberoptic bronchoscope. *Pediatr Clin North Am* 31:785, 1984.

13. Noviski N, Todres ID. Fiberoptic bronchoscopy in the pediatric patient. *Anesthesiol Clin North Am* 9:163, 1991.

14. Baker AS, Eavey RD. Adult supraglottitis (epiglottitis). *N Engl J Med* 314:1185, 1986.

15. Mayo Smith MF et al. Acute epiglottitis in adults. An eight-year experience in the state of Rhode Island. *N Engl J Med* 314:1133, 1986.

16. Faden HS. Treatment of *Haemophilus* influenzae type B epiglottitis. *Pediatrics* 63:402, 1979.

17. Kilham H, Gillis J, Benjamin B. Severe upper airway obstruction. *Pediatr Clin North Am* 34:461, 1987.

18. Jones R, Santos JI, Overall JB. Bacterial tracheitis. *JAMA* 242:721, 1979.

19. Rapkin RH. Nasotracheal intubation in epiglottitis. *Pediatrics* 56:110, 1975.

20. Cohen SR, Chai J. Epiglottitis, 20-year study with tracheotomy. *Ann Otol Rhinol Laryngol* 87:461, 1978.

21. Todres ID, Crone RK. Experience with a modified laryngoscope in sick infants. *Crit Care Med* 9:544, 1981.

22. Coté CJ et al. Cricothyroid membrane puncture. Oxygenation and ventilation in a dog model using an intravenous catheter. *Crit Care Med* 16:615, 1988.

23. Slutsky AS et al. Tracheal insufflation of O_2 at low flow rates sustains life for several hours. *Anesthesiology* 63:278, 1985.

24. Dajani AS, Asmar BI, Thirumoorthi MC. Systemic hemophilus influenzae disease: An overview. *J Pediatr* 94:355, 1979.

25. Friedman EM et al. Supraglottitis and concurrent Hemophilus meningitis. *Ann Otol Rhinol Laryngol* 94:470, 1985.
26. Kresch MJ. Pericarditis complicating hemophilus epiglottitis. *Pediatr Infect Dis* 4:559, 1985.
27. Molteni RA. Epiglottitis: Incidence of extra-epiglottic infection: Report of 72 cases and review of the literature. *Pediatrics* 58:526, 1976.
28. Walker SH. Influenza b epiglottitis and meningitis. *Pediatrics* 67:581, 1981.
29. Newth CJL, Levison H, Bryan HC. The respiratory status of children with croup. *J Pediatr* 81:1068, 1972.
30. Leipsig B et al. A prospective randomized study to determine the efficacy of steroids in treatment of croup. *J Pediatr* 94:194–196, 1979.
31. Jacobs S et al. Validation of a croup score and its use in triaging children with croup. *Anesthesia* 49:903–906, 1994.
32. Henry R. Moist air in the treatment of laryngotracheitis. *Arch Dis Child* 58:577, 1983.
33. Bourchier D, Dawson KP, Fergusson DM. Humidification in viral croup: A controlled trial. *Aust Paediatr J* 20:289–291, 1984.
34. Kairys SW, Olmstead EM, O'Conner GT. Steroid treatment of laryngotracheitis: A meta-analysis of the evidence from randomized trials. *Pediatrics* 83:683, 1989.
35. Super DM et al. A prospective randomized double-blind study to evaluate the effect of dexamethasone in acute laryngotracheitis. *J Pediatr* 115:323, 1989.
36. Freezer N, Butt W, Phelan P. Steroids in croup: Do they increase the incidence of successful extubation? *Anaesth Intensive Care* 18:224, 1990.
37. Editorial: Steroids and croup. *Lancet* 2:1134, 1989.
38. Tibballs J, Shann FA, Landau LT. Placebo controlled trial of prednisone in children intubated for croup. *Lancet* 340:745–748, 1992.
39. Klassen TP et al. Nebulized budesonide for children with mild-moderate croup. *N Engl J Med* 331:285–289, 1994.
40. Landau LT, Geelhoed GC. Aerosolized steroids for croup. *N Engl J Med* 331:322–323, 1994.
41. Fogel JM et al. Racemic epinephrine in the treatment of croup: Nebulization alone versus nebulization with intermittent positive pressure breathing. *J Pediatr* 101:1028, 1982.
42. Taussig LM et al. Treatment of laryngotracheobronchitis (croup): Use of intermittent positive pressure breathing and racemic epinephrine. *Am J Dis Child* 129:790, 1975.
43. Westley CR, Cotton EK, Brooks JG. Nebulized racemic epinephrine by IPPB for the treatment of croup; a double blind study. *Am J Dis Child* 132:484, 1978.
44. Skolnik NS. Treatment of croup: A critical review. *Am J Dis Child* 143:1045–1049, 1989.
45. Todres ID. Critical airway obstruction. In Tinker J, Zapol WM (eds): *Care of the Critically Ill Patient* (2nd ed). New York: Springer, 1992. P 1317.
46. Duncan PG. Efficacy of helium-oxygen mixtures in the management of severe viral and post-intubation croup. *Can Anaesth Soc J* 26:206, 1979.
47. Skrinkas GJ, Hyland RH, Hutcheon MA. Using helium-oxygen mixtures in the management of acute upper airway obstruction. *Can Med Assoc J* 128:555, 1983.
48. Friedman EM et al. Bacterial tracheitis: Two-year experience. *Laryngoscope* 95:9, 1985.
49. Han BK, Dunbar JS, Striker TW. Membranous laryngotracheobronchitis (membranous croup). *AJR* 133:53, 1979.
50. Jones R, Santos JI, Overall JC Jr. Bacterial tracheitis. *JAMA* 242:721, 1979.
51. Aytac A et al. Inhalation of foreign bodies in children: Report of 500 cases. *J Thorac Cardiovasc Surg* 74:145, 1977.
52. Blazer S, Navelo Y, Friedman A. Foreign body in the airway; a review of 200 cases. *Am J Dis Child* 134:68, 1980.
53. Cotton E, Yasuda K. Foreign body aspiration. *Pediatr Clin North Am* 31:937, 1984.
54. Strome M. Tracheobronchial foreign bodies: An updated approach. *Ann Otol Rhinol Laryngol* 86:649, 1977.
55. Lima JA. Laryngeal foreign bodies in children: A persistent life-threatening problem. *Laryngoscope* 99:415, 1989.
56. Friedman EM. Foreign bodies in the pediatric aerodigestive tract. *Pediatr Ann* 17:640, 1988.
57. Wolach B et al. Aspirated foreign bodies in the respiratory tract of children: Eleven years experience with 127 patients. *Int J Pediatr Otorhinolaryngol* 30:1, 1994.
58. Black RE, Johnson DG, Matlak ME. Bronchoscopic removal of aspirated foreign bodies in children. *J Pediatr Surg* 29:682, 1994.
59. Anas NG, Perkin RM. Aspiration of a balloon by a 3-month-old. *JAMA* 250:385, 1983.
60. Wiseman NE. The diagnosis of foreign body aspiration in childhood. *J Pediatr Surg* 19:531, 1984.
61. Heimlich HJ, Patrick EA. The Heimlich maneuver; best technique for saving any choking victim's life. *Postgrad Med* 87:38, 1990.
62. Haynes DE, Haynes BE, Yong YV. Esophageal rupture complicating Heimlich maneuver. *Am J Emerg Med* 2:507, 1984.
63. van der Ham AC, Lange JF. Traumatic rupture of the stomach after Heimlich maneuver. *J Emerg Med* 8:713, 1990.
64. Abman SH, Fan LL, Colton EK. Emergency treatment of foreign body obstruction of the upper airway in children. *J Emerg Med* 2:7, 1984.
65. Black RE et al. Bronchoscopic removal of aspirated foreign bodies in children. *Am J Surg* 148:778, 1984.
66. Cohen SR et al. Foreign bodies in the airway: Five year retrospective study with special reference to management. *Ann Otol Rhinol Laryngol* 89:437, 1980.
67. Hight DW, Phillipart AI, Hertzler JH. The treatment of retained foreign bodies in the pediatric airway. *J Pediatr Surg* 16:694, 1981.
68. Kosloske AM. Bronchoscopic extraction of aspirated foreign bodies in children. *Am J Dis Child* 136:924, 1982.
69. Hunsicker RC, Gartner WS Jr. Fogarty catheter technique for removal of endobronchial foreign body. *Arch Otolaryngol* 103:103, 1977.
70. Wood RE, Gauderer MW. Flexible fiberoptic bronchoscopy in the management of tracheobronchial foreign bodies in children: The value of a combined approach with open tube bronchoscopy. *J Pediatr Surg* 19:693, 1984.
71. Cotton RT. Pediatric laryngotracheal stenosis. *J Pediatr Surg* 19:699, 1984.
72. Loeff DS et al. Congenital tracheal stenosis: A review of 22 patients from 1965 to 1987. *J Pediatr Surg* 23:744, 1988.
73. O'Neill JA Jr. Experience with iatrogenic laryngeal and tracheal stenosis. *J Pediatr Surg* 19:235, 1984.
74. Benjamin B. Endoscopy in congenital tracheal anomalies. *J Pediatr Surg* 15:164, 1980.
75. Benjamin B, Pitkin J, Cohen D. Congenital tracheal stenosis. *Ann Otol Rhinol Laryngol* 90:364, 1981.
76. Grillo HC, Zannini P. Management of obstructive tracheal disease in children. *J Pediatr Surg* 19:414, 1984.
77. Akl BF, Yabek SM, Berman W Jr. Total tracheal reconstruction in a three-month old infant. *J Thorac Cardiovasc Surg* 87:543, 1984.
78. Sorensen HR, Holsteen V. Resection of congenital stenosis of the trachea in an infant. *Acta Paediatr Scand* 73:141, 1984.
79. Filler RM et al. Treatment of segmental tracheomalacia and bronchomalacia by implantation of an airway splint. *J Pediatr Surg* 17:597, 1982.
80. Idriss FS et al. Tracheoplasty with pericardial patch for extensive tracheal stenosis in infants and children. *J Thorac Cardiovasc Surg* 19:527, 1984.
81. Majeski JA et al. Tracheoplasty for tracheal stenosis in the pediatric burned patient. *J Trauma* 20:81, 1981.
82. Saad SA, Falla S. Management of intractable and extensive tracheal stenosis by implantation of cartilage graft. *J Pediatr Surg* 18:472, 1983.
83. Cogbill TH et al. Primary tracheomalacia. *Ann Thorac Surg* 35:538, 1983.
84. Sotomayor JL et al. Large-airway collapse due to acquired tracheobronchomalacia in infancy. *Am J Dis Child* 140:367, 1986.
85. Wiseman NE, Duncan PG, Cameron CB. Management of tracheo-

bronchomalacia with continuous positive airway pressure. *J Pediatr Surg* 20:489, 1985.

86. Vinograd I, Filler RM, Bahoric A. Long-term functional results of prosthetic airway splinting in tracheomalacia and bronchomalacia. *J Pediatr Surg* 22:38, 1987.

87. Piro AJ, Weiss DR, Hellman S. Mediastinal Hodgkin's disease: A possible danger for intubation anesthesia. Intubation danger in Hodgkin's disease. *Int J Radiat Oncol Biol Phys* 1:415, 1976.

88. Todres ID et al. Management of critical airway obstruction in a child with a mediastinal tumor. *Anesthesiology* 45:100, 1976.

89. Keon TP. Death on induction of anesthesia for cervical node biopsy. *Anesthesiology* 55:471, 1981.

90. Ferrari LR, Bedford RF. General anesthesia prior to treatment of anterior mediastinal masses in pediatric cancer patients. *Anesthesiology* 72:991, 1990.

Kristen Outwater

14 Asthma and Bronchiolitis

Asthma

Asthma is a reversible, obstructive, small airways disease. A National Institutes of Health (NIH) Expert Panel on Asthma agreed on a working definition: "Asthma is a lung disease with the following characteristics: (1) airway obstruction that is reversible (but not completely so in some patients) either spontaneously or with treatment; (2) airway inflammation; and (3) increased airway responsiveness to a variety of stimuli.[1] Status asthmaticus is an acute exacerbation of asthma that does not respond to appropriate drug therapy and may lead to progressive respiratory insufficiency and failure. Patients present with cough, wheezing, prolonged expiration, hypoxemia, and respiratory distress.

Epidemiology

Deaths from asthma appear to be on the increase, both in the United States and worldwide.[2] Approximately 5000 Americans, including children, die from asthma each year. Most of these deaths are preventable if treatment is instituted early and effectively.[3,4] In addition, uncontrolled asthma is responsible for serious chronic disability in the sufferer. There is an increased risk in ethnic and racial minorities who live in poor conditions.[5,6] Other risk factors associated with increased mortality include prolonged illness, increased bronchial reactivity, recurrent exacerbations of the illness, poor control of the asthma, marked oral steroid dependency, and poor compliance with medical therapy.

Pathophysiology

There are two recognizable patterns in asthma that, on the basis of pathophysiology, will present differently clinically (Fig. 14-1). Both may lead to respiratory failure and death from status asthmaticus.[7–9]

Characteristically, increased airflow obstruction gradually leads to progressive worsening of the asthma. This pattern accounts for the majority of severe attacks and mortality associated with asthma.[10] Airway inflammation and hyperresponsiveness are present in all of these patients with asthma, and when triggered by stimuli, the inflammatory response and airway smooth muscle constriction leads to airway obstruction.

Inflammatory mediators are released from inflammatory cells and eosinophils that have migrated to the airways. These mediators initiate inflammatory response, which leads to exudation of fluid into the airway mucosa, and stimulate excessive mucous secretion. The secretions are often thick and tenacious, consisting of cells, fibrin, and mucus.

The hallmark of asthma is increased airway resistance from bronchospasm, edema of the mucosa, and increased mucous secretions. Autopsy studies suggest that while bronchospasm may be the most important factor in the acute onset of a reversible attack, mucous plugging and airway edema become more important in a prolonged attack and may contribute to significant morbidity and mortality.[11]

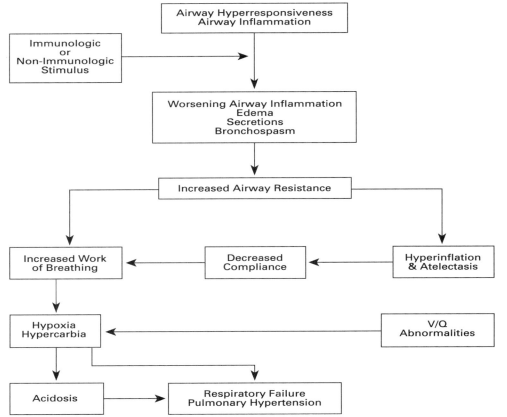

Figure 14-1. Pathophysiology of respiratory failure in asthma

Full airway obstruction leads to atelectasis; partial obstruction with a check-valve function (such that air enters but cannot exit distal airways) results in hyperinflation of distal alveoli. Decreased compliance and ventilation/perfusion mismatching result. An increase in minute ventilation compensates for the elevation in dead space, but the increased work of breathing, especially as oxygen consumption and carbon dioxide production rise, leads to respiratory muscle fatigue. Progressive inability to prevent hypoxemia, hypercarbia, and acidosis follows. Poor compliance also contributes to the increased work of breathing. Respiratory failure, in some cases accompanied by pulmonary hypertension and cardiac failure, may ensue.

A second pattern of presentation in the asthmatic patient which is less common is a rapid deterioration occurring without an apparent initiating incident or following a period of unstable asthma.[8] This rapid deterioration occurs secondary to severe bronchospasm. Neutrophils predominate in the airways, and there is little mucus associated with the attack. These patients may suffer a respiratory arrest within minutes of presentation, requiring urgent tracheal intubation and mechanical ventilation. They appear to have a bluntell perception of breathlessness and have been shown to have a significant reduction in chemoreceptor sensitivity to hypoxia.[12]

Clinical Presentation

Many patients will have a history of previous attacks, perhaps associated with allergen exposure, cold exposure, stress, or upper respiratory infection. A history of allergies in the patient or family, previous medication use at home, including steroids, and a history of previous hospitalizations should be obtained. The presence of fever may indicate a concurrent infection. Vomiting and decreased fluid intake during the current attack may result in dehydration.

The physical findings may reflect the severity of airway obstruction. Tachypnea, cyanosis on room air, prolonged expiratory time, and wheezes on inspiration and expiration that are aggravated by forced expiration may be present. The degree of wheezing does not necessarily reflect the severity of an attack. Decreased wheezing suggests poor air exchange in patients with severe distress. Use of accessory muscles should also be noted. Asymmetric breath sounds

suggest the presence of pneumothorax or foreign body. The patient should be examined for presence of subcutaneous emphysema, especially in the neck and upper thorax. As respiratory function becomes more severely compromised, a pulsus paradoxus will be present.

The differential diagnosis of asthma most commonly includes congenital malformations of respiratory, cardiovascular, and gastrointestinal systems; foreign body; cystic fibrosis; and infections, especially pneumonia, croup, and bronchiolitis.

Management

The goal of therapy in status asthmaticus is to reduce airway resistance and inflammation promptly by relieving bronchospasm, reducing mucosal edema, and helping to clear secretions, while supporting other vital organs. Oxygen is the most important agent that can be given. Most often, 40% oxygen will prevent hypoxemia. Continuous oxygen saturation monitoring is a valuable aid in adjusting oxygen therapy. Oxygen consumption is increased during status asthmaticus and may be exacerbated by use of sympathomimetic drugs; thus, the PO_2 is maintained at greater than 90 torr to prevent hypoxic/ischemic complications.

Many patients have had inadequate fluid intake during their illness, and fluid deficits are replaced to avoid hypovolemia. Once the fluid deficit has been replaced and the urine output has risen to greater than 1 ml/kg/hr, fluid balance is carefully monitored and excess fluid avoided. Large transpulmonary pressure swings and increased serum antidiuretic hormone may predispose patients to interstitial pulmonary edema during an acute asthmatic episode.[13,14]

Inhaled Bronchodilators

Beta-adrenergic agonists are potent bronchodilators and are often among the first agents that patients will receive in the emergency room (Table 14-1). Bronchodilation occurs by interaction of the drug at beta-adrenergic receptor sites on mast and smooth muscle cells with activation of adenyl cyclase activity and increased intracellular cAMP levels.

Table 14-1. Asthma medications in the intensive care setting

Drug	Dose	Comments
Albuterol	0.10–0.15 mg/kg (up to 5 mg) By continuous nebulization: 0.5 mg/kg/hr (up to 15 mg/hr)	Usually q2–4h May be used q20min for 1–2 hr Higher doses more likely to produce hypokalemia, tachycardia, hypotension dysrhythmias
Aminophylline	6 mg/kg IV—Loading dose Constant infusion rate: 1–6 mo 0.5 mg/kg/hr 6 mo–1 yr 1.0 mg/kg/hr 1–9 yr 1.5 mg/kg/hr 10–16 yr 1.2 mg/kg/hr	Adjust dose to achieve serum level of 5–15 μg/ml.
Methylprednisolone	1–2 mg/kg IV q6h	
Terbutaline	5–10 μg/kg IV over 10 min; then 0.1–0.4 μg/kg/min	May increase continuous infusion rate by 0.1 μg/kg/min every 15 min until clinical and ABG improvement seen. Monitor for hypokalemia, tachycardia, dysrhythmias, and hypotension.

Albuterol, a beta$_2$-agonist that may be delivered by nebulizer, is the initial recommended therapy for acute exacerbations of asthma in children. Guidelines issued by the NIH recommend doses of 0.15 mg/kg (maximum dose, 5 mg) as often as every 20 minutes if necessary.[1] The dose is based on studies demonstrating better clinical response without increased side effects when compared with lower doses.[15,16] NIH guidelines also recommend a dose of 0.5 mg/kg/hr (maximum dose, 15 mg/hr) if used by continuous nebulization, a dose extrapolated from the every-20-minute dose.[1] More recently, a study documented the safety and increased efficacy of 0.3 mg/kg as an occasional single dose of albuterol (maximum dose, 15 mg) compared with 0.15 mg/kg/hr.[17] However, hypokalemia occurs in 70% of patients receiving albuterol in doses of 0.05 to 0.15 mg/kg by nebulizer.[18] Lower doses of albuterol may be effective and have fewer side effects.

Metaproterenol and terbutaline also may be nebulized. The duration of action of metaproterenol is not as long as that of albuterol, and cardiovascular side effects may be more severe. Terbutaline by nebulizer is not recommended in the NIH guideline because a nebulizer solution is not available in the United States (although the injectable solution may be nebulized) and because it offers no advantage over albuterol.[1]

Corticosteriods

Corticosteroids reduce morbidity in acute asthma and are now used aggressively in children hospitalized with asthma.[19-21] In the patient with severe bronchospasm and impending respiratory failure, systemic steroids must be administered immediately, as the effect of the steroids may not be clinically apparent for 6 to 8 hours.[22,23] Methylprednisolone 1 to 3 mg/kg q6h is recommended. The steroids may be tapered rapidly as the patients respond to therapy. Frequently, the patients are treated at home with inhaled steroids, which should be continued. While the exact mechanisms of action are unknown, corticosteroids are thought to act by their effects on arachidonic acid metabolism and synthesis of leukotrienes and prostaglandins, by their prevention of inflammatory cell migration activation, and possibly by an increase in beta-receptor responsiveness in the smooth muscle of the airway.[1]

Intravenous Beta-Adrenergic Agonists

Most patients respond in the emergency room or in the hospital to nebulized bronchodilator, corticosteroid, and aminophylline therapy. A small portion will require admission to the intensive care unit (ICU) (Table 14-2) for persistent respiratory failure and will need more aggressive therapy. Intravenous (IV) terbutaline is now recommended if the patient does not respond adequately to aggressive nebulized albuterol therapy and corticosteroids. Isoproterenol is no longer recommended because other agents are as effective and less toxic.

The dose of terbutaline recommended by the NIH is 10 μg/kg

Table 14-2. Asthma: ICU admission criteria

Failure to respond to IV aminophylline and inhaled bronchodilators

Hypoxia (PO$_2$ < 60 torr) while on oxygen therapy

Pneumothorax/pneumomediastinum

PCO$_2$ > 40 torr in the presence of respiratory distress

Metabolic acidosis

IV over 10 minutes, followed by a continuous infusion of 0.4 μg/kg/min.[1] This dose was extrapolated from data about IV albuterol, since pharmacokinetics of albuterol and terbutaline are similar, although terbutaline is 40% to 50% as potent as albuterol. The only published report about IV terbutaline included only four children hospitalized with acute asthma; a dose of 2 μg/kg over 5 minutes followed by 4.5 μg/kg/hr (0.075 μg/kg/min) was used.[24]

Clearly, more work needs to be done before the optimal dose range of terbutaline is known. Until then, a conservative approach using a loading dose of 5 to 10 μg/kg IV over 10 minutes, followed by 0.1 to 0.4 μg/kg/min as a continuous infusion acknowledges the potential for hypokalemia, tachycardia, dysrhythmias, and hypotension while allowing for aggressive bronchodilation (see Table 14-1). The continuous infusion rate may be increased by 0.1-μg/kg/min increments until an improvement in clinical status and arterial blood gases occurs. Continuous monitoring of cardiopulmonary status, arterial blood pressure, and pulse oximetry are mandatory. In addition, oral terbutaline alters the metabolism of oral aminophylline when these drugs are used concomitantly.[25] Combination therapy may augment bronchodilation, and the clinical significance of a slight decrease in the aminophylline level is not known. The effect of IV terbutaline or IV aminophylline has not been studied but IV isoproterenol does influence serum theophylline levels.[26] Theophylline levels should be monitored when terbutaline is stopped to avoid a potentially toxic theophylline level. Whether cardiac-specific serum creatinine phosphokinase isoenzyme levels should be followed, as is recommended when isoproterenol is used, is not known.[27]

IV albuterol by continuous infusion is also effective in relieving bronchospasm.[28] Although not yet approved in the United States, a loading dose of 10 μg/kg of albuterol over 10 minutes, followed by an infusion of 0.2 μg/kg/min and adjusted by 0.1-μg/kg/min increments to clinical response, has been used safely. Side effects included a mild tachycardia in some patients. As with terbutaline, vasodilation may occur and patients should be normovolemic prior to beginning an albuterol infusion.

Other Medications

Upper respiratory infections are a common precipitant of an acute asthmatic episode. Most of these infections are caused by viruses, and no specific therapy is required. Mycoplasma should be considered. Antibiotic therapy is reserved for patients with signs and symptoms suggestive of a bacterial infection. Routine antibiotic therapy is not recommended.

The use of sodium bicarbonate therapy to correct the acidosis that is routinely found in patients during a severe asthmatic attack is controversial. The metabolic component of the acidosis may be a combined result of dehydration and hypoxemia. Acidosis may attenuate the catecholamine response and may result in refractory airway obstruction. Dehydration and hypoxemia are aggressively corrected. Correction of the metabolic component of the acidosis with sodium bicarbonate to raise the arterial pH to 7.3 or greater has been recommended.[21,29] Sodium bicarbonate therapy, however, may contribute to hypercapnia and result in hypernatremia, hypokalemia, and hyperosmolality. A study in a small group of patients with severe asthma documented the safety of tolerating a pH of 7.0 or greater and allowing gradual correction without use of sodium bicarbonate.[30]

Magnesium administration has been found to be effective as a bronchodilator in severe asthma in adults.[31] Its use in children has not been adequately evaluated to recommend its administration.

Cromolyn therapy is not appropriate for an acute severe attack of asthma. Anticholinergic agents may be recommended; for example, iprotropium bromide is generally reserved for moderate asthmatic attacks.

Mechanical Ventilation

Most patients with status asthmaticus will respond to the aggressive management approach just described. A small percentage will continue to develop progressive respiratory failure and will require mechanical ventilation (Table 14-3).

Tracheal intubation should be performed by the most experienced person available. The performance of tracheal intubation may lead to serious hemodynamic compromise. This occurs on the basis of (1) a reduction in venous return following intubation and positive pressure ventilation; (2) sedation for the procedure which may decrease endogenous catecholamines; and (3) preexisting acidosis and hypoxemia. A bolus of fluid administered prior to tracheal intubation may offset the development of hypotension.[32]

Usually, a rapid sequence intubation is performed with cricoid pressure (Sellick maneuver) to prevent pulmonary aspiration of gastric contents. Appropriate sedation medications include ketamine, fentanyl, midazolam, or thiopental. Ketamine has a potent bronchodilator effect on airway resistance and thus would appear to be a preferred choice in this situation. Whichever agent is employed, the drug should be titrated carefully to provide the desired effect and to minimize side effects.

Muscle relaxation is usually required for rapid-sequence intubation. The ideal agent is succinylcholine. Vecuronium, however, should be substituted if there is any concern regarding possible hyperkalemia, in which case succinylcholine may be contraindicated.

Volume ventilators capable of generating high inspiratory pressures are essential. An initial respiratory rate of 8 to 16 breaths/min with an I:E ratio of 1:2 or longer is usually required. The longer expiratory time allows adequate time for expiration and reduces air trapping. The initial effective tidal volume should be 8 to 10 ml/kg accompanied by high inspiratory flows.[33,34] Hypoventilation (permissive hypercapnia) with a PCO_2 of 50 to 60 torr or higher may be tolerated, if necessary, to minimize the peak inspiratory pressure (<40 cm H_2O) and reduce the incidence of barotrauma.[18,30,35] For further details on mechanical ventilation in these patients, see Mechanical Ventilation (by Kacmarek et al., this volume). (Young children may have significant pressure drops across narrow endotracheal tubes, and the peak inspiratory pressure may not reflect pressure in the lungs in this population.) Blood pressure, heart rate, and skin perfusion are checked immediately

after intubation because initiation of positive pressure ventilation may reduce venous return.

The use of positive end-expiratory pressure (PEEP) during ventilator therapy in patients with asthma is controversial.[36] Adding PEEP to an already hyperinflated lung, especially when the hypoxemia of asthma usually responds to moderate amounts of oxygen, seems counterproductive at first glance. To provide a rational approach to this situation, an assessment of the patient's auto-PEEP is important. A report on adult patients documented the adverse effects of PEEP on lung volumes, intrathoracic pressures, and hemodynamic status.[37] PEEP, however, may be useful in relieving atelectasis and improving ventilation-perfusion matching in ventilated patients who are recovering and no longer generating severely elevated peak pressures.[30] Ketamine also has been used effectively as a continuous infusion because of its bronchodilator effects.[38] Morphine produces mild histamine release, and for this reason some clinicians have avoided its use.

Sedation will be necessary in most patients in order to relieve anxiety, allow the patients to breathe in synchrony with the ventilator, reduce work of breathing and oxygen consumption, and decrease chest wall resistance. Sedative and anxiolytic agents should be used aggressively with muscle relaxation. Diazepam or midazolam may be used in conjunction with fentanyl.

In addition to sedation, muscle relaxants are required to facilitate ventilating those patients with marked increase in airway resistance. The nondepolarizing muscle relaxants, such as pancuronium bromide (0.1 mg/kg) or vecuronium (0.1 mg/kg), are commonly employed as either a bolus or continuous infusion. The amount of relaxants should be titrated to the desired effect (i.e., facilitating ventilation). This is evaluated either clinically or by performing nerve stimulation (see Muscle Relaxants, by Goudsouzian, this volume). The use of muscle relaxants in some asthmatic patients has been associated with a myopathy in the form of a prolonged period of muscle weakness.[39–42] The relaxants implicated have been those with a steroid-based nucleus (e.g., vecuronium).

Successful use of inhalation anesthetics (halothane, isoflurane) as bronchodilators in patients who continue to worsen despite other bronchodilator therapy and mechanical ventilation has been reported.[24,40–42] Myocardial depression, arrhythmias, and increased intrapulmonary shunting are side effects requiring close monitoring if these agents are used.

Most patients require mechanical ventilation for 24 to 72 hours.[18] Weaning may begin when bronchospasm has improved, inspiratory pressures are reduced, and arterial blood gases have normalized. Some patients, however, will require a more extended period of tracheal intubation and ventilation because of a more severe degree of pathology or because of muscle weakness. Complications of mechanical ventilation include barotrauma, endotracheal tube obstruction or malposition, and subglottic stenosis or granulation.

When the patient's condition deteriorates despite aggressive bronchodilator therapy and mechanical ventilation, extracorporeal membrane oxygenation (ECMO) has been a life-saving therapy.

Bronchiolitis

Bronchiolitis is an acute inflammatory disease of the lower airways that is common in infancy and is a major cause of morbidity in infants and children. The incidence of bronchiolitis peaks between November and March each year, and the attack rate has been

---

Table 14-3. Asthma: Criteria for initiating mechanical ventilation

Decreased respiratory effort due to progressive fatigue

Deterioration in mental status

Progressive respiratory acidemia and hypercarbia despite therapy

Cardiopulmonary arrest

Progressive hypoxemia with maximum oxygen therapy by mask

Overall clinical deterioration despite aggressive therapy

estimated to be as high as 30% for infants.[43] Respiratory syncytial virus (RSV) is the most common etiologic agent. Other viruses, such as adenovirus, parainfluenza, and influenza, are responsible for a smaller number of cases.

During the winter season, bronchiolitis is one of the major reasons for hospital admission of infants less than 1 year of age. Between 2% and 7% of hospitalized infants infected with RSV develop respiratory failure requiring mechanical ventilation.[44] Patients at high risk for requiring intensive care management of their bronchiolitis include infants less than 3 months of age, premature infants, and those with preexisting cardiopulmonary disease or compromised immune function. The mortality rate is estimated to be between 1% and 7%, with most fatalities occurring in infants less than 6 months of age. The mortality rate for infants with preexisting cardiac or pulmonary disease has been estimated to be as high as 37%, although a more recent study found a mortality rate of 2.5% in patients with congenital heart disease and less than 1% in patients acquiring the disease in the community.[45,46]

Pathophysiology

Viral infections of the lower respiratory tract lead to necrosis of the ciliated respiratory epithelium which impairs the infant's ability to handle secretions and debris (Fig. 14-2).[43] Subsequent proliferation of the epithelium produces cells without cilia. White cells invade the peribronchial tissues, and edema of the adventitia and submucosa occurs. Alveolar debris and fibrin strands cause plugs which form within the small airways and may partially or completely obstruct the airways, resulting in variable areas of atelectasis and hyperinflation. These alterations result in decreased compli-

ance and ventilation-perfusion abnormalities. Bronchiolitis invariably causes some degree of hypoxemia and increases the work of breathing. As the disease progresses and respiratory muscle fatigue ensues, untreated hypoxemia and hypercarbia lead to acidosis and respiratory arrest.

Clinical Presentation

Infants usually present with signs of an upper respiratory infection, including cough, sneezing, and rhinorrhea. Within a few days, the infant also has developed tachypnea, retractions, rales, nasal flaring, wheezing, lethargy, and poor feeding. Hyperinflation with or without areas of atelectasis or infiltrates is the hallmark of bronchiolitis on radiologic examination. Apnea may be a presenting sign of bronchiolitis in up to 20% of infants and may be secondary to respiratory muscle fatigue or to a direct effect of the RSV on central control of breathing.[47]

Hypoxemia is an almost universal finding in patients in respiratory distress with bronchiolitis. Pulse oximetry or arterial blood gas measurements are necessary to document the degree of hypoxemia and the response to oxygen, and in children with moderate to severe respiratory distress, arterial blood gas measurements are required to monitor PCO_2.

Management

All infants with bronchiolitis requiring hospitalization should be given oxygen. Preexisting fluid deficits should be replaced, and subsequent fluid administration should be controlled carefully to

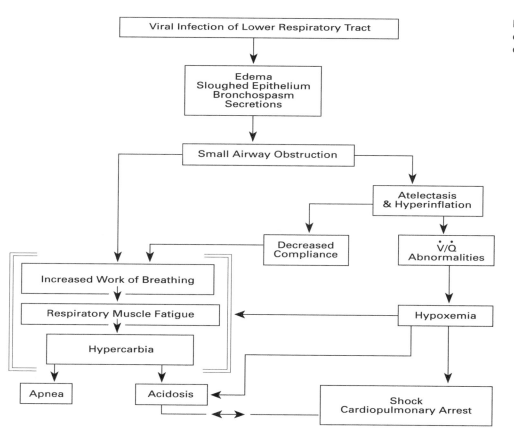

Figure 14-2. Pathophysiology of respiratory failure in bronchiolitis

guard against hypervolemia. Patients with reactive airways disease may be predisposed to develop pulmonary edema with or without elevated levels of antidiuretic hormone.[13,48]

Bronchodilators

The use of bronchodilators for bronchiolitis is controversial. Edema and obstruction of the airways from alveolar debris and fibrin result in wheezing that may not respond to bronchodilators. In addition, the presence and functional state of bronchiolar smooth muscle in infants has not been well studied. Engle noted that bronchiolar smooth muscle is present in the human fetus by 16 to 24 weeks of gestation but is only feebly developed by birth.[49] Lenney and Milner measured total respiratory resistance before and after albuterol therapy in 32 wheezing children aged 7 months to 3 years; no child under 18 months had a response to albuterol.[50] This study and others like it are flawed by the technique used for measuring respiratory resistance in the child and by the use of chloral hydrate in younger infants, which may decrease upper airway muscle tone and increase respiratory resistance.[51]

More recently, improvement has been shown in specific respiratory conductance after administration of aerosolized albuterol in infants with bronchiolitis.[52] In intubated infants, a drop in respiratory resistance can be documented after aminophylline use.[53] In addition, hypoxemia and wheezing in RSV infections are associated with the production of RSV-specific IgE and histamine found in nasopharyngeal secretion.[54] Histamine production may lead to release of arachidonic acid metabolites such as leukotrienes. These latter compounds cause reversible bronchospasm in asthmatics and may be expected to cause reversible bronchospasm in children with bronchiolitis.[55] Wheezing in RSV-infected patients has also been associated with the degree of the cell-mediated immune response.[56] Clinical improvement has been demonstrated after administration of nebulized albuterol (0.1–0.15 mg/kg) in patients with bronchiolitis.[57,58]

Children with bronchiolitis respond to one or more subcutaneous injections of epinephrine. Lowell et al. speculated that the beta-adrenergic activity reversed bronchospasm, while the alpha-adrenergic activity decreased edema.[59] Nebulized racemic epinephrine improves oxygen saturation, clinical scores, and lung function in children with bronchiolitis.[60–62] A study comparing racemic epinephrine and albuterol, both nebulized, claimed superiority of racemic epinephrine but used an albuterol dose of 0.03 mg/kg rather than the currently recommended dose of 0.15 mg/kg.[62]

The Expert Panel on Asthma at the NIH noted that even children a few weeks of age might have asthma.[1] Viral infections, most notably RSV, may precipitate asthma in the infant. Because symptoms of bronchiolitis and asthma may be almost identical in the infant, the panel recommended treating infants with the same drug regimen used in patients with asthma, including inhaled bronchodilator, corticosteroids, and in some patients, aminophylline.

Corticosteroids

The role of corticosteroids in treating infants with bronchiolitis is unknown. Thirty years ago, studies documented the lack of clinical efficacy of corticosteroids in children with bronchiolitis.[63] These studies were done prior to widespread use of aggressive bronchodilator therapy in children with bronchiolitis, use of higher-dose steroid therapy for asthma, and use of pulse oximetry and infant pulmonary function testing. These studies have not been repeated; as noted, however, the NIH guidelines endorsed use of corticosteroids in children with bronchiolitis who may have asthma (an impossible distinction in most cases!).[1] The lack of evidence supporting use of corticosteroids in these patients would instead argue for a more judicious approach while pursuing research to document efficacy.

Ribavirin

Ribavirin is a synthetic nucleoside that inhibits viral protein synthesis. Ribavirin was approved by the FDA for therapy of RSV infections and is delivered as an aerosol. Initial randomized, placebo-controlled clinical trials used water as the placebo.[64–66] Ribavirin-treated patients showed improvement in respiratory signs and symptoms scores, increases in oxygenation, and decreases in RSV titers at the end of therapy. These early studies involved only 10 to 20 patients in each treatment arm and did not address length of hospitalization or PICU stay, length of oxygen therapy, or days on a ventilator.

Ribavirin administration to 14 mechanically ventilated patients infected with RSV resulted in fewer days of mechanical ventilation and oxygen therapy, a shorter hospital stay, and a reduction in hospital costs compared to 14 placebo(water)-treated patients.[67] Several investigators have since questioned the use of water as a placebo and have suggested that aerosolized water may have worsened bronchospasm and biased studies in favor of ribavirin.[68–70]

An historical cohort study comparing 106 infants treated with ribavirin to 52 infants not treated with ribavirin failed to show a difference in length of hospital stay, days on oxygen therapy, and progression to ventilator status.[71] A randomized placebo(saline)-controlled study of mechanically ventilated infants with RSV showed no difference between 19 ribavirin-treated infants and 18 saline-treated infants in days on oxygen or mechanical ventilation, or in days in the PICU or in the hospital.[72] Another recent study did not show a reduction in length of stay when ribavirin was administered to 61 patients with RSV compared to 453 patients who did not receive ribavirin.[73] A prospective multi-institutional cohort study in previously well, mechanically ventilated infants showed increased days on the ventilator, in the PICU, and in the hospital in 84 ribavirin-treated infants compared to 128 patients who did not receive ribavirin.[74]

Little toxicity associated with ribavirin in pediatric patients has been documented, although in some patients, ribavirin seems to worsen bronchospasm. Significant adverse cardiopulmonary reactions have been reported in 3 patients.[75]

Teratogenicity has been observed in rodents but not in baboons. None has been reported in humans.[76] Ribavirin is concentrated in RBCs. In one study, ribavirin was not detected in the RBCs, plasma, or urine of nurses administering ribavirin aerosol.[77] Ribavirin exposure has been shown to be greater for nurses who were caring for patients receiving ribavirin through oxygen tents, compared with patients receiving ribavirin through mechanical ventilation.[78] Although only one nurse had a detectable level of ribavirin in one RBC sample, air samples estimated that a significant absorbed dose-per-work-shift was inhaled by nurses caring for patients receiving ribavirin through oxygen tents. Control systems have been designed to reduce aerosol emissions. These findings and the lack of reports of adverse fetal effects in humans suggest that the teratogenic risk of ribavirin is small.

Ribavirin appears to be safe, but expensive, and efficacy and effectiveness have not been clearly demonstrated in large randomized placebo-controlled trials. Routine use of ribavirin at this time cannot be recommended.

Intravenous Immunoglobulin

Recent studies in animals and infants suggest a role for intravenous IgG in the treatment of RSV infection.[79,80] Hospitalized RSV-infected infants were given intravenous immunoglobulin containing high levels of RSV-neutralizing antibodies. Significant reductions in serum neutralizing antibody titers and in nasal RSV titers occurred, as well as an improvement in pulse oximetry readings. Duration of hospitalization and clinical symptoms did not change in these 35 infants. Further studies in larger groups are underway.[81]

Parenteral RSV immune globulin has been used successfully to prevent severe lower respiratory tract infection in high-risk infants.[81,82]

Mechanical Ventilation

Criteria for initiating ventilator support include continued worsening of respiratory distress with or without signs of circulatory failure (metabolic acidosis, poor peripheral perfusion, tachycardia, lethargy, and poor muscle tone). In addition, hypoxia (PO_2 <60 mm Hg in 40% oxygen, or cyanosis in 100% oxygen), hypercarbia (PO_2 >60 mm Hg with or without respiratory acidosis), and apnea or bradycardia all warrant assisted ventilation.[44]

Various methods of respiratory support in infants with bronchiolitis have been described, including the use of continuous positive airway pressure (CPAP) and spontaneous breathing and the use of volume- or pressure-limited ventilators. Infants requiring mechanical ventilation for bronchiolitis are usually less than 10 kg in body weight, so we use pressure-limited ventilators rather than volume-limited ventilators because of the continuous-flow IMV characteristics as well as the dependence on pressure for determining delivered tidal volume.[44] In our experience, most patients require peak inspiratory pressures between 25 and 35 cm of H_2O to achieve adequate air movement and chest expansion and to maintain a PCO_2 less than 55 mm Hg. We also use PEEP to keep the small airways open throughout the respiratory cycle, theoretically reducing hyperinflation and gas trapping. Slow ventilatory rates and relatively long expiratory times are used to allow adequate time for expiration. Only rarely do patients require more than 60% oxygen to correct hypoxemia.

One study has documented the safety and efficacy of using CPAP and spontaneous breathing to avoid the need for mechanical ventilation.[83] We have not found CPAP alone to be effective in reducing the work of breathing and treating respiratory failure.

Most patients tolerate mechanical ventilation well with the use of sedative agents. Morphine or fentanyl in combination with midazolam may be used to prevent patients from becoming agitated or struggling against the ventilator. Neuromuscular blockade is usually not necessary.

Weaning from mechanical ventilation begins when the patient has clinically stabilized and improved. The peak inspiratory pressure may be lowered if lung compliance has improved, thus allowing adequate chest excursion and air exchange at a lower peak inspiratory pressure. The ventilator rate may be reduced gradually until the patient is breathing effectively without much help from the ventilator and with little or no respiratory distress.

When the patient's condition deteriorates despite aggressive medical and ventilation therapy, ECMO has been life-saving.

Prognosis and Outcome

Mortality rates for previously healthy patients with bronchiolitis should be extremely low. Mortality rates in patients with preexisting cardiopulmonary or immunologic diseases may be higher. In addition, several studies have documented chronic pulmonary changes after RSV infection.[84–86] An increased risk for the development of asthma after RSV infection has not been established.[87]

References

1. NHLBI National Asthma Education Program Expert Panel Report, U.S. Department of Health and Human Services. Bethesda, MD. Publication Number 91–3042, 1991.
2. Center of Disease Control. Asthma—United States, 1989–1987. *MMWR* 39:493, 1990.
3. Benatar SR. Fatal asthma. *N Engl J Med* 314:423, 1986.
4. British Thoracic Association. Deaths from asthma in two regions of England. *Br Med J* 285:1251, 1982.
5. Weiss KB, Wagener DK. Changing patterns of asthma mortality: Identifying target populations at high risk. *JAMA* 264:1683, 1990.
6. Marder D et al. Effect of racial and socioeconomic factors on asthma mortality in Chicago. *Chest* 101:427S, 1992.
7. Sur S et al. Sudden-onset fatal asthma. Editorial. *Mayo Clin Proc* 69:495, 1994.
8. Bellomo R et al. Asthma requiring mechanical ventilation. A low morbidity approach. *Chest* 105:891, 1994.
9. Wasserfallen JB et al. Sudden asphyxic asthma: A distinct entity? *Am Rev Respir Dis* 142:108, 1990.
10. Wasserfallen JB, Schaller MD, Perret CH. Life-threatening asthma with dramatic resolution. *Chest* 104:615, 1993.
11. Hogg JC. The pathophysiology of asthma. *Chest* 82(Suppl):85, 1982.
12. Kikughi Y et al. Chemosensitivity and perception of dyspnea in patients with a history of near-fatal asthma. *N Engl J Med* 330:1329, 1994.
13. Stalcup SA, Mellins RB. Mechanical forces producing pulmonary edema in acute asthma. *N Engl J Med* 297:592, 1977.
14. Szatalowicz VL, Goldberg JP, Anderson RJ. Plasma antidiuretic hormone in acute respiratory failure. *Am J Med* 72:583, 1982.
15. Robertson CF et al. Response to frequent low doses of nebulized salbutamol in acute asthma. *J Pediatr* 106:672, 1985.
16. Schuh S et al. High- versus low-dose, frequently administered, nebulized albuterol in children with severe, acute asthma. *Pediatrics* 83:513, 1989.
17. Schuh S et al. Nebulized albuterol in acute childhood asthma: Comparison of two doses. *Pediatrics* 86:509, 1990.
18. Stein R et al. Severe asthma in a pediatric intensive care unit: Six years experience. *Pediatrics* 83:1023, 1989.
19. Littenberg B, Gluck EH. A controlled trial of methylprednisolone in the emergency treatment of acute asthma. *N Engl J Med* 314:150, 1986.
20. Younger RE et al. Intravenous methylprednisolone efficacy in status asthmaticus of childhood. *Pediatrics* 80:225, 1987.
21. Section on Allergy and Immunology. Management of asthma. *Pediatrics* 68:874, 1981.
22. Hall JB, Wood LD. Management of the critically ill asthmatic patient. *Med Clin North Am* 74:779, 1990.
23. Kallenbach JM et al. Determinants of near fatality in acute severe asthma. *Am J Med* 95:265, 1993.
24. Fulsang G, Pedersen S, Borgstrom L. Dose-response-relationships of intravenously administered terbutaline in children with asthma. *J Pediatr* 114:315, 1989.
25. Danziger Y et al. Reduction of serum theophylline levels by terbutaline in children with asthma. *Clin Pharmacol Ther* 37:469, 1985.
26. O'Rourke PP, Crone RK. Effect of isoproterenol on measured theophylline levels. *Crit Care Med* 12:373, 1984.
27. Maguire JF, Geha RS, Umetsu DT. Myocardial specific creatine phosphokinase isoenzyme elevation in children with asthma treated with intravenous isoproterenol. *J Allergy Clin Immunol* 78:631, 1986.

28. Bohn D et al. Intravenous salbutamol in the treatment of status asthmaticus in children. *Crit Care Med* 12:892, 1984.

29. Menitove SM, Goldring RM. Combined ventilator and bicarbonate strategy in the management of status asthmaticus. *Am J Med* 74:898, 1983.

30. Dworkin G, Kattan M. Mechanical ventilation for status asthmaticus in children. *J Pediatr* 114:545, 1989.

31. Skobeloff EM et al. Intravenous magnesium sulfate for the treatment of acute asthma in the emergency department. *JAMA* 262:1210, 1989.

32. Cohen N, Janson S. Management of acute life-threatening asthma. In Parker MM, Shapiro MJ, Porembka DT (eds): *Critical Care: State of the Art.* Anaheim, CA. Society of Critical Care Medicine, 1995. Pp 115–142.

33. Schwartz DE et al. Succinylcholine-induced hyperkalemic arrest in a patient with severe metabolic acidosis. *Anesth Analg* 75:291, 1992.

34. Finfer SR, Garrard CS. Ventilatory support in asthma. *Br J Hosp Med* 49:357, 1993.

35. Darioli R, Perret C. Mechanical controlled hypoventilation in status asthmaticus. *Am Rev Respir Dis* 129:385, 1984.

36. Marinin JJ. Should PEEP be used in airflow obstruction? *Am Rev Respir Dis* 140:1, 1989.

37. Tuxen DV. Detrimental effects of positive end-expiratory pressure during controlled mechanical ventilation of patients with severe airflow obstruction. *Am Rev Respir Dis* 140:5, 1989.

38. Strube PH, Hallam PL. Ketamine by continuous infusion in status asthmaticus. *Anaesthesia* 41:1017, 1986.

39. Coakley JH et al. Prolonged neurogenic weakness in patients requiring mechanical ventilation for acute airflow limitation. *Chest* 101:1413, 1992.

40. Douglass JA et al. Myopathy in severe asthma. *Am Rev Respir Dis* 146:517, 1992.

41. Margolis BD et al. Prolonged reversible quadriparesis in mechanically ventilated patients who received long-term infusions of vecuronium. *Chest* 100:877, 1991.

42. Tanigaki T et al. Transient neuromuscular impairment resulting from prolonged inhalation of halothane and enflurane. *Chest* 98:1012, 1990.

43. Wohl MEB, Chernick V. Bronchiolitis. *Am Rev Respir Dis* 118:759, 1978.

44. Outwater KM, Crone RK. Management of respiratory failure in infants with acute viral bronchiolitis. *Am J Dis Child* 138:1071, 1984.

45. MacDonald NE et al. Respiratory syncytial viral infection in infants with congenital heart disease. *N Engl J Med* 307:397, 1982.

46. Moler FW et al. Respiratory syncytial virus morbidity and mortality estimates in congenital heart disease patients: A recent experience. *Crit Care Med* 20:1406, 1992.

47. Church NR et al. Respiratory syncytial virus-related apnea in infants. *Am J Dis Child* 138:247, 1984.

48. Rivers RPA, Forsling ML, Olver RP. Inappropriate secretion of antidiuretic hormone in infants with respiratory infections. *Arch Dis Child* 56:358, 1981.

49. Engle S. *Lung Structure.* Springfield, IL: Thomas, 1962.

50. Lenny W, Milner AD. At what age do bronchodilator drugs work? *Arch Dis Child* 53:532, 1978.

51. Hershenson MB et al. Effect of choral hydrate on genioglossus and diaphragmatic activity. *Pediatr Res* 18:516, 1984.

52. Soto ME et al. Bronchodilator response during acute viral bronchiolitis in infancy. *Pediatr Pulmonol* 2:85, 1985.

53. Schene JA, Crone RK, Thompson JE. The use of aminophylline in severe bronchiolitis. *Crit Care Med* 12:225, 1984.

54. Welliver RC et al. The development of RSV-specific IgE and the release of histamine in nasopharyngeal secretions after infection. *N Engl J Med* 305:841, 1981.

55. Griffin M et al. Effect of leukotriene D on the airways in asthma. *N Engl J Med* 308:436, 1983.

56. Welliver RC, Kaul A, Orga PL. Cell mediated immune response to RSV infection: Relationship to development of reactive airway disease. *J Pediatr* 94:370, 1979.

57. Schuh S et al. Nebulized albuterol in acute bronchiolitis. *J Pediatr* 117:633, 1990.

58. Klassen TP et al. Randomized trial of salbutamol in acute bronchiolitis. *J Pediatr* 118:807, 1991.

59. Lowell DI et al. Wheezing in infants: The response to epinephrine. *Pediatrics* 79:939, 1987.

60. Lodrup KC, Carlsen KH. The effect of inhaled nebulized racemic epinephrine upon lung function in infants and toddlers with acute bronchiolitis or asthma. *Am Rev Respir Dis* 143:A507, 1991.

61. Wennergren G et al. Nebulised racemic adrenaline for wheezy bronchitis. *Acta Paediatr Scand* 80:375, 1991.

62. Sanchez I et al. Effect of racemic epinephrine and salbutamol on clinical score and pulmonary mechanics in infants with bronchiolitis. *J Pediatr* 122:145, 1993.

63. Leer JA et al. Corticosteroid treatment in bronchiolitis. *Am J Dis Child* 117:495, 1969.

64. Hall CB et al. Aerosolized ribavirin treatment of infants with respiratory syncytial viral infection: A randomized double-blind study. *N Engl J Med* 308:1443–1447, 1983.

65. Taber LH et al. Ribavirin aerosol treatment of bronchiolitis associated with respiratory syncytial virus infection in infants. *Pediatrics* 72: 613–618, 1983.

66. Hall CB et al. Ribavirin treatment of respiratory syncytial viral infection in infants with underlying cardiopulmonary disease. *JAMA* 254: 3047–3051, 1985.

67. Smith DW, Frankel LR, Mathers LH. A controlled trial of aerosolized ribavirin in infants receiving mechanical ventilation for severe respiratory syncytial virus infection. *N Engl J Med* 325:24–29, 1991.

68. Moler FW, Bandy KP, Custer JR. Ribavirin for severe RSV infection. *N Engl J Med* 325:1884–5, 1991.

69. Wald E, Dashefsky B. Ribavirin Red Book Committee recommendations questioned. *Pediatrics* 93:672–3, 1994.

70. Krafte-Jacobs B, Holbrook PR. Ribavirin in severe respiratory syncytial virus infection. *Crit Care Med* 22:541–3, 1994.

71. Wheeler JG, Wofford J, Turner RB. Historical cohort evaluation of ribavirin efficacy in respiratory syncytial virus infection. *Pediatr Infect Dis J* 12:209–13, 1993.

72. Meert KL, Sarniak AP, Gelmini MJ, Lieh-Lai MW. Aerosolized ribavirin in mechanically ventilated children with respiratory syncytial virus lower respiratory tract disease: A prospective, double-blind, randomized trial. *Crit Care Med* 22:566–572, 1994.

73. Law BJ et al. Ribavirin does not reduce hospital stay in patients with respiratory syncytial virus lower respiratory tract infection. *Pediatric Research* 37:110A, 1995.

74. Moler FW and the Pediatric Critical Care Study Group. Effectiveness of ribavirin for well infants with RSV associated respiratory failure: A prospective multicenter cohort study. *Crit Care Med* 23:A225, 1995.

75. Eisenberg J. Hemodynamic alterations in patients treated with ribavirin. *Pediatr Infect Dis J* 9:S93–4, 1990.

76. Johnson EM. The effects of ribavirin on development and reproduction: a critical review of published and unpublished studies in experimental animals. *J Am Col Toxicol* 9:551–561, 1990.

77. Rodriguez WJ et al. Environmental exposure of primary care personnel to ribavirin aerosol when supervising treatment of infants with respiratory syncytial virus infections. *Antimicrob Ag Chemother* 31:1143–1146, 1987.

78. Harrison R et al. Assessing exposures of health-care personnel to aerosols of ribavirin—California. *MMWR* 37:560–2, 1988.

79. Hemming VG et al. Intravenous immunoglobulin treatment of respiratory syncytial virus infections in infants and young children. *Antimicrob Agents Chemother* 31:1882, 1987.

80. Hemming VG, Prince GA. Immunoprophylaxis of infections with respiratory syncytial virus: observations and hypothesis. *Reviews of Infectious Diseases* 12:S470, 1990.

81. Hemming VG, Prince GA, Groothuis JR, Siber GR. Hyperimmune globulins in prevention and treatment of respiratory syncytial virus infections. *Clin Microbiol Rev* 8(1):22–33, 1995.

82. Groothuis JR, Simoes EA, Hemming VG. Respiratory syncytial virus infection in preterm infants and the protective effects of RSV immune globulin. Respiratory Syncytial Virus Immune Globulin Study Group. *Pediatrics* 95(4):463–7, 1995.

83. Beasley JM, Jones SE. Continuous positive airway pressure in bronchiolitis. *Br Med J* 283:1506;1981.

84. Hall CB et al. Long-term prospective study in children after respiratory syncytial virus infection. *J Pediatr* 105:358, 1984.

85. Gurwitz D, Mindorff C, Levison H. Increased incidence of bronchial reactivity in children with history of bronchiolitis. *J Pediatr* 98:551, 1981.

86. Kransinski K. Severe respiratory syncytial virus infection: Clinical features, nosocomial acquisition and outcome. *Pediatr Infect Dis* 4:250, 1985.

87. Twiggs JT et al. Respiratory syncytial virus infection. *Clin Pediatr* 20:187, 1981.

John H. Fugate

15 Respiratory Failure

Respiratory failure is defined in terms of the primary function of the respiratory system, that is, to provide oxygen along with removal of carbon dioxide. When evaluating the respiratory system, the whole system is considered. This includes the integration of the respiratory control centers, nerve conduction pathways, myoneural junction, respiratory muscles, the thoracic cage, airways, and the lung parenchyma. Clinically, respiratory failure is seen when this integrated system fails to provide oxygenation adequately, as evidenced by low partial pressure of arterial oxygen (PaO_2) or when it fails to remove carbon dioxide, as evidenced by high elevated partial pressure of arterial carbon dioxide ($PaCO_2$). There are no fixed numbers that define respiratory failure, although general guidelines of PaO_2 less than 60 mm Hg or $PaCO_2$ greater than 50 mm Hg are frequently quoted numbers. The physiologic types of respiratory failure are defined in terms of gas exchange—ventilatory failure and oxygenation failure.

Ventilatory Failure

Ventilatory failure is defined as carbon dioxide retention. Carbon dioxide is eliminated from the body via gas exchange in the lungs and during expiration. It is transferred across the capillary-alveolar membrane by the pressure gradient between mixed venous PCO_2 and alveolar PCO_2 (normally a 6–8 mm Hg difference) and then exhaled. In the steady state, the amount of carbon dioxide that is eliminated by the lungs is equal to the amount produced by the body. This physiologic relationship is represented by the following formula:

$$PaCO_2 = \frac{Vco_2 \times K}{V_A} \qquad (1)$$

$PaCO_2$ is the arterial partial pressure of carbon dioxide in the blood. Vco_2 is the amount of carbon dioxide produced by the body, K is a constant, and V_A is alveolar ventilation (i.e., the amount of air that is breathed per minute that reaches the alveoli and participates in gas exchange). Thus, carbon dioxide elimination is directly proportional to carbon dioxide production and inversely proportional to alveolar ventilation. Carbon dioxide retention may be caused by increased production and/or decreased alveolar ventilation.

Two other physiologic parameters are important in understanding ventilatory failure. These are defined as follows:

$$V_A = V_E - V_D \qquad (2)$$

Alveolar ventilation is equal to minute ventilation (V_E) minus dead space ventilation (V_D). Minute ventilation is the amount of air moved in and out of the lungs each minute and is defined as the product of the frequency of breathing (breaths per minute) times the tidal volume (quantity of air in each breath). Dead space ventilation is the amount of air that does not take part in gas exchange each minute because it remains in the conducting airways or reaches alveoli that are not perfused and thus becomes wasted ventilation.

Thus, carbon dioxide retention may be caused by any process that decreases minute ventilation (either decreased respiratory frequency or tidal volume) or increases dead space ventilation. Because minute ventilation is clinically possible to assess by observing respiratory rate and measuring tidal volumes, it is easy to be trapped into believing that these observable parameters will equate to $PaCO_2$ levels. It is important, however, to remember that V_A is also dependent on dead space ventilation (Eq. 2), which may vary markedly in the patient, and that $PaCO_2$ is also dependent on carbon dioxide production (Eq. 1), which, too, can vary (e.g., fever, glucose load, activity level).

Clinically, carbon dioxide elevation (hypercapnia) is caused by two mechanisms: (1) hypoventilation and (2) increased dead space ventilation seen with ventilation-perfusion (V/Q) inequality. It must be remembered that decreased V_A by either mechanism causing hypercapnia is always relative to carbon dioxide production (Vco_2).

Hypercapnia Secondary to Hypoventilation

Pure hypoventilation is seen in a variety of conditions and is characterized by an increased $PaCO_2$, decreased PaO_2, and decreased P_AO_2 (alveolar partial pressure of oxygen). The alveolar-arterial (A-a) gradient is normal because there is no intrinsic lung disease or V/Q mismatch. There are many etiologies within the integrated respiratory system that will lead to a decrease in minute ventilation and cause hypercapnia. Table 15-1 gives examples of conditions that may cause hypoventilation within the respiratory system. Minute ventilation (V_E) is decreased in all of these clinical states by either decreased respiratory rate (e.g., apnea, depressed respiratory center from drugs, etc.) or decreased tidal volume (e.g., muscle dystrophies, weakness, Guillian-Barré, etc.). The severity of the hypoventilation will directly decrease oxygenation levels unless supplemental oxygen is administered.

Hypercapnia Secondary to Increased Dead Space

Hypercapnia may be caused by increased dead space ventilation, which may decrease alveolar ventilation if the patient cannot compensate by increasing minute ventilation. This is commonly seen in patients with restrictive lung diseases who exhibit rapid and shallow breathing. Shallow breathing causes a smaller percentage of the tidal volume to enter the alveoli, with a larger percentage of the tidal volume remaining in the conducting pathways, thus increasing dead space ventilation. Restrictive diseases include restricting thoracic wall abnormalities, either congenital or acquired, pleural diseases, or diseases that cause pulmonary fibrosis.

More commonly, increased dead space ventilation is seen in patients with V/Q inequality. In areas of low V/Q (poorly ventilated alveoli with normal or near-normal perfusion), both hypoxemia and hypercapnia occur. Generally, patients may compensate for hypercapnia by increasing respiratory rate or tidal volume (increasing V_E). By increasing minute ventilation to lung units of normal V/Q, the $PaCO_2$ is normal or even below normal. Because PaO_2 is dependent on the venous admixture of the combined hemoglobin saturations of the different lung units, it is usually significantly

Table 15-1. Common causes of hypoventilation

Area of respiratory system	Problems causing hypoventilation
Respiratory center (medulla)	Drug overdose (morphine, barbiturates) central apnea, encephalitis, hemorrhage, trauma, neoplasm
Spinal conducting pathways	Cervical cord injury, neoplasm, hemorrhage, poliomyelitis, amyotrophic lateral sclerosis
Peripheral nerves	Guillian-Barré syndrome, phrenic nerve palsy or injury
Myoneural junction	Myasthenia gravis, muscle relaxants
Respiratory muscles	Muscular dystrophies, myositis, limited diaphragmatic movement
Thoracic cage	Structural defects (e.g., Jeune's syndrome), severe scoliosis, flail chest
Airway obstruction	Congenital structural anomalies, infection, vocal cord palsy or injury, foreign body, obstructive sleep apnea

lower when there are many areas of low V/Q inequality. For this reason, it is not uncommon in patients with moderate V/Q mismatch to have a normal $PaCO_2$ while having a decreased PaO_2. With severe V/Q mismatch (low V/Q) the PCO_2 may rise above normal along with a low PaO_2. Also, if patients begin to tire in their work of breathing and are unable to have a compensated increased V_E, the $PaCO_2$ will increase above normal. These physiologic changes are common to obstructive diseases (asthma, bronchiolitis, bronchopulmonary dysplasia), pneumonias, interstitial lung diseases, and vascular problems leading to pulmonary edema.

Clinically, it may be useful to quantitate dead space ventilation by using the Bohr equation:

$$\frac{V_D}{V_T} = \frac{PaCO_2 - PeCO_2}{PaCO_2} \qquad (3)$$

V_D/V_T is the ratio of dead space ventilation to normal tidal volume, $PaCO_2$ is the arterial carbon dioxide pressure, and $PeCO_2$ is the mean expired carbon dioxide pressure that may be collected and measured. Normal $PeCO_2$ is approximately 28 mm Hg when $PaCO_2$ is 40 mm Hg.

$$\frac{V_D}{V_T} = \frac{40 - 28}{40} = 0.3$$

Thus the normal V_D/V_T or normal dead space ventilation is 30% of tidal volume.

Problems of Hypercapnia

Several problems arise from elevated $PaCO_2$ levels, although excessive carbon dioxide is not nearly as harmful as hypoxemia. As long as oxygen delivery is maintained, patients may tolerate very high levels of $PaCO_2$.[1] The major problems related to hypercapnia include low pH, low PaO_2, and decreased ventilatory reserve.

Decreasing pH levels occur with rising $PaCO_2$ levels, according to the Henderson-Hasselbach equation. The pH will decrease approximately 0.08 units for every 10-mm Hg rise of $PaCO_2$. As the pH decreases below 7.10, it should be considered potentially life-threatening.

Rising $PaCO_2$ levels will also decrease alveolar oxygen levels (P_AO_2) and therefore decrease PaO_2. This is evident in the alveolar oxygen equation:

$$P_AO_2 = F_iO_2 (P_B - 47) - \frac{PaCO_2}{R} \qquad (4)$$

where P_AO_2 equals alveolar oxygen pressure, F_iO_2 equals the fraction of inspired oxygen, P_B equals barometric pressure, and R equals respiratory quotient (normal, 0.8). Thus, as $PaCO_2$ rises, it may significantly decrease P_AO_2, especially in low fixed concentrations of inspired oxygen (e.g., room air).

As the $PaCO_2$ rises, the clinical status may become precarious in terms of ventilatory reserve. When alveolar ventilation (V_A) is plotted against $PaCO_2$ a hyperbolic relationship is seen (Fig. 15-1). In the hypercapneic patient, small decreases in alveolar ventilation will cause large increases in $PaCO_2$ with the concomitant decreases in pH and PaO_2. Thus the hypercapnic patient may deteriorate very quickly with only small changes in V_A. Clinically, it is not uncommon to observe a patient with a $PaCO_2$ of 55 to 60 rapidly develop very high levels of $PaCO_2$ (80–120 mm Hg) once small decreases in respiratory rate or tidal volume occur,

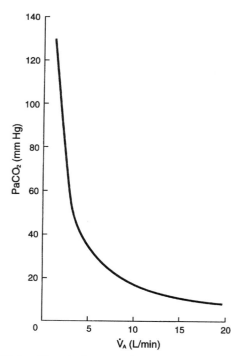

Figure 15-1. Hyperbolic curve of $PaCO_2$ versus V_A when carbon dioxide production is 200 cc/min. When $PaCO_2$ is 55 to 60 mm Hg, small decreases in V_A will dramatically increase $PaCO_2$.

either because lung mechanics change, the patient tires out, or intubated patients develop larger air leaks (e.g., positional, effect of muscle relaxants).

Generally, patients do not require artificial ventilation based on $PaCO_2$ alone. The patient's clinical condition, acute or chronic respiratory status, oxygen levels, buffering capacity, and other variables all contribute to the decision for the need for ventilatory assistance. Hypercapnia, when associated with any of the following problems, usually necessitates ventilatory assistance:

1. Worsening fatigue
2. Poor oxygenation
3. Acidosis
4. Poor mental status
5. Poor airway control or patency
6. Decreased cardiac output

Oxygenation Failure

Oxygenation failure is defined as the lack of normal oxygen gas exchange, resulting in hypoxemia. There are five etiologies of oxygenation failure:

1. Ventilation/perfusion inequality
2. Hypoventilation
3. Shunt
4. Diffusion impairment
5. Low FiO_2

Ventilation/Perfusion Inequality

Low ventilation/perfusion inequality is the most commonly encountered cause of hypoxemia in the ICU setting. Lung units that are poorly ventilated (e.g., atelectasis, obstruction, edema, etc.) and have normal or near-normal perfusion (low V/Q) will not have oxygen to saturate the hemoglobin in the adjacent capillary beds, and thus pulmonary venous blood returning from these lungs units will have the same hemoglobin saturation as when it arrived. PaO_2 is dependent on the mixture of blood returning from all of the lung units (venous admixture), which is determined by a mixture of hemoglobin that has been saturated. For example, a patient may be breathing a high FiO_2 (e.g., 0.8) and have only 50% normally ventilated lung units. In this situation, the P_AO_2 may be 400 mm Hg and the hemoglobin saturation 100% in these ventilated units, but other lung units, if totally nonventilated, would have a P_AO_2 of 40 and a hemoglobin saturation of 75%. The final arterial PO_2 will be 60 mm Hg because the mixed hemoglobin saturation (100% and 75%) will be 87.5% in this situation. Because of venous admixture in areas of low V/Q, hypoxemia readily develops.

In patients with diffuse lung diseases with significant atelectasis, pulmonary edema, inflammation, or obstruction, there will be marked low ventilation/perfusion inequality, leading to hypoxemia. Patients commonly present to the ICU with hypoxemia secondary to V/Q inequality from pneumonias, pulmonary edema, inflammatory disease of the lung, asthma, bronchiolitis, or bronchopulmonary dysplasia.

Hypoventilation

Hypoventilation was described in the previous section. With significant decreases in alveolar ventilation, there will be decreased PO_2 without change in the AaO_2 gradient.

Shunt

Shunt occurs when blood reaches the arterial system without passing through ventilated areas of the lung. Common nonpulmonary shunts include congenital and surgical right-to-left shunts associated with congenital heart disease and blood shunted across a patent foramen ovale with pulmonary hypertension. These types of shunts and their management are discussed in Intensive Care Following Cardiac Surgery by Lang et al., this volume. Pulmonary shunts occur in lung units of low V/Q.

Diffusion Impairment

Under the normal physiologic conditions of gas exchange between alveolar gas and capillary blood gas, there is plenty of reserve time for equilibration to occur. In some disease states, the blood-gas barrier has become thickened, and diffusion is significantly slowed so that normal equilibration may not occur. Most of these disease states are rare in pediatric patients. In patients with interstitial fibrosis, including sarcoidosis, diffuse interstitial diseases, severe pneumonia, collagen vascular diseases, rheumatoid lung, lupus erythematosus, Wagner's granulomatous disease, Goodpasture syndrome, this may occur.

Low Inspired Partial Pressure of Oxygen

Hypoxemia usually occurs in areas at high altitudes when there is a low inspired partial pressure of oxygen (P_IO_2). According to the alveolar oxygen equation (Eq. 4), P_AO_2 is directly proportional to the barometric pressure (P_B). It is not uncommon, therefore, to have a P_AO_2 of 60 mm Hg at elevations of 10,000 feet. Patients compensate for this by hyperventilating (Eq. 4) to increase P_AO_2 and thus PaO_2; hypoxemia may be severely exacerbated in patients with any type of parenchymal lung disease with low V/Q inequality.

Problems with Hypoxemia

Hypoxemia generally is much more serious than hypercarbia. Severe hypoxemia will lead quickly to cell injury and death in all organs, with the CNS being most sensitive. Severe hypoxemia is a medical emergency and must be treated urgently. Supplemental oxygen via nasal cannula, mask, or hood box is started in the patient who can ventilate normally. In patients who are unable to ventilate normally, artificial ventilation and oxygenation must be instituted rapidly. Long-term management of respiratory failure, either ventilatory failure or oxygenation failure, is discussed in Mechanical Ventilation by Kacmarek et al., this volume.

Reference

1. Goldstein B, Shannon DC, Todres ID. Supercarbia in children: Clinical course and outcome. *Crit Care Med* 18:166–168, 1990.

Thomas L. Truman
I. David Todres

15.1 Acute Respiratory Distress Syndrome

Historical Overview and Definitions

Acute respiratory distress syndrome (ARDS) describes a well-known constellation of clinical findings consisting of acute respiratory failure with significant hypoxemia, noncardiogenic pulmonary edema, and widespread infiltrates on chest radiograph that historically follow a pulmonary insult such as bacterial sepsis, gastric aspiration, or hypoxic/ischemic events. Although the pathologic scenarios were described by military surgeons following World War Two, it was in 1967 that Ashbaugh and colleagues first described the clinical and pathophysiologic features of ARDS in 12 trauma patients that exhibited respiratory failure 1 to 96 hours after injury, with a mortality rate of 58%.[1,2]

Initially termed *acute* respiratory distress syndrome because of its sudden onset and histologic similarity to neonatal RDS (hyaline membrane formation), *adult* respiratory distress syndrome has been the widely accepted term for many years. This is despite the presence of an 11-year-old in the original ARDS descriptive series.[1] Recently, it has become increasingly recognized that ARDS is a complex disorder where lung injury is typically associated with other organ dysfunction or failure, possibly a cause of, or component of, a systemic inflammatory response syndrome (SIRS).[3] For many years, the term *ARDS* has been imprecisely defined and has had a relatively heterogeneous group of etiologies, both of which are key factors contributing to the difficulty in conducting studies and developing effective therapies. An American-European Consensus Conference on ARDS in 1992 formulated definitions describing a wide clinical spectrum of respiratory failure, termed *acute lung injury* (ALI), while the term *ARDS* is reserved for the most severe forms of ALI.[4]

ALI is then defined as a syndrome of (1) acute-onset pulmonary inflammation and increased capillary permeability that is not on the basis of left atrial or pulmonary capillary hypertension (PCWP $\leq$ 18 mm Hg), (2) bilateral infiltrates on frontal chest radiograph, and (3) PaO_2/FiO_2 less than or equal to 300 mm Hg (regardless of PEEP). ARDS criteria consist of ALI, only with a PaO_2/FiO_2 less than or equal to 200 mm Hg (regardless of PEEP). Also agreed on at the conference was the change in terminology back to *acute respiratory distress syndrome* since it can be seen in patients of all ages.[4] The acute and diffuse involvement of the endothelial and epithelial surface of the lungs clinically characterized here refers to the **early** phase of ARDS, while the **late** phase refers to the clinical stage of ARDS in which the lung attempts to repair the initial or persistent injury to the respiratory units. Its histologic correspondent is termed *fibroproliferative phase*, which, if unhalted, leads to extensive fibrosis. This replacement of damaged epithelial cells with mesenchymal cells and their connective tissue products in the airspaces usually occurs by the second week of ARDS.[5–7]

Epidemiology/Morbidity and Mortality

It is estimated that the incidence of ARDS in the United States is approximately 150,000 cases per year in adults, but an accurate incidence of ARDS in the pediatric age group is unknown, most likely from inconsistent diagnostic criteria and inadequate reporting.[8,9] ARDS has been reported in essentially all age groups, including neonates.[10] Several reviews on pediatric ARDS report incidences ranging from 0.8% to 4.4% of all pediatric intensive care unit (PICU) admissions.[11,12] Despite the improved understanding of ARDS pathogenesis and numerous advances in ventilatory and nutritional support, the mortality rate in this syndrome has gone essentially unchanged from Ashbaugh's initial report of 58%. Most pediatric literature sites mortality rates in the range of 39% to 90%.[12,13]

It has become increasingly evident that associated pneumonia or sepsis implies a higher rate of mortality. Extremely poor prognosis has been reported with ARDS associated with malignancies and concomitant multiple organ dysfunction, and especially when following bone marrow transplantation.[14–18] Although fulminant sepsis with multiple organ dysfunction is a common cause of death during both the early and late phases of ARDS in adults, most late mortality is due to progressive pulmonary fibroproliferation and subsequent respiratory insufficiency.[7]

In attempts to further identify factors that accurately predict prognosis, an expanded definition of ARDS was formulated that assessed three clinical features: (1) severity of acute lung injury, (2) associated clinical disorders, and (3) systemic organ function. The severity of ALI is quantitatively obtained by the Lung Injury Score, which is based on a 4-point system including PaO_2/FiO_2 ratio, respiratory compliance, level of PEEP, and presence of consolidation on chest roentgenogram (Table 15.1-1). The associated clinical disorders describe the underlying etiology that predisposes the patient to ARDS, such as gastric content aspiration, sepsis, and trauma. Systemic organ function refers to the patient's acid-base status and any dysfunctioning organ systems, especially renal, hepatic, and cardiovascular.[19] Although still being actively researched and refined, the expanded definition of ARDS has been useful in that it provides the ability to follow the physiologic variables in patients with ALI (Lung Injury Score) and assists in identifying the patients at highest risk for mortality.

Future work on predicting prognosis will take key factors into account, such as acute underlying diagnosis, etiology of ARDS, severity of illness as measured by pulmonary and nonpulmonary factors, and comorbidities that affect immune status.[4] In those patients that do survive ARDS, there are usually persistent abnormalities in pulmonary function tests, but most have no severe pulmonary limitations.[20] With the new innovative treatments for childhood malignancies, expansions and advances in both solid organ and bone marrow transplants, and improved pediatric emergency services, it seems likely that the incidence of ARDS will increase and continue to be responsible for significant morbidity and mortality in the PICU.

Clinical Presentation/Differential Diagnosis

ARDS can present in the pediatric patient that has recently suffered a life-threatening event such as near drowning, multiple trauma, or an illness producing shock. The patient commonly exhibits signs and symptoms of respiratory difficulty, including tachypnea, grunting, nasal flaring, retractions, and the need for supplemental oxygen to sustain normal arterial oxygen saturations. Despite appropriate treatment(s) of underlying pulmonary insult, the disease process

Table 15.1-1. Components and individual values of the Lung Injury Score

		Value
1. Chest roentgenogram score		
No alveolar consolidation		0
Alveolar consolidation continued to 1 quadrant		1
Alveolar consolidation continued to 2 quadrants		2
Alveolar consolidation continued to 3 quadrants		3
Alveolar consolidation in all 4 quadrants		4
2. Hypoxemia score		
PaO_2/F_IO_2	300	0
PaO_2/F_IO_2	225–299	1
PaO_2/F_IO_2	175–224	2
PaO_2/F_IO_2	100–174	3
PaO_2/F_IO_2	100	4
3. PEEP score (when ventilated)		
PEEP	5 cm H_2O	0
PEEP	6–8 cm H_2O	1
PEEP	9–11 cm H_2O	2
PEEP	12–14 cm H_2O	3
PEEP	>15 cm H_2O	4
4. Respiratory system compliance score (when available)		
Compliance	>80 ml/cm H_2O	0
Compliance	60–79 ml/cm H_2O	1
Compliance	40–59 ml/cm H_2O	2
Compliance	20–39 ml/cm H_2O	3
Compliance	<19 ml/cm H_2O	4

The final value is obtained by dividing the aggregate sum by the number of components that were used.

	Score
No lung injury	0
Mild-to-moderate lung injury	0.1–2.5
Severe lung injury (ARDS)	>2.5

PaO_2/FiO_2, ratio of arterial oxygen tension to inspired oxygen concentration; PEEP, positive end-expiratory pressure.
Source: From Murray JF et al. An expanded definition of adult respiratory distress syndrome. *Am Rev Respir Dis* 138:720–723, 1988. With permission.

continues, and insufficiencies in both ventilation and oxygenation require tracheal intubation and mechanical ventilation with the addition of PEEP. Chest radiographs usually show a normal cardiac silhouette and the development of bilateral infiltrates suggestive of pulmonary edema within several days of the initial insult. Hemodynamic instability, ranging from tachycardia to frank shock, may be present. Other organ systems, such as the kidney, liver, and bone marrow/clotting mechanisms, may also dysfunction or fail.

While these are the classic signs and symptoms that accompany ARDS in the pediatric patient, other etiologies of severe respiratory distress and significant hypoxemia must be considered to diagnose correctly and avoid potential errors in management. Pulmonary embolism (PE), although uncommon in the pediatric population, must be entertained in the differential diagnosis, especially in (1) cases involving abdominal, pelvic, or lower extremity trauma, (2) older and obese children that are immobile, and (3) pediatric patients with disease processes that place them at higher risk for venous thrombosis, such as nephrotic syndrome, burns, autoimmune disease, and protein S, C, or antithrombin-3 deficiencies. PE differs from ARDS in that there is usually a very rapid deterioration of oxygenation without gross impairment of ventilation. The

chest radiographs are usually unremarkable in PE patients as opposed to ARDS. Left ventricular failure can also present with similar signs and symptoms of ARDS, but there is usually a history suggestive of progressive myocardial dysfunction, characteristic electrocardiographic changes, and elevated pulmonary capillary wedge pressures and decreased cardiac output. The history of a preceding global or pulmonary insult and the lack of data to support left ventricular failure or a PE usually forecasts ARDS.

Pathophysiology

The development of ARDS follows a clearly recognizable clinical predisposition, usually within 12 to 96 hours, that can be characterized as being a direct or indirect insult to the lungs. Examples of direct injury include aspiration of gastric contents, near drowning, inhalational injuries, and trauma. Indirect predispositions usually include overwhelming sepsis, SIRS, severe nonthoracic trauma, multiple blood-product transfusions, and pancreatitis (Table 15.1-2).[21] In recent years, the improved understanding of inflammatory cascade reactions and endothelial/epithelial injury models has suggested that common pathophysiologic mechanisms exist for both SIRS and ARDS. Hence, it is thought that SIRS can lead to ARDS, and ARDS can initiate SIRS.[3]

Whether ARDS is part of a SIRS or secondary to aspiration or near drowning, the pathologic sequelae are similar. Initially, there is a damage to the epithelial-lined alveoli and the endothelium-lined pulmonary capillary with accumulation of protein-rich fluid in both the interstitium and alveoli. This increased capillary permeability (noncardiogenic) edema most likely represents the effect of numerous inflammatory cells and the various cytokines and mediators they release.[22] The cytokines involved are best represented by tumor necrosis factor (TNF) and interleukin-1 (IL-1). They are produced by neutrophils, macrophages, as well as endothelial cells, and play a significant role in the hyperdynamic, hypercatabolic state of ARDS. Oxygen radicals are produced and are unstable, unpaired electron-possessing, toxic oxygen metabolites. Hydroxyl ion is the most damaging, with direct oxidation of epithelial/endothelial cells, alteration of the interstitial hyaluronic matrix, and fragmentation of basement membranes. Proteolytic enzymes, especially neutrophil-derived elastase, also have been found to be involved in damaging the alveolar-capillary barrier.[23] Platelet-activating factor (PAF), a mediator produced by neutrophils and endothelial cells, in addition to platelets, is released under the influence of phospholipase A_2 activation. PAF is respon-

Table 15.1-2. Major clinical predispositions to acute respiratory distress syndrome

Direct	Indirect
Aspiration of gastric contents	Bacterial sepsis
Infectious pneumonia	Trauma, nonthoracic
Inhalational of toxic gas or aerosol	Multiple blood transfusions
Near drowning	Pancreatitis
Lung contusion	Disseminated intravascular coagulation
	Systemic inflammatory response syndrome

Source: Adapted from Hyers TM. Predictions of survival and mortality in patients with ARDS. *New Horiz* 1(4):466–470, 1993. With permission.

sible for platelet and neutrophil aggregation, bronchoconstriction, and increased pulmonary and systemic vascular permeability.[24] There also is increased production of both cyclooxygenase and lipoxygenase products, namely thromboxane A_2, prostacyclin, and leukotrienes. Endotoxins, with origins from an infectious etiology or from the gut as a result of altered gut mucosal membrane function, also represent important activators of mediator release in the pathophysiology of ARDS.[25,26] Complement activation and its split-products C5a and C3a play important roles in the initiation and propagation of ARDS. Complement-related mediators have been found to be responsible for inducing the release of neutrophil mediators, increasing neutrophil aggregation and endothelial adherence, in addition to altering endothelial permeability.[27,28]

Once the predisposing factor and the ensuing inflammatory mediators have initiated the development of ARDS, the first 24 to 96 hours are associated with clinical signs of worsening respiratory distress and hypoxemia, which is termed the *acute or exudative phase* and correlates with the development of characteristic light microscopy changes in alveolar units. Engorgement of alveoli with neutrophils, RBCs, and proteinaceous fluid results in formation of obstructing hyaline membranes and decreased surfactant functions. There is obliteration of pulmonary capillaries with thrombi, fibrin, leukocyte, and platelet plugs. Accumulation of interstitial fluid and sloughing of type I pneumocytes, but not type II, also occurs during the early course of ARDS. The subacute or proliferative phase is typified by proliferation of type II pneumocytes and persistence of interstitial and alveolar fluid and lasts approximately 1 to 2 weeks. The last phase, referred to as the *chronic or fibrotic phase* is characterized by replacement of damaged epithelial cells by mesenchymal cells and their connective tissue products, resulting in relatively permanent obstruction of both alveoli and bronchoalveolar airspaces.[3,9]

Despite this initial diffuse alveolar damage with an overall increase in lung fluid, the ARDS process manifests itself in a heterogeneous pattern, from both a radiographic and mechanical standpoint. The once-thought-of "homogeneously diseased lungs" theory suggested by plain radiographs has been replaced by the "baby lungs" model, which accounts for the focal nature of lung injury and the remaining functionally normal small lung regions associated with ARDS. CT studies on adults with ARDS have demonstrated that dependent, posterior regions of diseased lungs are preferentially infiltrated, consolidated, and collapsed.[29] The lungs of ARDS patients are considered to have three pathologically separate areas: (1) loci of irreversible damage and alveolar collapse, (2) regions where compliance and ventilation are normal, and (3) mixed areas with both infiltration and consolidation, but with reversible degrees of atelectasis. The ARDS lung therefore can be viewed as heterogeneously diseased (infected, atelectatic, and noncompliant) with scattered areas of normal lung. As opposed to the diseased regions with large $\dot{V}/\dot{Q}$ mismatching, the normal regions are functionally small and usually demonstrate normal lung mechanics with well-matched ventilation and perfusion. These functionally small lungs (baby lungs) are approximately one third to one half the normal volume and must bear the entire burden of gas exchange.[29–31]

Management

Mechanical Ventilation

Traditionally, the goals of ventilatory management of ARDS in both children and adults have been to maintain normal arterial blood gases by utilizing relatively large tidal volumes with inherently high peak inspiratory pressures (PIPs), PEEPs of 5 to 15 cm H_2O, and high levels of FiO_2 via flow-controlled, volume-cycled ventilators with inspiration-expiration ratios of 1:2 to 1:5. The use of tidal volumes that are proportionally normal for nondiseased lungs (10–12 cc/kg) can result in alveolar overdistention and overventilation of the functionally normal baby lungs described in ARDS, and may expose endothelial and epithelial barriers to excessive stress. This ventilator-induced lung damage seen in ARDS is probably inflicted by several mechanisms, including (1) excessive transalveolar inflation pressures, (2) inappropriate tidal volumes, and (3) damaging sheer forces that arise from tidal opening and closing of susceptible alveoli when insufficient end-expiratory alveolar pressure is maintained. Data from both animal and human studies demonstrate that high PIPs result in exacerbation of both bronchial and parenchymal lung injury. At the alveolar level, the ventilator-induced lung injury is manifested by granulocyte infiltration, increased pulmonary vascular permeability, and production of proteinaceous alveolar edema leading to hyaline membrane formation. In addition to the microscopic evidence of lung injury, high peak inflation pressures can greatly increase the risk for catastrophic air leak syndromes.[32,33]

The adverse effects of large tidal volumes, high inflation pressures, and a better understanding of the heterogeneous distribution of lung injury interspersed with relatively normal lung regions (i.e., baby lungs) have resulted in a shift of attitudes in mechanical ventilation strategies. The mainstay of ARDS therapy is still supportive care, but we now focus on adequately ventilating the lung units that appear to have nearly normal gas-to-tissue ratios and well-preserved mechanical and gas-exchanging properties.[32,34]

Increasing amounts of data suggest that the most clinically beneficial and least injurious strategy of mechanically ventilating patients with ARDS, both adults and children, involves five major themes (Table 15.1-3): (1) limitation of the transalveolar pressure to no more than 35 cm H_2O (pressure-targeting mode); (2) PEEP at levels sufficient to obliterate any clear inflection point on the static pressure-volume curve (usually 7–15 cm H_2O); (3) reduction of minute ventilation by allowing PCO_2 to rise to 60 to 100, as long as serum pH is greater than 7.20 (permissive hypercapnia); (4) increasing inspiratory time and slowing the end-inspiratory flow (decelerating flow), allowing for better gas distribution to lung units with different time constants (inherently done with pressure-controlled ventilator); and (5) reduction of oxygen toxicity by lowering FiO_2 to less than 0.60.[32]

When worsening hypoxemia and high PIPs related to underlying ARDS are encountered in our PICU (Lung Injury Score of >1.0), volume-controlled conventional ventilation is replaced with the pressure-controlled, time-cycled mode of ventilation. We usually start by limiting the PIPs to 35 cm H_2O and begin with PEEP of

Table 15.1-3. Mechanical ventilatory strategy in children with ARDS

Pressure-controlled ventilation with limitation of PIP to 35 cm H_2O

PEEP of 7–15 cm H_2O—close monitoring of hemodynamics

Permissive hypercapnia—maintain pH > 7.20

Lengthening inspiratory time with decelerating inspiratory flow

FiO_2 < 0.6

---

6 cm H_2O, which is increased as needed to achieve greater than 90% arterial saturations while delivering less than 60% oxygen if possible. Because of the risks of cardiovascular compromise incurred with high levels of PEEP (12–15 cm H_2O), we elect to closely follow the intravascular volume status and left ventricular function by monitoring central venous pressure, pulmonary artery pressures, and left atrial filling pressures by pulmonary artery catheterization. Fluid is administered as boluses as needed to maintain an adequate cardiac output. If significant hypoxemia persists despite these measures, we then proceed to slowly increase the inspiratory time (normally 0.8–1.0 seconds) to 1.2 to 2.0 seconds, which usually corresponds to a duty cycle (% of total I/E time spent in inspiration) of 0.4 to 0.5. This accomplishes increased mean airway pressures without exceeding the PIP. Because lengthening the inspiratory time directly reduces the time allowed for exhalation, auto-PEEP is usually encountered, especially when underlying distal airway obstruction exists. Therefore, when prolonged inspiratory times are required or bronchospasm is evident, close attention is given to maintaining the **total** PEEP, which can be detected by measuring the end-exhalational pressure with the expiratory port occluded in the muscle-relaxed patient.[35] Under extreme cases, the inspiratory time can be prolonged such that inverse-ratio ventilation occurs. This type of ventilatory strategy can be helpful in improving oxygenation in that it increases lung volumes by recruiting alveoli for gas exchange.[32] Despite anecdotal reports on the employment of I:E ratios as high as 3:1 to 4:1, our experience is that the risks outweigh the benefits when greater than 2:1 ratios are used. The likelihood of barotrauma and the probable hemodynamic compromise associated with these high ratios usually preclude its use. Because of the nonphysiologic nature of this type of ventilation, heavy sedation and muscle relaxation are indicated to facilitate effective oxygenation and ventilation.

Decreases in minute ventilation are made by limiting PIP and increasing PEEP, hence dropping the tidal volume, as well as slowing the ventilator rate. PCO_2s are allowed to slowly rise to levels of 70 to 100 torr in a permissive manner to avoid acidemia, with goals of pH being greater than 7.20. Measures to buffer the increase in hydrogen ion associated with supranormal levels of PCO_2 include both bicarbonate or tromethamine administration. Like most medical therapies employed today, there are several limiting factors that we believe represent contraindications to the use of permissive hypercapnia. First, patients with increased intracranial pressures (i.e., patients with head injury or intracranial hemorrhage) can lose their cerebrovascular autoregulatory functions and may experience carbon dioxide narcosis and convulsions when subjected to hypercapnia. Second, patients with poor cardiac function may not tolerate the decreased myocardial contractility, vasodilation, and increased sympathetic activity with dysrhythmias that can occur with hypercarbia. Acute rises in PCO_2 without significant metabolic compensation can enhance hypoxic pulmonary vasoconstriction.[36,37] In extreme ARDS cases with profound ventilatory defects or in patients with contraindications to the use of permissive hypercapnia, extracorporeal carbon dioxide removal via a veno-venous circuit can be employed, but remains a tool to be used in special centers.

In addition to pressure-controlled ventilation, several "alternative" approaches and adjunctive therapies have emerged that attempt to reduce the high mortality rate in pediatric ARDS supported with conventional ventilatory techniques. Extracorporeal membrane oxygenation and high-frequency oscillatory ventilation head the list of alternative strategies of oxygenation and ventilation, while nitric oxide inhalation, surfactant replacement, and steroid administration remain the leaders of potentially useful adjunctive therapies for ARDS.

Extracorporeal Membrane Oxygenation

Extracorporeal membrane oxygenation (ECMO) obviates the need for barotraumatic ventilator support, thus allowing the acutely injured lungs to "rest" or heal (see Extracorporeal Life Support by Custer and Akingbola, this volume). ECMO has clear indications for use in the neonatal population with lung pathology, where the mortality rates of severe meconium aspiration pneumonitis, congenital diaphragmatic hernia, and overwhelming group B streptococceal (GBS) sepsis/pneumonia have been dramatically reduced. Several recent retrospective reports on experience with ECMO in pediatric ARDS have demonstrated that it may be a useful therapy with increased rates of survival when compared with survival of patients treated with conventional ventilatory strategies.[37–39] Currently, ECMO serves as our rescue therapy of choice for pediatric patients with severe ARDS that fails to respond favorably to pressure-control ventilator management and adjunctive therapies such as nitric oxide inhalation and surfactant administration. The likelihood that ECMO will improve outcome in a given case is probably maximized when (1) offered to patients without chronic pulmonary disease or preexisting malignancies, (2) instituted early in the course of acute lung injury before the onset of multiple-organ system organ failure, and (3) utilized with adjunctive therapies such as exogenous surfactant and inhaled nitric oxide. Because of the complications that potentially accompany extracorporeal life support (i.e., systemic anticoagulation with heparin, ligation of right common carotid artery, and exposure to foreign blood products), the early use of ECMO in pediatric ARDS must be formally evaluated and compared with other forms of therapy before becoming the primary mode of treatment. Until well-controlled, prospective, randomized studies are performed, ECMO will most likely remain a rescue form of treatment for a select subpopulation of children with ARDS.

High-Frequency Oscillatory Ventilation

Because of its success in treatment of severe neonatal RDS (HMD), high-frequency oscillatory ventilation technology has recently emerged in the PICU as a rescue-type therapy in patients with ALI/ARDS. It's ability to improve oxygenation and sustain ventilation at higher mean airway pressures, while avoiding the high PIPs, makes this a theoretically advantageous ventilatory alternative. Early reports on its use in pediatric patients with ARDS have indicated its apparent safety and potential benefits over both conventional ventilation and ECMO.[40–42]

When utilizing high-frequency oscillatory ventilation on pediatric patients (<35 kg) suffering from ARDS or persistent air leak syndrome, an aggressive approach of recruiting and maintaining optimal lung volumes has been outlined by Arnold et al. and seems the most efficacious.[40] Recommended initial settings and adjustments on the Sensormedics 3100 (Sensormedics, Yorba Linda, CA) are as follows: (1) FiO_2 1.0, wean to 0.3 to 0.4 after achieving optimal lung volumes; (2) operating frequency of 5 to 10 Hz, decrease by increments of 1 to 2 Hz if adequate ventilation is not possible with maximal pressure amplitudes; (3) mean airway pressure set 5 to 10 cm H_2O above that required on the previous mode of ventilation, and increased by 1 to 2 cm H_2O until chest x-ray film demonstrates optimal lung inflation (eight posterior ribs) or until oxygenation is adequate (arterial saturations >90%) and FiO_2 is 0.5; (4) inspiratory time of 33%, bias gas flow of greater than 18 liter/min; and (5) pressure amplitude is sufficient to result in adequate chest wall movement (subjectively assessed) and adjusted to achieve $PaCO_2$ values associated with a pH greater than 7.25. Once stable, the FiO_2 is reduced to less than 0.45 to limit possible oxygen toxicity. Mean arterial pressures and amplitude are then weaned slowly, with return to SIMV mode when mean arterial pressure is less than 12 to 14 cm H_2O and able to ventilate patient with PIP less than 35 cm H_2O and rate less than 25 to 30. Because of the ineffectiveness of spontaneous respirations during high-frequency oscillatory ventilation, patients are heavily sedated with opioid/benzodiazepine infusions and muscle-relaxed with nondepolarizing agents (tubocurare, if history of chronic steroid use). Although use of the Sensormedics 3100 on patients greater than 35 kg has occurred with reportedly mixed success, our current experience is limited to those pediatric patients less than 35 kg. High-frequency oscillatory ventilators designed to ventilate pediatric and adult patients greater than 35 kg are expected to be available for clinical use in the near future.

Avoidance of both barotraumatic PIPs and risks associated with ECMO makes high-frequency oscillatory ventilation an appealing mode of ventilation. At most centers, however, it currently remains a rescue therapy offered to patients failing the more conventional means of treatment until further studies demonstrating its efficacy have been completed.

Nitric Oxide

Nitric oxide (NO) is an endothelially derived relaxing factor that has a very short half-life (1–2 seconds) and whose mechanism of action is apparently dependent on the intracellular second messenger cGMP.[43] It has been found to have many diverse physiologic functions, including participation in immunoregulation, neurotransmission, inhibition of platelet adhesion, and smooth muscle relaxation.[44,45] Because of its small size, short half-life, and ability to be delivered via the inhalational route, Zapol et al. hypothesized that nitric oxide's vasodilatory properties may reduce the elevated pulmonary artery pressures frequently found in patients with ARDS.[46,47] Since then, many animal and human studies have demonstrated that inhaled nitric oxide decreases pulmonary artery hypertension without altering systemic vascular resistance. The ability to be selective for pulmonary vascular beds and not act peripherally at systemic vascular beds is because of its rapid inactivation by hemoglobin binding. A theoretical advantage offered by inhaled rather than systemic delivery of a vasodilating agent is that gas is distributed predominantly to well-ventilated regions as opposed to atelectatic or consolidated areas of the lung. Selective vasodilation of the vascular beds associated with the best ventilated alveoli should result in improvement of $\dot{V}/\dot{Q}$ mismatching that is responsible for hypoxemia in ARDS.[47] Because of these theoretical advantages and the encouraging results of nitric oxide use in persistent pulmonary hypertension of newborns, and both congenital and acquired heart disease, it is now being used in pediatric patients with ARDS.[48] Because nitric oxide remains an experimental therapy for children with pulmonary hypertension related to ARDS, we reserve its use for patients that are failing pressure-controlled ventilation. We start nitric oxide at 5 ppm and increase gradually up to maximum of 60 to 100 ppm. Most patients that respond to nitric oxide demonstrate a drop in pulmonary artery pressure and improved oxygenation at 10 to 40 ppm. After the patient is stable on FiO_2 of less than 0.5 for approximately 12 hours, the nitric oxide is slowly weaned to maintain saturations greater than 90%. In our experience, we have found that some patients that have received nitric oxide for greater than 72 to 96 hours require a slow wean (1–5 ppm every 12–24 hours). Close

and frequent monitoring of the inhaled concentrations are carried out with a electrochemical analyzer (Bedfont Sci. Ltd EC-90, Bedfont House, Kent, England) to ensure accurate delivery of nitric oxide. When nitric oxide combines with hemoglobin, methemoglobin is eventually formed, and therefore we follow daily serum methemoglobin levels. Although there have been no reported cases of severe methemoglobinemia associated with nitric oxide inhalation in adults or children, the infant's decreased intrinsic ability to reduce methemoglobin to hemoglobin (immaturity or lack of reducing enzymes), combined with increased usage of nitric oxide, suggests its inevitability.

Unfortunately, nitric oxide also is a well-known pollutant that exists in the atmosphere at levels of 10 ppb and is contained in cigarette smoke at concentrations of 400 to 1000 ppm.[49] Nitric oxide is oxidized by oxygen to nitric dioxide (NO_2), which is a known cytotoxin that subsequently is converted in aqueous solution to both nitric and nitrous acids, also cytotoxins.[50] The production of toxic gases produced when mixing nitric oxide and oxygen would seem to preclude its clinical use, but special ventilator circuits have been designed to mix the gases immediately prior to inhalation by the patient and therefore allow safe delivery. Guidelines on the safe delivery of nitric oxide have been outlined very well.[47] The long-term side effects of prolonged exposure to nitric oxide remain to be seen, but at this time its potential benefits seem to outweigh its known risks.

Exogenous Surfactant

Surfactant is a complex of 90% lipid (85% phospholipid) and 10% protein that is synthesized and stored in the type II pneumocytes and released into the alveolar space and distal small airways after adrenergic or prostaglandin stimuli.[51,52] Its function is to minimize alveolar collapse by decreasing the surface tension within alveoli, especially at low lung volumes (FRC) when prone to atelectasis. By maintaining alveolar integrity, it facilitates gas exchange and decreases the work of breathing.

When ARDS was first described, pathophysiologic findings of hyaline membranes, severe hypoxemia, decreased lung compliance, and surfactant dysfunction were very similar to those found in neonatal respiratory distress syndrome (NRDS). It is now known that the alveolar inflammatory reaction typical of ARDS results in recruited granulocytes releasing their contents and the production of reactive oxygen metabolites, which can inactivate the lungs' extracellular proteins, including elastase inhibitors and surfactant apoproteins. The pathophysiologic mechanisms thought to be responsible for the altered surfactant function in patients with ARDS are the following: (1) Type II pneumocytes are injured and do not produce sufficient phospholipid, apoprotein, or both; (2) surfactant turnover by type II pneumocytes is decreased; (3) normally produced surfactant is inactivated by alveolar flooding with inflammatory cells and protein fluid.[53]

Because exogenous surfactant administration has been found to reduce morbidity and mortality in NRDS, there may be a role for surfactant replacement for children and adults with ARDS. ARDS in animal models has been studied by utilizing various techniques to induce acute lung pathology, such as hyperoxic lung injury, bilateral vagotomy, saline-instilled lungs, and anti-lung serum.[54–57] These studies have demonstrated some benefit with surfactant administration. One study involving oleic acid–induced lung injury did not result in significant clinical benefits.[58] Surfactant dysfunction has been reported in patients with ARDS, and there have been several anecdotal reports on exogenous surfactant administration to patients with ARDS.[59–63] However, only one randomized, controlled study on the use of aerosolized surfactant in adult patients with sepsis-induced ARDS has been published.[64] This pilot study demonstrated its safety of administration and a possible trend of decreased mortality at admittedly low doses.

Because of the lack of adequate randomized, controlled studies demonstrating its efficacy, the use of exogenous surfactant must be limited to rescue therapy in severe cases of ARDS. Our experience with surfactant use in pediatric ARDS has been with patients who were (1) unresponsive to pressure-controlled ventilation and nitric oxide administration, (2) doing poorly on extracorporeal support, or (3) failing all measures but were not ECMO candidates, such as burn victims with recent grafts or patients with a preexisting malignancy. We use the surfactant preparation, Survanta (Ross Laboratories, Columbus, OH), because of its surface active proteins, SP-B and SP-C, in addition to the phospholipid contents. Our mode of administration is by direct bronchial instillation using a pediatric bronchoscope or instillation into the distal trachea via the infusion port of an in-line suction catheter with the patient in lateral decubital positions to facilitate mainstem bronchus delivery. There is a wide range of dosages quoted in animal studies and anecdotal human reports.[53] We use 0.3 to 0.5 cc/kg of Survanta (25 mg phospholipid/cc) per dose, divided between two lungs and infused over 5 minutes. Doses are administered every 24 hours while closely following pressure-volume loops, lung compliances, and FiO_2 requirements. Treatment courses are usually 2 to 7 days, with the treatment endpoint being sustained clinical improvement or the lack of positive response to two consecutive dosages (measured by changes in compliance, inflection point on P-V curve, or level of oxygenation). Most patients tolerated the surfactant instillations very well without any significant arterial desaturations or hemodynamic instability, while a few experienced apparent bronchospasm and significant desaturations requiring treatment with bronchodilators and increased FiO_2.

Steroids

Corticosteroids initially were thought to be helpful in early ARDS, but several well-controlled studies demonstrated their lack of efficacy and association with increased rates of ARDS in patients with sepsis.[65–68] The anecdotal use of corticosteroids in treating late-ARDS (>72 hours) has been reported to be helpful in both preventing the progression of the fibroproliferative stage and facilitating the improvement in gas exchange and static compliance, in addition to reducing mortality.[6,7,69] It is thought that the corticosteroids suppress cytokine release and halt ongoing lung injury.[6] Currently, we reserve the use of steroids in patients with ARDS for those who still require FiO_2 greater than 0.40, PIPs of greater than 30 cm H_2O, and presence of chronic infiltrates on chest radiographs after 7 to 10 days. We use methylprednisolone, 2 mg/kg/d, until extubation and then wean over a 2- to 4-week period. Although limited and purely anecdotal, our experience with corticosteroid use in late-ARDS has been favorable. Similar to ECMO, nitric oxide, and surfactant replacement, corticosteroids in late-ARDS remains a type of treatment whose efficacy needs to be properly demonstrated by well-controlled, randomized studies in both adult and pediatric populations.

Infections

The most common infection encountered in the pediatric patient with ARDS is bacterial pneumonia. These patients are at increased risk because of the bacterial colonization that is so frequent in intubated ICU patients and their associated impairment in immune defenses. Because the mortality rate is increased when secondary pulmonary infections exist, we closely follow the Gram stain and bacterial cultures of surveillance tracheal aspirates that are performed on these patients every other day. Keeping a high index of suspicion is very important, and early treatment of probable pneumonias with broad-spectrum antibiotics will usually prevent the spread of organisms and progression to sepsis. We utilize the combination of an antistaphylococcal penicillin with an aminoglycoside and third-generation cephalosporin to cover the most likely pathogens, *Staphylococcus aureus*, *Pseudomonas*, and other Gram-negative organisms. Close monitoring for possible fungal and viral infections is done in patients with profound immune compromise (i.e., bone marrow transplant and oncology patients). Patients with severe ARDS will require numerous indwelling catheters for both monitoring and nutrition, which predisposes these patients to line-related sepsis.

Nutrition

As with any critically ill pediatric patient, adequate nutrition is a key element in recovery. Caloric requirements are increased, especially if ARDS is accompanied by the sepsis syndrome. Parenteral nutrition is started after volume status and electrolytes are stable. Our goal is to supply 40 to 60 kcal/kg/d and prevent depletion of protein stores. This is usually achieved by providing 50% to 60% of total calories in the form of glucose, 1 to 3 g/kg/d of lipids, and 1 to 2 g/kg/d of protein. We avoid excessive fluid administration in order to reduce the development of pulmonary edema.

Administration of excess glucose calories may result in increased fat production in the liver (lipogenesis), which is associated with an increased respiratory quotient and production of carbon dioxide. Some ARDS patients with elevated PCO_2 production may require higher ventilatory settings and be unable to wean from mechanical ventilation. Slow infusions (over 20–24 hours) of 20% fat emulsions are used to prevent any hypoxemia or acutely elevated serum triglyceride levels. Metabolic cart studies may be helpful in determining the **increased** metabolic and caloric requirements seen in these patients.

Enteral feeds consisting of an age-appropriate formula are delivered via the nasogastric or nasojejunal route. We initiate enteral feeds as soon as possible, usually once the patient is hemodynamically stable and off vasoactive infusions.

References

1. Ashbaugh DG et al. Acute respiratory distress in adults. *Lancet* ii:319–323, 1967.
2. Petty TL. The acute respiratory distress syndrome: Historic perspective. *Chest* 105:44–47, 1994.
3. Costarino AT Jr. The systemic inflammatory response syndrome and the adult respiratory distress syndrome. *Curr Opin Anesthesiol* 6:981–992, 1993.
4. Bernard GR et al. The Consensus Committee. Report of the American-European Consensus Conference on ARDS: Definitions, mechanisms, relevant outcomes, and clinical trial coordination. *Am J Respir Crit Care Med* 149:818–824, 1994.
5. Meduri GU et al. Fibroproliferative phase of ARDS. Clinical findings and effects of corticosteroids. *Chest* 100:943–952, 1991.
6. Meduri GU. Late ARDS. *New Horiz* 1:563–577, 1993.
7. Meduri GU et al. Corticosteroid rescue treatment of progressive fibroproliferation of late ARDS—Patterns of response and predictors of outcome. *Chest* 105:1516–1527, 1994.

8. Andreadis N, Petty TL. Adult respiratory distress syndrome: Problems and progress. *Am Rev Respir Dis* 132:1344–1346, 1985.
9. Sarnaik AP, Lieh-Lai M. Adult respiratory distress in children. *Pediatr Clin North Am* 41:337–362, 1994.
10. Faix RG et al. Adult respiratory distress syndrome in fullterm newborns. *Pediatrics* 83:971–976, 1989.
11. Lyrene RK, Truog WE. Adult respiratory distress syndrome in a pediatric intensive care unit: Predisposing conditions, clinical course, and outcome. *Pediatrics* 67:790–795, 1981.
12. Davis SL, Furman DP, Costarino AT. Adult respiratory distress syndrome in children: Associated disease, clinical course, and predictors of death. *J Pediatr* 123:34–45, 1993.
13. Timmons OD, Dean JM, Vernon DD. Mortality rates and prognostic variables in children with adult respiratory distress syndrome. *J Pediatr* 119:896–899, 1991.
14. Krans PA et al. Acute lung injury at Baragwanath ICU. An 8 month audit and call for consensus for other organ failure in the adult respiratory distress syndrome. *Chest* 103:1832–1836, 1993.
15. Matthay MA. The adult respiratory distress syndrome. *Clin Chest Med* 11:575–580, 1990.
16. Suchyta MR et al. The adult respiratory distress syndrome. A report of survival and modifying factors. *Chest* 101:1074–1079, 1992.
17. Knaus WA et al. Evaluation of definitions for adult respiratory distress syndrome. *Am J Respir Crit Care Med* 150:311–317, 1994.
18. Nichols DG et al. Predictors of acute respiratory failure after bone marrow transplantation. *Crit Care Med* 22:1485–1491, 1994.
19. Murray JF et al. An expanded definition of the adult respiratory distress syndrome. *Am Rev Respir Dis* 138:720–723, 1988.
20. Morriss AH. Uncertainty in the management of ARDS: Lessons for the evaluation of a new therapy. *Intensive Care Med* 20:87–89, 1994.
21. Hyers TM. Prediction of survival and mortality in patients with ARDS. *New Horiz* 1:466–470, 1993.
22. Rinaldo JE, Christman JW. Mechanisms and mediators of the adult respiratory distress syndrome. *Clin Chest Med* ii:621–632, 1990.
23. Demling RH. Adult respiratory distress syndrome: Current concepts. *New Horiz* 1:388–401, 1993.
24. Koltai M et al. PAF: A review of its effects, antagonists and possible future clinical implications. *Drugs* 42:174–204, 1991.
25. Brigham KL, Bowers RE, Haynes J. Increased sheep lung vascular permeability caused by Escherichia coli endotoxin. *Circ Res* 45:292–297, 1979.
26. Parsons PE et al. The association of circulating endotox with the development of the adult respiratory distress syndrome. *Am Rev Respir Dis* 140:294–301, 1989.
27. Hammerschmidt DE et al. Association of complement activation and elevated plasma C-5a with ARDS. *Lancet* 1:947, 1980.
28. Duchateau J et al. Complement activation in patients at risk of developing the ARDS. *Am Rev Respir Dis* 130:1058–1064, 1984.
29. Gattinoni L et al. Relationships between lung CT density, gas exchange, and PEEP in acute respiratory failure. *Anesthesiology* 69:824–832, 1988.
30. Marini JJ. Lung mechanics in the adult respiratory distress syndrome: Recent conceptual advances and implications for management. *Clin Chest Med* 11:673–690, 1990.
31. Bone RC et al. Adult respiratory diffuse syndrome. Sequence and importance of development of multiple organ failure. *Chest* 101:320–326, 1992.
32. Marini JJ. New options for the ventilatory management of acute lung injury. *New Horiz* 1:489–503, 1993.
33. Hickling KG. Ventilatory management of ARDS: Can it affect the outcome? *Intensive Care Med* 16:219–226, 1990.
34. Hickling KG et al. Low mortality rate in adult respiratory distress syndrome using low-volume, pressure-limited ventilation with permissive hypercapnia: A prospective study. *Crit Care Med* 22:1568–1578, 1994.
35. Pepe PE, Marini JJ. Occult positive and expiratory pressure in mechanically ventilated patients with airflow obstruction: The auto-PEEP effect. *Am Rev Respir Dis* 126:166–170, 1982.

36. Kacmarek RM, Hickling KG. Permissive hypercapnia. *Respir Care* 38:373–387, 1993.
37. Tuxen DV. Permissive hypercapnic ventilation—clinical commentary. *Am J Respir Crit Care Med* 150:870–874, 1994.
38. Morton A et al. Extracorporeal membrane oxygenation for pediatric respiratory failure: Five year experience at the University of Pittsburgh. *Crit Care Med* 22:1659–1667, 1994.
39. Molar FW et al. Extracorporeal life support for severe pediatric respiratory failure: An updated experience 1991–1993. *J Pediatr* 124:875–880, 1994.
40. Arnold JH et al. High frequency oscillatory ventilation in pediatric respiratory failure. *Crit Care Med* 21:272–278, 1993.
41. Rosenberg RB et al. High frequency ventilation for acute pediatric respiratory failure. *Chest* 104:1216–1221, 1993.
42. Arnold JH et al. Prospective, randomized comparison of high frequency oscillatory ventilation and conventional mechanical ventilation in pediatric respiratory failure. *Crit Care Med* 22:1530–1539, 1994.
43. Rovira I et al. Increased plasma cGMP and pulmonary vasodilation with inhaled nitric oxide in an ovine ARDS model (abstr). *Am Rev Respir Dis* 147:A720, 1993.
44. Ignano LJ. Biological actions and properties of endothelium-derived nitric oxide formed and released from artery and vein. *Cir Res* 65:1–21, 1989.
45. Synder SH, Bredt DS. Biologic roles of nitric oxide. *Sci Am* 266:68–77, 1992.
46. Rossaint R et al. Inhaled nitric oxide for the adult respiratory distress syndrome. *N Engl J Med* 328:399–405, 1993.
47. Zapol WM, Hurford WE. Inhaled nitric oxide in the ARDS and other lung diseases. *New Horiz* 1:638–647, 1993.
48. Norman V, Keith C. Nitrogen oxides in tobacco smoke. *Nature* 205:915–916, 1965.
49. Abman SH et al. Acute effects of inhaled nitric oxide in children with severe hypoxemic respiratory failure. *J Pediatr* 124:881–888, 1994.
50. Stavert DM, Lehnert BE. Nitric oxide and nitrogen dioxide as inducers of acute pulmonary injury when inhaled at relatively high concentrations for brief periods. *Inhal Toxicol* 2:53–67, 1990.
51. Oyarzun MJ, Clements JA. Control of lung surfactant by ventilation, adrenergic mediators and prostaglandins in rabbits. *Am Rev Respir Dis* 117:879–891, 1978.
52. Wright JR, Clements JA. Metabolism and turnover of lung surfactant. *Am Rev Respir Dis* 135:425–432, 1987.
53. Lewis JF, Jobe AH. Surfactant and the ARDS. (State of the Art). *Am Rev Respir Dis* 147:218–233, 1993.
54. Holm BA et al. Pulmonary physiological and surfactant changes during injury and recovery from hypernoxia. *J Appl Physiol* 59:1402–1409, 1985.
55. Berry D, Ikegami M, Jobe A. Respiratory distress and surfactant inhibition following vagotomy in rabbits. *J Appl Physiol* 61:1741–1748, 1986.
56. O'Brodovich H, Hannam V. Exogenous surfactant rapidly increases PaO_2 in mature rabbits with lungs that contain large amounts of saline. *Am Rev Respir Dis* 147:1087–1090, 1993.
57. Lackman B, Hallman M, Bergmann KC. Respiratory failure anti-lung serum: Study or mechanisms associated with surfactant system damage. *Exp Lung Res* 12:163–168, 1987.
58. Zelter M et al. Effects of aerosolized artificial surfactant on repeated oleic acid injury in sheep. *Am Rev Respir Dis* 141:1014, 1990.
59. Pison U et al. Altered pulmonary surfactant in uncomplicated and septicemia—Complicated courses of anti respiratory failure. *J Trauma* 30:19–26, 1990.
60. Gregory TJ et al. Surfactant chemical composition and biophysical activity in acute respiratory distress syndrome. *J Clin Invest* 88:1976–1981, 1991.
61. Richman PS et al. The adult respiratory distress syndrome: First trials with surfactant replacement. *Eur Respir J* 2 (Suppl 3):109S–111S, 1989.
62. Lockmann B. Animal models and clinical pilot studies of surfactant replacement in adult respiratory distress syndrome. *Eur Respir J* 2(Suppl 3):98S–103S, 1989.

63. Chan CYJ, Barton TL, Rasch DK. Colfosceril in an infant with adult respiratory distress syndrome. *Clin Pharmacol* 11:880–882, 1992.

64. Weg JG et al. Safety and potential efficacy of an aerosolized surfactant in human sepsis-induced adult respiratory distress syndrome. *JAMA* 272:1433–1438, 1994.

65. Bernard GR et al. High dose cortico-steroids in patients with the adult respiratory distress syndrome. *N Engl J Med* 317:1565–1570, 1987.

66. Bone RC et al. Early methyl-prednisilone treatment for septic syndrome and the adult respiratory distress syndrome. *Chest* 92:1032–1036, 1987.

67. Luce JM et al. Ineffectiveness of high-dose methylprednisilone in preventing parenchymal lung injury and improving mortality in patients with septic shock. *Am Rev Respir Dis* 138:62–68, 1988.

68. Veterans Administration Systemic Sepsis Cooperative Study Group. Effect of high-dose glucocorticoid therapy on mortality in patients with clinical signs of systemic sepsis. *N Engl J Med* 317:659–665, 1987.

69. Hooper RG, Kearl RA. Established ARDS treated with a sustained course of adrenocortical steroids. *Chest* 97:138–143, 1990.

Robert Kacmarek

Joseph R. Custer

John H. Fugate

16 ▶ Mechanical Ventilation

A review of mechanical ventilation can be approached in many ways. One need only visit several different intensive care units (ICUs) in one's own institution to appreciate the varying degrees of parochialism and innovation in the provision of ventilatory support. Entire textbooks discuss ventilator design and function. An allied health profession, Respiratory Therapy, has evolved to care for patients who require mechanical ventilatory support. Devices that are microprocessor-controlled and servo-regulated, with a baffling array of modes of ventilation, are available. However, rarely has the introduction of novel or modified approaches to mechanical ventilation been preceded by prospective, let alone randomized, clinical trials. Valiant efforts to simplify a complex nomenclature and homogenize device descriptions have often led to increased complexity.[1,2] The ICU clinician must have not only a working knowledge of the scientific development of ventilators and circuit design, but also a sound basic knowledge of the physiology of gas exchange, pulmonary mechanics, and work of breathing, in order to optimally provide mechanical ventilatory support.

Goals of Ventilator Management

The overall goals of mechanical ventilation, regardless of to which age group applied, can be stated very simply. (1) Provide adequate alveolar ventilation, while avoiding respiratory acidosis or alkalosis. (2) Maximize ventilation to perfusion relationships, while ensuring optimal gas exchange. (3) Reduce work of breathing and enhance patient comfort, while avoiding detraining of the ventilatory muscles. (4) Accomplish the first three goals with minimal cardiovascular compromise and damage to the lung. These goals are central to the application of ventilatory support, regardless of the specific technology employed or the particular approach used to ventilate patients.

Indications for Mechanical Ventilation

Respiratory failure, defined as an inability to maintain adequate arterial oxygenation and carbon dioxide elimination, is the sole indication for mechanical ventilation. The actual level of abnormality consistent with failure has not been consistently defined; however, most would agree that a $PaCO_2$ of greater than 60 mm Hg with a pH less than 7.25 and a PaO_2 less than 60 mm Hg, a PaO_2/F_IO_2 less than 150, or an A-a gradient greater than 350 mm Hg defines failure.[3] From a pathophysiologic perspective, respiratory failure can be divided into two general categories: hypercapnic respiratory failure and hypoxic respiratory failure.

Hypercapnic Respiratory Failure

Alveolar ventilation is maintained by appropriate function of the ventilatory pump: the muscles, cartilage, and bones of the chest wall and abdomen along with the neuronetwork that maintains control of the pump. Failure of any part of this system results in the hallmark of hypercapnic respiratory failure, carbon dioxide retention. Three primary alterations of the normal pulmonary pump mechanism—(1) ventilatory muscle dysfunction, (2) altered central ventilatory drive, and (3) excessive ventilatory workload—singly or in combination, can lead to pump failure.[4]

Ventilatory Muscle Dysfunction

Numerous factors (Table 16-1) can alter ventilatory muscle function, leading to hypercapnic respiratory failure. In acute or chronically ill children without neuromuscular disease, asthma, or chronic pulmonary disease, metabolic disturbances are primary factors leading to respiratory failure. Deficiencies in potassium, magnesium, phosphate, or calcium can lead to muscle weakness.[5-7] Protein-caloric malnutrition leads to muscle atrophy and a reduction in ventilatory muscle strength and endurance, leading to failure.[8,9]

Children with asthma, bronchopulmonary dysplasia, or cystic fibrosis develop respiratory failure because airways obstruction results in hyperinflation and auto-PEEP, creating a mechanical disadvantage to ventilation and markedly increasing the work of breathing.[10] The altered length-tension relationship of the ventilatory muscles results in a decreased maximum inspiratory pressure and an increase in FRC.[11] Auto-PEEP also increases the gradient that must be overcome for gas movement to be established.[12] The result is increased patient effort to maintain alveolar ventilation, leading to a decrease in ventilatory reserve and an increased likelihood of failure.

Neuromuscular/neurologic disease markedly decreases the capacity of ventilatory muscles, leading to failure. Clinically, carbon dioxide retention does not occur until ventilatory muscle strength has decreased about 50%.[13] Thereafter, incremental decreases in ventilatory muscle strength result in proportional increases in $PaCO_2$. A number of drugs can directly affect the function of ventilatory muscles.[4] Adrenocorticosteroids can promote atrophy, while aminoglycoside antibiotics and calcium channel blockers can impair neuromuscular transmission.[14]

Inadequate Central Ventilatory Drive

Depression of the CNS by toxins, drugs, infection, trauma, or lesion can lead to ventilatory failure. Hypothyroidism and idiopathic central alveolar hypoventilation syndrome are causes of decreased ventilatory drive.[4] On the other hand, abnormal increases in ventilatory drive can also precipitate ventilatory failure when associated with already compromised inspiratory muscle

Table 16-1. Factors affecting ventilatory muscle function

Increased resistance/decreased compliance

Auto-PEEP

Neuromuscular/neurologic disease

Electrolyte balance, decreases in
  Potassium
  Calcium
  Magnesium
  Phosphate

Malnutrition

Drugs: adrenocorticosteroids, aminoglycoside antibiotics, calcium channel blockers

Disadvantaged length-tension relationship: Flattened diaphragm

Fatigue, disuse, detraining

function or an excessive workload. Metabolic acidosis, hepatic encephalopathy, and increased caloric consumption stimulate ventilatory drive.[15]

Excessive Workload

The altered pulmonary mechanics associated with both acute and chronic disease may result in an intolerable ventilatory load and precipitate failure.[3] Increased resistance to gas flow associated with secretions, edema, or bronchospasm may result in failure in individuals with already compromised ventilatory function. Decreased compliance elevates workload. Of particular concern is when altered pulmonary mechanics are associated with hyperinflation and auto-PEEP (Fig. 16-1). The elevated end-expiratory alveolar pressure with auto-PEEP results in a threshold load that must be overcome for ventilation to occur[11]; that is, if auto-PEEP is $+5$ cm H_2O, ventilatory muscles must create at least a 6-cm H_2O pressure gradient instead of the normal 1- or 2-cm H_2O gradient for ventilation to occur. This excessive workload, coupled with other factors affecting ventilatory muscle function, can precipitate failure (see section on Auto-PEEP).

Hypoxic Respiratory Failure

The most common form of respiratory failure is hypoxic respiratory failure, characterized by a decrease in PaO_2. Hypoxic respiratory failure may or may not be associated with hypercapnic respiratory failure; in fact, in most patients, hypoxic respiratory failure is associated with hyperventilation and respiratory alkalosis.[3] Hypoxemia is a result of one of five basic mechanisms: (1) ventilation/perfusion mismatch ($\dot{V}/\dot{Q}$ mismatch), (2) right-to-left shunt, (3) inadequate PiO_2, (4) alveolar hypoventilation, and (5) diffusion deficit.[4]

$\dot{V}/\dot{Q}$ Mismatch

The most common cause of hypoxemia is an alteration in the match between ventilation and perfusion ($\dot{V}/\dot{Q}$). Generally, $\dot{V}/\dot{Q}$ mismatch is a result of local pulmonary changes in compliance or resistance resulting in perfusion to a given lung unit being greater than ventilation. Frequently, this is referred to as a venous admixture producing a shunt-like effect. Contrary to true intrapulmonary shunts, however, hypoxemia caused by $\dot{V}/\dot{Q}$ mismatch can be corrected by increased FiO_2. Since increased FiO_2 allows the alveolar PO_2 to increase in areas poorly ventilated, hypoxemia resulting from $\dot{V}/\dot{Q}$ mismatch can be corrected by increased FiO_2[16] (Fig. 16-2).

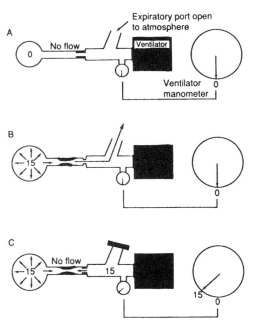

Figure 16-1. Relationship between alveolar, central airway, and ventilator circuit pressure **(A)** under normal conditions and in the presence of severe dynamic airway obstruction, **(B)** with expiratory port open, and **(C)** with expiratory port occluded. Auto-PEEP level is identified by creating an end-expiratory hold, allowing alveolar, central airway, and ventilator circuit pressure to equilibrate. Note that during equilibration, auto-PEEP level can be read on the system manometer. (With permission. Pepe PE, Marini JJ. Occult positive end-expiratory pressure in mechanically ventilated patients with airflow obstruction: The auto-PEEP effect. *Am Rev Respir Dis* 1982; 126:166–170.)

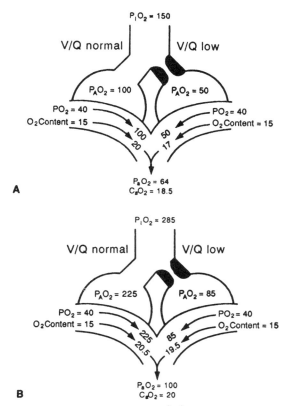

Figure 16-2. Hypoxemia due to $\dot{V}/\dot{Q}$ mismatch, showing the effect of supplemental O_2. $\dot{V}/\dot{Q}$ is normal on the left side of each idealized lung unit and low on the right. Only O_2 exchange is shown, and $P(A-a)O_2$ is assumed to be 0. **(A)** With room air, not enough O_2 reaches the poorly ventilated alveolus to fully saturate its capillary blood; **(B)** with 40% O_2, P_AO_2 in this alveolus is raised enough to make its capillary PO_2 nearly normal. Note that the P_AO_2 in the mixed effluent from the two capillaries is determined by the average of the O_2 contents of the two streams, not their PaO_2 values. (With permission. Pierson DJ, Kacmarek RM [eds]. *Foundations of Respiratory Care.* Churchill Livingston, New York, 1992.)

Right-to-Left Shunt

Hypoxemia occurs in this setting because venous blood directly mixes with arterialized blood, bypassing the lungs. Increasing FiO_2 has a minimal effect on hypoxemia caused by true shunts[16] (Fig. 16-3), because the majority of oxygen is carried attached to hemoglobin, and hemoglobin is 97% saturated in well-ventilated capillaries when the patient is breathing room air. Increasing FiO_2 only increases the oxygen dissolved in plasma in the non-shunt region: (0.003 ml O_2/ml plasma/mm Hg PaO_2 versus 1.34 ml O_2/g Hb at 100% saturation). Correction of the hypoxemia must be directed to the cause of the shunt. Application of PEEP and elevation of mean airway pressure ($\bar{P}aw$) assist in lung volume recruitment increasing the PaO_2.[16]

Inadequate PiO_2

An infrequent cause of hypoxic respiratory failure at sea level, but a primary cause of hypoxemia at higher altitudes, is an inadequate PiO_2. This cause of hypoxemia is easily corrected by administering oxygen.

Hypoventilation

Because alveolar PO_2 and alveolar PCO_2 are indirectly related, as indicated in the alveolar gas equation:

$$PaO_2 = (BP - PH_2O)(FiO_2) - PaCO_2\left(FiO_2 + \frac{1 - FiO_2}{R}\right)$$

where BP is barometric pressure, P_{H_2O} is the partial pressure of water vapor, and R is the respiratory exchange ratio (normal 0.8), hypoventilation results in hypoxemia. Correction of the hypoventilation also corrects the hypoxemia (Fig. 16-4).

Diffusion Deficit

Hypoxemia that is a result of incomplete equilibration of PO_2 across the alveolar capillary membrane is classified as a diffusion deficit. Incomplete equilibration can be caused by a thickening of the alveolocapillary membrane, a reduction in alveolar capillary

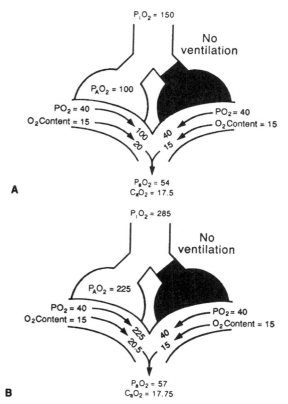

Figure 16-3. Alveolar-capillary diagram of intrapulmonary right-to-left shunt, showing why supplemental O_2 fails to correct the hypoxemia. Only O_2 exchange is shown, and P(A-a)O_2 is assumed to be 0. **(A)** With room air, although blood leaving the normal alveolar-capillary unit is normally saturated, blood passing the capillary on the right "sees" no O_2, because its alveolus is unventilated, and it leaves the unit desaturated. When the two effluent streams mix, the resulting PaO_2 is determined by the average of their O_2 contents, not by their PO_2 values. **(B)** Addition of 40% O_2 fails to correct the hypoxemia; because O_2 content is not significantly raised in the normal unit and capillary blood in the unventilated unit still "sees" no O_2, even 100% O_2 would not completely reverse the oxygenation defect in this example. [With permission. Pierson DJ, Kacmarek RM (eds). *Foundations of Respiratory Care.* Churchill Livingston, New York, 1992.]

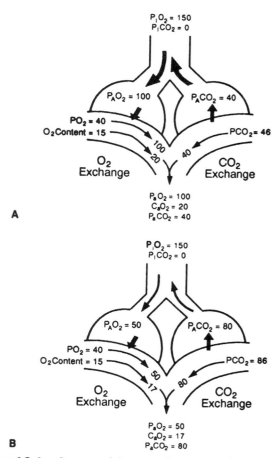

Figure 16-4. Conceptual diagram of hypoxemia due to alveolar hypoventilation. Both idealized lung units depict oxygenation on the left and ventilation on the right; P(A-a)O_2 is 0 in this example. **(A)** Normal alveolar gas exchange. **(B)** Alveolar hypoventilation, with V_A half of normal. (With permission. Pierson DJ, Kacmarek RM [eds]. *Foundations of Respiratory Care.* Churchill Livingston, New York, 1992.)

blood volume because of lung damage or destruction, an increased cardiac output or decreased mixed venous oxygen content, or a combination of these.[4] Increasing FiO_2, application of PEEP, and an increased $\bar{P}aw$ improve PaO_2; however, therapy is generally directed to the cause of the deficit.

Clinical Indications

From the perspective of clinical presentation, the indications for ventilatory support can be simply stated as (1) apnea, (2) acute ventilatory failure, (3) impending acute ventilatory failure, and (4) an oxygenation deficit.[17]

Acute Ventilatory Failure

Although some discussion over the exact level of $PaCO_2$ and pH change necessary to define acute ventilatory failure is common, most would agree that patients with a $PaCO_2$ greater than 60 mm Hg and a pH less than 7.25 require ventilatory support.

Impending Acute Ventilatory Failure

This is determined based on the clinical judgment of the clinician. Many patients are electively ventilated because they have not responded to more conservative therapy, and their clinical course indicates that they will continue to progress to failure. A good example is the patient with severe bilateral pneumonitis that demonstrates a pattern of worsening hypercarbia, acidosis, and hypoxemia along with a more rapid and shallow ventilatory pattern and increasing cardiovascular distress. The decision to ventilate may precede a clear definition of acute ventilatory failure. The decision to ventilate is based on clinical presentation; ventilatory failure is presumed imminent, considering the patient's clinical course.

Oxygenation

As stated earlier, hypoxic respiratory failure is the most common form of respiratory failure and normally can be treated effectively with oxygen or CPAP. There are patients, however, in whom work of breathing is so markedly elevated in spite of attempts to normalize PaO_2 that mechanical ventilation becomes necessary. The unloading of the work of breathing by mechanical ventilation can markedly decrease oxygen consumption and the work of the myocardium, resulting in improved oxygenation at the same FiO_2. In addition, tracheal intubation and ventilatory support make it much easier to titrate PEEP and $\bar{P}aw$ in the management of hypoxemia.

Modes of Mechanical Ventilation

Understanding the various, defined modes of mechanical ventilation currently available on new-generation mechanical ventilators is an overwhelming task. All of these conventional modes, however, can be classified as either volume- or pressure-targeted modes (Table 16-2).[18] This classification established the primary parameter that terminates the inspiratory phase and thus defines specific features of the approach to ventilatory support.

Volume-Targeted Modes

Modes of ventilation that are volume-targeted terminate the inspiratory phase when a preset tidal volume is delivered. This approach to cycling also defines the variable that must be set when adjusting the mechanical ventilator. The specific set of variables adjusted

Table 16-2. Pressure versus volume-targeted ventilation

	Volume Target	Pressure Target
Peak airway pressure	Variable	Constant
Peak alveolar pressure	Variable	Constant
Tidal volume	Constant	Variable
Minimum rate	Preset	Preset
Inspiratory time	Preset	Preset
Peak flow	Constant	Variable
Flow pattern	Preset	Decelerating

is dependent on manufacturer design; either V_T, peak flow, and flow waveform are selected, or V_T, flow waveform, and inspiratory time are adjusted. With some ventilators, minute volume, I:E ratio, and flow waveform need to be selected. Regardless of specific ventilator design, the clinician must select parameters that define volume delivered, time it takes to deliver the volume, and the flow waveform used during volume delivery. What is not programmed by the clinician is a pressure target. Those individuals that prefer volume-targeted ventilation have selected this approach based on their bias that controlling volume delivery, and thus, level of ventilation ($PaCO_2$), is more important than controlling peak airway and peak alveolar pressure.

Figure 16-5 illustrates the pressure, flow, and volume waveform established with typical volume-targeted, assist/control mode ventilation with a square waveflow pattern. Note the linearly increasing pressure and volume curves throughout the inspiratory phase. Because the flow pattern is square wave, the peak airway pressure reflects the amount of pressure necessary to overcome both compliance and resistance. To identify peak alveolar pressure, an end-inspiratory hold period (Fig. 16-6) must be programmed after the actual tidal volume delivery. Peak alveolar pressure is equal to airway pressure if system gas flow rate is 0 (end-inspiratory hold or plateau period).[19,20] Figure 16-7 also illustrates volume-targeted ventilation, but with a decelerating flow pattern and an end-inspiratory hold period. Note the difference between the pressure, volume, and flow waveforms in Figs. 16-5 and 16-7 during active gas delivery (before the end-inspiratory hold period). With decelerating flow, the majority of the tidal volume is delivered early in the inspiratory phase, thus the airway pressure pattern is more of a square wave. For the same tidal volume, inspiratory time, ventilatory rate, and I:E ratio, a decelerating flow pattern demonstrates a lower peak airway pressure and higher $\bar{P}aw$ than a square waveflow pattern, in spite of the fact that peak flow must be higher with a decelerating flow waveform.[21] However, the peak alveolar pressure will be the same, because the same volume is maintained in the airway at 0 flow. In Fig. 16-7, peak alveolar pressure is equal to the end-inspiratory plateau pressure established just before exhalation. There is evidence that gas exchange is improved with a decelerating flow pattern, as compared with other flow patterns (square, sine, decelerations).[22,23] Provided appropriate inspiratory time is maintained, none of the other inspiratory flow patterns show an advantage over the decelerating pattern.[24,25]

Pressure-Targeted Modes

Figure 16-8 depicts typical pressure-targeted, control mode ventilation. Note the similarities between Fig. 16-7 and 16-8B. With

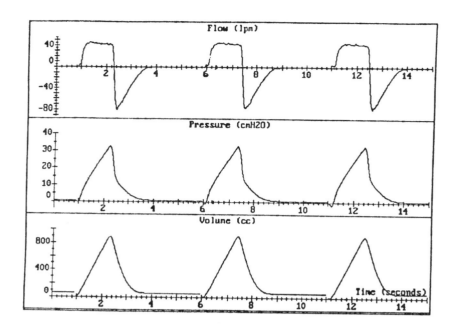

Figure 16-5. Pressure, flow, and volume versus time waveforms during volume-targeted assist/control ventilation. [With permission. Kacmarek RM, Hess D, Stoller JD. *Monitoring in Respiratory Care.* Mosby-Yearbook Medical Publishers, Chicago, 1993.]

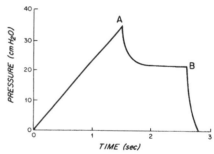

Figure 16-6. Idealized pressure-time waveform during volume-targeted, square flow waveform, controlled ventilation. Point *A* represents PIP; point *B* is P_{plat}. (With permission. Kacmarek RM, Hess D, Stoller JD. *Monitoring in Respiratory Care.* Mosby-YearBook Medical Publishers, Chicago, 1993.)

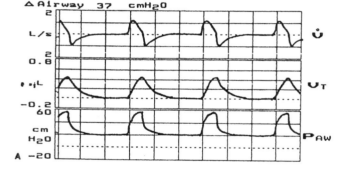

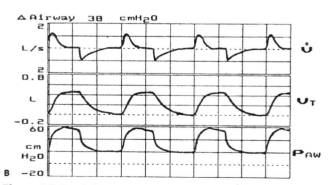

Figure 16-8. **(A)** Airway pressure (P_{AW}), flow ($\dot{V}$), and (V_T) waveforms during pressure-control ventilation. Note that inspiratory time is inadequate; flow rate has not returned to 0, nor is an inflation hold (zero flow period) observed. **(B)** Results of increasing inspiratory time. Now flow returns to 0 about midway through the inspiratory period. The remaining inspiratory time illustrates an end-inspiratory hold. (With permission. Kacmarek RM, Hess D, Stoller JD. *Monitoring in Respiratory Care.* Mosby-YearBook Medical Publishers, Chicago, 1993.)

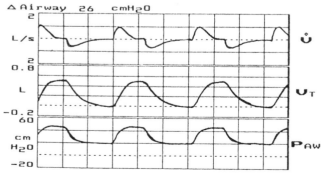

Figure 16-7. Airway (P_{AW}), flow ($\dot{V}$), and volume (V_T) waveforms during volume-targeted controlled ventilation, incorporating a decelerating flow waveform and inflation hold. (With permission. Kacmarek RM, Hess D, Stoller JD. *Monitoring in Respiratory Care.* Mosby-YearBook Medical Publishers, Chicago, 1993.)

pressure-targeted ventilation, the clinician sets the target pressure and inspiratory time, or I:E ratio. Because pressure is the target, tidal volume may vary from one breath to the next, because **it** is not targeted. Peak alveolar pressure, however, does not exceed the targeted pressure. Pressure-targeted ventilation, although appearing similar to volume-targeted decelerating flow, does differ in some fundamental aspects. With pressure control, the ventilator is designed to deliver enough gas flow at the onset of inspiration to rapidly pressurize the system to the target level, after which, the flow decreases, frequently exponentially, to maintain the target pressure. If inspiratory time is long enough and the impedance (resistance and compliance) of the system high enough, flow rate will reach 0 before the end of the inspiratory phase (Fig. 16-8B), thus the end-inspiratory pressure target level will be equal to the peak alveolar pressure. Those clinicians with a bias toward pressure-targeted ventilation are more concerned with maintaining a precise control over peak alveolar pressure and are willing to allow tidal volume and, as a result $PaCO_2$, to vary, dependent on changes in system impedance.

Tidal volume delivered in pressure-targeted ventilation is dependent on many variables. Any variable that affects the inspiratory pressure gradient or impedance of the system can alter V_T (Table 16-3). As illustrated in Fig. 16-8A, whenever inspiratory flow is greater than 0 at the end of inspiration, lengthening of the inspiratory time has the potential of increasing tidal volume (see Fig. 16-8B). The only setting where tidal volume would not increase is if lengthening inspiratory time caused auto-PEEP to develop. If there is a 0 flow period at the end of inspiration (see Fig.

Table 16-3. Factors affecting tidal volume during pressure-targeted ventilation

Pressure target level

Inspiratory time

Rate

Applied PEEP

Auto-PEEP

I:E ratio

Patient/ventilator system compliance

Patient/ventilator system resistance

16-8), lengthening of the inspiratory time will not increase V_T, but may result in a decrease in V_T if air trapping develops. Development of auto-PEEP during pressure-targeted ventilation always decreases V_T because the ventilator applies the pressure-targeted level above circuit baseline pressure (atm or PEEP). Because auto-PEEP is not recognized by the ventilator, its presence results in system pressure increasing immediately to the auto-PEEP level, essentially decreasing the applied inspiratory pressure gradient by a level equal to the auto-PEEP level. The result is always a decrease in V_T.

Applied PEEP in pressure-targeted ventilation may increase or decrease V_T, depending on whether it recruits lung units, improves compliance, or overdistends lung units, decreasing compliance.

Table 16-4. Pressure-targeted modes

Mode	Description	Advantages	Disadvantages
Pressure control	Complete control of ventilation; peak airway pressure constant, V_T variable; FVS only	Control over method of delivery except V_T, which may vary from breath to breath	Generally requires sedation, sedation/paralysis, or hyperventilation; spontaneously breathing patient may fight gas delivery
Pressure A/C	Pressure control; however, patient may increase rate of ventilation; pressure constant, V_T variable; FVS only	Patient may determine rate over set level; peak pressure constant; pressure control available with sedation, sedation/paralysis, or hyperventilation	May cause respiratory alkalosis, air trapping, auto-PEEP, cardiovascular compromise with high rates; V_T variable
Pressure support	Peak pressure set, otherwise all aspects of ventilation controlled by patient; PVS to FVS	Patient has control over process of ventilation; machine responds to patient demands; gas is delivered in response to patient desires; peak airway pressure set	V_T variable; no backup rate, continuous nebulizer therapy may cause hypoventilation; air trapping, auto-PEEP possible if rate high
Airway pressure release ventilation	Delivery of two levels of CPAP using continuous flow system; normally I/E ratio inversed; spontaneous breathing at each CPAP level possible; designed for use via artificial airway; PVS to FVS	Simple set up; airway pressure controlled; spontaneous breathing	V_T variable; increased WOB at inspiratory CPAP level, no alarms, no patient monitors
Bi-level CPAP	Delivery of two levels of CPAP (IPAP and EPAP) commercially available, designed for use via nasal mask; normal I/E ratio, patient can control rate, length of inspiration; PVS to FVS	Commercially available; airway pressure controlled; patient controls all aspects of ventilation except pressure level; designed for noninvasive use	V_T variable; no alarms, no patient monitors
MMV pressure limited	Ventilator maintains minimum minute volume by varying PSV level in response to patient's ability to maintain MMV level; PVS to FVS	Allows some patients to wean themselves; peak airway pressure maintained within specified range	Rapid shallow breathing can defeat goal of MMV; requires clinician to decrease MMV level if weaning is to continue; V_T variable

WOB, work of breathing; IPAP, inspiratory positive airway pressure; EPAP, expiratory positive airway pressure.
With permission. From Pierson DJ, Kacmarek RM (eds). *Foundations of Respiratory Care.* New York: Churchill Livingston, 1992. P 956.

Any factor that increases impedance (decreased compliance/increased resistance) to ventilation decreases V_T, and any factor that decreases impedance increases V_T.

Pressure- versus Volume-Targeted Ventilation

Considerable data have accumulated comparing pressure and volume-targeted ventilation.[26–33] The early data indicated pressure-targeted ventilation was superior to volume-targeted in reference to gas exchange and pulmonary mechanics; however, all of these studies[26–28] were uncontrolled case series, many of which were retrospective. More recently, numerous well-controlled prospective animal[29] and human[30–33] studies have demonstrated no difference in gas exchange or pulmonary mechanics when pressure and volume control were compared with total PEEP[28,30,32] (applied plus auto) or Paw[29] kept constant.

The decision to use either pressure or volume targeting is dependent on which of the following is of primary concern: (1) maintenance of V_T and $PaCO_2$ in spite of airway and alveolar pressure or (2) maintaining a pressure limit on peak alveolar and airway pressure, but allowing V_T and $PaCO_2$ to change based on system impedance. If volume control is selected, careful monitoring of peak airway pressure should be maintained, whereas with pressure targeting, careful monitoring of V_T/min volume must be maintained.

It is more difficult to identify acute changes in impedance with pressure targeting than with volume targeting. A decrease in impedance normally results in high-pressure alarms being activated, and if the change in impedance is progressive, as with a tension pneumothorax, the peak pressure alarm continues to activate as pressure continues to increase. With pressure targeting, an equilibrium between the peak airway pressure and the pressure inside the pneumothorax eventually occurs, limiting the change in impedance. Frequently, pneumothorax with pressure control is not identified until routine chest x-ray or by concern over acutely altered blood gases.

Volume and pressure targeting is available on most newly introduced mechanical ventilators. Either is available in assist (A), assist/control (A/C), control (C), intermittent mandatory ventilation (IMV), synchronized intermittent mandatory ventilation (SIMV), and mandatory minute ventilation (MMV).

Specific Modes

Tables 16-4 and 16-5 list the basic description, advantages, and disadvantages of the primary pressure- and volume-targeted modes of ventilation.[18] Historically, modes of mechanical ventilation have been classified as C, A/C, A, IMV, or SIMV. With control ventilation, regardless of whether it is pressure- or volume-targeted, the patient is unable to interact with the ventilator. The clinician determines all aspects of gas delivery. With A/C, however, the patient is able to control the initiation of the mechanical breath, provided it is at a rate greater than that programmed, but that is all. Every other aspect of gas delivery is determined by the clinician.

Table 16-5. Volume-targeted modes

Mode	Description	Advantages	Disadvantages
Volume control	Complete control of ventilation; patients unable to interphase with machine; V_T constant, peak pressure variable; FVS only	Control over minute volume and method of delivery	Patient unable to interact with machine; requires sedation, sedation/paralysis, or hyperventilation; spontaneously breathing patient fights ventilator; peak airway pressure variable
Volume A/C	Volume control, however, spontaneous breathing can increase rate; V_T constant, peak pressure variable; FVS only	Patients may determine rate over set level; control over minimum minute volume and delivery methodology can provide volume control with sedation, sedation/paralysis, or hyperventilation	May cause respiratory alkalosis, air trapping, auto-PEEP, cardiovascular compromise with high rates; peak airway pressure variable
IMV	Volume control with continuous flow in between control breaths allowing spontaneous breathing; PVS to FVS	Able to provide any level of ventilatory support; at low levels patient able to breath spontaneously; air trapping, auto-PEEP, and patient-induced respiratory alkalosis less likely than in volume A/C; can provide volume control with sedation, sedation/ paralysis, or hyperventilation; less cardiovascular compromise than volume control or A/C	Stacking of mechanical breaths on spontaneous breaths; increased work of breathing at low IMV mandatory rate; may cause respiratory alkalosis, air trapping, auto-PEEP at rapid spontaneous respiratory rates; peak airway pressure variable
SIMV	Volume A/C with demand spontaneous breathing in between A/C breaths; PVS to FVS	No stacking of mechanical breaths on spontaneous breaths; same as IMV	Same as IMV
MMV	Ventilator maintains minimum minute volume; may provide volume control, total spontaneous breathing, or anything in between dependent on patient's spontaneous minute ventilation; PVS to FVS	Allows some patients to wean themselves	Rapid shallow breathing when setting of MMV is low may prevent mandatory volume A/C breaths; increased WOB at low mandatory rate; requires clinician to decrease MMV if weaning is to continue; peak airway pressure variable

WOB, work of breathing.
With permission. From Pierson DJ, Kacmarek RM (eds). *Foundations of Respiratory Care*. New York: Churchill Livingston, 1992. P 957.

With volume-targeted ventilation, the assist mode is never used, whereas with pressure-targeted ventilation, the assist mode (pressure support) is commonly used.

Pressure Support Ventilation

Pressure support ventilation (PSV) is pressure-targeted assisted ventilation, but it does differ considerably from other pressure-targeted modes. The only variable set by the clinician is the pressure target; all other variables are patient-controlled. On a moment to moment basis, ventilatory rate, inspiratory time, I:E ratio, peak inspiratory flow, and V_T are patient-controlled and may change. In some ventilators, the clinician may also set the rise time or attack time, which is the amount of time it takes for the pressure target to be met. With some ventilators, target pressure can be achieved within 100 to 150 ms, whereas with others, the target pressure may not be achieved until the end of the inspiratory phase (Fig. 16-9).[34,35] Exhalation is initiated when peak flow has been reduced to some predetermined level, either a set flow (5 liters/min) or a percentage of peak flow (e.g., 25%). The ability to change the expiratory flow trigger is also possible in some ventilators. Confusion exists over the most appropriate rise time and expiratory trigger flow; ideally, both should be set to enhance patient comfort. The expiratory trigger should be adjusted so that a bump in pressure at end-exhalation is eliminated (Fig. 16-9).

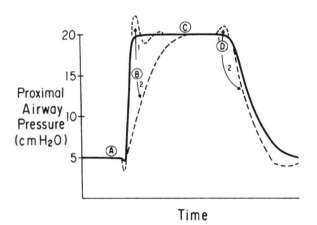

Figure 16-9. Design characteristics of a pressure-supported breath. In this example, baseline pressure (i.e., PEEP) is set at 5 cm H_2O and pressure support is set at 15 cm H_2O (PIP 20 cm H_2O). The inspiratory pressure is triggered at point A by a patient effort, resulting in an airway pressure decrease. Demand valve sensitivity and responsiveness are characterized by the depth and duration of this negative pressure. The rise to pressure (*line B*) is provided by a fixed, high initial flow delivery into the airway. Note that if flows exceed patient demand, initial pressure exceeds set level (B1), whereas if flows are less than patient demand, a very slow (concave) rise to pressure can occur (B2). The plateau of pressure support (*line C*) is maintained by servo control of flow. A smooth plateau reflects appropriate responsiveness to patient demand; fluctuations would reflect less responsiveness of the servo mechanisms. Termination of pressure support occurs at point D and should coincide with the end of the spontaneous inspiratory effort. If termination is delayed, the patient actively exhales (bump in pressure above plateau) (D1); if termination is premature, the patient will have continued inspiratory efforts (D2). (With permission. McIntyre N et al. The Nagoya conference on system design and patient-ventilator interactions during pressure support ventilation. *Chest* 1990; 97:1463–1466.)

This rise in pressure at end-exhalation is the result of recruitment of accessory muscles of exhalation to begin the expiratory phase. Rise time should be set to satisfy patient peak inspiratory demand. An initial "bump" in pressure above set pressure support level usually indicates that the rise time is too short, whereas a concave rise in initial airway pressure usually indicates the rise time is too long. The level of inspiratory work or effort performed by patients can be titrated with pressure support by altering the pressure support level.[36,37] With the newest mechanical ventilators, pressure support can be effectively applied even to very small pediatric patients ($\geq$ 7 kg).[38] Generally, pressure support level is set to produce a ventilatory pattern consistent with the expected pattern postextubation. Pressure support levels of between 5 and 15 cm H_2O are appropriate for most patients.

Intermittent Mandatory Ventilation

This approach to ventilatory support is a combination of control ventilation with spontaneous breathing (Fig. 16-10) and was introduced initially as a means of ventilatory support in infants[39,40] and to facilitate weaning in adults.[41] It can be applied with both volume- and pressure-targeted approaches[18] and has become the standard for the management of small infants. With IMV, a continuous flow of gas is maintained to allow spontaneous inspiration, and periodically a mandatory breath is delivered. SIMV is a variation of IMV. In SIMV, the mandatory breaths are assist/control, and the spontaneous breaths activate demand flow (Figs. 16-10 and 16-11). As a result, pressure support can be used in conjunction with either pressure- or volume-targeted SIMV. Of major concern with IMV or SIMV is asynchrony as a result of differing gas delivery patterns (i.e., mandatory breaths interspersed between spontaneous breaths).[42] Some patients tolerate IMV/SIMV poorly, especially at lower SIMV rates[43] (4–10/min, dependent on total respiratory rate;

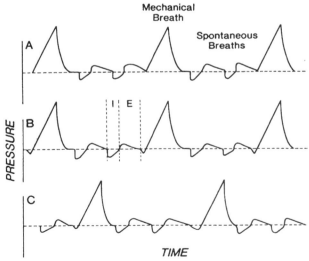

Figure 16-10. Pressure versus time waveforms during **(A)** IMV, **(B)** SIMV, and **(C)** volume-controlled MMV positive pressure ventilation. Note each spontaneous breath occurs between volume-targeted breaths. With IMV, mandatory volume breaths are controlled, while with SIMV, they are patient-triggered. MMV pressure waveforms are exactly the same as SIMV. Defections below baseline are created by patient inspiratory efforts. I, spontaneous inspiration; E, spontaneous expiration. (With permission. Pierson DJ, Kacmarek RM [eds]. *Foundations of Respiratory Care.* Churchill Livingston, New York, 1992.)

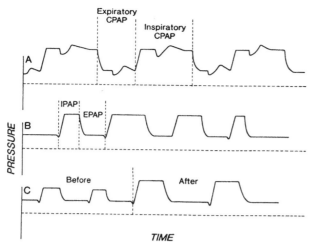

Figure 16-11. Pressure versus time waveforms during **(A)** airway pressure release ventilation (APRV), **(B)** bi-level CPAP, and **(C)** pressure-limited MMV. By design, APRV is usually adjusted with the inspiratory time longer than expiratory time, and it is expected that patients will superimpose a spontaneous breath at both the inspiratory and expiratory CPAP levels. With bi-level CPAP, normal application is via the timed/spontaneous mode (A/C), in which the patient is allowed to control all aspects of gas delivery except the IPAP (inspiratory positive airway pressure) and EPAP (expiratory positive airway pressure) levels. In pressure-limited MMV, the PSV level is periodically adjusted to ensure MMV. PSV levels are depicted before and after adjustment. (With permission. Pierson DJ, Kacmarek RM [eds]. *Foundations of Respiratory Care.* Churchill Livingston, New York, 1992.)

see section on Weaning). In addition, the work of breathing at low IMV/SIMV rates may be overwhelming and necessitate the addition of pressure support or a change of ventilation mode (see section on Work of Breathing).

Mandatory Minute Ventilation

This mode is a variation of SIMV wherein in addition to the normal settings in either pressure or volume targeting, a minimal minute ventilation is also set. Generally, with volume-targeted MMV, the mandatory rate is adjusted to ensure a minimum minute volume, whereas in pressure-targeted MMV, the pressure support or pressure control level is adjusted to ensure a minimal minute volume. This modification of SIMV was introduced to allow patients to "wean themselves"[44]; however, it has not performed as expected. Patients can satisfy the minute volume requirement by an unacceptable rapid and shallow breathing pattern.[45] The newer modes available on the Siemens 300 ventilator, volume support and pressure-regulated volume control, are a form of MMV. The concept of MMV is a reasonable extension of ventilator development; however, considerable refinement in the algorithms used is necessary before improved efficacy can be expected.

Airway Pressure Release Ventilation and Bi-level CPAP

These are very similar modes of pressure-targeted ventilation (see Fig. 16-11), and both can be considered a variation of pressure-targeted A/C ventilation. One of the major differences between airway pressure release ventilation (APRV)/bi-level CPAP and typical pressure-targeted ventilation is that a continuous flow of gas is maintained across the airway with APRV and bi-level CPAP.

Currently, bi-level CPAP is only available on portable home

mechanical ventilation units. It is essentially pressure support with CPAP. The patient may control all aspects of gas delivery except pressure levels, or an A/C minimum rate can be set. With some units, control ventilation can be provided. APRV is similar to IMV; patients are allowed to inspire spontaneously between mandatory increases in system pressure, but also can inspire at the upper level of pressure (see Fig. 16-11). APRV has been described as bi-level CPAP with spontaneous breaths allowed at each CPAP level. Bilevel CPAP is designed to be used at patient-selected I:E ratios,[46] whereas APRV is intended to be used at inverse ratios.[47–50] APRV is currently available on the Drager Irisa Ventilator. Most clinicians using this mode have developed homemade systems.[47]

The indications for APRV and bi-level CPAP diverge along different clinical routes. Proponents of APRV believe it is best used in intubated patients with mild-to-moderate acute ventilatory failure.[47–50] By contrast, bi-level CPAP has been designed for noninvasive ventilatory support through a nasal mask.[46,51] Its primary use is in patients with chronic ventilatory failure, who require nocturnal ventilatory muscle rest. However, bi-level CPAP also has been used to reverse acute ventilatory failure in patients with chronic ventilatory insufficiency[52] and as a transition from invasive mechanical ventilation,[53] again in those patients with chronic ventilatory failure.

Full Versus Partial Ventilatory Support

Controversy has long existed regarding the optimal mode of ventilation to employ during various phases of acute ventilatory failure. Regardless of the mode selected, however, ventilatory support can be categorized into two general approaches: (1) full ventilatory support (FVS) and (2) partial ventilatory support (PVS).[17] During FVS, the mechanical ventilator provides all, or nearly all, the effort required to maintain gas exchange. As will be noted later, many of the commonly available modes of ventilation can provide FVS, provided they are appropriately set and the patient is properly sedated.[16] FVS may also be provided in patients who trigger the ventilator, as long as the adjustment of gas delivery is consistent with patient demands.

Most patients requiring ventilatory support for acute respiratory failure present with hypercarbia, hypoxemia, acidosis, and either ventilatory muscle dysfunction or fatigue, and are commonly exhausted. For these reasons, FVS techniques are recommended during the first 24 to 72 hours of ventilatory support.

During partial ventilatory support, the patient provides a significant percentage of the effort required to maintain gas exchange. Partial ventilatory support can be provided by IMV, SIMV, PSV, APRV, bi-level CPAP, or MMV. Each of these approaches allows the clinician to titrate the level of support provided by the ventilator. With IMV, SIMV, or MMV, the frequency of the predetermined volume-limited breath can vary, allowing the patient to breathe spontaneously between the mandatory breaths. By contrast, PSV, APRV, and bi-level CPAP allow the clinician to select the level of ventilatory effort required of the patient for each breath by varying the pressure limit selected. Each of these modes (IMV, SIMV, PSV, MMV, APRV, and bi-level CPAP) allows various levels of patient-ventilator interaction, from almost completely spontaneous ventilation to FVS. PSV has the advantage of contouring the delivered flow of gas to meet the patient's demand to a greater extent than any of the other modes.[34,37]

Partial ventilatory support is a more physiologic approach to mechanical ventilation and a generally recommended approach to managing patients once they are past the acute phase of respiratory failure.[16–18] Allowing patients to play a more significant role in the process of ventilation normally improves $\dot{V}/\dot{Q}$ matching, decreases hemodynamic compromise, and may prevent further deterioration of diaphragmatic function. The key to appropriate application of PVS techniques is to titrate the level of patient-machine interaction so that active patient involvement is present but sufficient support is provided to prevent deterioration of ventilatory muscle function and overall cardiopulmonary status.[34,37,54] Because of the delicate balance required, FVS is generally easier to employ appropriately than PVS, with clinical judgment being the key to the optimal titration of PVS (see section on Weaning).

Pulmonary Mechanics

During normal daily activities, ventilation is maintained without conscious effort. At resting exhalation, a negative intrathoracic pressure of about 6 cm H_2O is established by the opposing recoil pressures of the lung and thorax. The 6-cm H_2O pressure gradient across the lungs (transpulmonary pressure) maintains the normal functional residual capacity. Midbrain respiratory centers, which receive input from stretch receptors, chemoreceptors, and in response to intracellular pH, initiate a breath. Timing of inspiration and the ventilatory pattern is defined by the midbrain and cortex. Arterial PCO_2 via pH change provides the primary stimulus for ventilation; hypoxemia is a distant secondary stimulus. Contraction of the diaphragm and external intercostal muscles decreases intrapleural pressure, creating a pressure gradient for air to move into the lungs. Gas movement and perfusion are generally matched. Blood flow and ventilation go to gravity (Fig. 16-12). Although overall $\dot{V}/\dot{Q}$ ratios are greater than 1.0 in the least gravity-dependent aspects of the lung and less then 1.0 in the most gravity-dependent areas[55]; the actual rate and distribution of alveolar filling is dependent on compliance, resistance, and tissue inertia. Venous return is facilitated during inspiration because of the lower intrathoracic pressure. Exhalation is passive, returning the lung to its end-expiratory resting position (FRC).

During controlled mechanical ventilation, the aforementioned processes become greatly altered (see Fig. 16-12).[56] As a result of PEEP, the resting intrathoracic pressure is closer to 0 or possibly positive. FRC is now determined by the interaction of the elastic recoil of the lungs and thorax as well as the applied PEEP and any auto-PEEP developed. During mechanical inspiration, the pressure in the lung and intrathoracic pressure become more positive instead of more negative. Ventilation is distributed primarily to the least gravity-dependent areas.[55] Perfusion is now dependent on the gradient between alveolar pressure, pulmonary artery pressure, and pulmonary venous pressure.[56] As a result, marked mismatching of ventilation and perfusion occur, increasing both dead space ventilation and shunting.[55] Because intrathoracic pressure is more positive during inspiration than exhalation, venous return is greatest during the expiratory phase. The elevated mean intrathoracic pressure, however, decreases venous return, decreasing cardiac output and systemic arterial pressure, and may increase or decrease pulmonary vascular pressure, depending on the system's ability to maintain flow. Because venous return is decreased, intracranial pressure is also increased (see section on Complications of Mechanical Ventilation).

With assisted ventilation, the patient participates to a varying degree in the process of ventilation; as a result, the process itself and the effects of $\dot{V}/\dot{Q}$ can span the spectrum from spontaneous unassisted ventilation to controlled ventilation. Regardless of whether assisted ventilation or controlled ventilation is applied, the compliance, resistance, and time constant of the total system, as well as individual lung units, can have a marked effect on the effort required to ventilate and on the distribution of both ventilation and perfusion.

Compliance

Compliance is a measure of the elastic recoil of the lung, thorax, or the lung-thorax system, and is affected not only by pathophysiology, but by the size of the lung. In large adolescents, compliance of the lung-thoracic system may reach that of an adult (70–100 ml/cm H_2O), whereas small pediatric patients may have a normal compliance of 3 or 4 ml/cm H_2O. Any factor that decreases the distensibility of the lung-thoracic system reduces compliance. During mechanical ventilation, estimates of total patient-ventilator system compliance can be made if the patient is passively ventilated, with volume-targeted square waveform ventilation. The term used to define compliance under these settings is *effective static compliance* (C_{ES}), because it is determined under less than ideal conditions and reflects the compliance of the total patient-ventilator system. C_{ES} is determined by dividing the measured exhaled, or corrected expired-mechanical V_T (V_{ET}), by the P_{plat} (the end-expiratory equilibration pressure) minus the total PEEP level (see Fig. 16-6).[57] A measured exhaled mechanical V_T is used because it is a more accurate estimation of the volume received on the previous breath than the machine volume setting. In addition, the exhaled volume, if measured other than at the patient endotracheal tube, must be corrected for compressible volume loss (i.e., the volume compressed in the ventilator circuit per delivered pressure [centimeters of water] [P_{plat} − total PEEP]). Compressible volume factors (CF) equal about 1 to 5 ml/cm H_2O for most ventilator circuits. Total PEEP is subtracted from the P_{plat} to reflect the true static pressure maintaining V_{ET} in the airway. Total PEEP is equal to the applied PEEP ($PEEP_A$) plus any auto-PEEP ($PEEP_I$) measured above the applied PEEP.

$$C_{ES} = \frac{V_{ET} - [(P_{plat} - PEEP_A - PEEP_I)\,(CF)]}{P_{plat} - PEEP_A - PEEP_I}$$

Many clinicians exclude the use of the CF because of consistent ventilator set-up, accepting a predictable and consistent error in the calculation.

$$C_{ES} = \frac{V_{ET}}{P_{plat} - PEEP_A - PEEP_I}$$

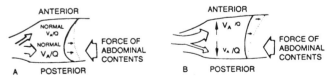

Figure 16-12. *(A)* Spontaneous breathing in the supine position is associated with greater posterior diaphragmatic and lung movement. Accordingly, $\dot{V}/\dot{Q}$ relationships here are more closely matched. Less ventilation and perfusion are present anteriorly. **(B)** When the diaphragm does not contract and the patient is mechanically ventilated, most ventilation is anterior (high $\dot{V}/\dot{Q}$), while most perfusion remains posterior (low $\dot{V}/\dot{Q}$). The result is a potentially significant alteration in normal overall $\dot{V}/\dot{Q}$. (With permission. Kirby RR, Banner JM, Downs JB [eds]. *Clinical Application of Ventilatory Support.* (2nd ed). Churchill Livingstone, New York, 1990.)

It is possible also to calculate chest wall and lung compliance in patients mechanically ventilated; however, both require the estimation of pleural pressure (placement of an esophageal balloon). Chest wall compliance (C_{TH}) can be measured in the passively ventilated patient and is determined by dividing the V_{ET} by the static end-inspiratory esophageal pressure. Lung compliance (C_L), however, can be measured only in the spontaneously breathing patient and is determined by dividing V_{ET} by the static end-inspiratory esophageal pressure. Obviously, it is difficult, if not impossible, to measure both C_{TH} and C_L in the same patient. With measurement of two of the three compliances, however, the third can be estimated.

$$\frac{1}{C_{ES}} = \frac{1}{C_L} + \frac{1}{C_{TH}}$$

A decrease in compliance indicates the system is "stiffer," and increases in compliance that the system is "less stiff." It is important to note that single values for C_{ES} have limited usefulness, although markedly decreased values do indicate a stiff system. More appropriately, the trend in C_{ES} should be followed.[58] If the C_{ES} is decreasing, the cause should be determined and appropriate action taken. When C_{ES} increases, appropriate steps to decrease therapy or level of support should be initiated. Determination of C_{ES} at different levels of PEEP or delivered V_T is useful in determining the proper settings for these variables.[59,60]

Resistance

Nonelastic resistance to ventilation, or patient-ventilator system resistance (R), can be estimated by dividing the difference between peak inspiratory pressure (PIP) and P_{plat} by the peak flow rate, provided the flow rate is delivered in a square wave pattern (see Fig. 16-6).[58] With a sine wave pattern, peak flow occurs at midinspiration, and with a decelerating pattern, peak flow occurs at the beginning of inspiration; thus the pressure differential (PIP − P_{plat}) may grossly underestimate the pressure necessary to overcome system resistance if a square waveform is not provided.

$$R = \frac{(PIP - P_{plat})}{\text{peak flow}}$$

Increases in R are caused by pathophysiologic changes that decrease airway lumen: edema, partial airway obstruction, or bronchospasm. Thus, bronchial hygiene therapy or aerosolized sympathomimetics may be indicated when estimates of R increase. PIP − P_{plat} may be reduced by decreasing peak flow rate or changing to a decelerating flow pattern.

Respiratory Time Constants

The respiratory time constant (TC) is a value that reflects the amount of time it takes the lung to return to baseline during passive exhalation. Thus, the time course of exhalation, as first described by Bergman in 1972 in anesthetized subjects,[61] is

$$V_{(t)} = Voe - \frac{(1)}{RC}t$$

where $V_{(t)}$ is the volume of gas remaining in the thorax at any time after the start of exhalation, Vo is the gas volume above resting FRC at the beginning of exhalation, e is the base of the natural logarithm, R is total resistance, C is total compliance, and t is time. The product RC is thus defined as the TC of the respiratory system.

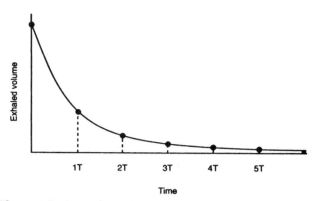

Figure 16-13. Relationship between volume passively exhaled and number of elapsed respiratory time constants (TC): 63%, 86.5%, 95%, 98.2%, and 99.3% of V_T is exhaled in one, two, three, four, and five TC, respectively. (With permission. Pierson DJ, Kacmarek RM [eds]. *Foundations of Respiratory Care.* Churchill Livingston, New York, 1992.)

(Resistance) (Compliance) = time
(cm H_2O/liters/sec) (liters/cm H_2O) = sec

If R and C are independent of volume, a finite time interval is necessary for complete passive exhalation (Fig. 16-13). In one TC, 63% of V_T is exhaled, and in 4 TC, 98% of V_T is exhaled.[17] Thus, unless 4 TC are available for passive exhalation, air trapping and auto-PEEP develop. TCs can be determined for the lung-thorax in total or for individual lung units. As has been illustrated in ARDS and chronic lung disease, individual lung units may have markedly different TCs as a result of the heterogeneity of the disease.[62,63] In all acute pulmonary pathology, there are some normal lung units, and with most diseases, there are both lung units with long and short time constants regardless of whether the global time constant of the lung is long, short, or normal. This realization can have important implications on management. For example, in ARDS, global time constants are short; however, normal and long time constant units prevent indefinite lengthening of inspiratory time because of air trapping and auto-PEEP.[64]

Auto-PEEP

Auto-PEEP is intrinsic PEEP or unidentified PEEP that develops as a result of incomplete emptying of local lung units and air trapping.[61] Two general settings increase the probability of the development of auto-PEEP: (1) acute or chronic pulmonary disease where dynamic airway compression is present and (2) a rapid respiratory rate with large V_T where expiratory time is inadequate.[65] As noted in Fig. 16-1, with auto-PEEP, central airway pressure and ventilator circuit pressure do not reflect the auto-PEEP level unless an end-expiratory hold is established.[66] Thus, unless auto-PEEP is sought, its presence is not identified. Auto-PEEP results in the same localized or global (if extensive) effects seen with PEEP,[66] except that it is established in lung units with high or normal compliance and high or normal airway resistance.[64] In the pediatric population, auto-PEEP is primarily a problem in children with bronchopulmonary dysplasia, asthma, cystic fibrosis, and pulmonary burns, and when inspiratory times are extensively lengthened.

Figure 16-14. Measurement of auto-PEEP (*arrow*) using an end-expiratory hold on the Servo 900C ventilator. Note that peak airway pressure is not affected on the inspiration following measurement since auto-PEEP is present, even though unnoticed, on every breath. (With permission. Pierson DJ, Kacmarek RM [eds]. *Foundations of Respiratory Care.* Churchill Livingston, New York, 1992.)

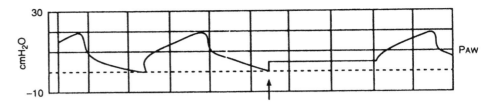

Identification of Auto-PEEP

Figure 16-14 illustrates auto-PEEP measurement in a patient wherein an end-expiratory hold is applied. The auto-PEEP reflected on the system manometer or the pressure waveform is the mean auto-PEEP level because it reflects the end-expiratory equilibration pressure within the patient-ventilator system; the maximum local auto-PEEP level always exceeds that measured.[64] Auto-PEEP measurement can occur only if no continuous system flow is present. Even systems utilizing low-level flow triggering must be turned off or the auto-PEEP level is overestimated. In noncontinuous flow systems, auto-PEEP can be identified but not quantified by evaluating end-expiratory flow (Fig. 16-15).[65] If end-expiratory flow has not reached 0 prior to the next inspiration, auto-PEEP is present. In patients with severe dynamic airway obstruction, however, the end-expiratory flow may be too slow to accurately measure by the crude flow measurement technology on ventilators. In patients with auto-PEEP, expiratory breath sounds continue until they are interrupted by inspiratory sounds, and physical examination and chest x-ray show hyperinflation. In spontaneously breathing patients, the only way to measure auto-PEEP accurately is to evaluate esophageal pressure change (Fig. 16-16) during inspiration at the same time airway opening pressure or flow is evaluated.[65] With auto-PEEP, a decrease in esophageal pressure occurs before flow is measured at the airway. The magnitude of the decrease is equal to the auto-PEEP level.

Because of the large intrathoracic pressure gradient that must be established to cause airflow and triggering of the ventilator in the presence of auto-PEEP, many patients are unable to trigger assisted breaths.[65] Whenever the patient's actual respiratory rate exceeds the ventilator response rate, auto-PEEP is present.

Management of Auto-PEEP

Table 16-6 lists the various techniques used to minimize the level of auto-PEEP. With dynamic airway compression or secretion accumulation, aggressive bronchial hygiene and aerosolized drugs should be employed. In addition, respiratory rate and tidal volume should be decreased and inspiratory time shortened to maximize expiratory time.[67] In spontaneously breathing patients, PEEP can be applied to balance the auto-PEEP; this allows alveolar, airway, and ventilator circuit pressures to equilibrate.[65,68] Provided the auto-PEEP is a result of dynamic airway obstruction and the applied PEEP does not exceed about 80% of the auto-PEEP, pulmonary mechanics should not be altered when PEEP is applied.[69] If peak and plateau pressure increase with volume-targeted ventilation, or if V_T decreases with pressure-targeted ventilation, the applied PEEP has caused greater overdistension.

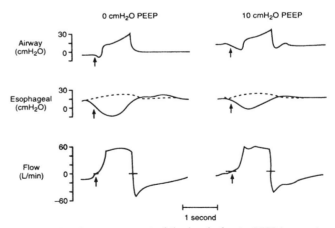

Figure 16-16. Assessment of the level of auto-PEEP in spontaneously breathing patients by evaluation of esophageal pressure change relative to either airway opening pressure or flow at airway opening. Arrows indicate pressure and flow change at airway opening. The change in esophageal pressure between baseline and the level that allows change in airway opening pressure or inflow is equal to the auto-PEEP level. Note the effect of 10 cm H_2O applied PEEP on the level of auto-PEEP (*left side*). (With permission. Smith TC, Marini JJ. Impact of PEEP on lung mechanics and work of breathing in severe airflow obstruction. *J Appl Physiol* 1988; 65:1499–1499.)

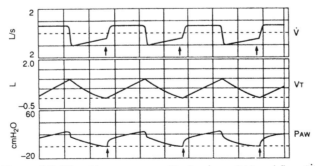

Figure 16-15. Airway pressure (P_{AW}) volume (V_T) and flow ($\dot{V}$) waveforms during volume-limited controlled ventilation in the presence of auto-PEEP. The initial airway pressure demonstrates a rapid initial increase (*arrow*), approximating the auto-PEEP level and then gradually increasing to peak airway pressure. Expiratory gas flow does not return to zero (*arrow*) in the presence of auto-PEEP. (With permission. Pierson DJ, Kacmarek RM [eds]. *Foundations of Respiratory Care.* Churchill Livingston, New York, 1992.)

Table 16-6. Approaches used to modify the level of auto-PEEP

Decrease dynamic airflow obstruction
  Aggressive bronchodilation
  Chest physical therapy
  Airway suctioning
  Large-size endotracheal tube
Normalize pH
  Administer $NaHCO_3$ during metabolic acidosis
  Avoid purposeful hyperventilation
Allow PCO_2 to rise > 60 mm Hg
  Decrease rate
  Decrease V_T
Modify ventilatory pattern
  Increase expiratory time
    Decrease rate
    Decrease V_T
  Decrease inspiratory time
    Increase peak inspiratory flow
    Use low compressible volume circuit
  Use low-rate SIMV
Apply PEEP/CPAP

Table 16-7. Factors that affect work of breathing

Improper setting of pressure triggers
Improper setting of flow triggers
Pressure triggers impose more work than flow triggers
Spontaneous breathing via endotracheal tubes
Low-rate SIMV via endotracheal tubes
Inadequate peak inspiratory flow with volume-targeted ventilation
Heat and moisture exchangers
Auto-PEEP

Work of Breathing

The assumption is frequently made that if mechanical ventilatory assistance is provided, work of breathing is markedly reduced. This assumption may be true in some settings, but many patients still perform a high level of work during assisted ventilation. Work is defined as force per unit area. When applied to the respiratory system, it is equal to the area of the pressure versus volume loop (Fig. 16-17A) established from V_T versus system pressure change. However, work of breathing may be a poor reflection of the total effort exerted by a patient, because for work to be performed, movement must occur.[65,68] In critically ill patients, large pressure changes may be established with little or no gas movement.

Classic calculations of lung work require the placement of an esophageal balloon to measure the transpulmonary pressure change during breathing. Even if work is not calculated, the magnitude of the esophageal pressure change reflects patient effort to breath.[70] A more common pressure tracing in critically ill patients that correlates with esophageal pressure change is the central venous pressure (CVP).[71] The inspiratory variation in the CVP is a qualitative, if not quantitative, reflection of patient effort. The greater the inspiratory deflection of CVP or esophageal pressure, the greater the effort and work performed by the patient.

Ventilatory circuit pressure change during triggering or spontaneous breathing only reflects the effort associated with activation of the ventilator system.[72] It does not reflect effort associated with the artificial airway or actual pulmonary pathology. Although, a large change in circuit pressure during triggering must reflect a large esophageal pressure charge, a large esophageal pressure change as seen with auto-PEEP (Fig. 16-17B) may not cause any change in ventilator circuit pressure.[65,68] During controlled ventilation, the pressure-volume loop created from the airway pressure and the V_T reflects the work required to ventilate the total patient-ventilator system.[73]

During mechanical ventilatory assistance, work of breathing or patient effort may be increased by the approach used to provide support (Table 16-7). The triggering mechanism for assisted ventilation may be either flow or pressure. When properly set, flow triggering imposes less work and patient effort than pressure triggering.[74,75] Flow triggers should be set at the lowest trigger flow that does not allow self-cycling. With pressure triggering, the sensitivity should be set at −0.5 to −1.0 cm H_2O. Because endotracheal tubes, especially nasal tubes, potentially impose work,[76,77] spontaneous breathing should be supported with low levels of pressure

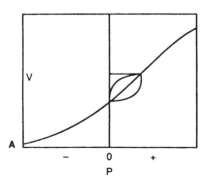 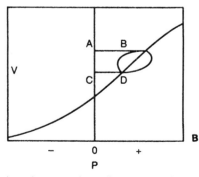

Figure 16-17. **(A)** Normal spontaneously breathing esophageal pressure-volume (*P-V*) loop. **(B)** Effect of auto-PEEP on area of P-V loop, reflecting marked increase in work of breathing as a result of the need to decompress the auto-PEEP prior to changing lung volume. Central airway pressure at end-exhalation is depicted by *C;* the pressure change from *C* to *D* must occur before gas movement to the lung perphiery is possible. The area of the rectangle CDBA represents the increased workload with auto-PEEP. (With permission. Otis AB. Work of breathing. In Finn WU, Rahn H [eds]: *Handbook of Physiology: The Respiratory System.* Vol 1. American Physiological Society, Washington, DC, 1964.)

support (5–8 cm H_2O).[78] Pressure support (5–8 cm H_2O) should also be set with SIMV, whenever the SIMV mandatory rate is set less than or equal to 4 to 10/min, depending on the size of the child.[54] In general, it is easier to ensure that the work of breathing is minimized with pressure-targeted ventilation than with volume-targeted ventilation, because the peak delivered flow with pressure-targeted ventilation varies with patient demand. Figure 16-18 illustrates pressure-volume loops during control and assist/control ventilation. If the ventilator were performing all of the work of breathing during assisted ventilation, the pressure-volume loop would be the same as during control ventilation.[79] During volume-targeted assist/control ventilation, peak flow should be set high enough to meet inspiratory demand, and inspiratory times short enough to match spontaneous breathing patterns. Whenever the airway pressure curve is concave during the initial part of inspiration, the patient is exerting a high level of effort. Heat and moisture exchangers (HME) impose a resistive load and should not be used during acute short-term ventilation in children[80]; this is especially true in infants with uncuffed airways.[81] The efficiency of the HME decreases if all exhaled gas does not pass through the device. During assisted ventilation, PEEP should be applied to balance auto-PEEP and minimize triggering effort (see Auto-PEEP section).

Management of Oxygenation

Oxygenation status, although dependent on FiO_2, is also intimately affected by the level of cardiopulmonary disease, PEEP, and $\bar{P}aw$. As discussed earlier, increased FiO_2 is the primary approach to management of hypoxemia that is a result of $\dot{V}/\dot{Q}$ mismatch and diffusion deficit, while appropriate level of ventilation corrects hypoxemia resulting from hypoventilation, and PEEP along with $\bar{P}aw$ adjustments are the primary approaches used to manage intrapulmonary shunt. Decreased cardiovascular function can extend

the hypoxemia resulting from any other cause. When cardiac output is low, tissue oxygen extraction rate is high and mixed venous PO_2 and oxygen content is low. When shunt, $\dot{V}/\dot{Q}$ mismatch, or diffusion deficit is present with low cardiac output, blood with a lower oxygen content from affected areas mixes with blood from unaffected lung units, resulting in a greater degree of hypoxemia than if cardiac output were higher. Regardless of the cause of hypoxemia or the approach used to manage it, for the most effective response to therapy, cardiovascular function must be optimized.

FiO_2

In general, the lowest FiO_2 that results in an acceptable PaO_2 should be set. Because of concerns regarding oxygen toxicity, however, FiO_2s above 0.6 for prolonged periods should be avoided. In healthy, small mammals, inspiration of 100% oxygen for about 24 hours results in structural changes at the alveolar-capillary membrane, pulmonary edema, atelectasis, and a decreased PaO_2.[82,83] In healthy humans, chest pain and tightness develops, but no edema, alectasis, or decreased PaO_2.[84] In the severely diseased lung, antioxidants capable of minimizing the effects of high FiO_2s may be induced allowing the lung to tolerate high FiO_2 without further damage.[85] Considering the potential damaging effects of high peak alveolar pressure (see Ventilator-Associated Lung Injury section), it is recommended that a higher FiO_2 be applied before the application of high peak alveolar pressure (>35 cm H_2O).[86–88]

In addition to the potential for oxygen toxicity, high FiO_2 may cause absorption atelectasis in poorly ventilated, unstable lung units due to denitrogenation. This does not mean that 100% oxygen should never be used. Whenever oxygenation status is in question or generalized cardiopulmonary instability occurs, 100% oxygen should be administered. FiO_2 should be reduced as rapidly as possible to more appropriate levels when the acute concerns have resolved. The use of 100% oxygen during patient transport, bronchoscopy, suctioning, chest physical therapy, and any other stressful procedure is also recommended. Unless the required FiO_2 is already established, 100% oxygen should be administered during initial ventilator set-up but quickly reduced when appropriate PaO_2/S_PO_2 levels are established.

PEEP

PEEP increases $\bar{P}aw$ and mean intrathoracic pressure affecting many other physiologic responses (Table 16-8). When applied to appropriate levels for the clinical setting, PEEP generally improves pulmonary mechanics and gas exchange, and may have varying effects on the cardiovascular system.[89]

Pulmonary Mechanics

PEEP increases FRC, regardless of the level applied or the setting used (Fig. 16-19). In acute lung injury where unstable lung units have collapsed, PEEP stabilizes functional lung units once expanded by preventing their collapse.[90] If recruitment of lung units is stabilized with PEEP, lung compliance improves (Fig. 16-20). Along with the improvement in compliance are a reduction in intrapulmonary shunt, an increase in PaO_2, and a decrease in work of breathing in spontaneously breathing patients.[91] Excessive PEEP further increases FRC, although at a smaller volume/unit pressure change because excessive PEEP places the lung on the flat portion of the compliance curve.[60] As a result, with pressure-

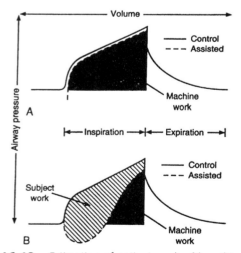

Figure 16-18. Estimation of patient work of breathing during assisted, volume-limited (square waveflow) ventilation. **(A)** Actual total work of breathing during controlled ventilation and ideal assisted ventilation. **(B)** Controlled ventilation compared with assisted ventilation. The hatched area represents work performed by a patient during assisted ventilation. (With permission. Marini JJ, Rodriguez M, Lamb V. The inspiratory workload of patient initiated mechanical ventilation. *Am Rev Respir Dis* 1986; 134:902–908.)

Table 16-8. Potential physiologic effects of appropriately and excessively applied PEEP

	Appropriate Level	*Excessive Level*
Intrapulmonary pressure	Increased	Increased
Intrathoracic pressure	Increased	Increased
FRC	Increased	Increased
Lung compliance	Increased	Increased or decreased
Closing volume	Decreased	Decreased
PaO_2	Increased	Increased or decreased
$PaCO_2$	No change or decreased	Increased
$\dot{Q}_s/\dot{Q}_T$	Decreased	Decreased or increased
$P(A-a)O_2$	Decreased	Decreased or increased
$C(a-\bar{v})O_2$	Decreased	Decreased or increased
$P\bar{v}O_2$	Increased	Increased or decreased
$PaCO_2\text{-}PETCO_2$	Decreased	Increased
V_D/V_T	Decreased	Increased
Work of breathing	Decreased	Increased
Extravascular lung water	No change or increased	No change or increased
Pulmonary vascular resistance	Increased	Increased
Total pulmonary perfusion	No change or decreased	Decreased
Cardiac output	No change or decreased	Decreased
Pulmonary artery pressure	No change or increased or decreased	Decreased
Pulmonary capillary wedge pressure	No change or increased or decreased	Decreased
Central venous pressure	No change or increased or decreased	Decreased
Arterial pressure	No change or increased or decreased	Decreased
Intracranial pressure	No change or increased	Increased
Urinary output	No change or decreased	Decreased

FRC, functional residual capacity; $\dot{Q}_s/\dot{Q}_T$, shunt fraction; $P(A-a)O_2$, alveolar-arterial O_2 pressure difference; $C(a-\bar{v})O_2$, arterial-mixed venous O_2 content difference; $P\bar{v}O_2$, mixed venous O_2 pressure; $PETCO_2$, end-tidal CO_2 pressure; V_D/V_T, dead space/tidal volume ratio.
With permission. From Pierson DJ, Kacmarek RM (eds). *Foundations of Respiratory Care.* New York: Churchill Livingston, 1992.

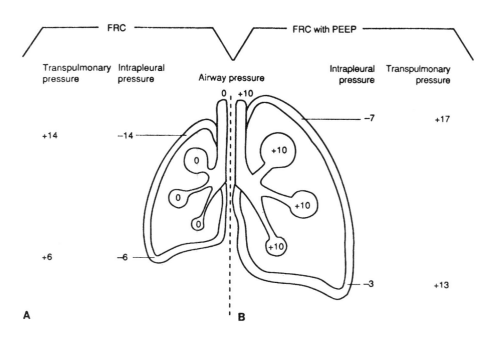

Figure 16-19. **(A)** Acute restrictive lung disease without PEEP results in greater than normal negative intrapleural pressures at functional residual capacity (*FRC*). **(B)** With 10-cm H_2O PEEP, more pressure is transmitted to the pleural space at the apex (7 cm H_2O transmitted) because of the normal apex-to-base variation in compliance than at the base (3 cm H_2O transmitted). Thus, transpulmonary pressure is increased by 7 cm H_2O at the base and only 3 cm H_2O at apex. (With permission. Shapiro, et al. *Clinical Applications of Respiratory Care.* [4th ed]. Mosby-YearBook Medical Publishers, St. Louis, 1990.)

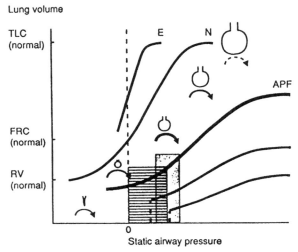

Lung volume

Figure 16-20. Family of regional pressure-volume curves of the respiratory system, in normal lungs (*N*) and in lungs of patients with emphysema (*E*) and acute pulmonary failure (*APF*). The whole lung APF curve is the sum of multiple regional compliance curves, some resembling normal and others very low compliance regions, two of which are shown in the diagram. Shaded areas show the pressure/volume relationship during the same tidal ventilation with and without PEEP. Broken vertical line denotes regional volume (*RV*) at which alveoli are unstable and readily "open" or "close." TLC, total lung capacity. (With permission. Suter PM, Fairley HB, Isenberg MD. Optimum end-expiratory airway pressure in patients with acute pulmonary failure. *N Engl J Med* 1975; 292:284–289.)

targeted ventilation, appropriate adjustment of PEEP can be expected to result in an increase in V_T, whereas, excessive application causes the V_T to decrease. While in volume-targeted ventilation, appropriate application of PEEP reduces peak alveolar and airway pressure, and excessive application increases peak alveolar and airway pressure.

Gas Exchange

In most clinical applications, PEEP is applied to improve arterial PO_2. This is accomplished primarily by preventing alveolar collapse and decreasing intrapulmonary shunt, although the elevation of $\bar{P}aw$ with the application of PEEP increases the gradient for oxygen movement into the blood, even when no recruitment occurs. Appropriate setting of PEEP usually results in increased PaO_2 and decreased intrapulmonary shunt.[91] PEEP also may improve the $PaCO_2$-$P_{ET}CO_2$ (end-tidal CO_2) difference and $PaCO_2$ by decreasing dead space.[92] Excessive PEEP, however, can decrease perfusion to well-ventilated areas, causing an increase in $PaCO_2$-$P_{ET}CO_2$ difference, $PaCO_2$ itself, and dead space.[92] Depending on the overall $\dot{V}/\dot{Q}$, excessive PEEP may or may not affect PaO_2 and shunt adversely.

Cardiovascular Function

The effect of PEEP on the cardiovascular system is dependent on the level of PEEP, the compliance of the lung-thorax system, and cardiovascular status. Because PEEP increases $\bar{P}aw$ and mean intrathoracic pressure, venous return and cardiac output may decrease as PEEP is applied.[93] PEEP has the greatest effect on cardiac output in a setting where lung compliance is high and thoracic compliance and cardiovascular reserve are low.[94] High levels of PEEP increase right ventricular afterload[95] (increased pulmonary

vascular resistance), which increases end-diastolic volume,[96] decreases ejection fraction,[97] and shifts the interventricular septum to the left.[98] This, along with a reduction in pericardial pressure gradient, limits left ventricular distensibility, reducing left ventricular end-diastolic volume and stroke volume.[99] Thus, both intrathorax and systemic vascular pressures are affected by PEEP. If flow is maintained when PEEP is applied, vascular pressures remain unchanged or increase. If pulmonary perfusion is decreased, however, vascular pressures generally decrease as PEEP is applied. The result is decreased cardiac output, arterial blood pressure, urine output, and tissue oxygenation. Thus, PEEP may increase arterial oxygenation but decrease tissue oxygenation.

Acute Lung Injury

The primary use of PEEP is in the management of acute lung injury. The pressure-volume curve of the lung-thorax system in acute lung injury is illustrated in Fig. 16-21.[100] This curve is characterized by a shift to the right, appearing as an inflection point, and marked hysteresis, when compared with normal pressure-volume curves. The inflection point on the curve represents a critical level of end-expiratory pressure. PEEP applied at or above this level prevents derecruitment of unstable lung units.[101] In adolescents and adults, the inflection point is reached with 10 to 12 cm H_2O PEEP. As noted by Gattinoni et al.[102] on serial CT scans of the chest with PEEP, the critical opening pressure of lung units is gravity-dependent. Thus, the inflection point can be expected to be below 10 cm H_2O in small infants and children.

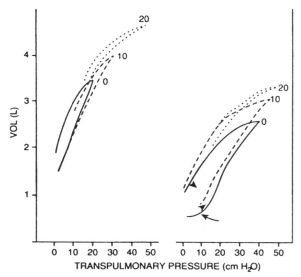

Figure 16-21. Static pressure-volume curves of the respiratory system for two patients at 0, 10, and 20 cm H_2O PEEP. The curves on the left are from a patient with a normal chest radiograph who was intubated for coma. There is little hysteresis, and the FRC is normal. The curves on the right are from a patient early in the course of ARDS. Without PEEP applied, the pressure-volume curve demonstrates marked hysteresis (*arrowheads*) and an inflection point on the inflation limb (*arrow, right*). At the highest level of PEEP (20 cm H_2O), the inflection point is lost and the pressure-volume curve assumes a monotonic profile with a P-V slope (compliance) similar to that of patients with normal lungs. (With permission. Benito S, Lemaine F. Pulmonary pressure-volume relationship in acute respiratory distress syndrome in adults: Role of positive end-expiratory pressure. *J Crit Care* 1990; 5:27–34.)

Generally, as PEEP is slowly titrated, a large improvement in gas exchange (>15-mm Hg increase in PO_2 or >2% increase in SaO_2) is observed and system compliance is improved as the inflection point is reached.[101,102] Once PEEP is above the inflection point, a linear relationship generally exists between PaO_2 and $\bar{P}aw$,[103] although the PaO_2 increase per cm H_2O $\bar{P}aw$ increase may be very small. In later stages of acute lung injury, marked consolidation and fibrosis are observed with a loss of the inflection point and grossly decreased lung volume; a PEEP level lower than that applied in early injury is frequently appropriate, although $\bar{P}aw$ may still have to be elevated.[102]

Mean Airway Pressure

$\bar{P}aw$ is the pressure applied to the lung over the entire ventilatory cycle. The magnitude of $\bar{P}aw$ is dependent on all of the factors that effect ventilation (Table 16-9). In acute lung injury, $\bar{P}aw$ and oxygenation are directly related if PEEP is applied above the inflection point on the pressure-volume curve.[102] Extending inspiratory time is a very useful method of increasing $\bar{P}aw$ without elevating peak alveolar pressure and of maintaining a constant level of ventilation.[102,104] This is true, provided no auto-PEEP develops. If auto-PEEP develops, either peak alveolar pressure or tidal volume is affected. With volume-targeted ventilation, auto-PEEP increases peak alveolar pressure because V_T is constant, while with pressure-targeted ventilation, tidal volume is decreased as auto-PEEP develops. Because peak airway pressure and peak alveolar pressure are kept constant with pressure-targeted ventilation, the pressure gradient establishing V_T decreases when auto-PEEP occurs. Auto-PEEP causes a less uniform distribution of PEEP and FRC than applied PEEP.[64] When heterogeneous lung disease is present, pulmonary time constants can vary considerably from one lung unit to another.[62,63] With auto-PEEP, FRC and total PEEP will be largest in the most compliant lung units (longest expiratory TC) and lowest in the least compliant lung units (shortest expiratory TC).[64] Limiting inspiratory time to the maximum that does not create auto-PEEP appears to be a reasonable approach.

Optimizing Oxygenation

Assuming appropriate cardiovascular function, increasing FiO_2 is the recommended first step in managing oxygenation. In acute lung injury, once FiO_2 exceeds 0.40, PEEP should be applied until the inflection point is exceeded. If oxygenation is still compromised, slowly increase the FiO_2 to 0.60, after which, increase the inspiratory time to further increase $\bar{P}aw$ until auto-PEEP develops. If further therapy is needed once inspiratory time is maximized,

either FiO_2 or PEEP should be increased further. It is at this point in the management of oxygenation when decisions regarding which maneuver is considered least detrimental—high FiO_2 or high peak alveolar pressure—must be made.

Ventilator-Induced Lung Injury

Mechanical ventilation is a nonphysiologic process. Pressure, volume, and FiO_2 beyond the levels that the lung normally tolerates are frequently used. As a result, lung injury may be caused or extended by the process of mechanical ventilation. Lung injury manifests itself in two forms: gross barotrauma (volutrauma) and parenchymal injury similar to ARDS (Table 16-10).

Barotrauma (Volutrauma)

The term *barotrauma* has been used to describe the gross air leak associated with mechanical ventilation. More recently, however, the term *volutrauma* has been preferred,[105] because it is now believed that the primary mechanical phenomenon that precipitates injury is localized overdistension of a lung, not pressure per se.[106] Three conditions must be present for volutrauma to develop: (1) disease, (2) high transpulmonary pressure, and (3) overdistension. The precise pressure and volume that increase the likelihood for volutrauma is unknown. Because the maximum transpulmonary pressure developed by healthy individuals is about 30 cm H_2O,[107] it seems reasonable to expect that the probability of volutrauma will increase if pressure is applied above this level.

Pneumothorax is the most commonly described acute complication of mechanical ventilation. In adult patients, the incidence varies from 0.5% to 44% of ventilated patients.[108] In pediatric populations, Pollack et al. have reported an incidence of 5.6%.[109]

Table 16-9. Factors affecting mean airway pressure

Applied PEEP

Auto-PEEP

Tidal volume

Pressure control level

Gas flow waveform*

Rate*

Inspiratory Time/I:E ratio*

---

*Do not increase peak alveolar pressure unless auto-PEEP develops

Table 16-10. The spectrum of lung injury induced by mechanical ventilation

Atelectasis

Alveolar hemorrhage

Alveolar neutrophil infiltration

Alveolar macrophage accumulation

Decreased compliance

Detachment of endothelial cells

Denuding of basement membranes

Emphysematous changes

Gross pulmonary edema

Hyaline membrane formation

Interstitial edema

Increased interstitial albumin levels

Interstitial lymphocyte infiltration

Intracapillary bleeding

Pneumothorax

Severe hypoxemia

Subcutaneous emphysema

Systemic gas embolism

Tension cyst formation

Modified from Kacmarek RM, Hickling KG. Permissive hypercapnia. *Respir Care* 38:373–387, 1993. With permission.

In pediatric ARDS patients, however, the incidence of air leak is 44%.[110] In a series of pediatric patients who underwent treatment with extracorporeal membrane oxygenation (ECMO) for severe respiratory failure, 80% suffered from air leak syndrome prior to meeting ECMO criteria.[111]

The consequences of air leak may be benign or catastrophic. Small air collections may be asymptomatic. Large collections of air may cause tamponade. The most dramatic and fatal air leak syndrome occurs with rupture into a bronchial vein, producing air embolism. Bronchopleural fistula occurs frequently if air leak persists for more than 24 hours.[108]

Precise guidelines for the avoidance of volutrauma are unavailable, although volutrauma is rare when PIP is less than 30 cm H_2O.[112] In an adult series, no patient whose peak airway pressure was less than 60 cm H_2O experienced an air leak, while a 44% incidence was observed when peak airway pressure exceeded 70 cm H_2O.[113] More recently, Hickling et al.,[114] reported no air leaks in a series of ARDS patients ventilated at PIP less than 45 cm H_2O. Darioli and Pervet[115] also reported a zero incidence of volutrauma in a series of 34 patients with severe asthma ventilated at PIP less than 60 cm H_2O. Both Hickling et al.[114] and Darioli and Perret[115] employed permissive hypercapnia. Analysis of this data makes it difficult to define a precise pressure limit because of the varying approaches used to ventilate patients. Some used volume-targeted ventilation with square waveforms; others, sine waveforms; and still others, pressure-targeted ventilation. The best information to date is that provided by American College of Chest Physicians, recommending limiting end-inspiratory plateau pressure to 35 cm H_2O.[116]

Parenchymal Lung Injury

Numerous animal studies (e.g., rats, sheep, dogs, and pigs) have demonstrated parenchymal damage (see Table 16-10) similar to acute lung injury after relatively short periods of mechanical ventilation when high peak airway pressures were maintained. Webb and Tierney[117] noted gross pulmonary edema and hemorrhage in rats after 60 minutes of ventilation with a peak inspiratory pressure of 45 cm H_2O. Similar results were reported by Hernandez et al[118] in rabbits following ventilation at peak inspiratory pressure of 45 cm H_2O. Kolobow et al.[119] ventilated normal sheep with 40% oxygen at peak airway pressures of 50 cm H_2O; all animals developed severe respiratory failure and at necropsy had pulmonary consolidation. Similar injury in rats was demonstrated by Dreyfuss et al.[106,120] (Fig. 16-22), who produced the same effect with equal levels of negative pressure ventilation.[106] Others have demonstrated attenuation of ventilator-induced parenchymal lung injury[106,117,121] when PEEP was applied above the inflection point on the compliance curve, or if the thorax was strapped (preventing hyperinflation because of decreased chest wall compliance).[106] The repetitive recruitment and subsequent derecruitment without the application of PEEP above the inflection point appears to extend the injury associated with localized overdistention.[121] The primary pressure associated with injury appears to be the peak alveolar distending pressure or transpulmonary pressure.[116,106] These data have led most authorities on mechanical ventilation to recommend limiting end-inspiratory plateau pressure, and thus the resulting inflation volume.

Based on the data from animal studies and the fact that during voluntary maximal inspiration, peak transpulmonary pressures are about 30 cm H_2O,[107] the American College of Chest Physicians,[116] as well as others, have recommended that the peak alveolar pressure be limited to a maximum of 35 cm H_2O.[86,104] It is understood that this level of alveolar pressure may compromise ventilation. When the targeted pressure is reached and gas exchange is still poor, a decision to exceed or not exceed this limit should be made based on the potential detrimental effects of elevated peak alveolar pressure versus permissive hypercapnia.

Gas Exchange Targets

Based on the probability of the development of ventilatory-induced lung injury, the concept of normal gas exchange during mechani-

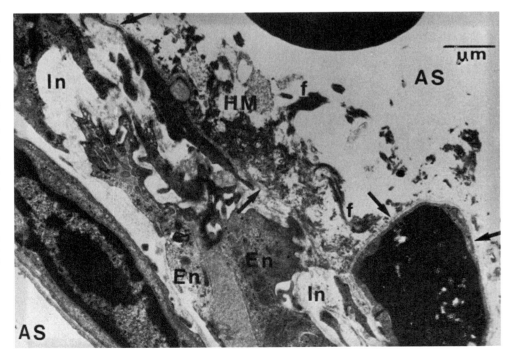

Figure 16-22. Alveolar septum with three capillaries of an adult rat after 20 minutes of ventilation at 45 cm H_2O. At the right side, the epithelial lining is destroyed, denuding the basement membrane (*arrows*). Hyaline membranes (*HM*) composed of cell debris and fibrin (*f*) are present. Two endothelial cells (*En*) of another capillary are visible inside the interstitium (*In*). At the lower left side, a monocyte fills the lumen of a third capillary with a normal blood–air barrier. (With permission. Dreyfuss D et al. Intermittent positive-pressure hyperventilation with high inflation pressure produces pulmonary microvascular injury in rats. *Am Rev Respir Dis* 1985; 132:880–884.)

cal ventilation is being challenged. Of particular concern are patients presenting with acute lung injury, asthma, or chronic lung disease with high impedance to ventilation.

Permissive Hypercapnia

Permissive hypercapnia is the deliberate limitation of ventilatory support to avoid alveolar overdistension (e.g., ARDS) or auto-PEEP (e.g., acute asthma).[122] As a result, $PaCO_2$ rises to levels greater than normal (50–100 mm Hg). Allowing the $PaCO_2$ to rise to these levels is considered when the only alternative is a potentially dangerous increase in peak alveolar pressure or auto-PEEP. The potentially adverse effects of an elevated $PaCO_2$ are listed in Table 16-11. Most of the more important clinical problems occur at $PaCO_2$ levels above 150 mm Hg.[86] Even small increases in $PaCO_2$ increase cerebral blood flow, however, and permissive hypercapnia is generally contraindicated when intracranial pressure is increased. Elevated $PaCO_2$ also stimulates ventilation, but patients are usually sedated and paralyzed in the settings where permissive hypercapnia is considered.

Permissive hypercapnia may adversely affect the oxygenation status of some patients. Elevated $PaCO_2$ and low pH shift the oxyhemoglobin dissociation curve to the right.[107] This decreases the affinity of hemoglobin for oxygen, decreasing oxygen loading in the lungs but facilitating the unloading of oxygen at the tissues.[107] As illustrated by the alveolar gas equation (see section on Hypoxic Respiratory Failure), an increase in the alveolar PCO_2 results in a decrease in alveolar PO_2. For each $PaCO_2$ rise of 1 mm Hg, the PaO_2 decreases by about 1 mm Hg.

The effect of carbon dioxide on the cardiovascular system is difficult to predict. As illustrated in Fig. 16-23, carbon dioxide elicits competing responses from the cardiovascular system.[123] Carbon dioxide directly stimulates or depresses specific aspects of the cardiovascular system, but opposite effects can occur via stimulation of the autonomic nervous system. It is thus difficult to predict the precise response of the cardiovascular system to permissive

Table 16-11. Potential adverse physiologic effects of permissive hypercapnia

Shift in the oxyhemoglobin dissociation curve to the right

Decreased alveolar PO_2

Both stimulation and depression of the cardiovascular system

CNS depression

Stimulation of ventilation

Dilation of vascular bed

Increased intracranial pressure

Narcosis ($PaCO_2 > 80$–100 mm Hg)

Decreased renal blood flow ($PaCO_2 > 150$ mm Hg)

Leakage of intracellular potassium ($PaCO_2 > 150$ mm Hg)

Alteration of the action of pharmacologic agents (result of intracellular acidosis)

hypercapnia in any given patient. The most common response, however, is an increase in pulmonary hypertension.[124] Dosages of pharmaceutical agents affecting the cardiovascular and autonomic nervous systems may need to be adjusted in the presence of permissive hypercapnia, as a result of acidosis.

The primary factor limiting permissive hypercapnia is the pH produced. Patients without primary cardiovascular disease or renal failure can usually tolerate a pH of 7.20 or greater, and some may tolerate an even lower pH.[86,88,114] The specific minimal pH acceptable needs to be determined on an individual patient basis. Allowing PCO_2 to rise gradually from the onset of ventilation, if necessary, allows gradual renal compensation, minimizing marked pH change. Abrupt changes in ventilator strategies that result in rapid and marked elevation of $PaCO_2$ are usually poorly tolerated.

Whether alkalinizing agents should be administered to manage the acidosis induced by permissive hypercapnia is debatable.[88,114]

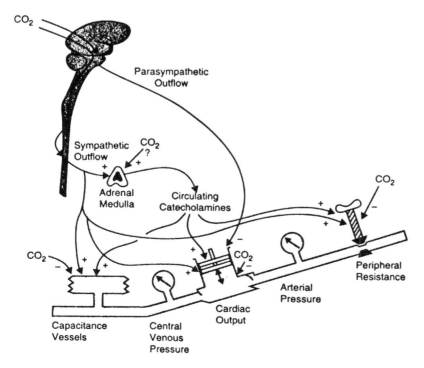

Figure 16-23. This diagram shows the complexity of the mechanisms by which carbon dioxide can influence the circulatory system. See text for details. (With permission. Nunn JF [ed]. *Applied Respiratory Physiology*, [2nd ed]. London: Butterworths & Co., 1977.)

Table 16-12. PaO$_2$ targets in acute lung injury

>80 mm Hg normal lungs
>70 mm Hg mild lung injury
>60 mm Hg moderate lung injury
>50 mm Hg severe lung injury

In the setting of hypoxic lactic acidosis, sodium bicarbonate administration may be detrimental because of the resulting increased intracellular acidosis.[125] Its use in permissive hypercapnia, however, has not been extensively studied. One can expect a short-term increase in carbon dioxide load when sodium bicarbonate is administered, which is exhaled over time if the level of ventilation is held constant. However, whether the use of alkalinizing agents has any effect on an overall tolerance of permissive hypercapnia is not known.

Oxygenation

Achievement of a normal PaO$_2$ ($\geq$80 mm Hg) is desired in all patients who are mechanically ventilated. The cost of maintaining this level of oxygenation, however, may exceed the benefit. Provided cardiovascular function is normal and adequate oxygen carrying capacity is present, a lower PaO$_2$ target becomes acceptable the more acutely ill the child. Table 16-12 summarizes the recommended targets.

Ventilatory Strategies

Three common categories of pediatric patients requiring ventilator support are (1) those with little or no lung disease with a loss of respiratory drive or airway control, (2) those with restrictive lung (low lung volume) disease, and (3) those with obstructive lung (high lung volume) disease.

Normal Lungs

General anesthesia, sedation, or overdose of many types of drugs may require short-term ventilation. Central hypoventilation, apnea, neuromuscular disease, coma, CNS infections, or congenital malformation of the airway are other common causes of ventilatory assistance. Usually, these patients present with a combination of hypercarbia and hypoxemia, with hypercarbia predominating but with hypoxemia being a major concern. This is especially of concern in patients with total loss of their respiratory drive or airway control. The aim of therapy for these children is to secure the airway and provide ventilation, avoiding either atelectasis or overdistension (Table 16-13). Full ventilatory support is needed in patients with total loss of respiratory drive. Partial ventilatory support may be appropriate in patients who are awake and able to participate in the ventilation process. Low inflation pressures because of normal lung compliance is the rule. Once patients are able to maintain the airway and demonstrate normal respiratory drive and function, they can readily be weaned and extubated.

Restrictive Lung Disease

Low lung volume disease is commonly encountered in the PICU setting. Children with pneumonia, interstitial disease, aspiration

Table 16-13. Ventilatory strategy: Normal lungs

Pressure or volume target acceptable
V$_T$ set at 12–15 ml/kg or
Pressure target set to allow V$_T$ of 12–15 ml/kg
Rate, age-dependent
F$_I$O$_2$ to keep PaO$_2$ > 80 mm Hg
Sensitivity set to ensure trigger pressure change < 1.5 cm H$_2$O
With volume target, set peak flow to prevent concave pressure waveform
Set inspiratory time < 1.0 sec
With SIMV, add 5–8 cm H$_2$O
Set PEEP 3–5 cm H$_2$O
Use partial ventilatory support if ventilatory drive intact
Keep plateau pressure < 35 cm H$_2$O

pneumonitis, near-drowning, and ARDS present with a restrictive lung disease characterized by a loss of FRC. These patients usually present with hypoxemia secondary to $\dot{V}/\dot{Q}$ mismatch and shunt and are frequently tachypneic.

The goal in treating these patients is to restore FRC and recruit underventilated areas, thus improving the $\dot{V}/\dot{Q}$ mismatch and oxygenation. This is accomplished by the application of PEEP and the management of P̄aw (Table 16-14). Increasing PEEP and P̄aw is not a benign process, and overdistension of nondiseased lung units may occur along with decreases in cardiac output and underperfusion of healthy lung units. The aim is to provide adequate oxygen delivery at the lowest FiO$_2$ and airway pressures possible. It is important for hemoglobin levels and cardiac output to be optimized.

With restrictive diseases, full ventilatory support with sedation and, occasionally, muscle relaxation is used initially. PEEP and FiO$_2$ are titrated to maintain target PaO$_2$. For children with severe acute lung injury, P̄aw is commonly increased by increasing inspiratory time, at times to the extent of equaling or inversing the I:E ratio. Cautious maintenance of peak alveolar pressure at 35 cm

Table 16-14. Ventilatory strategy: Restrictive lung disease

Pressure or volume target acceptable
Full ventilatory support during acute phase
Partial ventilatory support during recovery phase
V$_T$ set at 6–10 ml/kg
Pressure target set to allow V$_T$ of 6–10 ml/kg
Set rate according to age, avoid air trapping
Set PEEP at or above inflection point on P-V loop, 8–12 cm H$_2$O
Increase inspiratory time to increase P̄aw; avoid creating auto-PEEP
Adjust FiO$_2$ in conjunction with PEEP and P̄aw to keep PaO$_2$ 50–80 mm Hg, depending on severity
Keep peak alveolar pressure < 35 cm H$_2$O
Allow PCO$_2$ to rise > 60 mm Hg, if necessary
Set sensitivity to trigger at < 1.5 cm H$_2$O
With volume target, set peak flow to prevent concave pressure waveform
With SIMV, add PSV 5–8 cm H$_2$O

H_2O or lower is encouraged to prevent volutrauma and ventilator-induced lung injury. This is the primary patient population where permissive hypercapnia is commonly allowed. It is not uncommon for patients with severe acute lung injury to be maintained with $PaCO_2$ greater than 60 mm Hg and PaO_2 greater than 50 mm Hg. Appropriate sedation and paralysis is usually necessary with permissive hypercapnia.

Obstructive Lung Disease

Obstructive (high volume) lung diseases are encountered frequently in children presenting to the ICU. Most commonly, these patients have asthma, bronchiolitis, or bronchopulmonary dysplasia (BPD). Because of high airway resistance, gas trapping, and auto-PEEP, increased FRC and increased dead space are present. Ventilation-perfusion mismatch is further increased because of airway edema and mucous plugging. These pathophysiologic problems lead to hypoxemia and hypercapnia. Because of high airway resistance, respiratory TCs may be greatly lengthened.

The main strategy for ventilating children with obstructive disease is to provide adequate oxygenation and ventilation without further increasing air trapping and lung distension (Table 16-15). In children with severe asthma and overinflation, this frequently requires slow ventilator rates (6–10 range) and inspiratory times of 1 second or longer. This allows enough expiratory time to reduce air trapping, and the longer inspiratory times improve gas distribution. Permissive hypercapnia is the rule during the acute phase. Auto-PEEP should be monitored carefully throughout the ventilatory course. In patients who are breathing spontaneously, PEEP should be applied to reduce the effort necessary to overcome auto-PEEP.

In children with bronchiolitis, BPD, or less severe asthma, more rapid ventilator rates are frequently tolerated without worsening gas trapping. It is important to maintain airway pressure as low as possible to prevent volutrauma. Sedation and muscle relaxation may be needed, and permissive hypercapnia may be necessary.

Weaning

The ultimate goal of mechanical ventilatory support is ventilator discontinuation, and in the vast majority of patients, this is a simple process. About 75% to 80% of patients who are mechanically ventilated may have the ventilator discontinued when the physiologic reason for ventilatory support is reversed. Another 15% to 20% of ventilated children may require the use of a specific weaning protocol applied over an 8- to 72-hour period before discontinuation is possible. It is the remaining 5% of mechanically ventilated patients that require a gradual weaning, sometimes requiring weeks or months before discontinuation, that is the most problematic. This is the group where the term *weaning* is most properly applied. It should be realized that a very small percentage of these patients (<1.0%) may never be physiologically ready to wean and should be considered chronically ventilator-dependent.

Readiness to Wean

Before weaning is considered, the specific indication for ventilatory support must be reversed. The patient should be able to maintain a PaO_2 greater than or equal to 60 mm Hg with an FiO_2 less than or equal to 0.40 and PEEP less than or equal to 5 cm H_2O.[126] Excess minute ventilation during ventilatory support should not be required to maintain a normal $PaCO_2$. Generally, V_D/V_T should be less than 0.6. The child also must have an intact ventilatory drive. Cardiovascular function should be optimized, fever should be controlled, electrolytes balanced, nutritional status normalized, and all other major organ systems functioning appropriately. Without this level of readiness, wean trials frequently fail (Table 16-16).

Predictors of Weaning Outcome

Various indexes have been used to predict successful weaning outcomes. Unfortunately, few of these have demonstrated clinical efficacy. The single index that has demonstrated both sensitivity and specificity is the rapid/shallow breathing index (f/V_T) proposed by Yang and Tobin.[127] These authors compared the f/V_T to other traditional weaning indexes and found that f/V_T was the best predictor of weaning success, while the maximum inspiratory pressure measurement and the f/V_T were the best predictors of weaning failure. This evaluation was performed on adult patients in a medical ICU. Unfortunately, similar data are not available in pediatric patients. The f/V_T is evaluated 1 minute after both ventilation and oxygenation support are removed. An f/V_T of less than 100 is predictive of successful weaning.

Weaning Failure

One of the biggest mistakes made when weaning patients is to push patients to the point of exhaustion. When this occurs, weaning

Table 16-15. Ventilatory strategy: Obstructive lung disease

Pressure or volume target acceptable

Full ventilatory support first 24–72 hr

Thereafter, partial ventilatory support

V_T set at 8–12 ml/kg

Pressure target set to allow V_T of 8–12 ml/kg

Set rate according to time of expiratory "wheeze," but keep low 6–12/min to avoid auto-PEEP in most acute stage

Allow $PaCO_2$ to rise > 60 mm Hg, if necessary

Adjust FiO_2 to keep $PaO_2 \geq 60$ mm Hg

Keep peak alveolar pressure < 35 cm H_2O

Set sensitivity to trigger at < 1.5 cm H_2O

With volume target, set peak flow to prevent concave pressure waveform

Inspiratory time may need to be lengthened beyond 1.0 seconds

With SIMV, add PSV 5–8 cm H_2O

Table 16-16. Readiness to wean

Reversal of indication for ventilation

$PaO_2 \geq 60$ mm Hg with $FiO_2 \leq 0.40$ and PEEP ≤ 5 cm H_2O

Intact ventilatory drive

Cardiovascular stability

Electrolytes normal

Normal body temperature

Adequate nutritional status

Absence of other major organ system failures

Table 16-17. Common reasons for failure to wean

Weaning to exhaustion

Auto-PEEP

Excessive work of breathing

Poor nutritional status

Excess carbohydrate intake

Left heart failure

Decreased magnesium and phosphate levels

Infection/fever

Major organ system failure

Technical limitations, e.g., high airway resistance from small-diameter endotracheal tube

progress is always delayed. Although work of breathing is not a good predictor of weaning success, an excessive work load may be a primary reason why a patient fails a trial of weaning.[128] High airway resistance and low compliance contribute to the increased effort necessary to breathe. Aerosolized sympathomimetics, bronchial hygiene, and a normalized fluid balance assist in normalizing compliance, resistance, and work of breathing. In a large percentage of patients with chronic lung disease who require lengthy weaning periods, auto-PEEP is a primary problem.[129,130] If present, auto-PEEP increases the pressure gradient needed to inspire, regardless of whether patients are assisting breathing or breathing spontaneously. The use of CPAP/PEEP balances alveolar pressure with central airway pressure (see Auto-PEEP section).

Imbalance of electrolytes causes muscular weakness. Specifically, decreased potassium, magnesium, phosphate, and calcium levels impair ventilatory muscle function.[5-7] Patients with a negative nitrogen balance rarely are capable of weaning.[8] However, care should be exercised to avoid overfeeding because excessive carbohydrate ingestion markedly elevates carbon dioxide production. Failure of any other major organ system can precipitate weaning failure. Fever and infection are of particular concern, because both oxygen consumption and carbon dioxide production are thereby increased, resulting in an increased ventilatory requirement (Table 16-17).

Of particular concern in patients with cardiopulmonary disease is inadequately managed left heart failure.[131] A delicate balance between P̄aw and pulmonary hemodynamics may exist, which is easily disrupted by decreasing P̄aw during weaning trails. These patients may rapidly develop pulmonary edema during weaning. Appropriate management of cardiovascular status is necessary before weaning is successful.

Approaches to Weaning

In general, approaches to weaning can be grouped into three categories: (1) pressure support ventilation (PSV), (2) SIMV, or (3) T-piece/CPAP trials, although combinations of these are also employed.[126] In those patients requiring a lengthy period of weaning (more than 1 or 2 days), it is important to adjust ventilatory support to ensure ventilatory muscle rest at night and a good night's sleep. Successful weaning approaches appropriately mix work and rest periods and ensure proper nutrition and sleep.

Pressure Support

Many recommend the use of gradual reductions in the level of PSV, provided the patient can maintain a target respiratory rate and V_T, as the most appropriate approach to weaning.[36,37,54,132] The process is begun by setting the PSV at a level where a tidal volume and a respiratory rate consistent with the level expected on discontinuation is achieved. The minimum PSV level that prevents activation of accessory muscles is the most appropriate. PSV is then decreased on a regular basis (hours or days) until some minimum level (5–8 cm H_2O) is reached that unloads the work of breathing imposed by the ventilator/endotracheal tube system, provided the desired ventilatory pattern can be maintained. Once the patient is capable of maintaining the target ventilatory pattern and gas exchange at this minimal level, mechanical ventilation is discontinued.

Although this approach works well with most patients requiring short-term weaning (8–72 hours), it can be problematic in patients who require weeks to wean because it does not allow the patient to rest. Maintaining the level of ventilatory support at the minimal level necessary may not be appropriate in patients requiring lengthy weaning periods.[126]

Synchronized Intermittent Mandatory Ventilation

SIMV was introduced as a ventilatory mode to facilitate weaning.[41] Like PSV, a gradual reduction in SIMV rate to a predefined minimal level is commonly the approach used during weaning. Contrary to PSV, however, with SIMV two very distinct types of breaths are established: a pressure- or volume-targeted mandatory breath and an unassisted spontaneous breath. As a result, some patients may experience asynchrony with low SIMV rates.[133] As with PSV, an SIMV wean does not allow for rest periods at a level of support greater than the minimal set level. SIMV is most useful for the rapid weaning of short-term mechanical ventilation (e.g., postoperative, overdose). When SIMV is used during weaning of patients with longer ventilatory courses, it is essential that the level of ventilatory support be increased during the night to ensure rest and sleep.[57] Generally, at night an SIMV rate that provides nearly 100% support is recommended. Because of the work of breathing imposed by the ventilator and the endotracheal tube, patients should not be maintained on an SIMV rate of less than or equal to 4 to 10/min (dependent on age) without PSV unloading the spontaneous breaths.[54,57]

T-Piece/CPAP Trials

The classic approach to weaning is the T-piece or CPAP trial.[126] With this approach, increasing periods of unsupported spontaneous breathing are interspersed between periods of full ventilatory support. In long-term mechanically ventilated patients, the trial period may begin with periods as short as 5 minutes several times a day. The length of the trials is then increased over time as the patient's tolerance improves, always allowing periods of complete rest between trials and during the night. How long a spontaneous breathing trial should extend before ventilator discontinuation is dependent on the type of airway. In patients with tracheotomy tubes, T-piece/CPAP trials may extend for as much as 24 hours before ventilator discontinuation is complete. With endotracheal tubes, however, unsupported spontaneous ventilation for more than 60 to 90 minutes is poorly tolerated.[126] Patients with endotracheal tubes who can tolerate spontaneous breathing without blood gas or ventilatory pattern changes for 60 minutes should be considered weaned from ventilatory support and candidates for extubation.[126,127]

The Optimal Approach

Unfortunately, no single optimal approach to weaning has been defined. Recently, two multicenter, randomized, controlled weaning trials have been published,[132,134] with opposite results. In one,[135] PSV was considered the best approach, with shorter weaning periods than T-piece or SIMV. The second[136] demonstrated shorter weaning periods with T-piece weaning than with PSV or SIMV. Methologic concerns can be raised regarding both of these studies, but what these studies do demonstrate is that any weaning approach that is performed properly facilitates weaning, and those that are performed poorly lengthen it.

Complications of Ventilatory Support

As described earlier, mechanical ventilation is not a normal physiologic process and as a result may precipitate compromised function of many organ systems. Trauma to the lung as a result of the mechanical ventilation process is common and may manifest itself as an acute lung injury similar to respiratory distress syndrome or as gross volutrauma.

Hemodynamic Consequences of Positive Pressure

Spontaneous ventilation creates a negative pleural pressure, which in turn enhances blood return to the right ventricle. When positive pressure inflates the lung, venous return to the right heart decreases because of increased right ventricular afterload in direct proportion to the degree of lung volume increase.[95] The net effect on cardiac output in normovolemic patients with normal hearts and lungs is a reduction in cardiac output.[93] This occurs because venous return to the left heart diminishes, and encroachment of the right ventricular septum into the left ventricle, secondary to increases in right ventricular afterload,[98] limits left ventricular filling.

Effects on the left ventricle vary by condition. Spontaneous ventilation in normovolemic patients with normal hearts decreases ventricular transmural pressure, and cardiac output falls. Positive pressure may enhance left ventricular ejection in conditions of poor contractility by decreasing afterload.[135] Caution is required in interpreting this phenomenon clinically. An individual patient may have wide fluctuations in preload because of changes in vascular volume and may be ventilated with a combination of spontaneous and controlled mechanical breaths. Myocardial contractility can vary with changes in acid-base status or with infection.

Pulmonary blood flow is altered by positive pressure. Pulmonary blood flow is always greater to dependent areas of the lung, while positive pressure ventilation is preferentially distributed to nondependent zones. This increases $\dot{V}/\dot{Q}$ mismatch and increases the dead space to tidal volume ratio.[135,136] In clinical conditions with profoundly altered $\dot{V}/\dot{Q}$ states, positive pressure can be deleterious. In unilateral lung disease or in postunilateral lung transplant, positive pressure ventilation may exacerbate intrapulmonary shunt by overdistension of more compliant units, thus increasing dead space ventilation.[137,138] Kanarek and Shannon describe a 16-year-old patient with unilateral infiltrates in whom PaO_2 fell from 71 to 35 mm Hg with PEEP. Pulmonary blood flow to the diseased lung increased from 41% to 67% of a total flow, with PEEP increased incrementally from 0 to 15 cm H_2O.[139]

During spontaneous ventilation, distribution of ventilation and perfusion is optimal. Work of breathing, however, may be unacceptably high, and hypoxemia may occur as a result of loss of functional residual capacity. These latter sequelae are best improved with positive pressure ventilation. Thus, application of positive pressure is a trade-off of risks and benefits. Overzealous use of PEEP will depress cardiac output, increase dead space, increase pulmonary vascular resistance, and decrease compliance. Inadequate positive pressure will not recruit lung volume.

Many clinicians have long held to the caveat that poorly compliant lung will not allow transmission of airway pressure to the vascular bed. Data suggest, however, that airway pressure is transmitted to the heart through poorly compliant lungs.[139,140] Clinicians must consider pulmonary and hemodynamic events as a risk-benefit balance when contemplating or evaluating ventilation strategies.

A right heart flow-directed catheter is invaluable in monitoring the hemodynamic consequences when high levels of positive pressure ventilation are applied. Because blood volume status modifies the effects of positive pressure, especially end-expiratory pressure, determination of central venous and pulmonary artery occlusion pressures is helpful.[141] Pressor management may be better titrated by information gained from calculation of pulmonary and systemic vascular resistance. Dopamine, compared with dobutamine, produces a much higher wedge pressure in hypoxic respiratory failure.[142,143] Continuous monitoring of SVO_2 and calculations of oxygen delivery and extraction lend objectivity to transfusion decisions.[144] Thus, the right heart catheter with continuous SVO_2 monitoring is as close as technologically possible to definitive indexes of cell oxygenation. The judicious employment of these data allows clinicians to simultaneously consider hemodynamic and respiratory system events during ventilation.

Kidney and Water Balance

Application of PEEP has been demonstrated to decrease urine output, decrease sodium excretion[137,145] and cause a positive water balance. The administration of dopamine can modify these effects.[146,147] The causes are undoubtedly multifactorial. Decreased loss of water secondary to humidified air, decreased cardiac output, increased antidiuretic hormone secretion, altered intrarenal blood flow, and decreased atrial natriuretic peptides play a role.[146]

Research results have minimized the importance of increased antidiuretic hormone.[148] Atrial natriuretic peptide levels have been observed to triple with concomitant increases in urine output and sodium excretion following cessation for a brief period of ventilation.[149] Others have speculated that the observed shift in renal blood flow from cortical to juxtamedullary regions causes decreased renal function.[150]

Hepatic Function

The liver is an important organ in modulating host response to acute lung injury and is a target organ for cytokines released by lung inflammation.[151,152] Thus, it is difficult to separate the effects of positive pressure ventilation from host inflammatory effects when interpreting data from experimental models of liver dysfunction during ventilation. Positive pressure ventilation alters hepatic blood flow and distribution independent of static increases in intrathoracic pressure.[153]

Central Nervous System

A large percentage of pediatric critical care patients who require mechanical ventilation have sustained injury to the CNS from trauma, infection, and/or hypoxic, ischemic insults. Positive pressure ventilation exacerbates increased intracranial pressure. However, hyperventilation-induced hypocapnia is a major tool employed in the treatment of increased intracranial pressure.

Intrathoracic positive pressure impedes venous drainage from the cranial vault and increases intracranial blood volume. Cerebral perfusion pressure may also fall with a drop in arterial pressure subsequent to positive pressure ventilation, especially with the application of PEEP.[154] Transmission of intrathoracic pressure to the cerebral vault appears to be attenuated by decreased lung compliance.[155] In patients with normal lungs, an increase in intracranial pressure occurs with positive pressure ventilation. Also, when PEEP is discontinued abruptly in these patients, intracranial pressure rises dramatically, secondary to an increase in cardiac output.[155] Patients with altered neurologic status who require high PEEP and P̄aw are candidates for placement of devices to monitor intracranial pressure.

Nosocomial Pneumonia

Nosocomial infection is a commonly encountered problem with pneumonia, representing one third of all such infections in ventilated patients.[156] Research data indicate that contamination of the ventilator circuit, provided appropriate hand washing and universal precautions are maintained, is from the patient.[157,158] That is, the patient contaminates the circuit. It is reasonable to state, based on available evidence, that nosocomial pneumonias are a result of silent aspiration of gastric contents or oral secretions.[159,160] Prophylactic use of nonabsorbable antimicrobial agents has been shown to reduce both colonization and infection from Gram-negative organisms and yeast in intubated pediatric patients.[161] Because aspiration has been shown to occur frequently, even in intubated patients, these findings may have broad implications for the care of the compromised host.[159] Based on these and recent data on ventilator circuit change frequency, ventilator circuits need not be changed more frequently than once per week.[162,163]

Evaluating the Patient Who Becomes Acutely Hypoxemic

Hypoxemia can arise as a result of mechanical complications related to the ventilator or problems related to the patient. The safety of mechanical ventilation is determined as much by ICU design and staffing as by monitoring technology. Expensive bedside monitors of heart rate, respiratory rate, and SaO_2 alone are inadequate for the detection of ventilation-related incidents. Mechanical ventilators have multiple and often redundant alarms. Unless perceptive and well-trained pediatric-oriented respiratory therapy and nursing personnel are available, these alarms are often treated as a nuisance and ignored. An ICU design that allows for constant observation of the ventilated patient by nursing staff is crucial to the prevention and detection of mechanical mishaps.

Figure 16-24 is a conceptualized representation of the patient-ventilator system depicting the multiple technical or pathophysiologic complications that frequently develop during mechanical ventilation. Beginning with the ventilator, disruption of gas delivery, either oxygen or compressed air (1), prevents the ventilator from operating properly. Inadvertent adjustment of gas delivery

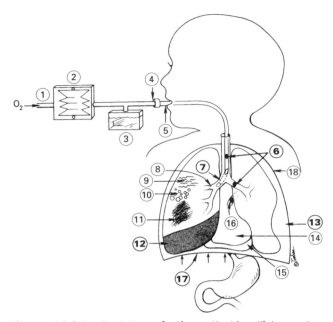

Figure 16-24. Depiction of zthe patient/ventilator system, highlighting those specific areas where technical and pathophysiologic complications of mechanical ventilation may occur. Note: Numbers in bold type (6, 7, 12, 13, 17) represent the most common complications clinically encountered in the patient. See text for details. Schematic illustration by I. David Todres.

variables or a disconnection of the inspiratory/expiratory circuit from the ventilator (2) may occur. The humidifier (3) is a potential location for many adverse events: disconnection, inadequate humidification, and excessive gas temperature. Disconnection of the ventilator circuit from the artificial airway (4) is a life-threatening complication of ventilatory support. Appropriate settings of both volume and pressure alarms are necessary to prevent a catastrophe, by rapid notification of a ventilator disconnection. During oral endotracheal intubation, kinking of the airway (5) is common in the active, alert child. Improper humidification, the administration of aerosolized ribavirin, and poor bronchial hygiene can precipitate obstruction of the endotracheal tube (artificial airway). A blood clot may obstruct the tube following a traumatic intubation (6). Major obstruction of the patient's natural airway may result from inadequate humidification and poor bronchial hygiene (6). Endobronchial intubation (7) is always a concern immediately postintubation and may also occur in patients who are active or require frequent repositioning. Inadvertent extubation may also occur. Bronchospasm and airway edema (8) compromise gas distribution and increase ventilating pressure. Pulmonary edema (9), interstitial air (10), pulmonary hemorrhage (11), and atelectasis (12) are all possible complications of mechanical ventilation. Pneumothorax (13) can develop in any ventilated patient but is a potentially greater problem with localized overdistention and high alveolar distending pressure. Cardiovascular compromise (14) due to decreased cardiac output leads to lower mixed venous PO_2 and potentially a lower PaO_2. Dissecting air as a result of gross air leak may enter the pericardium, producing cardiac tamponade (15). Major pulmonary embolus (16), although uncommon, is a possible cause of acute hypoxemia, secondary to embolization from long-standing central lines. In addition, pulmonary air embolus may follow accidental entry of air into the circulation. Abdominal distension (gastric dilation, ileus, ascites, peritoneal dialysis) (17) may impede diaphragmatic movement and thus effective ventilation. Chest wall restriction (18) from edema, splinting secondary to pain, and artificial binders may affect ventilation.

For immediate correction of the hypoxemic episode, the patient should be removed from the ventilator and "bagged" with 100% oxygen (ensuring that the oxygen is flowing to the resuscitation bag) and PEEP equivalent to the ventilator setting. This procedure eliminates any problems relating to the ventilator circuit (1–4). If the problem is not immediately resolved with "bagging," the problem is thus patient-related. The bold number's in Fig. 16-24 (i.e., 6, 7, 12, 13, 17) depict the most common causes of acute hypoxemia, and therefore management should immediately focus on these priorities. Endotracheal tube patency and positioning is of paramount importance. Immediate suctioning of the airway should be followed by confirming the correct positioning of the tube. This is done by checking for bilateral and equal chest expansion, both visually and on auscultation and, if necessary, performing a laryngoscopy to check for inadvertent extubation or malpositioning into a mainstem bronchus (markings on the tube will indicate the distance of the tube beyond the vocal cords). A tension pneumothorax should **always** be considered. If clinically suspected, needling of the chest should be performed, especially if desaturation is marked and accompanied by hemodynamic compromise. A chest x-ray should be carried out to further evaluate the problem (e.g., atelectasis, confirming the endotracheal tube position, and further evaluation of a possible pneumothorax). Further clinical evaluation includes assessment of abdominal distress as a possible cause of underventilation and acute hypoxemia. Placing a nasogastric tube or rechecking an existing one for proper positioning and patency is important in decompressing the abdomen.

References

1. Chatburn RL. A new system for understanding ventilators. *Respir Care* 36:1123–1155, 1991.
2. Hubmayr RD. Alternative modes of mechanical ventilation: On the aberration of inspiratory pressure and flow profiles. *Int Crit Care Dig* 9:28–30, 1990.
3. Stoller JK. Determining the need for mechanical ventilation. In Pierson DJ, Kacmarek RM (eds): *Foundations of Respiratory Care.* New York: Churchill Livingstone, 1992.
4. Aldrick TK, Prezant DJ. Indications for mechanical ventilation. In Tobin MJ (ed): *Principles and Practice of Mechanical Ventilation.* New York: McGraw-Hill, 1994.
5. Malloy DW, Dhingra S, Solven FS. Hypomagnesemia and respiratory muscle power. *Am Rev Respir Dis* 129:497–498, 1984.
6. Planus RF, McBrayer RH, Koen PA. Effect of hypophosphatemia on pulmonary muscle performance. *Adv Exp Med Biol* 151:283–290, 1982.
7. Aubier M et al. Effects of hypocalcemia on diaphragmatic strength generation. *J Appl Physiol* 58:2054–2061, 1985.
8. Pingleton SK. Nutritional support in the mechanically ventilated patient. *Clin Chest Med* 9:101–112, 1988.
9. Arora NS, Rochester DF. Effect of body weight and muscularity on human diaphragm muscle mass, thickness, and area. *J Appl Physiol* 52:64–70, 1982.
10. Petrof BJ et al. Continuous positive airway pressure reduces work of breathing and dyspnea during weaning from mechanical ventilation in severe COPD. *Am Rev Respir Dis* 141:281–289, 1990.
11. McCully KK, Faulkner JA. Length-tension relationship of mammalian diaphragm muscles. *J Appl Physiol* 54:1681–1686, 1983.
12. Smith TC, Marini JJ. Impact of PEEP on lung mechanics and work of breathing in severe airflow obstruction. *J Appl Physiol* 65:1488–1499, 1988.
13. Braun NMT, Arora NS, Rochester DF. Respiratory muscle and pulmonary function in polymyositis and other proximal myopathies. *Thorax* 38:616–623, 1983.
14. Aldrich TK, Prezant DJ. Adverse effects of drugs on the respiratory muscles. *Clin Chest Med* 11:177–189, 1990.
15. Talpers SS et al. Nutritionally associated increased carbon dioxide production: Excess total calories vs. high proportion of carbohydrate calories. *Chest* 102:551–555, 1992.
16. Pierson DJ. Respiratory failure: Introduction and overview. In Pierson DJ, Kacmarek RM (eds): *Fundamentals of Respiratory Care.* New York: Churchill Livingstone, 1992.
17. Shapiro BA et al. *Clinical Application of Respiratory Care* (4th ed). Chicago: Mosby, 1991.
18. Kacmarek RM. Methods of providing mechanical ventilatory support. In Pierson DJ, Kacmarek RM (eds): *Fundamentals of Respiratory Care.* New York: Churchill Livingstone, 1992.
19. Marcy T, Marini J. Inverse ratio ventilation: Rationale and implementation. *Chest* 100:494–504, 1991.
20. Ravenscraft S, Burke W, Marini J. Volume cycled, decelerating flow: An alternative form of mechanical ventilation. *Chest* 101:1342–1351, 1992.
21. Marcy T et al. Mean alveolar pressure is higher during ventilation with constant pressure than with constant flow or sinusoidal flow wave forms (abstr). *Am Rev Respir Dis* 141:A239, 1990.
22. Abraham E, Yoshihara G. Cardiorespiratory effects of pressure controlled ventilation in severe respiratory failure. *Chest* 98:1445–1449, 1990.
23. Al-Saady N, Bennett ED. Decelerating flow waveform improves lung mechanics and gas exchange in patients on intermittent positive pressure ventilation. *Intensive Care Med* 11:68–75, 1985.
24. Baker AB et al. Effects of varying inspiratory flow waveform and time in intermittent positive pressure ventilation. *Br J Anaesth* 49:1221–1233, 1977.
25. Baker AB, Restall R, Clark BW. Effects of varying inspiratory flow waveform and time in intermittent positive pressure ventilation: Emphysema. *Br J Anaesth* 54:547–554, 1982.
26. Tharratt R, Allen R, Albertson T. Pressure controlled inverse ratio ventilation in severe adult respiratory failure. *Chest* 94:755–762, 1988.
27. Gurevitch M et al. Improved oxygenation and lower peak airway pressure in severe adult respiratory distress syndrome: Treatment with inverse ratio ventilation. *Chest* 89:211–213, 1986.
28. Cole A, Weller S, Sykes M. Inverse ratio ventilation compared with PEEP in adult respiratory failure. *Intensive Care Med* 10:227–232, 1984.
29. Mang H et al. Cardiopulmonary effects of volume and pressure controlled CPPV at various I:E ratios in an acute lung injury model. *Am J Respir Crit Care Med* 151:731–736, 1995.
30. Lessard MRE et al. Effects of pressure-controlled with different I:E ratios versus volume-controlled ventilation on respiratory mechanics, gas exchange, and hemodynamics in patients with adult respiratory distress. *Anesthesiology* 80:983–991, 1994.
31. Munoz J et al. Pressure-controlled ventilation versus controlled mechanical ventilation with decelerating inspiratory flow. *Crit Care Med* 21:1143–1148, 1993.
32. Mercat A et al. Cardiorespiratory effects of pressure controlled ventilation with and without inverse ratio in the adult respiratory distress syndrome. *Chest* 104:871–875, 1993.
33. Brandolese R et al. Effects of intrinsic PEEP on pulmonary gas exchange in mechanically-ventilated patients. *Eur Respir J* 6:358–363, 1993.
34. MacIntyre NR et al. The Nagoya Conference on system design and patient-ventilator interactions during pressure support ventilation. *Chest* 97:1463–1466, 1990.
35. Hursh C, Kacmarek RM, Stanek K. Work of breathing during CPAP and PSV imposed by the new generation mechanical ventilators: A lung model study. *Respir Care* 36:815–828, 1991.
36. MacIntyre NR. Respiratory function during pressure support ventilation. *Chest* 89:677–683, 1986.

37. Brochard L et al. Pressure support prevents diaphragmatic fatigue during weaning from mechanical ventilation. *Am Rev Respir Dis* 139:513–521, 1989.

38. Nishimura M et al. Comparison of inspiratory work of breathing between flow-triggered and pressure-triggered demand flow systems in rabbits. *Crit Care Med* 22:1002–1009, 1994.

39. Kirby RR et al. A new pediatric volume ventilator. *Anesth Analg* 50:533–537, 1971.

40. Kirby RR et al. Continuous flow as an alternative to assisted or controlled ventilation in infants. *Anesth Analg* 18:179–189, 1972.

41. Downs JB, Klein EF, Desautels RA. Intermittent mandatory ventilation: A new approach to weaning patients from mechanical ventilation. *Chest* 64:331–335, 1973.

42. Luce JM, Pierson DJ, Hudson LD. Intermittent mandatory ventilation. *Chest* 79:678–685, 1991.

43. Marini JJ, Smith TC, Lamb VJ. External work output and force generation during synchronized intermittent mechanical ventilation: Effect of machine assistance on breathing effort. *Am Rev Respir Dis* 138:1169–1179, 1988.

44. Hewlett AM, Platt AS, Terry VG. Mandatory minute ventilation. *Anesthesiology* 32:163–169, 1977.

45. Chapin C et al. A new method of weaning from mechanical ventilation: CO2-regulated ventilation. *Presse Med* 12:495–497, 1983.

46. Hill NS et al. Efficacy of nocturnal mask ventilation in patients with restrictive thoracic disease. *Am Rev Respir Dis* 145:365–371, 1992.

47. Downs JB, Stock MC. Airway pressure release ventilation: A new concept in ventilatory support. *Crit Care Med* 15:459–461, 1987.

48. Räsänen J, Downs JB, Stock MC. Cardiovascular effects of conventional positive pressure ventilation and airway pressure release ventilation. *Chest* 93:911–915, 1988.

49. Valentine DP et al. Distribution of ventilation and perfusion with different modes of mechanical ventilation. *Am Rev Respir Dis* 143:1262–1266, 1991.

50. Cane RD, Peruzzi WT, Shapiro BA. Airway pressure release ventilation in severe acute respiratory failure. *Chest* 100:460–463, 1991.

51. Walham RE. Nocturnal nasal intermittent positive pressure ventilation with bilevel positive airway pressure (BiPAP) in respiratory failure. *Chest* 101:516–521, 1992.

52. Elliott MW et al. Domiciliary norturnal nasal intermittent positive pressure ventilation in hypercapnia respiratory failure due to chronic obstructive lung disease: Effects on sleep and quality of life. *Thorax* 47:342–348, 1992.

53. Restrick LJ et al. Nasal intermittent positive-pressure ventilation in weaning intubated patients with chronic respiratory disease from assisted positive-pressure ventilation. *Respir Med* 87:199–204, 1993.

54. Kacmarek RM. The role of pressure support ventilation in reducing the work of breathing. *Respir Care* 33:99–120, 1988.

55. Kirby RR, Banner JM, Downs JB (eds). *Clinical Application of Ventilatory Support* (2nd ed). New York: Churchill Livingstone, 1990.

56. Pingleton SK. Complications associated with mechanical ventilation. In Tobin MJ (ed): *Principles and Practice of Mechanical Ventilation*. New York: McGraw-Hill, 1994.

57. Kacmarek RM. Management of the patient's mechanical ventilator system. In Pierson DJ, Kacmarek RM (ed): *Foundations of Respiratory Care*. New York: Churchill Livingstone, 1992.

58. Bowe R. Monitoring ventilatory mechanics in acute respiratory failure. *Respir Care* 28:597–603, 1983.

59. Katz JA et al. Time course and mechanisms of lung-volume increase with PEEP in acute pulmonary failure. *Anesthesiology* 54:9–16, 1981.

60. Suter PM, Fairley HB, Isenberg MD. Optimum end-expiratory airway pressure in patients with acute pulmonary failure. *N Engl J Med* 292:284–289, 1975.

61. Bergman NA. Intrapulmonary gas trapping during mechanical ventilation at rapid frequencies. *Anesthesiology* 37:626–633, 1972.

62. Maunder RJ et al. Preservation of normal lung regions in the adult respiratory distress syndrome: Analysis by computed tomography. *JAMA* 255:2463–2465, 1986.

63. Gattinoni L et al. Pressure-volume curve of total respiratory system in acute respiratory failure: Computed tomographic scan study. *Am Rev Respir Dis* 136:730–736, 1987.

64. Kacmarek RM et al. The effects of applied vs auto-PEEP on local lung unit pressure and volume in a four-unit lung model. *Chest* 1995;108:1073–1079.

65. Smith TC, Marini JJ. Impact of PEEP on lung mechanics and work of breathing in severe airflow obstruction. *J Appl Physiol* 65:1488–1499, 1988.

66. Pepe PE, Marini JJ. Occult positive end-expiratory pressure in mechanically ventilated patients with airflow obstruction: The auto-PEEP effect. *Am Rev Respir Dis* 126:166–170, 1982.

67. Brown DG, Pierson DJ. Auto-PEEP is common in mechanically ventilated patients: A study of incidence, severity, and detection. *Respir Care* 31:1069–1074, 1986.

68. Petrof BJ et al. Continuous positive airway pressure reduces work of breathing and dyspnea during weaning from mechanical ventilation in severe COPD. *Am Rev Respir Dis* 141:281–289, 1990.

69. Ranieri VM et al. Physiologic effects of positive end-expiratory pressure in patients with obstructive pulmonary disease during acute ventilatory failure and controlled mechanical ventilation. *Am Rev Respir Dis* 149:5–13, 1993.

70. Field S, Sanci S, Grassino A. Respiratory muscle oxygen consumption estimated by the diaphragm pressure-time index. *J Appl Physiol* 57:44–51, 1984.

71. Hylkema BS et al. Central venous versus esophageal pressure changes for calculation of lung compliance during mechanical ventilation. *Crit Care Med* 11:271–275, 1983.

72. Christopher KL, Neff TA, Bowman JL. Demand and continuous flow intermittent mandatory ventilation systems. *Respir Care* 33:625–630, 1984.

73. Marini JJ, Capps JS, Culver BH. The inspiratory work of breathing during assisted ventilation. *Chest* 87:612–618, 1985.

74. Sassoon CSH et al. Inspiratory muscle work of breathing during blow-by, demand-flow, and continuous-flow systems in patients with chronic obstructive pulmonary disease. *Am Rev Respir Dis* 148:1219–1222, 1992.

75. Sassoon CSH et al. Inspiratory work of breathing on flow-by and demand-flow continuous positive airway pressure. *Crit Care Med* 17:1108–1119, 1989.

76. Shapiro W, Wilson RK, Casar G. Work of breathing through different sized endotracheal tubes. *Crit Care Med* 14:1028–1031, 1986.

77. Wright PE, Marini JJ, Bernard GR. In vitro versus in vivo comparison of endotracheal tube airflow resistance. *Am Rev Respir Dis* 140:10–16, 1989.

78. Brochard L et al. Inspiratory pressure support compensates for the additional work of breathing caused by the endotracheal tube. *Anesthesiology* 75:739–745, 1991.

79. Marini JJ, Rodriguez M, Lamb V. The inspiratory workload of patient-initiated mechanical ventilation. *Am Rev Respir Dis* 134:902–909, 1986.

80. Polysongsang Y et al. Effect of flow rate and duration of use on the pressure drop across six artificial noses. *Respir Care* 34:902–907, 1989.

81. Branson RN et al. AARC Guidelines: Humidification during mechanical ventilation. *Respir Care* 37:887–890, 1992.

82. Bryan CC, Jenkinson SG. Oxygen toxicity. *Clin Chest Med* 9:141–152, 1988.

83. Duane P. Pulmonary insults due to transfusion radiation and hyperoxia. *Semin Respir Infect* 3:240–246, 1988.

84. Comroe JH et al. The effect of inhalation of high concentrations of oxygen for 24 hours on normal men at sea level and at a simulated altitude of 18,000 ft. *JAMA* 128:710–717, 1945.

85. Lodata RF. Oxygen toxicity. In Tobin MJ (ed): *Principles and Practice of Mechanical Ventilation*. New York: McGraw-Hill, 1994.

86. Kacmarek RM, Hickling K. Permissive hypercapnia. *Respir Care* 38:373–387, 1993.

87. Marini J, Kelsen S. Re-targeting ventilatory objectives in adult respiratory distress syndrome. *Am Rev Respir Dis* 146:2–3, 1992.

88. Hickling K. Ventilatory management of ARDS: Can it affect outcome? *Intensive Care Med* 16:219–226, 1990.

89. Hurford WE, Teboul JL. Cardiovascular function during acute respiratory failure. In Zapol WM, Lemaire F (eds): *Adult Respiratory Distress Syndrome.* New York: Marcel Dekker, 1991.

90. Kumar A et al. Continuous positive-pressure ventilation in acute respiratory failure. *N Engl J Med* 273:1430–1436, 1970.

91. Kirby RR et al. Cardiorespiratory effects of positive end-expiratory pressure. *Anesthesiology* 43:533–539, 1975.

92. Murray IP et al. Titration of PEEP by the arterial minus end-tidal CO_2 gradient. *Chest* 85:100–104, 1984.

93. Qvist J et al. Hemodynamic responses to mechanical ventilation with PEEP. *Anesthesiology* 42:45–49, 1975.

94. Marini JJ, Wheeler AP. *Critical Care Medicine: The Essentials.* Baltimore: Williams & Wilkins, 1989.

95. Hobelmann CF et al. Hemodynamic alterations with positive end-expiratory pressure: The contribution of the pulmonary vasculature. *J Trauma* 15:951–959, 1975.

96. Fewell JE, Abendschein DR, Carlson CJ. Mechanism of decreased right and left ventricular end-diastolic volumes during continuous positive-pressure ventilation in dogs. *Circ Res* 47:467–473, 1980.

97. Lenfant C, Howell BJ. Cardiovascular adjustment in dogs during continuous positive-pressure breathing. *J Appl Physiol* 15:425–432, 1960.

98. Robotham JL et al. The effects of positive end-expiratory pressure on right and left ventricular performance. *Am Rev Respir Dis* 121:677–684, 1980.

99. Dorinsky PM, Whitcomb ME. The effects of PEEP on cardiac output. *Chest* 84:210–218, 1983.

100. Benito S, Lemaire F. Pulmonary pressure-volume relationship in acute respiratory distress synchrome in adults: Role of positive end-expiratory pressure. *J Crit Care* 5:27–34, 1990.

101. Pesenti A et al. Mean airway pressure vs positive end-expiratory pressure during mechanical ventilation. *Crit Care Med* 13:34–37, 1985.

102. Gattinoni L et al. Regional effects and mechanism of positive end-expiratory pressure in early adult respiratory distress syndrome. *JAMA* 269:2122–2127, 1993.

103. Ciszek T et al. Mean airway pressure: Significance during mechanical ventilation in neonates. *J Pediatr* 99:121–126, 1981.

104. Marcy TW. Inverse ratio ventilation. In Tobin MJ (ed): *Principles and Practices of Mechanical Ventilation.* New York: McGraw-Hill, 1994.

105. Dreyfuss D, Saumon G. Ventilator induced injury. In Tobin MJ (ed): *Principles and Practices of Mechanical Ventilation.* New York: McGraw Hill, 1994.

106. Dreyfuss D et al. High inflation pressure pulmonary edema: Respective effects of high airway pressure, high tidal volume and positive end-expiratory pressure. *Am Rev Respir Dis* 137:1159–1164, 1988.

107. West JB. *Respiratory Physiology: The Essentials* (4th ed). Baltimore: Williams & Wilkins, 1990.

108. Tobin MJ, Dantzker DR. Mechanical ventilation and weaning. In Dantzker DR (ed): *Cardiopulmonary Critical Care.* Orlando: Grune and Stratton, 1986.

109. Pollack MM, Fields AI, Holbrook PR. Pneumothorax and pneumomediastinum during pediatric mechanical ventilation. *Crit Care Med* 7:536–541, 1979.

110. Timmons OD, Dean JM, Vernon DD. Mortality rates and prognostic variables in children with adult respiratory distress syndrome. *J Pediatr* 119:896–899, 1991.

111. Moler FW, Palmisano J, Custer JR. Extracorporeal life support for pediatric respiratory failure: Predictors of survival from 220 patients. *Crit Care Med* 21:1604–1611, 1993.

112. Hillman K. Pulmonary barotrauma. *Clin Anesthesiol* 3:777–782, 1985.

113. Cullen DJ, Caldera DL. The incidence of ventilator induced pulmonary barotrauma in critically ill patients. *Anesthesiology* 50:185–190, 1979.

114. Hickling KG et al. Low mortality rate in adult respiratory distress syndrome using low-volume, pressure-limited ventilation with permissive hypercapnia: A prospective study. *Crit Care Med* 22:1568–1578, 1994.

115. Darioli A, Perret C. Mechanical controlled hypoventilation in status asthmaticus. *Am Rev Respir Dis* 129:385–387, 1984.

116. Slutsky AS. Mechanical ventilation: ACCP Concensus Conference. *Chest* 104:1833–1859, 1993.

117. Webb HH, Tierney DF. Experimental pulmonary edema due to intermittent positive pressure ventilation with high inflation pressure: Protection by positive end-expiratory pressure. *Am Rev Respir Dis* 110:556–565, 1974.

118. Hernandez LA et al. Chest wall restriction limits high airway pressure-induced lung injury in young rabbits. *J Appl Physiol* 66:2364–2368, 1989.

119. Kolobow T et al. Severe impairment in lung function induced by high peak airway pressure during mechanical ventilation: An experimental study. *Am Rev Respir Dis* 135:312–315, 1987.

120. Dreyfuss D et al. Intermittent positive-pressure hyperventilation with high inflation pressure produces pulmonary microvascular injury in rats. *Am Rev Respir Dis* 132:880–884, 1985.

121. Muscedere JG et al. Tidal ventilation at low airway pressure can augment lung injury. *Am J Respir Crit Care Med* 149:1327–1334, 1994.

122. Hickling KG, Henderson SJ, Jackson R. Low mortality associated with low volume, pressure limited ventilation with permissive hypercapnia in severe adult respiratory distress syndrome. *Intensive Care Med* 16:372–377, 1990.

123. Nunn JF. Carbon dioxide. In Nunn JF (ed): *Applied Respiratory Physiology* (2nd ed). London: Butterworths, 1977. Pp 334–374.

124. Puybasset L et al. Inhaled nitric oxide reverses the increase in pulmonary vascular resistence induced by permissive hypercapnia in patients with acute respiratory distress syndrome. *Anesthesiology* 80:1254–1267, 1994.

125. Graf H, Leach W, Arieff AI. Evidence for a detrimental effect of bicarbonate therapy in hypoxic lactic acidosis. *Science* 227:754–756, 1991.

126. Tobin MJ, Alex CG. Discontinuation of mechanical ventilation. In Tobin MJ (ed): *Principles and Practices of Mechanical Ventilation.* New York: McGraw-Hill, 1994.

127. Yang K, Tobin MJ. A prospective study of indexes predicting outcome of trials of weaning from mechanical ventilation. *N Engl J Med* 324:1445–1450, 1991.

128. Fiastro JF et al. Comparison of standard weaning parameters and mechanical work of breathing in mechanically ventilated patients. *Chest* 94:232–238, 1988.

129. Tobin MJ. Respiratory muscles in disease. *Clin Chest Med* 9:263–286, 1988.

130. Rochester DF, Braun NMT. Determinants of maximal inspiratory pressure in chronic obstructive pulmonary disease. *Am Rev Respir Dis* 132:42–47, 1985.

131. Lemaire F et al. Acute left ventricular dysfunction during unsuccessful weaning from mechanical ventilation. *Anesthesiology* 69:171–179, 1988.

132. Brochard L et al. Comparison of three methods of gradual withdrawal from ventilatory support during weaning from mechanical ventilation. *Am J Respir Crit Care Med* 150:896–903, 1944.

133. Heenen TJ et al. Intermittent mandatory ventilation: Is synchronization important? *Chest* 77:598–602, 1980.

134. Esteban A, Frutos F, Tobin MJ. A comparison of four methods of weaning patients from mechanical ventilation. *N Engl J Med* 332:345–350, 1995.

135. Hubmayer RD, Abel MD, Rehder K. Physiologic approach to mechanical ventilation. *Crit Care Med* 18:103–113, 1990.

136. Snyder JV, Carroll GC, Schuster DP. Mechanical ventilation: Physiology and application. *Curr Probl Surg* 21:40–45, 1984.

137. Froese SD, Bryan SC. Effects of anesthesia and paralysis on diaphragmatic mechanics in man. *Anesthesiology* 41:242–247, 1974.

138. Tyler DC. Positive end-expiratory pressure: A review. *Crit Care Med* 11:300–308, 1983.

139. Kanarak DJ, Shannon DC. Adverse effect of positive end-expiratory pressure on pulmonary perfusion and arterial oxygenation. *Am Rev Respir Dis* 112:456–459, 1975.

140. Cabrera MR, Nokamure GE, Montague DA. Effect of airway pressure on pericardial pressure. *Am Rev Respir Dis* 50:630–636, 1989.

141. Venus B, Cohen LE, Smith RA. Hemodynamic and intrathoracic pressure transmission during controlled mechanical ventilation and positive end-expiratory pressure in normal and low compliance lungs. *Crit Care Med* 16:686–692, 1988.

142. Luce JM. The cardiovascular effects of mechanical ventilation and positive end-expiratory pressure. *JAMA* 252:807–811, 1984.

143. Molloy WD et al. Hemodynamic management in clinical acute hypoxemic respiratory failure: Dopamine vs dobutamine. *Chest* 89:636–640, 1986.

144. Lucking SE, Pollock MM, Fields A. Shock following generalized hypoxic ischemic injury in previously health infants and children. *J Pediatr* 108:359–363, 1986.

145. Mink RB, Pollock MM. Effect of blood transfusion on oxygen consumption in pediatric septic shock. *Crit Care Med* 18:1087–1091, 1987.

146. Morquez JM et al. Renal function and cardiovascular responses during positive airway pressure. *Anesthesiology* 50:393–398, 1979.

147. Hemmer M, Suter PM. Treatment of cardiac and renal effects of PEEP with dopamine in patients with acute respiratory failure. *Anesthesiology* 50:399–403, 1979.

148. Priebe HJ, Heiman JC, Hedley-White J. Mechanism of renal dysfunction during positive end-expiratory pressure ventilation. *J Appl Phys Respir Environ Exercise Physiol* 50:643–648, 1981.

149. Payen DM, Farge D, Beloucif S. No involvement of antidiuretic hormone in acute antidiureses during PEEP ventilation in humans. *Anesthesiology* 66:17–25, 1987.

150. Ivariba H, Kohno M, Matsuura T. Circulating atrial natriuretic peptides during weaning from mechanical ventilation. *Chest* 91:797–804, 1987.

151. Strieter RM et al. Host responses in mediating sepsis and ARDS. *Semin Respir Infect* 5:233–247, 1990.

152. Kunkel S, Strieter RM. Cytokine networking in lung inflammation. *Hosp Pract* 34:63–76, 1990.

153. Matuschak BM, Pinsky MR. Effects of positive pressure ventilatory frequency on hepatic blood flow and performance. *J Crit Care* 4:153–165, 1989.

154. Aidinis S, Lefferty J, Sapiro HM. Intracranial responses to PEEP. *Anesthesiology* 45:275–286, 1976.

155. Huseby JS, Paulin EG, Butter J. Effect of positive end-expiratory pressure on intracranial pressure in dogs. *J Appl Physiol* 44:25–27, 1978.

156. Tobin MJ, Grensik A. Nosocomial lung infection and its diagnosis. *Crit Care Med* 12:191–196, 1984.

157. Craven DE et al. Nosocomial pneumonia: Epidemiology and infection control. *Intensive Care Med* 18:S3–S9, 1992.

158. Torres A et al. Gastric and pharyngeal flora in nosocomial pneumonia acquired during mechanical ventilation. *Am Rev Respir Dis* 148: 352–357, 1993.

159. Browning DH, Graves SA. Incidence of aspiration with endotracheal tubes in children. *J Pediatr* 102:582–585, 1983.

160. Kingston GW, Phang PT, Leathley MJ. Increased incidence of pneumonia in mechanically ventilated patients with subclinical aspiration. *Am J Surg* 161:589–592, 1991.

161. Zobel G et al. Reduction of colonization and infection rate during pediatric intensive care by selective decontamination of the digestive tract. *Crit Care Med* 19:1242–1245, 1991.

162. Dreyfuss D et al. Prospective study of nosocomial pneumonia and of patients and circuit colonization during mechanical ventilation with circuit changes every 48 hours versus no change. *Am Rev Respir Dis* 143:738–743, 1991.

163. Hess D et al. Weekly ventilator circuit changes: A strategy to reduce cost without affecting pneumonia rates. *Anesthesiology* 82;903–911, 1995.

Joseph R. Custer
Olugbenga A. Akingbola

17 Extracorporeal Life Support

Extracorporeal life support (ECLS) has undergone an interesting evolution, and a history of its development is invaluable to understanding the rationale for the reemergence of interest in clinical trials. The technology and equipment used in this therapy were designed in the early 1950s for use in cardiac surgery. The first successful membrane oxygenators were developed in the early 1950s by Clowes et al.[1] Successful and efficient oxygenators for commercial use, these could be adapted for long-term use. The roller pump, still in use today, was developed over 40 years ago. Bartlett[2] has reviewed the development of extracorporeal support in detail.

In the early 1960s, experiments employing long-term bypass in animals were carried out in many laboratories.[3,4] These laboratories set the stage for allowing safe short-term bypass for the burgeoning field of cardiovascular surgery. Early problems that limited the application of this technology were hemolysis, increased capillary permeability, and multiple organ failure.[5] These problems were eventually solved. However, the major limitation, then and now, has been bleeding induced by the need for anticoagulation.

A crucial early clinical contribution in basic research use of ECLS was the observation of Bartlett et al.[6,7] that small doses of heparin could decrease bleeding and still prevent clotting in the circuits. Without the ability to manage and monitor heparin effects, bleeding in patients would have prevented clinical trials of long-term bypass.

In 1972, Hill et al.[8] reported the first successful use of protracted ECLS in a motorcycle accident victim. Bartlett and colleagues[9] rescued a neonate with ECLS and presented their results in 1975. These reports occurred simultaneously with the recognition of nearly uniform fatality in surgical patients who developed what was coined "shock lung," a form of hypoxemic respiratory failure now recognized as adult respiratory distress syndrome (ARDS). In 1975, a National Institutes of Health (NIH)–sponsored extracorporeal membrane oxygenation (ECMO) trial for the treatment of ARDS was begun, and the results were reported in 1979.[10] This ambitious feasibility trial of a complex technology (with death as an outcome) interpreted ECMO as a failure. The study was planned for 300 patients, but was stopped after 92 patients when survival in both ECMO and control groups was found to be 8%. Modern insight into the study reveals many problems. Many of the centers participating in the study had no experience with ECLS. Thus, learning-curve patients were included in the data analysis. A nationwide epidemic of severe influenza B was in progress, and these patients dominated the trial. Many of these patients would not be candidates for ECMO today. Bleeding losses per day were 10 times higher than that observed today and contributed to excessive mortality in the ECMO group. The contribution of high airway pressure to lung pathology is now well accepted. In the trial, however, ECMO patients remained on 100% oxygen and high inflation pressures; therefore, no ECMO patient was provided lung rest, which is now known to be the primary benefit of ECMO therapy. Overinterpretation of the results and lack of an understanding of the pathophysiology of barotrauma led to a moratorium in applied ECMO research in the United States.

Two investigators continued clinical investigations. The pioneering work of Bartlett and Gattinoni has led to a renaissance in clinical research. Bartlett and colleagues[11] recognized that new-born respiratory failure was temporary. If gas exchange could be supported without the toxicity of mechanical ventilation, the neonate could survive. Indeed, by 1981, 45 cases of neonatal respiratory failure, with 25 babies surviving, were reported. Bartlett began holding seminars to disseminate the technology in 1979. As more experience accumulated, a registry was established to collect data from all patients. By 1986, 715 cases, with an 80% survival rate, had been reported.[12] These results were sensational because the general perception at the time was that these infants met 90% mortality criteria.

By 1995, ECMO has been utilized in 10,391 cases of neonatal respiratory failure with an 80% survival rate. In pediatric patients aged 1 month to 17 years, 982 ECMO cases have been reported with 53% surviving.

Several pathways of investigation have led to this "propagation" of ECLS technology in the pediatric patient. The success observed in the neonatal age group led many centers to attempt ECLS in an older age group. Eighty-one centers have reported 5683 neonatal cases to the registry, with a survival rate of 83%.[13] A further stimulus to the use of ECMO in children was the cumulative experience in Europe and, to a lesser extent, in Japan in using ECMO in adults who met 90% mortality criteria generated from the first NIH trial. Gattinoni, in 1986, reported a 50% survival in 43 patients from Monza, Italy.[14] Other European investigators, including Lennartz in Marburg, Falke in Dusseldorf, and Bindslev in Stockholm, have similar results, with more than 50% survival in more than 300 patients. Nearly the same success was observed by Morioka in Japan.[2]

As centers accumulated experience with neonates and adults, the extension of this technology to children was natural and inevitable. Anderson et al., from the University of Michigan, reported 33 pediatric-age patients from 1971 to 1989.[15] Seventeen patients with primary respiratory disease had a survival of 47%. Mechanical complications included membrane lung failure, tubing rupture, and pump failure, none of which contributed to mortality. The major cause of death was irreversible lung injury or brain death.

Steinhorn and Green reported a single institution's experience in the use of venoarterial (V-A) bypass for support of respiratory syncytial virus (RSV) bronchiolitis in children unresponsive to conventional ventilator management. The survival rate was 58% in 12 patients. This is one of the few reports on the use of ECMO in a relatively homogeneous (single etiology of respiratory failure) population. Preexisting chronic lung disease did not predict survival.[16] These results are similar to those in a national report. Moler et al. reported the national experience in ECLS management of RSV-associated respiratory failure. By 1992, 53 patients were tested with ECMO and 49% survived.[17] Adolph and others reported their results in New Orleans at the Ochsner Clinic in the treatment of nonneonatal respiratory failure with extracorporeal membrane oxygenation.[18] The authors treated 22 patients ranging in age from 1 to 105 months and in weight from 3 to 35 kg. Eighteen of these patients met criteria for ARDS, two had RSV pneumonia, and one had severe barotrauma complicating the management of reactive airway disease. All patients were considered to be failing conventional management as evidenced by hypoxia, hypercarbia, excessive ventilatory pressures, or progressive barotrauma. All were considered likely to die with conventional management. Sixteen of the 22 patients had complications (73%), but one half of the most recent ten patients had no complications. Hemorrhagic complications predominated. Mechanical complications were common, but not related to patient morbidity. Eleven of 22 patients survived (50%), and nine of the most recent 12 patients survived. The authors suggest that ECMO is a useful technique for pediatric respiratory failure. This experience agrees with that noted in the ELSO registry, where 672 patients in this age group have been reported with a survival rate of approximately 50%. The increased survival rate in the most recent 12 patients could reflect better selection and exclusion of patients, less risk taking on the part of the authors, or improvement in a learning curve gained from previous experience. The survivors and deaths were similar in $PA-aO_2$. Oxygenation index was lower in the survivors, and a crested "respiratory severity index" was lower in the survivors. The survivors also had a lower mean airway pressure (MAP) and a lower peak inspiratory pressure (PIP). Prior to going on bypass, the survivors had a higher PO_2 and a slightly higher PCO_2.

These data raise several questions. In considering ECMO as an efficacious treatment for pediatric respiratory failure, what are appropriate selection and exclusion criteria? What is a reasonable expected mortality rate for severe respiratory failure, and are there morbidity predictors for respiratory failure in the childhood age group using conventional medical management? More data must be collected to document the natural history of morbid childhood lung disease. This is important to evaluate not only ECMO, but also conventional and novel therapies, such as new ventilators, surfactant, nitric oxide, and antiinflammatory agents.

Physiologic Assumptions

The current use of ECLS technology is based on several assumptions, clinical experience, and laboratory data. The purpose of mechanical ventilation is to remove carbon dioxide. Oxygenation can be preserved in most cases with alveolar inflation alone. An artificial lung can remove carbon dioxide. Peak and mean airway pressures can be reduced to safer levels while preserving enough alveolar volume to maintain oxygenation and prevent atelectasis, thus allowing "pulmonary rest."

Terminal respiratory failure is precipitated only if several events coexist. First, there must be an inciting injury such as sepsis, hypoxia, trauma, shock, or pneumonia. Second, the original insult must be followed by a massive host inflammatory response. These humoral and cellular interactions lead to accumulation of mesenchymal cells in alveoli, fibroproliferation, and, eventually, fibrosis. Platelets, leukocytes, and macrophages interact with the endothelium, damaging the alveolar capillary membrane. This damage is mediated by cytokines, including platelet activating factor, tumor necrosis factor, interleukins, and neutrophil chemotactic factor.[19,20]

It is now clear that, following these first two insults, mechanical ventilator-induced lung injury can produce a third, irreversible lung insult. Ventilator-induced airway pressure may play a major role in terminally damaging the lung. This key observation provides the fundamental hypothesis justifying the use of ECMO in patients with respiratory failure. If barotrauma is a major cause of terminal lung injury, and ECMO can support gas exchange while the lungs are rested (spared high-pressure ventilation), then ECMO will improve survival if it is employed prior to the initiation of ventilator-induced fibrosis.

Many laboratories have demonstrated the toxicity of mechanical ventilation. Greenfield et al.[21] ventilated normal dogs at peak airway pressures of 32 cm H_2O and observed changes consistent with ARDS. Barsch et al.[22] caused terminal lung failure in dogs ventilated at 34 cm H_2O airway pressure. Webb and Tierney[23] and Parker et al.[24] demonstrated that pulmonary edema could be created merely by ventilating animal lungs at high airway pressures. Dreyfus et al.[25,26] noted that high pressure and large tidal volumes were injurious to the lung. Both large tidal volumes and high airway pressures cause injury, even if negative-pressure ventilation is used. In an injured lung, cycling from high to low pressure worsened edema in a canine acid aspiration model.[27]

Early critics of conclusions drawn from these studies observed that low alveolar PCO_2 may have caused vasoconstriction and an ischemic injury. Kolobow et al.,[28] however, produced terminal respiratory failure in sheep ventilated with and without 4% carbon dioxide in the ambient air, but at high airway pressures, and produced ARDS pathology.

Reports of improved survival in adult ARDS when airway pressures are limited or controlled substantiate the conclusions of the laboratory data. Hickling et al.[29] observed a 16% mortality in ARDS patients for whom predicted mortality was 40% when peak airway pressures were limited to 40 cm H_2O and patients purposefully hypoventilated. Suchyta et al.[30] reported a 45% survival rate in a group of 178 ARDS patients, 51 of whom met the 90% mortality criteria used in the 1975 NIH trial. The patients were managed using a computer-driven algorithm that used pressure-controlled inverse ratio ventilation.

Moler et al.[31] have reported a survival rate of 70% in 57 pediatric respiratory failure patients who had a predicted mortality of 90%. These patients are placed on ECMO if 40 cm of H_2O pressure fails to support gas exchange adequately, and the A-a DO_2 is greater than 500 mm Hg despite maneuvers such as positive end-expiratory pressure (PEEP), reversed I:E ratio, and oscillation.

Gattinoni et al.[14] attributed the dramatic improvement they reported in ARDS survival to the lung rest and inflation-pressure limitation that could occur when an extracorporeal circuit was used to remove carbon dioxide. Kolobow[32] has summarized the data and mechanism of ventilator-induced lung injury in an insightful editorial.

Gattinoni et al.[33,34] noted a 70% reduction in lung volume available for recruitment maneuvers with airway pressure when compliance is less than 30 ml/cm H_2O. Thus, the tidal volume and airway pressure of a patient with ARDS are distributed to only 20% to 30% of the lung volume, producing overdistension and tissue destruction. Thus, a small remnant of normal lung, if ventilated at normal full tidal volume, will be drastically overdistended.

An understanding of these assumptions is necessary as patient selection criteria are developed. The optimal timing of ECMO in acute lung injury is before fibrosis occurs. In this light, this technology is not a rescue therapy, a therapy for multiple organ failure, or a therapy for chronic lung conditions. It is rather a complex method of providing for gas exchange without the hazards ensuant to positive-pressure ventilation.

Selection of Patients for ECLS Management: Pre-ECLS Management

Selection criteria for ECLS should not be discussed without an understanding of principles employed in the management of severe respiratory failure. Most centers of excellence and experience with the treatment of severe respiratory failure have embraced some or all of these precepts.[35]

The major common features include limited inflation pressures less than 40 cm H_2O, permissive hypercapnea so that PCO_2 is regulated only to keep pH above 7.2. The titration of oxygen, PEEP, and MAP is done by measuring pulmonary venous oxygen saturation continuously and maximizing oxygen delivery. Most centers aggressively attempt to minimize the effects of pulmonary edema by achieving dry weight. An appreciation of these concepts is needed to understand current selection criteria for ECLS, as patients must be rigorously managed in a prospective manner before ECLS is instituted.

At the University of Michigan, directors of the Adult Surgical and Critical Care Units have agreed on principles of respiratory failure management. These are summarized in Table 17-1. An agreed-on approach to patient management by conventional means allows development of institution-wide consensus for the criteria of ECLS use and new therapeutic strategies. Figure 17-1 represents a generic algorithm.

Patient Selection

Indications for ECLS therapy are based on historical data. In the 1975–1979 adult trial, the assumption was made that patients with a PaO_2 of 60 mm Hg or less, in an ambient FiO_2 of 0.6 or greater, had a predicted mortality of 90%. Today, there are no generally accepted inclusion criteria among the many centers that have entered data in the ELSO registry. Particularly disputed is the assumption that the blood gas criteria of the NIH trial, which were gathered historically, predict mortality accurately. A review of pediatric and adult ARDS survival data reflects current controversies in determination of mortality prediction and, consequently, the dilemmas encountered in devising criteria for use of this technology.

Suchyta reported increased survival of conventionally managed adult ARDS patients with severe hypoxemia when the 1979 NIH ECMO Trial Criteria were employed.[30] From 1975 to 1979, patients with severe hypoxemia who met the blood gas criteria defined by the NIH trial had a reported survival of 11%.[36] They speculated that numerous advances and evolutions in technology may have altered survival; the authors prospectively evaluated morbidity in ARDS patients meeting these older blood gas criteria. They studied 178 ARDS patients prospectively. Fifty-one of those patients met

Table 17-1. Management of severe respiratory failure

1. Breathing and ventilation is for CO_2 removal; inflation is for oxygenation.

2. Normalize O_2 delivery, not just PaO_2.

3. Oxygenation management (FiO_2, position, suction, PEEP, inotropes) is based on SvO_2.

4. In apnea, hypoxemia is fatal in minutes. Hypercarbia alone is never fatal.

5. Increasing FiO_2 decreases alveolar nitrogen and causes atelectasis.

6. Mechanical ventilation does more harm than good at high PIP and high FiO_2.

7. Never exceed PIP (plateau) over 40 cm H_2O. Hypercarbia is safer than PIP > 40.

8. Ventilation management (rate, pressure, volume) is based on $PaCO_2$ or end-tidal CO_2.

9. Achieve and maintain dry weight.

10. Don't confuse pulmonary capillary wedge pressure and hydration status.

the older NIH ECMO trial criteria. A 45% survival rate was observed with conventional ICU management. There were no obvious differences in etiology, APACHE 2 scores, organ system failure, or the incidence of sepsis between the survivors and nonsurvivors. The authors conclude that survival of ARDS patients meeting the older ECMO criteria was higher in this hospital than that previously reported in other centers. The authors have suggested that conventional ventilator management done in a protocolized manner may result in a much higher survival rate than that observed in 1979. In designing prospective trials to assess the effectiveness of ECMO as it influences survival in ARDS, these authors suggest that a survival rate on conventional management in 1991 may be closer to 45% than the previously reported 15%. The authors cite three explanations for the increased survival in their institution: (1) patient selection, (2) changes in medical technology in patient management, and (3) hospital-specific reasons. In this study, the patients were older than in the previous studies reported by Zapol et al. in the 1979 trial, and in the extracorporeal carbon dioxide removal trial of Gattinoni et al. There was, however, a common predominant risk factor for ARDS (i.e., pneumonia) in all of the studies. The study was prospective and reduced selection bias. The authors speculated that advances in medical technology, including antimicrobial agents, cardiac assist devices, organ transplantation, and nutritional support, all contribute to an increased survival in the modern era. They point out that evolutions in the use of such modalities as steroids and changes in fluid management are different now than 10 or 15 years ago. They suggest that permissive hypoventilation allowing hypercapnia by the use of smaller tidal volumes may lead to less diffusely damaged lungs in ARDS patients. Could the observations of this study have been hospital-specific? The authors' institution was at this time in a randomized trial aimed at the "Development of Detailed Computerized Protocols for the Management of Oxygenation in ARDS Patients." The authors speculate that interest and commitment to the ARDS patient may have increased significantly and, therefore, effected increased survival.

Three papers have studied the prediction of mortality in pediatric respiratory failure. Rivera et al. reported "predictors of mortality in children with respiratory failure" aimed at developing objective predictors of death with conventional management.[37] Globally agreed-on predictors of mortality with conventional therapy would make design of randomized trials and implementation of ECMO therapy more precise. To determine the predictors of death, the authors retrospectively evaluated the charts of 42 children, aged 1 month to 18 years, admitted to the Intensive Care Unit at Royal Children's Hospital in Parkfield, Victoria, Australia. All children were ventilated for more than 12 hours, received greater than 90% oxygen, had a PIP greater than 25 cm H_2O, and had no preexisting neurodevelopmental handicap. The authors developed a combination variable reflecting ventilation and another variable reflecting oxygenation, which reliably predicted death. A ventilation index greater than 40 and an oxygenation index greater than 0.4 was associated with a 77% chance of mortality. This produced a sensitivity of 65% and a specificity of 74%. A combination of PIP greater than 40 cm H_2O and an A-aDO_2 greater than 580 mm Hg had a specificity of 79%. The study excluded children who died from neurologic sequelae after hypoxic ischemic or septic insult. The authors defined ARDS as a syndrome of low lung compliance with hypoxia and diffuse alveolar and interstitial lung disease radiographically. The oxygenation index was defined as the MAP times the FiO_2 divided by the PaO_2. The ventilation index was defined as the respiratory rate times the PCO_2 times the peak inspiratory

Figure 17-1. Michigan Respiratory Failure Algorithm. SaO₂, arterial oxygen saturation; TV, tidal volume; PIP, peak inspiratory pressure; SVO₂, mixed venous oxygen saturation; CO, cardiac output; PRBC, packed red blood cells; PCWP, pulmonary capillary wedge pressure; PCIRV, pressure control inverse ratio ventilation. (Modified from Bartlett RH. *Critical Care Handbook* [11th ed]. Surgical Critical Care Program, Department of Surgery, University of Michigan, 1993. With permission.)

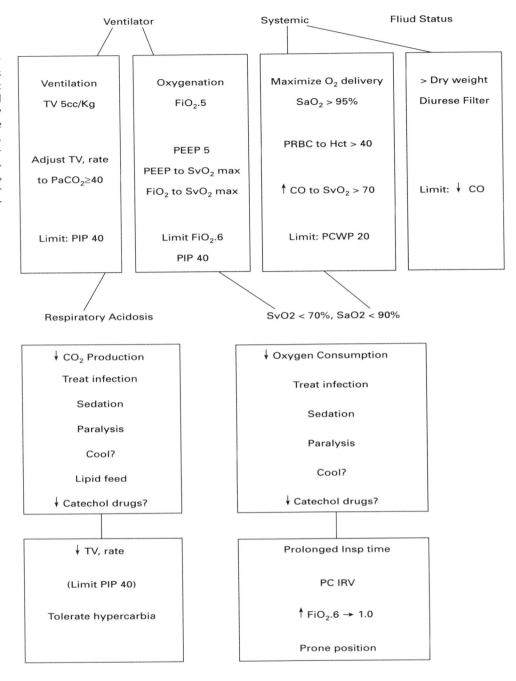

pressure, divided by 1000. Receiver operating curves were constructed for each of the clinical predictors.

Tamburro et al., from the University of Tennessee, evaluated the use of the alveolar-arterial oxygen gradient as a predictor of outcome in patients with nonneonatal pediatric respiratory failure.[38] The authors performed a 4-year observational descriptive study of all patients admitted with respiratory failure to the LeBonheur Children's Medical Center Pediatric Intensive Care Unit. During that time, 4800 patients were admitted to the unit. The first two and a half years of this study were retrospective, while the last year and a half was prospective. Patients with acute lung disease who required mechanical ventilation with a PaO₂ of less

than 60 mm Hg, while receiving an FiO₂ of greater than 0.5, were eligible. Patients with any pathologic process other than acute lung disease, such as chronic lung disease, congenital heart disease, neuromuscular disease, and severe head injury, were excluded. Also excluded were patients with severe hypoxic-ischemic encephalopathy or terminal disease. The study did not include patients less than 1 month of age. The authors identified 37 patients that met entrance criteria. Five of these were excluded because they died before completion of the 48-hour study period. Of the remaining 32 patients, 18 survived. Thirteen survivors and ten nonsurvivors were studied retrospectively; five survivors and four nonsurvivors were studied prospectively. Of the 14 deaths, 93%

(13) resulted from cardiorespiratory failure as a result of lung injury, while one death was caused by a hemothorax. An A-aDO$_2$ of greater than 450 mm Hg for 16 hours predicted death with 86% sensitivity, 100% specificity, and a P value less than .01, and was associated with a 100% mortality rate.

Timmons et al. reported a retrospective chart review of mortality rates and prognostic variables in children with ARDS.[39] In this review of cases from 1987 to 1990, the authors attempted to identify physiologic variables predictive of death. They identified 44 children, with a mortality rate of 75%. Significant differences between survivors and nonsurvivors were found in intrapulmonary venous admixture, MAP, A-aDO$_2$ gradient, oxygenation index, and PIP. Shunt fraction greater than 0.5, MAP greater than 23 cm H$_2$O, and alveolar arterial oxygen difference of more than 470 mm Hg were 93%, 90%, and 81% predictors of death, respectively. Sensitivity and specificity were enhanced when multiple predictors were linked. In this study, the oxygenation index was the airway pressure multiplied by the FiO$_2$ times 100, divided by the arterial partial pressure of oxygen. Notably, data included patients with near-drowning, asphyxia, and sudden infant death syndrome. Thus, patients with a high mortality rate from another related disease were included. For example, septic patients (mortality rate of 70%) and drowning patients (90% mortality) were included. There were three patients with sudden infant death syndrome who had a 100% mortality. One would assume the mortality rate in these patients would be extraordinarily high with or without respiratory failure.

Of note, in all three of these studies the survival rate from pediatric ARDS is still quite dismal (e.g., mortality rate in the Timmons' paper is 75%), thus, no improvement over data reported 10 years ago. The Tennessee study showed 18 survivors out of 32 patients. The Australian study had 23 deaths and 19 survivors. As opposed to adult ARDS survival data, the predominant cause of death in these studies was progressive respiratory failure. Adult data are not consistent with that observation, where patients tend not to die of respiratory failure but of multisystem organ failure or late-occurring sepsis.

Moler et al. have recently analyzed available data in the ELSO registry in an attempt to discover predictors of survival from hyoxic respiratory failure for children with ECMO therapy. Data from that study are seen in Tables 17-2 and 17-3. Stepwise multivariate logistic regression modeling found age and days of mechanical ventilation to correlate with survival.[40]

The same investigators have suggested that predictors of outcome can be drawn from existing data, such as in the ELSO Registry. The authors examined all cases of RSV-induced respiratory failure treated with ECLS. Fifty-three patients who reported to the ELSO Registry through June of 1992 were evaluated. The patient age was 5 months; duration of mechanical ventilation prior

Table 17-2. Survival trend by age groups in 220 pediatric respiratory failure patients receiving ECLS

Age Group	Total	Survived	% Survived
1 mo to 1 yr	99	60	60.6
1–2 yrs	46	18	39.1
2–8 yrs	50	19	38.0
Greater than 8 yrs	25	5	20.0

Data from Moler et al.[40]

Table 17-3. Survival trend of duration of mechanical ventilation prior to ECLS in 220 pediatric respiratory failure patients receiving ECLS

Mechanical ventilation duration before ECLS	Total	Survival %
0–3 d	86	54
4–6 d	52	52
7–10 d	50	44
Greater than 10 d	32	22

Data from Moler et al.[40]

to ECLS was 8 days. Forty-nine percent survived to discharge. Multivariate logistic regression analysis revealed four variables to be predictive of nonsurvival: male gender, duration of ventilation in days prior to bypass, PIP, and lower PaO$_2$/FiO$_2$ ratio.

Receiver operator characteristic curve analysis at a cutoff point of $r = 0.5$ revealed 92% sensitivity and 81% specificity. Thus, historical controls provide some insight into the development of criteria for ECLS therapy.[17] Wide alveolar-arterial gradients for oxygen have been observed to be associated with nonsurvival in several reports of pediatric hypoxic respiratory failure treated with mechanical ventilation. Moler et al. compared a group of pediatric patients managed with ECMO at the University of Michigan Medical Center. In 36 patients whose P(A-a)O$_2$ gradient would have predicted death, a 61% survival to discharge was observed.[41] Selection criteria in use at the University of Michigan are given in Table 17-4.

Experience has taught that exclusion criteria are at least as important as inclusion criteria. ECLS therapy is attractive because of its high technology. In the best of hands, however, the mortality rate is still 30% to 50%. Further, there inevitably exists a situation in which one is tempted to employ ECMO as rescue therapy for compassionate reasons. Given the current state of the art, rigid exclusion criteria are appropriate. This will avoid needless, yet agonizing, labor-intensive prolongation of death at great cost. The

Table 17-4. Eligibility criteria for ECMO

Age	Days of ventilation
<2 yrs	≤10
2–8 yrs	≤8
>8 yrs	≤6
Respiratory failure	
PEEP > 8 cm H$_2$O × 12 hours	
FiO$_2$ > .8 × 12 hours	
PaO$_2$/FiO$_2$ < 150	
P(A-a)O$_2$ > 450 mm Hg	
Respiratory acidosis	
pH < 7.28 with	
Peak inspiratory pressure 40 cm H$_2$O or airleak syndrome	
Maximal minute ventilation without air trapping	
Reasonable medical certainty of quality of life	

Table 17-5. Exclusion criteria for ECMO

Age	Days of ventilation
<2 yrs	≥10
2–8 yrs	≥8
>8 yrs	≥6
Major hemorrhage	
Immunosuppression	
Cardiac arrest with neurologic impairment	
Recent cerebral-vascular accident	
Certainty of low quality of life	

exclusion criteria at the University of Michigan are listed in Table 17-5.

Physiology of Gas Exchange

The spiral coil membrane lung, designed by Kolobow and others, is the predominant type of oxygenator used in ECLS. Membrane lungs (as opposed to bubble oxygenators) prevent exposure of air to blood and allow construction of noncompliant circuits. The membrane material is dimethylpolysiloxone, or silicon rubber. This material allows the diffusion of oxygen and carbon dioxide. Excellent gas exchange properties are achieved with low priming volumes at a cost, however, of high perfusion pressures. As blood flows over the membrane, oxygen diffuses into the blood as a result of the pressure gradient differences between 100% oxygen in the gas phase and the lower partial pressure of oxygen in the venous blood. Because a usual value for the venous PO_2 would be 40 mm Hg, the gradient, or driving force, for oxygen into the blood would be approximately 700 mm Hg. Simultaneously, carbon dioxide diffuses out of the blood because of the driving pressure difference between a venous PCO_2 of approximately 45 mm Hg

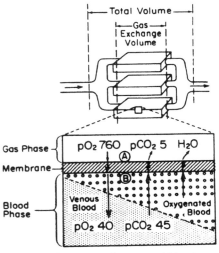

Figure 17-2. Partial pressures for gas and blood compartments in an artificial lung. (With permission from Chapman RA, Bartlett RH. *Extracorporeal Life Support Manual for Adult and Pediatric Patients.* ECMO Department, University of Michigan Medical Center, 1990.)

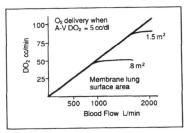

Figure 17-3. The total oxygen delivery is limited by oxygen-carrying capacity of the blood and flow through the artificial lung. When capacity for blood flow is exceeded, oxygenation efficiency decreases, as inadequate time for gas exchange occurs. This flow rate is termed the "rated" flow of the membrane lung. (With permission from Chapman RA, Bartlett RH. *Extracorporeal Life Support Manual for Adult and Pediatric Patients.* ECMO Department, University of Michigan Medical Center, 1990.)

and a partial pressure of 0 for carbon dioxide in the gas phase. These are summarized in Fig. 17-2.

As flow increases, oxygen transfer is increased proportionally. This is maximal when blood leaving the oxygenator is 95% saturated. Increasing flow beyond this point will actually overwhelm the time and membrane diffusion constants for a given lung, and blood will leave the lung desaturated. The flow rate that achieves maximal oxygen transfer is called "rated flow" (Fig. 17-3).

Carbon dioxide transfer through silicone rubber is 6 times greater than that for oxygen. Limitations for carbon dioxide transfer include the narrow gradient for carbon dioxide between venous blood and the gas phase, and commercially feasible membrane thickness. Most devices are capable of 200 ml/min/m² of carbon dioxide transfer. This is more efficient than oxygen transfer, so much so that carbon dioxide frequently needs to be added to the gas phase to prevent hypocapnea during clinical use.

The clinician should understand from this description two important facets of gas exchange with artificial membrane lungs. Oxygen transfer is flow dependent, and carbon dioxide removal is surface area dependent. Carbon dioxide removal is a more sensitive indicator of membrane function.

CO₂ Removal	Oxygen Transfer
Independent of blood flow membrane thickness	Independent of sweep gas flow
Dependent on gas diffusion gradient sweep gas flow membrane surface area	Dependent on membrane diffusion blood film thickness flow rate

Techniques and Physiology of Prolonged Bypass

The most common form of bypass for prolonged support is veno-arterial (V-A), or V-A bypass. Blood is drained from the internal jugular alone or in combination with a femoral vein. Because oxygenation is flow dependent, and flow is limited primarily by the internal diameter of the drainage cannula, adequate drainage is crucially dependent on site selection and catheter size.[42,43] The femoral vessels are usually inadequate as a sole source of blood in children. Blood is drained passively (by gravity) to a compliant

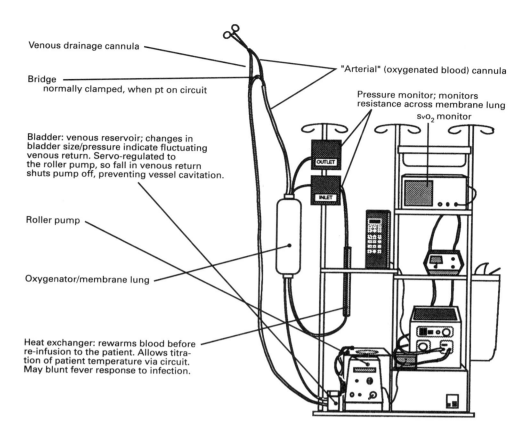

Venous drainage cannula

Bridge
normally clamped, when pt on circuit

"Arterial" (oxygenated blood) cannula

Pressure monitor; monitors
resistance across membrane lung
$S_{v}O_2$ monitor

Bladder: venous reservoir; changes in
bladder size/pressure indicate fluctuating
venous return. Servo-regulated to
the roller pump, so fall in venous return
shuts pump off, preventing vessel cavitation.

OUTLET

INLET

Roller pump

Oxygenator/membrane lung

Heat exchanger: rewarms blood before
re-infusion to the patient. Allows titration of patient temperature via circuit.
May blunt fever response to infection.

Figure 17-4. A typical ECLS circuit. (With permission from Chapman RA, Bartlett RH. *Extracorporeal Life Support Manual for Adult and Pediatric Patients.* ECMO Department, University of Michigan Medical Center, 1990.)

bladder. The bladder is attached to a servo-regulated micro switch so that if the bladder collapses, the pump will cut out, preventing cavitation. Blood is pumped with a rotor pump into the artificial lung. Pressures are monitored both proximal and distal to the membrane lung. Blood requires rewarming with a water jacket heat-exchanger device and is then returned to the descending aortic arch, utilizing the right carotid artery. A typical circuit is depicted in Fig. 17-4.

Total bypass is physiologically not achieveable in clinical circumstances; thus, the native heart continues to pump some blood through the damaged lung. When the lung is severely diseased, left ventricular blood will then have the same PaO_2 as the right atrium. This deoxygenated blood is added to blood returning from the oxygenator circuit in the descending aorta. This has two consequences. The coronary arteries are perfused with relatively deoxygenated blood. The oxygen content in the patient's aorta is a combination of poorly oxygenated blood from the native lung combined with the 100% saturated blood from the circuit. The resultant systemic oxygen content is thus given by the formula:

$$\text{Perfusate oxygen content} \times \frac{\text{extracorporeal circuit flow}}{\text{combined blood flow}}$$

$$+ \text{ Left ventricle oxygen content} \times \frac{\text{native lung flow}}{\text{combined flow}}$$

The dilemma of an accurate measure of oxygen delivery and consumption is met by monitoring the venous oxygen content ($S_{v}O_2$) continuously in the venous drainage circuit. An increase (or a decrease) in the patient's oxygen consumption can be detected instantly. Arterial blood samples reflect a mixture of oxygen content from both native heart and artificial lung. At normal conditions

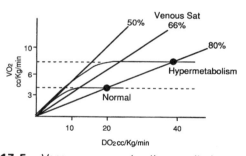

Figure 17-5. Venous oxygen saturation monitoring provides a continuous reflection of a patient's oxygen consumption. (With permission from Chapman RA, Bartlett RH. *Extracorporeal Life Support Manual for Adult and Pediatric Patients.* ECMO Department, University of Michigan Medical Center, 1990.)

of tissue oxygen delivery and consumption, 4 times more oxygen is delivered than consumed. As is seen in Fig. 17-5, These conditions correlate directly with an $S_{v}O_2$ of 75%. When delivery falls, or consumption rises, $S_{v}O_2$ will decrease. Thus continuous $S_{v}O_2$ measurements monitor adequacy of tissue oxygen delivery.

The ECMO patient is monitored to maintain an $S_{v}O_2$ of approximately 70%. Because combined pump and cardiac output is relatively fixed at high pumping rates, a low venous saturation may reflect inadequate hemoglobin, flow inadequate to meet increasing oxygen demand, inadequate flow, or a hypermetabolic state in the patient. As can be seen in Fig. 17-5, a seizure in a patient would increase oxygen consumption and $S_{v}O_2$ would decrease, whereas a maneuver that increases native cardiac output, such as a transfu-

Table 17-6. Major differences between V-A and V-V ECLS

Hemodynamics	Veno-arterial ECLS	Veno-venous ECLS
Systemic perfusion	Circuit flow and cardiac output	Cardiac output only
Arterial BP	Pulse contour damped	Pulse contour full
CVP	Not very hepful	Accurate guide to volume status
Pulmonary artery pressure	Decreased proportionally to circuit flow	Not affected by flow
Effect of R → L shunt	Mixed venous/perfusate blood	None
Effect of L → R shunt	Pulmonary hyperperfusion; may require increased flow	No effect on circuit flow; usual PDA physiology
Selective R arm/brain perfusion	Occurs	Does not occur
Gas Exchange		
Blood flow for full gas exchange	80–100 cc/kg/min	100–120 cc/kg/min
Arterial oxygenation	O_2 sat. controlled by circuit flow	80–95% sat. common at max flow
CO_2 removal	Depends on sweep gas and membrane lung size	Same as V-A
Oxygenator size	0.4 or 0.6	0.6 or 0.8
Decrease initial vent settings	Rapidly	Slowly

sion or addition of an inotrope, would add desaturated blood to the descending aorta as pulmonary blood flow through a dysfunctional native lung would increase. Conversely, a decrease in native heart function, secondary to myocardial stun or tamponade, would have the effect of decreasing the proportion of desaturated blood coming from the native lung. The majority of blood would come from the extracorporeal circuit, which is 100% saturated with oxygen. Because combined output (cardiac plus pump) is reduced, the patient's PaO_2 would increase but the S_vO_2 would fall (decreased oxygen delivery).

As the contribution to total flow from the circuit is increased, more blood is "stolen" from the right heart, native cardiac output drops, and the pulse contour will be damped. In normal circumstances, approximately 80% of the total flow is from the ECLS circuit, with the balance coming from the native heart. Thus, "total" bypass is never achieved.

Veno-venous (V-V) bypass has several advantages over V-A circuits. The carotid artery is not utilized; the native lung acts as a filter for air and thrombus, thus preventing arterial embolization to the brain and other vital organs. Perfusate blood is returned to the venous circulation, and the native heart pumps blood through the lung. Thus, the myocardium must be normal. Because total venous and arterial blood volumes are unaffected by circuit flow, unlike the situation encountered in V-A bypass, venous, pulmonary, and systemic pressures accurately reflect the patient's preload and cardiac output in a conventional manner. Interpretation of adequacy of oxygenation is, however, complicated by the presence of inevitable recirculation. Most of the well-oxygenated blood returning from the artificial lung passes into the right atrium. Some of this well-oxygenated blood, however, is siphoned into the venous drainage cannula, thus falsely elevating the PvO_2 in the venous drainage catheter. The circuit S_vO_2 (measured in the venous drainage catheter) may reflect 10% to 30% recirculation of well-oxygenated blood, while the systemic saturation in the descending aorta reflects a combination of mixing in the venous circulation and a contribution of variably oxygenated blood from the (diseased) native lung. A consequence of total perfusion of the native lung is that alveolar recruitment and oxygenation

in the native lung might contribute to the total oxygen content. The balance of oxygenation is achieved by use of the native lung at "safe" distending pressures. When relatively low flow rates are used in the circuit, 30% to 50% of total estimated blood flow support, the system is described as extracorporeal carbon dioxide removal (ECCOR), as defined by Gattinoni in Italy.[14] Within limits, adequate systemic oxygen delivery can be accomplished. Because systemic blood flow is determined totally by the patient's cardiac output, oxygen delivery can be enhanced by inotropes, increased preload, and elevated arterial oxygen content achieved by increasing the hemoglobin. Alternatively, consumption of oxygen could be reduced by decreasing temperature, treating sepsis, and control of seizures. Table 17-6 summarizes differences between V-A and V-V bypass.

Results of Extracorporeal Life Support

Six hundred seventy-two cases of pediatric respiratory failure were reported to the ELSO registry between 1981 and April 1994, with an overall survival rate of 55% from 55 centers. Pediatric cases show a wide variety of survival when separated by diagnosis (Table 17-7). The University of Michigan group has reported a single institution case experience.[31,44]

Twenty-five pediatric patients with severe pulmonary failure

Table 17-7. Pediatric respiratory cases by diagnosis

Diagnosis	Total	% Survivors
Bacterial pneumonia	51	47
Viral pneumonia	200	51
Pulmonary hemorrhage	10	70
Aspiration	69	64
Pneumocystis	10	40
Hypoxic respiratory failure	414	47

were managed with ECLS at the University of Michigan from 1982 to May 1991. Sixty percent (15/25) survived their life-threatening respiratory failure and were eventually weaned from mechanical ventilation. The mean patient age was 4.1 years (± 5.0). Sixty-eight percent (17/25) of the patients were male. The mean days of mechanical ventilation prior to ECLS was 5.9 days (± 4.4). The mean duration of ECLS for all patients was 12.6 days (± 8.6). In 15 survivors, the mean time from decannulation to extubation was 6.0 days (± 5.4).

Patient diagnoses and outcome are summarized in Table 17-8. Diagnoses were heterogeneous. The most common diagnoses prior to ECLS were ARDS, secondary to various etiologies (five patients), and presumed viral pneumonia (ten patients). Examination of patients from the perspective of certainty of diagnosis revealed three patients with unconfirmed diagnoses of viral pneumonia or ARDS and three patients with immunocompromised state. None of these six patients survived. When specific etiologies for respiratory failure could be documented before ECLS, however, 14 of 18 patients survived.

Survivors and nonsurvivors were compared by age, sex, duration of mechanical ventilation prior to ECLS, and duration of V-V ECLS (Table 17-9). Only age was statistically associated with outcome, with younger patients more likely to survive. There existed no relationship between PaO_2, $PaCO_2$, $P(A-a)O_2$, or FiO_2 and patient outcome. A significant association between patient out-

come and ventilator pressure did exist, with those having lower pressures (PIP, MAP, and PEEP) more likely to survive.

In 15 additional patients managed from 1991 through 1994, 84% were referred after conventional ventilator management failed over 5.8 ± 2.7 days. Prior to the initiation of bypass, the patients were morbidly ill. The PaO_2 was 56 ± 20 mm Hg in an FiO_2 of 0.98, with an alveolar-arterial oxygen gradient of 572 ± 81 mm Hg (MAP of 21.6 ± 6.2 cm H_2O and PEEP of 11.0 ± 4.3 cm H_2O). The patients also could not be adequately ventilated because $PaCO_2$ was 46 ± 17 mm Hg, with PIPs of 46 ± 10 cm H_2O. This latter group of 15 was compared to the patients treated since 1991. The characteristics of the two cohorts are summarized in Tables 17-10 and 17-11.

The duration of ECLS therapy was 373 ± 259 hours. The survival of 88% was significantly different when compared with the pre-1991 treated cohort with a 58% survival. Younger ages had higher survival. Infants under 1 year have a 100% survival in our experience.

Experience in adult respiratory failure continues to accumulate. Gattinoni et al.[45] have summarized the European experience. A total of 327 patients have been treated in a variety of centers, with a 47% observed survival rate and a predicted survival of 10%.

Gattinoni et al.[45] have treated 99 patients with ARDS. The etiologies were pneumonia in 63%, trauma in 21%, and embolism and sepsis in 16%. The overall survival rate is 45%. In the most

Table 17-8. Diagnoses before ECLS and outcome of 25 pediatric ECLS patients from the University of Michigan

Primary diagnosis	Total	Survivors	Nonsurvivors
ARDS			
Cold-water near-drowning	1	1	0
Collagen vascular disease[a,b]	1	0	1
Hydrocarbon pneumonitis	1	1	0
Gastric aspiration	1	0	1
Viral pneumonia			
RSV bronchiolitis	3	3	0
Bronchiolitis, probable RSV	1	1	0
Parainfluenza	1	1	0
Varicella	1	1	0
Unknown[b]	2	0	2
Cancer			
Wilm's tumor with chemotherapy and chest irradiation, ? viral pneumonia (u + i)	1	0	1
Lymphoma post BMT, ? viral pneumonia[a,b]	1	0	1
Unexpected pulmonary sarcoma, ? ARDS[b]	1	0	1
Bacterial pneumonia			
Staphylococcal and influenza A	1	1	0
Streptococcal	1	1	0
Pulmonary contusion	3	1	2
Idiopathic pulmonary hemorrhage	2	2	0
Pulmonary infarct, SCA	1	0	1
Pulmonary alveolar proteinosis	1	1	0
Congenital cystic adenomatoid malformation and CMV pneumonia[b]	1	1	0

[a]Immunocompromised.
[b]Unknown respiratory failure etiology.
For patients with known pulmonary insults and without immunocompromised state, 14/18 survived.
ECLS, extracorporeal life support; ARDS, adult respiratory distress syndrome; RSV, respiratory syncytial virus; BMT, bone marrow transplant; SCA, sickle cell anemia; CMV, cytomegalovirus; ?, pressured diagnosis not established.
Data from Moler et al.[44]

Table 17-9. Comparison of survivors and nonsurvivors by arterial blood gas values and mechanical ventilation parameters immediately before extracorporeal life support (ECLS) (mean ≠ SD)

	Survivors (n = 15)	Nonsurvivors (n = 10)	P value[a]
PaO₂ (torr)	71.1 (±53.3)	64.5 (±53.4)	0.716
(kPa)	9.5 (±7.1)	8.6 (±7.1)	
PaCO₂ (torr)	42.0 (±9.7)	44.8 (±11.5)	0.520
(kPa)	5.6 (±1.3)	6.0 (±1.5)	
P(A-a)O₂ (torr)[b]	552 (±70.3)	579 (±23.3)	0.257
(kPa)	73.6 (±9.4)	77.1 (±3.1)	
FiO₂ × 100	97 (±9.3)	99 (±3.2)	0.429
PIP (cm H₂O)	43.1 (±11.5)	57.9 (±18.9)	0.025
MAP (cm H₂O)	18.4 (±6.3)	27.1 (±11.9)	0.024
PEEP (cm H₂O)	8.1 (±4.0)	12.1 (±1.5)	0.006

[a]Independent sample t-test
[b]Estimated $P(A-a)O_2 = [FiO_2(P_{BH_2O}) - PaCO_2/0.8 - PaO_2]$ where P_B assumed to be 746 torr, P_{H_2O} assumed to be 46 torr, and respiratory quotient 0.8.
P(A-a)O₂, alveolar-arterial oxygen difference; PIP, peak inspiratory pressure; PEEP, positive end-expiratory pressure; MAP, mean airway pressure.
Data from Moler et al.[44]

Table 17-10. Descriptive information of patients treated with extracorporeal life support before and after May 1991 at the University of Michigan Hospitals

	Before May 1, 1991	Since May 1, 1991	P
Patients (no.)	24	25	
Age (mo)	50±61 [25; 1–204]*	60±75 [18; 1–196]*	0.912
Weight (kg)	19.1±18.0 [11.2; 2.8–63.3]*	23.6±24.8 [10.5; 2.2–71.3]*	0.469
Gender male (%)	63	44	0.195
Duration of mechanical ventilation prior to bypass (d)	6.1±4.2	5.8±2.7	0.755
Initial cannulation route veno-venous (%)	12/24 (50)	12/25 (48)	0.889
Duration of extracorporeal life support (hr)	313±202 [278; 71–853]*	373±259 [282; 115–1052]*	0.509
Survived (%)	14/24 (58%)	22/25 (88%)	0.018

*Median; range
Data from Moler et al.[31]

recent 32 patients who survived, the mean age was 39 years, and the PaCO₂ 90 mm Hg prior to bypass.

Falke[46] has emphasized that ECLS should be viewed as part of a continuum of excellent management of respiratory failure. Of 54 patients referred for severe ARDS, 30 responded to aggressively proscribed conventional management protocols featuring vigorous diuresis and pressure-controlled ventilation. Twenty-four patients either failed this management protocol or were moribund on admission; these were placed on V-V ECLS. These 24 patients had a 60% survival rate. However, the overall survival rate for the 54-patient group of severely ill patients managed with ECLS as part of the protocol was 80%. Anderson et al.[37] have summarized the University of Michigan Medical Center experience. He reported a Phase I trial completed in patients with a predicted mortality of 90% (from historical controls). Of these patients, 45% survived. The entire U.S. experience is 95 patients, with a large array of cardiac and septic etiologies. Of the 25 patients with ARDS, the survival matches the European reports of 56%.

Management of Patients on Extracorporeal Membrane Oxygenation

Control of bleeding is the major limiting factor in use of ECLS, and bleeding is the major complication.[47] Because exposure of blood to the foreign surface of the circuit promotes binding of blood proteins to the surface, thrombosis occurs unless heparin is utilized. Bound fibrinogen activates platelets, complement, and WBCs, and the coagulation cascade is initiated. Anticoagulation is maintained by continuous infusion of heparin at a rate that produces an activated whole-blood clotting time of 180 to 200 seconds. The range of heparin dose required is on the order of 15 to 60 units/kg/hr. Obviously, the patient so heparinized is vulner-

Table 17-11. Comparison of ventilator parameters and arterial blood gas values 24 hours before extracorporeal life support in patients treated before May 1, 1991, and since May 1, 1991, at the University of Michigan.

	Before *May 1, 1991*	*Since* *May 1, 1991*	P
PaO$_2$ torr (kPa)	79 ± 56 (10.5 ± 7.4)	57 ± 15 (7.7 ± 2.0)	0.169
SaO$_2$ (%)	90 ± 9	87 ± 10	0.219
PaCO$_2$ (torr) (pKa)	40 ± 11 (5.3 ± 1.5)	48 ± 17 (6.3 ± 2.2)	0.034
HCO$_3^-$ (mEq/liter)	25.7 ± 6.6	27.6 ± 4.8	0.224
pH	7.42 ± 0.11	7.39 ± 0.09	0.197
FiO$_2$	0.88 ± 0.18	0.82 ± 0.17	0.086
Ventilation rate (bpm)	52.1 ± 82.0	29.4 ± 13.6	0.654
PIP (cm H$_2$O)	46.3 ± 13.5	41.3 ± 12.4	0.245
PEEP (cm H$_2$O)	9.0 ± 5.5	10.0 ± 3.7	0.181
MAP (cm H$_2$O)	—	—	
PaO$_2$/FiO$_2$ (pKa)	485 ± 135 (64.7 ± 18.0)	456 ± 133 (60.8 ± 17.7)	0.419
PaO$_2$/FiO$_2$	95.7 ± 76.1	74.6 ± 30.7	0.455
OI	—	—	

SaO$_2$, arterial oxyhemoglobin saturation; kPa, kilopascal; HCO$_3^-$, bicarbonate; PIP, peak inspiratory pressure; PEEP, positive end-expiratory pressure; MAP, mean airway pressure; OI, oxygenation index;—, insufficient data for MAP and OI because referring pediatric intensive care units did not obtain this information.
Data from Moler et al.[31]

able to bleeding. Extraordinary care by surgical and medical personnel is required to supervise this degree of anticoagulation. No procedure is conducted without surgical personnel present. This restricts such common intensive care unit procedures as the placement of chest tubes, central venous catheters, and so on. Blood loss is replaced with packed RBCs, and the hematocrit is maintained at 35% to 45%. Platelets are consumed continuously and require replacement, generally to maintain platelet count at 100,000/μL or greater. Hypocalcemia is common, and ionized calcium is monitored frequently, especially when large volumes of citrated blood products are administered.[48]

Pesenti et al.[49] have reported nearly total reduction of catheter-site bleeding with the use of percutaneously placed catheters. Bleeding from cutdown cannulation formerly contributed as much as 50% to total blood loss in heparinized patients. The experience at the University of Michigan Medical Center is identical; cannula-site bleeding is no longer a problem when percutaneously placed catheters can be used. The typical patient on V-V bypass has jugular and femoral catheters placed by guide wires percutaneously. Blood loss at the catheter site is negligible, even with bypass times in excess of 400 hours.

Bleeding has been the major limitation in application of ECLS, and blood loss remains the source of most morbidity. ECLS centers of experience have reported innovations that have minimized this problem. In the original NIH trial, blood loss per patient was in excess of 2 liters per day of bypass. In many centers, blood loss per patient has been reduced to an easily manageable 360 ml/d or less.

Heparin has long been used in bypass. Heparin titration by use of activated clotting time remains the standard practice. In 1992, Pesenti et al.[49] began trials with heparin-coated tubing, cannulae,

and oxygenator lungs. Adult patients still require some heparin—20,000 to 30,000 units per day—to maintain activated clotting times of 160 to 180 seconds. Bleeding was reduced by one third, and heparin doses were significantly decreased. Surface-heparinized circuits that minimize blood loss due to anticoagulation have undergone extensive testing in Europe and preliminary trials in the United States.

At the University of Michigan Medical Center, blood loss has been reduced to 300 ml/d from 2/liters/d by using a protocolized approach to conventional heparin use. Heparin is titrated to achieve an activated clotting time in whole blood of 160 to 190. Platelets are maintained at 100,000/μL. If bleeding is encountered, definitive correction of surgical site bleeding is performed. Heparin is decreased to achieve an activated clotting time of 140 to 170, and platelet concentration is increased to 125,000/μL. If further bleeding is intractable, heparin is reduced to maintain an activated clotting time of 120 to 150, and platelet concentration is increased to 150,000. Because these maneuvers predispose the circuit and artificial lung to clot, flow must be maintained at greater than 100 ml/kg. As a further precaution, a spare circuit is placed in immediate readiness, should the artificial lung clot. A circuit can be changed completely in approximately 3 minutes. Other methods to minimize anticoagulation risks have been employed. Koul et al.[50] and Whittlesey et al.[51] have reported success with conventional circuits run at high flow with no heparin. In European centers, antithrombin-3 is administered routinely to ECLS patients.[45] Some U.S. centers have published improvement in coagulation-related complications by the use of aminocaproic acid.

Patients tend to retain fluid either from their primary disease or as a result of the effects of extracorporeal circulation. The renal response to reduced pulsatility is to activate the renin angiotensin system. ARDS and pneumonia often lead to increases in extravascular lung water. Patients usually require diuretics when body weight increase exceeds 10% of the pre-ECMO dry weight. Adequate diuresis is maintained with usual doses of loop diuretics. If extravascular lung water is deemed to be present and diuretics fail, slow continuous ultrafiltration is used to maintain weight within 5% of dry weight. This is often done as a clinical trial in conjunction with measurements of lung compliance to document and limit the effects of noncardiogenic edema on pulmonary function.

Hepatosplenomegaly is commonly noted and is felt to be caused by the accumulation of effete RBCs and platelets in the reticuloendothelial system. The hepatic enzymes are usually normal. All patients are placed on central venous hyperalimentation.

The lung is placed at rest settings during V-A bypass. This is interpreted practically as employing "nontoxic" levels of peak airway pressure and inspired oxygen. Pressure control ventilation is used. Generally, PIP is set at 30 to 35 cm H_2O, FiO_2 at 0.4, end-expiratory pressure at 5 to 10 cm H_2O, and inspiratory time at 0.6 to 1.0 seconds, at 10 bpm. Static compliance is serially monitored. Increase in specific compliance to greater than 2 ml/cm H_2O/kg indicates improvement. Roto or circle beds are used in the older patient to prevent atelectasis and the development of consolidation in the lung. Measurements of mid-volume expiratory resistance are used to guide therapy with bronchodilators. Flexible bronchoscopy is used to ensure patency of airways, to obtain material for culture and cytology, and for lavage, either therapeutic or diagnostic. Routine radiographs are used to follow degree of aeration, detect airleaks, and ensure endotracheal, chest tube, and cannulae position.

Patients on V-V support will require more vigorous ventilation as the native lung contributes to oxygenation. Thus, higher MAPs are used to maintain alveolar distension. An FiO_2 of approximately 0.5 to 0.6 is generally used in these patients. PEEP of 5 to 15 cm of H_2O is utilized to maintain lung volume, and a rate of 10 to 15 bpm at peak pressures of 35 cm H_2O is used to ventilate.

The patient is weaned from V-A bypass by gradual reduction in circuit flow, and decannulation is considered when satisfactory gas exchange is possible on modest ventilator settings and the ECLS circuit provides 50% or less of total support. Circuit flow may be reduced to levels that allow clots to form, so flow cannot be weaned completely prior to trials of ECLS support. The mixed venous oxygen saturation is the best indicator of weaning success. Temporary trials of ECLS support for minutes to hours allow preservation of the circuit, maintenance of anticoagulation, and adequate gas exchange prior to decannulation.

Complications

Long-term follow-up data of pediatric respiratory cases is unavailable. Of nearly 70 patients from the University of Michigan, one patient remains dependent on oxygen by nasal cannulae and diuretic therapy 3 years following therapy, and one patient has significant sensorimotor hearing loss. The only patient with developmental delay had a history of extreme prematurity prior to ECLS therapy.

Heulitt et al. reported a small but well-studied group of 15 pediatric patients treated with ECMO for respiratory failure. The overall survival was 68%. All patients were prospectively evaluated for pediatric cerebral performance category and pediatric overall performance category scales; the evaluations were repeated at discharge. Only one survivor had moderate disability, and one had severe disability. The authors conclude that disability is rare in survivors.[52,53]

The same authors performed a similar evaluation of patients with severe respiratory failure treated with conventional ventilatory techniques. Thirty-five (46%) of 76 patients survived. The majority of the survivors were left with significant disability.

In ECLS centers with experience in managing at least 25 cases, circuit complications rarely lead to major morbidity. Patient death usually results from preexisting multisystem organ failure, especially neurologic injury or pulmonary end-organ failure.

The Michigan group has reported complications observed in 7550 hours of bypass in 25 patients.[44] Oxygenator failure requiring replacement occurred on nine occasions in six patients. The second most common circuit complication was raceway rupture, which occurred in four patients. Pump failure occurred on three occasions and power failure once. The frequency of significant circuit complications was 19 events during 7550 hours of ECLS, or one event per 16.6 days. Fourteen patients had no circuit complications. Mortality was 36% in those without complications and 45% in those with one or more complications.

Surgical site bleeding, often minor, occurred in 14 patients. Four of 13 V-V bypass patients were converted to V-A bypass for better cardiac and perfusion support (one survived). Pneumothorax during ECLS was a reported complication in five patients. Five patients had hemothoraxes, which required therapy. Three of these patients had chest trauma with secondary pulmonary contusions, one had a chest tube placed for a pneumothorax just prior to heparinization for ECLS, and one had definitive surgery for congenital adenomatoid malformation while on ECLS. Other complications included cardiopulmonary resuscitation (6), cardiac tamponade (3), probable seizure (3), hemolysis (2), sepsis (1), hypertension (3), gastrointestinal hemorrhage (1), and intracranial hemorrhage (1). Three patients had no complications. Survival was 100% in those without complications and 55% in the 22 patients with one or more complications. This was not statistically significant.

The ELSO Registry documents complications in all participating centers. These data are useful to developing programs as a barometer of progress and to existing programs for quality assurance activities. The future of ECLS in the pediatric patient is dependent on the development and standardization of entry criteria for ECLS. This will require a multicenter data collection.

Study development is hampered by the unavailability of data describing the natural history of pediatric respiratory failure. Logical spin-off from ECLS research will include development of novel approaches to anticoagulation and fibrinolytic therapy, the development of heparin-coated circuitry, and an implantable artificial lung. Advances in the use of such novel therapies has fostered research in novel approaches to conventional ventilation and to our understanding of the natural history of acute lung injury.

References

1. Clowes GHS, Hopkins AL, Neville WE. An artificial lung dependent upon diffusion of oxygen and carbon dioxide through plastic membranes. *J Thorac Surg* 32:630–637, 1956.
2. Bartlett RH. Extracorporeal life support for cardiopulmonary failure. *Curr Probl Surg* 27:623–705, 1990.
3. Kolobow T, Zapol W, Pierce J. High survival and minimal blood damage in lambs exposed to long term (1 week) veno-venous pumping

with a polyurethane chamber roller pump with and without a membrane blood oxygenator. *ASAIO Trans* 15:172–177, 1969.

4. Bartlett R, Isherwood J, Moss RA. A toroidal flow membrane oxygenator: Four day partial bypass in dogs. *Surg Forum* 20:152–143, 1969.

5. Bartlett RH, Fong SW, Bruns NE. Prolonged partial venoarterial bypass: Physiologic biochemical, and hematologic responses. *Ann Surg* 180:850–856, 1974.

6. Bartlett RH, Kittredge D, Noyes FS Jr. Development of a membrane oxygenator: Overcoming blood diffusion limitation. *J Thorac Cardiovasc Surg* 58:795, 1969.

7. Bartlett RH et al. The toroidal membrane oxygenator: Design, performance and bypass testing of a clinical model. *ASAIO Trans* 18: 369–373, 1972.

8. Hill JD, O'Brien TG, Murray JJ. Extracorporeal oxygenation for acute post traumatic respiratory failure (shock-lung syndrome): Use of the Bramson Membrane Lung. *N Engl J Med* 286:629–634, 1972.

9. Bartlett RH, Gazzaniga AB, Jeffries R. Extracorporeal membrane oxygenation (ECMO) cardiopulmonary support in infancy. *ASAIO Trans* 22:80–88, 1976.

10. Zapol WM, Snider MT, Hill JE. Extracorporeal membrane oxygenation in severe respiratory failure. *JAMA* 242:2193–2196, 1979.

11. Bartlett RH et al. Extracorporeal membrane oxygenation (ECMO) for newborn respiratory failure: 45 cases. *Surgery* 92:425–433, 1982.

12. Toomasian JM, Snedecor M, Cornell R. National experience with extracorporeal membrane oxygenation (ECMO) for neonatal respiratory failure. *ASAIO Trans* 23:140–1147, 1988.

13. ECMO Registry Report of the Extracorporeal Life Support Organization. Ann Arbor, MI: ELSO, 1993.

14. Gattinoni L, Pesenti A, Mascherone D. Low frequency positive pressure ventilation with extracorporeal CO$_2$ removal in severe acute respiratory failure, *JAMA* 256:881–885, 1986.

15. Anderson HL et al. Extracorporeal membrane oxygenation for pediatric cardiopulmonary failure. *J Thorac Cardiovasc Surg* 99:1011, 1990.

16. Steinhorn RH, Green TP. Use of extracorporeal membrane oxygenation in the treatment of respiratory syncytial virus bronchiolitis: The national experience, 1983 to 1988. *J Pediatr* 116:338, 1990.

17. Moler FW et al. Predictors of outcome of severe respiratory syncytial virus associated respiratory failure treated with ECMO. *J Pediatr* 123;46–52, 1993.

18. Adolph V et al. Extracorporeal membrane oxygenation for nonneonatal respiratory failure. *J Pediatr Surg* 26:326, 1991.

19. Snyder LS. Failure of lung repair following acute lung injury. *Chest* 98:733–738, 1990.

20. Strieter RM, Standiford TJ, Rolfe MW. Cytokines in pulmonary injury. In Kunkel SL, Remick DG (eds): *Cytokines in Health and Disease.* New York: Marcel Dekker, 1992. Pp 397–412.

21. Greenfield LJ, Ebert PA, Benson DW. Effect of positive pressure ventilation on surface tension properties of lung extracts. *Anesthesiology* 25:312–316, 1964.

22. Barsch J, Birbara C, Eggers GWN. Positive pressure as a cause of respiratory failure induced lung disease. *Ann Intern Med* 72:810, 1970.

23. Webb HH, Tierney OF. Experimental pulmonary edema due to intermittent positive pressure ventilation with high inflation pressure: Protection by positive end expirtory pressure. *Am Rev Respir Dis* 110:556–571, 1974.

24. Parker JD, Hernandez LA, Longnecker GL. Lung edema caused by high peak inspiratory pressure and permeability. *Am Rev Respir Dis* 142:321, 1990.

25. Dreyfus D, Soler P, Basset G. High inflation pressure pulmonary edema: Respective effects of high airway pressure, high tidal volume, and positive end expiratory pressure. *Am Rev Respir Dis* 137: 1159–1164, 1988.

26. Dreyfus D, Basset G, Soler P. Intermittent positive pressure hyperventilation with high inflation pressures produces pulmonary microvascular injury in rats. *Am Rev Respir Dis* 132:880–884, 1988.

27. Corbridge TL, Wood LDH, Crawford GP. Adverse effects of large

28. Kolobow T, Moretti MD, Fumagalli R. Severe impairment in lung function induced by high peak airway pressure during mechanical ventilation: An experimental study. *Am Rev Respir Dis* 135:312–315, 1987.

29. Hickling KG, Henderson SJ, Jackson R. Low mortality associated with low volume pressure limited ventilation with permissive hypercapnea in severe ARDS. *Intensive Care Med* 16:372–377, 1990.

30. Suchyta MR et al. Increased survival of ARDS patients with severe hypoxemia (ECMO criteria). *Chest* 99:951–955, 1991.

31. Moler F, Custer J, Palmisano J. Extracorporeal life support for severe pediatric respiratory failure: An updated experience 1991–1993. *J Pediatr* 124:875–880, 1994.

32. Kolobow T. Acute respiratory failure: On how to injure healthy lungs and prevent sick lungs from recovery. *ASAIO Trans* 34:31–34, 1988.

33. Gattinoni L, Pesenti A, Avalli L. Pressure volume curves of the total respiratory system in respiratory failure. *Am Rev Respir Dis* 136:730–736, 1987.

34. Gattinoni L, Pesenti A, Bambino M. Relationship between lung computed tomographic density gas exchange and PEEP in acute respiratory failure. *Anesthesiology* 69:824–832, 1988.

35. Bartlett RH. Use of the mechanical ventilator. In Holcroft T (ed): *Care of the Surgical Patient*, Vol I. (2 ed). New York: Scientific American, 1993.

36. Zapol W, Snider M, Hill J. Extracorporeal membrane oxygenation in severe acute respiratory failure: A randomized prospective study. *JAMA* 242:2193, 1979.

37. Rivera RA, Butt W, Shann F. Predictors of mortality in children with respiratory failure: Possible indications for ECMO. *Anaesth Intens Care* 18:385, 1990.

38. Tamburro RF, Bugnitz MC, Stidham G. Alveolar-arterial oxygen gradient as a predictor of outcome in patients with nonneonatal pediatric respiratory failure. *J Pediatr* 119:935, 1991.

39. Timmons OD, Dean JM, Vernon DD. Mortality rates and prognostic variables in children with adult respiratory distress syndrome. *J Pediatr* 26:326, 1991.

40. Moler FW, Palmisano JM, Custer JR. Extracorporeal life support for pediatric respiratory failure: Predictors of survival from 220 patients. *Crit Care Med* 21:1604–1611, 1993.

41. Moler FW, Palmisano JM, Custer JR. Alveolar-arteriolar oxygen gradients before extracorporeal life support for severe pediatric respiratory failure: Improved outcome for ECLS patients? *Crit Care Med* 22:620–625, 1994.

42. Montoya JP, Merz SI, Bartlett RH. A standardized system for describing flow/pressure relationships in vascular access devices. *ASAIO Trans* 37:60, 1991.

43. Sinard JM, Merz S, Bartlett R. A standardized system for describing flow/pressure relationships in vascular access devices. *ASAIO Trans* 37:4, 1991.

44. Moler FW, Custer JR, Bartlett RH. Extracorporeal life support for pediatric respiratory failure. *Crit Care Med* 20:1112–1118, 1992.

45. Gattinoni I, Pesenti A, Barabino M. Role of extracoroporeal circulation in ARDS management. *New Horiz* 1:603–612, 1993.

46. Falke KJ. Reduced mortality rates in severe adult respiratory distress syndrome. Annual Meeting, Extracorporeal Life Support Organization, Dearborn, Michigan, October 1993.

47. Sell LL, Cullen ML, Whittlesey GC, et al. Hemorrhagic complications during extracorporeal membrane oxygenation: Prevention and treatment. *J Pediatr Surg* 21:1087, 1986.

48. Meliones JN et al. Hemodynamic instability after the initiation of extracorporeal membrane oxygenation: Role of ionized calcium. *Crit Care Med* 19:1247, 1991.

49. Pesenti A, Gattinoni L, Barabino M. Long term extracorporeal respiratory support: 20 years of progress. *Intens Crit Care Digest* 12:15–18, 1993.

50. Koul B et al. Twenty four hour heparin free ventricular ECMO. *Ann Thorac Surg* 53:1046–1051, 1992.

51. Whittlesey G, Drucker O, Sally S. ECMO without heparin, clinical and laboratory experience. *J Pediatr Surg* 118:117–120, 1991.

52. Heulitt M, Moss M, Schexnader S. Morbidity and mortality in pediatric patients with acute respiratory failure supported with extracorporeal life support. Extracorporeal Life Support Organization Fifth Annual Meeting, Dearborn, Michigan, 1993.

53. Heulitt M, Moss M, Walker W. Morbidity and mortality in pediatric patients with severe respiratory failure. Extracorporeal Life Support Organization Fifth Annual Meeting, Dearborn, Michigan, 1993.

Steve Kurachek

◆18◆ Pulmonary Artery Hypertension

Pulmonary artery hypertension (PAH) is a common pathophysiologic finding among infants and children with critical illness. A variety of congenital heart defects, chronic pulmonary conditions, and acute lung injury are complicated by elevations in pulmonary artery pressure (PAP). Minor elevations of PAP (mean: 20–30 mm Hg) as occur with childhood pneumonia are likely to pass unnoticed, whereas acute elevations to systemic levels or higher that may precipitously occur in postoperative congenital heart patients are potentially life-threatening.[1,2] Recognition of PAH is likely to modify the approach to basic management issues such as fluid balance, acid-base direction, inotrope/vasodilator support, and ventilator strategy. Seemingly simple procedures, such as endotracheal suctioning or tube retaping, as well as more complex tasks, such as endotracheal intubation or bedside bronchoscopy, are risky procedures when performed in the face of PAH. Whenever possible, therapy for PAH is directed at the underlying cause. If recent studies are any indication, nitric oxide has emerged as a relatively nontoxic, specific pulmonary artery vasodilator applicable in the setting of reversible pulmonary vasospasm.

Developmental Aspects

In the first few weeks of gestation, the primitive lung receives blood from vessels off the dorsal aorta that involute and disappear by the sixth week. Interestingly, persistence of one or more of these primitive vessels may give rise to the phenomenon of sequestration. Pulmonary arteries and arterioles are conveniently divided into preacinar and intraacinar regions. The preacinar arteries consist of conventional vessels that tightly parallel airway formation in a 1:1 fashion. Supernumerary vessels are additional pulmonary artery branches that exceed the branching number of airways. According to the laws of lung development, pulmonary artery and airway growth occurs "side-by-side" until completion of airway branching by the sixteenth week. The growth of intraacinar vessels parallels the appearance of alveoli and takes place through the first 8 years of life, with the majority of vessels appearing in the first 3 years.[3–5]

Pulmonary blood flow in the fetus is limited as oxygenated blood from the placenta streams through the foramen ovale to the left heart, and blood that enters the right heart from the superior vena cava bypasses the lungs through a patent ductus arteriosus. At birth, expulsion of fetal lung fluid, chest wall expansion, and alveolar opening distend pulmonary vessels, abruptly reducing pulmonary vascular resistance and prompting venous return to the right heart to participate in gas exchange through the lung. Ultimately, the fetal ductuses functionally and then anatomically close, fetal muscularization of the pulmonary arteries regresses, and the pulmonary vascular circuit is transformed into a low-pressure, high-flow, noncapacitance system.

The progressive appearance of intraacinar vessels through early childhood is accompanied by considerable remodeling of the entire pulmonary vasculature. At birth, small resistance arteries are characterized by exuberant medial hypertrophy, with the wall to external diameter ratio being larger than at any time during life. Except in pathologic states such as persistent PAH of the newborn, immediate preacinar and acinar vessels are relatively free of muscularization. With age, the pulmonary arteries lengthen and the wall to external diameter ratio decreases. This "thinning" process occurs in conjunction with alveolar multiplication and extension of muscularization into the alveolar region of the adult lung.[6] Downstream from the acinus, the venous side of the circuit undergoes change as well. New vessel formation can take place here, and similar changes in muscularization are observed with pathologic states (congenital heart disease), at times resulting in exaggerated hypertrophy.

The newborn and early childhood lung might best be thought of as both vulnerable and, at the same time, resilient. The lung is vulnerable in the sense that pathologic processes can interrupt the normal developmental program, particularly as it relates to ongoing vascular remodeling. On the other hand, early lung injury might in some ways be better accomodated, as the window for compensatory lung growth, particularly with regard to acinar development, is open only during infancy and early childhood. Moderate-to-severe bronchopulmonary dysplasia, for example, is perhaps universally accompanied by an oxygen-responsive increase in PAP. Nonetheless, long-term follow-up of these patients suggests that despite the necessity of considerable acinar remodeling, as well as variable amounts of airway distortion, pulmonary vascular and lung function—albeit not normal—are well preserved. Pulmonary vascular changes, however, due to increases in flow and pressure that occur with left-to-right cardiac shunts, are characterized by excessive arterial muscularization. The strategy to correct congenital heart lesions, such as VSDs and PDAs early in life to permit normal pulmonary and acinar development, is unfortunately not always successful. Some patients develop exuberant muscularization of peripheral arteries and severe PAH leading to right heart failure and death in the first year of life.[7,8] Analogously, bronchopulmonary dysplasia (BPD) patients unresponsive to oxygen therapy have a poor prognosis.[9] Why these patients are apparently permanently derailed from normal pulmonary vascular and acinar development is unclear.

Pulmonary Blood Flow

The pulmonary circuit accepts the entire cardiac output. Pressure across the circuit is relatively low compared with the systemic circulation, with the normal mean PAP approximately 15 mm Hg (inflow pressure) and the mean left atrial pressure 5 mm Hg (outflow pressure). Beyond infancy, normal pulmonary arterial vessels are relatively thin-walled compared with their systemic counterparts. The pulmonary vessels display less smooth muscle and greater distensibility. A hallmark of a variety of PAH states is the extension of excessive smooth muscle into the acinus or beyond. In a parallel sense, similar differences between the pulmonary and arterial circuits are reflected in the structures of the right and left ventricles. The former is small and thin-walled compared with the latter, and chronic elevation of PAP results in right ventricular hypertrophy, diminished chamber compliance, and ventricular dysfunction.

Pulmonary blood flow is defined through the hydraulic equivalent of Ohm's law, which states that flow is determined by the difference between inflow and outflow pressures divided by resistance. Applying an electrical model to a vascular system is cumbersome in that vascular resistance changes with flow for reasons other than the pressures that engage the circuit. Vessel distensibility, for example, alters and is altered by moment-to-moment changes in flow, and the system itself is similar to a Starling resistor in that alveolar pressure can effectively become the outflow pressure, especially under conditions of positive pressure ventilation. Blood flow through the lung is governed by a complex interplay between cardiac output and both passive (cross-sectional vascular anatomy, gravity, lung volume, blood viscosity) and active variables (e.g., vascular tone, hypoxic vasoconstriction) that are individually or in combination disrupted in disease states.

Diagnosis and Hemodynamic Consequences

PAH is associated with a variety of disorders (Table 18-1) that raise mean PAP above 20 mm Hg. Pediatric patients at risk for PAH

Table 18-1. Conditions associated with PAH

Heart Disease
  Increased pulmonary blood flow
    Ventricular or atrial septal defect, patent ductus arteriosus, a-v canal, a-p window, transposition of great arteries, truncus arteriosus, anomalous pulmonary veins
  Left-sided obstructive disease
    Pulmonary vein stenosis, veno-occlusive disease, cor triatriatum, mitral stenosis or atrial myxoma, LV dysfunction, subaortic stenosis, aortic stenosis, coarctation of aorta
  Miscellaneous
    Pericarditis, pulmonary atresia, and uncorrected TOF (collateral systemic vessels)
Thromboembolic Disorders
  Coagulopathic deficiencies
    Protein s, antithrombin 3, plasminogen
  Hemoglobinopathies
    Sickle cell, hereditary spherocytosis, thalassemia
  Platelet disorders
    S/p splenectomy (thrombocytosis), platelet storage pool disease
  Catheter-associated
    Ventriculo-atrial shunt, indwelling central line (broviac), transvenous pacemaker
  Miscellaneous
    Acute or chronic thromboembolic disease, tumor emboli, schistosomiasis, antiphospholipid antibody syndrome
Respiratory Conditions
  Upper airway obstructive defects
    Macroglossia, obstructive sleep apnea, Pierré Robin, tonsillar hypertrophy, vocal cord paresis, craniofacial dysostosis
  Lower airway obstructive defects
    Bronchopulmonary dysplasia, cystic fibrosis, COPD, asthma
  Restrictive defects
    Pulmonary hypoplasia (d. hernia, oligohydramnios, hydrops) kyphoscolisis, neuromuscular disorders, obesity, interstitial fibrosis, sarcoid, primary and metastatic neoplastic disease, scleroderma, rheumatic lung, mixed connective tissue disease, dermatomyositis, acute parenchymal disorders, ARDS, b. pertussis, pneumonia, others
  Vasculitis
    Lupus, Takayasu's disease
Primary Pulmonary Hypertension
Other Disorders
  AIDS, toxin-induced (aminorex, rapeseed oil, chemotherapy, native teas) pulmonary hilar fibrosis, amyloidosis, capillary hemangiomatosis, portal hypertension with or without cirrhosis, cirrhosis, birth control pills

include individuals afflicted by congenital heart disease and a variety of acute and chronic lung disorders. Many of the conditions listed in Table 18-1, including primary PAH, however, are not common in the pediatric population, and their de novo appearance in the pediatric intensive care unit (PICU) is likely to be unexpected and sometimes dramatic. History may suggest the diagnosis of PAH. Exertional dyspnea and fatigue are the hallmarks of clinically significant PAH. Dyspnea at rest, chest pain, and syncope or near-syncopal episodes signify more progressive disease. The infant/childhood equivalent of these symptoms includes poor activity tolerance, sluggish feeding sessions, diminished curiosity and exploratory behavior, irritability, and pallor or grey spells that abruptly interrupt a child's focus or play. Acute right ventricular failure in the PICU, however, tends to affect particular children at risk who have some degree of baseline pulmonary vascular disease and may additionally have cor pulmonale and/or ventricular dysfunction for other reasons, most notably congenital heart disease (discussion to follow). Nasopharyngitis in the undiagnosed obstructive sleep apnea child or pneumonia in an infant with severe BPD are conditions that are likely to expose underlying pulmonary vascular pathology. Physical examination findings (Table 18-2) and cardiopulmonary diagnostics (Table 18-3) will confirm the presence of PAH. When the etiology of PAH is obscure, an extensive laboratory evaluation may be necessary (Table 18-4).

Table 18-2. Physical exam findings in PAH

Cardiac findings

Jugular venous distension

Congestive organomegly

Parasternal heave

Fixed or reverse splitting S2

Palpable P2 (infants)

Right-sided gallop rhythm

Diastolic murmurs (pulmonary or tricuspid insufficiency)

Table 18-3. Cardiopulmonary diagnostic tests in PAH

CXR
  Cardiomegaly (R ventricular pattern)
  Dilated pulmonary arteries
  Oligemic lung fields
EKG
  Right axis
  Right atrial enlargement
  Right ventricular hypertrophy
  Right bundle branch block
ECHO
  RA/RV enlargement
  Pulmonary and/or tricuspid insufficiency
  Leftward atrial septal bowing
  RV dyskinesia
  Doppler findings of PAH
Catheterization
  Elevated PAP
  Elevated RV and RA pressures
  Pruning of pulmonary vessels
  Decreased cardiac index

Table 18-4. Diagnostic evaluation of PAH of unclear etiology

Cardiac evaluation
  CXR, EKG, ECHO, CATH

Thromboembolic disorders
  V̇/Q̇ scan, doppler for DVT, protein S, protein C, antithrombin 3, plasminogen antigen and function, peripheral blood smear, Hgb electrophoresis, Doppler for catheter-related thrombus, antiphospholipid antibody

Respiratory disorders
  Pulmonary functions, sleep evaluation, ESR, u/a, ANA, anti-smooth muscle ab, anti-cardiolipin ab, RNP, C3, C4, anti-DNA ab, BUN, creatinine

Other
  Toxicology hx, HIV eval, b. pertussis screen and culture, liver function studies

Table 18-6. Potential triggers of reactive PAH in the PICU

Hypoxemia
  Atelectasis
  Barotrauma
  ETT displacement
  Prolonged suctioning

Acidosis
  Hypovolemia
  Hypoglycemia
  Low cardiac output

Hypercapnia
  Inadequate ventilation
  Dead-space ventilation

Inadequate sedation
  Suctioning
  Bedside procedures

Inadequate analgesia

Dysrhythmias

Temperature instability

The hemodynamic consequences of PAH are well known. The partially conditioned or unconditioned right ventricle is morphologically vulnerable to increases in PAP, particularly when a mean level of 40 mm Hg or higher occurs acutely. The thin-walled chamber is exquisitely sensitive to increases in afterload (PVR), promptly reducing stroke volume and increasing right ventricular end-diastolic volume. Predictably, left ventricular preload falls. The pressure- and volume-loaded right ventricle displaces the interventricular septum into the body of the left ventricle. As a consequence of diminished preload and interventricular shift, output from the left ventricle decreases. To reverse the potentially lethal combination of acute PAH and systemic hypotension, the events precipitating PAH must be recognized and reversed, volume and metabolic support appropriate, and inotropic/vasodilator assistance provided as necessary.

Acute Pulmonary Artery Hypertension in the Postoperative Surgical Patient

In one study, acute PAH crisis accompanied by desaturation and systemic hypotension occurring in the postoperative congenital heart patient has a mortality rate of 50%.[10] Children at risk (Table 18-5) have flow-induced medial muscularization of precapillary

Table 18-5. Postoperative patients with congenital heart disease at risk for PAH crisis

Left-to-right shunts with preoperative increase in PAP
  Ventricular septal defect
  Aortopulmonary window
  Patent ductus arteriosus
  Atrial septal defect

Left-sided obstructive diseases
  Coarctation of the aorta
  Aortic stenosis
  Mitral stenosis
  Cor triatriatum
  Total anomalous pulmonary drainage

Complex congenital heart lesions
  Atrioventricular canal
  Transposition of the great arteries
  Double-outlet right ventricle

pulmonary vessels or, less commonly, persistence of fetal muscularization. At this stage, the process is reversible and the vasculature prone to vasospasm. Intimal proliferation develops if flow injury is not interrupted, ultimately leading to the plexiform arteriopathy of irreversible obliterative pulmonary vascular disease.[11] Children with trisomy 21 and congenital heart disease appear to develop PAH and pulmonary vascular obstructive disease at an earlier age than individuals with a similar heart defect but no chromosomal abnormality.[12] Postoperatively, these at-risk children share the potential to develop paroxysmal pulmonary vasospasm in response to a triggering event (Table 18-6) that is often identifiable. The triggers listed in Table 18-6 are in large part avoidable phenomenon. If children at risk are clearly identified and educational measures undertaken to create a PICU staff sensitized to the potential for crisis, perhaps the majority of events can be avoided.

Common Respiratory Conditions Associated with Pulmonary Artery Hypertension

A wide variety of pediatric conditions associated with a critical reduction in the cross-sectional area of the upper airway (above the carina) can result in PAH. Acute upper airway disorders are oftentimes dramatic in their presentation (see Acute Upper Respiratory Distress Syndrome by Truman and Todres, this volume) and pose less diagnostic than interventional difficulty. Chronic conditions, however, that ostensibly impair respiration only during sleep periods are more insidious and oftentimes pass unnoticed until advanced symptoms become manifest. Obstructive sleep apnea resulting in nocturnal hypoventilation, hypercapnia, respiratory acidosis, and hypoxia, regardless of the cause, results in pulmonary arteriolar constriction. Repetitive and prolonged periods of obstructive sleep apnea over months results in abnormal muscularization of small pulmonary arteries, PAH, cor pulmonale, and, eventually, right ventricular failure if the condition passes undiagnosed and untreated. Not uncommonly, an acute respiratory infection exposes the chronic pulmonary vascular irregularity by projecting symptoms and signs out of proportion to the acute illness. In such instances, additional history reveals nocturnal breathing concerns or chronic progressive symptoms, including daytime somnolence, irritability, failure to thrive, hyperphagia, easy fatigue, developmental regression, or other behavioral difficulties. Patients with chronic upper airway obstruction, evidence of PAH, and an acute respiratory infection are legitimate PICU patients, as respiratory failure is likely to occur at an accelerated rate. Additionally, postoperative patients treated for surgically remedial upper airway obstruction who have preoperative evidence of PAH require PICU care, as edema from the surgical procedure may temporarily increase airway obstruction, and the vagaries of individualized analgesia, oxygen supplementation, and pulmonary toilet must be closely monitored to avoid triggering acute PAH.[13]

Children with moderate-to-severe BPD often have oxygen-responsive PAH. Cardiac catheterization studies of children with BPD reveal that PAH is universally present if the baseline $PaCO_2$ is greater than or equal to 50 mm Hg.[9,14] PAH in this population is not due only to pulmonary arterial muscularization but also to the systemic pressure contribution of aortic collaterals that may have invaded the lung at the hilum. BPD patients with PAH unresponsive to oxygen therapy have a poor prognosis. Respiratory decompensation due to infection, gastroesophageal reflux, and airway reactivity acutely increases oxygen requirements and decreases ventilatory efficiency, resulting in hypoxemia, hypercapnia, and respiratory acidosis. These changes, of course, increase PAH and accelerate the progression to acute respiratory failure. Apart from appropriate ventilatory support, decompensated BPD patients require an aggressive approach to pulmonary toilet, bronchodilators, antimicrobial agents, and nutritional supplementation.

Children with chronic progressive respiratory conditions such as cystic fibrosis, interstitial pneumonia, primary PAH, bronchiolitis obliterans, and so on, share a progressive reduction in the cross-sectional area of the pulmonary vascular bed. Additionally, systemic collaterals may augment pulmonary blood flow, contributing to PAH, or precipitously result in pulmonary hemorrhage. At any point in the disease process, an acute respiratory decompensation may result in a PICU admission, and pre-illness documentation of PAH suggests at least moderately severe progression of any chronic pulmonary disease. Additionally, pre-illness pulmonary function history, formal pulmonary function testing, and acute illness severity provide some, albeit not complete, insight into reversibility. Ventilatory requirements may in some circumstances be met noninvasively with curass ventilation, BIPAP, or CPAP. Pulmonary toilet, tempering airway reactivity, antibiotics when indicated, nutritional balance, and psychological support are of paramount importance to caring for these individuals. Many of these patients may additionally require right heart support or vasodilator therapy, given the prolonged nature of their disorder and progressive ventricular dysfunction due to PAH.

Management

The presence of PAH will launch a thorough investigation into the vast array of disorders associated with the condition. The situation may be obvious when PAH accompanies congenital heart disease or a chronic pulmonary disorder, though it is always valuable to intellectually entertain other considerations in order not to miss the unusual appearance of a secondary or tertiary diagnosis.[15,16] PICU patients with less common, if not rare, conditions, such as thromboembolic disease, mixed connective tissue disease, or capillary hemangiomatosis, are diagnostically challenging, and therapy for such disorders includes agents as diverse as anticoagulants, cytotoxic drugs, and alpha interferon. Regardless of the cause,

however, acute PAH leading to right heart failure or PAH exacerbated by respiratory infection often requires intensive care.

Acute interventions are directed at improving cardiac output. This goal merits emphasis, as it is altogether an oversimplification and potentially disastrous to attempt to address the PAP "number" alone. Critical cardiopulmonary failure in the pediatric patient with or without PAH is likely to begin with securing the airway and initiating mechanical ventilation. Approriate monitoring includes arterial, central, and pulmonary catheters, with the latter being placed when the loading and inotropic conditions of the heart lack clarity after initial volume resuscitation and vasotonic therapy. The importance of avoiding a pulmonary vasospastic crisis due to a predictable trigger (see Table 18-6) cannot be overemphasized. In postoperative patients, for example, fentanyl may be necessary to block bronchocarinal stimulation attendant to endotracheal suctioning.[17] Hyperinflation and atelectasis, the extremes of the lung volume curve, will contribute to PAH, the former by compressing intraacinar capillaries, the latter by effecting larger extraacinar vessels. Normocarbia or hypocarbia and normoxemia are maintained to avoid abrupt increases in PAH. Mechanical ventilation, as reviewed by Pinsky, has a variety of effects on cardiac function.[18] On one hand, it may serve as an effective afterload reducer of the left ventricle and, depending on the magnitude of negative intrapleural pressure swings and the reduction of functional residual capacity accompanying respiratory disease, may improve right ventricular function as well. On the other hand, positive-pressure ventilation tends to reduce right ventricular function by decreasing venous return and increasing right ventricular afterload by compressing acinar vessels. Yet again, mechanical ventilation can preserve cardiac output "lost" to the laboring respiratory muscles. The complexity of changes that occurs in the somersault from labored spontaneous breathing to positive-pressure artificial ventilation are in the balance salutory when applied for cardiopulmonary failure characterized by PAH.

Inotropic support is likely to be necessary for a variety of reasons. Myocardial depression is commonplace following open heart surgery. Patients with chronic pulmonary disease with PAH who decompensate with respiratory infection may have biventricular dysfunction on the basis of PAH as outlined earlier. In either setting, dopamine may be disadvantageous due to its alpha-agonist activity, whereas dobutamine and amrinone provide mild pulmonary artery vasodilation as well inotropic support. Combinations of vasotonic medications such as dobutamine/amrinone or dopamine/nitroprusside are often attempted to strike a balance between the major determinants of cardiac output—inotropy, preload, and afterload—depending on patient need. Other vasodilators (Table 18-7) have been tried in both the acute and chronic settings with variable success. Calcium channel blockers, for example, have found a role in the care of patients with chronic PAH, but these agents are likely to be dangerous in the setting of ventricular failure. Ultrashort-acting agents such as acetylcholine, prostacyclin, and PGE_1 may be used as trial medications to determine the potential reversibility of PAH, but the absence of oral analogues limits their long-term usage.[15,19] With the possible exception of nitric oxide, all agents have potentially adverse systemic or myocardial effects, and no single intravenous agent has found universal favor in treating acute PAH.

Nitric oxide is a ubiquitous biologic mediator and in 1987 was identified as the major endothelium-derived relaxing factor.[20] Nitric oxide is synthesized from arginine by nitric oxide synthases, which are found in a variety of tissues, including endothelium,

Table 18-7. Vasodilators used for PAH

Low-flow continuous oxygen

Hydralazine

Nitroprusside

Nitroglycerine

Tolazaline

Isoproterenol

Nifedipine

Diltiazem

Adenosine

Prostacyclin

PGE_1

Acetylcholine

Nitric oxide

Table 18-8. Biologic effects of nitric oxide

Arterial vasodilation (basal tone)

Smooth muscle relaxant

Inhibition of platelet aggregation

Lymphocyte regulation

Macrophage activation (?)

Inhibition of renin release

CNS effects

myocardium, platelets, central and peripheral neurons, macrophages, and others. The half-life of nitric oxide is measured in milliseconds. Hemoglobin catalyses the agent into nitrite and nitrate ions as well as methemoglobin. Nitric oxide activates cyclic guanosine monophosphate, altering intracellular calcium flux and cell function.

Nitric oxide is produced continually in the lung. Expiratory gas nitric oxide in normal adults is approximately ten parts per billion.[21] Nitric oxide has numerous biologic effects (Table 18-8) and appears to be responsible for basal vascular tone in the pulmonary circulation and likely contributes to normal ventilation/perfusion matching on a regional basis. Fronstell et al. determined that inhaled nitric oxide effectively and selectively reduces hypoxic pulmonary vasoconstriction and does not alter either pulmonary or systemic hemodynamics in normoxic volunteers.[22] Furthermore, inhalation of nitric oxide by patients with severe adult respiratory distress syndrome not only reduces PAP but also improves ventilation/perfusion matching by augmenting blood flow only to well-ventilated alveoli.[23] Similar to other nitrates, nitric oxide is a bronchodilator, and inhalation likely improves regional ventilation by decreasing airway resistance.[24]

As a selective pulmonary vasodilator with seemingly limited adverse effects, nitric oxide is rapidly finding a place in the PICU. Studies have demonstrated its efficacy in selectively reducing PAP in patients with congenital heart disease.[25,26] In infants with postoperative PAH, Journois et al. demonstrated selective reduction in mean PAP ($35\% \pm 21\%$) with a concomitant improvement in oxygen arterial saturation ($9.7\% \pm 12\%$) and mixed venous oxygen-

ation ($37\% \pm 28\%$).[27] Patients with Fontan procedures in whom small elevations in pulmonary vascular resistance are critical have been managed successfully with nitric oxide.[28,29] Pediatric patients with adult respiratory distress syndrome, lung transplantation, and a variety of neonatal lung diseases benefit from inhaled nitric oxide.[30–32] Toxic effects of nitric oxide can be minimized with meticulous attention to in-line monitoring of nitric oxide and nitrogen dioxide, serial methemoglobin levels, and adherence to published standards of drug delivery.[33,34] The clinical future of nitric oxide rests with investigative work that clarifies indications for use, optimal and strategic dosing formulas, improved delivery systems, and safer monitoring devices.

References

1. Jun-Bao D et al. Doppler echocardiographic evaluation of pulmonary artery pressure in pneumonia of infants and children. *Pediatr Pulmonol* 10:296–298, 1991.
2. Wheller J et al. Diagnosis and management of post-operative pulmonary hypertensive crisis. *Circulation* 60:1640–1644, 1979.
3. Hislop A, Reid L. Intrapulmonary arterial development during fetal life-branching pattern and structure. *J Anat* 113:35–48, 1972.
4. Hislop A, Reid L. Pulmonary arterial development during childhood: Branching pattern and structure. *Thorax* 28:129–135, 1973.
5. Hislop A, Reid L. Development of the acinus in the human lung. *Thorax* 29:90–94, 1974.
6. Haworth SG, Hislop AA. Pulmonary vascular development: Normal values of peripheral vascular structure. *Am J Cardiol* 52:578–583, 1983.
7. Sreeram N et al. Progressive pulmonary hypertension after the arterial switch procedure. *Am J Cardiol* 73:620–621, 1994.
8. Hall S, Haworth SG. Onset and evolution of pulmonary vascular disease in young children: Abnormal postnatal remodelling studied in lung biopsies. *J Pathol* 166:183–193, 1992.
9. Goodman G et al. Pulmonary hypertension in infants with bronchopulmonary dysplasia. *J Pediatr* 112:67–72, 1988.
10. Hopkins RA et al. Pulmonary hypertensive crises following surgery for congenital heart defects in young children. *Eur J Cardiothorac Surg* 5:628–634, 1991.
11. Rabinovitch M et al. Lung biopsy in congenital heart disease: A morphometric approach to pulmonary vascular disease. *Circulation* 58:1107–1122, 1978.
12. Clapp S et al. Down's syndrome, complete atrioventricular canal, and pulmonary vascular obstructive disease. *J Thorac Cardiovasc Surg* 100:115–121, 1990.
13. Rosen GM et al. Post-operative respiratory compromise in children with obstructive sleep apnea syndrome: Can it be anticipated? *Pediatrics* 93:784–788, 1994.
14. Berman W et al. Evaluation of infants with bronchopulmonary dysplasia using cardiac catheterization *Pediatrics* 70:708–712, 1982.
15. Rider L, Clarke WR, Rutledge J. Pulmonary hypertension in a seventeen-year-old boy. *J Pediatr* 120:149–159, 1992.
16. Perkin MP, Anas NG. Pulmonary hypertension in pediatric patients. *J Pediatr* 105:511–522, 1984.
17. Hickey PR et al. Blunting of stress response in the pulmonary circulation of infants by fentanyl. *Anesth Analg* 64:1137–1142, 1985.
18. Pinsky MR. The effects of mechanical ventilation on the cardiovascular system *Crit Care Clin* 6:663–678, 1990.
19. Bush A et al. Does prostacyclin enhance the selective pulmonary vasodilator effect of oxygen in children with congenital heart disease? *Circulation* 74:135–144, 1986.
20. Palmer RM, Ferrige AG, Moncada S. Nitric oxide release accounts for the biologic activity of endothelium derived relaxing factor. *Nature* 327:524–526, 1987.
21. Trolin G, Anden T, Hedenstierna G. Nitric oxide in expired air at rest and during exercise. *Acta Physiol Scand* 151:159–163, 1994.

22. Fronstell CG et al. Inhaled nitric oxide selectively reverses human hypoxic pulmonary vasoconstriction without causing systemic vasodilation. *Anesthesiology* 78:427–435, 1993.

23. Rossaint R et al. Inhaled nitric oxide for the adult respiratory distress syndrome. *N Engl J Med* 328:399–405, 1993.

24. Dupuy PM et al. Bronchodilator action of inhaled nitric oxide in guinea pigs. *J Clin Invest* 90:421–428, 1992.

25. Winberg P, Lundell BPW, Gustafsson LE. Effect of inhaled nitric oxide on raised pulmonary vascular resistance in children with congenital heart disease. *Br Heart J* 71:282–286, 1994.

26. Roberts JD et al. Inhaled nitric oxide in congenital heart disease. *Circulation* 87:447–453, 1993.

27. Journois D et al. Inhaled nitric oxide as a therapy for pulmonary hypertension after operations for congenital heart defects. *J Thorac Cardiovasc Surg* 107:1129–1135, 1994.

28. Yahagi N et al. Inhaled nitric oxide for the postoperative management of fontan-type operations *Ann Thorac Surg* 57:1369–1374, 1994.

29. Miller OI, James J, Elliott MJ. Intraoperative use of inhaled low-dose nitric oxide. *J Thorac Cardiovasc Surg* 105:550–551, 1993.

30. Leclerc F et al. Inhaled nitric oxide for a severe respiratory syncytial virus infection in an infant with BPD. *Intensive Care Med* 20:511–512, 1994.

31. Adatia L et al. Inhaled nitric oxide in the treatment of postoperative graft dysfunction after lung transplantation. *Ann Thorac Surg* 57:1311–1318, 1994.

32. Finer NN et al. Inhaled nitric oxide in infants referred for extracorporeal membrane oxygenation: Dose response. *J Pediatr* 124:302–308, 1994.

33. Miller OI et al. Guidelines for the safe administration of nitric oxide. *Arch Dis Child* 70:F47–49, 1994.

34. Foubert L et al. Safety guidelines for use of nitric oxide. *Lancet* 339:1615–1616, 1992.

Elizabeth A. Catlin

19 Bronchopulmonary Dysplasia

Bronchopulmonary dysplasia (BPD) is an important chronic lung disorder of infancy, described initially by Northway et al. in 1967.[1] BPD is characterized by specific histologic changes in both airways and lung tissue, with varying degrees of clinical respiratory insufficiency. In practical terms, BPD is the most common chronic lung disease of infants, and these patients have a significant rehospitalization rate during the first several years of life; thus, a finite number of children admitted to pediatric intensive care units (PICUs) carry this diagnosis, and a working knowledge of the disease is required of caregivers.

Epidemiology and Pathophysiology

Our current understanding supports a multifactorial etiology for BPD. Goetzman has proposed that the development of BPD may be dissected into four contributing components: (1) the susceptible host, (2) acute lung injury, (3) secondary lung injury, and (4) abnormal healing of lung tissue.[2] Prematurely born neonates are at highest risk for this lung disease,[3] but there are also family histories of airway hyperreactivity in some children with BPD.[4] A 1987 survey documented that significant differences in the incidence of BPD occur in a category of very low birth weight babies (birth weights from 700 to 1500 g) between major North American neonatal centers, with the highest incidence approaching 35%.[5] Analysis of 1776 babies in this weight range, born in 1983–1984, confirmed significant variability in outcomes between institutions with an overall survival rate of 85% and a 30% incidence of chronic lung disease.[6]

Respiratory distress syndrome (RDS, synonymous with hyaline membrane disease) is the most common lung condition predisposing to BPD and is characterized by immature lungs with insufficient pulmonary surfactant. RDS is the most frequent cause of acute lung injury in the neonate, and its presence is progressively more likely with decreasing gestational age. Similarly, the incidence of BPD increases dramatically in extremely premature babies.[7] Antenatal treatment with betamethasone and ritodrine can decrease mortality, morbidity, and RDS in premature babies[8]; surfactant replacement therapy may improve neonatal outcome using a combined measure of survival and BPD, although a single dose of bovine surfactant does not alter the incidence of BPD.[9–11] Less frequently, other neonatal lung diseases such as meconium aspiration and bacterial pneumonitis provide the acute lung insult preceding the development of BPD. Barotrauma appears to greatly increase the incidence of BPD development in infants mechanically ventilated for RDS.[12] Necrosis of alveolar epithelium has been shown to occur within minutes of commencement of positive-pressure ventilation in animal models with insufficient surfactant and seems to relate directly to the occurrence of barotrauma.[13] That positive-pressure ventilation itself, in the premature respiratory tract, may contribute to the development of BPD is suggested by reports of BPD in infants ventilated for apnea[14] and by the marked decrease in BPD development in a neonatal intensive care unit (NICU), systematically minimizing mechanical ventilation and relying on nasal CPAP.[5]

Oxygen toxicity plays a role in the lung injury leading to BPD. Premature survivors of RDS treated with high oxygen concentrations without mechanical ventilation have small airway abnormalities 10 years after therapy similar to babies ventilated for RDS with high FiO_2.[15] The term *diffuse alveolar damage* has been coined to describe the histologic changes induced by hyperoxia, and these include an exudative stage followed by a proliferative stage.[16] Prolonged exposure to high concentrations of oxygen first damages capillary endothelial cells, producing leakage of serum proteins and fluid.[17] Direct oxidant damage with supplemental oxygen exposure impairs ciliary motion, and indirect oxidant damage occurs from cellular release of oxygen radicals[18,19] (Fig. 19-1). Enzymatic replacement, using bovine superoxide dismutase (a free oxygen radical scavenger), has been reported to reduce the inci-

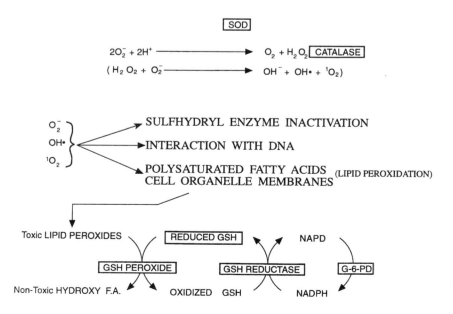

Figure 19-1. Oxygen free radicals and antioxidant defense systems. Illustrated are the highly reactive O_2 metabolites: O_2^-, superoxide anion; $OH^·$, hydroxyl radical; H_2O_2, hydrogen peroxide; and $^1O_2$, singlet oxygen. Also shown are the antioxidant enzyme defense systems: SOD, superoxide dismutase; catalase; and, glutathione (GSH) peroxidase, glutathione (GSH) reductase, and glucose-6-phosphate dehydrogenase (G-6-PD). These enzymes function to protect the cell from the types of damaging biochemical interactions with oxygen radicals listed: critical sulfhydryl oxidations; DNA scism, alteration; membrane lipid peroxidations. The reaction between H_2O_2 and O_2^- to form other toxic oxygen metabolites is the so-called Haber-Weiss reaction (in parentheses). This reaction requires trace amounts of metals such as iron. (From L Frank, D Massaro. Oxygen toxicity. *Am J Med* 69:117–126, 1980. With permission.)

dence of BPD.[20] The presence of a patent ductus arteriosus (PDA) in infants later developing BPD has been proposed as aggravating its development via increased pulmonary edema. A trial of very early prophylactic PDA ligation in tiny premature neonates demonstrated no decrease in the incidence of BPD.[21] In a case-control study of antecedents of BPD, however, patients with BPD received greater quantities of crystalloid, colloid, and total fluids per day than control infants in the first 4 days of life, and more often were given a clinical diagnosis of PDA.[22]

Abnormal healing is thought to contribute to the development of this chronic lung disease of infancy for the following reasons: The bronchoalveolar lavage from babies who later develop BPD contains polymorphonuclear leukocytes, proteolytic enzymes, and evidence of fibrosis by the end of the first week compared with the predominance of macrophages, antiproteolytic enzymes, and evidence of tissue regeneration in infants who do not develop BPD.[18] By 2 to 3 weeks of age, tracheal lavage fibronectin (fibronectin is a glycoprotein important in cell adhesion and proliferation of fibroblasts in areas of lung damage) is much higher in infants who develop BPD and remains elevated 30 days after birth.[23] Vitamin A deficiency may contribute to the abnormal healing of lung and airway tissue in BPD. A study of 40 very low birth weight babies receiving either placebo or supplemental vitamin A (retinyl palmitate, 2000 IU) for a 28-day course revealed statistically much less BPD in the vitamin A group.[24] This work supports the contention that promoting regenerative healing of lung and airway tissues diminishes the incidence of infant chronic lung disease.

Pathologically, BPD is a disease of airways and lung parenchyma.[1] In early stages of diffuse alveolar damage, hyaline membranes, atelectasis, and permeable capillary epithelium leading to pulmonary edema are present, similar to findings in RDS; dilatation of pulmonary lymphatics is also present.[25] Epithelial desquamation and necrosis precede widespread mucosal metaplasia. O'Brodovich and Mellins have pointed out that much of the pathologic information available on BPD is based on autopsy material[26]; thus, the most severe cases of BPD have supplied the majority of the histologic data, presenting perhaps a skewed picture of the disease. Fibrotic healing of necrotizing bronchiolitis occurs with obliteration of lumens and results in interstitial fibrosis. Areas of emphysematous alveoli develop which alternate with atelectatic lung in more advanced BPD. Adjacent bronchioles are surrounded by hypertrophied peribronchial smooth muscle. Pulmonary hypertension with medial muscular hypertrophy of pulmonary vasculature is not an infrequent finding in severe BPD with progression to cor pulmonale in a smaller subset of patients.

Clinical Presentation

Current clinical diagnostic criteria for BPD include lung dysfunction on and after 28 days of life following acute neonatal lung injury, with clinical respiratory distress, chronic chest x-ray abnormalities, and requirement for supplemental oxygen.[26] The chest x-ray features of BPD require special mention. The four stages of progression of BPD initially described[1] are uncommonly seen at present.[27] While the cystic "bubbly" chest film appearance of previously seen Stage IV BPD is still seen at times, much more commonly hyperinflation with milder evidence of chronic, bilateral, fine, lacy densities is now seen (Fig. 19-2). The typical chest radiograph of BPD, seen more recently, shows milder, more homogenous pulmonary parenchymal changes with infrequent cardiomegaly.

Pulmonary function early in the course of BPD is characterized

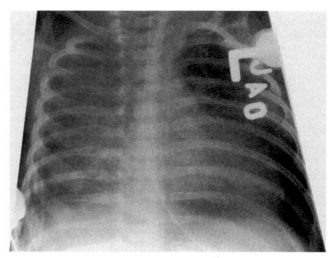

Figure 19-2. AP chest radiograph of 5½-week-old infant with oxygen- and diuretic-dependent BPD. Note the bilateral hyperinflation and lacy densities.

by increased airway resistance and abnormal gas exchange, evidenced by decreases in arterial oxygen tensions and elevations in carbon dioxide levels. Lung compliance in BPD is much below normal early on but improves gradually over the first years of life in some patients.[28] Airway hyperreactivity has been demonstrated in the first several weeks of postnatal life in very premature babies with BPD, and their bronchospasm often responds to inhaled bronchodilators with marked improvement in expiratory flows[29]

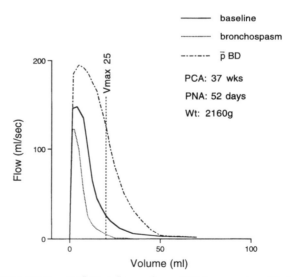

Figure 19-3. Deflation flow-volume (DFV) curves in a 52-day-old premature infant in respiratory failure with BPD who had apparent bronchospasm following endotracheal suctioning after the baseline DFV curves had been obtained. There was a marked reduction in both forced vital capacity (FVC) (-50%) and Vmax$_{25}$ (-80%). The infant responded promptly to a bronchodilator (BD); Vmax$_{25}$BD increased 4.7-fold from baseline, and FVC returned to baseline level. The descending portion of DFV curve after BD is less concave to the volume axis, indicating an increase in upstream conductance. (From EK Motoyama et al. Early onset of airway reactivity in premature infants with bronchopulmonary dysplasia. *Am Rev Respir Dis* 136:50–57, 1987. With permission.)

(Fig. 19-3). Both early and later in the course of BPD, infants have shown improvement in respiratory system resistance and compliance with bronchodilator treatment.[30] Certain pulmonary function measurements show near normalization, specifically FRC and pulmonary conductance, over the first 3 years of life, although minute ventilation and work of breathing remain elevated.[28] Abnormal gas exchange and airway obstruction persist at school age in some patients, as well as a significant incidence of exercise-induced bronchospasm.[31] In other infants, lung mechanics and gas exchange normalize early in infancy, with little or no residual dysfunction later in childhood.

Children with BPD may be admitted to the PICU as a direct consequence of their respiratory disease or because of another problem requiring intensive care.[32] In our PICU at the Massachusetts General Hospital, the majority of BPD patients admitted are postoperative or have acute infectious exacerbations of their lung disease; less frequently, infants are transferred from NICUs for chronic ventilatory management. Infants with BPD have an increased incidence and severity of subsequent lower respiratory disease,[33] and in the first 2 years following discharge, their rehospitalization rate may approach 50%.[15,34]

Management

Intensive care management of the BPD patient must focus on (1) nutritional support, (2) fluid balance, and (3) respiratory management; these three elements are highly interrelated.

Nutritional Support

A number of infants with BPD have elevated metabolic rates; this increase in oxygen consumption (VO_2) is only partially explained by increased work of breathing.[35] In the postoperative patient, tissue loss (catabolism) is occurring, even following elective surgery. During "stressed starvation," autocannibalism may deplete nutritional reserves quickly, and so ventilatory demands increase significantly.[36] Nutritional depletion has been associated with easier muscle fatigue, which may be reversed with nutritional repletion.[37] The metabolic demands imposed by surgery, infection/sepsis, childhood (i.e., energy required for growth above basal requirements), and by BPD compel the intensivist to address nutritional support on admission to the PICU.

The enteral route is far superior to the parenteral route for alimentation; it is physiologic and low risk. The patient must be stable, adequately oxygenated, and perfused, with a benign abdominal examination and normal bowel sounds before reinstituting enteral feedings. Gastroesophageal reflux (GER) has been variously thought to occur more commonly in BPD patients; a recent small study found less GER in BPD infants than in a control group.[38] Caloric requirements should be calculated ideally using measured oxygen consumption (VO_2) and carbon dioxide production (VCO_2). Estimates of daily caloric requirements (including tissue growth) for infants with BPD range from 100 to 160 kcal/kg, with the higher energy requirements in those infants with growth failure.[39] Intolerance of large fluid volumes often necessitates increasing formula caloric density to 30 kcal/oz and above, using additional carbohydrate and fat.

If enteral alimentation is not possible, parenteral feeding is indicated. Peripheral hyperalimentation solutions of glucose, amino acids, trace elements, and vitamins are available with dextrose concentrations of up to 12.5%. Intravenous lipids should also be given to provide essential fatty acids and to augment caloric

intake. Nonprotein energy sources must meet total metabolic expenditure to prevent weight loss. In the occasional BPD patient requiring long-term parenteral alimentation, central hyperalimentation using dextrose in concentrations up to 25% as tolerated combined with lipids provides for caloric needs; amino acids are added to provide for nitrogen needs at approximately 25 mg/kcal. Certain patients with compensated respiratory acidosis may not tolerate increased carbohydrate loads because of high VCO_2, and ideally their VO_2 and VCO_2 should be measured and alimentation tailored to meet their specific needs. It seems prudent to avoid extremes, keeping in mind that a range of fuel mixtures (combinations of nonprotein calorie sources) can maintain protein balance in the patient with chronic lung disease.[40]

Fluid Balance

Striking a balance between fluid inadequacy and fluid overload in the child with BPD may be a difficult task. These children are often maintained as outpatients on diuretics and fluid restriction. Intraoperative fluid administration or fluid boluses in the emergency department may result in pulmonary edema evidenced in the PICU. Acute pulmonary edema in these patients is manifest as dyspnea, cyanosis, rales, respiratory acidosis, and bilateral opacities on chest radiograph. Therapy consists of supplemental oxygen, diuretic administration, fluid restriction, and mechanical ventilation, if indicated. CVP measurement may be helpful in assessing fluid administration needs in the critically ill BPD patient. Maintenance fluids in normal children greater than 10 kg are estimated based on body surface area (BSA) nomograms using as a total 1500 ml/m^2 BSA/24 hr. Fluid requirements for normal infants less than 10 kg may be estimated at 100 ml/kg/d, with somewhat higher amounts of 125 ml/kg in the first few months of life. There are no strict guidelines for calculating maintenance fluids for infants with BPD except that administration of usual maintenance fluid volumes to these infants often results in increased respiratory distress with pulmonary edema. Thus, fluid restriction is empiric; 80% of usual maintenance estimates is not unusual. It is worth mentioning that humidification of inspired oxygen is a significant fluid source because the autohumidification (an insensible fluid loss) of inspired gas normally accounts for approximately 15% of total fluid losses per day.

Diuretic therapy is frequently a mainstay of treatment in BPD. Furosemide has been shown to acutely decrease airway resistance,[41] and with prolonged therapy, to improve dynamic compliance and resistance in BPD.[42] The improved lung function has been associated with earlier weaning from ventilatory support and supplemental oxygen.[43] Furosemide is usually given intravenously at 1 mg/kg every 12 hours or enterally at 2 mg/kg every 12 hours. Side effects include calciuria with bone demineralization and nephrolithiasis, and volume and salt depletion. Alternate-day furosemide therapy in BPD has been shown to minimize alterations in electrolyte and mineral balance.[44] Other diuretic agents have been tried with variable results, and a trial assessing lung function, 1 and 8 days after spironolactone-hydrochlorothiazide in infants with BPD, found no improvement in lung mechanics or oxygenation.[45]

Respiratory Management

The **respiratory management** of the BPD patient, admitted to the PICU, centers on oxygen supplementation, mechanical ventilation, diuretic use, bronchodilator therapy, and, when indicated, steroid therapy. Oxygen administration (FiO_2) should be monitored in the acute stabilization period by arterial blood gas (ABG) and continuous Hgb-O_2 saturation measurements (SaO_2, pulse oximetry). Transfer of stable BPD patients into the PICU (e.g., for chronic ventilator management), however, need not be accompanied by aggressive ABG determinations; continuous oxygen saturation measurement combined with the physical examination supplemented by infrequent ABGs is sufficient. Recommended guidelines for oxygen therapy in these patients include maintaining the PaO_2 from 55 to 65 mm Hg or SaO_2 from 90% to 92% to prevent hypoxemia and long-term cor pulmonale[46] and to minimize oxygen toxicity. Many BPD patients will have significant reductions in their pulmonary artery pressures with oxygen administration; by decreasing pulmonary vascular resistance, improvement in gas exchange may occur. Those patients with fixed pulmonary hypertension have a poor long-term prognosis.[47]

Mechanical ventilation management may be divided into acute, subacute (or transitional), and weaning phases.[48] During acute management, initial stabilization of all organ systems, including the respiratory system, is addressed aggressively to achieve a stable airway, adequate cardiac performance, and correction of oxygenation and ventilation. Tracheal intubation should be accomplished in the safest, most controlled manner with adequate pre-oxygenation and pre-medication, rapid laryngoscopy and endotracheal tube placement, and careful securing of the airway once in proper position. BPD patients less than 10 kg requiring mechanical ventilator support are ventilated with time-cycled, pressure-limited units. Volume ventilators (volume-limited, or time-cycled, volume-limited) are used in children larger than 10 kg. The ventilator should provide for all of the patient's ventilation needs during stabilization, thus allowing for diaphragm rest and recovery. Sedation may be appropriate during this early stage, being careful not to sedate a patient whose agitation stems from hypoxemia. Oxygen administration should be titrated to achieve hemoglobin-oxygen saturations of approximately 90% to 92%; although oxygen toxicity contributes to the development of BPD, it is also a cornerstone of its therapy. Erring on the side of liberal oxygen administration during acute management is preferable to undertreatment resulting in hypoxemia.

Based on the earlier discussion of pulmonary function abnormalities in BPD patients, it is apparent that mechanically ventilating these patients will present specific challenges. Because of the high airway resistance in BPD, the time constants (tau = resistance × compliance) for alveoli will be prolonged, resulting in slow expansion and emptying of alveolar units.[48] Therefore, adequate inspiratory and expiratory times must be set; 3 to 5 time constants are required for complete filling or emptying of alveoli. For example, short expiratory times in BPD patients may result in incomplete expiration, with progressive gas trapping leading to increased auto-positive end-expiratory pressure (PEEP) and inadequate ventilation. Appropriate inflating pressures and tidal volumes must be determined for each patient. In general, with their high airway resistance and decreased compliance, these patients will require increased pressures for adequate air entry and chest expansion. Careful hand-controlled ventilation with an in-line manometer to prevent delivery of excessive inflating pressures[49] (Fig. 19-4) should be used in concert with the physical examination (i.e., visualization of bilateral chest movements and auscultation of breath sounds!) to guide initial ventilator settings. Thereafter, ABGs and oxygen saturations will help guide ventilator and oxygen therapy. One key difference in the mechanical ventilation of BPD patients, compared with other children with acute lung disease, is that the

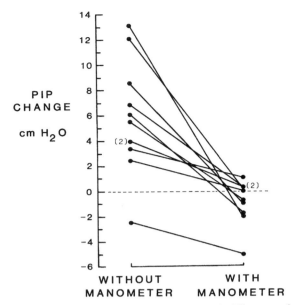

Figure 19-4. Peak inspiratory pressure (PIP) differences from mechanical ventilation PIP in 11 neonates during hand-regulated ventilation without and with manometers inline; $P = 0.00047$ (From B Goldstein et al. The role of in-line manometers in minimizing peak and mean airway pressure during the hand-regulated ventilation of newborn infants. *Respir Care* 34[1]:23–27, 1989. With permission.)

overall time from acute stabilization through subacute/transitional phase and finally to the weaning phase is a much slower process in the child with BPD.[32]

Weaning the BPD patient from assisted ventilation may be potentially achieved using one of several types of schedules. The two most widely used methods for weaning are (1) intermittent mandatory ventilation (IMV) and (2) CPAP trials.[48] Occasionally, we have used pressure-support ventilation for weaning from assisted ventilation in young toddlers with chronic lung disease, but there are negligible data on this method in young children. Once the child has achieved stability in oxygenation and ventilation, a "transition phase" exists where acute derangements (in organ function, metabolism, etc.) reach homeostasis. Weaning programs may thereafter be initiated. As mentioned earlier, nutritional adequacy is very important for successful weaning programs. The IMV form of weaning uses progressively increased numbers of spontaneous breaths taken by the patient while concomitantly decreasing the number of breaths delivered by the ventilator. CPAP weaning programs utilize initially short periods of totally spontaneous breathing that are gradually lengthened, supported only by CPAP. Many, if not most, mechanically ventilated BPD patients in the PICU are infants, and so will not generally be capable of meeting criteria for ventilator weaning used in adults and older pediatric patients (i.e., negative inspiratory force of greater than 30 mm Hg, vital capacity over 10–15 ml/kg, etc.). Therefore, weight gain, oxygen saturations, respiratory effort, and occasional blood gas determinations are used to evaluate the success of decreasing mechanical support. The process of weaning from mechanical support in some infants with severe BPD may have to be very gradual, requiring weeks or even many months until extubation. Although decisions regarding tracheostomies should be individualized to a degree for each patient, strong consideration for placing

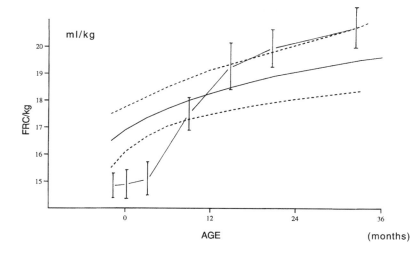

Figure 19-5. Sequential measurement of functional residual capacity per kilogram in infants with chronic lung disease (mean ± SE, *heavy line*). Measurements were shifted to left to correct for lower gestational age. For comparison, the curve for normal infants *(thin line)* and its 95% confidence limits *(dashed lines)* are shown. (From T Gerhardt et al. Serial determination of pulmonary function in infants with chronic lung disease. *J Pediatr* 110[3]: 448–456, 1987. With permission.)

a tracheostomy and gastrostomy tube should be given when a weaning course of several months is anticipated.

Bronchodilators have been found to have a place in the pulmonary management of BPD patients. Inhaled beta-2 agonists have been demonstrated to increase compliance and decrease respiratory system resistance in ventilator-dependent babies[30] as well as improve pulmonary function in spontaneously breathing subjects. BPD patients admitted to the PICU with acute respiratory decompensation with bronchospasm should be treated initially with nebulized bronchodilator followed by aminophylline infusion (with careful monitoring of serum levels to achieve and maintain theophylline levels of 10–20 mg/liter) if necessary. In both intubated and spontaneously breathing patients, albuterol (Ventolin) at 0.05 mg/kg up to 0.15 mg/kg may be delivered every 20 minutes or every 2 to 4 hours, and if necessary, even continuously (0.4–0.6 mg/kg/hr).[46,50]

Corticosteroids appear to improve lung function in mechanically ventilated infants with BPD.[51] A small study concluded that a 42-day course of dexamethasone accelerated weaning from mechanical ventilation and supplemental oxygen.[52] The Collaborative Dexamethasone Trial Group studied a group of approximately 3-week-old BPD patients treated for 1 week with 0.6 mg/kg/d of dexamethasone, with or without a second 9-day tapering course, and found significant reduction in duration of mechanical ventilation when compared with placebo-treated infants.[53] Therefore, steroid treatment may be indicated in certain BPD patients to accelerate initial ventilator weaning. Additionally, older BPD patients presenting acutely with severe bronchospasm may benefit from a short course of steroids, as prompt treatment of acute asthma in emergency settings significantly improves lung function and reduces the number of hospitalizations[54] (reactive airway disease may affect up to 50% of adolescents and young adults following BPD in infancy[55]).

Prognosis

A number of infants with BPD will enter their school years with normal or near normal pulmonary function (Fig. 19-5). For a smaller group of BPD patients, the long-term prognosis must be considered guarded, as they may show persistent impairments in pulmonary function, have poor growth, and exhibit developmental or motor delays.[56] Unexpected, sudden death can occur in BPD patients, particularly those that have been mechanically ventilated

for longer than 2 months,[57] despite in-hospital cardiopulmonary monitoring and rapid institution of resuscitative measures. Information on the prognosis for supplemental oxygen-dependent BPD patients with pulmonary hypertension has been collected using cardiac catheterization; lack of normalization of pulmonary artery pressures with oxygen administration seems to bode poorly for survival in these patients.[47] Northway et al. have reported that many adolescents and young adults who have had the diagnosis of BPD during infancy demonstrate persisting pulmonary function abnormalities, including airway obstruction, reactive airway disease, and hyperinflation.[55] Whether the introduction of corticosteroid therapy in infantile BPD will alter long-term outcome requires further study.

References

1. Northway WH Jr, Rosan RC, Porter DY. Pulmonary disease following respirator therapy of hyaline-membrane disease. *N Engl J Med* 276:357–368, 1967.
2. Goetzman BW. Understanding bronchopulmonary dysplasia. *Am J Dis Child* 140:332–334, 1986.
3. Hakulinen A et al. Occurrence, predictive factors and associated morbidity of bronchopulmonary dysplasia in a preterm birth cohort. *J Perinatol Med* 16:437–446, 1988.
4. Nickerson BG, Taussig LM. Family history of asthma in infants with bronchopulmonary dysplasia. *Pediatrics* 65:1140–1144, 1980.
5. Avery ME et al. Is chronic lung disease in low birth weight infants preventable? A survey of eight centers. *Pediatrics* 79:26–30, 1987.
6. Horbar JD et al. Variability in 28 day outcomes for very low birth weight infants: An analysis of 11 neonatal intensive care units. *Pediatrics* 82:554–559, 1988.
7. Tooley WH. Epidemiology of bronchopulmonary dysplasia. *J Pediatr* 95:851–858, 1979.
8. Papageorgiou AN et al. Reduction of mortality, morbidity and respiratory distress syndrome in infants weighing less than 1,000 grams by treatment with betamethasone and ritodrine. *Pediatrics* 83:493–497, 1989.
9. Merritt TA et al. Prophylactic treatment of very premature infants with human surfactant. *N Engl J Med* 315:785–790, 1986.
10. Horbar JD et al. A multicenter randomized, placebo-controlled trial of surfactant therapy for respiratory distress syndrome. *N Engl J Med* 320:959–965, 1989.
11. Lang MJ et al. A controlled trial of human surfactant replacement therapy for severe respiratory distress syndrome in very low birth weight infants. *J Pediatr* 116:295–300, 1990.

12. Moylan FMB et al. The relationship of bronchopulmonary dysplasia to the occurrence of alveolar rupture during positive pressure ventilation. *Crit Care Med* 6:140–142, 1978.

13. Lachmann B et al. Modes of artificial ventilation in severe respiratory distress syndrome: Lung function and morphology in rabbits after wash-out of alveolar surfactant. *Crit Care Med* 10:724–732, 1982.

14. Fitzhardinge PM et al. Mechanical ventilation of infants of less than 1,501 gm birth weight: Health, growth, and neurologic sequelae. *J Pediatr* 88:531–541, 1976.

15. Coates AL et al. Oxygen therapy and long term pulmonary outcome of respiratory distress syndrome in newborns. *Am J Dis Child* 136:892–895, 1982.

16. Lodato RF. Oxygen toxicity. *Crit Care Clin* 6:749–765, 1990.

17. Massaro D. Oxygen: Toxicity and tolerance. *Hosp Prac* 21:95–101, 1987.

18. Sinkin RA, Phelps DL. New strategies for the prevention of bronchopulmonary dysplasia. *Clin Perinatol* 14:599–620, 1987.

19. Frank L, Massaro D. Oxygen toxicity. *Am J Med* 69:117–126, 1980.

20. Rosenfeld W et al. Prevention of bronchopulmonary dysplasia by administration of bovine superoxide dismutase in preterm infants with respiratory distress syndrome. *J Pediatr* 105:781–785, 1984.

21. Cassady G et al. A randomized controlled trial of very early prophylactic ligation of the ductus arteriosus in babies who weighed 1000 g or less at birth. *N Engl J Med* 320:1511–1516, 1989.

22. Van Marter LJ et al. Hydration during the first days of life and the risk of bronchopulmonary dysplasia in low birth weight infants. *J Pediatr* 116:942–949, 1990.

23. Gerdes JS et al. Tracheal lavage and plasma fibronectin: Relationship to respiratory distress syndrome and development of bronchopulmonary dysplasia. *J Pediatr* 108:601–606, 1986.

24. Shenai JP et al. Clinical trial of vitamin A supplementation in infants susceptible to bronchopulmonary dysplasia. *J Pediatr* 111:269–277, 1987.

25. Taghizadeh A, Reynolds EOR. Pathogenesis of bronchopulmonary dysplasia following hyaline membrane disease. *Am J Pathol* 82:241–257, 1976.

26. O'Brodovich HM, Mellins RB. State of the art: Bronchopulmonary dysplasia. *Am Rev Respir Dis* 132:694–709, 1985.

27. Edwards DK. Radiographic aspects of bronchopulmonary dysplasia. *J Pediatr* 95:823–829, 1979.

28. Gerhardt T et al. Serial determination of pulmonary function in infants with chronic lung disease. *J Pediatr* 110:448–456, 1987.

29. Motoyama EK et al. Early onset of airway reactivity in premature infants with bronchopulmonary dysplasia. *Am Rev Respir Dis* 136:50–57, 1987.

30. Wilkie RA, Bryan MH. Effect of bronchodilators on airway resistance in ventilator-dependent neonates with chronic lung disease. *J Pediatr* 111:278–282, 1987.

31. Bader D et al. Childhood sequelae of infant lung disease: Exercise and pulmonary function abnormalities after bronchopulmonary dysplasia. *J Pediatr* 110:693–699, 1987.

32. Katz R, McWilliams B. Bronchopulmonary dysplasia in the pediatric intensive care unit. *Crit Care Clin* 4:755–787, 1988.

33. Myers MG, McGuinness GA, Lachenbruch PA. Respiratory illness in survivors of infant respiratory distress syndrome. *Am Rev Respir Dis* 133:1011–1018, 1986.

34. Katz RW, Samet J. Longitudinal study of respiratory morbidity of infants with bronchopulmonary dysplasia (abstract). *Am Rev Respir Dis* 137(Suppl):A235, 1988.

35. Kurzner SI, Garg M, Bautista DB. Growth failure in bronchopulmo-

nary dysplasia: Elevated metabolic rates and pulmonary mechanics. *J Pediatr* 112:73–80, 1988.

36. Shayevitz JR, Weissman C. Nutrition and metabolism in the critically ill child. In Rogers MC (ed): *Textbook of Pediatric Intensive Care.* Baltimore: Williams & Wilkins, 1987. Pp 943–978.

37. Jeejeebhoy KN. Nutrition in critical illness. In Shoemaker WC (ed): *Critical Care Medicine: State of the Art.* Fremont, CA: Society of Critical Care Medicine, 1984.

38. Sindel BD, Maisels MJ, Ballantine TVN. Gastroesophegeal reflux to the proximal esophagus in infants with bronchopulmonary dysplasia. *Am J Dis Child* 143:1103–1106, 1989.

39. Kurzner SI et al. Growth failure in infants with bronchopulmonary dysplasia: Nutrition and elevated resting metabolic expenditure. *Pediatrics* 81:379–384, 1988.

40. Wilson DO, Rogers RM, Hoffman RM. State of the art: Nutrition and chronic lung disease. *Am Rev Respir Dis* 132:1347–1365, 1985.

41. Kao LC et al. Furosemide acutely decreases airways resistance in chronic bronchopulmonary dysplasia. *J Pediatr* 103:624–629, 1983.

42. Engelhardt B, Elliott S, Hazinski TA. Short- and long-term effects of furosemide on lung function in infants with bronchopulmonary dysplasia. *J Pediatr* 109:1034–1039, 1986.

43. McCann EM et al. Controlled trial of furosemide therapy in infants with chronic lung disease. *J Pediatr* 106:957–962, 1985.

44. Rush MG et al. Double-blind, placebo-controlled trial of alternate-day furosemide therapy in infants with chronic bronchopulmonary dysplasia. *J Pediatr* 117:112–118, 1990.

45. Engelhardt B et al. Effect of spironolactone-hydrochlorothiazide on lung function in infants with chronic bronchopulmonary dysplasia. *J Pediatr* 114:619–624, 1989.

46. Blanchard PW, Brown TM, Coates AL. Pharmacotherapy in bronchopulmonary dysplasia. *Clin Perinatol* 14:881–910, 1987.

47. Goodman G et al. Pulmonary hypertension in infants with bronchopulmonary dysplasia. *J Pediatr* 112:67–72, 1988.

48. McWilliams BC. Mechanical ventilation in pediatric patients. *Clin Chest Med* 8:597–609, 1987.

49. Goldstein B et al. The role of in-line manometers in minimizing peak and mean airway pressure during the hand-regulated ventilation of newborn infants. *Respir Care* 34:23–27, 1989.

50. Schuh S et al. High- versus low-dose, frequently administered, nebulized albuterol in children with severe, acute asthma. *Pediatrics* 83:513–518, 1989.

51. Ng PC. The effectiveness and side effects of dexamethasone in preterm infants with bronchopulmonary dysplasia. *Arch Dis Child* 68:330–336, 1993.

52. Cummins JJ, D'Eugenio DB, Gross SJ. A controlled trial of dexamethasone in preterm infants at high risk for bronchopulmonary dysplasia. *N Engl J Med* 320:1505–1510, 1989.

53. Collaborative Dexamethasone Trial Group. Dexamethasone therapy in neonatal chronic lung disease: An international placebo-controlled trial. *Pediatrics* 88:421–427, 1991.

54. Littenberg B, Gluck EG. A controlled trial of methylprednisolone in the emergency treatment of acute asthma. *N Engl J Med* 314:150–152, 1986.

55. Northway WH Jr et al. Late pulmonary sequelae of bronchopulmonary dysplasia. *N Engl J Med* 323:1793–1799, 1990.

56. Berman W et al. Long-term follow-up of bronchopulmonary dysplasia. *J Pediatr* 109:45–50, 1986.

57. Abman SH et al. Late sudden unexpected deaths in hospitalized infants with bronchopulmonary dysplasia. *Am J Dis Child* 143:815–820, 1989.

James W. Ziegler

◆20◆ Near-Drowning

Epidemiology

Drowning is a major cause of death in children and is second only to motor vehicle accidents as a cause of accidental death.[1,2] In the United States, between 5,000 and 10,000 people die each year from drowning, and though these statistics are impressive, they do not reflect the delayed mortality and long-term morbidity associated with near-drowning.

There are two major groups within the pediatric age range that are at highest risk.[3–8] The first is the infant and toddler. In this group, the majority of drowning and near-drowning events occur in private swimming pools, usually owned by the immediate family. Most victims in this group are White males, and lack of adequate adult supervision is the major contributing factor. The second high-risk group consists of the late childhood to adolescent age range; again males predominate, with Blacks accounting for a disproportionately high percentage of cases. Common locations include lakes, ponds, canals, and the ocean, and alcohol use becomes increasingly more common as age increases (Table 20-1).

Virtually any body or container of water can result in drowning and near-drowning. Although swimming pools are the most common site overall,[8,9] wading pools, hot tubs, bath tubs,[10] and even buckets of water[11] can be potential sources. In all except bathtub drownings, males predominate in a ratio of approximately 3:1.[12] In most series, freshwater drownings and near-drownings greatly outnumber salt water cases, even in states bordering the ocean.

A few subpopulations deserve special mention.[8] Several reports of submersion accidents in epileptic patients have been described. In addition, mentally retarded patients and diabetics should be considered at increased risk. Although swimming should not be discouraged in these individuals, adequate adult supervision assumes paramount importance, as it does in the toddler age range.

Definitions

Before proceeding, a few terms need to be defined. *Drowning* refers to submersion resulting in death either while submerged or within 24 hours of the epidode. *Near-drowning* refers to a submersion episode significant enough to warrant medical attention, but if death occurs, it occurs greater than 24 hours after the submersion event. *Wet drowning* (85% of cases) refers to cases where significant aspiration occurs, whereas *dry drowning* (15% of cases) implies minimal fluid aspiration, with the cause of death being intractable laryngospasm with resulting asphyxia. *Secondary drowning*, or the acute respiratory distress syndrome (ARDS), occurs in patients who have been resuscitated, and after a latent period of minutes to hours develop progressive dyspnea and respiratory failure.[13,14] *Hyperventilation-submersion syndrome* occurs in older males who hyperventilate before an attempted underwater endeavor.[15,16] With loss of the hypercarbic drive to breathe, hypoxemia severe enough to cause unconsciousness occurs while underwater. Most of these patients die.[17]

The immediate cause of death in drowning victims is cardiorespiratory arrest refractory to resuscitative efforts. Most late morbidity and mortality results from anoxic damage to the CNS. As many as one third of all survivors of near-drowning accidents are profoundly neurologically damaged.[18]

Pathophysiology

The following course of events is thought to occur in patients who suffer significant submersions (Fig. 20-1). Initially there is a period of struggling with voluntary breathholding. As time progresses, one of three things occurs. First, the victim may swallow large amounts of water with subsequent vomiting and aspiration of swallowed water and stomach contents. Second, gasping may occur with direct aspiration of water into the tracheobronchial tree. Last, and least common, persistent largyngospasm may occur with minimal aspiration. The end result of any of these three pathways is asphyxia with anoxic damage to various organ systems.

In experimental studies,[19,20] the tonicity of the fluid aspirated results in different physiologic changes (Table 20-2). Because of its hypotonicity relative to plasma, fresh water enters the bloodstream, causing hemodilution, hyponatremia, and fluid overload with a resultant increase in central venous pressure. Also, RBC lysis with hyperkalemia, hemoglobinemia, and hemogolbinuria occurs. Salt water, because it is hypertonic relative to plasma, causes opposite changes and osmotically "pulls" fluid from the intravascular compartment into the lungs, resulting in hemoconcentration, hypernatremia, and a decreased central venous pressure. Clinically, these changes are rarely seen in the human near-drowning victim, except in exceptional cases such as submersions in the Dead Sea.[21] Most likely, humans resuscitated from submersion episodes do not aspi-

Table 20-1. Risk groups for near-drowning in pediatric population

	Infants and toddlers	*Older children*
Sex	Males >>> females	Males >>> females
Location	Pools	Open bodies of water
Risk factors	Inadequate supervision Inadequate barrier	Inadequate supervision "Showing off" Hyperventilation-submersion
Special considerations	Child neglect Child abuse	Substance abuse Head and neck injuries

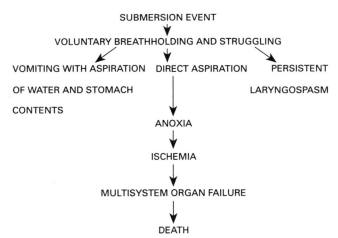

Figure 20-1. Sequence of events occurring during submersion.

rate large enough volumes of fluid to manifest the changes noted in experimental settings.[5,22,23]

The pathophysiology of the pulmonary injury in near-drowning patients does differ depending on whether fresh or salt water is aspirated.[19,24] Fresh water causes inactivation and washout of surfactant with a subsequent change in the surface tension properties of alveoli, resulting in atelectasis and disruption of the alveolar-capillary membrane. Salt water directly damages the alveolar-capillary membrane and causes alveolar "flooding" with exudative fluid. Of the two, fresh water appears to be more damaging, probably because it destroys surfactant to a greater degree than does salt water.[25,26] The end result of both processes is pulmonary edema and atelectasis resulting in diminished lung compliance, ventilation/perfusion mismatch, an increased alveolar-arterial oxygen gradient, and hypoxemia. Other factors may augment the pulmonary injury. Pneumonia occurs in up to 50% of near-drowning patients, sometimes with unusual organisms.[27,28] In addition, stomach contents and other debris may be aspirated into the tracheobronchial tree.[29] Complications of therapy, including barotrauma and oxygen toxicity, may also potentiate lung damage.

Although arrhythmias may occur in the near-drowning patient, they are usually secondary to hypoxemia, acidosis, hypothermia, or electrolyte changes, and resolve as the underlying abnormality is corrected.[30] Persistent cardiac dysfunction usually occurs only in severe cases and is secondary to hypoxic-ischemic injury. Late hemodynamic instability suggests sepsis. Metabolic acidosis is noted frequently in near-drowning victims and usually resolves by optimizing cardiac output and oxygen delivery.

Cerebral injury results from hypoxemia and hypoperfusion. Subsequent tissue anoxia causes impaired neuronal metabolism, depletion of ATP stores, loss of membrane stability, and the development of cytotoxic cerebral edema. Reperfusion injury and the loss of cerebral autoregulation may also be contributing factors. In any patient whose submersion was precipitated by trauma or a possible diving accident (or if events surrounding the submersion event are unknown), **cervical spine injury and operable intracranial lesions should be considered and ruled out.**

Other organ systems may be involved. Disseminated intravascular coagulation has been reported rarely and occurs secondary to hypoxemia, shock, or sepsis.[31,32] Renal failure also occurs in both fresh and salt water submersions; the usual etiology is hypoxemia and hypoperfusion.[33]

Ice Water Submersions

In discussing the pathophysiology of near-drowning, one subgroup needs to be discussed separately—the victims of ice water submersion. It is in this group of near-drowning patients that remarkable recoveries have been described following prolonged submersions. It is important to realize, however, that "hypothermic protection" is the exception rather than the rule; that is, most prolonged submersions in ice water still result in death. Also, hypothermia during resuscitation in the absence of submersion in frigid water negatively correlates with survival.

In Orlowski's review of the world's literature regarding prolonged ice water submersion greater than 15 minutes, 17 cases with full recovery were identified.[34] Thirteen of the 17 cases were persons less than 19 years old, with the average age being 10. All pediatric cases were male. In this review, the longest submersion recorded was 40 minutes.[35] Since then, a 2-year-old girl survived 66 minutes of submersion in ice water with complete neurologic recovery.[36]

Studies suggest that the dive reflex, which consists of peripheral vasoconstriction with preferential maintenance of cerebral and cardiac perfusion, is probably not active in humans.[37,38] Hypothermia, however, is known to be protective of the brain, primarily by dramatically decreasing cerebral metabolism and energy requirements. In rhesus monkeys slowly cooled to 20°C, complete cardiopulmonary arrest for up to 75 minutes was tolerated with complete recovery, and in 7 of 8, postmortem exams revealed normal brain histopathology.[39] It is probably rapid body cooling, causing metabolic rate to fall before hypoxia becomes critical, that affords protection to some children suffering ice water submersions.[40]

Because hypothermia below 29°C may slow down cerebral metabolism enough to mimic brain death and cause profound sinus bradycardia, it is very important that resuscitation efforts proceed until core temperature reaches 32°C or higher. The dictum that "nobody is dead until they are warm and dead" has been borne out by experience.[34]

Therapy
Initial Management

Minimizing the period of hypoxemia suffered by the near-drowning patient after a significant submersion is critical, and on-the-scene management is the most important phase of treatment. Early CPR provides the best possibility of a successful outcome.[41-43] It should be initiated as soon as possible and continued until the patient reaches the emergency room. Some propose performance of the Heimlich maneuver before the initiation of standard CPR.[44] Because many victims swallow large quantities of water, however, and because direct abdominal pressure may potentiate reflux and aspiration, this practice cannot be recommended as routine. It should be attempted if a clear airway cannot be obtained by other means or if there is no response to CPR.[45-47] Other early maneuvers include cervical spine immobilization and, as soon as possible, the provision of 100% oxygen. During transport to the hospital by paramedical personnel, optimization of oxygenation and hemodynamic stability should be the major focus. All near-drowning victims should be transported to the hospital and admitted for at least 24 hours.

Because treatment of the near-drowning patient is mostly supportive, careful monitoring of the adequacy of oxygenation, ventilation, and perfusion is very important. Heart rate, respiratory rate, ECG, BP, urine output, and, in the more unstable patient, central venous pressure (CVP) or pulmonary capillary wedge pressure (PCWP) should be followed continuously. Arterial blood gases, electrolytes, BUN, creatinine, and repetitive neurologic assessments using the Glasgow Coma Scale (GCS) (Table 20-2) should be checked frequently. A urinalysis, clotting profile, complete blood count with differential, and chest radiograph should be obtained on admission and repeated as necessary based on the patient's clinical status. In the unconscious patient, a Foley catheter and nasogastric tube should be placed. Immediate measures to restore body temperature should begin so that specific therapy can be directed at the major organ systems involved.

Treating Hypothermia

The approach to the hypothermic near-drowning victim should be individualized, bearing in mind that in the presence of hypothermia, clinical scoring systems (e.g., GCS) fail to predict the presence or absence of neurologic derangement.[48] It is also unclear when CPR is indicated in the presence of severe hypothermia (<28°C). The presence of any respirations and heart rate, no matter how slow, is probably sufficient, and because CPR may promote the development of ventricular fibrillation in this setting, it should probably be withheld until rewarming begins.[40]

Rewarming the hypothermic near-drowning victim should begin in the intensive care unit (ICU) after cardiac monitoring has been instituted. Hypothermia is associated with large fluid shifts, and profound hypotension may accompany rewarming. Close attention to BP, preferably with an indwelling arterial line, is very important.[49] In addition, because the hypothermic heart is very prone to develop ventricular arrhythmias, continous ECG monitoring is essential.[50] The method of rewarming depends on both the patient's core temperature and clinical state (Table 20-3).[50,51]

Table 20-2. Pediatric Coma Scale

Eyes	Open spontaneously	4
	Open to speech	3
	Open to pain	2
	Not open	1
Motor	Obeys commands	6
	Localizes pain	5
	Flexion to pain	4
	Decorticate posturing	3
	Decerebrate posturing	2
	No reaction	1
Verbal	Obeys commands	5
	Says words	4
	Vocalizes	3
	Cries	2
	No sounds	1
"Normal" score for age:	0–6 mo	9
	6–12 mo	11
	1–2 yrs	12
	2–5 yrs	13
	Over 5 yrs	14

Table 20-3. Treatment of hypothermia

Rectal temperature	Therapeutic interventions
≥32°C	External warming measures
29–32°C and hemodynamically stable	External warming measures Gastric and colon lavage Warmed IV fluids Heated, humidified air
<29°C or hemodynamically unstable	Above methods Peritoneal dialysis Direct mediastinal lavage Cardiopulmonary bypass

Patients with a rectal temperature greater than 32°C usually are hemodynamically stable and can be warmed slowly with external methods such as warmed blankets and radiant heat lamps. In hemodynamically stable patients with a rectal temperature between 29°C and 32°C, active rewarming with gastric and colonic lavage, warmed intravenous fluids, and heated, humidified air (enriched with oxygen) should begin. Fluids used for lavage and intravenous administration should be warmed to 35°C to 40°C. Patients with a temperature less than 29°C are at high risk for the development of ventricular arrhythmias and should be rewarmed rapidly with the aforementioned methods. In addition, techniques such as peritoneal dialysis, hemodialysis, or direct mediastinal lavage should be considered, especially if ventricular fibrillation intervenes. DC cardioversion and antiarrhythmics are usually not effective with a hypothermic, fibrillating heart.[51]

The previously mentioned child who suffered a 66-minute ice water submersion had a rectal temperature of 19°C at one point in her course.[36] Extracorporeal rewarming was utilized via the femoral artery and vein using a warming gradient of 10°C between the perfusate and the patient's temperature. Total bypass time was 53 minutes. Extracorporeal rewarming has the advantage of maintaining perfusion regardless of the patient's cardiac rhythm. Because of this and the rapidity with which normothermia can be achieved, extracorporeal rewarming is advocated by several authors for the patient with hypothermia to less than 29°C associated with asystole or ventricular fibrillation.[38] This modality is limited to certain tertiary centers.

Pulmonary Management

The pulmonary injury resulting in pulmonary edema, atelectasis, diminished lung compliance, and intrapulmonary shunt ultimately leads to hypoxemia and if severe enough, hypercarbia. Thus, the mainstay of therapy consists of effective airway control and the maintenance of adequate oxygenation and ventilation. Guidelines for intubation include the requirements of an FiO_2 greater than 0.60 to maintain a PaO_2 greater than 70 mm Hg, hypercarbia, and the inability to adequately protect and maintain the airway secondary to neurologic compromise.

Positive-pressure ventilation provides inflation of atelectatic and fluid-filled alveoli. Positive end-expiratory pressure (PEEP) restores functional residual capacity, decreases $\dot{V}/\dot{Q}$ mismatch and intrapulmonary shunt, and improves arterial oxygenation. Because high levels of PEEP impede venous return and cardiac output, fluid replacement to optimize cardiac filling pressures and placement of a thermodilution pulmonary artery catheter to monitor cardiac output may be required. The "optimum" PEEP that maximizes oxygen delivery should then be sought. After optimizing PEEP, incremental lowering of the FiO_2 (to < 0.60) should proceed before withdrawing PEEP.

Most patients recover gradually from the pulmonary injury over a period of several days, and radiographic clearing of infiltrates is usually noted by the fourth or fifth day. In the patient who requires prolonged ventilatory support or experiences a sudden respiratory deterioration, one must remain cognizant of potential complicating factors. As mentioned, pneumonia is not uncommon, and in the intubated patient, routine surveillance tracheal aspirates for Gram stain and culture along with daily CBCs and CXRs should be followed. A high index of suspicion for superimposed pulmonary infection needs to be maintained, as pneumonia on top of acute or chronic lung injury greatly increases morbidity and mortality. Prophylactic antibiotics have not proven beneficial in preventing pneumonia, and in some studies, their use has adversely affected outcome.[30,52] When utilized, antibiotics should be targeted at specific organisms based on the clinical setting and the results of laboratory evaluations. There are a few situations in which specific coverage is indicated. If the near-drowning episode occurred in a hot tub, *pseudomonas* is a likely infectious agent, and anti-pseudomonal therapy is indicated. Streptococcal pneumonia can cause superimposed pneumonia and sepsis within the first 24 hours of admission to the hospital, and if early signs of sepsis develop, this pathogen should be covered.[53] Foreign body aspiration should be suspected in the patient with asymmetric pulmonary disease that does not improve on chest radiographs; if a diagnostic possibility, bronchoscopy should be performed. ARDS may occur following a near-drowning episode (usually within the first 48 hours) and necessitate the use of prolonged and intensive cardiorespiratory support. When acute changes in the near-drowning patient's respiratory status occur, one should consider mechanical problems related to the ventilator and endotracheal tube or the development of a pnemothorax or pneumomediastinum.

Steroids were previously thought to modify the respiratory failure associated with near-drowning. In a dog model, however, treatment with methylprednisolone had no effect on arterial blood gas or intrapulmonary shunt fraction values, and survival was not altered.[54] Human studies have shown no benefit from the use of steroids in treating the pulmonary injury associated with near-drowning. Because of their potential side effects and lack of proven benefit, they are not indicated.

Cardiovascular Management

Most arrhythmias in the near-drowning victim are secondary and resolve with treatment of the primary disorder (i.e., hypoxemia, acidosis, hyperkalemia, hypothermia). Persistent hemodynamic instability usually implies marked hypoxemic-ischemic damage to the myocardium, and because these patients also require high levels of PEEP and mean airway pressure to maintain adequate oxygenation, placement of a CVP or pulmonary artery catheter may be helpful. Optimizing cardiac filling pressures and the use of inotropic agents may then proceed rationally.

The hypothermic patient is usually relatively hypovolemic and may become hypotensive on rewarming. This "rewarming shock" responds to fluid replacement, although in some patients, vasopressors are required to maintain BP. Continued cardiovascular monitoring throughout the rewarming period is essential.

Brain Injury Management

Whereas irreversible CNS damage usually occurs with greater than 5 minutes of submersion in warm water, the heart can tolerate much longer periods of total ischemia. Thus, as CPR and other supportive measures have improved, a large group of patients now survive the initial submersion episode only to become profoundly brain damaged. Because of this, in the late 1970s Conn et al. recommended intense cerebral resuscitative techniques, including intracranial pressure (ICP) monitoring, steroids, barbiturate coma, and controlled hypothermia, in treating the severely comatose, near-drowning victim.[55] It was felt that by decreasing cerebral metabolic rate, controlling ICP, and protecting the brain from developing any further oxygen debt that one could prevent ongoing injury to already damaged neurons and, perhaps, provide recovery to some. Unfortunately, although theoretically sound, this approach has not decreased the morbidity of near-drowning. In addition, many of these therapeutic modalities have untoward side effects[56] and their routine use in the near-drowning patient has been abandoned in most centers. The following discussion outlines why these modalities are no longer favored.

One of the major goals in cerebral resuscitation is controlling ICP and optimizing cerebral perfusion pressure; thus, direct measurement of ICP rationally became a standard part of therapy. Its positive value has been documented in head injury and other forms of nonischemic causes of elevated ICP where control of ICP greatly improves intact survival.[57,58] Its usefulness in near-drowning (and other forms of global anoxic CNS injury), however, is questionable for two reasons: (1) In near-drowning patients, when ICP is elevated, it is associated universally with either death or profound brain damage,[59,60] and normalizing ICP in this setting does not improve neurologic outcome[58,61]; and (2) many patients have no elevation in their ICP despite profound CNS hypoxic-ischemic injury. The absence of a raised ICP, therefore, does not guarantee a good outcome.[56,59,60,62]

Steroids are thought to be efficacious in brain lesions with localized edema, such as tumors and abscesses. They have never proven beneficial in hypoxic-ischemic injury,[63] however, and because they increase the susceptibility to infection and have other associated side effects, their use cannot be justified.

Barbiturates have many effects that should be advantageous to the damaged brain. When given intravenously in large doses, they modulate cerebral blood flow, decrease metabolic requirements, and decrease cerebral oxygen consumption.[64] At these doses, they also impair cardiac output and adversely affect oxygen delivery. The premise of their protective effect is that they will selectively lower cerebral oxygen consumption more than cerebral oxygen delivery. Several studies have investigated the efficacy of barbiturates in treating hypoxic-ischemic encephalopathy, including near-drowning. The results of these studies have revealed that barbiturates increase the degree of hemodynamic instability and do not alter outcome.[65–69]

As mentioned ealier, hypothermia can be "cerebro-protective" and decrease the brain's susceptibility to hypoxic-ischemic damage. Because of this, controlled hypothermia became a routine part of cerebral resuscitative techniques in the near-drowning patient. Hypothermia also affects other organ systems, some adversely. In animal studies, it reduces the number of circulating polymorphonuclear leukocytes and interferes with their release from bone marrow.[70] Clinically, this has proven true in humans, and an increased incidence of sepsis and multisystem organ failure occurs in patients treated with controlled hypothermia to 32°C. For this reason and because it has not been shown to improve neurologic recovery, hypothermia is no longer routinely employed.

In conclusion, it seems that present methods of intense cerebral resuscitation do not significantly affect outcome in the near-drowning victim who has suffered a prolonged submersion. Perhaps newer therapies such as calcium channel blockers, free radical scavengers, and excitotoxin antagonists, which attempt to reverse the physiology of the primary and secondary injuries, will prove more useful.[64] For the present, therapy should concentrate on optimizing oxygen and substrate delivery, maintaining normothermia, avoiding acidosis, and providing essential supportive care.

Management of Other Organ Systems

Renal failure is usually secondary to hypoperfusion and is treated by optimizing renal perfusion through volume infusions (avoiding hypervolemia) and the administration of dopamine. If urinalysis reveals hemoglobinuria or myoglobinuria, forced diuresis with furosemide and mannitol with alkalinization of the urine should proceed. Inappropriately high volumes of dilute urine may occur in the face of high-output, acute tubular necrosis or diabetes insipidus.

Disseminated intravascular coagulation should be treated with platelet and clotting factor replacement. Sepsis is a common complicating factor in near-drowning patients, and treatment with antibiotics should be initiated if suspicion is high or as guided by culture results.

Epithelial sloughing of the gastrointestinal mucosa has been found frequently in autopsy studies. This finding probably portends a dismal prognosis; if bloody stools are noted, however, enteral feeds should be held and total parenteral nutrition started. Nutritional replacement in the near-drowning patient is key, as in any critically ill patient.

Special Considerations in Therapy

Drowning and near-drowning may be an extreme form of child abuse. This crime usually occurs in infants and toddlers in an unwitnessed setting, usually within the home. Abuse should be suspected in the near-drowning victim with other unexplained injuries or if the history surrounding the event is inconsistent. Often there is a preceding history of child abuse or drug and alcohol use in the perpetrator.[71]

Alcohol and drug use should be considered in older near-drowning victims, and blood alcohol and toxicology screens should be obtained. In one series, all near-drowning patients over 18 years of age had ingested alcohol.[52]

In older children who suffer diving accidents or other trauma associated with the submersion event, one needs to rule out cervical spine injury and intracranial hemorrhage. The neck should be immobilized until cleared by appropriate radiologic studies.

Prognosis

If one could predict accurately on admission those patients with a hopeless outcome, one might then be able to justify withholding resuscitation from that group of patients. With this in mind, several studies have attempted to prognosticate based on clinical and laboratory data, and thus separate patients into two groups: those who recover and those who die or suffer permanent neurologic damage.[4-6,42,52,67,72-77] Different studies have evaluated different parameters, including age of patient, estimated length of submersion, depth of coma, need for CPR on admission to the emergency department, presence of fixed and dilated pupils, period of time before initiation of CPR, and initial arterial pH. From these studies, a few important points can be made.

Patients who arrive at the emergency room noncomatose or in lighter stages of coma (i.e., GCS > 5) with spontaneous cardiac activity have a reasonably good prognosis, and most of these patients should survive neurologically intact.

It is impossible to predict with 100% accuracy those patients who will not recover. Several patients suffering warm water submersions have arrived at the emergency room asystolic and have survived neurologically intact. Therefore, although some authors disagree,[75,76] resuscitation should proceed on all near-drowning patients presenting to the emergency room regardless of the initial clinical state.[74,77] In the nonhypothermic patient presenting with asystole despite aggressive resuscitative efforts in the field, the period of resuscitation should not be prolonged.

Observing patients over time may be a more accurate method of predicting outcome. In one study, all patients whose neurologic status improved over the 2 hours between arrival at the emergency department and admission to the pediatric ICU survived neurologically intact.[78] In another study, all patients arriving in the ICU with a GCS of 5 or greater experienced full recovery regardless of their initial clinical state. Likewise, no patient arriving in the ICU with a GCS of 3 survived neurologically intact.[74]

Prevention

As in other forms of accidental death and injury, the real key to decreasing the morbidity and mortality of submersion episodes lies in preventing their occurrence. An adequate barrier between swimming pools and toddlers would lower substantially the incidence of drowning in that age group.[9,79] Older children need to be trained in water safety and warned of the danger of mixing alcohol with swimming. All pool owners should be proficient in CPR. By promoting stronger legislation mandating these goals, health care professionals could take an active role in reducing the number of submersion injuries and deaths in children.

References

1. Orlowski JP. Drowning, near drowning, and ice water drowning. *JAMA* 260:390–391, 1988.
2. Baker SP, O'Neill B, Karpf RS. Drowning. In *The Injury Fact Book.* Lexington, MA: Lexington Books, 1984. Pp 155–165.
3. Rowe MI, Arango A, Allington G. Profile of pediatric drowning victims in a water oriented society. *J Trauma* 17:587–591, 1977.
4. Fandel I, Bancalari E. Near drowning in children: Clinical aspects. *Pediatrics* 58:573–579, 1976.
5. Peterson B. Morbidity of childhood near drowning. *Pediatrics* 59:364–370, 1977.
6. Dean JM, Kaufman ND. Prognostic indicators in pediatric near-drowning: The Glasgow Coma Scale. *Crit Care Med* 9:536–539, 1981.
7. Dietz PE, Baker SP. Drowning, epidemiology and prevention. *Am J Public Health* 64:303–312, 1974.
8. Brooks JG. The child who nearly drowns. *Am J Dis Child* 135:998–999, 1981.
9. Wintemute GJ et al. Drowning in childhood and adolescence: A population based study. *Am J Public Health* 77:830–832, 1987.

10. Peam JH et al. Bathtub drownings: Report of seven cases. *Pediatrics* 64:68–70, 1979.

11. Scott PH, Eigen H. Immersion accidents involving pails of water in the home. *J Pediatr* 96:282–284, 1980.

12. Levin DL. Near-drowning. *Crit Care Med* 8:590–595, 1980.

13. Fine NL et al. Near drowning presenting as the adult respiratory distress syndrome. *Chest* 65:347–349, 1974.

14. Peam JH. Secondary drowning in children. *Br Med J* 281:1103–1105, 1980.

15. Craig AB. Summary of 58 cases of loss of consciousness during underwater swimming and diving. *Med Sci Sports* 8:171, 1976.

16. Craig AB. Causes of loss of consciousness during underwater swimming. *J Appl Physiol* 16:583–586, 1961.

17. Gonzalez-Rothi RJ. Near drowning: Consensus and controversies in pulmonary and cerebral resuscitation. *Heart Lung* 16:474–482, 1987.

18. Cavalier S. Drownings. In *National Pool and Spa Safety Conference.* Washington, DC: U.S. Consumer Product Safety Commission 1985:9–12.

19. Giammona ST, Modell JH. Drowning by total immersion: Effects on pulmonary surfactant of distilled water, isotonic saline, and sea water. *Am J Dis Child* 114:612–616, 1967.

20. Modell JH et al. The effects of fluid volume in seawater drowning. *Ann Intern Med* 67:68–80, 1967.

21. Yagil Y et al. Near drowning in the Dead Sea: Electrolyte imbalances and therapeutic implications. *Arch Intern Med* 145:50–53, 1985.

22. Modell JH. Serum electrolyte changes in near drowning victims. *JAMA* 253:557, 1985.

23. Modell JH et al. Blood gas and electrolyte changes in human near-drowning victims. *JAMA* 203:337–343, 1968.

24. Modell JH et al. Effects of ventilatory patterns on arterial oxygenation after near-drowning in sea water. *Anesthesiology* 40:376–384, 1974.

25. Orlowski JP, Medhat MA, Phillips JM. Effects of tonicities of saline solutions on pulmonary injury in drowning. *Crit Care Med* 15:126–130, 1987.

26. Greenburg MI et al. Effects of endotracheally administered distilled water and normal saline on the arterial blood gases of dogs. *Ann Emerg Med* 11:600–604, 1982.

27. Rosenthal SL, Zuger JH, Apollo E. Respiratory colonization with pseudomonas putrafascens after near drowning in salt water. *Am J Clin Pathol* 64:382–384, 1975.

28. Kelly MT, Avery DM. Lactose-positive vibrio in seawater, a cause of pneumonia and septicemia in a drowning victim. *J Clin Microbiol* 11:278–280, 1980.

29. Hoff BH. Multisystem failure: A review with special reference to drowning. *Crit Care Med* 7:310–320, 1979.

30. Modell JH, Graves SA, Ketover A. Clinical course of 91 consecutive near drowning victims. *Chest* 70:231–238, 1976.

31. Culpepper RM. Bleeding diasthesis in fresh water drowning. *Ann Intern Med* 83:675, 1975.

32. Ports TA, Deuel TF. Intravascular coagulation in fresh water submersion. *Ann Intern Med* 87:60–61, 1977.

33. Grauze H, Amend WJ, Earley LE. Acute renal failure complicating submersion in sea water. *JAMA* 217:207–209, 1971.

34. Orlowski JP. Drowning, near drowning, and ice water submersions. *Pediatr Clin North Am* 34:75–92, 1987.

35. Siebke H et al. Survival after 40 minutes submersion without cerebral sequellae. *Lancet* i:1275–1277, 1975.

36. Bolte RG et al. The use of extracorporeal rewarming in a child submerged for 66 minutes. *JAMA* 260:377–379, 1988.

37. Ramey CA, Ramey DN, Hayward JS. Dive response of children in relation to cold-water near-drowning. *J Appl Physiol* 63:665–668, 1987.

38. Hayward JS et al. Temperature effect on the human dive response in relation to cold water near-drowning. *J Appl Physiol* 56:202–206, 1984.

39. Kopf GS, Mirvis DM, Myers RE. Central nervous system tolerance to cardiac arrest during profound hypothermia. *J Surg Res* 18:29–34, 1975.

40. Corneli HM. Accidental hypothermia. *J Pediatr* 120:671–679, 1992.

41. Torphy DE, Minter MG, Thompson BM. Cardiorespiratory arrest and resuscitation of children. *Am J Dis Child* 138:1099–1102, 1984.

42. Quan L et al. Outcome and predictors of outcome in pediatric submersions receiving prehospital care in King County, Washington. *Pediatrics* 86:586–593, 1990.

43. Kyriaccou DN et al. Effects of immediate resuscitation on children with submersion injury. *Pediatrics* 94:137–142, 1994.

44. Patrick EA. Heimlich maneuver removes water from respiratory tract of near-drowning victim. *Emergency* 13:44, 1981.

45. Wilder RJ, Wedro BC. "Heimlich maneuver" for near-drowning questioned (letter). *Ann Emerg Med* 11:111, 1982.

46. Orlowski JP. "Heimlich maneuver" for near-drowning questioned (letter). *Ann Emerg Med* 11:111–113, 1982.

47. Modell JH. Near drowning. *Circulation* 74 (Suppl IV):IV-27–IV-28, 1986.

48. Fox JB et al. A retrospective analysis of air-evacuated hypothermia patients. *Aviat Space Environ Med* 59:1070–1075, 1988.

49. Nugent SK, Rogers MC. Resuscitation and intensive care monitoring following immersion hypothermia. *J Trauma* 20:814–815, 1980.

50. Maclean D. Emergency management of accidental hypothermia: A review. *J R Soc Med* 79:528–531, 1986.

51. Treatment of hypothermia. *Med Lett* 28:123–124, 1986.

52. Oakes DD et al. Prognosis and management of victims of near-drowning. *J Trauma* 22:544–549, 1982.

53. Vernon DD et al. *Streptococcus pneumiae* bacteremia associated with near-drowning. *Crit Care Med* 18:1175–1176, 1990.

54. Calderwood HW, Modell JH. The ineffectiveness of steroid therapy for treatment of fresh-water near-drowning. *Anesthesiology* 43:642–650, 1975.

55. Conn AW, Edmonds JF, Barker GA. Cerebral resuscitation in near-drowning. *Pediatr Clin North Am* 26:691–701, 1979.

56. Bohn DJ et al. Influence of hypothermia, barbiturate therapy, and intracranial monitoring on morbidity and mortality of near drowning. *Crit Care Med* 14:529–534, 1986.

57. Marshall LF, Smith RW, Shapiro HM. The outcome with aggressive treatment in severe head injuries; the significance of intracranial pressure monitoring. *J Neurosurg* 50:20–25, 1979.

58. LeRoux PD et al. Pediatric intracranial pressure monitoring in hypoxic and nonhypoxic brain injury. *Childs Nerv Syst* 7:34–39, 1991.

59. Nussbaum E, Galant SP. Intracranial pressure monitoring as a guide to prognosis in the nearly drowned, severely comatose child. *J Pediatr* 102:215–218, 1983.

60. Dean JM, McComb JG. Intracranial pressure monitoring in severe pediatric near-drowning. *Neurosurgery* 9:627–630, 1981.

61. Connors R et al. Relationship of cross-brain oxygen content difference, cerebral blood flow, and metabolic rate to neurologic outcome after near-drowning. *J Pediatr* 121:839–844, 1992.

62. Frewen TC et al. Cerebral resuscitation therapy in pediatric near-drowning. *J Pediatr* 106:615–617, 1985.

63. Anderson DC, Cranford RE. Corticosteroids in ischemic stroke. *Stroke* 10:68–72, 1979.

64. Rogers MC, Kirsch JR. Current concepts in brain resuscitation. *JAMA* 261:3143–3147, 1989.

65. Conn AW. Freshwater drowning and near drowning: An update. *Can Anesth Soc J* 31:S38–S44, 1984.

66. Rogers MC. Near drowning: Cold water on a hot topic. *J Pediatr* 106:603–604, 1985.

67. Nussbaum E, Maggi JC. Pentobarbital therapy does not improve neurologic outcome in nearly drowned, flaccid-comatose children. *Pediatrics* 81:630–634, 1988.

68. Frewen TC et al. Outcome in severe Reye syndrome with early pentobarbital coma and hypothermia. *J Pediatr* 100:663–665, 1982.

69. Grisvold SE et al. Thiopental treatment after global brain ischemia in pigtailed monkeys. *Anesthesiology* 60:88–96, 1984.

70. Biggar WD, Bohn DJ, Kent G. Neutrophil circulation and release from bone marrow during hypothermia. *Infect Immunol* 40:708–712, 1983.

71. Griest KJ, Zumwalt RE. Child abuse by drowning. *Pediatrics* 83:41–46, 1989.
72. Nussbaum E. Prognostic variables in nearly drowned, comatose children. *Am J Dis Child* 139:1058–1059, 1985.
73. Frates RC. Analysis of predictive factors in the assessment of warm-water near-drowning in children. *Am J Dis Child* 135:1006, 1981.
74. Lavelle JM, Shaw KN. Near drowning: Is emergency department cardiopulmonary resuscitation or intensive care unit cerebral resuscitation indicated? *Crit Care Med* 21:368–373, 1993.
75. Nichter MA, Everett PB. Childhood near-drowning: Is cardiopulmonary resuscitation always indicated? *Crit Care Med* 17:993, 1989.
76. Biggart MJ, Bohn DJ. Effect of hypothermia and cardiac arrest on outcome of near-drowning accidents in children. *J Pediatr* 117:179–183, 1990.
77. Allman FD et al. Outcome following cardiopulmonary resuscitation in severe pediatric near-drowning. *Am J Dis Child* 14:571–575, 1986.
78. Turner GR, Levin DL. Improvement of neurologic status after pediatric near-drowning accidents (letter). *Crit Care Med* 13:1080, 1985.
79. Milliner N, Pearn J, Guard R. Will fenced pools save lives?: A 10 year study from Mulgrave Shire, Queensland. *Med J Aust* 2:510–511, 1980.

III Cardiovascular System

Peter Lang

Lars C. Erickson

E. Marsha Elixson

Alejandro López

Gus J. Vlahakes

21 Intensive Care Following Cardiac Surgery

The care of patients who are critically ill with congenital heart disease (CHD) often begins before physicians involved in critical care medicine are physically introduced to the patient. Fetuses identified in the emerging area of prenatal screening are brought to the attention of practitioners far in advance of their arrival to the hospital.[1-5] It is clear that the ultimate outcome of patient management is dependent on the wisdom of the recommendations made during these earliest encounters. Although dramatic, prenatal diagnosis is only one of the recent advances that have dramatically altered the care of infants and children with CHD. It is only during the past 15 years that invasive hemodynamic monitoring, two-dimensional echocardiography, palliative prostaglandin E-1 (PGE$_1$), and the surgical techniques that allow reparative surgery to be performed on the smallest infants have emerged as the standard of care in the treatment of children with CHD.

The development of two-dimensional echocardiography as an accurate and reliable diagnostic tool has altered the approach to children suspected of having congenital cardiac disease.[6-8] Infants can be reliably screened for suspected cardiac problems at virtually no risk. Cardiac catheterization, if indicated, can be planned in a rational fashion, minimizing the risk to the patient and maximizing the efficiency of the procedure. In many cases, echocardiography has replaced cardiac catheterization as the primary preoperative diagnostic tool (Fig. 21-1)[9-13] with comparable results (Fig. 21-2).[12]

The emergence of PGE$_1$ as a powerful pharmacologic agent for the treatment of children with cardiac disease has been equally dramatic. Following the administration of PGE$_1$, newborns with ductus arteriosus-dependent pulmonary or systemic blood flow[14-17]

can often be resuscitated and stabilized easily prior to cardiac catheterization and corrective surgery.

Advances in pediatric cardiac surgery have been no less dramatic. Whenever possible, primary repair in young infants has replaced palliative surgery.[18-22] The use of hypothermic circulatory arrest, low-flow cardiopulmonary bypass, and cardioplegia has enabled surgeons to operate on the smallest of infants with results not obtainable 10 years ago. In addition, patients with "uncorrectable" diseases are now undergoing "reparative" operations,[18,23-25] and patients with "inoperable" lesions are undergoing palliative surgery.[26,27]

Critical reevaluation of standard forms of treatment is a demonstration of the flexibility with which pediatric cardiologists and pediatric cardiac surgeons approach patients. An example of this trend has been the abandonment of the "accepted" operations for treatment of transposition of the great arteries.[28-31] Although these earlier operations were life-saving and afforded thousands of patients with years of symptom-free growth and development, after careful follow-up, long-term prognosis was suboptimal.[32] Accordingly, anatomic repair, initially performed amid much controversy, has become the standard of care because of its potential for improved long-term cardiac performance.[18,30,31,33,34]

Equally dramatic has been the emergence of therapeutic cardiac catheterization as a treatment option for many forms of CHD.[35] Just as with patients undergoing surgical procedures, the management of patients during and following these interventions often requires the collaborative efforts of a skilled team. Thus, as the intensive care unit (ICU) has become an extension of the operating room, it must also coordinate efforts with the cardiac catheterization laboratory.

What follows in this chapter is an approach to the care of infants and children with CHD that has developed over the past 15

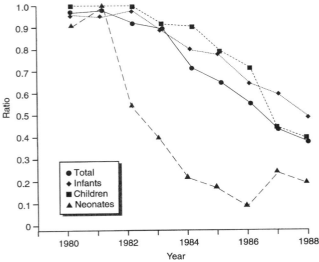

Figure 21-1. Ratios of cardiac catheterizations to operations for congenital heart disease in newborns, infants, and children. (From N Sreeram et al. Changing role of noninvasive investigation in the preoperative assessment of congenital heart disease: A nine year experience. *Br Heart J* 63:345–349, 1990. With permission.)

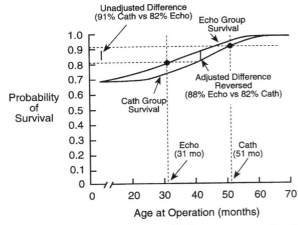

Figure 21-2. Probability of survival following surgery after diagnosis by echocardiography alone versus cardiac catheterization. (From JC Huhta et al. Surgery without catheterization for congenital heart defects: Management of 100 patients. *J Am Coll Cardiol* 9:823–829, 1987. With permission.)

years. It should be stressed that it represents an approach that has developed at several institutions during that time frame. Surely, other approaches can work just as well. The overall principles that have been employed in the care of children with CHD have been an aggressive approach to a complete anatomic and physiologic diagnosis, complete repair of cardiac defects whenever possible, and a self-critical attitude if problems persist following intervention. The last point is critical. If a child is not doing well following a therapeutic intervention, surgery, catheter-directed treatment, or pharmacologic therapy, the initial impulse must be to aggressively reassess the situation. It is important to question the accuracy of the original diagnosis or the conduct of the therapeutic procedure; failure of therapeutic management is not the fault of the patient.

General Considerations

Diagnosis of Congenital Heart Disease

Accuracy of diagnosis is fundamental to successful cardiac care in infants. A careful physical examination in conjunction with the ECG and chest x-ray will lead to the detection of CHD in the vast majority of affected children. In the critically ill infant, however, two-dimensional echocardiography and cardiac catheterization are often necessary to characterize the hemodynamic issues. On occasion, as in the case of an isolated coarctation of the aorta or a more complex lesion such as total anomalous pulmonary venous return, surgery can be planned based solely on the echocardiographic findings. Reports have been published of fairly large series of infants who have undergone corrective surgery without cardiac catheterization,[9] although in the majority of cases the benefits of cardiac catheterization are felt to outweigh the risks. In general, decisions regarding preoperative catheterization should be individualized based on the status of the patient, the conditions present in a particular institution, and the nature of the proposed surgery.

Transportation of Newborns with Congenital Heart Disease

The transportation of children requiring critical care can be fraught with hazards. Monitor batteries become depleted, catheters become dislodged, and inadvertent discontinuation or boluses of medications occur. The switch from mechanical ventilation to hand ventilation can lead to hemodynamic changes in many patients.

For these reasons, the safe transportation of a critically ill child into or out of the ICU requires advance planning and personnel with the prerequisite skills. A nurse familiar with the patient should be included in the transport team. If the child is receiving respiratory support, a respiratory therapist familiar with the child's respiratory status might accompany the team as well. Finally, sufficient personnel must accompany the child so that someone is available to open doors, call elevators, or call for help as required.

When necessary, changing intravenous infusions from one set of equipment to another for transport must be done with care so that a constant infusion rate is maintained. Equipment must be available to allow bag-valve-mask ventilation of the child should the endotracheal tube become dislodged. Monitors and infusion pumps must have batteries that are fully charged, and air and oxygen tanks must have sufficient reserve to allow for substantial delays over the course of transportation. In the event that a monitor fails in the course of the transport, a finger on the pulse can

provide a considerable amount of information about the cardiac rhythm, rate, and BP.

Techniques of Cardiac Surgery

Closed Procedures (Non-Pump)

Cardiac procedures that do not require exposing the interior of the heart to air or cardiopulmonary bypass are termed *closed* surgery. These include most instances of ligation of the ductus arteriosus, pulmonary artery banding, the Blalock-Hanlon atrial septectomy,[36] systemic-to-pulmonary shunts such as the Blalock-Taussig shunt,[37] and some cases of repair of coarctation of the aorta later in childhood. Because there is no use of cardiopulmonary bypass (CPB) or hypothermic arrest (HA), there is very little, if any, myocardial dysfunction following closed procedures.

Inflow Occlusion

In the case of inflow occlusion, venous return from the inferior vena cava (IVC) and superior vena cava (SVC) is temporarily occluded, the heart is opened and an intracardiac procedure is performed, the heart is closed and inflow occlusion is released. This approach is appropriate for very short operations such as aortic or pulmonary valvotomy or a right atrial thrombectomy.

Cardiopulmonary Bypass

CPB was first described by Gibbon in the 1930s,[38] who also performed the first successful CPB operation in 1953.[39] In 1954 Warden et al.[40] reported a series of children operated on with CPB using a parent as the "oxygenator" (controlled cross-circulation), and in 1955 the first successful case of CPB using a pump oxygenator was performed.[41]

CPB involves the placement of cannulae in the heart which receive the venous return, usually in the SVC and IVC, and a cannula in the ascending aorta to provide arterial flow. Alternatively, a single cannula may be placed in the right atrium or right atrial appendage for venous return. The heart continues to receive blood flow via the coronary arteries unless the ascending aorta is clamped (cross-clamped) proximal to the aortic cannula (Fig. 21-3). The blood from the venous cannulae is pumped through a membrane oxygenator and heat exchanger then returned to the aortic cannulae at a flow rate and pressure sufficient to meet the metabolic demands of the body.

CPB may be used at normal body temperatures, but in practice is almost always used in combination with moderate core cooling, which allows a lower flow rate due to reduced oxygen consumption. For example, the cerebral oxygen consumption falls roughly ninefold as the body temperature is reduced from 37°C to 18°C (Fig. 21-4).[42]

Frequent problems following CPB include increased capillary permeability (capillary leak), edema, fever, vasoconstriction or dilation, mild renal dysfunction, and hemolysis. These problems are often lumped together under the term *post-pump syndrome* and may be related to complement activation and a total-body inflammatory response. Much less frequent are severe renal, neurologic, and coagulation disorders. These complications can be attributed largely to injury to the formed blood elements within the bypass circuit.

Younger children with longer bypass times appear to be at greater risk for more severe complications (Fig. 21-5).[43] The risk of severe complications of CPB appears to increase after 80 to 120 minutes of bypass. Patients who are cyanotic prior to CPB appear to be at greater risk, particularly for bleeding complications.

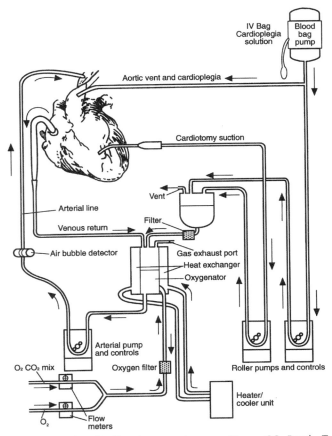

Figure 21-3. Cardiopulmonary bypass. (From CC Reed, T Stafford. *Cardiopulmonary Perfusion* [2nd ed]. Houston: Texas Medical, 1985. With permission.)

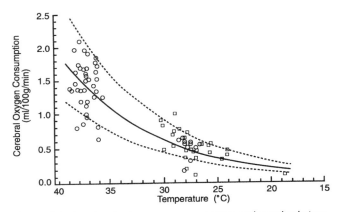

Figure 21-4. Cerebral oxygen consumption and core body temperature. (From N Croughwell et al. The effect of temperature on cerebral metabolism and blood flow in adults during cardiopulmonary bypass. *J Thorac Cardiovasc Surg* 103:549, 1992. With permission.)

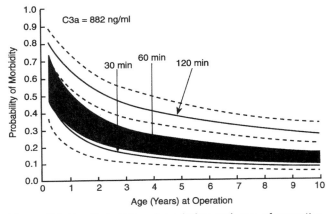

Figure 21-5. Probability of morbidity and age of operation. (From JK Kirklin et al. Complement and the damaging effects of cardiopulmonary bypass. *J Thorac Cardiovasc Surg* 86:845, 1983. With permission.)

Deep Hypothermic Circulatory Arrest

Because the metabolic demands of the body are lowered substantially at very low body temperatures,[44,45] it is possible to arrest the heart for purposes of open-heart surgery using cooling alone. The technique of HA was developed by Bigelow[45,46] and was first used in humans in 1953.[47,48] Current practice usually involves CPB with a cooled perfusate (core cooling) down to a core temperature of at most 16°C, after which CPB is stopped so that the cannulae in the vena cavae may be removed to allow easier access to the heart. The improved access to the interior of the heart during deep HA allows surgery on smaller infants with more complex lesions. HA times of up to about 50 to 60 minutes are considered relatively safe, although injury to the brain, heart, and kidneys continues to represent a small but significant risk.

Cardiac Effects of Cardiopulmonary Bypass and Hypothermic Arrest

CPB is associated with myocardial ischemia and injury in children.[49] Peak CPK cardiac isoenzyme elevations occur between 8 and 24 hours following the start of bypass in both adults and children,[50] and both postoperative cardiac output and survival are inversely related to the degree of myocardial injury.[51] Prolonged aortic cross-clamp time and HA further increase the likelihood of myocardial injury.

The results of myocardial injury secondary to CPB and HA include tissue death (infarction), depression of myocardial contractility, and myocardial edema.

The extent of myocardial tissue injury associated with CPB is related to the duration of ischemia,[52] the effectiveness of measures to protect the myocardium during bypass, the conditions of reperfusion,[53,54] and the metabolic demands placed on the myocardium following bypass. A significant reduction in myocardial injury has resulted from the development of cold potassium cardioplegia, which causes a rapid cessation of cardiac contraction, reducing the metabolic demands of the ischemic myocardium. In addition, myocardial injury in the immediate postoperative period can be limited by minimizing the metabolic demands of the heart. The use of catecholamines[55,56] and failure to support an adequate core temperature both increase the metabolic demands of the heart.

Myocardial depression following CPB or HA appears to follow the same time course as myocardial injury.[50,57] Systolic dysfunction usually peaks around 8 to 24 hours after surgery but may continue to progress for 2 to 3 days. Signs of depressed systolic function include decreased cardiac output, deteriorating perfusion, and decreasing urine output.

Optimally, any measures chosen to support failing systolic function should avoid increasing the metabolic demands of the myocardium, which might in turn lead to increased myocardial injury. Afterload reducing agents and the intraaortic balloon pump may, for example, improve systolic function without increasing myocardial oxygen consumption. In practice, inotropic agents and pressors are frequently required following CPB, but the additional risk of myocardial injury they entail must be weighed against their advantages.

Myocardial edema during and following CPB may be related to altered membrane permeability leading to increased interstitial water, as well as swelling of the myocytes themselves. Cardiac edema has two disadvantages: cardiac compression due to swelling of the myocardium, and reduced compliance. Manifestations occur between 6 and 12 hours following surgery and may include decreasing cardiac output and increasing filling pressures. Increased inotropic support (e.g., dopamine) and intravascular volume replacement may be required during this period. By the morning following surgery, any myocardial dysfunction is usually improving.

The increased volume of an edematous myocardium leaves less room in the pericardial sac for cardiac filling and may contribute to a degree of cardiac tamponade physiology. When severe myocardial edema is noted, or expected, the sternum may be left open for 1 or more days until the edema has subsided. When there is evidence of cardiac tamponade following CPB, the volume status has been optimized, and there are no signs of blood accumulation in the pericardial space, consideration should be given to reopening the chest because there are no other interventions that are likely to be effective in the setting of tamponade secondary to myocardial edema.

When the myocardium becomes edematous, it is also "stiffer," or less compliant.[58] Consequently, the heart requires a higher filling pressure for the same filling volume. This phenomenon is referred to as "diastolic dysfunction" and is common in the postoperative setting. The time course of diastolic dysfunction is similar to that of systolic dysfunction (see earlier discussion) and tends to compound the resulting fall in cardiac output, because a failing myocardium generally requires higher filling volumes than usual. The result of diastolic dysfunction is less cardiac filling at a given venous pressure. As the venous pressure increases to maintain the cardiac output, pulmonary and peripheral edema, as well as effusions, may develop. This is particularly a problem in the setting of a cavopulmonary anastomosis in which the venous pressure and pulmonary blood flow can be reduced significantly in the setting of an elevated ventricular end-diastolic pressure (see section on Fontan Procedure).

The treatment for diastolic dysfunction is difficult, both because there are few effective interventions and because the effects of diastolic dysfunction are difficult to separate from those of systolic dysfunction in the clinical setting. A falling cardiac output, or the need for increased filling pressures, could be the result of either or both. Intravascular volume expansion may be required to maintain an acceptable cardiac output, and any measure that improves systolic function will tend to allow lower filling pressures and fewer complications related to diastolic dysfunction. The use of diuretics and fluid restriction, if tolerated, may lower right atrial pressure and hasten resolution of myocardial edema. Similarly, it is important to maintain the osmotic pressure of the plasma to help reduce accumulation of fluid in the myocardium.

Types of Incisions

Median Sternotomy

The majority of open-heart procedures are performed through a midline sternotomy incision. This incision, which splits the sternum longitudinally (Fig. 21-6), provides excellent access to all intrapericardial structures as well as the main pulmonary artery, vena cavae, and ascending aorta. The descending aorta also can be approached with additional mediastinal dissection, but collateral vessels arising from the descending aorta can be very challenging to reach.

At closing, the sternum is closed with stainless steel wires, the twisted ends of which are buried in the front table of the sternum. The skin is usually closed with subcuticular sutures, and mediastinal tubes are placed to drain the pericardial space. If the pleural spaces have been entered, pleural drains are placed as well. Separate closure of the pericardium may minimize risk of injury of the anterior structure of the heart at future surgeries. If there is significant risk of bleeding or myocardial edema, however, the pericardium is left open to avoid tamponade.

There appears to be less postoperative pain following a median sternotomy than other types of thoracic incisions; this may be related to the fact that the incision in the sternum is not subjected to strain during voluntary respiration, and no accessory muscles are divided. Local anesthetics such as bupivicaine may be injected into the wound at the time of surgical closure to minimize pain in the early hours after surgery.

Inframammary Incision

The inframammary incision is a variant of the midline sternotomy and attempts to improve the cosmetic results of healing in female patients. The incision in the skin follows the transverse inframammary fold, a location that may provide an improved cosmetic result. The sternum may be opened transversely or vertically, although the latter requires mobilization of a large tissue flap. This incision is not suitable for very young patients.

Lateral Thoracotomy

The left or right lateral thoracotomy incision is used when access to predominantly extrapericardial structures is required and CPB is not anticipated. Surgery in the posterior mediastinum or far into

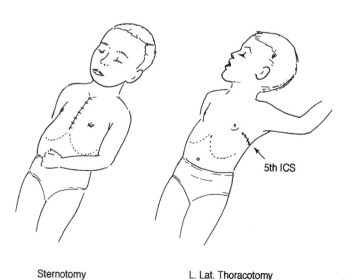

Sternotomy   L. Lat. Thoracotomy

Figure 21-6. Incisions. L.Lat., left lateral; ICS, intercostal space.

the pulmonary hilum, including repair of coarctation of the aorta, ligation of a patent ductus arteriosus, ligation of aortopulmonary collaterals, or placement of a Blalock-Taussig shunt are usually performed from a lateral approach. There may be one thoracostomy tube or none at all.

Recovery from a lateral thoracotomy is complicated by a greater degree of pain associated with division of accessory muscles and stretching the incision site with each breath. "Splinting" during inhalation can lead to atelectasis and poor expectoration of pulmonary secretions. Adequate pain management, possibly including epidural analgesia, early mobilization, and aggressive pulmonary toilet may help prevent pulmonary complications related to pain at the incisional site.

The Open Chest

Following CPB, the heart and mediastinal structures may become sufficiently edematous that the sternum cannot be closed without compressing the heart. Even if the heart is not compressed, systolic dysfunction following surgery may mandate a greater end-diastolic volume during recovery than preoperatively. Consequently, the sternum must occasionally be left open after surgery to allow the heart to fill sufficiently; otherwise, mechanical tamponade may result.

The sternum may be left open with or without closure of the skin. When the skin is left open, a membrane of synthetic material may be sutured to the margins of the wound to preserve sterility within the mediastinum. Until the chest is closed, most patients will require sedation and muscle relaxants to prevent ineffective spontaneous respiration. When the child has had sufficient resolution of edema and improvement in cardiac function, a brief second procedure, often in the ICU, is required for surgical closure of the chest.

Clinical Estimation of Cardiac Output

Despite the expanding technical resources available in a modern ICU, the physical examination remains the most reliable indicator of the patient's clinical status.

Clinical indicators of cardiac output can be roughly divided into signs of central perfusion or signs of peripheral perfusion. As the cardiac output falls relative to the metabolic demands of the body, the peripheral perfusion falls first, followed by a fall in perfusion to such essential organs as the kidneys, heart, and brain.

In the awake child, mental status is a sensitive indicator of central perfusion. An inadequate cardiac output may be heralded by combative behavior, confusion, or somnolence. Patients may complain of low energy or a sensation of coldness.

Urine output is a fairly reliable measure of central perfusion in the absence of medications with diuretic effects. A urine output of 1 ml/kg/hr is considered a minimum below which concern over adequate cardiac output should be raised. This measure cannot be used in children with acute renal failure.

Peripheral perfusion refers to the extent of blood flow to the skin and extremities. One measure of peripheral perfusion is relative skin temperature. As perfusion falls below the minimum required to meet the needs of the body, the distal extremities become cool. The soles of the feet are the first to lose their warmth, then the feet and ankles, and so on up the leg. A patient who is warm above the ankles is usually doing well, whereas a child who is cool to above the knees usually has significantly reduced cardiac output. The reduction in peripheral perfusion can be severe enough to impair the patient's ability to exchange heat, resulting

in an elevated core temperature (central fever) with very cool extremities. This clinical sign does have caveats: A child mounting a genuine febrile response will also have cool extremities regardless of the cardiac output. Also, a child with an inappropriate reduction in systemic vascular resistance (e.g., septic shock) may have warm extremities in the presence of a BP that is inadequate to meet the perfusion demands of the body.

Capillary refill time (CRT) is another measure of peripheral perfusion. Pressing firmly against the skin and then releasing pressure will leave a blanched area. The time required for the blanched area to return to the color of the surrounding skin is the CRT. CRTs in the 1- to 2-second range suggest an adequate perfusion pressure. Prolonged CRTs suggest reduced perfusion.

Measures of peripheral perfusion, such as extremity temperature and CRT, along with signs of organ perfusion such as mental status and urine output are often more meaningful than "quantitative" measures such as BP. One must often decide whether a given BP is sufficient based on clinical information.

Monitoring

Caveats

Despite their usefulness in the critical care setting, electronic monitoring devices have a great potential to lead the clinician astray. Electrodes lose skin contact, probes fall off, calibrations drift, and catheters thrombose, change position, and become disconnected. **When the monitor suggests a problem, it is essential to confirm the finding by examining the patient before taking action.** If there is a discrepancy between the clinical evaluation and the monitoring data, the data and equipment must be carefully examined. A falling BP in a patient with good pulses and perfusion may represent disconnection of a monitoring catheter or malposition of the transducer. If discrepancies persist, other means of evaluation, such as cuff plethysmography, echocardiography, or even cardiac catheterization, should be considered.

Preoperative Monitoring

Prior to cardiac surgery, newborn infants are admitted to the ICU and, depending on the degree of hemodynamic compromise, may have external cardiac, respiratory, pulse oximetry, and often end-tidal carbon dioxide monitors in place. Very often, indwelling monitoring catheters are also indicated, including peripheral, central and/or umbilical venous catheters, and peripheral or umbilical arterial catheters. Other children who are hemodynamically unstable prior to surgery may require invasive monitoring prior to surgery as indicated. Children who have undergone cardiac catheterization just prior to surgery also may have had central vascular catheters left in place. Any catheters placed preoperatively may be used at the time of surgery for monitoring and vascular access. Barring hemodynamic compromise or other accepted indications for invasive monitoring, however, most children can be comfortably followed prior to cardiac surgery with, at most, an external cardiac monitor and pulse oximetry.

Postoperative Monitoring

The monitoring plan for children after cardiac surgery should follow the needs of the patient based on the diagnosis, the type of surgery performed, and the clinical condition (Table 21-1). While they are often critical in the management of postoperative cardiac patients, intracardiac catheters, especially when placed transthoracically, must be handled carefully and according to accepted nursing guidelines if complications are to be minimized.[59] All patients should have the position of any intracardiac catheter

Table 21-1. Typical postoperative courses

Defect	CPB DHA NP	Incision	CT	NG	Foley	Monitor	Mech vent	Pacer wires	Stay in ICU	Monitoring catheters
PDA	NP	LLTX	+/−		+	+			6–24	
ASD 2	CPB	ST	+	+/−	+	+	+		6–24	RA
VSD	CPB DHA	ST	+	+	+	+	+	+	24–48	RA, LA, PA, ART
Coarct	NP	LLTX	+	+	+	+	Only infants		6–24	ART
TOF	CPB DHA	ST	+	+	+	+	+	+	24–48	RA, LA, PA, ART
dTGA	CPB DHA	ST	+	+	+	+	+		48–72	RA, LA, PA, ART
CAVC	CPB DHA	ST	+	+	+	+	+	+	48–72	RA, LA, PA, ART
TAC	CPB DHA	ST	+	+	+	+	+	+	48–72	RA, LA, PA, ART
TAPVR	CPB DHA	ST	+	+	+	+	+		48–96	RA, LA, PA,ART
Fontan	CPB DHA	ST	+	+	+	+	+	+	72–96	RA, ART
Pulm valvotomy	NP or CPB	ST	+	+	+	+	+	+	6–24	RA, ART
DORV	CPB DHA	ST	+	+	+	+	+	+	24–48	RA, LA, PA, ART
HLHS	DHA	ST	+	+	+	+	+		>1 week	RA, ART × 2

ART, peripheral arterial catheter; ASD 2, secundum atial septal defect; CAVC, complete atrioventricular canal; Coarct, coarctation of the aorta; CPB, cardiopulmonary bypass; CT, chest tubes; DORV, double-outlet right ventricle; dTGA, d-transposition of the great arteries; HA, hypothermic cardiac arrest; HLHS, hypoplastic left heart syndrome; ICU, intensive care unit; LA, left atrial catheter; LLTX, left lateral thoracotomy; Mech vent, mechanical ventilation; NG, nasogastric tube; NP, non-pump; PA, pulmonary arterial catheter; PDA, patent ductus arteriosus; RA, right atrial catheter; ST, sternotomy; TAC, truncus arteriosus communis; TAPVR, total anomalous pulmonary venous return; TOF, tetralogy of Fallot; VSD, ventricular septal defect; PA/IVS, pulmonary atresia with intact ventricular septum.

confirmed by chest x-ray and waveform analysis prior to infusing through it.

For children who have undergone repair of simple defects such as a patent ductus arteriosus, no extensive monitoring is required. Infants with such diagnoses can return from the operating room with a peripheral intravenous line alone. Children who have undergone more extensive surgery are more fully monitored. A reasonable general approach is to take advantage of as much information as can safely be obtained. Thus, a child who has undergone repair of a ventricular septal defect or tetralogy of Fallot will return from the operating room with a right atrial monitoring catheter, a left atrial catheter, a pulmonary artery catheter, and an arterial line placed in a peripheral systemic artery. In newborns, the use of umbilical vessels can provide atraumatic venous and arterial access. If the possibility of low cardiac output is suspected, a thermistor placed transthoracically in the pulmonary artery or a flow-directed thermodilution catheter introduced via a central venous sheath allows measurement of cardiac output. These catheters allow complete monitoring of hemodynamic status and afford a means of assessing the adequacy of the repair.

Noninvasive Monitoring

A considerable amount of information regarding the well-being of pediatric cardiac patients can be obtained with little or no risk through noninvasive monitoring techniques.

Pulse Oximetry and Capnography (See Respiratory Monitoring with Pulse Oximetry and Capnography by Arguin, this volume.)

Invasive Monitoring

Despite the importance of the physical examination, as mentioned earlier, the era of infant heart surgery has made invasive monitoring in the postoperative period a necessity. Most children returning from the operating room will have in place between one and three hemodynamic monitoring catheters (Fig. 21-7). Often these catheters are placed through the chest wall at the time of surgery. Transthoracic intracardiac catheters (TIC) are generally 3.4 F in diameter and are sutured to the chest wall. There is a considerable amount of evidence to suggest that TICs are generally safe when handled appropriately.[60]

The Right Atrial Catheter/Central Venous Pressure Route

Unless a right atrial central venous catheter has been placed preoperatively, a right atrial catheter may be placed at the time of surgery. Frequently a triple-lumen catheter is introduced into the right atrium trancutaneously via the internal jugular vein. Alternatively, a TIC may be placed in the right atrium via the right atrial appendage.

Access

The right atrial catheter is useful for routine blood sampling and intravenous infusions. In the past, the right atrial catheter was used

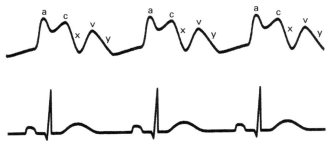

Figure 21-8. Right atrial wave (schematic).

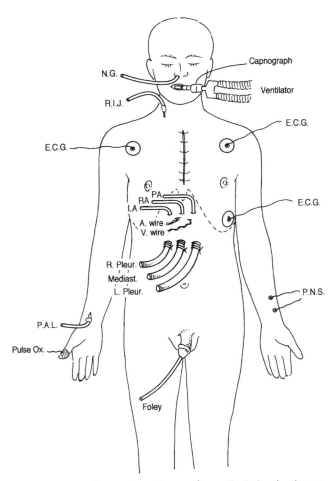

Figure 21-7. The postoperative cardiac patient. A. wire, temporary atrial pacing wires; E.C.G., cardiorespiratory monitoring leads; L. Pleur., left pleural thoracostomy tube; LA, left atrial transthoracic intracardiac monitoring catheter; Mediast., mediastinal thoracostomy tube; N.G., nasogastric tube; P.A.L., peripheral arterial catheter; P.N.S., peripheral nerve stimulator; PA, pulmonary arterial transthoracic intracardiac monitoring catheter; Pulse Ox., pulse oximetry saturation monitoring lead; R. Pleur., right pleural thoracostomy tube; R.I.J., right internal jugular monitoring catheter; RA, right atrial transthoracic intracardiac monitoring catheter; V. wire, temporary ventricular pacing wires.

for the assessment of right-to-left shunting by means of contrast echocardiography. Color flow imaging has, for the most part, superceded the need for this technique.

Waveforms

The right atrial waveform consists of three positive deflections (Fig. 21-8): The a wave follows the P wave on the ECG and corresponds to the pressure generated when the atrium contracts. The c wave is thought to represent bulging of the tricuspid valve into the right atrium during the beginning of systole. The v wave corresponds to atrial filling with a closed tricuspid valve. An increase in the a wave amplitude may be evidence of poor right ventricular compliance, or diastolic dysfunction. This may, in turn, result from myocardial stiffness after CPB, volume overload of the right ventricle, or pressure overload of the right ventricle. An elevated a wave may also result from tricuspid stenosis.

An increase in the v wave may be the result of tricuspid insufficiency. This can be important following repair of Ebstein's anomaly, pulmonary atresia with intact ventricular septum, or endocardial cushion defects such as a primum atrial septal defect or a complete atrioventricular canal.

A "cannon wave" is a very tall atrial pressure wave and is the result of simultaneous atrial and ventricular contraction. This can result from any of many causes of atrioventricular discordance, including heart block, ventricular premature beats, and electronic cardiac pacing.

Pressures

The right atrial catheter allows accurate measurement of systemic venous pressure. In situations where the right-sided filling pressures are likely to be higher than those on the left side (such as with severe right ventricular hypertrophy), the mean right atrial pressure serves as the measure of intravascular volume. Elevated right atrial pressures may also be associated with intravascular volume overload, tricuspid regurgitation or stenosis, Ebstein's anomaly, pulmonary stenosis, elevated pulmonary artery pressure, right-sided congestive heart failure, or pericardial tamponade.

Saturations

In the absence of an atrial-level shunt, the right atrial saturation can be a rough guide to mixed venous saturation, and thus the cardiac output, using the Fick formula and the arterial saturation. Right atrial saturations can be quite variable, however, because of streaming from the hepatic veins and coronary sinus. A pulmonary artery saturation or, in the presence of intracardiac shunting, an SVC saturation, provides a better estimation of the mixed venous saturation. The mixed venous saturation early in the postoperative course correlates with the risk of cardiac death in the postoperative period (Fig. 21-9).[61]

Complications

As with most catheters, right atrial catheters have a host of potential complications. If the right and left circulations are completely separated, air or thrombi introduced through a right atrial catheter may embolize only to the pulmonary circulation where all but the largest of emboli are usually reabsorbed. Many children, however, have potential sites of "paradoxical" embolization from the right-to-left circulation, either as a result of structural heart disease with a continuous right-to-left shunt or because of potential shunts at the ventricular or atrial level. The consequences of embolization to the systemic circulation include stroke, myocardial infarction, and ischemic injury to any organ in the body.

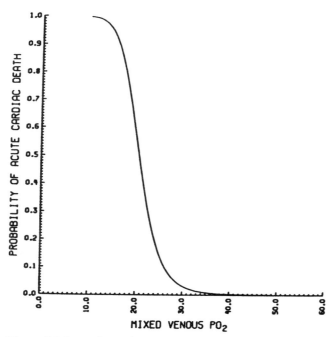

Figure 21-9. Relationship of mixed venous PO₂ and acute cardiac death. (From GV Parr, EH Blackstone, W Kirklin. Cardiac performance and mortality early after intracardiac surgery in infants and young children. *Circulation* 51:867–874, 1975. With permission.)

Chronically indwelling right atrial catheters may be the site for intravascular thrombus formation.[62–64] Such thrombi are also sources of emboli, or may themselves disrupt cardiac function by obstructing the tricuspid valve, causing tricuspid regurgitation, or by obstructing systemic venous return.

Infection of intracardiac catheters is a well-documented risk, particularly following cardiac surgery when the risk of infection of the operated tissue is great. Certain organisms are of particular concern, including *Staphylococcus aureus* and *Candida albicans*.[65]

Perforation of the heart or vessels occurs occasionally and may result in hemothorax, hemopericardium, or extravasation of catheter fluids into either space.[66] Fluid in the pleural or pericardial spaces should always be examined for sugar concentration since most intravenous fluids will have 5% to 10% dextrose, giving a fluid concentration well over 1000 mg/dl.

Catheters that fail to draw blood back should be suspected of malposition or perforation, but this is often not the case. Catheters may be subject to a "ball-valve" effect if the lumen is adjacent to the wall of the vessel. Chronically indwelling catheters may also develop a fibrinous sheath that may extend beyond the tip of the catheter. Infusion of fluids may be unimpeded, but with negative pressure, the wall of the sheath may be drawn against the lumen, preventing withdrawal of blood. Following removal of an intravascular catheter, the fibrous sheath may remain, mimicking a retained catheter fragment, or may embolize to downstream structures and even form a nidus for thrombus formation (personal observation, LCE).

Other risks of all intracardiac catheters include malposition,[64,67] arrhythmias,[64,68] injury to the conduction system,[63] fragmentation, or retention of the catheter.[60]

Removal

Following surgery, the right atrial catheter is usually the last to be removed, due to its suitability for vascular access. In the case of transthoracic right atrial catheters, care must be exercised when removing the sutures securing the catheter to the chest, because, if handled roughly, the plastic catheters may fragment at the suture site. Clinically, significant bleeding is very rare following removal of the right atrial catheter as long as there is no associated bleeding disorder or systemic anticoagulation.[60]

The Left Atrial Catheter
Route

Most transthoracic left atrial catheters that are placed surgically enter the left atrium via the right upper pulmonary vein and lie across the back wall of the left atrium.

Access

The left atrial catheter is rarely used for routine blood sampling or infusions because of the additional risks that potential catheter-related emboli carry on the systemic side of the circulation. This catheter may be useful for performing contrast echocardiography in children suspected of having residual left-to-right shunts.

Waveform

The left atrial waveform, as with the right atrial pressure, is characterized by an a wave (atrial contraction), a c wave (mitral valve closure), and a v wave (systolic atrial filling). The atrial a wave may be increased dramatically in mitral stenosis, while a very prominent v wave may be a sign of mitral regurgitation. As with the right atrial waveform, artificial pacing may lead to very elevated left atrial pressure waves (cannon waves) as the atrium contracts against a closed mitral valve during a paced ventricular contraction.

Pressures

In the majority of patients, the left atrial pressure (LAP) is higher than the right atrial pressure. In this setting, the mean left atrial catheter serves to monitor volume status. The mean LAP is also a measure of left ventricular diastolic function: A rising LAP suggests that the left ventricular myocardium may be impaired (requiring higher filling pressures for the same output) or stiffer (from volume overload, tamponade, or myocardial edema following CPB).

Saturations

The left atrial catheter serves as a source of pulmonary venous blood, which is helpful for differentiating pulmonary venous desaturation from residual right-to-left shunting at the ventricular or great vessel level.

Complications

The potential complications of the left atrial catheter include most of those mentioned for the right atrial catheter. As mentioned, however, the risks of embolization of thrombi, air, and catheter fragments to the systemic circuit are far more severe than those posed by a right heart catheter. For this reason, the left atrial catheter is usually removed very early following surgery. In addition, the risk of bleeding may be increased with left atrial catheter removal[60] because of the relatively higher pressures in the left atrium.

Removal

Because of the somewhat increased risk of bleeding, left atrial catheters are usually removed while the thoracostomy and pericardial drains are still in place. Otherwise, the same procedure is used as was outlined for the right atrial catheter.

The Pulmonary Artery Catheter

Route

The pulmonary artery catheter can be introduced via a peripheral vein or transthoracically via the right atrium or right ventricular outflow tract.

Access

Pulmonary artery catheters are used occasionally for routine infusions and blood sampling, because they have about the same risks related to embolization and infection as a right atrial catheter.

Waveform

The pulmonary artery waveform in most children is characterized by a rapid upstroke in systole followed by the peak systolic pressure. The pressure begins to fall near the end of systole. Closure of the pulmonary valve is associated with a brief increase in pressure in the pulmonary artery (the dichrotic notch), after which the pressure falls continuously until the beginning of the next cardiac cycle.

In children with separated circulations, an increase in pulmonary vascular resistance will lead to an increased systolic and diastolic pressure (discussion to follow). Children with a large left-to-right shunt (atrial septal defect, ventricular septal defect) or a "run off" lesion (e.g., pulmonary arteriovenous malformation, pulmonary regurgitation) may have an elevated systolic pressure but a low or normal diastolic pressure.

Patients with significant pulmonary regurgitation, or who have no pulmonary valve at all (after pulmonary valvectomy or tetralogy of Fallot repair with an outflow tract patch), will have pulmonary artery waveforms similar to that of the right ventricle, with a diastolic pressure close to 0 and no dichrotic notch.

Patients who have undergone cavopulmonary anastomoses (e.g., cavopulmonary shunt, Fontan procedure) will have a pulmonary artery waveform similar to that of the right atrium. This type of "pulmonary artery tracing" is usually obtained from a catheter in the SVC or right atrium.

Pressures

The mean pulmonary artery pressure is useful for assessing the status of the pulmonary vascular bed in patients who have had pulmonary artery hypertension prior to repair. Children with Down's syndrome[69,70] or who have had to accommodate to high pulmonary artery pressures or flows (large ventricular septal defect, truncus arteriosus communis, total anomalous pulmonary venous return) may have very reactive pulmonary vascular beds in the postoperative period. Such children are prone to "pulmonary hypertensive crises" characterized by acute elevations in the pulmonary artery pressure, right ventricular failure, and reduced cardiac output. A measure of the mean pulmonary artery pressure can afford an advanced warning of a pulmonary hypertensive crisis and provide an indication for intervention.

Another very useful purpose of the pulmonary artery catheter is to evaluate the success of repair of obstructions to the right ventricular outflow tract, particularly following repair of tetralogy of Fallot. When the catheter is introduced through the right atrium or right ventricular outflow tract, one may record a pressure tracing as the catheter is pulled back from the pulmonary artery to the right ventricle as the catheter is removed. This "minicatheterization" affords collection of a substantial amount of hemodynamic information in the immediate postoperative period, particularly regarding the presence or absence of residual defects at the ventricular level and the adequacy of right ventricular outflow tract reconstruction.[60]

Saturations

In the absence of left-to-right intracardiac shunting, the pulmonary artery saturation is the most reliable measure of mixed venous saturation and is therefore very useful in the estimation of cardiac output. Although an absolute value of cardiac output cannot be obtained without measuring oxygen consumption, trends can be followed closely. It is unusual to have a mixed venous oxygen shunt of 65% or greater in the presence of low cardiac output. Similarly, a mixed venous oxygen saturation lower than 50% is reasonable evidence of low cardiac output.

An additional important use of the pulmonary artery saturation has been to assess left-to-right shunting at the atrial or ventricular level. Following repair of ventricular septal defect, tetralogy of Fallot, or more complicated lesions, a pulmonary artery oxygen saturation of less than 80% on FIO$_2$ 0.40 with normal pulmonary artery pressure virtually rules out the presence of a significant left-to-right shunt.[71]

Complications

Transthoracic intracardiac pulmonary artery catheters have a slightly increased incidence of complications, compared with right and left atrial catheters, particularly when introduced transthoracically via the right ventricular outflow tract.[60] In addition to the complications previously discussed, pulmonary artery catheters may be associated with an increased incidence of associated arrhythmias and bleeding.[60,72,73]

Occasionally, a pulmonary artery catheter will pass through a patent ductus arteriosus into the descending aorta, even if a ligature was placed on the ductus. If the pulmonary artery pressure is near systemic levels, confirmation of catheter position by chest x-ray and oxygen saturations may help identify this situation.

Thermodilution Catheters in Children

The use of a thermodilution catheter allows accurate measurement of cardiac output in the immediate postoperative period. The use of a small thermistor placed through the right atrium may be preferable to a large flow-directed catheter placed through a central vein. Small thermistor catheters can easily be placed in the operating room, and the right atrial catheter can serve as the injection site. The small intralumenal displacement of the right atrial catheter allows for injections of iced saline of only 1 ml per injection. Thus, multiple determinations of cardiac output can be performed without volume-overloading the smallest of infants.

Thoracostomy Tubes

A chest tube, or thoracostomy tube, is utilized for drainage of blood, fluid, or air from the pleural and mediastinal cavities. The chest tube is connected to a chest drainage system with an underwater seal and 20 cm of negative pressure.

Route

Chest tubes are placed after CPB prior to chest closure. In the case of a median sternotomy, both anterior and posterior mediastinal tubes may be used, as well as pleural tubes when the pleural cavity has been entered. In closed cases (non-pump) where surgery has been approached via a thoracotomy, a pleural tube alone may be used, or none at all.

Kelly clamps must be kept at the bedside to temporarily occlude the chest tube to prevent pneumothorax if accidental disconnection occurs. If the patient is intubated and receiving positive-pressure ventilation at the time of accidental chest tube disconnection, atmospheric pressure does not enter the chest, lessening the chance of a pneumothorax. If the patient is waking and taking spontaneous breaths, however, accidental chest tube disconnection can still result in pneumothorax. Reexpansion of the lung can be determined on the chest x-ray and by noting diminished bubbling through the water seal chamber of the drainage system. A persistent air leak will result in continuous bubbling through the water seal chamber.

Management

Chest tubes must remain patent. The tubing should not be kinked, clamped, or elevated above the patient's torso, or drainage will be hindered. Large amounts of fluid in the dependent tubing will alter the pressures or may clot and obstruct flow. Frequent milking or stripping of the chest tubes is necessary to maintain patency. Clots or fibrin should be stripped or evacuated. Some institutions report suctioning or using a Fogarty catheter to unclog a clotted chest tube.

Drainage is assessed visually and recorded every 30 to 60 minutes on the ICU flow sheet. Anticipated drainage is less than 2 ml/kg/hr after the first few hours, assuming effective heparin reversal with protamine has been attained and circulating platelets are adequate. Fresh frozen plasma, platelets, and DDAVP may be used to correct excessive bleeding. A rough guideline regarding the volume of drainage contained in the drainage system is as follows: Each chest tube contains 5 to 10 ml of drainage, and the rubber connecting tube between chest tube and drainage system contains about 1 ml of fluid per centimeter length. Chest tubes should not be hidden or covered with blankets because an abrupt, acute deluge of chest drainage may reflect dehiscence or rupture at a suture line. Generally, 10 ml/kg/hr or more warrants a return to the operating room for reexploration.

Autotransfusion or reinfusion of collected bloody drainage can be one way of providing readily available volume and lessening the risks associated with blood bank transfusions. Many types of commercial collection systems are available. The recent use of aprotinin has resulted in a significant reduction in postoperative bleeding, presumably related to a reduction in platelet glycoprotein receptor damage associated with CPB.[74]

Removal

Chest tubes are removed when there is decreased-to-minimal drainage, coagulation status is normalized, and transthoracic monitoring lines have been removed. Usually this is accomplished on the first postoperative day. Chest tube removal can be painful, and additional analgesia is often required.

Ventilation Management

Most infants and children require assisted ventilation following cardiac surgery. The exceptions to this rule are term infants with patent ductus arteriosus, infants with uncomplicated coarctation of the aorta, some children with atrial septal defects, and many of the children who undergo palliative operations such as Blalock-Taussig shunts or pulmonary artery bands.

The duration of assisted ventilation should be minimized to the extent possible, but there are important situations in which premature ventilatory weaning is contraindicated. Children prone to pulmonary hypertensive crises may require sedation and mechanical ventilation for 24 hours or more following surgery to avoid the discomfort and respiratory acidosis that may trigger such crises. Fentanyl combined with a muscle relaxant has particularly beneficial effects in infants with extremely reactive pulmonary vascular beds, leading to its use as a first-line sedation agent in many centers.[75,76] The combination of morphine and a muscle relaxant is a very effective alternative and may be preferable when weaning from the muscle relaxant because of the small, but significant, risk of muscular rigidity associated with the use of fentanyl.

Many small infants are relatively malnourished at the time of surgery as a result of chronic congestive heart failure. Such children often require prolonged periods of ventilation following repair while their nutritional and pulmonary status is allowed to improve.

It is preferable to employ intermittent mandatory ventilation (IMV) as soon as there is any spontaneous respiratory activity, and extubation is usual the day following surgery unless pulmonary complications occur. It is unusual for an infant to require peak inspiratory pressures greater than 30 cm H_2O following corrective cardiac surgery.

There are situations, however, wherein excessive extravascular pulmonary water and chest wall edema may lead to the need for inspiratory pressures far in excess of the values expected. The peak inspiratory pressure required to maintain a normal tidal volume usually increases somewhat during the night following surgery, and there are times when vigorous ventilation, even including the use of neuromuscular blockade, may be required for adequate ventilation.

Positive end-expiratory pressure (PEEP) may help reduce pulmonary lung water in children with persistent pulmonary venous hypertension after surgery, improving oxygenation and lung compliance. The deleterious hemodynamic effects of PEEP, however, must be taken into account whenever it is employed. Patients with venopulmonary anastomoses (e.g., cavopulmonary shunts, Glenn shunts) as their only source of pulmonary blood flow may become more cyanotic with positive-pressure ventilation in general and PEEP in particular. Following the Fontan operation, systemic cardiac output may drop with increasing mean airway pressure.[77] It is important to extubate patients after such procedures as early as possible in the postoperative period after returning from the operating room.

Oxygen Therapy

The use of supplemental oxygen in patients with CHD may have a direct impact on their cardiac physiology. Oxygen is a potent pulmonary vasodilator and can result in a significant reduction in pulmonary vascular resistance. In patients with excessive pulmonary blood flow due to interventricular communications, such a reduction in pulmonary vascular resistance can result in a further increase in pulmonary blood flow and aggravation of congestive heart failure. The extreme example of this phenomenon is in patients with hypoplastic left heart syndrome. On the other hand, supplemental oxygen can have a pronounced beneficial role in patients who require pulmonary vasodilation, such as following a cavopulmonary shunt or Fontan procedure, or in children following surgical closure of a ventricular septal defect in whom the pulmonary vascular bed may be very sensitive to factors that promote vasoconstriction.

Fluid Management and Nutrition

Fluid management in the immediate postoperative period must, of course, be tailored to meet the needs of the individual patient. In general, fluids should be limited to approximately 50% to 60% of maintenance requirements during the initial 24 hours after surgery involving CPB. Dextrose 5% in 0.25 normal saline is usually effective. In newborns and malnourished older infants, dextrose 10% is more appropriate, because this group of patients may be at risk for hypoglycemia following the period of relative hyperglycemia usually seen immediately after CPB. If an infant is not receiving enteral nutrition by the second postoperative day, electrolytes are usually added to the intravenous fluid.

Adequate nutrition is exceedingly important during recovery from preexisting cardiac failure and the stress of cardiac surgery. In the infant who cannot be extubated within 24 hours of surgery, feedings with the child's usual formula, often supplemented with additional caloric content, may be started via nasogastric tube. For infants who do not tolerate enteral feeding, parental alimentation should be started. The importance of an adequate caloric intake and positive nitrogen balance as soon after surgery as possible cannot be overstated. The right atrial or pulmonary artery catheter can serve for the delivery of parenteral nutrition if necessary.

Vasoactive Agents

Vasoactive agents, usually infusions (drips), are the hallmark of a cardiac ICU. There is a large selection of these medications from which to choose, and for most indications there may be several effective agents (Table 21-2). Rather than attempt to use every vasoactive agent available, it is probably safer and more practical to define a handful of commonly used agents and develop a personal and institutional experience with their use and side effects.

Inotropic Agents

If a cardiac defect has been repaired adequately, it is unusual for an infant to require significant prolonged inotropic support after

Table 21-2. Inotropic agents and vasopressors

Agent	Dosages (IV)	Peripheral vascular effect*	Cardiac effect*	Conduction system effect
Digoxin TDD is given as follows: ½ TDD followed by ¼ TDD × 2 q8h	20 μg/kg premature 30 μg/kg neonate (0–1 mo) 40 μg/kg infant (<2 yr) 30 μg/kg child (2–5 yr) 20 μg/kg child (>5 yr)	Increases peripheral vascular resistance 1–2 +; acts directly on vascular smooth muscle	Inotropic effect 3–4 + acts directly	Slows sinus node Decreases AV conduction
Maintenance	5–10 μg/kg/d divided q12h			

Calcium:
  Chloride
  Gluconate
	10–20 mg/kg/dose (slowly)
	30–60 mg/kg/dose (slowly)
		Variable; probably depends on serum ionized Ca++ level	Inotropic effect 3 +; depends on ionized Ca−−	Slows sinus node

Amrinone	0.3–1.0 mg/kg/loading 5–20 μg/kg/min	Vasodilator	Positive inotrope	Side effect: arrhythmia

		Peripheral vascular effect			Cardiac effect*		
Agent	Dosage range	Alpha	Beta₂	Delta	Beta₁	Beta₂	Action and comments
Phenylephrine	0.1–0.5 μg/kg/min	4 +	0	0	0	0	Increases systemic resistance, no inotropy; may cause renal ischemia
Isoproterenol	0.1–0.5 μg/kg/min	0	4 +	0	4 +	4 +	Strong inotropic and chronotropic agent; peripheral vasodilator; reduces preload, pulmonary vasodilator
Norepinephrine	0.1–0.5 μg/kg/min	4 +	0	0	2 +	0	Increases systemic resistance; mildly inotropic; may cause renal ischemia
Epinephrine	0.1 μg/kg/min 0.2–0.5 μg/kg/min	2 + 4 +	1–2 +	0 0	2–3 + 4 +	2 + 3 +	Beta₂ effect with lower doses; best for supporting blood pressure in anaphylaxis and drug toxicity
Dopamine	2–4 μg/kg/min 4–8 μg/kg/min >10 μg/kg/min	0 0 2–4 +	0 2 + 0	2 + 2 + 0	0 1–2 + 1–2 +	0 1 + 1 +	Splanchnic and renal vasodilator; may be used with isoproterenol; increasing doses produce increasing alpha effect
Dobutamine	2–15 μg/kg/min	1 +	2 +	0	3–4 +	1–2 +	Less chronotropy and arrhythmias at lower doses. Effects vary with dose similar to dopamine

*Magnitude of peripheral vascular effects and cardiac effects is noted on a scale of 0 to 4 +, estimating the strength of the effect.
AV, atrioventricular; TDD, total digitalizing dose.
From Coté CJ, Ryan JF, Todres ID, Goudsouzian NG. *A Practice of Anesthesia for Infants and Children* (2nd ed). Philadelphia: Saunders, 1993. With permission.

surgery. Should such support be needed, the choice of agents depends on the nature of the underlying condition.

Dopamine is an excellent first choice as a primary inotropic agent.[78,79] At low doses (2–5 µg/kg/min), it increases renal blood flow, whereas at somewhat higher doses (5–15 µg/kg/min), the beta effects become more prominent, resulting in increased inotropic and chronotropic effects. As the administered dose increases (>15 µg/kg/min), alpha effects begin to predominate, leading to peripheral vasoconstriction. An initial dose of 5 µg/kg/min is often effective, although the rate may be increased to 25 µg/kg/min or more if needed. Infusion rates in excess of 30 µg/kg/min will not provide significant additional inotropic effects.

Other inotropic agents also have specific indications. **Dobutamine** may be preferable in settings in which an elevated systemic vascular resistance may be disadvantageous, such as cardiomyopathy or mitral regurgitation. **Isoproterenol** may be a preferred inotrope for use in pediatric patients with bronchospasm, bradycardia, a highly reactive pulmonary vascular bed, or when minimal elevations in pulmonary arteriolar resistance may be important, despite its relatively disadvantageous effects on the myocardial oxygen supply-demand ratio.

Chronotropic Agents

Agents that increase the heart rate are necessary occasionally in the ICU setting, particularly in children with increased vagal tone. Elevated vagal tone is often seen in children who have had oropharyngeal procedures, or who have instrumentation of the oropharynx (e.g., nasogastric or endotracheal tubes), or with the administration of certain sedatives, including fentanyl. Children with Down's syndrome often seem to have unusually high vagal tone, as manifested by inappropriate bradycardia, or even asystole, in response to stressful stimulation. The most useful chronotrope in the setting of increased vagal tone and minimal hemodynamic compromise is isoproterenol, because of the ease with which the dose can be titrated for its effect on heart rate.

In the setting of bradycardia with significant hemodynamic compromise, epinephrine and atropine each have a very rapid onset. Paradoxical bradycardia has been reported in infants receiving atropine at less than the minimum recommended dose of 0.1 mg. Because this often represents a large dose on a per-kilogram basis for infants, atropine can lead to a prolonged period of tachycardia, which may be detrimental to the patient recovering from heart surgery.

Chronotropic agents also may be used in the management of bradycardia secondary to sinus node dysfunction or conduction disorders, although other interventions also may be appropriate (see section on Arrhythmias).

Systemic Vasodilators

The use of vasodilator therapy has proved to be beneficial following cardiac surgery. In this setting, low cardiac output secondary to myocardial failure may be improved by a reduction in systemic vascular resistance as long as intravascular volume is adequate. Effective afterload reduction is usually judged clinically through signs of improved perfusion.

Sodium nitroprusside is an extremely valuable and selective afterload-reducing agent.[80] It is given as a constant infusion and must be protected from light. It is usually started at 0.5 µg/kg/min and titrated for effective vasodilation. Doses exceeding 10 µg/kg/min should be avoided.[81]

Nitroprusside must be given cautiously in settings of impaired hepatic function, and in all patients, cyanide levels must be followed closely if the agent is used for more than 24 hours. Cyanide poisoning, a potential side effect of nitroprusside therapy, is manifested by a metabolic acidosis and an increase in mixed venous saturation.

Amrinone is a very effective vasodilator and offers the additional benefit of inotropic support as a nonglycoside, noncatecholamine inotropic agent.[82] In children, a loading dose of 1.5 mg/kg is administered over 30 minutes, with close monitoring of the BP. Following this, an infusion of 5 to 10 µg/kg/min is initiated. If further afterload reduction is required, an additional 1.5-mg/kg bolus may be given for a total loading dose of 3 mg/kg.

Pulmonary Vasodilators

Reactive pulmonary hypertension may be a management problem in the postoperative period following correction of certain congenital cardiac defects. Although many agents have been investigated as specific pulmonary vasodilators, few have been very effective and specific. The exceptions are inhaled oxygen, inhaled nitric oxide, and prostacyclin. Prostacyclin is an agent given via continuous infusion and may reduce long-term risk of sudden death in patients with primary pulmonary hypertension,[83] but it is not generally useful in the ICU setting.

Oxygen is an extremely effective pulmonary vasodilator. Although most clinicians feel that fractions of inhaled oxygen over 0.5 to 0.6 are toxic, the damaging effects probably occur over relatively long periods. Consequently, oxygen has become the preferred pulmonary vasodilator in the early postoperative setting wherein short-term treatments are often sufficient.

Nitric oxide is an agent that has recently been shown to be an effective and highly specific pulmonary vasodilator in certain groups of children and adults[84–88] (Fig. 21-10).[85] Doses of 20 to 80 ppm of inhaled gas are usual, and patients must be followed closely for methemaglobinemia. Although nitric oxide has been used for periods up to 50 to 60 days in infants, the long-term safety profile in children has not been well established.

Vasoconstrictors

Vasoconstricting agents are rarely required in the pediatric ICU. Exceptions include settings in which pulmonary blood flow depends largely on systemic BP, such as single ventricle with severe pulmonary stenosis and systemic-to-pulmonary shunts (e.g., Blalock-Taussig shunts). Children with tetralogy of Fallot may require vasoconstricting agents, particularly during a hypercyanotic spell and especially if other interventions have been ineffective. Also, children with dynamic subaortic stenosis, as with idiopathic hypertrophic subaortic stenosis (IHSS), may require vasoconstrictors to increase afterload and ameliorate the dynamic obstruction. Selective vasoconstrictors are preferred in these settings because the inotropic effects of combination agents may actually worsen the dynamic subpulmonary stenosis seen in tetralogy of Fallot and the subaortic stenosis associated with IHSS. In the setting of pathologically decreased systemic vascular resistance, as with septic shock or toxic ingestion, selective vasoconstrictors are also indicated.

Children with severely impaired cardiac output may require vasoconstrictors to maintain an adequate BP, although this should be considered a last resort after inotropic agents and intravascular volume expansion. All children should have at least a normal intravascular volume as indicated by clinical examination or central venous pressure monitoring. Because vasoconstrictors tend to

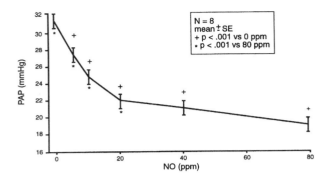

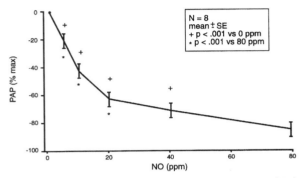

Figure 21-10. Mean pulmonary artery pressure and inhaled concentration of nitric oxide. %max, percent of maximum; mm Hg, millimeters of mercury; NO, nitric oxide; PAP, pulmonary artery pressure; ppm, parts per million. (From C Frostell et al. Inhaled nitric oxide: A selective pulmonary vasodilator reversing hypoxic pulmonary vasoconstriction. *Circulation* 83:2038–2047, 1991. With permission.)

increase cardiac work, these children fare better with agents with both vasoconstrictor activity and inotropic effects.

The most selective of the vasoconstrictors are phenylephrine and methoxamine, both of which are exclusively alpha-1 adrenergic agents. Ephedrine and norepinephrine are predominantly alpha-1 agents, but the former also has modest degrees of beta-2 activity and the latter has a small amount of both beta-1 and beta-2 adrenergic action.

Combination agents with significant inotropic effects include dopamine and epinephrine. These agents are discussed in more detail elsewhere (see Table 21-2 and Pharmacological Support of the Circulation by Ziegler, Englander, and Fugat, this volume).

Congestive Heart Failure

The fundamental function of the heart is to pump a sufficient volume of blood at a sufficient pressure to meet the metabolic demands of the body. As the demands of the tissues increase, a number of compensatory mechanisms come into play: The heart rate increases under the influence of neural and humoral input. The venous capacitance vessels constrict, and the kidneys retain intravascular volume, increasing venous pressure, which, in turn, results in increased filling of the heart and an increased stroke volume. In this fashion, changes in demand result in changes in cardiac output.

As the demand placed on the heart increases (e.g., a large

intracardiac shunt), or the ability of the heart to meet that demand falls (e.g., ventricular dysfunction following surgery), these mechanisms fail. It is easiest to break down the manifestations of ventricular failure into several categories:

heart rate

Starling curve

LaPlace Law

Over a certain optimal heart rate, any further increase results in a net decrease in cardiac output because of inadequate diastolic filling. Similarly, an impaired heart may not be able to respond to increases in diastolic filling in a normal fashion, and venous pressure will continue to rise in response to an inadequate cardiac output until the familiar signs of venous congestion become manifest: tachypnea, rales, hepatomegaly, ascites, and so on. Eventually, an adequate cardiac output may not be possible, even at the limit of physiologically supportable venous pressures, and as ventricular function deteriorates further, the cardiac output will fall.

Pulmonary Hypertension

In certain groups of patients, the arteriolar musculature in the pulmonary vascular bed is extremely reactive. Children with elevated pulmonary blood flow or pressure and children with Down's syndrome are particularly prone to pulmonary vasospasm in response to hypoxia, acidosis, and perhaps hypercarbia. When the pulmonary and systemic circulations are separated, pulmonary vasospasm results in pulmonary hypertension. In addition, children with excessive pulmonary flow or pressure, or elevated pulmonary venous pressure (pulmonary vein obstruction, mitral stenosis or regurgitation, elevated left ventricular filling pressures), may develop a component of chronic reactive pulmonary hypertension over months or years.

Pulmonary hypertension is particularly detrimental in the immediate postoperative period because it places an increased strain on the right ventricle, which already may have been adversely affected by a ventriculotomy, CPB, HA, or pulmonary regurgitation. In addition, pulmonary artery hypertension increases myocardial oxygen consumption and may interfere with left ventricular diastolic function. Pulmonary artery hypertension may predispose to postoperative bleeding through right-sided suture lines and catheter insertion sites.

Pulmonary hypertension can be attenuated, or avoided, through the use of sedation, supplemental oxygen, and alkalinization of the blood. Hyperventilation has been shown to reduce pulmonary artery pressure in children following cardiac surgery (Fig. 21-11).[84] In addition, nitric oxide is evolving into a very effective, specific pulmonary vasodilator. When severe pulmonary hypertension becomes life-threatening, as it may in the postoperative period, extracorporeal membrane oxygenation (see Extracorporeal Life Support by Custer and Akingbola, this volume.) may provide short-term relief when it is expected that the cause of the pulmonary hypertension will resolve within a few days (e.g., following surgery when there has been chronic pulmonary venous hypertension).

Pleural Effusions

Pleural effusions are not uncommon following cardiac surgery in children. Pleural fluid accumulations, or persistent chest tube drainage, can be the result of changes in the hydrostatic or osmotic

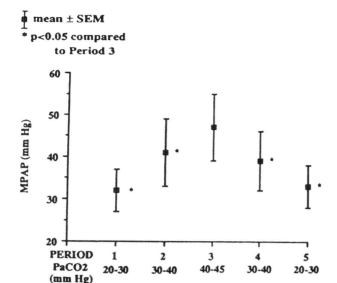

Figure 21-11. Mean pulmonary artery pressure and PCO$_2$. MPAP, mean pulmonary artery pressure; mm Hg, millimeters of mercury; PaCO$_2$, partial pressure of CO$_2$. (From JP Morray, AM Lynn, PB Mansfield. Effect of pH and PCO$_2$ on pulmonary and systemic hemodynamics after surgery in children with congenital heart disease and pulmonary hypertension. *J Pediatr* 113:474–479, 1988. With permission.)

balance in the pleura (transudates),[89] inflammation of the pleura (exudates),[89] or persistent leakage of structures within the chest (injury to the thoracic duct, perforation of vessels by indwelling catheters, transudation of fluid through Gortex grafts).

Transudates

Transudates are the result of an alteration in the mechanical factors influencing the formation or reabsorption of pleural fluid.[90] Following cardiac surgery, there can be acute changes in the capillary osmotic pressure, hydrostatic pressure, and membrane permeability.

Following CPB, the replacement of lost blood with crystalloid solutions may result in a relative hypoproteinemia. This phenomenon may be aggravated by relative undernourishment and poor protein stores in children who had been suffering from congestive heart failure in the preoperative period. Hypoproteinemia in the postoperative period can result in lower intracapillary osmotic pressure and decreased reabsorption of fluid from the pleural space. Volume replacement with blood products or an albumin solution can help reduce this problem.

It is common for the capillary hydrostatic pressure to be increased following CPB. Elevated venous pressures are the result of reduced systolic function, requiring higher filling pressures, and some degree of stiffening of the myocardium (diastolic dysfunction) due to myocardial edema. In the early postoperative period, aggressive treatment with diuretics may result in a reduced central venous pressure and help reverse the course of an accumulating pleural effusion, but only at the price of a reduced cardiac output.

The systemic venous pressure also may be increased dramatically following venopulmonary anastomoses such as the cavopulmonary and Glenn shunts,[91–95] the fenestrated Fontan procedure,[92,96–99] and the Fontan procedure.[23,100–109] In this setting, the acutely increased capillary pressures can result in refractory pleural, and even pericardial, effusions. Maneuvers that reduce the pulmonary vascular resistance, including supplemental oxygen, hyperventilation, and alkalinization, will tend to ameliorate the elevation in systemic venous pressure. During mechanical ventilation, any reduction in the mean airway pressure, and particularly the end-expiratory pressure, will also allow adequate pulmonary blood flow at lower systemic venous pressures.

Exudates

An exudate is the result of inflammation or other diseases of the pleural surface (tuberculosis, pneumonia, malignancy, etc.). Light et al. showed that a pleural fluid-serum ratio of greater than 0.5, a pleural fluid LDH of greater that 200 IU, or a pleural-serum ratio of greater than 0.6 are indicative of a pleural exudate rather than a transudate.[110] Evidence of an exudative process mandates close scrutiny of the fluid for signs of an infectious process. Similarly, any evidence of an infectious process in the presence of a pleural effusion warrants diagnostic pleurocentesis to rule out an empyema.

Chylothorax

Chylothorax is not uncommon following certain types of cardiac surgery in children. Accumulation of chyle in the pleural space is likely related to increased central venous pressure (e.g., with congestive heart failure or secondary to diastolic dysfunction after CPB) as well as to trauma to lymphatic vessels (thoracic duct) or damage to tiny lymphatic channels in the mediastinum and pleura. Chylothorax is particularly prevalent following surgery in the vicinity of the thoracic duct (Blalock-Taussig shunt). It is also frequent following venopulmonary shunts such as the Fontan procedure or other cavopulmonary anastomoses, after which the central venous pressure is often quite elevated, although in most patients of this type a pleural effusion is more likely to be a transudate than chylous.

The cellular elements in a chylous effusion are generally almost exclusively lymphocytic. The absolute number of lymphocytes in a chylous effusion may be quite variable and tends to drift downward as the total population of lymphocytes becomes depleted by persistent drainage. Enteral administration of fatty food (e.g., cream) may cause a clear chylous effusion to become acutely milky, thus aiding in the diagnosis.

Treatment of chylous effusions is directed at reduction in lymphatic flow and replacement of elements lost in the drained chyle, when possible. Elimination of enteral fat, particularly long-chain triglyerides, is often sufficient in reducing chylous drainage, although complete elimination of enteral intake is necessary occasionally. Formulas that are low in long-chain triglycerides include Pregestamil and Portagen. Albumin supplementation is required frequently in refractory chylous effusions. Some centers have experimented with reinfusion of drained chyle that has been collected in a sterile fashion. Note that intravenous lipids will not result in clouding of a chylous effusion because chyle is the result of lymphatic drainage of the gut.

Other Causes of Pleural Effusions

Some types of synthetic materials used in the repair of CHD are composed of a mesh or weave. The gaps between the strands of material usually fill quickly with clot, which, as it organizes, helps create a surface onto which the developing endothelial membrane can adhere. Occasionally, however, persistent "weeping" may occur through these openings during the postoperative period.

In this situation, the chemical characteristics (albumin, glucose, LDH) of the fluid recovered from the pleural space are generally identical to those of serum.

Occasionally, a central vascular catheter will erode through, or become dislodged from, the vascular system, resulting in an infusion of exogenous fluids into the pleural or pericardial space. Because they are often quite hyperosmolar, exogenous fluids drained into the pleural space may draw a considerable volume of transudate into the pleural space as well. Pleural fluid with a very high glucose concentration suggests an effusion of exogenous origin. Catheters that fail to "draw" blood back should be suspected of extravascular placement, but this is not always the case.

Arrhythmias

A majority of arrhythmias seen in the pediatric postoperative period are related to underlying abnormalities of the conduction system, damage to the conduction system at surgery, or changes in the myocardial conduction and repolarization properties during and following surgery. Most of the arrhythmias mentioned here are covered in considerably more detail in Cardiac Arrhythmias in the Intensive Care Unit by Walsh and Liberthson, this volume. Only those features peculiar to the **postoperative period** will be discussed in detail in the sections that follow.

Sick Sinus Syndrome

Sick sinus syndrome, or tachycardia-bradycardia syndrome, is felt to be the result of injury to the sinus node, either due to mechanical injury or through interruption of the sinus node artery. Damage to the sinus node is more common following extensive atrial surgery, such as with the Mustard, Senning, or Fontan procedures, or following some types of repair for sinus venosus atrial septal defects. The sinus node artery may be interrupted during surgery involving the coronary arteries, as with the Jatene arterial switch procedure, or may be involved in coronary artery aneurysms following the Kawasaki syndrome.

The features of sick sinus syndrome include atrial tachyarrhythmias, such as ectopic atrial tachycardia and atrial fibrillation, alternating with sinus bradycardia. Because most medications effective in suppressing abnormal atrial rhythms also aggravate sinus bradycardia, implantation of an artificial pacemaker is often necessary when treating this disorder medically.

Bradycardias
Sinus Bradycardia
The diagnosis of sinus bradycardia is based on a few basic criteria: a heart rate that is lower than normal for age (Table 21-3), a P wave before every QRS with a normal axis, a variable beat-to-beat interval, and a normal QRS complex. Sinus bradycardia is a common occurrence following pediatric heart surgery. In the majority of cases, it is related to an administered medication, an electrolyte imbalance, or increased vagal tone in the patient.

Medications may cause sinus bradycardia through their action on adrenergic receptors, as in the case of beta-blockers, or may increase vagal tone through a variety of mechanisms. Fentanyl, for example, is sometimes associated with sinus bradycardia. Similarly, many other medications, including some antiseizure medications, may be associated with sinus bradycardia.

Some electrolyte disorders can be associated with decreased automaticity of the sinoatrial node, leading to sinus bradycardia. Hyperkalemia and hypocalcemia are the most common. Associated findings include widening of the QRS complex, a long QT interval, and, in severe cases, ventricular arrhythmias.

Table 21-3. Normal heart rates in infants and children

Age	Mean heart rate (beats/min)
0–24 hrs	120
1–7 d	135
8–30 d	160
3–12 mo	140
1–3 yrs	125
3–5 yrs	100
8–12 yrs	80
2–16 yrs	75

From D Todres. *A Practice of Anesthesia for Infants and Children* (2nd ed). Philadelphia: Saunders, 1993. With permission.

Finally, many children have elevated vagal tone in the postoperative period. Nasopharyngeal instrumentation may cause increased vagal stimulation, and bradycardia is frequent following placement of nasogastric tubes or suctioning of endotracheal tubes. However, bradycardia may signal serious hypoxemia. Central nervous system abnormalities, either predating surgery or complicating the postoperative course, also are associated with increased vagal tone and sinus bradycardia. Sinus bradycardia associated with hypertension is classically associated with raised intracranial pressure. Children with Down's syndrome appear to have unusually high vagal tone and can have severe sinus bradycardia with noxious stimulation.

The approach to sinus bradycardia in the postoperative period is aimed at discerning the likely etiology and treating only when necessary. Acute intervention should be reserved for the relatively unusual patients with hemodynamic compromise. In most patients, the etiology for sinus bradycardia is vagal, and vagolytic medications such as atropine are very effective. In fact, atropine is often too effective, resulting in a prolonged period of marked tachycardia with a concomitant increase in myocardial oxygen consumption. Isoproterenol has the advantage of allowing careful control. Although it also results in increased myocardial oxygen consumption, very low doses may be sufficient in the treatment of bradycardia. If sinus bradycardia is associated with severe hemodynamic compromise, temporary atrial pacing using the transvenous, external, or esophageal route may be indicated.

Complete Heart Block
Complete heart block may follow surgical repair of CHD as a result of direct injury to the conduction fibers or because of edema in the vicinity of the conduction system. Particularly in the latter case, complete heart block may be heralded by increasing degrees of second-degree heart block. In many cases, heart block may be transient, although block persisting after 7 to 10 days is unlikely to resolve.

The treatment of complete heart block in the immediate postoperative period is temporary pacing (see pacing section of Medical Issues for the Cardiac Patient by Erickson and Elixson, this volume.)

Narrow Complex Tachycardias
Sinus Tachycardia
Sinus tachycardia is diagnosed on the basis of a heart rate higher than expected for the patient's age, a P wave before every QRS with a normal axis, beat-to-beat variability, and normal QRS mor-

phology. Sinus tachycardia is a common occurrence following pediatric heart surgery and is usually related to an administered medication, hemodynamic insufficiency, or patient discomfort or fear. The approach to sinus tachycardia in the postoperative period is aimed at discerning the likely etiology.

Medications may cause sinus tachycardia through direct chronotropic effects, as in the case of catecholamines, xanthine derivative, and vagolytics, or may cause tachycardia indirectly through negative inotropic effects or vasodilation, as with nitroprusside.

Sinus tachycardia, however, is often a normal physiologic response to the hemodynamic consequences of cardiac surgery. Tachycardia is the first response to an insufficient cardiac output and will usually precede a fall in BP or urine output. Myocardial failure, intravascular volume depletion, volume overload, residual intracardiac lesions, and pericardial tamponade may all present first with sinus tachycardia. In addition, any disorder that increases the metabolic demands of the body, such as infection, may lead to sinus tachycardia. Seizure activity also is associated with sinus tachycardia, possibly centrally mediated.

Supraventricular Tachycardia

Supraventricular tachycardia is not uncommon in the postoperative period. Its features include an abrupt onset and cessation, a fixed cycle length, and a normal QRS complex (except in the case of aberrancy). Supraventricular tachycardia requires a specific physiologic substrate, but, because of the numerous changes in myocardial conduction and repolarization, many children who develop this arrhythmia in the postoperative period may never have had it prior to surgery.

The treatment of supraventricular tachycardia depends on the severity of the hemodynamic consequences. One concerning result of supraventricular tachycardia is increased metabolic demands on the myocardium, which is often reason enough to attempt termination of the rhythm. Other results of supraventricular tachycardia include congestive heart failure and low cardiac output.

Supraventricular tachycardia may be terminated through vagal maneuvers, pharmacologic agents, or overdrive pacing. Digoxin is effective in controlling supraventricular tachycardia, but may take considerable time to terminate the rhythm. For this reason, digoxin is often used in combination with adenosine or overdrive atrial pacing. Many medications that are effective in terminating supraventricular tachycardia are relatively potent negative inotropic agents and are avoided in the postoperative patient when possible. These agents include beta-blockers, verapamil, and, to a lesser extent, procainamide.

Termination of supraventricular tachycardia may be achieved by pacing through transthoracic or transvenous atrial pacing wires, or via a transesophageal pacing catheter. Ideally, a programmable electronic stimulator can introduce a single premature beat shorter than the cycle length of the reentrant rhythm. When a programmable stimulator is not available, a pacer can be used to introduce a short burst of atrial pacing at a rate slightly higher than that of the supraventricular tachycardia. Rarely, rapid atrial pacing can lead to atrial, or even ventricular, arrhythmias. Consequently, a synchronized cardioversion unit must be available immediately before overdrive pacing is attempted.

Junctional Ectopic Tachycardia

Junctional ectopic tachycardia (JET) is an abnormal automatic junctional rhythm that seems to occur almost exclusively in the postoperative period. Its features include tachycardia (usually 200–240 BPM), absent or retrograde P waves, and a normal QRS

complex (except in the case of bundle branch block or aberrancy). An esophageal lead or an atrial wire (when available) added to the ECG can be very helpful in differentiating sinus tachycardia from JET. JET seems to occur more frequently following surgical repair of large ventricular septal defects, but may complicate any intracardiac surgery.

At sufficiently high heart rates, JET may result in congestive heart failure, low cardiac output, and increased metabolic demands on the myocardium. Like most automatic rhythms, however, it can be very difficult to treat. Most effective regimens include the combination of core cooling to 33°C and either digoxin or diphenylhydantoin. Fortunately, most cases of JET resolve spontaneously after 1 to 3 days.

Occasionally, JET may take a less severe form with a heart rate in the 170 to 200 range and more variability in rate. This variant may be called an "accelerated junctional rhythm" and usually results in less serious hemodynamic consequences.

Postoperative Bleeding

Bleeding from small vessels and sternal marrow in the operative field, as well as from suture lines, may continue for several hours following surgery and may be aggravated by diminished clotting factors and platelets secondary to CPB. Patients who are chronically polycythemic or cyanotic prior to surgery have a secondary platelet disorder and are at increased risk of serious postoperative bleeding. Preoperative phlebotomy to reduce the hematocrit to 65% may help reduce the risk of perioperative bleeding. Patients who have had a previous operation are also at increased risk for postoperative bleeding because of adhesions and an increased need for dissection of the mediastinal structures. Finally, there is an increased risk of bleeding in patients who are hypertensive following surgery.

Chest tubes can be kept patent of clotted blood by "milking" them away from the patient at regular intervals. Systemic and pulmonary hypertension should be controlled to reduce bleeding at suture lines. In the patient who had been chronically cyanotic in the preoperative period, platelet transfusions may have some benefit in reducing hemorrhage. Bleeding in excess of 10 ml/kg/hr after the first few hours is considered excessive and may warrant reexploration to control the source of bleeding. The use of fresh whole blood, compared with banked blood, may reduce the risk of clotting abnormalities. If possible, reoperation should be undertaken before administration of large volumes of banked blood becomes necessary.

Anemia

Anemia results in decreased oxygen delivery to the tissues and requires an increased cardiac output from the recovering heart to meet metabolic demands. In addition, anemia can result in hypoxemia in children in whom the systemic and pulmonary venous return mixes prior to being pumped to the body. For these reasons, a low hemoglobin level should be particularly avoided in the postoperative period.

When large amounts of blood are required, a metabolic acidosis may result, requiring administration of sodium bicarbonate. In addition, the citrate in banked blood chelates ionized calcium. A reasonable rule of thumb is that 200 mg of calcium gluconate will generally offset the calcium loss caused by chelation from 100 ml of any blood product. It is generally safe to raise the hemoglobin level to 13 to 15 gram%, particularly if the total number of donor units can be reduced by transfusing several times with the same unit in a small child.

Sedation and Pain Management

Sedation is a "two-edged sword" when considered for use in the postoperative surgical patient. Administration of sedatives can result in a reduction in endogenous catecholamine production and aggravation of congestive heart failure in children with CHD. In addition, sedatives may mask important changes in the patient's level of consciousness or pain. On the other hand, pain and the inability to rest are inhumane to the patient, increase the metabolic demands of the heart, and predispose to hypertension and postoperative bleeding. Consequently, it is essential that sedatives and sedating analgesic medications be provided, but be limited to what is necessary to provide rest and relief from pain (Table 21-4).

Following most open procedures, heavy sedation and pharmacologic muscle relaxation are continued through the night following the surgery when postoperative bleeding is more likely, and then weaned the following morning. Morphine or fentanyl are favored narcotic agents because of their combined sedative and analgesic effect. Midazolam is a potent sedative with the additional advantageous effect of amnesia.

Infection

Infants who undergo cardiac surgery are often susceptible to infection because of poor preoperative nutrition, increased metabolic demands, and edematous lungs. This issue often is further complicated by an increased incidence in fever immediately following surgery, probably related to atelectasis and the release of pyrogens from leukocytes injured during bypass and sequestered blood within the surgical site.

Prophylactic antibiotics are generally used for a 24- to 48-hour period following surgery, and are usually continued until the central venous pressure monitoring catheter is removed. The usual protocol includes a cephalosporin, such as cefazolin (25 mg/kg IV q8°), with the addition of vancomycin (15 mg/kg/dose IV q12°) in the case of a prosthetic valve replacement. No regimen, however, has been objectively evaluated in the pediatric population.

Neurologic Problems after Surgery

Obtundation and Coma

Obtundation and coma can be related to several factors in the postoperative period, including neurologic injury, inadequate metabolic substrate, and oversedation. Severe neurologic injury may occur in as many as 1% to 2% of children undergoing open heart surgery. A majority of patients in this category have undergone HA with arrest times in excess of 45 minutes.[111] Many of these children also will be affected by seizures and chorioathetoid movement disorders.

Whenever neurologic function is not normal after cardiac surgery, the adequacy of metabolic substrate must be confirmed. Low cardiac output, hypoxemia, and hypoglycemia can lead to obtundation or coma. Hypercarbia also may cause depression in mental status.

A common cause of depressed neurologic function in the immediate postoperative period, however, is oversedation. Very large doses of narcotics are often used in pediatric cardiac anesthesia, and narcosis can persist for many days, contrary to the expected half-life for these agents. Persistent narcotization is suggested by obtundation without evidence of focal neurologic injury, particularly in the presence of miosis. Because of the rapid onset of physiologic dependence on agents such as fentanyl and the adverse effects of abrupt opiate withdrawal on pulmonary vascular resistance (not to mention patient comfort), the use of opiate receptor blocking agents such as naloxone should be avoided if possible.

Seizures

Seizures may occur in as many as 10% of children following HA. The majority of postoperative seizures in this group are transient.[112–114] Unfortunately, recent evidence suggests that late neurologic sequellae may be a problem in this group of children, so long-term follow-up may be appropriate.[115]

Chorioathetosis

A very small fraction of children will develop chorioathetosis during the first week following HA.[111,116–118] This unfortunate disorder appears to be rare following arrest times of less than 30 minutes and particularly common following arrest times greater than 60 minutes.[111] Its etiology is not clear, although lactic acidosis,[117] occlusion of the cerebral microcirculation[119–122] and hypothermia[123] have been proposed as causes of neurologic injury. In some children, this movement disorder may resolve, particularly when mild in severity, but in others it may be permanent.

Renal Complications following Cardiac Surgery

Low urinary output following cardiac surgery may be related to prerenal, renal, or (rarely) postrenal factors. In the setting of a normally functioning kidney, the urine output is a sensitive indi-

Table 21-4. Sedatives and analgesics

Agent	PO	IM	IV	Comments
Morphine		0.1 mg/kg	0.1 mg/kg	May be given SQ
Fentanyl		1–2 µg/kg	1–2 µg/kg	
Acetaminophen	15 mg/kg			
Diazepam			0.1–0.2 mg/kg	May be given PR
Midazolam	0.3–0.75 mg/kg	0.02–0.03 mg/kg	0.02–0.03 mg/kg	
Chloral hydrate	100 mg/kg minus 100 mg*			Less effective PR Max. dose 1000 mg

*Example: A 10-kg child would receive (100 mg/kg × 10 kg) − 100 mg = 900 mg.

cator of cardiac output. When the urine output falls below 1 ml/kg/hr, it suggests a suboptimal renal blood supply. For this reason, urine output is a favorite clinical indicator of cardiac output in the immediate postoperative period. It follows that a drop in urine output, which is considered to be secondary to decreased cardiac output, should be addressed by treating the low cardiac output. In general, decreased urine output secondary to reduced renal blood flow is associated with urine that is concentrated with a reduced sodium concentration, a normal protein concentration, and very few erythrocytes or leukocytes. Modestly elevated blood urea nitrogen (BUN) and creatinine concentrations are also usual but rapidly return to normal with restoration of normal renal blood flow.

Injury to the kidney itself can be the result of HA,[114] or injury can result from any cause of severely reduced renal blood flow, such as low cardiac output or renal artery thrombosis. Acute tubular necrosis resulting from ischemic injury to the kidney is manifested by large numbers of erythrocytes and red cell casts in the urine, as well as proteinuria. A variable degree of oliguria to anuria may be present initially (oliguric phase). If the kidney is damaged severely, peritoneal dialysis or hemodialysis may be required. In most children, renal function slowly returns after several days to several weeks, often heralded by a period of abnormally, and sometimes inappropriately, increased urine output (polyuric phase). A small number of children may not recover adequate renal function. In addition to possible dialysis, treatment of acute tubular necrosis is not different from the management of other types of renal failure, including fluid restriction as appropriate to prevent volume overload and careful monitoring of serum electrolytes and serum levels of drugs known to be nephrotoxic.

Rarely, oliguria may be the result of urinary obstruction in the ICU. Foley catheters may become obstructed by blood or sediment in the urine or by a kink in the lumen of the catheter.

In children who do not have an indwelling urinary catheter, oliguria and anuria may be the result of detrusor spasm, which can be the result of pain or injury to the bladder. In addition, following the administration of narcotics, many children are unable to relax the detrusor sufficiently to allow urination. Signs of detrusor spasm include agitation, often refractory to sedation, and oliguria.

Temperature Control Following Surgery

Heat loss following CPB is significant, despite rewarming at the end of hypothermic bypass.[124] A considerable fraction of this heat loss is due to convection and evaporation, factors that are more significant in infants and children.

Recovery of core temperature demands an increase in the metabolic demands of the patient, putting an additional strain on the cardiovascular system. Consequently, it is important to supply exogenous heat to patients who have a reduced core temperature following surgery. Rewarming in the ICU can be achieved with warming blankets, which use circulating warmed water, or with warming lamps. Exposure must be monitored when using lamps to prevent thermal injury.

Cardiac Assist Devices

Extracorporeal Membrane Oxygenation

Extracorporeal membrane oxygenation (ECMO) can be conducted using venoarterial or veno-venous circuits. Both have a place in the support of children during recovery from cardiac surgery.

In venoarterial ECMO, a fraction of the returning systemic venous blood is removed via a cannula in the right atrium or SVC, oxygenated, and added back to the systemic arterial system via a carotid artery, which must often be sacrificed. As with CPB, which venoarterial ECMO resembles in many ways, oxygenated blood is delivered to the systemic circulation bypassing the heart and lungs. This is an effective support modality when the lungs are incapable of adequate gas exchange, or when the pulmonary vascular resistance is sufficiently high that the right ventricle cannot pump a cardiac output through them. In general, a postoperative patient who has severe pulmonary hypertension and low cardiac output, with or without pulmonary venous hypoxemia, may be a candidate for venoarterial ECMO. Newborns with severe lung disease and CHD may be candidates for venoarterial ECMO prior to surgery as well, if their lung disease places them at unacceptable risk for surgery.

In veno-venous ECMO, a fraction of the returning systemic venous blood is removed, oxygenated, and added back to the systemic venous system. The saturation of the returning systemic venous blood is increased, but pulmonary blood flow is not reduced. This is an effective support modality in patients who have mixing of the systemic and pulmonary venous returns and are severely cyanotic due to insufficient pulmonary blood flow (e.g., pulmonary atresia, clotted Blalock-Taussig shunt) or inadequate mixing of the venous returns (e.g., transposition of the great arteries). Veno-venous ECMO will not be effective for patients with severe pulmonary artery hypertension unless there is right-to-left shunting at some level (atrial septal defect, ventricular septal defect, or patent ductus arteriosus).

ECMO is, at best, a temporary measure. Because it requires systemic anticoagulation and a membrane oxygenator, the morbidity of the procedure increases with the duration of support. ECMO carries a very high risk when used for a condition that will not improve over a week or so. Veno-venous ECMO has somewhat less risk of hemorrhage and has the additional advantage that it does not require sacrifice of a major artery. Recently, however, techniques to repair the artery may avoid sacrificing it.

Intraaortic Balloon Pump

Intraaortic balloon pumping (IABP)[125,126] employs a pneumatically driven balloon placed in the descending aorta to reduce the systolic afterload by eliminating some of the work of pumping the arterial blood and to augment systemic, and particularly coronary, blood flow during diastole. IABP is effective in patients who have a low cardiac output following surgery despite other efforts to optimize the circulation, including catecholamines. It has been used in children and adults following surgery for ischemic, valvular, and CHD.[127] Because the use of catecholamines can often be reduced with the use of IABP, it is possible that this modality also could help reduce the extent of myocardial injury following major cardiac operations.

The technique of IABP insertion is generally percutaneous or by cutdown. The introducer sheath should be placed in the common femoral artery just below the inguinal ligament. Once the balloon is positioned in the descending aorta (confirmed by x-ray), counterpulsation can begin. The diastolic balloon inflations are timed electronically using ventricular systole on the electrocardiographic or arterial pulse tracing. Immediate improvement in cardiac function and perfusion is often apparent.

In most cases, IABP is continued for only 12 to 48 hours. The support is then weaned and the balloon is removed. Pressure is applied to the groin for at least an hour to facilitate sealing of the anterior arterial puncture. If bleeding persists, or a hematoma develops, surgical exploration is indicated to repair the artery. The use of IABP in children is limited by the size of the child, particularly with respect to the size of the common femoral artery.

Management of Prosthetic Valves in Children

Children who receive a mechanical valve at the aortic or mitral position require lifelong anticoagulation. Oral warfarin is begun about 24 hours following extubation at about 0.1 mg/kg in a daily dose up to an initial dose of 5 mg. Heparin may be used for anticoagulation temporarily if there is a delay removing the chest tubes and transcutaneous monitoring catheters. The warfarin dose is titrated according to daily prothrombin times until a stable value of about 1.5 to 2.0 times control is achieved. Where available, an alternative standardized index of anticoagulation is the INR, which should be maintained at 2 and 3.

It is important to note that warfarin affects a number of factors, which vary in their time to respond to a change in dose between 1 and 4 days.[128] Consequently, it is essential that the warfarin dose should be titrated in small steps. Any medication administered in conjunction with warfarin must be checked for possible dosage interactions. Warfarin is a known teratogen and must be discontinued prior to conception in any patient who may become pregnant.

Warfarin poses special risks of bleeding for children in whom it is difficult to limit activity. For this reason, homografts and autografts are preferable when practical in pediatric patients. After initial stabilization of the dose, it is necessary to check the prothrombin time every week for several weeks, then monthly for several months, and every 2 to 3 months thereafter to maintain the dose in the therapeutic range.

Surgical Repair Procedures

Postoperative Care: General Considerations

Before discussing the postoperative care following a number of representative surgical procedures, it is helpful to review the general course following surgery after closed procedures, routine open procedures, and open procedures that are likely to be complicated by pulmonary hypertension.

General Course Following Closed Procedures (e.g., patent ductus arteriosus, pulmonary artery band) and Minor Open Procedures (atrial septal defect, pulmonary stenosis).

The patient's hemodynamic status must be assessed immediately on arrival in the ICU. A quick check of the heart rate and rhythm, BP, perfusion, core temperature, and auscultation of the heart and lungs is necessary prior to transferring the child, and the accompanying equipment, into the ICU bed space. The external monitors and intravascular catheters are switched over from the transportation monitoring system to the ICU monitoring system (these should preferably be compatible). Chest tube drainage systems, if present, are attached to wall suction, and drainage levels are marked. If the core temperature is low, a heating blanket and/or heating lamps are set up.

Once the child is settled into the ICU bedspace, a hemoglobin level and chest x-ray are checked. Electrocardiography may be reserved for patients with a suspected conduction disorder. The heart rate, rhythm, and pulse oximetry are monitored continuously.

As the child awakens from sedation and begins spontaneous respiration, mechanical ventilatory support is weaned. If not performed in the operating room, extubation is usually accomplished within a few hours of admission to the ICU. Postoperative myocardial edema and systolic dysfunction are not to be expected in children following most closed procedures, and the use of supplemental inotropic agents is rarely indicated. Analgesic agents should be limited to what is sufficient to manage expected postoperative pain.

Enteral feeding is started as soon as bowel sounds are present. Clear liquids, such as dextrose water, are attempted first. If the gag and swallow mechanisms are intact, the diet should be advanced rapidly to a full caloric intake. Oral medications, if necessary, can be started at this point as well.

By 6 to 24 hours following surgery, most children are extubated, awake, hemodynamically stable, feeding well, and have had their chest tube removed. At this point, they are transferred to the ward.

General Course Following Longer Open Cases (tetralogy of Fallot repair, arterial switch operations, atrioventricular canal repair).

Open cases, whether involving CPB alone or with HA, require more cautious treatment because of the risks of myocardial injury and significant bleeding. Although relatively short operations, such as atrial septal defect closure, may be managed much as with a closed procedure, most patients who have had a significant course of CPB or HA benefit from heavy sedation and muscle relaxants during the night following surgery. This approach reduces oxygen consumption and BP fluctuations, minimizing aggravation of myocardial injury and making significant suture line bleeding or patch dehiscence less likely.

Many children who require open heart operations have had excessive pulmonary artery flow and/or pressure (ventricular septal defect, complete atrioventricular canal) and are particularly prone to reactive vasoconstrictive "spells" in response to a variety of stimuli. Patients with Down's syndrome are also more likely to have pulmonary hypertensive episodes than other children.

Acute pulmonary hypertension can be difficult to reverse; it is important to identify an upward trend in pulmonary artery pressure as early as possible and correct the cause. Pulmonary hypertensive episodes can be be triggered by fear, pain, hypoxemia, or acidosis and can lead to right heart failure, venous congestion, and low cardiac output. Acute pulmonary artery hypertension episodes can be minimized by heavy sedation (especially during the first night following surgery), mild hyperventilation (pH > 7.45), and a modest amount of supplemental oxygen (FiO_2 between 0.35 and 0.45). If these measures are not effective in reducing an elevated pulmonary artery pressure, one must consider structural and functional disorders of the heart such as ventricular dysfunction, mitral regurgitation, and pulmonary vein obstruction, which can also lead to elevated pulmonary artery pressure. These types of problems are usually associated with an elevated pulmonary arterial wedge pressure or left atrial pressure as well as pulmonary artery hypertension.

Postoperative myocardial edema and systolic dysfunction often gradually worsen over the first 6 to 12 hours following surgery. Manifestations may include diminished cardiac output and increasing filling pressures. Increased inotropic support (e.g., dopamine) and intravascular volume expansion may be required during this period.

By the early morning following surgery, myocardial function is usually already improving. Muscle relaxants can be discontinued at this point, and analgesic agents are weaned to a level sufficient to manage expected postoperative pain. As the child awakens from sedation and begins spontaneous respiration, mechanical ventilatory support is weaned, aiming for conciousness with an intact respiratory drive by the midmorning. Extubation is best performed early in the day to allow close monitoring by the staff most familiar with the patient. Extubation is usually accomplished on the day following surgery.

The left atrial and pulmonary artery catheters are removed the day following surgery if the patient is hemodynamically stable. These catheters are removed before the chest tubes so that bleeding from the catheter sites can be monitored. The chest tubes can be removed the day following surgery if chest tube drainage is not significant.

About 12 to 24 hours following surgery, peripheral edema has usually peaked. Urine output often increases at this point as the extra water in the tissues begins to mobilize back into the intravascular space. If venous filling pressures are elevated, this process may be accelerated through the judicious use of a diuretic (e.g., furosemide).

As with closed procedures, enteral feeding is started as soon as possible. Most patients are awake and ready to take oral feedings within 6 to 8 hours following extubation. If oral feedings are not appropriate because of continued mechanical ventilation, sedation, or neurologic complications, nasogastric feedings should be considered. Oral medications can be started at this point. Most children require at least a few months of oral digoxin and furosemide following CPB and HA, although some do well without any long-term pharmacologic support.

By 24 to 48 hours following surgery, most children are extubated, awake, hemodynamically stable, feeding well, and have had their left atrial catheter, pulmonary arterial catheter, and chest tubes removed. At this point, they are transferred to the ward. The peripheral arterial catheter and right atrial catheter are discontinued at this point. Transcutaneous pacing wires usually are left in place until shortly before discharge from the hospital to guard against the event of late occurrence of atrioventricular block secondary to edema.

General Course Following Venopulmonary Connections (Glenn shunt, cavopulmonary shunt, hemi-Fontan procedure, and Fontan procedure).

Procedures that include an anastomosis between a systemic vein and the pulmonary artery require low resistance in the pulmonary circuit for blood to flow to the lungs. In addition to the issues discussed earlier for open cases, these patients require special efforts to maintain the pulmonary vascular resistance as low as possible. One clinical measure often used to estimate the resistance of the pulmonary vascular circuit is the difference between the pulmonary artery pressure (often measured in the SVC) and the LAP. A difference of 6 to 9 mm Hg with saturations greater than 85% suggests a reasonably low pulmonary vascular resistance. A second important indicator in these patients is the absolute central venous (and hence pulmonary artery) pressure: Most patients can tolerate a mean pulmonary arterial pressure of up to 18 to 20 mm Hg. If a patient requires a higher pressure, there is often an associated decrease in pulmonary pressure, and therefore systemic blood flow and signs of venous congestion, such as edema or effusions, will increase.

Many factors impact on the resistance to flow through the pulmonary vascular system. Obstruction in the pulmonary arteries themselves can result from congenital small size, surgical scarring, or thrombosis. Pulmonary arteriolar resistance can be elevated secondary to reactive vasoconstriction or pulmonary vascular occlusive disease. Pulmonary venous pressure can be elevated secondary to pulmonary vein stenosis or obstruction or left atrial hypertension, which may, in turn, be caused by mitral valve stenosis, regurgitation, or elevated ventricular diastolic pressure. The last factor is particularly important in the postoperative period because the transient ventricular dysfunction that results from CPB and HA may result in a significantly increased ventricular end-diastolic pressure. For example, it is fairly common for the patient to have higher mixed venous saturations immediately after surgery, when oxygen consumption is low and the effects of CPB on the myocardium have not yet peaked. Over the ensuing 6 to 12 hours, as systolic and diastolic dysfunction become more significant, the saturations may decrease as pulmonary blood flow decreases in response to the elevated pulmonary venous pressure. Then, during the gradual recovery from bypass, the mixed venous saturation slowly rises once again.

Postoperative myocardial edema and systolic dysfunction often become gradually worse over the first 6 to 12 hours following surgery. Manifestations may include falling cardiac output and increasing filling pressures. Increased inotropic support (e.g., dopamine) and intravascular volume administration may be required during this period. The need for additional intravascular volume may be more than usual because of the additional capacitance of the systemic venous system. Some dilation of these veins is expected because they will very likely be under higher pressure than preoperatively. Because of the increased systemic venous pressure, systemic edema may be more marked than in children undergoing CPB for other indications.

By the morning following surgery, however, myocardial function is usually already improving. Muscle relaxants can be discontinued and analgesic agents are weaned to a level sufficient to manage expected postoperative pain. As the child awakens, care must be taken to wean the mechanical ventilation carefully to avoid periods of hypoventilation, which might result in an elevated pulmonary vascular resistance. In addition, the FiO_2 must be weaned very gingerly, particularly below a fraction of 0.4 to 0.5, where the toxic effects of oxygen are probably minimal. Any metabolic acidosis should be corrected to minimize the requirement for additional ventilation to maintain an alkaline pH.

The left atrial catheter is removed the day following surgery if the patient is hemodynamically stable. These catheters are removed before the chest tubes so that bleeding from the catheter sites can be monitored. To ensure that pleural fluid accumulation will not be a problem, the chest tubes may be left in place for a couple of days until enteral feeds have begun.

By 24 to 72 hours following surgery, most children are ready for transfer to the ward. There are a significant number, however, who require longer ICU admissions because of persistent effusions or myocardial dysfunction.

Patent Ductus Arteriosus

Diagnosis

The diagnosis of patent ductus arteriosus is made clinically.[129] In term infants, the diagnosis is usually not made until the infant is several weeks old and pulmonary vascular resistance has fallen to a level to allow sufficient left-to-right shunting to permit detection. Two-dimensional echocardiography may confirm the absence of significant intracardiac defects. If the clinical presentation is unusual, such as severe congestive heart failure at a very early age or an unusual location of the murmur, cardiac catheterization may be indicated to rule out lesions that mimic the presentation of patent ductus arteriosus, such as coronary artery-to-right ventricular fistulas or an aortopulmonary window. In preterm infants, one also relies on clinical evaluation to make the diagnosis of patent ductus arteriosus. It should be stressed that the presence of a patent ductus arteriosus in a preterm infant is not by itself an indication for surgery. There should be evidence of hemodynamic compromise or potentiation of respiratory problems before surgery is undertaken.

Nonsurgical Options

The efficacy of closure of a patent ductus arteriosus with catheter-delivered devices has been demonstrated.[130–135] As with several of the new catheter-directed treatment modalities, short periods of anesthesia may be required to ensure patient stability and immobility during placement of occluder devices. Consequently, a short period of recovery in an ICU unit may be indicated. Following recovery from anesthesia, however, many patients may be candidates for discharge the day of the procedure or the following morning.

Few problems have been encountered following catheter-directed closure of patent ductus arteriosus. Embolization of the occluder devices has occurred, usually while the patient is in the catheterization laboratory. Embolization immediately following the procedure is an indication for a return to the catheterization laboratory for percutaneous retrieval of the device and, if indicated, a further attempt at closure.

Postoperative Care

The surgical repair is usually via a left lateral thoracotomy without CPB. Infants generally arrive from the operating room intubated, whereas older children are frequently extubated in the operating room. There may be one chest tube, or none, and transthoracic monitoring catheters are not used. In fact, often only a peripheral intravenous catheter is necessary. Cardiorespiratory and pulse oximetry monitors will be present. Usually, there are no medications being infused at the time of transfer to the ICU.

Careful palpation of the femoral pulses and pulse oximetry of the lower extremity rule out accidental ligation of the aortic isthmus, a rare occurrence. Symmetric pulmonary blood flow on chest x-ray rules out accidental ligation of the left branch pulmonary artery (further discussion follows). The absence of the continuous "machinery-type murmur" of a patent ductus arteriosus makes either of these complications very unlikely. The chest tube, if present, can be removed the evening of surgery if the chest tube drainage is not significant.

Problems

Significant problems after surgery for patent ductus arteriosus are rare. The first indication that something may be amiss can occur in the operating room if the surgeon fails to find a patent ductus arteriosus. In such a situation, the surgeon has the option of exploring for other problems that may have mimicked the clinical presentation. An alternative approach, and perhaps a wiser one, is to discontinue the operative procedure and recommend the child for whatever diagnostic tests, including cardiac catheterization, are necessary for complete anatomic diagnosis.

An equally unusual circumstance is incomplete closure of the ductus if ligation without division is performed.[136] This can be recognized after surgery by persistence of a murmur and clinical evidence of patency of the ductus, such as a hyperactive left ventricular impulse and bounding peripheral pulses. In this situation, cardiac catheterization should be undertaken to fully assess the situation before further surgery is contemplated.

Injury to the recurrent laryngeal nerve can result in vocal cord paralysis or paresis and hoarseness.

More significant problems can occur. The left pulmonary artery can be mistaken for the ductus arteriosus, and it can be ligated.[137] In that situation, there is persistence of the cardiac murmur and other evidence of a persistently patent ductus arteriosus. In addition, a chest film may show diminished pulmonary blood flow to the left lung. A radionuclide scan will confirm the absence of flow to the left pulmonary artery. Immediate reparative measures should be undertaken to restore continuity of the left pulmonary artery. A more serious (and fortunately unusual) complication is the ligation of the descending thoracic aorta. Such a circumstance should be apparent immediately by the absence of lower extremity pulses following surgery and hypoxemia of the lower extremities if the ductus is left patent. Immediate reoperation is indicated.

It is not unusual to see a mild degree of systemic arterial hypertension following ligation of a ductus arteriosus. It has been speculated that the etiology of this condition is persistence of the preoperative hypervolemia. There is usually a rapid diuresis, and antihypertensive medication is not required.

Secundum Atrial Septal Defect

Diagnosis

The diagnosis of a secundum-type atrial septal defect is rare in infancy. With the increase in frequency of echocardiography being performed for a variety of indications, however, an increasing number of patients are being identified with this condition. Infants with atrial septal defects rarely have significant left-to-right shunts because right ventricular compliance does not accommodate large left-to-right shunts until pulmonary vascular resistance has fallen and hypertrophy of the right ventricular muscle has regressed in relation to the left ventricle. If an infant with an atrial septal defect presents with significant congestive heart failure, questions must be raised as to the reason for this highly unusual presentation. Consideration must be given to the presence of mitral valve disease, left ventricular hypoplasia or dysfunction, or left ventricular outflow tract obstruction. These conditions can lead to elevated pulmonary venous pressure with resultant large left-to-right shunts at the atrial level. Closure of atrial septal defects in these circumstances may decrease the pulmonary blood flow, but problems of pulmonary hypertension may be exacerbated by the absence of a means of decompressing the left atrium.

Cardiac catheterization often is not necessary in the preoperative evaluation of a patient with a secundum atrial septal defect.[11] Catheterization may be undertaken, however, if questions regarding the anatomy persist following echocardiography, or if there is consideration of catheter-directed closure of a secundum atrial septal defect.

Nonsurgical Options

Catheter-directed occluder devices in various stages of clinical testing have enabled many patients to have atrial septal defects closed on an ambulatory basis, obviating the need for ICU management.[138,139] As with any new treatment modality, the full range of complications is not yet known. The very real problems of device embolization and arrhythmias have already been seen.

Postoperative Care

The surgical repair is via a median sternotomy, usually using CPB alone, although in very small infants HA may be required.

In infants whose indication for closure included congestive heart failure, a more aggressive postoperative course, with a full array of monitoring catheters, is indicated. Most children, however, are repaired after early infancy and require minimal monitoring.

The child often will be extubated in the operating room or soon after arrival in the ICU. The surgeon will usually have placed chest tubes to drain the mediastinum and, if necessary, the pleural space. Usually, a central venous pressure catheter is placed in the operating room. Transthoracic monitoring catheters are usually not required. In fact, a cardiorespiratory monitor, pulse oximetry monitor, and arterial and venous access may be all the monitoring and access needed. A Foley catheter may be in place if the child is still asleep. Usually, there are no medications being infused at the time of transfer to the ICU. The chest tubes can be removed the day of surgery or the following morning if the drainage is not significant.

Problems

Infants who require early surgical treatment of atrial septal defects often have a variety of associated cardiac problems, and thus issues of pulmonary dysfunction and congestive heart failure may lead to a longer and more involved stay in the ICU.

Ventricular Septal Defect

Diagnosis

Cardiac catheterization remains the mainstay for the accurate, complete diagnosis of infants with ventricular septal defect. Although two-dimensional echocardiography has proved valuable in screening these infants, it has been disappointing in its ability to identify infants with multiple defects, particularly defects in the muscular septum. Recent studies, however, have been more encouraging. Color flow imaging has enhanced our ability to detect multiple defects but has not persuaded us from performing cardiac catheterization on virtually all infants considered for surgical closure of the ventricular septal defects. In addition, cardiac catheterization provides invaluable information concerning pulmonary artery pressure and pulmonary vascular resistance.

An intriguing recent development has been the combination of catheter-directed treatment and surgical closure for infants with multiple ventricular septal defects. Large midmuscular and apical ventricular septal defects may be closed effectively in the cardiac catheterization laboratory preceding surgical closure of defects in the outlet septum. Employing such techniques may shorten the surgical procedure, avoid ventriculotomies, and minimize the possibility of a residual shunt, thus obviating the need for multiple operations.

Postoperative Care

The surgical repair is via a median sternotomy using CPB. The child will arrive in the ICU following surgery intubated and mechanically ventilated with deep sedation and pharmacologic muscle relaxation. The surgeon will usually have placed two to three chest tubes to drain the pleura and mediastinum. Transthoracic right atrial, left atrial, and pulmonary artery monitoring catheters usually will have been placed in the operating room, although a transcutaneous central venous catheter may be used instead of a right atrial catheter. In addition to these, cardiorespiratory,

peripheral arterial, and pulse oximetry monitors will be present. A bladder catheter will be in place.

Medications being infused at the time of transfer to the ICU will vary depending on the patient's condition. Dopamine or dobutamine may be used to improve ventricular function during recovery from CPB, and nitroprusside or another afterload reducing agent may be necessary to reduce the systemic BP. It is particularly important to avoid systemic hypertension, because the additional strain caused by elevated left ventricular pressures can contribute to disruption of the sutures securing the ventricular septal defect patch.

Problems

Residual Ventricular Septal Defect

If an infant returns from the operating room after closure of a ventricular septal defect and continues to have a pansystolic murmur, the question of persistent patency of the ventricular septal defect must be raised. A second undetected defect also must be suspected. Measurement of oxygen saturation in blood samples from the right atrial (or central venous) and pulmonary artery catheters may confirm this suspicion. In general, a pulmonary artery oxygen saturation above 80% will indicate significant persistent shunting.[60]

The use of the left atrial catheter for the performance of contrast two-dimensional echocardiography and the use of color flow mapping can also be useful. It should also be stressed that the latter is a nonquantitative evaluation. If the residual left-to-right shunting is significant enough to contribute to an inability to discontinue assisted ventilation, cardiac catheterization should be undertaken to confirm the diagnosis, locate the site of the residual defect, and quantitate the flow across any defect. It has been our experience that residual shunts with a pulmonary-systemic flow ratio of greater than 2 are not well tolerated in the immediate postoperative period. In such a situation, a second operation should be contemplated.

Pulmonary Hypertension

Following surgical repair of a ventricular septal defect, many patients have unusually reactive pulmonary vascular beds and may develop severe reactive pulmonary hypertension and right heart failure in response to pain, hypercarbia, or hypoxemia. This is particularly prevalent in patients who are repaired later in infancy.

Pulmonary Problems

Infants who require surgery for a ventricular septal defect often suffer from recurrent pulmonary infections and bronchospasm and may have failed to thrive to the point of cachexia. Frequently, they have significant pulmonary artery hypertension. Thus, it is not unusual for them to require a relatively long period of ventilatory support. Preoperative atelectasis and bronchospasm often are exacerbated in the immediate postoperative period. If the defect has been completely closed, a very patient attitude toward weaning from assisted ventilation is indicated. The use of inhaled or parenteral bronchodilators may be necessary. In infants who have had marked failure to thrive, it may be necessary to continue assisted ventilation for many days while a positive nitrogen balance is established by enteral or even parenteral feeding.

Persistent Congestive Heart Failure

Following closure of a large ventricular septal defect, particularly if a ventriculotomy was required, congestive heart failure is the rule rather than the exception. Digoxin and diuretics should be instituted immediately after surgery.

Endocardial Cushion Defect

Diagnosis

Diagnosis of the various forms of endocardial cushion defect (primum atrial septal defect, transitional atrioventricular canal, and complete atrioventricular canal) traditionally depended on the combined use of two-dimensional echocardiography and cardiac catheterization. As with other lesions, however, there has been a recent trend toward relying solely on noninvasive diagnostic measures.

There is an anatomic continuum among the varied forms of endocardial cushion defect, from primum atrial septal defect to complete atrioventricular canal. The postoperative course may, however, depend more on associated factors than the underlying diagnosis. Mitral regurgitation following surgical repair, for example, is a strong determinant of the postoperative hemodynamic status, as is mild hypoplasia of the left ventricle.

There has been an increasing trend toward repair of endocardial cushion defects early in infancy, primarily in an effort to avoid the development of pulmonary vascular obstructive disease. Vascular disease may be accelerated in this defect because of the combined effects of excessive pulmonary blood flow and pulmonary venous hypertension caused by atrioventricular valve regurgitation. Eighty percent of children with endocardial cushion defects also have Down's syndrome; in these children, pulmonary vascular occlusive disease may occur even earlier than in other children. These factors, and others, have pushed the desirable operation age for complete atrioventricular canal back to 3 to 6 months of age, or earlier. Although the immature valve tissue in some young infants may compromise the integrity of the repair if performed very early in infancy, fewer and more predictable problems with management of pulmonary artery hypertension may make the perioperative period less turbulent in this group.

Postoperative Care

The surgical repair is via a median sternotomy using CPB and occasionally HA, depending on the size of the infant. The child will arrive in the ICU following surgery intubated and mechanically ventilated with deep sedation and pharmacologic muscle relaxation. The surgeon will have placed two to three chest tubes to drain the pleura and mediastinum. Transthoracic right atrial, left atrial, and pulmonary artery monitoring catheters usually will also have been placed in the operating room, although a transcutaneous CVP catheter may be used, if available, instead of a right atrial catheter. In addition to these, cardiorespiratory, peripheral arterial, and pulse oximetry monitors will be present. A bladder catheter will also be in place.

Medications being infused at the time of transfer to the ICU may include inotropic agents and systemic vasodilators as needed. It is particularly important to avoid systemic hypertension, because the additional strain caused by elevated left ventricular pressures can lead to disruption of the sutures securing the patch covering the defect or the sutures securing the atrioventricular valves to the patch.

Following surgical repair of a complete atrioventricular canal, many patients have unusually reactive pulmonary vascular beds. This is particularly the case in children with Down's syndrome. Such patients may develop severe reactive pulmonary hypertension and right heart failure in response to awakening, pain, hypercarbia, or hypoxemia.

Problems

Mitral Regurgitation

Because some degree of mitral regurgitation is the rule rather than the exception after repair of complete common atrioventricular canal, the left atrial catheter is perhaps the most useful monitoring catheter in this condition because it allows the assessment of the degree of mitral regurgitation (Fig. 21-12). The position of the left atrial catheter should be assessed carefully. If it is near the orifice of the mitral valve, falsely high pressures and abnormal waveforms may be recorded.

The patient's response to mitral regurgitation is more important than the absolute pressure recorded from the left atrial catheter. If the patient tolerates the mitral regurgitation well, as evidenced by an ability to wean from assisted ventilation, there is no absolute value of left atrial hypertension that mandates further intervention. If, on the other hand, the child is not making satisfactory progress following surgery, the left atrial catheter serves as a valuable diagnostic tool in estimating the contribution of mitral regurgitation to such failure to progress. Monitoring of pulmonary artery pressure can prove to be useful as a way of measuring the secondary effects of pulmonary venous hypertension. Doppler echocardiography further enhances noninvasive assessment of mitral regurgitation.

It should be noted that patients with a primum type of atrial septal defect with cleft mitral valve may tolerate moderate degrees of mitral regurgitation less well after closure of the atrial septal defect than before. This probably is the result of the inability to decompress the left atrium through a newly closed atrial septal defect.

The use of systemic vasodilators can prove useful in allowing patients with significant mitral regurgitation to wean from assisted ventilation. A full trial of medical management usually is indicated prior to recommending complete hemodynamic evaluation by cardiac catheterization and/or further surgery.

The degree of mitral regurgitation may increase following surgery. While the closure of the anterior mitral valve cleft may limit regurgitation by enhancing coaptation of mitral valve leaflets, the restriction to valve mobility created by some reconstructive efforts may lead to greater regurgitation or even a degree of mitral stenosis.

Mitral Stenosis

The preoperative anatomy of the common atrioventricular valve, as well as the papillary muscle configuration, may rarely lead to

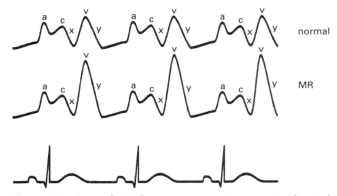

Figure 21-12. Left atrial pressure tracing in a patient with mitral regurgitation (schematic). Note the accentuation of the v peaks corresponding to the increase in LAP secondary to the regurgitant flow.

postoperative mitral stenosis. This is more common in children with complete atrioventricular canal of the Rastelli type A, because the surgeon has less latitude in reconstructing the mitral component of the valve.

The use of the new modality of transesophageal echocardiography has led to some encouraging experiences. Intraoperative monitoring after discontinuation of CPB has identified persistent problems with valve function and directed immediate surgical management in selected circumstances.

Persistent Congestive Heart Failure
Residual left-to-right shunts may be the cause of persistent congestive heart failure following repair of endocardial cushion defects. Residual shunts of hemodynamic significance should be suspected if there is elevated pulmonary artery oxygen saturation (>80%) and elevated pulmonary artery pressure.

Respiratory Difficulties
Patients with trisomy 21 (Down syndrome) and endocardial cushion defect often have significant pulmonary problems prior to surgery. These problems do not disappear on repair of their cardiac lesions. It is the rule, rather than the exception, to see significant atelectasis and pulmonary venous desaturation following surgery in these patients. In addition, pulmonary edema, hypoventilation, and airway obstruction often lead to pulmonary artery hypertension in the postoperative period. It is occasionally necessary to perform cardiac catheterization to adequately differentiate pulmonary problems from residual left-to-right shunting or significant mitral regurgitation.

Tricuspid Regurgitation
Tricuspid regurgitation is rarely a problem after repair of a complete common atrioventricular canal. It is the usual surgical practice to employ that portion of the common atrioventricular valve that is necessary to assure mitral valve competence and reconstruct the tricuspid portion of the valve with whatever tissue is left. Thus, some tricuspid regurgitation is the rule rather than the exception. If there is relatively normal pulmonary artery pressure, and therefore low right ventricular pressure, tricuspid regurgitation is not a significant problem. In the less usual circumstance of persistent right ventricular hypertension, tricuspid regurgitation may not be well tolerated. Anticongestive measures with digoxin and diuretic therapy are often adequate for handling such problems.

Special Consideration
Complete Atrioventricular Canal with Tetralogy of Fallot
The circumstance in which the common atrioventricular canal accompanies tetralogy of Fallot deserves special mention. Residual right ventricular hypertension is more likely to accompany this lesion because of right ventricular outflow tract hypoplasia. Elevated right ventricular systolic pressure may lead to a troublesome degree of tricuspid regurgitation. Further, the presence of significant pulmonary valve regurgitation (which may follow from transannular right ventricular outflow tract reconstruction) is likely to put further demands on the tricuspid valve.

d-Transposition of the Great Arteries

Diagnosis
Although d-transposition of the great arteries is accurately diagnosed by two-dimensional echocardiography, we still employ car-

diac catheterization as part of our routine preoperative evaluation. The purpose of cardiac catheterization is to confirm the presence or absence of an associated ventricular septal defect(s), to localize the defect if it is present, to assess the left ventricular outflow tract, to define the coronary artery distribution, and to perform a balloon atrial septostomy (Rashkind procedure). Additional information can be gained concerning the competence of the mitral and tricuspid valves and left and right ventricular function. In older children, assessment of the pulmonary vascular bed is essential. Until recently a balloon atrial septostomy was performed routinely in all children with d-transposition of the great arteries. As more centers are performing primary repair in the newborn period with an arterial switch procedure, the need for septostomy is declining.

Arterial Switch Operation (Jatene Procedure)

Postoperative Care
The surgical repair is via a median sternotomy using CPB.[30,31,140] The child will arrive in the ICU following surgery intubated and mechanically ventilated with deep sedation and pharmacologic muscle relaxation. Cardiorespiratory, peripheral arterial, and pulse oximetry monitors will be present. A bladder catheter also will be in place. The surgeon will usually have placed chest tubes to drain the pleura and mediastinum. Transthoracic right atrial, left atrial, and pulmonary artery monitoring catheters usually will have also been placed in the operating room, although a transcutaneous CVP catheter may be used if available. Medications being infused at the time of transfer to the ICU may include inotropic agents and systemic vasodilators as needed. The left atrial catheter can be exceedingly useful in assessing left ventricular filling pressure as an indication of ventricular performance. This is critically important if ventricular function is impaired because of compromised coronary artery flow or in the presence of a potentially unprepared left ventricle, or if left ventricular outflow tract obstruction is a problem.

Problems
Obstruction at the Great Artery Anastomoses
Pulmonary artery obstruction at the site of a pulmonary artery reconstruction can lead to persistent right ventricle hypertension. Because infants with transposition of the great arteries have had systemic pressure in the right ventricle prior to surgery, even severe obstruction is well tolerated for a significant period. Obstruction at the aortic anastomotic site is unusual.

Systemic Ventricular Dysfunction
Following the arterial switch procedure, the left ventricle is required to work against a higher resistance (the systemic circuit) than it had preoperatively (the pulmonary circuit). In addition, the arterial switch procedure usually requires a relatively longer CPB time. Consequently, the postoperative myocardial injury and edema are often more severe and persist longer than in most other types of infant heart surgery. As a result of these two factors, the degree and duration of depressed systolic function and systemic edema are often greater in this group of patients, as is the need for inotropic and intravascular volume support.

In addition, one must be aware of the possibility of coronary artery insufficiency resulting from kinking or occlusion of the coronary arteries during transfer to the "neoaorta" (former pulmonary outflow tract). Ligation of coronary artery branches may be necessary to transfer the coronaries without kinking. Fortunately, kinking is unusual, but when it occurs it can be catastrophic. Often the ECG is not as helpful as one might expect, because infants following the arterial switch procedure often have little or no left ventricular forces on electrocardiography even when the coronary artery circulation is intact. Severe myocardial dysfunction earlier than 4 to 6 hours following surgery, or failure of myocardial function to begin to improve after 12 to 18 hours should cause concern over the status of the coronary arteries. Cardiac catheterization is the only reliable means of ensuring coronary artery patency.

Atrial Switch Operations (Senning and Mustard Procedures)

In most medical centers, the **arterial** switch operation has supplanted the use of **atrial** switch operations—the Mustard and Senning procedures. There are instances, however, when arterial switch operations are inappropriate and atrial procedures are used to redirect venous pathways and physiologically correct the circulation. In addition, there are many patients who have previously undergone atrial switch operations who have recurrent problems with rhythm disturbance, ventricular function, or residual and/or recurrent hemodynamic problems. Thus, an understanding of the problems encountered after such operations is helpful.

Postoperative Care

The surgical repair is via a median sternotomy using CPB and HA. The child will arrive in the ICU following surgery intubated and mechanically ventilated with deep sedation and pharmacologic muscle relaxation. Often, a transcutaneous SVC catheter may be placed to monitor and detect occlusion of the SVC in the postoperative period. Medications being infused at the time of transfer to the ICU may include inotropic agents and systemic vasodilators as needed.

Problems
Obstruction to Venous Return

Obstruction to systemic venous return is an uncommon problem following either the Mustard or Senning procedure. SVC obstruction is more common than IVC obstruction. The cardinal sign of SVC obstruction is facial plethora and edema. Hepatomegaly and lower extremity edema can be seen with obstruction of the IVC. A mild degree of peripheral edema is not at all uncommon following uncomplicated surgery, so it is the severity and persistence of edema rather than its appearance that should alert one to a potential problem. Echocardiography should be performed, and, if that is suggestive of a significant narrowing, cardiac catheterization should be undertaken. Chylothorax, as a reflection of elevated systemic venous pressure, is not an unusual manifestation of obstruction at the superior margin of the interatrial baffle.

Pulmonary venous obstruction also can be seen. Pulmonary venous congestion on the chest film is often the first indication that there is a problem. Some degree of congestion is not uncommon in uncomplicated cases; it is the severity and persistence of evidence of pulmonary venous congestion that should alert the physician to a problem. Echocardiography can serve as a screening test, to be followed by cardiac catheterization, if there is evidence of obstruction.

Recent advances in catheter-directed therapy have changed both the short- and long-term approaches to problems of obstruction to venous return. Balloon dilation of systemic venous obstruction,

with or without stent placement, has proved to be an effective method in most cases. The procedure cannot be undertaken until there has been healing and "maturation" of the suture lines. Thus, acute obstruction to caval pathway flow in the immediate postoperative period must be dealt with surgically, unless it can be deferred for 6 weeks. There has been successful treatment by balloon dilation of obstruction to pulmonary venous return, but this problem may prove to be more difficult to handle both because of difficulty in access to the pulmonary venous pathway with dilation catheters and because pulmonary venous obstruction is very frequently recurrent despite dilation and/or stent placement.

Arrhythmias

Disorders of sinus node function are not uncommon after interatrial baffle placement in transposition of the great arteries. The most common arrhythmia is sinus bradycardia with a junctional escape rhythm. This rhythm disturbance is most often of no consequence in the immediate postoperative period. If significant bradycardia is a problem, temporary pacing should be instituted. Supraventricular tachyarrhythmias are far less common in the ICU setting and should be handled by the usual pharmacologic means.

Long-term problems with heart rhythm are common for patients undergoing atrial switch procedures. Sinus node dysfunction is an almost inevitable outcome of the extensive atrial baffling procedures. The susceptibility to both tachyarrhythmias and bradyarrhythmias makes management of this problem difficult. Pharmacologic treatment of the tachycardic component of the arrhythmias may exacerbate bradycardia. For this reason, patients with symptomatic "sick sinus syndrome" in the setting of atrial baffling procedures may require placement of pacemakers as part of management of their rhythm disturbances.

Persistent Congestive Heart Failure

Persistent congestive heart failure following repair of transposition of the great arteries usually has an anatomic basis. Isolated right- or left-sided congestive heart failure is often a manifestation of obstruction to the venous pathway flow. In a child with an associated ventricular septal defect, if a significant murmur persists following surgery, the persistence of an interventricular shunt must be suspected. Tricuspid valve regurgitation (the systemic atrioventricular valve in transposition of the great arteries following an atrial switch procedure) is another potential cause of congestive heart failure following transatrial closure of ventricular septal defects associated with d-transposition of the great arteries. The valve may have intrinsic abnormalities or may be damaged during surgery. Another potential cause of congestive heart failure is right ventricular dysfunction. This can be the consequence of closure of a ventricular septal defect via a right ventriculotomy.

An increasing minority of patients who have undergone atrial switch procedures for transposition of the great arteries are developing evidence of right ventricular dysfunction leading to congestive heart failure. Initial management of these patients is inotropic support of the right ventricle as well as afterload reduction. Because a second ventricle (the anatomic left ventricle) usually has good function, consideration may be given toward a delayed, secondary arterial switch operation. If such a procedure is anticipated, the "preparedness" of the left ventricle must be considered. Staged operations to prepare the left ventricle (usually a pulmonary artery banding operation followed by an arterial switch procedure) are necessary in patients with normal pulmonary artery pressure.

Tetralogy of Fallot

Diagnosis

The diagnosis of tetralogy of Fallot is based on clinical, echocardiographic, and cardiac catheterization findings. At this time, infants with this defect probably should not undergo reparative surgery without a cardiac catheterization. Information that is essential for complete assessment is best evaluated at cardiac catheterization. This includes the distal distribution of the coronary arteries, the location of multiple ventricular septal defects, and the evaluation of the distal pulmonary arteries for peripheral stenoses.

Several variations in the surgical approach depend on the anatomical details of the defect. Children with a large coronary artery passing across the right ventricular outflow tract and supplying the left anterior descending coronary artery cannot have the right ventricular outflow tract incised, and may require a conduit from the right ventricle to the main pulmonary artery or a more limited transatrial and transarterial outflow tract resection, rather than an outflow tract patch. Generally, the foramen ovale is left open to allow some decompression of the hypertensive right ventricle, particularly during the immediate postoperative period when right ventricular systolic function is likely to be depressed secondary to CPB and a right ventriculotomy. Similarly, the ventricular defect may be left open, or closed with a perforated patch, to allow right ventricular decompression if the pulmonary arteries are hypoplastic and inadequate to carry a normal cardiac output. In such circumstances, the ventricular defect can be closed secondarily with a second operation or a catheter-directed technique after the pulmonary vasculature has developed.

Postoperative Care

The surgical repair is via a median sternotomy using CPB and HA. The child will arrive in the ICU following surgery intubated and mechanically ventilated with deep sedation and pharmacologic muscle relaxation.

Medications being infused at the time of transfer to the ICU may include inotropic agents and systemic vasodilators. It is particularly important to avoid systemic hypertension, because the additional strain caused by elevated left ventricular pressures can lead to disruption of the sutures securing the ventricular septal defect patch.

Problems

Residual Ventricular Septal Defect or Right Ventricular Outflow Obstruction

Within the first 24 hours following surgery, a saturation is drawn from the pulmonary arterial catheter followed by a pressure pullback tracing recorded as the pulmonary artery catheter is withdrawn from the pulmonary artery to the body of the right ventricle (Fig. 21-13). If the pulmonary artery oxygen saturation is less than 80%, there is little chance of a significant residual ventricular septal defect (Fig. 21-14).[60] If a significant ventricular septal defect or significant right ventricular outflow obstruction is detected, catheterization must be considered to confirm and further define such residual problems. An aggressive approach is appropriate in the setting of residual hemodynamic problems in tetralogy of Fallot; it is well documented that they are poorly tolerated.

Persistent Hypoxemia

Patients can have persistent hypoxemia following repair of tetralogy of Fallot for several reasons. First, if there is a pulmonary problem leading to pulmonary venous desaturation, there will be systemic hypoxemia. The chest x-ray and left atrial oxygen saturation will help define this problem.

A second source of hypoxemia is right-to-left shunting at the atrial level. This is more common when the foremen ovale has been left open, allowing right-to-left shunting when the right ventricular filling pressure is greater than on the left. Generally, right atrial decompression through a persistent patent foremen ovale is very well tolerated and alleviates some of the signs of systemic venous congestion and low cardiac output that result from right ventricular dysfunction after right ventriculotomy. Color flow mapping or Doppler echocardiography can confirm right-to-left atrial shunting as the cause of hypoxemia.

Third, patients with a residual ventricular septal defect and persistent obstruction to the right ventricular outflow tract can have persistent hypoxemia due to right-to-left shunting at the ventricular level. This is an infrequent problem, but should be considered in a patient with hypoxemia and elevated right ventricular pressure. As mentioned, under some circumstances, the ventricular septal defect may be left open intentionally to allow right-to-left shunting when the pulmonary arterial tree is anatomically inadequate.

Congestive Heart Failure

Patients with tetralogy of Fallot will very frequently develop some degree of congestive heart failure following surgical repair. The most likely explanations include right ventricular dysfunction secondary to a fibrotic, noncompliant hypertrophied right ventricle; systolic dysfunction due to the effects of CPB and a ventriculotomy; and volume overload due to pulmonary regurgitation when a transannular outflow tract reconstruction has been performed. Mild congestive heart failure is well tolerated and easily managed by anticongestive medications. If congestive heart failure is not well tolerated or persists beyond the first few months after surgery, a structural basis should be sought. A residual ventricular septal

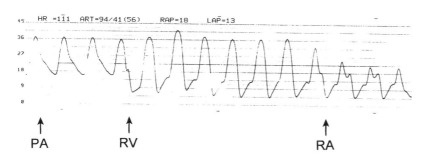

HR =111   ART=94/41 (56)   RAP=18   LAP=13

PA   RV   RA

Figure 21-13. Pulmonary artery pull-back. Continuous BP tracing recorded from a transthoracic pulmonary arterial catheter as it is withdrawn from the pulmonary artery to the right ventricle and into the right atrium. PA, pulmonary artery; RA, right atrium; RV, right ventricle.

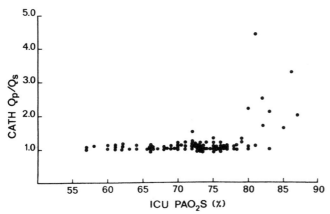

Figure 21-14. Pulmonary artery saturation and residual ventricular septal defect. Relationship of pulmonary artery oxygen saturation in the immediate postoperative period in the ICU to the pulmonary-to-systemic flow ratio at catheterization 1 year after surgery in patients with tetralogy of Fallot. CATH, catheterization; ICU, intensive care unit; PAO_2S, pulmonary artery oxygen saturation; Q_p/Q_s, pulmonary-to-systemic flow ratio. (From Lang P, Chipman CW, Siden H, Williams RG, Norwood WI, Castañeda AR. Early assessment of hemodynamic status after repair of tetralogy of Fallot: a comparison of 24 hour (intensive care unit) and 1 year postoperative data in 98 patients. *Am J Cardiol* 50:795–799, 1982. With permission.)

defect is probably the most common cause. Infants tend to have a higher left atrial pressure than right atrial pressures in the postoperative period than do older children following surgical repair of tetralogy of Fallot. This may reflect the absence of right ventricular dysfunction (mentioned earlier) because of repair at an earlier age. Recent studies also suggest that left ventricular function is significantly better when tetralogy is repaired in infancy rather than in early childhood.

Truncus Arteriosus Communis

Diagnosis
The diagnosis of truncus arteriosus is based on clinical, echocardiographic, and cardiac catheterization findings. Children with this defect probably should not undergo reparative surgery without a cardiac catheterization. Several variations in the surgical approach depend on the anatomic details of the defect. Particularly important, and difficult to assess echocardiographically, are the anatomies of the pulmonary arteries, aortic arch, and coronary arteries.

The pulmonary arteries may arise as a common pulmonary artery from the aorta, or their origins may be separated by a small or great distance. Each of these circumstances requires a slightly different surgical approach. Rarely, one pulmonary artery may not connect to the truncus (hemitruncus) and may be fed from the ductus arteriosus or one or more systemic collateral vessels. Retrograde angiography of the pulmonary vein on the affected side may reveal the location of the missing pulmonary artery or branches.

The truncal valve is often abnormal, consisting frequently of more than three leaflets. It may be stenotic or regurgitant. Occasionally, the truncal valve may require replacement at the time of surgery. The ascending and transverse aortic arch may be hypoplastic, or there may be a coarctation or interruption of the aortic

arch, a condition that may account for as many as 12% of cases of truncus arteriosus communis. The coronary arteries may arise anomalously in as many as 8% of patients with truncus arteriosus communis. This information may be difficult to obtain through echocardiographic examination.

Repair of truncus arteriosus communis requires closure of the subtruncal ventricular septal defect so that only the left ventricle ejects to the truncus. The pulmonary arteries are excised from the truncus and connected via a conduit or a homograft to the right ventricle. Thus, the truncus becomes the neoaorta.

Postoperative Care
The surgical repair is via a median sternotomy using CPB with hypothermia. The child will arrive in the ICU following surgery intubated and mechanically ventilated with deep sedation and pharmacologic muscle relaxation. Medications being infused at the time of transfer to the ICU may include inotropic agents and systemic vasodilators as needed. It is particularly important to avoid systemic hypertension, because the additional strain caused by elevated left ventricular pressures can lead to disruption of the sutures securing the ventricular septal defect patch.

Problems
Residual Ventricular Septal Defect or Right Ventricular Outflow Obstruction
Within the first 24 hours following surgery, a saturation is drawn from the pulmonary arterial catheter followed by a pressure pullback tracing recorded as the pulmonary artery catheter is withdrawn from the conduit serving as the main pulmonary artery to the body of the right ventricle. If the pulmonary artery oxygen saturation is less than 80%, there is little chance of a significant residual ventricular septal defect.[60]

Persistent Hypoxemia
Patients can have persistent hypoxemia following repair of truncus arteriosus for several reasons. If there is a pulmonary problem leading to pulmonary venous desaturation, there will be systemic hypoxemia. The chest x-ray and left atrial oxygen saturation will help define this problem.

A second source of hypoxemia is right-to-left shunting at the atrial level. This is more common when the foremen ovale has been left open, allowing right-to-left shunting when the right ventricular filling pressure is greater than on the left. Generally, right atrial decompression through a persistently patent foremen ovale is very well tolerated and alleviates some of the signs of systemic venous congestion and low cardiac output that result from right ventricular diastolic dysfunction after right ventriculotomy. Color flow mapping or Doppler echocardiography can confirm right-to-left atrial shunting as the cause of hypoxemia.

Patients with a residual ventricular septal defect and persistent obstruction to the right ventricular outflow tract can have persistent hypoxemia due to right-to-left shunting at the ventricular level. This is an infrequent problem, but should be considered in a patient with hypoxemia and elevated right ventricular pressure.

Pulmonary Hypertension
Following surgical repair of truncus arteriosus, many patients have unusually reactive pulmonary vascular beds and may develop severe reactive pulmonary hypertension and right heart failure in response to awakening, pain, hypercarbia, or hypoxemia. This is particularly prevalent in patients who are repaired later in infancy

and has been a significant factor in surgical morbidity and mortality.

Congestive Heart Failure

Patients with truncus arteriosus will often develop some degree of congestive heart failure following surgical repair. The most likely explanations include right ventricular dysfunction secondary to a fibrotic, noncompliant, hypertrophied right ventricle, systolic dysfunction due to the effects of CPB and a ventriculotomy, and incompetence of the truncal valve. Mild congestive heart failure is well tolerated and easily managed by anticongestive medications. If congestive heart failure is not well tolerated or persists beyond the first few months after surgery, a structural basis should be sought. Residual ventricular septal defects, truncal valve regurgitation, branch pulmonary artery stenosis, and homograft valve stenosis or insufficiency are possible causes of congestive heart failure following truncus arteriosus communis repair.

Aortic Stenosis

Diagnosis

Aortic stenosis of significant enough degree to cause congestive heart failure during infancy has been called "critical" aortic stenosis. There are instances wherein systemic cardiac output is so limited by varying combinations of left ventricular dysfunction and aortic stenosis that the systemic circulation can be maintained only by right-to-left shunting through a persistently patent ductus arteriosus. This situation differs significantly from the course of aortic stenosis in older children and young adults, in whom it is exceedingly unusual to see compromised cardiac output. The physical examination is usually highly suggestive in the case of aortic stenosis. The definitive diagnosis can usually be made on the basis of two-dimensional echocardiography. Infants in extremis have undergone urgent cardiac surgery on the basis of echocardiography alone. More recently, therapeutic treatment in the cardiac catheterization laboratory has become an option resulting in the reinstitution of cardiac catheterization for almost all children with aortic stenosis.

Infants who are dependent on the ductus arteriosus for systemic cardiac output benefit from the administration of PGE_1 to assure a reliable right-to-left shunt, so that the right ventricle can provide systemic output.

Postoperative Care

Surgery to correct aortic stenosis varies from simple commissurotomy to valve replacement with or without widening of the left ventricular outflow tract (Konno procedure[141,142]). Children who require aortic valve replacement may receive a mechanical valve, a bioprosthetic valve, a homograft, or even a pulmonary artery autograft. Mechanical valves include the St. Jude valve and Carbomedics bileaflet valves. Bioprosthetic valves are made from animal valve tissue or pericardium that has been mounted on a rigid mechanical strut. Homograft valves are human valves that have been harvested from cadavers and cryopreserved. It is even possible to remove the patient's own pulmonic valve and implant it in the aortic position, replacing the native pulmonic valve with a homograft (Ross procedure[143]). In contrast to mechanical valves, bioprosthetic, homograft, and autograft valves do not require lifelong systemic anticoagulation.

As the surgical procedures become more elaborate, the postoperative course becomes more complex. Consequently, it is difficult to predict a "usual" postoperative course, and individual variations are likely to be marked.

The surgical repair is via a median sternotomy using CPB and, in the case of the newborn, HA. The child will arrive in the ICU following surgery intubated and mechanically ventilated with deep sedation and pharmacologic muscle relaxation. A thermistor catheter in the pulmonary artery may be used to aid in monitoring cardiac output. Medications being infused at the time of transfer to the ICU may include inotropic agents and systemic vasodilators as needed.

In the case of a mechanical aortic valve replacement, warfarin anticoagulation is usually begun 18 to 24 hours following surgery. The patient's prothrombin time should be followed daily until a stable value in the therapeutic range is achieved. (see Medical Issues in the Cardiac Patient by Erickson and Elixson, this volume.)

Problems

Congestive Heart Failure

There are several possible etiologies for persistent congestive heart failure following aortic valve treatment (surgical or catheter-directed) for critical aortic stenosis. The first to be considered is persistent obstruction of the left ventricular outflow tract. The aortic valve in infants with critical aortic stenosis is frequently thickened and cartilaginous, and relief of commissural fusion does not always lead to relief of obstruction. It should be remembered, however, that a relatively small increase in the orifice size will lead to a marked improvement in cardiac output. In situations in which adequacy of surgery is under question, reinvestigation with either echocardiography or cardiac catheterization may be necessary. If persistent obstruction is documented, a decision must be made as to whether a second attempt at a valve intervention will be rewarding. In this situation, one runs the risk of causing a large degree of aortic regurgitation for a small improvement in gradient. Unfortunately, placement of a prosthetic aortic valve in infants with critical aortic stenosis is often impossible because of the small size of the aortic annulus. Placement of a left ventricular-to-descending aortic conduit is an option that has met with mixed results.

Another cause of persistent congestive heart failure following aortic valvuloplasty is the presence of severe aortic regurgitation. As noted earlier, an excessive attempt to relieve aortic stenosis can result in severe aortic regurgitation. In this unusual situation, there is no completely satisfactory alternative. If an infant or young child cannot tolerate the degree of aortic regurgitation that is present, consideration must be given to attempt surgical reconstruction of the aortic valve (unfortunately, the stenosis might be recreated) or aortic valve closure and the placement of a left ventricle-to-ascending aortic conduit.

A more common cause of persistent congestive heart failure after aortic valvuloplasty is left ventricular myocardial or endocardial disease. A subset of patients with critical aortic stenosis have severe left ventricular dysfunction secondary to endocardial fibroelastosis. Once the adequacy of initial treatment has been documented by echocardiographic or catheterization techniques, one can support such patients only with anticongestive regimens.

Finally, patients with critical aortic stenosis can have a significant degree of mitral regurgitation secondary to either left ventricular dilatation or associated mitral valve anomalies. If the degree of mitral regurgitation is unmanageable by medical means, consideration must be given to mitral valve reconstruction or replacement.

Coarctation of the Aorta

Diagnosis

The diagnosis of an isolated coarctation of the aorta can be made accurately on clinical grounds supported by a high-quality two-dimensional ECG to rule out the presence of significant intracardiac defects or complex aortic arch hypoplasia. An infant in severe distress, with low cardiac output, may have a relatively small pressure gradient between upper and lower extremities because of the low flow across the coarctation. Thus, the severity of the lesion may be underestimated in the presence of congestive heart failure (critical coarctation). Cardiac catheterization remains an important diagnostic procedure for children with associated defects or when the anatomic and/or physiologic definition is incomplete on echocardiographic evaluation.

Newborns with critical coarctation may benefit from the administration of PGE_1, which may relax contractile tissue in the aortic arch that can contribute to obstruction. In addition, a patent ductus arteriosus can provide supplemental blood flow to the descending aorta, which, although desaturated, will provide some additional oxygen to the postductal tissues.

Nonsurgical Options

Balloon dilation of coarctation of the aorta during cardiac catheterization is being used with increasing frequency to eliminate simple, discrete native (previously unoperated) coarctation in selected patients. Although intensive care management of patients in the period immediately following dilation is usually not necessary, concern regarding the integrity of the aortic arch may lead to higher levels of patient care monitoring than is available on many patient floors.

Newborns are in a special situation. The size of the femoral vessels may make the likelihood of femoral artery injury during a percutaneous intervention more likely. The integrity of the aortic arch itself may be compromised more easily. There is also the possibility that persistent or recurrent aortic obstruction may be more prevalent because of the distensibility of ductal tissue in the newborn.

Less controversial than the dilation of native coarctation is the use of transcutaneous balloon dilation of late recurrent or residual postoperative coarctation of the aorta. Management of patients following balloon dilation in this setting usually has been handled outside the ICU setting. The procedures can be undertaken with the usual catheterization laboratory sedation, obviating the need for general anesthesia and the use of the ICU for recovery. For unknown reasons, the postoperative problems of paradoxical hypertension, with its accompanying abdominal pain syndrome, have been rare. Intensive care has been required in the setting of femoral artery injury, an uncommon but important complication of this new form of therapy.

Postoperative Care

The surgical repair is usually via a left lateral thoracotomy, although occasionally a median sternotomy may be used in complex cases. Most cases are performed without CPB. Newborns with critical coarctation generally arrive from the operating room intubated, whereas older children are frequently extubated in the operating room. There will usually be one chest tube, and transthoracic monitoring catheters are usually not used. Cardiorespiratory, peripheral arterial, and pulse oximetry monitors will be present.

A bladder catheter will also be in place. Usually, there are no medications being infused at the time of transfer to the ICU, although some children may require nitroprusside and beta-blockade to reduce postoperative hypertension.

An essential feature of monitoring is the measurement of simultaneous upper and lower extremity BPs as soon after surgery as possible. This will assess the adequacy of repair. Once again, the measured gradient must be interpreted in light of the estimated cardiac output. In an infant with clinical evidence of a low cardiac output, the measured gradient across the arch repair may be lower than one would expect from the actual degree of obstruction. Taking this into account, the magnitude of the gradient should govern whether further diagnostic procedures are necessary. Some centers recommend against the presence of indwelling umbilical artery catheters in infants after repair of coarctation of the aorta. The low flow to the lower body, both prior to surgery and during aortic cross-clamping, may exacerbate umbilical artery catheter complications, including thrombus formation and necrotizing enterocolitis. If an umbilical artery catheter is used prior to surgery for stabilization and monitoring of the patient, it should be replaced with a right radial artery line as soon after surgery as feasible if prolonged BP monitoring is needed.

If not performed in the operating room, extubation is usually accomplished within a few hours of admission to the ICU, unless there was severe congestive heart failure preoperatively. The chest tube can be removed the day following surgery if the chest tube drainage is not significant. Postoperative myocardial edema and systolic dysfunction are uncommon in children who do not require CPB.

Caution must be exercised when restarting feedings following coarctation repair. Some children will develop abdominal discomfort or ileus (discussion follows) and may require 1 or more days of bowel rest.

Problems

Persistent Hypertension

The most frequent problem encountered in infants and small children after repair of coarctation of the aorta is persistent hypertension. Of primary importance is the ruling out of significant residual obstruction. If a residual narrowing of the aortic arch is suspected, the magnitude of the obstruction can be accurately diagnosed by upper and lower extremity BPs. Injection of contrast material into a right radial artery catheter with the performance of angiography has proved to be a valuable diagnostic tool in locating the site of obstruction, particularly in infants.

In addition to a residual aortic obstruction, hypertension may be a component of the syndrome of paradoxical hypertension following repair of coarctation of the aorta. Briefly, the initial period of hypertension is secondary to increased circulating catecholamines. This lasts for approximately 36 hours and is followed by a period of hyperreninemia. Although this syndrome is seen more commonly in adults and older children, it can be seen occasionally in small infants. Therapy is directed at the underlying mechanisms of the hypertension. If there is significant hypertension immediately after surgery, the response to increased levels of circulating catecholamines can be blunted through the use of intravenous propranolol. Sodium nitroprusside can be used as a second medication, and labetolol as a third in severe cases. If the hypertension persists more than a few days, an ACE inhibitor such as captopril, perhaps supplemented by a beta-blocker if necessary, becomes the treatment of choice.

Abdominal Discomfort

A degree of abdominal discomfort, with absent bowel sounds, vomiting, and even mesenteric arteritis, can occur following surgery for coarctation of the aorta. Although this has been reported in adults and older children, the incidence in infants is low.

Persistent Congestive Heart Failure

Persistent congestive heart failure following repair of coarctation of the aorta is usually a manifestation of previously undetected associated heart disease. Aortic valve disease, mitral valve anomalies, or primary left ventricular disease should be suspected in infants who have persistent congestive heart failure following adequate repair of coarctation of the aorta.

Pulmonary Stenosis

Diagnosis

Isolated valvar pulmonary stenosis is generally diagnosed and treated in a straightforward manner. Usually, the diagnosis can be made on clinical grounds, confirmed by echocardiography and evaluated and treated in the cardiac catheterization laboratory with catheter-directed balloon pulmonary valvotomy. When valvar pulmonary stenosis is complicated by an associated atrial septal defect, surgery is usually performed (although it is likely that catheter-directed treatment of the stenotic pulmonary valve and catheter-delivered occluder atrial septal defect closure will replace surgery in the future).

Pulmonary stenosis is called critical when the degree of obstruction to pulmonary blood flow is so severe that neonates are dependent on the ductus arteriosus to supply pulmonary blood flow. These infants require stabilization with PGE_1 and relatively urgent treatment. Catheter-directed therapy has become the standard of care for this group of patients as well as older children. The postoperative course described next applies to patients in whom catheter-directed therapy was not selected for a variety of reasons, or in whom balloon dilation was not successful. In this setting, the surgeon will frequently opt for surgical valvotomy or excision of an often severely dysplastic pulmonary valve.

Postoperative Care

Pulmonary valvotomy or valvectomy is performed via a median sternotomy using CPB. The child often will be extubated in the operating room prior to arrival in the ICU. Otherwise, he or she will be mechanically ventilated with deep sedation. Transthoracic monitoring catheters may not be used, as the operation is generally very short and extensive monitoring is not as necessary as with longer, more complicated procedures. Postoperative vasoactive medications are rarely required.

Postoperative myocardial edema and systolic dysfunction are uncommon following a pulmonary valvotomy because of the short normothermic CPB.

Problems

Persistent Hypoxemia

PGE_1 is routinely discontinued at the time of surgical or catheter-directed pulmonary valvotomy. Infants with severe or critical pulmonic stenosis associated with hypoxemia due to atrial-level shunting often remain fairly hypoxemic following their valvotomies. It is not unusual for these children to have a systemic arterial PO_2 of below 30 torr following surgery. This is the result of continued right-to-left atrial shunting, which will resolve over the ensuing weeks as the right ventricular hypertrophy resolves and right ventricular compliance improves, allowing closure of the foramen ovale.

Occasionally, there is an infant with a severely hypoplastic right ventricle who may require augmentation of pulmonary blood flow by a systemic-to-pulmonary artery shunt following valvuloplasty. It must be remembered that the degree of right-to-left shunting at the atrial level is directly proportional to the functional impairment of flow through the right ventricle and pulmonary arterial tree. With a knowledge of the expected degree of hypoxemia, physicians are more able to refrain from unnecessary intervention. If patience on the part of the physician is not rewarded by an increased arterial oxygen saturation, then echocardiography and cardiac catheterization should be undertaken to be certain that the initial obstruction has been adequately relieved.

Pulmonary Atresia with Intact Ventricular Septum

Diagnosis

Pulmonary atresia with intact ventricular septum is characterized by total obstruction to right ventricular outflow. Severe hypoplasia of the right ventricle is the rule rather than the exception in this defect, although normal, or even large, right ventricular cavities may be present. There are instances in which echocardiography cannot always differentiate between pulmonary atresia with intact ventricular septum and critical pulmonary stenosis. For that reason, cardiac catheterization may be required for the accurate diagnosis. These infants are ductus arteriosus-dependent for pulmonary blood flow and require PGE_1 for initial stabilization or surgery. The rare infant with a relatively large right ventricle can be managed in a fashion similar to that outlined for critical pulmonary stenosis. The more usual infant requires a systemic-to-pulmonary artery shunt in addition to relief of the right ventricular outflow tract obstruction. The right ventricle in this condition often is a severely hypertrophied noncompliant chamber, which can serve as an obstruction between the right atrium and the main pulmonary artery. There often is significant hypoplasia and stenosis of the tricuspid valve. A complicating feature can be an aneurysm of septum primum, which can obstruct the orifice of the mitral valve, leading to low cardiac output and death. Such an aneurysm is best diagnosed by two-dimensional echocardiography. If it is recognized, an atrial septectomy should be performed as part of the initial surgery.

A potentially lethal complication to this condition is the presence of sinusoid connections between the right ventricular cavity and the coronary arterial bed. Under these circumstances, portions of the myocardium may receive their blood supply from the right ventricle rather than from the aortic root. Under these circumstances, if the right ventricular hypertension is relieved, the area of myocardium supplied by these blood vessels may be compromised. Accordingly, complete evaluation of coronary arteries is necessary before intervention can be undertaken.

Postoperative Care

The surgical repair is via a median sternotomy using CPB and possibly HA. The child will arrive in the ICU following surgery intubated and mechanically ventilated with deep sedation and pharmacologic muscle relaxation. Because the patients are invariably newborns, an umbilical central venous catheter is often present, making a percutaneous or transthoracic CVP catheter unnecessary. Medications being infused at the time of transfer to the ICU may include inotropic agents and systemic vasodilators as needed.

Problems
Subpulmonary Stenosis

Following relief of right ventricular outflow tract obstruction, the hypertrophic right ventricular myocardium may obstruct the subpulmonary region dynamically during systole, a phenomenon known as "suicide right ventricle." If hypoxemia persists following reconstruction of the right ventricular outflow without placement of a systemic-to-pulmonary artery shunt, consideration must be given to the adequacy of relief of obstruction and to the role of the right ventricle or tricuspid valve size in preventing adequate pulmonary blood flow. If severe hypoxemia develops, a shunt is indicated. If the ductus arteriosus has not been ligated at the time of surgery, PGE_1 can be reinstituted to stabilize the patient prior to surgery. If a systemic-to-pulmonary artery shunt has been performed in addition to right ventricular outflow tract reconstruction, and there is persistent severe hypoxemia, consideration must be given to the adequacy of the shunt. Often, cardiac catheterization is required to sort out the various factors in the persistently cyanotic infant following surgery for pulmonary atresia with intact ventricular septum.

In the rare instance in which there is an obstructive interatrial communication as well as obstruction to flow across the tricuspid valve and right ventricle, significant right atrial hypertension can develop. Relief of the obstruction to right-to-left atrial flow should be undertaken.

Total Anomalous Pulmonary Venous Return

Diagnosis

An accurate, complete diagnosis of total anomalous pulmonary venous return can usually be made by two-dimensional echocardiography.[144,145] Indeed, this diagnostic modality can be superior to cardiac catheterization when attempting to sort out those difficult cases in which the anomalous veins return through several channels.[146] In most circumstances, however, cardiac catheterization is a helpful adjunct to assess left ventricular size and function and to evaluate pulmonary artery pressure and resistance.

Postoperative Care

The surgical repair is via a median sternotomy using CPB and usually HA. The child will arrive in the ICU following surgery intubated and mechanically ventilated with deep sedation and pharmacologic muscle relaxation. The surgeon will usually have placed chest tubes to drain the pleura and mediastinum. Transthoracic right atrial, left atrial, and pulmonary artery monitoring catheters usually will have also been placed in the operating room, although a transcutaneous CVP catheter may be used if available. Medications being infused at the time of transfer to the ICU may include inotropic agents and vasodilators as needed.

The left atrial and pulmonary artery catheters are removed the day following surgery if the patient is awake and hemodynamically stable. These catheters are usually removed before the chest tubes so that bleeding from the catheter sites can be monitored. Usually a pressure pull-back tracing is recorded during withdrawal of the left atrial catheter to identify any obstruction across the anastomosis between the common pulmonary venous chamber and the left atrium.

Problems
Pulmonary Venous Hypertension

The presence of pulmonary venous hypertension after repair of total anomalous pulmonary venous connection can be suspected on the basis of pulmonary congestion or a "white-out" appearance on chest x-ray. If such an appearance is seen, it should raise the question of a narrow anastomosis between the common pulmonary vein and the left atrium. Echocardiography has been helpful in defining the postsurgical anatomy.[144] If the infant's clinical condition is not improving, a complete cardiac catheterization should be performed to assess the situation. If a significant obstruction exists, it should be relieved promptly. In cases of mixed pulmonary venous return, it is not unusual for part of the pulmonary venous connection to be relatively obstructed. Such conditions are tolerated fairly well, presumably because of interlobar pulmonary venous anastomoses.

Low Cardiac Output

Low cardiac output is tolerated very well following repair of total anomalous pulmonary venous return. If obstruction at the anastomotic site is ruled out, patience is warranted. Very severe hypoplasia of the left atrium, mitral valve, and left ventricle may result in severe, low cardiac output with pulmonary venous hypertension in the absence of obstruction. Over a period of several months, however, there may be growth of the entire left side of the heart to near-normal size, with resultant marked clinical improvement.

Palliative Surgery
Pulmonary Artery Banding

Despite the general preference for reparative surgery, there are a number of patients with complicated CHD with excessive pulmonary blood flow whose anatomy does not lend itself to physiologic repair early in life; such defects include single ventricle without restriction to pulmonary blood flow or large ventricular septal defects in premature infants. In these situations, when uncontrolled congestive heart failure is present in association with pulmonary artery hypertension, some limitation of pulmonary flow can be accomplished with pulmonary artery banding.

In the past, banding of the pulmonary artery was performed with an eye toward a good clinical result. In the modern era, in addition to a satisfactory clinical course, the pulmonary artery architecture must be preserved and the pulmonary arteriolar bed must be protected. These considerations have reached a degree of importance because of the advent of the Fontan procedure and its modifications. Virtually all children with complex CHD should be considered as potential candidates for some form of reparative surgery in the future. Infants who are potential candidates for Fontan-type operations will remain so only if their pulmonary artery architecture and pulmonary vascular bed grow and develop in a suitable fashion.

Diagnosis

All infants with complex disease who require pulmonary artery banding are in need of complete evaluation by two-dimensional echocardiography and cardiac catheterization. Although there is a tendency to rely solely on echocardiography for infants who will require only pulmonary artery banding, cardiac catheterization is usually necessary to be certain that the pulmonary vascular bed is completely defined before surgical procedure. If there is associated pulmonary venous obstruction as a contributor to pulmonary hypertension, the obstruction must be relieved to assure the normal development of the pulmonary vascular bed. In addition, branch pulmonary arteries often are not well seen by echocardiographic imaging, and angiography may unmask previously unrecognized areas of distal obstruction.

Postoperative Care

Pulmonary artery banding is a closed procedure. The approach may utilize a median sternotomy or an anteriolateral thoracotomy, depending on the specific anatomy of the patient.

The child may be extubated in the operating room or soon after arrival in the ICU. The surgeon will likely have placed chest drainage tubes, depending on the incision and condition of the operative field at the end of the case.

Transthoracic monitoring catheters are usually not required. A peripheral arterial catheter, cardiorespiratory monitor, pulse oximetry monitor, and a peripheral IV may be all the monitoring and access needed. In children with a complete mixing lesion (single ventricle, etc.), the percent saturations following pulmonary artery band are typically in the 70s to 80s.

A bladder catheter may be in place if the child is still asleep. Usually, there are no medications being infused at the time of transfer to the ICU. Intravenous fluids are restarted at a full maintenance rate following surgery.

Postoperative myocardial edema and systolic dysfunction are rarely a problem following closed surgery of this type. As the child awakens from sedation and begins spontaneous respiration, mechanical ventilatory support is weaned, if the child has not already been extubated. The chest tubes can be removed the day of surgery or the following morning if the drainage is not significant.

Problems

Excessive Pulmonary Blood Flow

If there is excessive pulmonary blood flow, resulting in congestive heart failure or pulmonary artery hypertension, one must make a judgment whether the situation is tolerable. Will the child "grow into" the band with time? If the degree of excessive blood flow is so great that there is either unmanageable congestive heart failure or an unprotected pulmonary vascular bed, then reoperation and band adjustment is indicated.

Hypoxemia

If there are excessive hypoxemia and decreased pulmonary blood flow on chest film, it is likely that the pulmonary artery band is "too tight." It must be recognized that a degree of pulmonary venous desaturation is likely to follow the surgical procedure, so the oxygen saturation in the hours immediately after surgery is often misleading.

Branch Pulmonary Artery Obstruction

Improper placement or postoperative distal migration of pulmonary artery bands can obstruct one or both of the branch pulmonary arteries. In such a situation, there will be an unequal distribution of pulmonary blood flow. This can lead to distortion of pulmonary artery architecture and the possible development of pulmonary vascular obstructive disease in the unprotected lung.

Congestive Heart Failure

The most likely cause of persistent congestive heart failure after pulmonary artery banding is an inadequate pulmonary artery band-

ing or an uncorrected associated defect. Whatever diagnostic tests are required to differentiate the two must be undertaken so that remedial measures can be undertaken before irreparable damage has been done to the pulmonary vasculature.

Systemic-to-Pulmonary Artery Shunts

Occasionally, infants with severe hypoxemia and diminished pulmonary artery blood flow require systemic-to-pulmonary artery shunts if a reparative operation cannot be safely undertaken because of either hemodynamic instability, small size of the patient, or other factors (Fig. 21-15).

The evolution of the systemic-to-pulmonary shunt has been a long and rocky one. Historically, initial palliation of severe cyanosis due to reduced pulmonary blood flow was attempted by anastomosing the ascending aorta side-to-side to the right pulmonary artery (Waterston shunt) or the descending aorta side-to-side to the back of the left pulmonary artery (Potts shunt). Both of these techniques allowed little room for error and often resulted in an ineffective shunt with persistent cyanosis or too much pulmonary blood flow, increasing the risk of pulmonary vascular occlusive disease. Also, iatrogenic stenosis or late occlusion of the branch pulmonary arteries was common.

The classical Blalock-Taussig shunt involves mobilization and division of the subclavian artery with reanastomosis of the distal end to the branch pulmonary artery. Because the caliber of the subclavian artery serves to regulate pulmonary blood flow, acceptable results tend to be the rule. More often, a Gore-Tex conduit is substituted for the subclavian artery (modified Blalock-Taussig shunt). The Blalock-Taussig shunt, or modified Blalock-Taussig shunt, is associated with a low incidence of early occlusion, and in newborns the ductus arteriosus is often not ligated to preserve the option of opening the ductus with PGE_1 in the event of acute shunt occlusion.

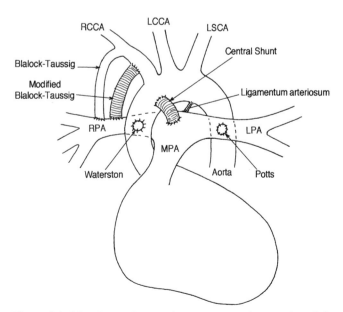

Figure 21-15. Systemic-to-pulmonary artery shunts. LCCA, left common carotid artery; LPA, left pulmonary artery; LSCA, left subclavian artery; MPA, main pulmonary artery; RCCA, right common carotid artery; RPA, right pulmonary artery.

A final type of systemic-to-pulmonary shunt consists of a small conduit that connects the ascending aorta to the main pulmonary artery or proximal branch pulmonary artery. This "central shunt" has the disadvantages that it requires opening the pericardium and is generally shorter than the Blalock-Taussig shunt, resulting in even more pulmonary blood flow. It is frequently convenient, however, in conjunction with other intrapericardial procedures.

Diagnosis

An accurate anatomic diagnosis with particular attention to the aortic arch and its branches and the pulmonary artery architecture is essential for the performance of a systemic-to-pulmonary artery shunt. Because the aortic arch and distal pulmonary arteries often are not well seen utilizing echocardiography, cardiac catheterization is frequently indicated.

Many anatomic features of the aortic arch impact on the design of a systemic-to-pulmonary shunts: A left or right aortic arch, as well as missing or anomalous bracheocephalic vessels, may rule for or against certain shunt configurations. For example, a modified Blalock-Taussig shunt is performed optimally on the side opposite the arch because of the decreased risk of kinking at the systemic end.

Significant peripheral pulmonary artery stenosis can lead to insufficient or asymmetric pulmonary blood flow following placement of a systemic-to-pulmonary shunt. In the case of asymmetric pulmonary blood flow, the potential exists for the development of pulmonary vascular disease in one lung or the other.

Postoperative Care

Systemic-to-pulmonary artery shunts can be performed as closed procedures when the anatomy does not require interruption of pulmonary blood flow. Otherwise, a short run of CPB is often required. The surgical procedure is via a median sternotomy (central shunt) or lateral thoracotomy (Blalock-Taussig shunt and its modifications).

The child may be extubated in the operating room or soon after arrival in the ICU. The surgeon may have placed a chest drainage tube depending on the incision and condition of the operative field at the end of the case.

Transthoracic monitoring catheters are usually not required. In fact, a peripheral arterial catheter, cardiorespiratory monitor, pulse oximetry monitor, and a peripheral IV may be all the monitoring and access needed. A bladder catheter may be in place if the child is still asleep. Usually, there are no medications being infused at the time of transfer to the ICU.

Problems

Excessive Pulmonary Blood Flow

Patients with excessive pulmonary blood flow following a systemic-to-pulmonary shunt may develop congestive heart failure. This is a particularly common problem with the modified Blalock-Taussig shunt in a small newborn, because a larger-than-necessary conduit is required initially to prevent early redevelopment of cyanosis during the rapid growth of the infant.

Congestive heart failure secondary to excessive pulmonary blood flow may require anticongestive therapy, increased PEEP, and minimization of FiO_2 as interim measures. One must recognize, however, that prolonged excessive pulmonary blood flow can lead to pulmonary vascular disease and ventricular dysfunction secondary to volume overload. Fortunately, in the case of the modified Blalock-Taussig shunt, pulmonary blood flow is reduced in a relative way as

the child grows, making pulmonary vascular disease less of a concern. Long-term excessive pulmonary blood flow is more of a concern with the Waterston and Potts shunts and with other modified aortopulmonary shunts that may have a larger diameter or are shorter than the usual modified Blalock-Taussig shunt.

Persistent Hypoxemia

If there is persistent hypoxemia after the creation of a systemic-to-pulmonary artery shunt, then adequacy and patency of the shunt must be questioned. Because the pulmonary blood flow is dependent on the systemic BP, hypotension must be managed aggressively. Echocardiography and cardiac catheterization have a role in the investigation of suspected shunt malfunction, although the latter tends to provide better images and more quantitative information. If the ductus arteriosus has not been ligated at the time of the initial procedure in a newborn, PGE_1 can be reinstituted to relieve severe hypoxemia while appropriate diagnostic tests are performed.

Many centers advocate the use of low-dose aspirin (5 mg/kg/ 24 hr) in the first few months following construction of systemic-to-pulmonary artery shunts to minimize the risk of thrombosis.

Venopulmonary Shunts

Although very useful in the newborn period, systemic-to-pulmonary artery shunts have serious drawbacks: Because a fraction of the blood being circulated to the lungs has already been oxygenated, systemic-to-pulmonary shunts increase the amount of blood pumped by the heart, creating an additional volume load for the ventricle. Systemic-to-pulmonary shunts can also expose the pulmonary vascular bed to flows, pressures, and oxygen saturations that are greater than normal, increasing the risk of pulmonary vascular occlusive disease. For these reasons, there is an advantage to using a systemic vein, usually the SVC, to supply pulmonary blood flow instead of a systemic artery. This approach is workable, however, only when the resistance of the pulmonary vascular circuit is low. Systemic-to-pulmonary artery shunts are generally still required in infants during the first 4 to 6 months of life and in other patients with elevated pulmonary vascular resistance.

There are several commonly used venopulmonary shunts. The first is the classical Glenn shunt, in which the SVC and right pulmonary artery are severed and anastomosed to one another (Fig. 21-16). A second is the cavopulmonary shunt, also called a "bidirectional Glenn," in which the severed SVC is anastomosed to the top of the right pulmonary artery without detaching the latter from the rest of the pulmonary arterial tree.[91,93–95,147,148] These procedures may be performed on the left in the case of a left SVC, and a cavopulmonary shunt may be bilateral when two SVCs are present.

The cavopulmonary shunt often is performed as the initial stage of a Fontan procedure (discussion follows). In this case, a modified cavopulmonary shunt may be performed that involves anastomosing both the proximal and distal SVC to the pulmonary artery, then applying a patch to the orifice of the SVC at the right atrium. This procedure, often called a "hemi-Fontan," simplifies completion of the Fontan at a later stage.[91,149,150]

Diagnosis

Before a venopulmonary anastomosis can be contemplated, it must be certain that an adequate pulmonary blood flow can be driven at pressures generated by a venous bed. This is particularly true

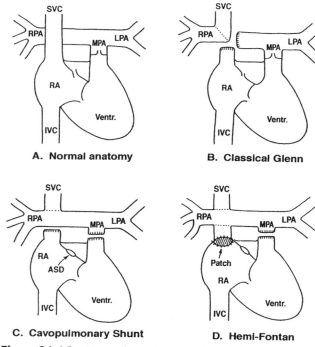

Figure 21.16. Venopulmonary shunts. IVC, inferior vena cava; LPA, left pulmonary artery; MPA, main pulmonary artery; RA, right atrium; RPA, right pulmonary artery; SVC, superior vena cava; Ventr., ventricle.

when the entire pulmonary blood flow will be delivered via the systemic vein, as with the cavopulmonary shunt or hemi-Fontan. In this setting, relative contraindications to the procedure include small or stenotic branch pulmonary arteries, elevated pulmonary vascular resistance, pulmonary vein obstruction, and elevated LAP from a variety of causes (e.g., mitral stenosis, mitral regurgitation, and ventricular dysfunction).

Because much of this information cannot be derived from non-invasive studies, cardiac catheterization is generally required prior to any venopulmonary anastomosis.

Postoperative Care

With the exception of the Glenn shunt, which can be performed from a lateral thoracotomy, the majority of venopulmonary anastomoses are performed via a median sternotomy. The procedure can be performed without CPB if the anastomosis can be accomplished without completely interrupting pulmonary blood flow, although CPB is usually required. A central venous catheter is placed in the SVC, and a transcutaneous monitoring catheter is placed in the left atrium.

These patients require special efforts to maintain the pulmonary vascular resistance as low as possible. Elevation of the head of the bed by 30 degrees helps promote pulmonary blood flow by increasing SVC pressure. It is possible to get a general idea of the changes in pulmonary vascular resistance by monitoring the arterial saturation and the transpulmonary pressure gradient (the difference between the pulmonary artery and left atrial mean pressures). The saturation will decline as the pulmonary resistance increases and pulmonary blood flow decreases, while the transpulmonary gradient will increase as the resistance increases. These

two measures are mutually dependent: If the resistance of the pulmonary vascular bed increases, the saturation may be reduced, the transpulmonary gradient may increase, or both. In general, an oxygen saturation greater than or equal to 75% and a transpulmonary gradient of less than 6 to 9 mm Hg suggest reasonable pulmonary vascular resistance. A second important indicator is the absolute pulmonary artery pressure: Most patients can tolerate a mean pulmonary arterial pressure of up to 18 to 20 mm Hg, but as the pressure rises, the pulmonary blood flow will fall and signs of venous congestion, such as edema or effusions, will increase.

Many factors impact on the resistance to flow through the pulmonary vascular system. Obstruction in the pulmonary arteries themselves can result from congenital small size, surgical scarring, or thrombosis. Pulmonary arteriolar resistance can be elevated secondary to reactive vasoconstriction or pulmonary vascular occlusive disease. Pulmonary venous pressure can be elevated secondary to pulmonary vein stenosis or obstruction or left atrial hypertension, which may, in turn, be caused by mitral valve stenosis, regurgitation, or elevated ventricular diastolic pressure. The last factor is particularly important in the postoperative period because the transient ventricular dysfunction that results from CPB and HA may result in a significantly increased ventricular end-diastolic pressure. For example, it is not unusual for the patient to have fairly high saturations immediately after surgery, when oxygen consumption is low and the myocardium has yet to "feel the effects" of CPB. Over the ensuing 6 to 12 hours, as systolic and diastolic dysfunction become more significant, the saturations may decrease as pulmonary blood flow falls in response to the elevated pulmonary venous pressure. Then, during the gradual recovery from bypass, the saturations slowly increase once again.

Postoperative myocardial edema and systolic dysfunction often gradually worsen over the first 6 to 12 hours following surgery. Manifestations may include falling cardiac output and increasing filling pressures. Increased inotropic support (e.g., dopamine) and volume replacement may be required during this period. The need for additional intravascular volume may be more than usual because of the additional capacitance of the systemic venous system. Some dilation of these veins is expected because they will very likely be under higher pressure than preoperatively. Also, because of the increased systemic venous pressure, peripheral edema may be more marked than in children undergoing CPB for other indications.

Early extubation may reduce the adverse effects of elevated systemic venous pressures because positive-pressure ventilation adds to the pressure required for venous blood to enter the chest. Analgesic agents are weaned to a level sufficient to manage expected postoperative pain. As the child awakens, care must be taken to wean the mechanical ventilation carefully to avoid periods of hypoventilation that might result in an elevated pulmonary vascular resistance. In addition, the FiO$_2$ must be weaned very gingerly, particularly below a fraction of 0.4 to 0.5, where the toxic effects of oxygen are probably minimal. Any metabolic acidosis should be corrected, if possible, to minimize the requirement for additional ventilation to maintain an alkaline pH. Extubation is often accomplished by late in the day of surgery.

Problems
Hypoxemia
With the exception of the Glenn shunt, most venopulmonary shunts are used in children without a functional pulmonary outflow tract. In fact, the main pulmonary artery is often ligated at

the time of a cavopulmonary shunt or a hemi-Fontan. Of necessity, therefore, whatever systemic venous return is not shunted to the pulmonary arteries must mix with the pulmonary venous return and get recirculated to the body. Therefore, following the cavopulmonary shunt or its variants, all children have some degree of desaturation.

The degree of hypoxemia in children with "mixing" circulations, such as following a cavopulmonary shunt, depends on the ratio of pulmonary venous return to systemic venous return. Because most patients will maintain a fairly constant systemic cardiac output if they can, this ratio varies primarily according to the pulmonary blood flow, which is subject to many factors.

Most children will have relatively good saturations immediately following surgery, often in the 80% to 90% range. Following a course of CPB, however, the ventricle may have diminished contractility and compliance, leading to an elevated end-diastolic pressure. Because any flow though the lungs must ultimately push against the ventricular end-diastolic pressure in order to flow into the atrium, ventricular dysfunction can lead to reduced pulmonary blood flow and hypoxemia. Hypoxemia secondary to ventricular dysfunction can be treated with inotropic agents if it is severe, although more often a lower saturation is accepted for several days if this is known to be the cause. A variety of other causes of increased resistance to flow in the pulmonary vascular circuit can also result in hypoxemia, as outlined in Table 21-5.

Alveolar hypoxia and acidosis are reversible causes of hypoxemia in this setting. Structural obstructions to pulmonary blood flow are rare but potentially catastrophic complications. Some centers advocate the use of antiplatelet agents for a variable period following venopulmonary anastomoses to reduce the risk of thrombosis. Whenever unexplained hypoxemia is present following a venopulmonary anastomosis, immediate echocardiography and possibly cardiac catheterization are indicated to look for a correctable cause.

Other causes of hypoxemia following surgery of this type include a variety of pulmonary disorders, including pneumonia, atelectasis, pulmonary edema, and pleural effusions. Chest radiography is always indicated in the setting of progressive or unexplained hypoxemia.

Finally, hypoxemia can be caused by anemia in children in whom the systemic and pulmonary venous return mix prior to being pumped to the body. A low concentration of hemoglobin in the blood can result in excessive extraction of oxygen by the body from the hemoglobin that is available. Returning systemic venous blood with a very low oxygen saturation then mixes with the pulmonary venous return, lowering the saturation of the mixture that is pumped back to the systemic arterial system. For this reason, and because anemia mandates a higher cardiac output from the recovering heart, a low hemoglobin level should be avoided. It is generally safe to raise the hemoglobin level to 13 to 15 gram%, particularly if the total number of donor units can be reduced by transfusing several times with the same unit in a small child.

Pleural Effusions

Because of the elevation in systemic venous pressure following venopulmonary shunts, transudative pleural effusions are particularly prevalent in this group of patients. The course of most pleural transudates follows that of systemic edema and should begin to resolve within a few days of surgery. Patients often have pleural chest tubes placed at the time of surgery, even if the pleural space has not been entered because of the risk of effusion formation.

Chylothorax

The increased incidence of chylothoraces following cavopulmonary shunt is probably related to at least three factors:

1. increased systemic venous pressure in the upper compartment (drained by the SVC), leading to raised hydrostatic lymphatic pressure
2. injury to small lymphatic vessels in the mediastinal and pleural spaces
3. possible injury to the thoracic duct

Treatment of postoperative chylothoraces was discussed earlier in this chapter. Following a venopulmonary shunt, however, more aggressive and prolonged therapy may be required. As the ventricular end-diastolic pressure falls during recovery, the tendency toward accumulation of effusion and/or chyle in the pleural space should resolve.

Table 21-5. Factors associated with increased pulmonary vascular resistance

Pulmonary vascular reactivity
  Alveolar hypoxia
  Arterial acidosis
    Metabolic acidosis
    Respiratory acidosis
Structural obstruction to pulmonary blood flow
  Thrombosis or stenosis of SVC
  Thrombosis or stenosis of pulmonary arteries
  Hypoplasia of pulmonary arteries
  Pulmonary vein obstruction (stenosis, cor triatriatum)
Causes of left atrial hypertension
  Atrioventricular valve stenosis
  Atrioventricular valve regurgitation
  Ventricular dysfunction (elevated EDP)

SVC, superior vena cava; EDP, end-diastolic pressure.

Table 21-6. Defects suitable for the Fontan procedure

Single ventricle
Hypoplastic right ventricle
  Tricuspid atresia
  Pulmonary atresia/intact ventricular septum
Hypoplastic left ventricle
  Mitral atresia
  Hypoplastic left heart syndrome
Double-inlet left ventricle
Heterotaxy (some forms)
Double-outlet right ventricle (some forms)
Double-inlet left ventricle
Complete atrioventricular canal
  Straddling or hypoplastic atrioventricular valve
  Hypoplastic ventricle
Ventricular septal defects
  "Swiss cheese septum"
  Straddling atrioventricular valves

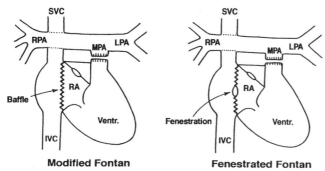

Figure 21-17. Fontan procedure. IVC, inferior vena cava; LPA, left pulmonary artery; MPA, main pulmonary artery; RA, right atrium; RPA, right pulmonary artery; SVC, superior vena cava; Ventr., ventricle.

Fontan Procedure

Many types of CHD preclude any surgical repair featuring two functioning ventricles (Table 21-6). The principle behind the Fontan procedure is that all systemic venous return can be redirected directly to the pulmonary arterial system without the use of a pulmonary ventricle. The systemic venous pressure propels the blood through the lungs, and the ventricle or ventricles are left only to pump blood to the body (Fig. 21-17). Although it predated the operation historically, the Fontan can be considered an extension of the cavopulmonary shunt. Converting a cavopulmonary shunt to a Fontan may require only baffling of the IVC flow to the pulmonary arteries.

As with venopulmonary shunts, however, the Fontan procedure is workable only when the resistance of the pulmonary vascular circuit is low. The stakes are higher with the Fontan procedure, however: If the pulmonary vascular resistance is temporarily increased in the case of a cavopulmonary shunt, less blood will flow to the pulmonary vascular bed and more will return to the heart via the IVC. The patient will have to tolerate an increased degree

of hypoxemia, but there will be relatively little impact on cardiac output. In the case of the Fontan procedure, however, there is no alternate pathway for systemic venous blood in the case of a temporary increase in pulmonary vascular resistance. The consequent fall in cardiac output is often poorly tolerated.

Because of the increased risk of the Fontan procedure, a number of factors have been identified that distinguish poor candidates for the procedure. Prior to the staged approach, children under 2 years of age were considered at unacceptably high risk. Since the advent of the two-stage Fontan, using the cavopulmonary shunt or hemi-Fontan as an initial step in infancy, the procedure has had good success with children between 12 and 24 months of age. Also, the same risk factors noted for the cavopulmonary shunt regarding pulmonary artery anatomy, atrioventricular valve function, and ventricular function, are even more important in the planning of a Fontan procedure.

Children who are not considered ideal candidates for the Fontan procedure may be candidates for a fenestrated Fontan, in which a hole is placed in the patch baffling the IVC to the pulmonary arteries (Fig. 21-18). This hole serves as a pop-off for the systemic venous pressure if the resistance of the pulmonary circuit becomes unacceptably high, reducing the risk of impaired cardiac output. Bridges et al.[96,98] and Kopf et al.[151] have described a fenestrated Fontan procedure in which the hole in the baffle was routinely closed using a catheter-delivered umbrella device following recovery from surgery (Fig. 21-19). Other approaches have included patch fenestrations that could be closed by applying tension on a drawstring following recovery from surgery.

Diagnosis

Before a Fontan procedure can be contemplated, one must be certain that an adequate pulmonary blood flow can be driven at pressures generated by the systemic venous system. Relative contraindications to the procedure include small or stenotic branch pulmonary arteries, elevated pulmonary vascular resistance, pulmonary vein obstruction, and elevated left atrial pressure from a variety of causes (e.g., atrioventricular valve stenosis or regurgitation and ventricular dysfunction). Because much of this

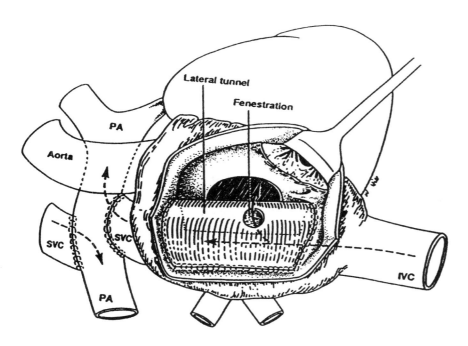

Figure 21-18. Fenestrated Fontan procedure. IVC, inferior vena cava; PA, pulmonary artery; SVC, superior vena cava. (From GS Kopf et al. Fenestrated Fontan operation with delayed transcatheter closure of atrial septal defect: Improved results in high-risk patients. *J Thorac Cardiovasc Surg* 103: 1039–1048, 1992. With permission.)

Figure 21-19. Transcatheter closure of the ASD in a fenestrated Fontan. IVC, inferior vena cava; LA, left atrium; RA, right atrium. (From GS Kopf et al. Fenestrated Fontan operation with delayed transcatheter closure of atrial septal defect: Improved results in high-risk patients. *J Thorac Cardiovasc Surg* 103: 1039–1048, 1992. With permission.)

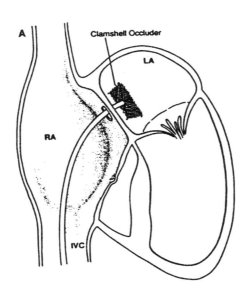
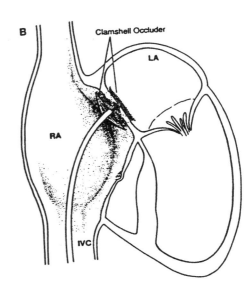

information cannot be derived from noninvasive studies alone, both echocardiography and cardiac catheterization are required prior to a Fontan procedure.

Postoperative Care

The procedure is performed using CPB via a median sternotomy. The child will arrive in the ICU following surgery intubated and mechanically ventilated with deep sedation and pharmacologic muscle relaxation.

The postoperative physiology following a Fontan procedure is unique. Because the systemic veins have a limited capacity to increase pulmonary artery pressures, any factor that elevates the resistance of the pulmonary circuit is likely to result in a decrease in pulmonary blood flow. Because there is no other route for systemic venous return, a fall in pulmonary blood flow will result in a fall in cardiac output. As a result, the principles that govern the postoperative management of the Fontan patient include (1) keeping the resistance of the pulmonary circuit as low as possible, (2) avoiding high LAPs, and (3) maintaining the intravascular volume so that the systemic veins can maintain an adequate pulmonary artery pressure.

The difference between the mean pulmonary arterial and left atrial mean pressures (the transpulmonary gradient) is monitored closely as a measure of pulmonary resistance. Increases in the transpulmonary gradient often are the result of hypoxemia or acidosis, both of which are potent pulmonary vasoconstrictors. Consequently, adequate oxygen and ventilation are critical in the immediate postoperative period. An arterial pH of 7.45 to 7.50 is usually sufficient to minimize the pulmonary vascular resistance. The FiO_2 must be weaned very gingerly, particularly below a fraction of 0.4 to 0.5, where the toxic effects of oxygen are probably minimal. The lowest PEEP tolerated and a short inspiratory time will optimize systemic venous return. Any metabolic acidosis should be corrected, if possible, to minimize the requirement for additional ventilation to maintain an alkaline pH. Sedation also can have a potent effect of pulmonary vascular resistance, and deep sedation is generally required through the night following surgery.

Any elevation in the LAP could be evidence of ventricular failure. A modest rise in left atrial is expected over the 6 to 12 hours after surgery secondary to myocardial edema and tissue injury resulting from CPB. Manifestations may include falling cardiac output and increasing filling pressures. Increased inotropic support (e.g., dopamine) and volume administration may be required during this period. Excessive or acute increases in LAP could be evidence of a catastrophic injury to the myocardium or acute atrioventricular valve regurgitation.

The need for additional intravascular volume may be more than usual because of the additional capacitance of the systemic venous system. Some dilation of these veins is expected because they will very likely be under higher pressure than preoperatively. The left atrial pressure as well as clinical indicators of cardiac output (peripheral coolness, urine output, etc.) are the best indicators of volume status. Also, because of the increased systemic venous pressure, systemic edema may be more marked than in children undergoing CPB for other indications.

By the morning following surgery, myocardial function is usually improving. Muscle relaxants can be discontinued, and analgesics are weaned to a level sufficient to manage expected postoperative pain. As the child awakens from sedation, mechanical ventilatory support is weaned; careful attention must be paid to the transpulmonary mean pressure gradient because the pulmonary vascular resistance may increase as a result of decreased ventilation and discomfort. Some elevation in the pulmonary artery pressure is to be expected, but evidence of falling cardiac output may suggest that a slower withdrawal of sedation and ventilatory support is indicated. Nonetheless, extubation is usually accomplished on the first or second day following surgery.

The left atrial catheter is removed a day or two following surgery if the patient is hemodynamically stable and has weaned successfully from the ventilator. The chest tubes may be removed after a day of full enteral feedings if there is no evidence of pleural effusions or chylothorax.

Problems

Hypoxemia

A modest degree of desaturation is the rule following the Fontan procedure. In many patients, the right atrial baffle is constructed so that the coronary sinus and/or some of the hepatic veins drain to the systemic atrium, resulting in a small right-to-left shunt and systemic saturations in the mid-90s.

In addition, pulmonary autoregulation appears to be impaired following a Fontan procedure. Consequently, there can be some degree of hypoxemia due to ventilation/perfusion mismatch and pulmonary venous desaturation. As the child recovers from surgery, there is likely to be improvement in atelectasis and some loss of excess pulmonary water, making ventilation/perfusion mismatch less of a clinical issue.

Despite these factors, however, most children following a Fontan procedure will have saturations in the 90% to 96% range. Significant hypoxemia below this range warrants investigation into pulmonary and cardiac causes.

Pulmonary causes of persistent hypoxemia include endotracheal tube or bronchial obstruction, ventilator malfunction, pulmonary effusions, chylothorax, atelectasis, infiltrates, and phrenic nerve injury. Endotracheal tube position and patency must be confirmed clinically and radiographically. Often, hand ventilation will provide a lot of information regarding endotracheal tube function, airway resistance, and lung compliance. Ultrasound or fluoroscopy may be required to evaluate diaphragmatic function.

Cardiac causes of persistent hypoxemia are usually attributable to a persistent right-to-left shunt other than those mentioned earlier. Two possibilities include disruption of the atrial baffle and significant systemic venous collaterals to the left side of the heart. Because the systemic venous pressure may be much higher than the pulmonary venous pressure, especially immediately following surgery, there is a tendency for small collaterals to dilate to accommodate larger flow. For example, systemic venous collaterals to the hepatic venous system may allow a pop-off through hepatic veins that sometimes are left draining to the pulmonary venous side of a Fontan procedure. Often, cardiac catheterization is required to identify cardiac causes of hypoxemia.

Elevated Pulmonary Artery Pressure

A variety of causes of increased resistance to flow in the pulmonary vascular circuit also can result in elevated pulmonary artery pressure and impaired cardiac output, as outlined in Table 21-5. As noted, alveolar hypoxia, acidosis, anxiety, and pain are reversible causes of elevated pulmonary artery pressure in this setting. An elevated transpulmonary gradient that does not reverse with sedation, supplemental oxygen, and hyperventilation mandates echocardiographic evaluation, and possibly cardiac catheterization, to rule out rare, but potentially catastrophic, structural obstructions to pulmonary blood flow. Structural problems may include pulmonary venous obstruction, a restrictive atrial septal communication (in mitral valve obstruction), subaortic obstruction, and intracardiac thrombus formation. Some centers advocate the use of antiplatelet agents for a variable period following the Fontan procedure to reduce the risk of thrombosis of the pulmonary arteries.

Pleural Effusions

Because of the elevation in systemic venous pressure following the Fontan procedure, transudative pleural effusions are particularly prevalent in this group of patients. The course of most pleural transudates follows that of systemic edema and should begin to resolve within a few days after surgery, but may persist in some patients.

Chylothorax

The pathophysiology, diagnosis, and treatment of postoperative chylothoraces have been discussed earlier. Following a Fontan procedure, however, more aggressive and prolonged therapy may be required. As the ventricular end-diastolic pressure decreases during recovery, the tendency toward accumulation of chyle in the pleural space should resolve.

Congestive Heart Failure

Because the systemic venous pressure is very likely to be elevated following the Fontan procedure, some indicators of congestive heart failure (jugular venous distension, hepatomegaly) may be misleading. Nonetheless, congestive heart failure with ventricular dilation and elevated end-diastolic pressure should not be a feature of the postoperative recovery following the Fontan procedure unless an unusually long CPB time is required for the repair. More often, congestive heart failure is the result of an anatomic problem with the repair. Subaortic obstruction (discussion follows), atrioventricular valve regurgitation, coronary artery occlusion, and certain arrhythmias can cause signs of congestive heart failure and must be ruled out. Echocardiography, a 12-lead ECG, and, frequently, cardiac catheterization are likely to be required to completely evaluate these issues.

In the less common patient, whose Fontan procedure included a ventriculotomy, who required a longer-than-usual CPB time, or who developed complete heart block during or after surgery requiring pacing, congestive heart failure may be the result of ventricular dysfunction or loss of atrioventricular sequential contraction, with no other contributing factors. In this setting, support with inotropic agents may be necessary for relatively prolonged periods. When pacing is necessary, sequential atrioventricular pacing may be important in promoting pulmonary blood flow.

Aortic Obstruction

It is not unusual for patients who have had no obstruction to aortic flow prior to a Fontan procedure to develop acute subaortic stenosis immediately after surgery.[152–154] This is probably more likely to occur when the aorta arises from a hypoplastic ventricle or when there is subaortic conus or abnormal atrioventricular valve tissue (Table 21-7). Subaortic obstruction must be suspected in patients who have a new, loud murmur following surgery, especially in the setting of congestive heart failure. In this situation, an aggressive approach toward diagnosis, often with cardiac catheterization, and reoperation is appropriate.

Table 21-7. Incidence of subaortic stenosis following the Fontan procedure

Type of heart	No. of Fontan operations	No. with postop SAS
Tricuspid atresia	92	0
Tricuspid atresia and TGA	23	1
Single LV and TGA	106	6
Single RV	35	3
AV and VA discordance with RV, hypoplasia	2	1
Pulmonary atresia intact septum	10	1
Others	38	0

SAS, subaortic stenosis; TGA, transposition of the great arteries; LV, left ventricle; RV, right ventricle; AV, atrioventricular; VA, ventriculoarterial.
From AJ Razzouk et al. The recognition, identification or morphologic substrate, and treatment of subaortic stenosis after a Fontan procedure. *J Thorac Cardiovasc Surg* 104:938–944, 1992. With permission.

References

1. Benacerraf BR, Sanders SP. Fetal echocardiography. *Radiol Clin North Am* 28:131–147, 1990.

2. Benacerraf BR, Pober BR, Sanders SP. Accuracy of fetal echocardiography. *Radiology* 165:847–849, 1987.

3. Bromley B et al. Fetal echocardiography: Accuracy and limitations in a population at high risk and low risk for heart defects. *Am J Obstet Gynecol* 166:1473–1481, 1992.

4. Brown DL et al. Sonography of the fetal heart: Normal variants and pitfalls. *AJR* 160:1251–1255, 1993.

5. Cullen S et al. Potential impact of population screening for prenatal diagnosis of congenital heart disease. *Arch Dis Child* 67:775–778, 1992.

6. Sanders SP. Echocardiography and related techniques in the diagnosis of congenital heart defects. Part I: Veins and atria. *Echocardiography* 1:250–332, 1984.

7. Sanders SP. Echocardiography and related techniques in the diagnosis of congenital heart defects. Part II: Atrioventricular valves and ventricles. *Echocardiography* 1:333–386, 1984.

8. Sanders SP. Echocardiography and related techniques in the diagnosis of congenital heart defects. Part III: Conotruncus and great arteries. *Echocardiography* 1:443–493, 1984.

9. Stark J et al. Surgery for congenital heart defects diagnosed with cross-sectional echocardiography. *Circulation* 68:II129–II138, 1983.

10. Leung MP et al. The role of cross sectional echocardiography and pulsed Doppler ultrasound in the management of neonates in whom congenital heart disease is suspected: A prospective study. *Br Heart J* 56:73–82, 1986.

11. Freed MD et al. Is routine preoperative cardiac catheterization necessary before repair of secundum and sinus venosus atrial septal defects? *J Am Coll Cardiol* 4:333–336, 1984.

12. Huhta JC et al. Surgery without cathterization for congenital heart defects: Management of 100 patients. *J Am Coll Cardiol* 9:823–829, 1987.

13. Sreeram N et al. Changing role of non-invasive investigation in the preoperative assessment of congenital heart disease: A nine year experience. *Br Heart J* 63:345–349, 1990.

14. Lang P et al. Use of prostaglandin E1 in infants with d-transposition of the great arteries and intact ventricular septum. *Am J Cardiol* 44:76–81, 1979.

15. Indeglia RA et al. Treatment of transposition of the great vessels with an intra-atrial baffle (Mustard procedure). *Arch Surg* 101:797–805, 1970.

16. Elliott RB, Starling MB, Neutze JM. Medical manipulation of the ductus arteriosus. *Lancet* 1:140–142, 1975.

17. Lang P et al. The use of prostaglandin E1 in an infant with interruption of the aortic arch. *J Pediatr* 91:805–807, 1977.

18. Castañeda AR et al. Transposition of the great arteries and intact ventricular septum: Anatomical repair in the neonate. *Ann Thorac Surg* 38:438–443, 1984.

19. Joshi SV, Brawn WJ, Mee RB. Pulmonary atresia with intact ventricular septum. *J Thorac Cardiovasc Surg* 91:192–199, 1986.

20. Murphy JD et al. Hemodynamic results after intracardiac repair of tetralogy of Fallot by deep hypothermia and cardiopulmonary bypass. *Circulation* 62:I168, 1980.

21. Norwood WI et al. Reparative operations for interrupted aortic arch with ventricular septal defect. *J Thorac Cardiovasc Surg* 86:832–837, 1983.

22. Sell JE et al. The results of a surgical program for interrupted aortic arch. *J Thorac Cardiovasc Surg* 96:864–877, 1988.

23. Fontan F, Baudet E. Surgical repair of tricuspid atresia. *Thorax* 26:240–248, 1971.

24. McGoon DC et al. Correction of complete atrioventricular canal in infants. *Mayo Clin Proc* 48:769–772, 1973.

25. Moulton AL, Bowman FO. Primary definitive repair of type B interrupted aortic arch, ventricular septal defect, and patent ductus arteriosus. *J Thorac Cardiovasc Surg* 82:501–510, 1981.

26. Lang P, Norwood WI. Hemodynamic assessment after palliative surgery for hypoplastic left heart syndrome. *Circulation* 68:104–108, 1983.

27. Norwood WI et al. Experience with operations for hypolastic left heart syndrome. *J Thorac Cardiovasc Surg* 82:511–519, 1981.

28. Senning A. Surgical correction of transposition of the great vessels. *Surgery* 45:966, 1959.

29. Mustard WT. Successful two-stage correction of transposition of the great vessels. *Surgery* 55:469, 1964.

30. Castañeda AR et al. The early results of treatment of simple transposition in the current era. *J Thorac Cardiovasc Surg* 95:14–28, 1988.

31. Quaegebeur JM et al. The arterial switch operation: An eight-year experience. *J Thorac Cardiovasc Surg* 361:384, 1986.

32. Graham TP et al. Abnormalities of right ventricular function following Mustard's operation for transposition of the great arteries. *Circulation* 52:678–684, 1975.

33. Jatene AD et al. Successful anatomic correction of transposition of the great vessels. A preliminary report. *Arq Bras Cardiol* 28:461–464, 1975.

34. Wernovsky G et al. Midterm results after the arterial switch operation for transposition of the great arteries with intact ventricular septum: Clinical, hemodynamic, echocardiographic, and electrophysiologic data. *Circulation* 77:1333–1344, 1988.

35. Lock JE et al. Transcatheter closure of atrial septal defects: Experimental studies. *Circulation* 79:1091–1099, 1989.

36. Blalock A, Hanlon CR. The surgical treatment of complete transposition of the aorta and the pulmonary artery. *Surg Gynecol Obstet* 91:1, 1950.

37. Blalock A, Taussig HB. The surgical treatment of malformations of the heart in which there is pulmonary artery stenosis or pulmonary atresia. *JAMA* 128:189, 1945.

38. Gibbon JH Jr. The maintenance of life during experimental occlusion of the pulmonary artery followed by survival. *Surg Gynecol Obstet* 69:602, 1939.

39. Gibbon JH Jr. Application of a mechanical heart and lung apparatus to cardiac surgery. In *Recent Advances in Cardiovascular Physiology and Surgery.* Minneapolis: University of Minnesota, 1953. Pp 107–113.

40. Warden HE et al. Controlled cross circulation for open intracardiac surgery. *J Thorac Surg* 28:311, 1954.

41. Kirklin JW et al. Intracardiac surgery with the aid of a mechanical pump-oxygenator system (Gibbon type): Report of eight cases. *Proc Staff Meet Mayo Clin* 30:201, 1955.

42. Croughwell N et al. The effect of temperature on cerebral metabolism and blood flow in adults during cardiopulmonary bypass. *J Thorac Cardiovasc Surg* 103:549, 1992.

43. Kirklin JK et al. Complement and the damaging effects of cardiopulmonary bypass. *J Thorac Cardiovasc Surg* 86:845, 1983.

44. Ross DN. Hypothermia. II. Physiological observations during hypothermia. *Guy's Hosp Rep* 103:116, 1954.

45. Bigelow WG et al. Oxygen transport and utilization in dogs at low body temperatures. *Am J Physiol* 160:125, 1950.

46. Bigelow WG, Lindsay WK, Greenwood WF. Hypothermia—Its possible role in cardiac surgery: An investigation of factors governing survival in dogs at low body temperatures. *Ann Surg* 132:849, 1950.

47. Lewis FS, Taufic M. Closure of atrial septal defects with the aid of hypothermia: Experimental accomplishments and the report of one successful case. *Surgery* 33:52, 1953.

48. Swan H et al. Surgery by direct vision in the open heart during hypothermia. *JAMA* 153:1081, 1953.

49. Neutze JM et al. Serum enzymes after cardiac surgery using cardiopulmonary bypass. *Am Heart J* 88:425, 1974.

50. Pagliero M, Blackstone EH, Kirklin JW. Myocardial protection during cardiac surgery with cardiopulmonary bypass. In Kirklin JW, Barratt-Boyes BG (eds): *Cardiac Surgery.* New York: Churchill Livingstone, 1986. Pp 84–86.

51. Pagliero M, Blackstone EH, Kirklin JW. Myocardial protection during cardiac surgery with cardiopulmonary bypass. In Kirklin JW, Barratt-

Boyes BG (eds): *Cardiac Surgery.* New York: Churchill Livingstone, 1986. P 85.

52. Jennings RB et al. Myocardial necrosis induced by temporary occlusion of a coronary artery in the dog. *Arch Pathol Lab Med* 70:82, 1960.
53. Follette DM et al. Reducing reperfusion injury with hypocalcemic, hyperkalemic, alkalotic blood during reoxygenation. *Surg Forum* 29:284, 1978.
54. Martin AM Jr, Hackel DB. An electron microscopic study of the progression of myocardial lesions in the dog after hemorrhage shock. *Lab Invest* 15:243, 1966.
55. Mueller HS, Evans R, Ayers SM. Effect of dopamine on hemodynamics and myocardial metabolism in shock following acute myocarial infarction in man. *Circulation* 57:361, 1978.
56. Piscatelli RL, Fox LM. Myocardial injury from epinephrine overdosage. *Am J Cardiol* 21:735, 1968.
57. Casale AS et al. Progression and resolution of myocardial reflow injury. *J Surg Res* 37:94, 1984.
58. Follette DM et al. Prolonged safe aortic clamping by combining membrane stabilization, multidose cardioplegia and appropriate pH reperfusion. *J Thorac Cardiovasc Surg* 74:682, 1977.
59. Elixson EM. Hemodynamic monitoring modalities in pediatric cardiac surgical patients. *Crit Care Nurs Clin North Am* 1:263–273, 1989.
60. Gold JP et al. Transthoracic intracardiac monitoring lines in pediatric surgical patients: A ten-year experience. *Ann Thorac Surg* 42:185–191, 1986.
61. Parr GV, Blackstone EH, Kirklin JW. Cardiac performance and mortality early after intracardiac surgery in infants and young children. *Circulation* 51:867–874, 1975.
62. Williams EC. Catheter-related thrombosis. *Clin Cardiol* 13: VI34–VI36, 1990.
63. Fenn JE, Stansel HC Jr. Certain hazards of the central venous catheter. *Angiology* 20:38–43, 1969.
64. Langston CS. The aberrant central venous catheter and its complications. *Diagn Radiol* 100:55–59, 1971.
65. Dato V, Dajani A. Candidemia in children with central venous catheters: The role of catheter removal and Amphotericin B treatment. *Pediatr Infect Dis J* 9:309–314, 1990.
66. Mariano BP Jr, Roper CL, Staple TW. Accidental migration of an intravenous infusion catheter from the arm to the lung. *Radiology* 86:736–738, 1966.
67. Hausdorf G et al. Intra-atrial malpositions of Silastic catheters in newborns. *Crit Care Med* 15:308–309, 1987.
68. Conwell JA, Cocalis MW, Erickson LC. EAT to the beat: "Ectopic" atrial tachycardia caused by catheter whip. *Lancet* 342:740, 1993.
69. Chi TL, Krovetz LJ. The pulmonary vascular bed in children with Down syndrome. *J Pediatr* 86:533–538, 1975.
70. Wilson SK, Hutchins GN, Neill CA. Hypertensive pulmonary vascular disease in Down syndrome. *J Pediatr* 95:722–726, 1979.
71. Vincent RN et al. Assessment of hemodynamic status in the intensive care unit immediately after closure of ventricular septal defect. *Am J Cardiol* 55:526–529, 1984.
72. Geha DG, Davis NJ, Lappas DG. Persistent atrial arrhythmias associated with placement of a Swan-Ganz catheter. *Anesthesiology* 39: 651–653, 1973.
73. Elliott CG, Zimmerman GA, Clemmer TP. Complications of pulmonary artery catheterization in the care of critically ill patients: A prospective study. *Chest* 76:647–652, 1979.
74. Royston D. High-dose aprotinin therapy: A review of the first five years' experience. *J Cardiothorac Vasc Anesth* 6:76–100, 1992.
75. Hickey PR et al. Blunting of stress responses in the pulmonary circulation of infants by fentanyl. *Anesth Analg* 64:1137–1142, 1985.
76. Hickey PR et al. Pulmonary and systemic hemodynamic responses to fentanyl in infants. *Anesth Analg* 64:483–486, 1985.
77. Williams DB et al. Hemodynamic response to positive end-expiratory pressure following right atrium-pulmonary artery bypass (Fontan procedure). *J Thorac Cardiovasc Surg* 87:856–861, 1984.

78. Outwater KM et al. Renal and hemodynamic effects of dopamine in infants following cardiac surgery. *J Clin Anesth* 2:253–257, 1990.
79. Lang P et al. The hemodynamic effects of dopamine in infants after corrective cardiac surgery. *J Pediatr* 96:630–634, 1980.
80. Appelbaum A et al. Afterload reduction and cardiac output in infants early after intracardiac surgery. *Circulation* 39:445–451, 1977.
81. Ivankovich AD. Sodium nitroprusside: Metabolism and general considerations. *Int Anesthesiol Clin* 16:1, 1978.
82. Levy JH, Bailey JM. Amrinone: Pharmacokinetics and pharmacodynamics. *J Cardiothorac Anesth* 3(Suppl 2):10–14, 1989.
83. Rubin LJ et al. Treatment of primary pulmonary hypertension with continuous intravenous prostacyclin (Epoprostenol): Results of a randomized trial. *Ann Intern Med* 112:485–491, 1990.
84. Morray JP, Lynn AM, Mansfield PB. Effect of pH and PCO$_2$ on pulmonary and systemic hemodynamics after surgery in children with congenital heart disease and pulmonary hypertension. *J Pediatr* 113:474–479, 1988.
85. Frostell C et al. Inhaled nitric oxide: A selective pulmonary vasodilator reversing hypoxic pulmonary vasoconstriction. *Circulation* 83: 2038–2047, 1991.
86. Roberts JD Jr et al. Inhaled nitric oxide in congenital heart disease. *Circulation* 87:447–453, 1993.
87. Rossaint R et al. Inhaled nitric oxide for the adult respiratory distress syndrome. *N Engl J Med* 328:399–405, 1993.
88. Roberts JD Jr et al. Inhaled nitric oxide in persistent pulmonary hypertension of the newborn. *Lancet* 340:818–819, 1992.
89. Paddock FK. The diagnostic significance of serous fluids in disease. *N Engl J Med* 223:1010–1015, 1940.
90. Agostoni E, Tagleitti A, Setnikar I. Absorption force of the capillaries of the visceral pleura in determination of the intrapleural pressure. *Am J Physiol* 191:277–282, 1957.
91. Lamberti JJ. Palliation of the uni-ventricular heart without increasing ventricular work. *Ann Thorac Surg* 510:882–883, 1991.
92. Laks H. The partial Fontan procedure: A new concept and its clinical application. *Circulation* 82:1866–1867, 1990.
93. Bridges ND et al. Bidirectional cavopulmonary anastomosis as interim palliation for high-risk Fontan candidates: Early results. *Circulation* 82:IV170–IV176, 1990.
94. Trusler GA et al. The cavopulmonary shunt: Evolution of a concept. *Circulation* 82:IV131–IV138, 1990.
95. Bridges ND et al. Bidirectional cavopulmonary anastomosis as interim palliation for high-risk Fontan candidates. Early results. *Circulation* 82:IV170–IV176, 1990.
96. Bridges ND, Lock JE, Castañeda AR. Baffle fenestration with subsequent transcatheter closure: Modification of the Fontan operation for patients at increased risk. *Circulation* 82:1681–1689, 1990.
97. Laks H et al. Partial Fontan: Advantages of an adjustable interatrial communication. *Ann Thorac Surg* 52:1084–1095, 1991.
98. Bridges ND et al. Effect of baffle fenestration on outcome of the modified Fontan operation. *Circulation* 86:1762–1769, 1992.
99. Bridges ND, Castañeda AR. The fenestrated Fontan procedure. *Herz* 17:242–245, 1992.
100. Mair DD et al. Early and late results of the modified Fontan procedure for double-inlet left ventricle: The Mayo Clinic experience. *J Am Coll Cardiol* 18:1727–1732, 1991.
101. Sanders SP et al. Clinical and hemodynamic results of the Fontan operation for tricuspid atresia. *Am J Cardiol* 49:1733–1740, 1982.
102. Mayer JE et al. Extending the limits for modified Fontan procedures. *J Thorac Cardiovasc Surg* 92:1021–1028, 1986.
103. Farrell PE Jr et al. Outcome and assessment after the modified Fontan procedure for hypoplastic left heart syndrome. *Circulation* 85:116–122, 1992.
104. Cohen AJ et al. Results of the Fontan procedure for patients with univentricular heart: *Ann Thorac Surg* 52:1266–1271, 1991.
105. Lamberti JJ et al. The Damus-Fontan procedure. *Ann Thorac Surg* 52:676–679, 1991.
106. Choussat A et al. Selection criteria for Fontan's procedure. In Ander-

son RH, Shinebourne EA (eds): *Pediatric Cardiology 1977.* Edinburgh: Churchill Livingstone, 1978. Pp 559–566.

107. O'Brien P, Elixson EM. The child following the Fontan procedure: Nursing strategies. *AACN Clin Issues Crit Care Nurs* 1:46–58, 1990.

108. Mayer JE Jr et al. Extending the limits for modified Fontan procedures. *J Thorac Cardiovasc Surg* 92:1021–1028, 1986.

109. Jonas RA, Castañeda AR. Modified Fontan procedure: Atrial baffle and systemic venous to pulmonary artery anastomotic techniques. *J Cardiol Surg* 3:91–96, 1988.

110. Light RW et al. Pleural effusions: The diagnostic separation of transudates and exudates. *Ann Intern Med* 77:507–513, 1972.

111. Stewart RW, Blackstone EH, Kirklin JW. Neurological dysfunction after cardiac surgery. In Parenzan L, Crupi G, Graham G (eds): *Congenital Heart Disease in the First Three Months of Life. Medical and Surgical Aspects.* Bologna, Italy: Patron Editore, 1981. P 431.

112. Barratt-Boyes BG et al. Repair of ventricular septal defect in the first two years of life using profound hypopthermic-circulatory arrest techniques. *Ann Surg* 184:376, 1976.

113. Belsey RHR, Keen G, Skinner DB. Profound hypothermia in cardiac surgery. *J Thorac Cardiovasc Surg* 56:497, 1968.

114. Venugopal P et al. Early correction of congenital heart disease with surface-induced deep hypothermia and circulatory arrest. *J Thorac Cardiovasc Surg* 66:375, 1973.

115. Newburger JW et al. A comparison of the perioperative neurologic effects of hypothermic circulatory arrest versus low-flow cardiopulmonary bypass in infant heart surgery. *N Engl J Med* 329:1057–1064, 1993.

116. Clarkson PM et al. Developmental progress following cardiac surgery in infancy using profound hypothermia and circulatory arrest. *Circulation* 62:855, 1980.

117. Brunberg JA, Reilly EL, Doty DB. Central nervous system consequences in infants of cardiac surgery using deep hypothermia and circulatory arrest. *Circulation* 49:II11, 1973.

118. Bergouignan M et al. Syndromes choreiformes de l'enfant au décours d'interventions cardiochirurgicales sous hypothermie profonde. *Rev Neurol (Paris)* 105:48, 1961.

119. Chiang J et al. Cerebral ischemia. III. Vascular changes. *Am J Pathol* 52:455, 1968.

120. Hallenbeck JM, Bradley ME. Experimental model for systematic study of impaired microvascular reperfusion. *Stroke* 8:23, 1977.

121. Hallenbeck JM. Prevention of postischemic impairment of microvascular perfusion. *Neurology* 27:3, 1977.

122. Olsson Y, Hossmann KA. The effect of intravascular saline perfusion on the sequelae of transient cerebral ischemia. *Acta Neuropathol* 17:68, 1971.

123. Egerton N, Egerton WS, Kay JH. Neurologic changes following profound hypothermia. *Ann Surg* 157:366, 1963.

124. Davis FM, Parinelazhagan KN, Harris EA. Thermal balance during cardiopulmonary bypass with hypothermia in man. *Br J Anaesth* 49:1127, 1977.

125. Moulopoulos SD, Topaz S, Kolff WJ. Diastolic balloon pumping (with carbon dioxide) in the aorta—A mechanical assistance to the failing circulation. *Am Heart J* 63:669, 1962.

126. Kantrowitz A et al. Initial clinical experience with intraaortic balloon pumping in cardiogenic shock. *JAMA* 203:113, 1968.

127. Downing TP et al. Use of the intra-aortic balloon pump after valve replacement. Predictive indices, correlative parameters, and patient survival. *J Thorac Cardiovasc Surg* 94:210, 1986.

128. Corrigan JJ Jr. Coagulation disorders. In Miller DR, Baehner RL (eds): *Blood Diseases of Infancy and Childhood* (6th ed). St. Louis: Mosby, 1989. P 885–887.

129. Ellison RC et al. Evaluation of the preterm infant for patent ductus arteriosus. *Pediatrics* 71:364–372, 1983.

130. Schenck MH et al. Transcatheter occlusion of patent ductus arteriosus in adults. *Am J Cardiol* 72:591–595, 1993.

131. Rashkind WJ et al. Nonsurgical closure of patent ductus arteriosus: Clinical application of the Rashkind PDA occluder system. *Circulation* 75:583–592, 1987.

132. Latson LA et al. Transcatheter closure of patent ductus arteriosus in pediatric patients. *J Pediatr* 115:549–553, 1989.

133. Lloyd TR et al. Transcatheter occlusion of patent ductus arteriosus with Gianturco coils. *Circulation* 88:II1412–II1420, 1993.

134. Bridges ND et al. Transcatheter closure of a large patent ductus arteriosus with the clamshell septal umbrella. *J Am Coll Cardiol* 18:1297–1302, 1991.

135. Rao PS et al. Transcatheter occlusion of patent ductus arteriosus with adjustable buttoned device: Initial clinical experience. *Circulation* 88:1119–1126, 1993.

136. Jones JC. Twenty-five years' experience with the surgery of patent ductus arteriosus. *J Thorac Cardiovasc Surg* 50:149–165, 1965.

137. Fleming WH et al. Ligation of patent ductus arteriosus in premature infants: Importance of accurate anatomic definition. *Pediatrics* 71:373–375, 1983.

138. Lloyd TR et al. Atrial septal defect occlusion with the buttoned device (a multi-institutional U.S. trial). *Am J Cardiol* 73:286–291, 1994.

139. Rome JJ et al. Double-umbrella closure of atrial defects: Initial clinical applications. *Circulation* 82:751–758, 1990.

140. Jatene AD et al. Anatomic correction of transposition of the great vessels. *J Thorac Cardiovasc Surg* 72:364–370, 1976.

141. Konno S et al. A new method for prosthetic valve replacement in congenital aortic stenosis associated with hypoplasia of the aortic valve ring. Early and late results of aortic valvotomy. *J Thorac Cardiovasc Surg* 70:909, 1975.

142. Misbach GA et al. Left ventricular outflow enlargement by the Konno procedure. *J Thorac Cardiovasc Surg* 84:696, 1982.

143. Ross D. Replacement of the aortic valve with a pulmonary autograft: The "switch" operation. *Ann Thorac Surg* 52:1346–1350, 1991.

144. van der Velde ME et al. Two-dimensional echocardiography in the pre- and postoperative management of totally anomalous pulmonary venous connection. *J Am Coll Cardiol* 18:1746–1751, 1991.

145. Sreeram N, Walsh K. Diagnosis of total anomalous pulmonary venous drainage by Doppler color flow imaging. *J Am Coll Cardiol* 19:1577–1582, 1992.

146. Goswami KC et al. Echocardiographic diagnosis of total anomalous pulmonary venous connection. *Am Heart J* 126:433–440, 1993.

147. Pearl JM et al. Total cavopulmonary anastomosis versus conventional modified Fontan procedure. *Ann Thorac Surg* 52:189–196, 1991.

148. Lamberti JJ et al. The bidirectional cavopulmonary shunt. *J Thorac Cardiovasc Surg* 100:22–30, 1990.

149. Douville EC, Sade RM, Fyfe DA. Hemi-Fontan operation for single ventricle: A preliminary report. *Ann Thorac Surg* 51:893–900, 1991.

150. Douville EC, Sade RM, Fyfe DA. Hemi-Fontan operation in surgery for single ventricle: A preliminary report [see comments]. *Ann Thorac Surg* 51:893–900, 1991.

151. Kopf GS et al. Fenestrated Fontan operation with delayed transcatheter closure of atrial septal defect: Improved results in high-risk patients. *J Thorac Cardiovasc Surg* 103:1039–1048, 1992.

152. Razzouk AJ et al. The recognition, identification or morphologic substrate, and treatment of subaortic stenosis after a Fontan procedure. *J Thorac Cardiovasc Surg* 104:938–944, 1992.

153. Coté CJ, Ryan JF, Todres ID, Goudsouzian NG. *A Practice of Anesthesia for Infants and Children* (2nd ed). Philadelphia: Saunders, 1993.

154. Reed CC, Stafford T. *Cardiopulmonary Perfusion* (2nd ed.). Houston: Texas Medical, 1985.

Lars C. Erickson

E. Marsha Elixson

22 ▷ Medical Issues for the Cardiac Patient

Congestive Heart Failure

The fundamental function of the heart is to pump a sufficient volume of blood at a sufficient pressure to meet the metabolic demands of the body. As the demands of the tissues increase, a number of compensatory mechanisms come into play: (1) The heart rate increases under the influence of neural and humoral input; (2) the contractility of the ventricle increases in response to circulating catecholamines and autonomic input; (3) the venous capacitance vessels constrict; and (4) the kidneys retain intravascular volume, increasing venous pressure, which, in turn, results in increased filling of the heart and an increased stroke volume. In this fashion, changes in demand result in changes in cardiac output.

As the demand placed on the heart increases (as with a large intracardiac shunt), or the capacity of the heart to meet that demand falls (as with ventricular dysfunction following surgery), the heart rate and venous pressure continue to rise, leading to signs and symptoms of venous congestion, or "compensated" congestive heart failure. As further increases in demand overwhelm these compensatory mechanisms, cardiac output cannot be increased to meet the needs of the body. This represents "decompensated" congestive heart failure.

To understand the features of congestive heart failure and its treatment, it is necessary to explore a few basic concepts in cardiac function.

Starling Relationship

The Starling relationship states that the heart contracts more vigorously when filled with a larger volume of blood. This feature of myocardial contractility is crucial in allowing the heart to respond to the changing needs of the circulation. The Starling relationship can be graphically presented if a measure of myocardial contractility (e.g., end-systolic pressure) is plotted against a measure of ventricular filling (e.g., end-diastolic volume). Over the range of physiologic values, this relationship is essentially a straight line (Fig. 22-1).

The Starling relationship is essentially an expression of the systolic function, or contractility, of the ventricle. If the myocardium is weakened, there will be less vigorous contraction for a given degree of ventricular filling. The line representing the Starling relationship will be lower.

LaPlace's Law

LaPlace's Law is a function describing the stress on the wall of a chamber that is resisting pressure.

$$\text{Wall Stress} = \frac{(\text{Pressure} \times \text{Radius})}{(2 \times \text{Wall Thickness})}$$

Wall stress is a measure of how much force the walls of a chamber can exert and is independent of loading conditions. One of the features of LaPlace's Law is that as a chamber's radius gets larger, the walls exert less pressure on its contents. A practical example of this is a toy balloon, which is very hard to inflate when it is just beginning to fill, but very easy to inflate as it gets bigger. The application of this law to the heart suggests that as the heart dilates, its ability to pump is reduced (Fig. 22-2).

LaPlace's Law suggests that the Starling relationship cannot be linear indefinitely; increased filling will lead eventually to an increasing mechanical disadvantage for the ventricle as it dilates. The phenomenon of failing cardiac function when filling is increased beyond a certain point is often called "falling off the Starling Curve." In fact, it can be largely explained on the basis of LaPlace's Law. This relationship is also the reason that decreasing preload (e.g., with diuretics) can result in an increase in cardiac output when the heart is dilated.

Diastolic Function

Another factor that plays an important role in congestive heart failure is diastolic function, or the compliance of the ventricle. Compliance is a measure of how much something will stretch for an increase in tension:

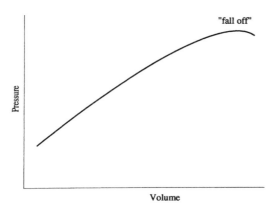

Figure 22-1. Starling relationship.

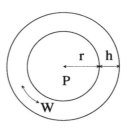

$$W = Pr/2h$$

W   wall stress
P   pressure
r   radius
h   wall thickness

Figure 22-2. LaPlace's law. W, wall stress; P, pressure; r, radius; h, wall thickness.

$$\text{Compliance} = \frac{\text{Change in Dimension}}{\text{Change in Tension}}$$

For a filling ventricle, for example:

$$\text{Compliance} = \frac{\text{Change in Volume}}{\text{Change in Diastolic Pressure}}$$

The heart is basically a sack made up of a material that is somewhat elastic. Like a rubber band, the heart can be stretched rather easily up to a point, but as its limit of distensibility is approached, more and more effort is required to stretch it further. In other words, the more dilated a heart becomes, the harder it is to fill further. This is graphically represented in Fig. 22-3. Venous pressure can only rise so high, usually 25 to 30 mm Hg, before further increases in pressure result in transudation of intravascular fluid and venous dilation. Consequently, there is a limit to how much preload can be increased to augment cardiac output.

Course of Congestive Heart Failure

Congestive heart failure occurs when the demands on the heart to pump blood exceed its capacity. As the demand increases, compensatory mechanisms that come into play ultimately reach their limit of effectiveness and cardiac output slips behind demand.

The first compensatory mechanism that comes into play is an increase in heart rate. Cardiac output is the product of heart rate and stroke volume. As long as there is sufficient time for ventricular filling during diastole, an increase in heart rate is a very effective way to compensate for an inadequate cardiac output. There is always an optimal maximum heart rate, however, beyond which there is insufficient time for ventricular filling during diastole. Further increases in heart rate beyond the optimal rate will result in a drop in stroke volume and decreased, rather than increased, cardiac output. The optimal heart rate varies with each patient and depends on myocardial contractility and loading conditions. For those patients in whom the heart rate is under pharmacologic (e.g., isoproterenol) or electrical (e.g., electronically paced) control, the optimal heart rate may be determined by experimentation.

As the demands on the heart increase relative to its capacity, increases in heart rate may no longer result in an adequate cardiac output. Constriction of the venous capacitance vessels and retention of fluid by the kidney result in an increased preload, stimulating an increased cardiac output, according to the Starling relationship. As the venous pressure rises, however, signs and symptoms of venous congestion become apparent (Table 22-1).

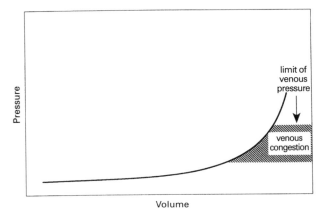

Figure 22-3. Diastolic function.

Table 22-1. Signs and symptoms of congestive heart failure

Tachycardia
Venous congestion
  Right-sided
    Hepatomegaly
    Ascites
    Pleural effusions
    Edema
    Jugular venous distension
  Left-sided
    Tachypnea
    Retractions
    Nasal flaring
    Rales
    Pulmonary edema
Low cardiac output
  Fatigue, low energy
  Pallor
  Sweating
  Cold extremities
  Feeling of coldness
  Poor growth
  Dizziness
  Obtundation
  Syncope

Right-sided congestive heart failure results in elevated systemic venous pressure. In infants, this is manifested by hepatomegaly, which can progress to congestive hepatic dysfunction when present chronically. Right-sided venous congestion also can result in pleural, pericardial, and ascitic effusions. Edema may be present in older children and in the fetus that develops congestive heart failure in utero (fetal hydrops), but is uncommon in infants except in the setting of infection or hypoproteinemia, or after cardiopulmonary bypass or deep hypothermic arrest.

Left-sided venous congestion results in transudation of fluid into the pulmonary parenchyma. The earliest manifestation of this is tachypnea, followed by rales and a radiographic appearance of pulmonary edema.

Right- and left-sided venous congestion may be hard to separate in the analysis of a child with congestive heart failure. Elevated pulmonary venous pressure can lead to pulmonary artery hypertension and right-sided congestive heart failure. In addition, right-sided congestive heart failure with right ventricular dilation can actually impair left ventricular filling due to mechanical distortion of the ventricle in diastole.

Eventually, elevation of venous pressure reaches its limit, and any further increase does not result in increased cardiac output. This can be related to the mechanical disadvantage caused by ventricular dilation (LaPlace's Law) or simply because the venous system cannot generate a higher pressure because of capillary leak and vessel dilation. By the time this stage is reached, the patient usually appears ill.

As the compensatory mechanisms near their maximum, the cardiac output begins to fall, resulting in "decompensated" congestive heart failure. A fall in cardiac output triggers an increase in sympathetic autonomic activity and circulating catecholamines, which help preserve myocardial contractility. The increase in catecholamines may produce sweating in infants and adults, and in the former, sweating may be particularly prominent during feeding when the demand on the heart is increased.

The signs of an inadequate cardiac output in infants include cool extremities, pallor, and irritability. Failure to gain weight (failure to thrive) is common in severe congestive heart failure. Symptoms of an inadequate cardiac output in older children and adults include cool extremities (or a general feeling of coldness), dizziness, confusion, and syncope. The complaints of fatigue and "low energy" are common as well.

Treatment of Congestive Heart Failure

The treatment of congestive heart failure relies on (1) improving cardiac contractility, (2) reducing cardiac work, and (3) relieving venous congestion.

Improving Contractility

As mentioned, myocardial contractility can be improved with a variety of inotropes, including cardiac glycosides, catecholamines, and amrinone. Each inotropic agent has unique advantages and disadvantages that must be considered.

Digoxin

The only practical oral inotrope is digoxin, a cardiac glycoside. Although it produces a relatively weak inotropic effect compared with the other agents discussed in this section, digoxin is available as an oral preparation and is not associated with clinically significant side effects at nontoxic serum levels. The average half-life of digoxin in children and adults is approximately 34 hours,[1] but can be quite variable. The half-life of digoxin in premature infants may be much longer,[2] possibly because of reduced renal function in this group of patients.

Because of a large volume of distribution, a loading dose of digoxin is required if therapeutic serum levels are required within a short period (Table 22-2). In obese patients, lower loading doses may be required, because digoxin is not significantly absorbed by adipose tissue. Alternatively, many physicians prefer to start with the maintenance dose without a loading dose in the non-urgent setting, realizing that a therapeutic serum level will develop slowly. This approach is justifiable in that most episodes of digoxin toxicity occur in association with the loading dose.[3] Serum levels of digoxin are of limited usefulness because they tend to be inaccurate using current assays, and in children with normal renal function, it may be reasonable to forgo serum testing. When following serum levels, values of 1.1 to 1.7 ng/ml are appropriate for all ages.[4–7]

Table 22-2. Digoxin dosing

	Total oral digitalizing dose ($\mu g/kg$)*	Maintenance oral dose ($\mu g/kg/d$)
Premature newborn (<37 wk)	20–25	5
Full-term infant	30	8–10
Infant (<2 yr)	30–40	8–10
Child (>2 yr)	30–40	8–10
Maximum dose	1 mg total	0.250 mg total

*In myocarditis, digitalizing dose is reduced by 25%.
IV dose = 75% PO dose.
From Garson et al,[91] P 2017. Reprinted with permission.

In addition to the initial loading period, digoxin toxicity may occur in association with renal failure (often secondary to low cardiac output and/or the effects of diuretics) or overdose. Digoxin toxicity can also be precipitated by alterations in intestinal flora, such as during the administration of antibiotics, or by concomitant use of agents known to decrease the renal excretion of digoxin, such as amiodarone, quinidine, and verapamil.

The signs of digoxin toxicity in infants and children include poor feeding, gagging, and vomiting. Older children may complain of visual disturbances. Typical electrocardiographic signs of digoxin toxicity include decreased automaticity (e.g., sinus bradycardia) and conduction abnormalities (2-degree and 3-degree heart block), although nearly any rhythm disturbance should raise suspicion of digoxin toxicity in patients taking this medication.

Initial steps in managing digoxin toxicity include discontinuation of digoxin and admission to an intensive care facility in which continuous cardiac monitoring and emergency pacing equipment are available. Hypokalemia can increase the potential for arrhythmias in the setting of digoxin toxicity and must be identified and treated if present. In the presence of life-threatening arrhythmias, treatment with digoxin antibody fragments (Fab) may be necessary. It is important to recognize, however, that treatment with Fab may result in complete withdrawal of digoxin effect and may precipitate acute congestive heart failure in patients who are very dependent on inotropes. Digoxin is not efficiently dialyzed from the serum.

Catecholamines

Intravenous catecholamines generally have a more rapid onset of action and allow greater control than other classes of inotropes. Dobutamine and dopamine are the catecholamines most frequently used for the management of congestive heart failure in an intensive care setting. Both have favorable effects in addition to inotropy: Dobutamine also results in a decrease in systemic vascular resistance, reducing the work of the heart. Dopamine increases flow to the kidneys at low doses, leading to a favorable diuretic effect. For either agent, an initial dose of 5 $\mu g/kg/min$ is often effective, although the rate may be increased to 25 $\mu g/kg/min$ or more if needed. It is unusual that infusion rates in excess of 30 $\mu g/kg/min$ will provide significant additional inotropic effects.

In the presence of bronchospasm, bradycardia, a highly reactive pulmonary vascular bed, or when minimal elevations in pulmonary arteriolar resistance may be important, isoproterenol may be a preferred inotrope, despite its relatively disadvantageous myocardial oxygen supply-demand ratio.

Epinephrine is rarely used for congestive heart failure except in the setting of severely reduced cardiac output and shock. Although it is an excellent inotrope, it has disadvantages that outweigh its advantages in patients who could be managed with other agents. Epinephrine causes a markedly increased peripheral vascular resistance, increasing the work of the heart. It also results in an increased oxygen demand, which may result in further myocardial dysfunction or injury.

Diuretics

Diuretics serve two roles in the management of congestive heart failure in children: They reduce symptomatic venous congestion and help improve ventricular function by reducing ventricular dilation. Diuretics, however can have serious drawbacks in the intensive care unit (ICU) setting. The use of diuretics in patients who are dependent on preload may result in an acute drop in cardiac output. In any patient in whom congestive heart failure is severe, diuretics should be used in combination with an inotrope to help them adapt to any drop in preload that may result. Also, the management of severe congestive heart failure with high doses of diuretics may lead to renal injury or failure or severe electrolyte abnormalities. Specific diuretics have additional risks. Consequently, diuretics must be used with care.

Furosemide is the primary diuretic used in the management of pediatric congestive heart failure. The preferred route is oral, because high serum levels, which are more common with intravenous administration, may be associated with injury to the auditory nerve, resulting in hearing loss. The usual initial dose is 1 mg/kg/dose qd or bid, but doses up to 2 mg/kg/dose tid or qid have been used. At doses in excess of 2 mg/kg/d, it becomes necessary to add spironolactone 1 to 2 mg/kg PO qd to offset some of the potassium-wasting effects of furosemide. Electrolytes and renal function must be followed regularly in all patients receiving more than 2 mg/kg/d of furosemide. A severe metabolic alkalosis is an indication of total body potassium depletion and indicates that additional spironolactone or supplemental potassium chloride may be necessary. Unfortunately, oral potassium supplements are sufficiently unpleasant-tasting that they result in feeding problems in many young children.

More than a modest rise in the blood urea nitrogen (BUN) and creatinine suggests that the drop in preload caused by the use of diuretics is resulting in a drop in peripheral perfusion. These laboratory values should be used to adjust the dose of diuretic to avoid significant renal impairment.

Vasodilators

Agents that reduce systemic vascular resistance decrease the effective pressure that the ventricle must generate for a given stroke volume, resulting in a benefit in congestive heart failure. Vasodilators have an advantage in patients with mitral regurgitation or a ventricular septal defect in that they may allow a decrease in shunt fraction.

Evaluation of the Hypoxemic Newborn

Hypoxemia in the newborn has many possible etiologies, some of which represent medical emergencies. Consequently, timely diagnosis is critical. Most children with hypoxemia present with cyanosis, but it is important to remember that not all children with cyanosis are hypoxemic, and not all hypoxemic children are cyanotic: The perception of cyanosis is less closely related to the arterial oxygen saturation than to the absolute concentration of deoxygenated hemoglobin in the capillary bed, generally between 3 and 5 g/dl, depending on the level of experience of the observer. The result is that infants who are polycythemic may appear cyanotic at relatively high oxygen saturations, whereas very anemic babies may not become cyanotic despite very low oxygen concentrations (Table 22-3).

Furthermore, with reduced blood flow through a capillary bed, the saturation of the capillary blood may be lower than usual, so that children with peripheral vasoconstriction due to low cardiac output, a cold environment, or during the rising phase of a fever can all appear peripherally cyanotic.

Babies who appear cyanotic, dusky, or pale should have a pulse oximeter oxygen saturation or arterial PaO_2 measured for a more quantitative estimate of tissue oxygen levels. Pulse oximetry should be checked in at least two locations: on the ear (optimally) or right hand (preductal) and on a foot (postductal) because a right-

Table 22-3. Cyanosis and hemoglobin levels

Patient	Hemoglobin (gram%)	Approximate arterial saturation below which cyanosis occurs (%)
Anemic	6	33
Normal newborn	15	73
Polycythemic	25	84

Assumes that an observer is able to detect cyanosis at a desaturated hemoglobin level of 4 g/dl and peripheral perfusion is normal.

to-left shunt at a patent ductus arteriosus can present with hypoxemia of the postductal distribution only.

The causes of hypoxemia in newborns can be broadly divided into a few major groups: hemoglobin disorders, pulmonary diseases, and cardiac malformations. Hypoxemia secondary to disorders of hemoglobin is the result of abnormal hemoglobin oxygen affinity and is rare. Pulmonary hypoxemia is the result of deoxygenated blood returning to the heart from the pulmonary veins and may be the result of a mismatch of ventilation and perfusion (e.g., respiratory distress syndrome, atelectasis, pneumonia, right mainstem bronchus intubation). Cardiac hypoxemia is caused by shunting of desaturated blood from the systemic venous return to the systemic output (e.g., right-to-left shunting via atrial or ventricular septal defects or across a patent ductus arteriosus).

Classically, pulmonary hypoxemia has been differentiated from cardiac hypoxemia by examining the response of the arterial PaO_2 to inhaled 100% oxygen (the hyperoxic test). Usually hypoxemia secondary to pulmonary disease will correct to a much greater extent than hypoxemia secondary to cardiac malformations, and in general a PaO_2 greater than 225 mm Hg in 100% oxygen is a strong indication that there is no significant intracardiac right-to-left shunting.

Unfortunately, there are many caveats to this approach. In the case of severe lung disease, even a patient with purely pulmonary hypoxemia may "fail" the hyperoxic test by failing to achieve the cutoff PaO_2. Similarly, PaO_2 may rise considerably in some children with congenital heart disease and right-to-left shunting because of an increase in pulmonary blood flow induced by inhaled oxygen, a potent pulmonary vasodilator. A few patients with intracardiac mixing and enormous pulmonary blood flow (e.g., hypoplastic left heart syndrome) may even achieve oxygen tensions close to the cutoff of 225 mm Hg. Also, intracardiac right-to-left shunting is not always the result of structural heart disease: Severe pulmonary artery hypertension secondary to pulmonary disease (e.g., persistent pulmonary hypertension of the newborn) may result in right-to-left shunting at the foramen ovale and/or ductus arteriosus. Finally, pulmonary "disease" can be the result of an underlying cardiac disorder: Pulmonary venous hypertension secondary to pulmonary vein or mitral valve obstruction can lead to severe pulmonary hypertension and pulmonary edema. Hypoxemia in this setting may be responsive to increased inspired oxygen to the same extent as "primary" pulmonary processes.

Because of all of these limitations to the hyperoxic test, it is important to gather additional information in every child, regardless of the results. A careful physical examination, ECG, chest x-ray, and four-extremity BPs are important in screening for cardiac disease. Echocardiography is a very sensitive test for structural heart disease and can provide information regarding pulmonary artery pressure and intracardiac shunting secondary to pulmonary disease.

Even when no heart disease is suspected on the basis of these tests, it is important to keep in mind that congenital heart disease often becomes hemodynamically significant late in the postnatal period (e.g., ventricular septal defect, patent ductus arteriosus) or may actually develop late (e.g., aortic and pulmonary stenosis, coarctation of the aorta). If a child is not progressing as expected, a second investigation into the possibility of heart disease may be warranted.

The Management of Acute Cardiac Hypoxemia

It is fortunate that most children with cyanotic heart disease have arterial saturations that are compatible with life. Nonetheless, there are certain situations in which cyanosis can be severe enough to endanger the life of the patient. Such situations occur in newborns with transposition of the great arteries, pulmonary atresia, or pulmonary venous obstruction, as well as in older children with acute obstruction to pulmonary blood flow, such as during a hypercyanotic spell in tetralogy of Fallot.

The primary risk of hypoxemia is failure of oxygen delivery to meet the tissue demands. As tissue demands outstrip oxygen delivery, anaerobic metabolism ensues, leading to an accumulation of metabolic acid in the blood. When the tissues run out of substrate for anaerobic metabolism, tissue death ensues. The heart and brain are particularly susceptible to injury by severe hypoxemia.

Fortunately, there are several ways in which to compensate for hypoxemia and maintain a sufficient oxygen supply to the tissues. Oxygen delivery (O_2 Del) is a function of cardiac output (CO) and the oxygen content (O_2 Cont) of the blood:

$$O_2 \text{ Del (ml/min)} = CO \text{ (liter/min)} \times O_2 \text{ Cont (ml/liter)}.$$

It is possible to compensate for hypoxemia to some extent by increasing cardiac output, but the utility of this measure is probably limited for several reasons. In the newborn, there is limited capacity for increasing cardiac output, and in most other patients in whom cyanosis is a problem, increasing the metabolic requirements of the heart by trying to increase output may be detrimental. In life-threatening situations, however, it is appropriate to attempt to increase the cardiac output, preferably using an inotropic agent with predominantly beta effects, such as dobutamine. Agents such as dopamine or epinephrine with prominent alpha effects may reduce tissue perfusion at high doses and further increase the metabolic demands on the heart. In addition to improving oxygen delivery, measures that increase the cardiac output may also result in an increase in systemic venous saturation because of decreased extraction by the tissues. Because cardiac cyanosis is the result of mixing of the systemic and venous returns, any increase in the systemic venous return will result in some increase in the systemic arterial saturation.

Oxygen content can be increased by increasing oxygen carrying capacity or increasing the affinity of hemoglobin for oxygen. Oxygen affinity is described by the oxygen dissociation curve and is a function of hemoglobin phenotype and a variety of physiologic variables, none of which are within the physician's direct control. In response to chronic hypoxemia, the dissociation curve shifts to the left, allowing a higher hemoglobin saturation for a given PaO_2. Newborn infants tolerate hypoxemia remarkably well, largely because of their adaptation to the relative hypoxia of the uterine environment: The systemic arterial saturation of the fetus is about 60%.[8] High levels of fetal hemoglobin, which is also characterized by a leftward shift in the oxygen dissociation curve, in addition to

a relatively high hemoglobin concentration, allow the newborn to tolerate hypoxemia far more readily than a patient with adult hemoglobin and a normal hemoglobin concentration.

Despite its limited usefulness to the physician, hemoglobin type and oxygen affinity are important issues in judging the impact of hypoxemia on a given patient. Shifts in the oxygen dissociation curve due to chronic hypoxemia or high levels of fetal hemoglobin will be diluted by any blood that is transfused into the patient. It should be anticipated that a child with chronic cyanosis, particularly a newborn, will tolerate hypoxia less well in the event of a significant transfusion, even if the hemoglobin concentration remains constant. This fact must be taken into consideration if exchange transfusion, cardiopulmonary bypass, extracorporeal membrane oxygenation (ECMO), or even frequent diagnostic phlebotomy are being considered in the course of therapy.

The primary method under the control of the physician for helping a patient compensate for hypoxemia is by increasing the potential oxygen content of the blood. Oxygen content (O_2 Cont, ml/liter) is chiefly determined by hemoglobin concentration:

$$O_2 \text{ Cont} = [1.36 \times \text{hgb} \times 10 \times \%\text{sat}] + [0.003 \times PaO_2]$$

where hgb is hemoglobin concentration (g/dl) and %sat is percent saturation (expressed as a decimal, e.g., 0.85). The first element of the equation represents the amount of oxygen bound to hemoglobin. The second element of the equation represents the small amount of oxygen dissolved in the serum, where PaO_2 is the partial pressure of oxygen in the serum. This additional oxygen is negligible in room air, but can represent an important contribution to oxygen content in enriched oxygen environments. For the purposes of the following examples, however, the dissolved oxygen can be assumed to be insignificant.

For example, a patient with an arterial oxygen saturation of 100% and a hemoglobin of 15 g/dl (a hematocrit of about 45%) will have an arterial oxygen content of

$$O_2 \text{ Cont} = 1.36 \times 15.0 \times 10 \times 1.00$$
$$= 204 \text{ ml/liter}$$

whereas the same patient with an oxygen saturation of 70% will have an oxygen content of

$$O_2 \text{ Cont} = 1.36 \times 15.0 \times 10 \times 0.70$$
$$= 143 \text{ ml/liter}$$

Hypoxemia is a potent stimulus for erythrocyte production and generally results in a degree of polycythemia proportional to the extent of desaturation. For the patient in this example to achieve the same oxygen carrying capacity with a saturation of 70%, he would have to increase his hemoglobin concentration to 21.4 g/dl, a hematocrit of about 64%.

$$O_2 \text{ Cont} = 1.36 \times 21.4 \times 10 \times 0.70$$
$$= 204 \text{ ml/liter}$$

Because of their reliance on an increased hemoglobin concentration to maintain oxygen delivery, children with hypoxemia must not be allowed to become anemic. Particularly in the ICU, where the metabolic demands of the tissues may be increased by intercurrent illness or recovery from surgery, hemoglobin concentration must be kept at an optimum level. For children with saturations greater than 85%, a hemoglobin level of 14 g/dl is probably sufficient if the patient is not unduly stressed. For saturations of 75% to 85%, a hemoglobin of 16 g/dl is indicated, while saturations of 60% to 75% may require hemoglobins of 18 g/dl or more. The exact hemoglobin concentration required by an individual child will vary considerably according to the factors outlined here.

As with an increase in cardiac output, increasing the hemoglobin concentration in hypoxemic patients may also result in an increase in their arterial saturation. An elevated hemoglobin concentration allows delivery of the necessary oxygen to the tissues with less desaturation of the returning venous hemoglobin.

Despite optimization of oxygen carrying capacity and cardiac output, there are patients in whom the metabolic demands of the tissues cannot be met due to severe hypoxemia. In this setting, it is critical to reduce the metabolic demands of the body. Heavy sedation and muscle relaxants with mechanical ventilation may reduce oxygen consumption and should be considered in any patient with an evolving metabolic acidosis in the face of severe hypoxemia.

Consequences and Complications of Chronic Hypoxemia

During the past few decades there has been a dramatic decrease in the number of patients with chronic hypoxemia, chiefly due to advances in the surgical management of congenital heart disease. For the few remaining patients with chronic hypoxemia, however, there are a number of important issues.

Chronic hypoxemia results in polycythemia (secondary to increased erythropoietin production in the kidney). This is an appropriate compensatory mechanism aimed at increasing oxygen carrying capacity. Above a hematocrit of approximately 70%, however, the increasing viscosity of the blood becomes an impediment to flow through the circulation, increasing the work of the heart and decreasing oxygen delivery. Headache and fatigue are common consequences. Polycythemia also appears to be associated with a bleeding diathesis related to platelet dysfunction and an increased risk of stroke and brain abscess.

In patients with a hematocrit greater than 70%, the consequences of increased viscosity and the bleeding diathesis can be treated with plasmapheresis or phlebotomy, with replacement of removed blood with albumin in saline. It is important to maintain a constant intravascular volume during either procedure, particularly in patients who depend on their systemic pressure to maintain pulmonary blood flow (e.g., tetralogy of Fallot, Blalock-Taussig shunt). The patient's hematocrit should be lowered no more than 10% to avoid a significant decrease in oxygen carrying capacity. As a rule, the hematocrit should be reduced to below 70% in any chronically hypoxemic patient scheduled for surgery or any other procedure that might be complicated by bleeding.

In addition to bleeding diathesis, children with chronic hypoxemia may be hypercoagulable. This state is thought to be related to the increased viscosity of the blood associated with a "relative" iron-deficiency anemia, which may be present despite a hemoglobin concentration at or above normal. Cerebrovascular accidents may occur in these patients and may be secondary to arterial or venous thromboembobli as well as venous thrombosis. In addition, they may be a direct result of hypoxic injury to the brain.

Brain abscesses also occur in patients with chronic hypoxemia, and may present with headache, seizures, or focal neurologic findings. The suspicion for brain abscess must be high, because polycythemia alone may present with headache, confounding the clinical presentation.

Scoliosis is a well-described complication of congenital heart disease and is more prevalent among patients with chronic hypoxemia. Scoliosis may affect as many as 1% to 6% of these patients.

Special Issues for Children with Tetralogy of Fallot

Physiology

Children with tetralogy of Fallot have a large ventricular septal defect and "dynamic" obstruction to the pulmonary artery caused by bundles of muscle below the pulmonary valve (Fig. 22-4). If the degree of pulmonary obstruction is mild, pulmonary blood flow may be normal, or even increased, an arrangement referred to as "pink" tetralogy of Fallot. Alternatively, if the pulmonary obstruction is more severe, "blue blood" from the right ventricle may pass instead into the aorta, causing systemic cyanosis. Pulmonary obstruction also leads to a decrease in pulmonary blood flow and diminished pulmonary venous return, further increasing the fraction of aortic flow that comes from the desaturated systemic venous return. In general, the more severe the pulmonary obstruction, the more severe the hypoxemia.

Hypercyanotic "Tet" Spells

Fortunately, most children with tetralogy of Fallot have only moderate pulmonary obstruction most of the time, resulting in safe systemic saturations. Of more concern than their baseline saturations, however, is the potential for hypercyanotic "tetralogy" spells. These spells can occur at any time but become increasingly likely starting in the second half of the first year of life. They are characterized by constriction of the subpulmonary muscle bundles, causing acute severe hypoxemia due to reduced pulmonary blood flow and increased right-to-left shunting at the ventricular septal defect. Clinical signs include severe cyanosis associated with deep, rapid respirations. Children may be irritable or somnolent. The harsh murmur of subpulmonary stenosis may become shorter, or even inaudible. Hypercyanotic spells often are precipitated by pain, anger, or situations that result in a drop in systemic vascular resistance, such as a warm bath or awakening in the morning.

Although most hypercyanotic spells resolve within 5 to 20 min-

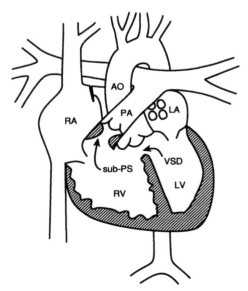

Figure 22-4. Tetralogy of Fallot. AO, aorta; LA, left atrium; LV, left ventricle; PA, main pulmonary artery; RA, right atrium; RV, right ventricle; sub-PS, subvalvar pulmonary stenosis; VSD, anterior malalignment ventricular septal defect.

utes without obvious sequellae, it is possible for them to lead to severe hypoxemia and even death. In addition, frequent episodes of severe hypoxemia may contribute to major organ injury, including damage to the central nervous system. Consequently, parents and ICU personnel alike must be instructed carefully on the management of hypercyanotic spells. Because surgical repair of tetralogy of Fallot is possible even in the newborn period, it is rarely necessary to delay surgery once a child has demonstrated the capacity to "spell."

The management of hypercyanotic spells centers around reducing subpulmonary muscle spasm, increasing systemic venous return, increasing systemic vascular resistance, maintaining oxygen delivery, and, in the more severe episodes, reducing oxygen demand. In older children, a hypercyanotic spell often can be aborted by squatting, which abruptly increases the systemic vascular resistance and systemic venous return, factors that promote pulmonary blood flow. Otherwise, children with hypercyanotic spells require a step-wise approach (Table 22-4).

Early in a hypercyanotic spell, comforting a baby by putting him or her on a parent's abdomen or over the shoulder in a knee-chest position may be all that is required. The most important factor is comfort, because circulating catecholamines may precipitate or aggravate the subpulmonary constriction. In the hospital, oxygen may be administered to the extent that it does not irritate the patient. Intramuscular or subcutaneous morphine is a well-described specific treatment of hypercyanotic spells and may be tried if more conservative measures do not result in immediate improvement in oxygenation. Cardiorespiratory and saturation monitors are indicated in a child suspected of having hypercyanotic spells.

If hypoxemia persists despite less intrusive measures, it becomes necessary to start a peripheral intravenous catheter. It is critical that this procedure be as nontraumatic as possible, and the most skilled personnel should perform it. Subcutaneous lidocaine may help prevent undue discomfort associated with a difficult procedure. Once the IV is in place, the morphine dose may be repeated IV.

Table 22-4. Management of hypercyanotic spells in tetralogy of Fallot

Stage 1
  Knee-chest position
  Comfort
  Oxygen
  Morphine 0.1 mg/kg IM or SQ
  Cardiac monitor
  Pulse oximeter

Stage 2
  Start a peripheral IV
  Morphine 0.1 mg/kg IV
  Propranolol 0.05–0.10 mg/kg IV (up to 1 mg)
  Normal saline 10 ml/kg IV
  Sodium bicarbonate 1 mEq/kg IV

Stage 3
  Phenylephrine 0.01 mg/kg/min IV infusion
  PRBCs 10 ml/kg IV

Stage 4
  General anesthesia
  Emergency surgical intervention

Propranolol is another specific remedy for hypercyanotic spells, but must be given with some caution. Usually 0.05 mg/kg IV can be given in a bolus, and another 0.05 mg/kg IV given over 3 to 5 minutes if improvement in oxygenation is not immediately evident. Propranolol may reduce subpulmonary spasm directly and will also result in a lower heart rate, leading to increased filling of the heart, which reduces subpulmonary obstruction indirectly. Intravenous volume (saline or blood) can also increase filling. Sodium bicarbonate may be administered as well in any hypercyanotic spell that has gone on longer than 10 minutes, because a metabolic acidosis often develops early in hypercyanotic spells.

If these measures have not been effective in reducing hypoxia, a specific systemic vasoconstrictor, such as phenylephrine, should be added to try to force pulmonary blood flow, and packed RBCs should be administered to increase oxygen carrying capacity. By this stage, preparations should be initiated for transfer of the patient to the ICU and possible emergency surgical repair or palliation of the tetralogy of Fallot.

Finally, if all else fails and severe cyanosis cannot be corrected, general anesthesia may be necessary. Anesthesia may reverse severe subpulmonary obstruction, and it will reduce oxygen demand in a severely hypoxemic child. One hundred percent oxygen and a combination of a potent narcotic (e.g., fentanyl) and a muscle relaxant often are used in this setting. Anesthesia generally is followed by emergency surgical repair or palliation with a systemic-to-pulmonary shunt.

Cardiac Catheterization in Tetralogy of Fallot

Cardiac catheterization is often necessary prior to surgical correction of tetralogy of Fallot to rule out peripheral pulmonary stenoses, additional ventricular septal defects, and important coronary artery anomalies. Unfortunately, hypercyanotic spells are particularly prevalent during and following cardiac catheterization. Contributing factors may include stress, increased catecholamine production, dehydration, and direct irritation of the pulmonary outflow tract with catheter manipulation.

Children with tetralogy of Fallot who are admitted for cardiac catheterization should have a peripheral IV started the day before the procedure and receive continuous maintenance fluids during the night prior to catheterization. Sedation should be as effective as possible to prevent a surge in circulating catecholamines during the move to the catheterization laboratory. Although morphine may have a specific benefit in reducing the risk of hypercyanotic spells, it may not be effective as a sole sedative agent.

While in the catheterization laboratory, the patient must be kept well sedated. Morphine is often used, usually in conjunction with a benzodiazepine (e.g., midazolam). The patient must be kept warm, as core cooling results in increased catecholamine production. Some cardiologists prefer to administer propranolol prior to catheterization to reduce the likelihood of a hypercyanotic spell.

Following catheterization, the child may continue to require sedation if expected to stay flat in bed for 4 to 6 hours to promote hemostasis. Cardiorespiratory and saturation monitors must be utilized during the day following catheterization because this is a period during which hypercyanotic spells are common.

Should a spell occur, it should be managed in the fashion outlined previously, although other causes of cyanosis must also be considered. Pericardial tamponade or internal hemorrhage can also make a child ill, and must not be overlooked in the enthusiasm to treat a hypercyanotic spell.

Patent Ductus Arteriosus in the Newborn

Patent ductus arteriosus is a major complicating factor in the management of newborns born prematurely. The incidence of patent ductus arteriosus may be up to 77% of human neonates born at 28 to 30 weeks' gestation,[9] whereas it is rarely an important problem in term infants. The increased incidence of patent ductus arteriosus may be the result of a diminished contractile response of the ductus arteriosus with decreasing gestational age.[10] The clinical impact of a patent ductus arteriosus is aggravated by the sensitivity of the premature lung to left-to-right shunting and the harmful effects of prolonged mechanical ventilation and supplemental oxygen. The result is an increased incidence of chronic lung disease and retinal oxygen toxicity[11,12] in premature infants with patent ductus arteriosus.

Diagnosis

The signs of patent ductus arteriosus in the newborn include an increase in arterial pulse pressure, tachypnea or increased respiratory support, cardiomegaly, and a murmur. All of these findings can be variable or nonspecific, however. A wide pulse pressure with bounding pulses can also be a sign of infection, as can respiratory distress. Cardiomegaly may not be apparent early in the course of a patent ductus arteriosus because of fluid restriction and reduced cardiac filling secondary to positive-pressure ventilation. The murmur of patent ductus arteriosus in newborns can be nonspecific: Often, the typical diastolic component of a ductal "machinery-like" Gibson murmur[13] is absent. Consequently, a high degree of suspicion is required to identify a patent ductus arteriosus in a premature infant, who may well benefit from early intervention.

To make matters more complicated, the ductus arteriosus is comprised of contractile tissue and is suspected of transient closure (winking) in some infants with classic signs of patent ductus arteriosus but no echocardiographic evidence of left-to-right flow on a single examination. A murmur and bounding pulses that come and go, associated with rapid fluctuations in requirements for ventilator support, may be related to this phenomenon.

The standard diagnostic tool used in the diagnosis of patent ductus arteriosus is two-dimensional echocardiography with color Doppler mapping. Unfortunately, even direct imaging of the ductus arteriosus is not always as revealing as one might like. Although left-to-right flow may be detected, the hemodynamic significance of such flow cannot be estimated reliably.[14] Even infants without evidence of a large shunt appear to be at risk of severe pulmonary impairment. With the exception of a "trial of closure," there is no reliable indicator of the significance of a patent ductus arteriosus.

Management

Management of a patent ductus arteriosus in a premature infant includes mild fluid restriction, as long as the urine output remains acceptable. There is some concern that a patent ductus arteriosus may contribute to the risk of necrotizing enterocolitis in premature infants, so feedings are often held. Positive-pressure ventilation may be used to reduce the pulmonary edema that results from the increase in pulmonary artery pressure. Supplemental oxygen and mechanical ventilation should not be increased beyond what is necessary to maintain an acceptable arterial blood gas, as both excess oxygen and mechanical ventilation can be harmful to the premature infant and may aggravate the left-to-right shunt by reducing pulmonary vascular resistance.

There is little evidence that the administration of digoxin is of benefit in infants with hemodynamically significant patent ductus arteriosus, particularly when ventricular function is not impaired.[15] Diuretics, (e.g., furosemide) are often used to reduce cardiac filling pressures and may reduce signs of pulmonary congestion. In general, however, diuretics havem any side effects (renal, auditory, and metabolic) that may outweigh their benefits if used continuously. Furthermore, there is evidence to suggest that furosemide may increase the production of endogenous prostaglandins[16] and may be associated with an increased incidence of patent ductus arteriosus in premature infants.[17] Ironically, furosemide may help ameliorate some of the harmful effects of other medications used in the management of patent ductus arteriosus (discussion follows).

There is evidence that a patent ductus arteriosus that has not closed by 3 days of age is unlikely to close spontaneously.[18] Closure of a patent ductus arteriosus in premature infants has been shown to reduce the requirement for supplemental oxygen and mechanical ventilation, and is associated with a reduced risk of chronic lung disease and retinopathy, particularly when performed during the first 10 days of life.[19–21] These benefits may be increased with "routine" pharmacologic closure of the ductus arteriosus at 3 days of life.[19,22] Consequently, it may well be reasonable to consider pharmacologic or surgical closure in any premature infant with continuing respiratory difficulties who has evidence of a patent ductus arteriosus at 3 days of age.

Pharmacologic closure of a patent ductus arteriosus may be attempted through the use of indomethacin, an inhibitor of prostaglandin synthesis through its effect on cyclooxygenase. Dosing regimens vary by weight and age (Table 22-5). A plasma level of about 0.5 μg/ml is probably sufficient to suppress prostaglandin synthesis in premature infants,[23] although many centers do not find it helpful to follow plasma levels because of the brevity of the course of treatment. The success of a course of indomethacin is usually measured in terms of the reduction in supplemental oxygen and respiratory support that ensues. Because the recurrence rate for patent ductus arteriosus is fairly high after pharmacologic closure, particularly in very low birth weight infants, repeat evaluation, and possibly a second course of indomethacin, is indicated if significant improvement is not forthcoming.

Indomethacin is associated with several significant side effects in preterm infants. The most concerning complication is a depression of renal function, characterized by a reduced urine output and an increase in serum creatinine. The renal effects of indomethacin may be related to interference with the action of PGE_2,[24–26] which has a protective effect on urine output in the presence of reduced intravascular volume. The impact of indomethacin on renal function may last up to 14 days,[27] and may be at least partly reversed through the concurrent administration of furosemide.[28]

Indomethacin also reduces platelet function,[29] leading to a pro-

Table 22-5. Dosing regimen for indomethacin in newborns

Age	Dose (mg/kg) q12° IV		
	No. 1	No. 2	No. 3
<48 hrs	0.20	0.10	0.10
2–7 d	0.20	0.20	0.20
>7 d	0.20	0.25	0.25

longation of bleeding time in premature infants.[30] Nonetheless, the administration of indomethacin to premature infants has not been linked to an increase in hemorrhagic complications, including intraventricular hemorrhage.[21,31–33]

In general, up to two courses of three doses of indomethacin may be given, either because the first course was ineffective or because the signs of a patent ductus arteriosus recurred following initial improvement. If evidence of a significant patent ductus arteriosus persists, surgical ligation of the ductus arteriosus may be indicated.[34] Because of the difficulties involved in transporting a very small premature infant to the operating room, this procedure is carried out in the neonatal ICU at many centers.[35] Surgical ligation can be accomplished without an increased risk of intraventricular hemorrhage,[36] but extreme care is necessary to prevent blood pressure swings during and after the procedure. The surgical management of patent ductus arteriosus is discussed in detail in Intensive Care of the Infant and Child Following Cardiac Surgery by Lang, Erickson, Elixson, Vlahakes and Lopez.

Acquired Heart Disease

Myocarditis

The term *myocarditis* describes an extremely broad group of processes, all of which have in common inflammation of the myocardium. The reported incidence is low, although the true incidence may be higher than suspected due to an unknown number of clinically unsuspected cases.[37] Although Coxsackie virus B is the most commonly identified agent, myocarditis can be associated with many infectious agents, including viruses, bacteria, rickettsia, fungi, and protozoa. Toxic myocarditis may result from exposure to a large number of drugs and other agents. Furthermore, it is seen complicating autoimmune and other systemic illnesses. Despite the plethora of known etiologies, however, the responsible agent is identified in less than half of diagnosed cases of myocarditis.[38–42]

The diagnostic approach to myocarditis is outlined in Table 22-6. The clinical presentation of myocarditis can be variable. There is often a prodrome characterized by fever and nonspecific signs of a viral illness, which may include congestion, cough, rash, vomiting, and diarrhea. Subsequent signs of myocardial involvement range from subclinical to fulminant congestive heart failure. In infants, tachypnea, irritability, lethargy, poor feeding, and failure to thrive are common, and fever may be present in up to half. In older children, fever, listlessness, abdominal pain, dizziness, and decreased exercise tolerance have been described. Rapidly fulminant disease is characterized by respiratory distress, cyanosis, fatigue, arrhythmias, and syncope.

The course of myocarditis is variable. Infants have a very poor prognosis, with a mortality of up to 75%.[43] Older children may have a mortality of up to 25%. Another 25% have chronic residua, and the remaining 50% have apparent full recovery,[44] although even asymptomatic patients may have limited exercise tolerance.[45] Finally, residual scarring and fibrosis may predispose to ectopy and arrhythmias in children who recover. It has been postulated that a considerable fraction of patients with dilated cardiomyopathy suffered a prior episode of myocarditis.

The physical examination may reveal tachycardia, tachypnea, and respiratory distress. The extremities may be cool and clammy with a thready pulse in severe cases. The precordium is quiet. A gallop rhythm may be present. The pulmonary component of the second heart sound may be loud if pulmonary artery hypertension is present. The first heart sound may be softer than usual. There

Table 22-6. Diagnostic approach to myocarditis

Past medical history
  Rheumatic fever
  Systemic lupus erythematosis
  Ulcerative colitis

History
  Prior illnesses
  Toxic exposures
    Scorpion sting
  Drug exposures
    Acetazolamide
    Amphotericin B
    Cyclophosphamide
    Indomethacin
    Isoniazid
    Methyldopa
    Neomercazole
    Penicillin
    Phenylbutazone
    Phenytoin
    Sulfonamides
    Tetracycline
  Travel history
    Coccidiomycosis
    Parasitic/protazoal infections
    Lyme disease

Physical exam
  Fever
  Blood pressure and pulsus paradoxus
  Tachycardia
  Tachypnea
  Respiratory distress
  Perfusion
  Hepatomegaly
  Pulses
  Precordial activity
  Gallop rhythm
  Pericardial rub
  Murmur of mitral insufficiency
  Evidence of infection
  Evidence of connective tissue disorders
  Evidence of autoimmune disorders

Electrocardiogram

Chest x-ray

Echocardiogram

Laboratory tests
  Pharyngeal, rectal, urine, and blood viral cultures
  Urine and blood bacterial and fungal cultures
  Viral titers
  Stool ova and parasite examination
  Electrolytes, BUN, and creatinine
  Glucose
  Calcium
  Complete blood cell count with differential
  Erythrocyte sedimentation rate
  Liver function tests (SGOT, SGPT, CPK, LDH)
  Biopsy
    Histopathology
    Viral, bacterial, fungal cultures
    Immunofluorescent staining for viral antigens
    Electron microscopy for infectious agents?
    Viral PCR

may be a murmur of mitral regurgitation, depending on the degree of left ventricular dilation. Pulmonary rales and hepatomegaly are common.

A chest x-ray will almost always reveal cardiomegaly. Electrocardiography may reveal tachycardia, low-amplitude QRS and T waves, ST segment depression, and inversion of the T waves in the leftward leads (V5 and V6). Arrhythmias may include atrial premature beats, ventricular premature beats, and varying degrees of heart block. Conduction disorders are particularly prevalent in the case of diphtheroid myocarditis and portend a poor outcome.[46] Similarly, a poor prognosis is associated with supraventricular tachycardia (usually an automatic atrial tachycardia such as multifocal atrial tachycardia).[47]

The diagnosis of myocardial dysfunction is confirmed by echocardiography, which may reveal dilation of all four chambers and poor contractility of the ventricles. A pericardial effusion suggests the diagnosis of concurrent pericarditis, an often-associated condition that must be ruled out because it may lead to pericardial tamponade.

Because of the broad range of possible etiologies, some of which are treatable, every effort must be made to identify the agent responsible for any case of myocarditis. A careful history is required to identify possible medicine or toxic exposures, infections, or other preceding illnesses. Blood, urine, pharyngeal, and stool cultures for bacteria and viruses are indicated. Acute and convalescent viral antibody titers may also be helpful in establishing the diagnosis. Liver function tests may be elevated in any systemic viral illness, although elevated transaminases are particularly suggestive of diphtheria infection.

Cardiac catheterization is helpful in confirming the diagnosis of myocarditis through endomyocardial biopsy. Tissue can be tested for histopathology, culture, and PCR screening. The fraction of positive biopsies may be enhanced by prior screening with Gallium 67 MRI scanning to identify the presence of myocardial inflammation.[48] In some cases, myocarditis can be difficult to distinguish from other types of dilated cardiomyopathy, which share the features of ventricular dysfunction but are not characterized by myocardial inflammation. Cardiac catheterization may be necessary to make this distinction, particularly in a child without fever or other signs of systemic inflammation.

Treatment of myocarditis is aimed at maintaining cardiac function and, when possible, eradication of the responsible agent. Antibiotics should be withheld unless a specific bacterial agent is suspected except in the case of cardiovascular collapse or in the newborn, settings in which sepsis may be fulminant and difficult to rule out in a timely fashion. Intravenous immunoglobulin infusion has been shown to be of benefit to children with myocarditis. To date, there have been no controlled studies in humans that support the use of immunosuppressive agents in myocarditis.

The supportive therapy for myocarditis is essentially the management of congestive heart failure. A useful caveat is that patients with myocarditis are often much more compromised than they appear by physical examination. In addition, their cardiovascular reserve is often so impaired that even mild oral sedation can tip them over into cardiovascular collapse. Consequently, admission to an ICU with cardiorespiratory and BP monitoring is appropriate. Frequent physical examinations may be a more reliable measure of cardiac function than that from the monitors. Respiratory rate, peripheral perfusion, mental status, and urine output should be checked frequently.

The management of congestive heart failure is discussed in detail at the beginning of this chapter, but several caveats bear mentioning with respect to managing patients with myocarditis. Because of the potential pitfalls of diuretics, intravascular volume expansion, and afterload reducing agents, the first medication instituted in the ICU is usually an inotrope. In the acute setting, dobutamine (5–20 μg/kg/min) may be the best choice both because it has relatively little chronotropic effect and because it has the additional benefit of peripheral vasodilation. Agents such as epinephrine, isoproterenol, and dopamine, which may aggravate the underlying tachycardia, must be used with caution because any further increase in heart rate may lead to a decrease in cardiac output. If hypotension is present, dopamine (3–10 μg/kg/min) may be used initially, and dobutamine added when the BP is stable.

Patients with myocarditis may be very sensitive to increases in intravascular volume owing to severe dilation of the ventricle, which, in turn, leads to poor ventricular compliance. In the setting of poor perfusion or an inadequate BP, isotonic volume should be administered gingerly (3–5 ml/kg over 5–10 minutes). In severe cases, patients with myocarditis may require intracardiac monitoring with a thermodilution (Swan-Ganz) catheter.

Diuretics may result in a marked improvement in cardiac output to the extent that they reduce ventricular dilation and restore the mechanical advantage of a smaller ventricle. They must be used with caution, however, as some patients with myocarditis may require considerably elevated filling pressures to generate an adequate output. An initial dose of furosemide may be tried, with close attention to clinical signs of cardiac output (perfusion, BP, urine output). If perfusion appears to suffer rather than improve, intravenous administration of isotonic fluids is indicated.

If perfusion continues to be poor despite inotropes and diuretics, an afterload reducing agent such as nitroprusside (0.5–6.0 μg/kg/min) or amiodarone may be indicated. The use of these agents requires a stable, adequate BP, and additional intravascular volume may be required to compensate for the effects of venodilation.

There is increasing evidence that in cases of severe left ventricular dilation there may be a benefit to catheter-directed atrial septostomy (CDAS). By opening a hole in the atrial septum, the left atrial pressure is reduced and the left ventricle may "decompress," improving ventricular function because of a smaller end-diastolic volume and an improved LaPlace relationship (Congestive Heart Failure). CDAS may also reduce pulmonary artery hypertension by eliminating pulmonary venous hypertension, thus improving signs of right-sided congestive heart failure. Finally, CDAS may reduce the risk of intracardiac thrombosis in children with myocarditis requiring ECMO support whose aortic valves do not open against the artificially maintained arterial pressure.

Following initial stabilization, an oral regimen of digoxin, diuretics, and afterload-reducing agents is initiated. Because the inflamed myocardium may be particularly sensitive to digoxin, this medication is generally used in lower-than-usual loading doses. Oral digitalization is preferred, at about 75% of the usual digitalizing dose, followed by the usual maintenance dose (see Table 22-2). Furosemide may be given up to 4 times per day (1.0–1.5 mg/kg/dose PO), with the concomitant administration of spironolactone (1–2 mg/kg/d PO divided bid or qd) if more than twice-a-day furosemide is required. Captopril (0.1–0.5 mg/kg/dose q8° in infants, 0.1–1.0 mg/kg/dose q8° in older children, maximum dose 25 mg PO q8°) or Enalapril (0.08 mg/kg/dose q12°–24° for older children) may be of benefit for long-term maintenance as well.

Any arrhythmias that present during the management of patients with myocarditis must be treated aggressively (see Management of Cardiac Arrythmias by Walsh and Liberthson). Antiarrhythmic agents with potent negative inotropic effect, such as beta-blockers and procainamide, should be avoided if alternative medical regimens are available.

Cardiomyopathy

Cardiomyopathy is a heterogeneous collection of conditions in which there is derangement of myocardial structure or function. (Cardiomyopathies secondary to inflammation are discussed in the section, Myocarditis.) Cardiomyopathies are associated with a wide variety of metabolic, genetic, environmental and other conditions. Some of the more common etiologies are listed in

Table 22-7, although in a large fraction of cases no cause can be deduced.

Cardiomyopathies can be divided into three distinct physiologic and clinical categories: (1) dilated, (2) hypertrophic, and (3) restrictive. The most common type of cardiomyopathy in children is the dilated variety. Most cases of dilated cardiomyopathy may be secondary to myocarditis or a "burned-out" inflammation of the myocardium, although other etiologies include carnitine deficiency, Duchenne's muscular dystrophy, Friedreich's ataxia, and anthracycline administration. Structural heart disease (e.g., aortic stenosis or coarctation) may result in severe myocardial dysfunction, as may chronic arrhythmias such as paroxysmal supraventricular tachycardia or ventricular tachycardia.

Dilated cardiomyopathy is characterized by impaired ventricular systolic function with dilation of the ventricle, congestive heart

Table 22-7. Primary and secondary causes of cardiomyopathy

Diseases related to energy creation or utilization
  Fatty acid transport
    Primary carnitine deficiency
      Biosynthetic defect
      Absorption defect
      Excessive urinary loss
    Secondary carnitine deficiency
      Dietary deficiency
      Excessive urinary losses
      Liver disease
      Dehydrogenase enzyme deficiencies
      Organic acidurias
        Blutaric aciduria type II
        Isovaleric aciduria
        Methylmalonic aciduria
        Propionic aciduria
        Homocystinuria
      Other metabolic disorders
        Cytochrome disorders
        Kearns-Sayre
        X-linked mitochondrial disease
  Transferase enzyme disorders
  Glucose utilization
    Glycolysis
    Glycogenolysis
      Glycogen storage disease type 2 (Pompe's)
      Normal acid maltase, "type 2-like disease"
      Cardiac phosphorylase kinase deficiency
      Glycogen storage disease, type 3 (Cori)
    Glycogen synthesis
      Glycogen storage disease, type 4 (Anderson's)
  Protein metabolism
    Amino acid degradation
    Beta-ketothiolase deficiency
Disorders of mitochondrial function
  Fatty acid oxidation
    Short-chain acyl CoA dehydrogenase deficiency
    Medium-chain acyl CoA dehydrogenase deficiency
    Long-chain acyl CoA dehydrogenase deficiency
    Multiple-chain acyl CoA dehydrogenase deficiency
      Glutaric aciduria type II
  Pyruvate metabolism
    Pyruvate dehydrogenase complex disorder
    Pyruvate carboxylase deficiency
    Leigh's disease
  Citric acid cycle

  Oxidative phosphorylation
    Complex 1 deficiency
    Complex 2 deficiency
    Complex 3 (cytochrome C reductase) deficiency
      Histiocytoid cardiomyopathy
    Complex 4 (cytochrome C oxidase) deficiency
  Idiopathic (suspected mitochondrial) "cardiomyopathy plus syndromes"
    X-linked inheritance
    Congenital cataract
    Ophthalmoplegia
    Brain infarcts
    Vermal atrophy/lactic acidosis
    Skeletal muscle weakness
    Oncocytic
Disorders of lysosomal enzymes
  Mucopolysaccharidoses
    Type 1H Hurler
    Type 1S Scheie
    Type 1 S/H Hurler-Scheie
    Type 2 Hunter
    Type 4 Morquio
    Type 6 Maroteaux-Lamy
    Type 7 Sly
  Mycolipidoses
    Type 2 1-cell disease
    Type 3 pseudo-Hurler polydystrophy
  Glycoproteinoses
    Fucosidosis
    Aspartylglycosaminuria
    Sialidosis
    Mannosidosis
  Ceramidase deficiency
    Farber's lipogranulomatosis
  Sphingomyelin lipidoses
    Niemann-Pick disease
  Glucosylceramide lipodoses
    Gaucher's disease
  Gangliosidoses
    G_{M1} gangliosidoses
    G_{M2} gangliosidoses
      Tay-Sachs
      Sandhoff's
Other metabolic disorders
  Ethanolaminosis
  Phytanic acid storage disease (Refsum's)

continued

Table 22-7. Continued

Infectious	Collegen
Viral	Lupus erythematosus
Septicemia	Drugs/Toxins
Postmyocarditis	Anthracyclines
Acquired immune deficiency syndrome	Steroids/ACTH
Nutritional	Catecholamines
Thiamine deficiency	Iron overload
Kwashiorkor	Other
Pellagra	Beckwith-Wiedemann syndrome
Selenium deficiency	Noonan syndrome
Endocrine	Multiple lentigines
Hypo- and hyperthyroidism	Epidermolysis bullosa
Hypoparathyroidism	Turner syndrome
Pheochromocytoma	Kawasaki
Infant of a diabetic mother	Rheumatic fever
Hypoglycemia	Chronic arrhythmias
Tyrosinemia	

Modified from Moller JH et al. *Fetal, Neonatal, and Infant Cardiac Disease.* Appleton-Lange, East Norwalk, CT, 1990. With permission.

failure, and deterioration in cardiac output. Symptoms of fatigue, chest pain, and shortness of breath are common. The physical examination may reveal tachypnea, tachycardia, pulmonary rales, hepatomegaly, and cool extremities. There may be a gallop rhythm, although a murmur is generally absent. The treatment for dilated cardiomyopathy parallels that of congestive heart failure.

Hypertrophic cardiomyopathy may be familial or sporadic and has a particularly poor prognosis when it presents in infancy. One exception to that rule is the hypertrophic cardiomyopathy that affects infants of diabetic mothers and resolves during infancy. Hypertrophic cardiomyopathy is characterized by localized or generalized thickening of the ventricular wall, leading to impaired diastolic function and increased venous pressures without dilation. Cardiac output may fall secondary to insufficient filling of the ventricle. Ventricular ejection fraction may be increased, particularly if ventricular filling is impaired. The hypertrophy may also result in obstruction to the left ventricular outflow tract (hypertrophic obstructive cardiomyopathy, idiopathic hypertrophic subaortic stenosis). Subendocardial ischemia may occur secondary to impaired perfusion of the innermost regions of the myocardium. Symptoms of hypertrophic cardiomyopathy may include shortness of breath, fatigue, chest pain, or syncope.

When signs of symptomatic left ventricular outflow tract obstruction or low cardiac output are present, the acute management of hypertrophic cardiomyopathy includes negative inotropes such as beta-blockers or verapamil. Esmolol, a short-acting beta-blocker, may allow improved ventricular filling and reduce subaortic obstruction, and has the additional advantage it can be titrated to effect in patients with low cardiac output. Volume administration will also increase ventricular filling and reduce subaortic obstruction, but may also increase venous pressure and should be avoided in the presence of pulmonary edema. Inotropes should be avoided because they may worsen subaortic obstruction and have no beneficial effects on diastolic function in patients who already have normal or hyperdynamic systolic function.

Restrictive cardiomyopathy is unusual in children and is most often associated with endomyocardial fibrosis or Löffler's disease. Restrictive cardiomyopathy is characterized by poor ventricular diastolic compliance without hypertrophy and with normal systolic function. It chiefly affects the left ventricle, and the right ventricle is often hypertensive due to elevated pulmonary venous pressures. The ventricular chambers may be normal or small, but the atria are often very dilated. Signs of pulmonary edema may be present. Symptoms include shortness of breath, chest pain, and fatigue. The examination may reveal edema, jugular venous distension, hepatomegaly, tachypnea, a gallop rhythm, and occasionally the blowing holosystolic murmur of mitral regurgitation. Cardiomegaly on chest x-ray may be caused by atrial dilation, although pericardial effusions sometimes occur. Restrictive cardiomyopathy is generally diagnosed echocardiographically and must be distinguished from constrictive pericardial disease and pericarditis. It is not clear whether there is any effective treatment for restrictive cardiomyopathy, short of heart transplantation.

Pericardial Disorders

Mechanics of Pericardial Tamponade

The pericardial sac encloses the heart as well as the origins of the great arteries and the vena cavae. Under normal circumstances it contains only a small amount of fluid, which serves to lubricate the surfaces of the visceral and parietal pericardium. Under a variety of abnormal conditions, however, large amounts of fluid can accumulate within this space, leading to tamponade of cardiac filling.

As the pericardium fills with fluid, it is able to distend a certain amount without significantly impairing cardiac filling. The mechanical properties of the pericardial sac are such that acute accumulations of fluid may lead to tamponade at relatively low volumes, whereas slow accumulations may allow gradual distention of the pericardial sac to quite a large size. Eventually, however, the limit of pericardial compliance is approached and the intrapericardial pressure begins to rise. Because venous return to the heart must overcome the intrapericardial pressure in order to enter the heart, filling pressures begin to rise. When intrapericardial pressure exceeds the baseline ventricular diastolic pressure, atrial and ventricular diastolic pressures on both the left and right side of the heart come to equal the intrapericardial pressure. In fact, equalization of the left and right atrial pressures is one of the hallmarks of pericardial tamponade. Further elevation of the intrapericardial pressure results in elevated left- and right-sided venous pressure with jugular venous distension, hepatomegaly, and tachypnea.

Under normal circumstances, venous return to the right and left heart varies considerably with the respiratory cycle. Pulmonary venous return falls during inspiration due to an increase in the volume of the pulmonary vascular bed, leading to a mild drop in stroke volume and systolic BP. This drop is usually no more than 10 mm Hg and is associated with an increase in heart rate. Conversely, systemic venous return and right heart filling are increased during inspiration due to transmission of negative intrathoracic pressure to the right atrium and vena cavae, in effect drawing systemic venous blood into the chest. During pericardial tamponade, the total volume of the cardiac chambers is essentially fixed. Consequently, the increase in right ventricular filling during inspiration results in mechanical compression of the left ventricle and a further reduction in left ventricular filling, stroke volume, and systolic pressure than normal.[49] *Pulsus paradoxus*[50] refers to a fall in systolic BP during inspiration of more than 10 mm Hg.[51] The term derives from the fact that the pulse may become unpalpable during inspiration, giving the false impression of a slowing of the heart rate during inspiration rather than the usual acceleration. In this sense, the term is a misnomer, but it has been retained for historical interest.

Once the pericardium becomes filled to the limit of its distensibility, further increases in intrapericardial volume increasingly restrict cardiac filling. As filling drops off, the heart rate increases, the stroke volume and BP pressure fall, and pulsus paradoxus becomes more marked. At the limit of pericardial distensibility, small changes in pericardial volume can result in a dramatic fall in BP: A patient may tolerate a long period of slowly increasing pericardial effusion, then develop tamponade leading to death in less than an hour.

The procedure for pericardiocentesis is described in detail in *Cardiac Procedures* by Erickson and Elixson, this volume.

Infectious Pericarditis

Pericarditis, or inflammation of the pericardium, can be caused by a wide range of disorders. Most commonly, the cause of pericarditis is not determined, although the majority of cases are thought to be viral in origin. Many other etiologies have been described (Table 22-8).

Most patients who present with pericarditis should be hospitalized. Because the onset of pericardial tamponade can be abrupt, frequent examinations and close monitoring are necessary until the course of the illness has been characterized: Patients with large or rapidly accumulating effusions may require invasive monitoring and/or pericardiocentesis.

The presenting clinical features of pericarditis are fever and chest pain, with or without signs of pericardial tamponade. The chest pain is typically left-sided and sharp and may be positional and/or pleuritic. The pain may be reduced when leaning forward and aggravated when supine.

The physical examination may reveal a pericardial friction rub, even in the presence of a large effusion. The heart sounds may be muffled. If tamponade is present, venous congestion, tachycardia, and a pulsus paradoxus may be evident.

The electrocardiographic signs of pericarditis evolve with time. Findings early in the course are present in all leads except aVR and the rightward precordial leads (V1 and sometimes V2). Initially, there is ST segment elevation with a "concave upward"

Table 22-8. Etiologies of pericarditis

Idiopathic
Viral
Bacterial
Mycobacterial
Fungal
Parasitic
Neoplastic
Uremic
Radiation
Autoimmune
Drugs
Post-hemorrhagic
Traumatic/Surgical

configuration to the ST segment. In addition, PR segment depression may be present in a large fraction of patients during this stage. After a period of days, the ST segment elevation resolves, followed by inversion of the T waves. As the pericardial inflammation resolves, the T waves revert to normal.

The chest x-ray may reveal an enlarged "water bottle" cardiac silhouette if a large pericardial effusion is present. In addition, there may be a pleural effusion, which is present in a significant fraction of patients with pericarditis.

Echocardiography is the standard technique for the identification and quantification of pericardial effusions (Fig. 22-5). In addition, echocardiographic evidence of early pericardial tamponade may precede clinical signs. Finally, echocardiography is helpful in planning the site for pericardiocentesis when indicated.

Pericardiocentesis is probably not indicated in all patients with pericarditis unless there is a threat of pericardial tamponade or there is an urgent need to establish an etiologic agent. The need for a diagnosis may be particularly pressing in the case of a suspected

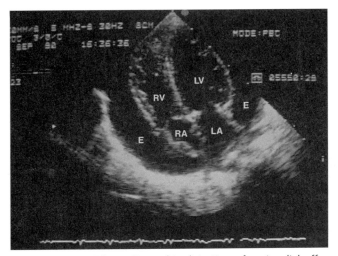

Figure 22-5. Echocardiographic detection of pericardial effusion. E, effusion; LA, left atrium; LV, left ventricle; RA, right atrium; RV, right ventricle.

bacterial pericarditis, during which most patients are gravely ill, or a suspected malignancy.

Other tests that may be appropriate in patients with pericarditis include complete blood cell count, BUN, creatinine, erythrocyte sedimentation rate, blood cultures, viral cultures and titers, HIV testing, tuberculosis skin testing, cold agglutinins, thyroid function tests, ASO titer, antinuclear antibody, and rheumatoid factor.

The treatment for pericarditis should be aimed primarily at eradicating the etiologic agent, if known, and relieving pericardial tamponade when present. Otherwise, bed rest and pain management are recommended. Nonsteroidal antiinflamatory drugs (NSAIDS) such as aspirin or indomethacin are generally effective for pericardial pain, although high-dose corticosteroids may be required for short periods. Antiinflamatory agents are rarely required for more than a week and may be tapered as the pain resolves.

Noninfectious Pericardial Effusions

Noninfectious pericarditis can be secondary to uremia, neoplasia, radiation, autoimmune and immune disorders (lupus erythematosis, acute rheumatic fever, drug allergy), or myocardial injury after infarction (Dressler Syndrome) or cardiac surgery (postpericardiotomy syndrome). Of these, postpericardiotomy requires special vigilance because of its relatively high incidence.

Postpericardiotomy syndrome occurs in roughly a third of patients who undergo surgery involving the myocardium and may also complicate other types of injury to the heart, such as blunt trauma and perforation of the heart during cardiac catheterization. Postpericardiotomy syndrome presents with fever, chest pain, irritability, and pericardial and/or pleural effusions, usually between 1 and 3 weeks after the myocardial insult. Examination may reveal dullness over the lung fields, muffled heart sounds, a pericardial rub, signs of left- or right-sided venous congestion, and/or a pulsus paradoxus. Chest x-ray may reveal pleural effusions or enlargement of the cardiac silhouette. Electrocardiographic changes generally include nonspecific ST and T wave changes. In the absence of a communication between the pericardium and pleural space, echocardiography will reveal a pericardial effusion, with or without evidence of tamponade.

The course of postpericardiotomy syndrome, in the absence of pericardial tamponade, usually leads to spontaneous resolution over 1 to 3 months or longer. Treatment relies on antiinflamatory agents. Usually an NSAID such as aspirin (60 mg/kg/d divided qid) is tried initially, and corticosteroids (prednisone 1 mg/kg qd) may be added if NSAIDs are ineffective. Large effusions, or effusions with evidence of tamponade, require percutaneous drainage.

Myocardial Infarction

Myocardial infarction is an unusual, albeit possibly underdiagnosed, entity in childhood. The most common causes of childhood myocardial infarction are illicit drug use, anomalous origin of the left coronary artery,[52,53] other coronary artery anomalies,[54] perinatal asphyxia, myocarditis, obstruction of the coronary arteries following cardiac surgery, and Kawasaki syndrome.[55,56] Air and thromboemboli may be introduced into the coronary circulation at the time of intravascular instrumentation or surgery. In addition, accelerated atherosclerosis may become an important cause of premature coronary artery disease in children who have undergone cardiac transplantation or who have had coronary artery inflammation secondary to vasculitic syndromes.

Besides coronary artery problems, myocardial infarction can result from any global ischemic injury. Severely impaired cardiac output or hypoxemia can result in injury to any tissue, including the myocardium. A variable degree of myocardial injury results from deep hypothermic arrest and, to a lesser extent, cardiopulmonary bypass.

Presentation

The clinical presentation of myocardial ischemia and infarction in childhood varies depending on the age of the child. Newborns and infants present with nonspecific signs such as pallor, diaphoresis, irritability, vomiting, diarrhea, and lethargy. When the degree of myocardial dysfunction is significant, cyanosis, tachypnea, poor feeding, and respiratory distress may be prominent signs of congestive heart failure. Many infants present with these signs right after feeding, a feature that helps distinguish the usual degree of fussiness or colic of the newborn from signs of ischemia.

Older children who are capable of verbalizing their symptoms may complain of chest or abdominal pain that is usually prolonged, nonpleuritic, and cannot be reproduced by compression of the chest. Chest pain may be sharp or dull, and may or may not be associated with exertion. Pallor, nausea, vomiting, and anxiety are also common signs and symptoms.

Physical Examination

The physical examination may reveal pallor or a mottled appearance. Tachycardia and tachypnea are early signs of myocardial dysfunction, while cyanosis, poor perfusion, hypotension, and other signs of congestive heart failure may be associated with more severe myocardial injury. The cardiac examination may reveal a gallop as well as the regurgitant murmurs of mitral or tricuspid insufficiency. In the presence of severe left ventricular failure and pulmonary artery hypertension, there may be a murmur of pulmonary insufficiency (Graham Steell's murmur). Occasionally, a pericardial friction rub may be present. Some coronary artery abnormalities, such as anomalous origin of the left coronary artery and coronary artery fistulae, may produce a continuous murmur similar to that of a patent ductus arteriosus.

Electrocardiography

There is an enormous amount of material written on the electrocardiographic changes characteristic of myocardial ischemia and infarction,[57–60] most of which is far beyond the scope of this chapter. Subendocardial and papillary muscle infarction is more likely in the setting of severe ventricular hypertrophy,[61–65] and has a distinctive electrocardiographic presentation.

Initial myocardial ischemia is associated with inversion of the T waves in the leads overlying the affected myocardium, except in the case of subendocardial ischemia, in which the T waves in these leads are upright but unusually tall. The QT_c may become prolonged, as the ischemic tissue is slower to repolarize than the normal tissue. As the ischemic myocardium becomes injured, a continuous electrical "leak" from the cells in the injured tissue results in elevation of the ST segments in the leads overlying the region of injury. Once again, the case of subendocardial injury is unusual and is characterized by ST segment depression over the affected myocardium.

As injury evolves into tissue death, the area becomes electrically "silent." Leads overlying the affected area are characterized by wide Q waves produced as the wave of depolarization moves around and away from the infarcted tissue. Note, however, that narrow Q waves (less than 30 ms) in the leftward and inferior leads (I, II, III, aVF, V5, V6) are normal and represent septal depolarization. In addition, patients with Kawasaki syndrome may have unusually deep Q waves within the first 2 weeks of the onset of the illness without evidence of myocardial ischemia. Abnormal Q waves that develop more than 2 weeks after onset are more likely to represent myocardial infarction.[55]

Global or severe myocardial injury may be present following severe perinatal asphyxia, after sudden occlusion of the left coronary artery, during myocarditis, or after a very long period of deep hypothermic arrest. Under these circumstances, the ECG may reveal severely reduced, or even absent, ventricular forces. The T waves may be very flat as well. Occasionally, the combination of nearly absent ventricular forces and a very elevated ST segment may mimic a wide-complex tachycardia.

As recovery proceeds, the T wave inversion and ST segment elevation resolve, signifying healing of the ischemic and injured tissue. The Q waves that remain represent regions of myocardial tissue death.

Chest X-Ray

The chest x-ray is not a sensitive screening test for myocardial ischemia. Cardiac dilation secondary to myocardial dysfunction may be a prominent feature of myocardial infarction, particularly when it is chronic, as with congenital anomalies of the coronary arteries. Pulmonary edema may be present in an acute infarction.

Echocardiography

One of the earliest signs of myocardial ischemia is loss of contractile function. Consequently, echocardiography can be extremely valuable in identifying ischemic regions through their abnormal contractility. It also may identify atrioventricular valve regurgitation, papillary muscle rupture, and, rarely, a ventricular septal defect resulting from septal infarction. Echocardiography also may identify the giant coronary artery aneurysms of Kawasaki syndrome, as well as thrombi and/or stenoses within the aneurysms.

Exercise Stress Testing

Exercise stress testing is particularly helpful in distinguishing chest pain of an ischemic nature from the benign chest wall pain typical of children and teenagers[66,67] who have otherwise normal ECGs.

Myocardial Nuclear Scans

Technetium pyrophosphate and thallium nuclear medicine studies are tests of myocardial perfusion. The latter is commonly performed at rest and during exercise.

Cardiac Catheterization

Selective coronary artery angiography is the optimal method for identification of anomalous coronary arteries and coronary artery obstruction. In addition, left ventriculography may help identify regions of poor contractility secondary to ischemia, or aneurysms secondary to prior infarctions. Direct measurement of the ventricular filling pressures also may supply an index to the severity of myocardial dysfunction.

In the case of coronary artery stenosis or thrombosis, interventional techniques are available in the catheterization laboratory to open occluded vessels. Balloon dilation or stenting of stenotic vessels may be appropriate under certain circumstances, particularly when surgery is not felt to be a safe alternative. Direct infusion of thrombolytic agents such as streptokinase, urokinase, and tPA

are also possible and may be more effective, with fewer side effects, than systemic thrombolysis.

Kawasaki Syndrome

Kawasaki syndrome is an inflammatory illness of unknown etiology, consisting of acute, subacute, and chronic phases.[68–71] The diagnosis is usually established in the acute phase on the basis of fever, typical rash, swelling and induration of the palms and soles, lymphadenopathy, stomatitis, and conjunctivitis (Table 22-9). The rash often begins in the perineal region and is accentuated in the skin folds. Other findings typical for Kawasaki syndrome include urethral meatitis and a sterile monocytic pyurea. Examination of the anterior chamber of the eye may reveal a very subtle anterior uveitis. Extreme irritability is usually present. Echocardiography may reveal myocardial dysfunction and insufficiency at the aortic and/or mitral valves. Unfortunately, infants and older children often present without all criteria, so an increased level of suspicion is required in these groups.

The subacute phase begins when the signs of acute inflammation are waning. The conjunctivitis and stomatitis become less prominent, as do the swelling and induration of the palms and soles. There is usually desquamation of the skin on the hands and

Table 22-9. Kawasaki criteria

A. Principal symptoms
1. Fever persisting 5 days or more
2. Changes of peripheral extremities:
   [Initial stage]: reddening of palms and soles, indurative edema
   [Convalescent stage]: membranous desquamation from fingertips
3. Polymorphous exanthema
4. Bilateral conjunctival congestion
5. Changes of lips and oral cavity: reddening of lips, strawberry tongue, diffuse injection of oral and pharyngeal mucosa
6. Acute nonpurulent cervical lymphadenopathy

B. Other significant symptoms or findings
   The following symptoms and findings should be clinically considered:
1. Cardiovascular: auscultation (heart murmur, gallop rhythm, distant heart sounds), ECG changes (prolonged PR-QT intervals, abnormal Q wave, low voltage, ST-T changes, arrhythmias), chest x-ray findings (cardiomegaly), 2-D echo findings (pericardial effusion, coronary aneurysms), aneurysm of peripheral arteries other than coronary (axillary, etc.) angina pectoris or myocardial infarction
2. GI tract: diarrhea, vomiting, abdominal pain, hydrops of gallbladder, paralytic ileus, mild jaundice, slight increase of serum transaminase
3. Blood: leukocytosis with shift to the left, thrombocytosis, increased α2-globulin, slight decrease in erythrocyte and hemoglobin levels
4. Urine: proteinuria, increase of leukocytes in urine sediment
5. Skin: redness and crust at the site of BCG inoculation, small pustules, transverse furrows of the fingernail
6. Respiratory: cough, rhinorrhea, abnormal shadow on chest x-ray
7. Joint: pain, swelling
8. Neurological: pleocytosis of mononuclear cells in CSF, convulsion, unconsciousness, facial palsy, paralysis of the extremities

With at least five of the six principal symptoms, or four associated with coronary lesions confirmed by two-dimensional echocardiography or angiography, diagnosis of MCLS can be established.
From J Fukushige, MR Nihill. Kawasaki disease. In A Garson Jr, JT Bricker, DG McNamara (eds): *The Science and Practice of Pediatric Cardiology.* Philadelphia: Lea & Febiger, 1990. Pp 1542–1560. With permission.

feet, generally beginning around the nail beds. Examination of the peripheral blood smear will reveal a marked thrombocytosis.

The most concerning aspect of the acute and subacute phases of Kawasaki syndrome, however, is the formation of dilated aneurysms of medium-sized systemic arteries. The coronary arteries are the most worrisome target of this phenomenon and are involved in 15% to 25% of untreated cases.[72] The coronary arteries may be dilated in a fusiform fashion (coronary ectasia) and subsequently recover their normal configuration. Less frequently, they may develop markedly dilated aneurysms with abrupt transition points from normal-sized arteries ("giant" coronary aneurysms). The combination of relatively slow flow through these large aneurysms and the thrombocytosis present in most children with Kawasaki syndrome may lead to thrombosis of the coronary artery. In addition, as recovery from the acute inflammatory phase progresses, stenoses may form at the transition points between normal-sized coronary artery and aneurysm. Either mechanism can lead to coronary artery occlusion and myocardial ischemia or infarction.

The chronic phase of Kawasaki syndrome is characterized by complete resolution of all inflammatory findings, with the exception of arterial aneurysms in a fraction of patients. The subsequent risk for coronary artery insufficiency or occlusion has been recently stratified according to the degree and severity of coronary artery involvement in the early stages of the illness.[73]

The treatment for Kawasaki syndrome is still undergoing investigation and revision (Table 22-10).[73] Aspirin is administered in antiinflammatory doses during the acute phase, and then in antiplatelet doses during the subacute phase when thrombocytosis is likely. The incidence of giant coronary artery aneurysms can be reduced three- to fivefold when a course of intravenous IgG is administered during the acute phase of the illness.[72]

Table 22-10. Acute treatment for Kawasaki syndrome

Diagnosis
    Examination
    Chest x-ray
    Electrocardiogram
    CBC with differential and platelets
    ESR
    Electrolytes, BUN, creatinine
    Mg, glucose
    LFTs
    Urinalysis with spun sediment stained for monocytes
    Cultures of urine, blood, and throat
    Echocardiogram
    Slit-lamp examination if uveitis suspected
    Abdominal ultrasound if LFTs abnormal or evidence of gall stones
Consultations
    Pediatric Cardiology
    Pediatric Infectious Diseases
Management
    IV IgG 2.0 g/kg IV administered over 10–12 h
    Aspirin 100 mg/kg/d PO divided q6° for 14 days
    Aspirin 5 mg/kg/d PO given qd for 28 days (if no aneurysms)
    If there is no evidence of coronary artery aneurysms on the initial echocardiogram, patient may be discharged after evaluation and administration of IV IgG
Follow-up
    Repeat echocardiogram at 10–14 days
    Repeat echocardiogram at 6 weeks
    Repeat echocardiogram at 6 months

Children who develop giant coronary artery aneurysms require chronic systemic anticoagulation with warfarin. Evidence of acute myocardial ischemia or infarction is an indication for cardiac catheterization to confirm the diagnosis and guide further therapy. In the presence of acute thrombosis of the coronary artery, systemic thrombolysis or selective administration of thrombolytic agents into the affected coronary artery may be a life-saving intervention. Coronary artery bypass grafting may be required in selected patients. Long-term treatment of Kawasaki syndrome depends on the number and size of coronary artery aneurysms.[73] Patients with significant coronary artery involvement may require additional pharmacologic management (e.g., warfarin, verapamil) and restriction in physical activity.

Infective Endocarditis

Infectious endocarditis is an unusual occurance in pediatric patients with congenital heart disease, although the incidence may be increasing among children without congenital heart disease, particularly children who require chronic indwelling catheters. Infectious endocarditis will not be discussed in great detail here except to say that children with congenital heart disease may have a very fulminant course, especially when infected with *Staphylococcus aureus*. Children with artificial material are particularly at risk, including children with shunts, conduits, patches, catheter-implanted devices, and prosthetic cardiac valve replacements. Any child with congenital heart disease who develops a new murmur with a fever must be considered at risk for infectious endocarditis and evaluated immediately.

Infectious endocarditis may be caused by infection with bacterial, fungal, or other pathogens. It presents with fever and may or may not be associated with splinter hemorrhages, Osler nodes, Janeway lesions, or splenomegaly. Blood cultures are positive in up to 90% of cases, the remainder having been diagnosed after echocardiographic identification of intracardiac vegetations or findings at surgery.

When infectious endocarditis is suspected, it is generally recommended that, when possible, six sets of blood cultures be drawn from different sites. Very careful sterile technique is indicated, because contamination of the culture could unnecessarily mandate a prolonged course of intravenous antibiotics. Antimicrobial therapy should be directed by specialists in pediatric cardiology and infectious diseases. Additional support may be required for congestive heart failure and other systemic effects of sepsis.

Cardiac Trauma

As with adult patients, cardiac trauma is often unsuspected in children. Serious cardiac injury may exist in the absence of significant injury to the chest wall. Nonpenetrating injuries to the chest are the most frequent cause of cardiac trauma in children, and are often the result of a motor vehicle accident or a fall with direct trauma to the chest. Indirect injury to the heart also may result from a severe blow to the abdomen with transmission of sudden high pressure along the major vessels. Penetrating cardiac trauma due to stab wounds and gunfire are occurring with increasing incidence, particularly in urban areas.

Pediatric patients with cardiac trauma may suffer injury or rupture of the pericardium, cardiac contusion or rupture, or injury to the cardiac valves or coronary arteries. Injury to the pericardium, myocardium, or other intrathoracic structures may result in hemopericardium with tamponade. Arrhythmias may be associated with any of these injuries or may be the sole manifestation of cardiac trauma.

Following a traumatic event, cardiac trauma must be considered in any patient who has evidence of injury to the chest (chest wall injury, rib fractures, pulmonary contusion or effusion, cardiomegaly) or who has sustained a significant impact (fall, automobile accident, explosion), regardless of whether the chest was involved. The physical exam, chest x-ray, and ECG may be nonspecific, although tachycardia out of proportion to other injuries, or any other type of arrhythmia (including frequent ventricular premature beats), should raise the suspicion of cardiac injury. Widening of the mediastinum suggests aortic rupture. Laboratory studies have been disappointing in identification of myocardial injury, including CPK cardiac isoenzymes and nuclear myocardial scans. Echocardiography and radionucleotide angiography may be helpful in identification of systolic dysfunction and regional wall motion abnormalities. Echocardiography will also identify intracardiac thrombus formation, valve rupture, traumatic septal defects, ventricular aneurysms, hemopericardium, and tamponade.

The treatment for penetrating cardiac trauma or nonpenetrating injury with hemopericardium is immediate surgical repair. Pericardiocentesis may provide temporary relief of tamponade, but may be difficult due to clotting of blood within the catheter. Patients who present with the penetrating object in place should not have it removed except at surgery in order to prevent aggravation of intrathoracic hemorrhage. Patients with suspected aortic rupture or dissection require emergency aortography and/or surgical repair.

In the absence of injuries requiring emergency surgical intervention, stabilization of patients with cardiac trauma includes the administration of inotropes, diuretics, and afterload-reducing agents for congestive heart failure as needed and pharmacologic management of arrhythmias that are judged to have a negative impact on cardiac function. Bed rest is indicated during the acute phase to reduce myocardial work.

Any patient with penetrating injury requires prophylactic antibiotics to prevent infectious endocarditis and pericarditis. Echocardiographic evidence of intracardiac thrombi raises the issue of systemic anticoagulation, although this issue is complicated by concerns over hemorrhage related to trauma. Valve injury or septal defects may require surgical intervention depending on their severity.

Late complications of cardiac trauma can include arrhythmias, ventricular aneurysm and pseudoaneurysm formation, late rupture, or septal defect formation due to break down of injured tissue. Rupture may occur as late as 2 weeks following the initial injury. Serial echocardiographic observations for aneurysm for about 6 months are indicated to rule out aneurysm formation. Postpericardiotomy syndrome may follow penetrating or nonpenetrating cardiac injury by up to several months. Late dissection of the aorta may be identified years after the traumatic event, and may present with back pain or rupture of a dissecting aneurysm. Fistulas involving the coronary arteries may form as a result of trauma and present late with a continuous "machinery-type" murmur.

Management Following Cardiac Catheterization

The objects of cardiac catheterization include the diagnosis of structural abnormalities, evaluation of hemodynamics, and catheter-directed intervention. The procedure takes place in a specially equipped catheterization laboratory utilizing sterile field technique.

The femoral, axillary, or umbilical artery may be used for percutaneous arterial access. Favored venous sites include the femoral, subclavian, brachial, internal jugular, and umbilical veins. In addition to the diagnostic procedures performed in the catheterization laboratory, many interventional procedures are now possible using transcutaneous methods (Table 22-11).

With or without catheter-directed interventional procedures, cardiac catheterization entails a small risk of serious complications (Table 22-12). Many of these complications are recognized in the catheterization laboratory, while others become apparent later. In addition, cardiac catheterization can be a significant stressor to children with and without preexisting cardiovascular compromise, aggravating any underlying disorders (e.g., congestive heart failure) that might otherwise have been well compensated.

On arrival in the ICU, following catheterization, the patient should be examined immediately. Intravenous access and cardiorespiratory monitoring are appropriate for every patient recovering

Table 22-11.　Catheter-directed interventions

Balloon dilation of stenotic valves

Balloon dilation of peripheral pulmonary arteries

Balloon dilation of coarctation of the aorta

Balloon dilation of systemic venous return

Stenting of stenotic vessels

Coronary artery angioplasty

Balloon atrial septostomy (Rashkind)

Blade atrial septostomy

Closure of patent ductus arteriosus

Closure of atrial septal defect (some types)

Closure of ventricular septal defect (some types)

Occlusion of arteriovenous malformations

Occlusion of collateral vessels

Table 22-12.　Complications of cardiac catheterization

Embolism of air, thrombus, implanted devices, catheter fragments, guidewires, or other foreign material, possibly resulting in stroke, myocardial infarction, injury to any organ, or even loss of life

Excessive bleeding, either during the procedure or after leaving the catheterization suite, requiring transfusion or leading to shock

Perforation of the vascular space, leading to significant hemorrhage, hematoma, pericardial tamponade, or hemothorax

Occlusion or injury of the peripheral vessels used for vascular access

Injury to the conduction system of the heart, leading to heart block, bundle branch block, or arrhythmias

Injury to the valve apparatus, leading to valvar incompetence

Dissection of the vessel wall by high-pressure contrast injection ("staining")

Volume overload secondary to crystalloid used for flush and hypertonic intravenous contrast agents

Respiratory compromise due to sedation

Hypercyanotic spells in patients with subpulmonary stenosis (e.g., tetralogy of Fallot)

from cardiac catheterization in the ICU. Bleeding or hematoma at the catheterization sites may develop after hemostasis has been obtained in the catheterization laboratory. Patency of the peripheral arteries should be confirmed by identification of the pulse and examination of the peripheral perfusion distal to the percutaneous entry site. Evidence of a poor cardiac output (hypotension, tachycardia, cool extremities, obtundation) mandates an immediate investigation into the cause, including a careful examination, hematocrit, a chest x-ray, and possibly an ECG to rule out pericardial tamponade.

Following an uncomplicated catheterization, the patient is encouraged to rest flat in bed for at least 4 to 6 hours following any catheterization involving arterial access. Purely venous studies may not require as long a period of bed rest. Small children who would rather thrash and scream than lay flat in bed should be allowed to lie in a parent's lap, because thrashing and screaming do little to prevent rebleeding at the catheterization sites. Vital signs are taken every 15 minutes for the first hour, with examination of the dressings and peripheral pulses. Hourly vital signs are taken for the following few hours. Clear liquids may be taken when the patient is awake, but retching and vomiting, side effects of some sedatives and anesthetics, must be avoided. A hematocrit is taken at 4 hours following the end of the catheterization to rule out occult hemorrhage. The pressure dressings may be removed the day following the catheterization.

Bleeding

Bleeding or hematoma formation may follow cardiac catheterization, particularly when arterial access is required. Hemostasis can generally be obtained by firm, constant pressure on the puncture site, keeping in mind that the puncture in the vessel may be several centimeters cephalad to the skin puncture. It is important to keep the pressure firm, but not painfully so, and to avoid excessive movement while holding the site: A lot of wiggling, adjusting, and peeking on the part of the holder discourages hemostasis and causes a considerable amount of pain for the patient. Position the hand applying the pressure so that the palm is resting on a stable surface, and try to avoid checking for hemostasis more often than every 5 minutes. Try to maintain just enough pressure to prevent bleeding or hematoma formation, but not so much that the vessel is completely occluded for a long period. Occasionally, additional sedation may be required for smaller patients.

If bleeding cannot be stopped with these measures, a vessel tear must be suspected, and local surgical exploration may be required. Continued oozing may be a sign of insufficient platelets or clotting factors, or excessive heparin effect. Heparin given in the catheterization may be reversed with protamine. This is not often done in children, however, because the heparin effect has usually worn off by the end of the case, and because thrombosis of vessels and artificial shunts is generally a more difficult management problem in children than is bleeding.

Thrombosis

Thrombosis of the femoral artery is rarely as dangerous in children as it can be in adults, and in most cases there is no evidence of significant tissue ischemia. However, there are important reasons to try to reestablish patency in the femoral artery in children. Arterial occlusion may result in leg-length discrepancies later in life among children who have not completed their growth at the

Table 22-13. Protocol for the acutely thrombosed femoral artery following cardiac catheterization

Cardiorespiratory monitor

Vital signs q1 hour

Heparin 100 μ/kg loading dose (if > 3 hours from last dose)

Heparin 20 μ/kg/hr (adjust dose to keep q6 hour PTT at 1.5 times baseline)

If pulse is still absent after 24 hours, add a thrombolytic agent such as urokinase or streptokinase for an additional 24–48 hours.
If bleeding occurs, stop all anticoagulants and thrombolytics and apply pressure.

If at any time the perfusion to the distal extremity appears inadequate, consult a vascular surgeon regarding the advisability of a surgical thrombectomy.

---

time of cardiac catheterization. In addition, there are relatively few sites for arterial access in children, and occlusion of the femoral artery may significantly diminish the odds of a successful cardiac catheterization in the future for a child who may require repeated studies. Consequently, when arterial occlusion is suspected on the basis of an absent distal pulse following cardiac catheterization, most centers follow a protocol aimed at restoring patency through the use of anticoagulants, thrombolytics, and, if necessary, surgical thrombectomy (Table 22-13).

Occasionally, thrombosis of the femoral vein occurs following cardiac catheterization. The affected leg may appear dusky and mottled for a short period, but eventually the vein recanalizes, or collateral vessels dilate and signs of venous congestion resolve. Other veins used for access, including the subclavian and internal jugular, may also thrombose on occasion. Although systemic venous occlusion may limit the sites for intravascular access during future catheterizations, treatment with anticoagulants and thombolytics is not generally indicated.

Sedation and Pain Control in Children with Congenital Heart Disease

There are several issues peculiar to children with congenital heart disease who require sedation and pain control in the ICU, including congestive heart failure, tetralogy of Fallot, and hypertrophic obstructive cardiomyopathy.

Children with severe congestive heart failure may be dependent on endogenous catecholamines to maintain an effective cardiac output. Such children are generally tachycardic and tachypneic at rest and require multiple anticongestive medications. Sedation in these children may result in aggravation of congestive heart failure and an acutely depressed cardiac output. Sedation of such children requires close observation and the availability of emergency medical support. In many cases, sedation is most safely accomplished in the ICU with intravenous access. The agents of choice include an opioid (e.g., morphine or fentanyl) and a benzodiazepine (e.g., midazolam). For short procedures, an ultra-short-acting agent (e.g., propofol or ketamine) may be more appropriate. Potent negative inotropes (e.g., inhalational anesthetic agents) should be avoided when possible.

In children with tetralogy of Fallot, catecholamine release may precipitate or aggravate a hypercyanotic spell. Pretreatment with EMLA cream and morphine (0.1 mg/kg SQ) may reduce catecholamine release when starting an IV for more effective sedation or general anesthesia. Agents that result in systemic venous or arterial dilation may aggravate cyanosis as well, and may require concomitant administration of intravascular volume. Ketamine has the advantage that it is associated with an increase in systemic vascular resistance and may favor pulmonary blood flow.

Children with hypertrophic obstructive cardiomyopathy may have aggravation of subaortic obstruction if they are allowed to become dehydrated. Intravenous hydration is mandatory if a child will be NPO prior to a procedure requiring an empty stomach.

Anticoagulation and Thrombolysis

Intravascular Thrombi

Thrombi and thromboemboli are difficult management issues in the pediatric patient population. In addition, infants have unique characteristics of their coagulation and thrombolytic systems that make the prevention and treatment of intravascular thrombi more challenging.[74]

Intravascular thrombi can form as a result of stasis (e.g., catheter occlusion of a vessel, atrial fibrillation, intracardiac tumor), endothelial abnormalities (injury or foreign material used in surgery[75]), foreign bodies (usually catheters), or a coagulopathy (DIC, thrombocytosis, or a congenital disorder of the coagulation system). In children, most intravascular thrombi are associated with chronically indwelling catheters.[76] Most are located in the systemic venous system (innominate vein, superior vena cava, or inferior vena cava), although in newborns with umbilical arterial catheters, there appears to be a significant incidence of aortic thrombus formation.[77–79] Thrombi may be adherent to the catheter itself, a fibrinous sheath surrounding the catheter or the wall of a vessel or cardiac chamber.[80] Most intracardiac thrombi involve the right atrium, although any chamber of the heart may be involved. Many are identified serendipitously in the course of echocardiography for other purposes.

Intracardiac thrombi are associated with several risks: embolization to the pulmonary or systemic circulation, interference with cardiac function, and infection. Embolization to the systemic circulation can be a catastrophic complication, leading to strokes, myocardial infarction, or injury to any tissue in the body. Embolization to the pulmonary circuit may, if sufficiently large, result in obstruction to pulmonary flow. Cardiac thrombi may interfere with cardiac function by creating a physical obstruction to flow through valves or by preventing valves from closing competently, leading to regurgitation.

Intracardiac thrombi are frequently associated with sepsis, particularly catheter-related sepsis. Often it is difficult to discern whether the thrombus is the cause of the sepsis or the result, and it can be quite difficult to be sure whether the thrombus itself is actually infected at all, although, in the case of a gas-forming organism, one can occasionally identify the formation of gas pockets within the thrombus by CT scan.

Once identified, the treatment of intracardiac thrombi is directed at elimination of the thrombus with a minimum of risk. Because of the complexities of the pediatric hemostatic mechanisms, a pediatric hematology expert should direct the treatment process if possible. Initially, heparin is used to prevent further thrombosis and allow the endogenous thrombolytic system to lyse the thrombus. Heparin acts with the cofactor antithrombin III to inactivate thrombin and other activated enzymes (IXa and XIa). It is degraded by the liver and has a half-life of about 30 minutes in the newborn and 60 minutes in the adult. An initial bolus of

50 to 75 U/kg IV is followed by a continuous infusion of 10 to 25 U/kg/hr. The infusion is titrated to maintain the prothrombin time at 1.5 to 2.0 times the patient's own control value. If uncontrollable bleeding occurs, heparin can be neutralized with protamine (1 mg/100 U heparin).[81]

If there is no reduction in the size of the thrombus after 24 hours of heparin therapy, direct lysis of the thrombus can be attempted.[82] Thrombolytic agents include streptokinase, urokinase, and tissue-type plasminogen activator (tPA). Streptokinase is the most commonly used of the three, although urokinase is probably equally effective and may have fewer side effects. Streptokinase can be diluted at 250,000 units in 250 ml D5W to give a concentration of 1000 U/ml. A bolus of 1000 U/kg over 20-minute IV is followed by a continuous infusion of 400 to 1400 U/kg/min.[81,82] The bolus can be repeated if a thrombin time 4 hours after the last bolus is not elevated. The thrombin time, fibrinogen, and fibrin split products should be followed at 4 hours, 8 hours, then every 12 hours thereafter. Thrombolysis with streptokinase or urokinase should result in a prothrombin time of 1.5 to 2.0 times baseline and fibrin split products that are elevated (>40 μg/ml).[83] The fibrinogen should remain greater than 100, although infants may have an isoform of fibrinogen that is not detected by commercial assays, leading to a spuriously low fibrinogen value.

Streptokinase is relatively contraindicated in patients with known trauma, fresh surgery, or a known sensitivity to streptokinase. Streptokinase may increase the risk of intracranial hemorrhage in newborns, particularly premature infants. The streptokinase infusion should be stopped in case of hypotension, bronchospasm, bleeding (including occult blood in the stool or urine), a fibrinogen that is less than 100, clot lysis, or if there is no effect after 48 hours. When it occurs, bleeding can be corrected with cryoprecipitate and FFP. Other side effects of streptokinase include rash and fever.

Because urokinase is an endogenous substance, there may be fewer immune-related side effects and complications associated with its use.[84] The usual systemic thrombolytic dose for urokinase is a loading dose of 4400 U/kg IV over 20 minutes, followed by between 4000 and 20,000 U/kg/hr.[81,82] The same contraindications and monitoring hold for urokinase as for streptokinase. There is relatively little experience using tPA as a thrombolytic in children.

When practical, thrombolytics can be administered locally via an indwelling catheter using a much lower dose. A continuous infusion of streptokinase at 50 U/kg/hr has been used successfully in infants with thrombi in the aorta, inferior vena cava, and Blalock-Taussig shunt.[85] Local thrombolysis may require up to 72 hours or longer.

In general, thrombolytic agents are used for 24 to 72 hours. If there has been no diminution in the size of the thrombus by that time, and the dosage used has been therapeutic according to the aforementioned guidelines, it is unlikely that continued administration will be of benefit. At that point, it may be reasonable to try a different agent, or stop thrombolysis. In a patient who may experience severe complications from thrombus propagation, heparin may be continued according to individual physician judgment.

Surgical thrombectomy may be indicated in a small fraction of patients in whom thrombolytic therapy has been unsuccessful and in whom (1) the thrombus is causing hemodynamic compromise due to interference with cardiac function or (2) bacteremia associated with a presumed infected thrombus cannot be cleared with antibiotics. Surgical intervention in this setting may carry a significant risk, often because of underlying medical problems that may have predisposed to thrombus formation initially.

Management of Thrombosed Intravascular Catheters

As thrombus forms on the tip and inner surface of an intravascular catheter, it can become more and more difficult to infuse fluids through it. Such partially thrombosed catheters can often be cleared by instilling 5000 units of urokinase into the catheter and letting it sit for 30 to 60 minutes, after which the catheter is flushed. If the catheter still presents increased resistance to flow, a second dose of 10,000 units may be used. When two urokinase boluses fail to clear an occluded catheter, a continuous infusion of 200 U/kg/hr may reestablish patency over 24 to 48 hours without significantly affecting systemic coagulation parameters.[86]

Intravascular catheters frequently develop a fibrinous "sheath," which is often noted on echocardiography as a thin structure with a lumen where a catheter had previously been removed. This sheath may extend beyond the tip of the catheter, creating a ball-valve effect that prevents fluid from being withdrawn, leading to concern that the catheter is occluded or has eroded through the vessel wall. Although such concerns are always valid, the intravascular placement of such a catheter can be confirmed with relative ease by contrast echocardiography, thus avoiding an unnecessary catheter removal in patients in whom intravascular access is difficult and crucial.

Anticoagulation of Prosthetic Valves

Both mechanical and bioprosthetic valves are associated with a significant risk of acute or gradual thrombosis. In the aortic position, the resulting aortic obstruction and/or insufficiency can represent a very significant hemodynamic burden. Mitral obstruction can be rapidly fatal. Consequently, antithrombotic therapy is recommended for all patients undergoing valve replacement with the exception of those who receive human homograft or autograft valves.

In children with mechanical valve prostheses, a low dose of heparin (to keep PTT at upper limit of normal) is initiated 6 hours following surgery, then increased to therapeutic doses following removal of thoracostomy tubes (to keep PTT 1.5 to 2.0 times upper limit of normal).[87] When medicines can be taken orally, warfarin is begun at a dose sufficient to maintain the PT at 1.5 to 2.0 times control.[88,89] A good starting dose of warfarin is 0.1 mg/kg/d, not to exceed 10 mg.[81] Aspirin (5 to 10 mg/kg/d) or dipyridamole (3 to 7 mg/kg/d)[91] may be added to warfarin, particularly for mechanical valves in the mitral position. Anticoagulation is continued indefinitely in patients with mechanical valves.

Bioprosthetic (xenograft) valves are infrequently used in the pediatric population because of their relative lack of durability in children. When a bioprosthetic valve is used in the aortic position, therapeutic doses of heparin are continued for 7 to 10 days, then the child is switched over to aspirin at 5 to 10 mg/kg/d. For bioprosthetic mitral valve replacements, the perioperative heparin is again used, followed by warfarin (PT 1.5–2.0 times control) for 3 months, followed by aspirin at 10 mg/kg/d.

The risks of mechanical valve replacements in children include both hemorrhage secondary to anticoagulation, which can be life-threatening, and noncompliance with the anticoagulant therapy, resulting in thrombosis of the valve, frequently leading to severe hemodynamic consequences. The family of any child who requires a mechanical valve prosthesis must be carefully and repeatedly informed of the importance of compliance with the medical regimen. Coagulation studies must be checked regularly and without exception, usually on a monthly basis.

References

1. Doherty JE. The clinical pharmcology of digitalis glycosides: A review. *Am J Med Sci* 255:382, 1968.
2. Lang D, von Bernuth G. Serum concentration and serum half-life of digoxin in premature and mature newborns. *Pediatrics* 59:902, 1977.
3. Hastreiter AR, van der Horst RL, Chow-Tung E. Digitalis toxicity in infants and children. *Pediatr Cardiol* 5:131, 1984.
4. Wettrell G. Optimum therapy of digoxin for low-birth-weight infants. *Pediatrics* 70:1010, 1982.
5. Rutkowski MM, Cohen SN, Doyle EF. Drug therapy of heart disease in pediatric patients. *Am Heart J* 86:270, 1973.
6. Park MK. Use of digoxin in infants and children, with specific emphasis on dosage. *J Pediatr* 108:871, 1986.
7. Pinsky WW et al. Dosage of digoxin in premature infants. *J Pediatr* 96:639, 1979.
8. Rudolph AM. Distribution and regulation of blood flow in the fetal and neonatal lamb. *Circ Res* 57:811, 1985.
9. Siassi B et al. Incidence and clinical features of patent ductus arteriosus in low-birthweight infants: A prospective analysis of 150 consecutively born infants. *Pediatrics* 57:347, 1976.
10. McMurphy DM et al. Developmental changes in constriction of the ductus arteriosus: Responses to oxygen and vaso-active agents in the isolated ductus arteriosus of the fetal lamb. *Pediatr Res* 6:231, 1972.
11. Cotton RB et al. Medical management of small premature infants with symptomatic patent ductus arteriosus. *J Pediatr* 92:467, 1978.
12. Gersony WM et al. Effects of indomethacin in premature infants with patent ductus arteriosus: Results of a national collaborative study. *J Pediatr* 102:895, 1983.
13. Gibson GA. Persistence of the arterial duct and its diagnosis. *Edinburgh Med J* 8:1, 1900.
14. Valdez-Cruz LM, Dudell GG. Specificity and accuracy of echocardiographic and clinical criteria for diagnosis of patent ductus arteriosus in fluid-restricted infants. *Pediatrics* 98:298–305, 1981.
15. Berman W et al. Digoxin therapy in low-birth-weight infants with patent ductus arteriosus. *J Pediatr* 93:652, 1978.
16. Friedman Z et al. Urinary excretion of prostaglandin E following the administration of furosemide and indomethacin to sick low birth weight infants. *J Pediatr* 93:512, 1978.
17. Green TP et al. Furosemide promotes patent ductus arteriosus in premature infants with the respiratory distress syndrome. *N Engl J Med* 308:743, 1983.
18. Dudell GG, Gersony WM. Patent ductus arteriosus in neonates with severe respiratory distress. *J Pediatr* 104:915, 1984.
19. Merritt TA et al. Early closure of the patent ductus arteriosus in very low birth-weight infants: A controlled trial. *J Pediatr* 99:281, 1981.
20. Yeh TF et al. Intravenous indomethacin therapy in premature infants with persistent ductus arteriosus—A double blind controlled study. *J Pediatr* 98:137, 1981.
21. Peckham GJ et al. Clinical course to 1 year of age in premature infants with patent ductus arteriosus: Results of a multicenter randomized trial of indomethacin. *J Pediatr* 105:285, 1984.
22. Cotton RB, Hickey D, Stahlman MT. Management of premature infants with symptomatic patent ductus arteriosus. In Stern L, Bard H, Friis-Hansen B (eds): *Intensive Care of the Newborn* (4th ed). New York: Masson, 1983.
23. Syberth HW et al. Introduction of plasma indomethacin level monitoring and evaluation of an effective threshold level in very low birthweight infants with symptomatic patent ductus arteriosus. *Eur J Pediatr* 141:71, 1983.
24. Cifuentes RF et al. Indomethacin and renal function in premature infants with persistent patent ductus arteriosus. *J Pediatr* 95:583, 1979.
25. Millard RW, Baig H, Vatner SF. Prostaglandin control of the renal circulation in response to hypoxemia in the fetal lamb in utero. *Circ Res* 45:172, 1979.
26. Catterton Z, Sellers B, Gray B. Insulin clearance in the premature infant receiving indomethacin. *J Pediatr* 96:737, 1980.

27. Halliday HL, Hirata T, Brady JP. Indomethacin therapy for large patent ductus arteriosus in the very low birthweight infant: Results and complications. *Pediatrics* 64:154, 1979.

28. Yeh TF et al. Furosemide prevents the renal side-effects of indomethacin therapy in premature infants with patent ductus arteriosus. *J Pediatr* 101:433, 1982.

29. Friedman Z et al. Indomethacin disposition and indomethacin-induced platelet dysfunction in premature infants. *J Clin Pharmacol* 18:272, 1978.

30. Corazza MS et al. Prolonged bleeding time in preterm infants receiving indomethacin for patent ductus arteriosus. *J Pediatr* 105:292, 1984.

31. Ment LR et al. Randomized indomethacin trial for prevention of intraventricular hemorrhage in very low birth weight infants. *J Pediatr* 107:937, 1985.

32. Gerson WM et al. Effects of indomethacin in premature infants with patent ductus arteriosus: Results of a national collaborative study. *J Pediatr* 102:895, 1983.

33. Setzer ES et al. Prophylactic indomethacin and intraventricular hemorrhage in the premature (abstract). *Pediatr Res* 18:345A, 1984.

34. Cotton RB et al. Randomized patent ductus arteriosus in small preterm infants. *J Pediatr* 93:647, 1978.

35. Eggert LD et al. Surgical treatment of patent ductus arteriosus in preterm infants: Four year experience with ligation in the newborn intensive care unit. *Pediatr Cardiol* 2:15, 1982.

36. Strange MJ et al. Surgical closure of patent ductus arteriosus does not increase the risk of intraventricular hemorrhage in the preterm infant. *J Pediatr* 107:602, 1985.

37. Noren GR et al. Occurrence of myocarditis in sudden death in children. *J Forensic Sci* 22:188–196, 1978.

38. Haynes RE et al. Echo virus type 3 infection in children: Clinical and laboratory studies. *J Pediatr* 80:589–595, 1972.

39. Berkovich S, Rodriguez-Torres R, Lin JS. Virologic studies in children with acute myocarditis. *Am J Dis Child* 115:207, 1968.

40. Verlinde JD, Van Tongeren HAE, Kret A. Myocarditis in newborns due to Coxsackie B virus: Viral studies. *Ann Pediatr* 187:113, 1956.

41. Schmidt NJ, Magoffin RL, Lennette EH. Association of group B coxsackieviruses with cases of pericarditis, myocarditis or pleurodynia by demonstration of the immunoglobulin M antibody. *Infect Immun* 8:341–348, 1973.

42. Hirschman ZS, Hammer SG. Coxsackie virus myopericarditis: A microbiological and clinical review. *Am J Cardiol* 34:224–232, 1974.

43. Kibrick S, Benirschke K. Severe generalized disease (encephalohepatomyocarditis) occuring in the newborn period and due to infection with coxsackievirus group B. Evidence of intrauterine infection with this agent. *Pediatrics* 22:857–874, 1958.

44. Hastreiter AR, Miller RA. Management of primary endomyocardial disease: The myocarditis-endocardial fibroelastosis syndrome. *Pediatr Clin North Am* 11:401–430, 1964.

45. Bengtssen E, Lamberger B. Five year follow-up study of cases suggestive of acute myocarditis. *Am Heart J* 72:751, 1966.

46. Tahernia AC. Electrocardiographic abnormalities and transaminase levels in diphtheritic myocarditis. *J Pediatr* 75:1008–1014, 1969.

47. Begg MD. Diphtheritis myocarditis—EKG study. *Lancet* 1:857, 1937.

48. O'Connell JB et al. Gallium-67 imaging in patients with dilated cardiomyopathy and biopsy proven myocarditis. *Circulation* 70:58–62, 1984.

49. Settle HP et al. Echocardiographic study of cardiac tamponade. *Circulation* 56:951, 1977.

50. Kussmaul A. Ueber schwieglige Mediastino-perikarditis und der paradoxen Puls. *Klin Wochenschr* 10:443, 1873.

51. Golinko RV, Kaplan N, Rudolph AM. The mechanism of pulsus paradoxus during acute pericardial tamponade. *J Clin Invest* 42:229, 1963.

52. Franciosi RA, Blanc WA. Myocardial infarcts in infants and children. I: A necropsy study in congenital heart disease. *J Pediatr* 73:309, 1968.

53. Edwards JE. The direction of blood flow in the coronary arteries arising from the pulmonary trunk. *Circulation* 29:163, 1964.

54. Hubbard JF et al. Right ventricular infarction with cardiac rupture in an infant with pulmonary valve atresia with intact ventricular septum. *J Am Coll Cardiol* 2:363, 1983.

55. Fujiwara H et al. Clinicopathologic study of abnormal Q waves in Kawasaki disease (MCLNS): An infantile cardiac disease with myocarditis and myocardial infarction. *Am J Cardiol* 45:797, 1980.

56. Fukushige J, Nihill MR, McNamara DG. Spectrum of cardiovascular lesions in MCLNS: Analysis of 8 cases. *Am J Cardiol* 45:98, 1980.

57. Garson A. *The Electrocardiogram in Infants and Children: A Systematic Approach*. Philadelphia: Lea & Febiger, 1983.

58. Gault MH, Usher R. Coronary thrombosis with myocardial infarction in a newborn infant: Clinical, electrocardiographic and post-mortem findings. *N Engl J Med* 263:379, 1960.

59. Chou TC. *Electrocardiography in Clinical Practice*. New York: Grune & Stratton, 1979.

60. Mariott H. *Practical Electrocardiography* (7th ed). Baltimore: Williams & Wilkins, 1986.

61. Vincent WR, Buckberg GD, Hoffman JIE. Left ventricular subendocardial ischemia in severe valvar and supravalvar aortic stenosis: A common mechanism. *Circulation* 49:326, 1974.

62. Bialostozky D et al. Coronary insufficiency in children. *Am J Cardiol* 36:509, 1975.

63. Buckberg G et al. Ischemia in aortic stenosis: Hemodynamic prediction. *Am J Cardiol* 35:778, 1975.

64. Lewis AB et al. Evaluation of subendocardial ischemia in valvar aortic stenosis in children. *Circulation* 449:978, 1974.

65. Moller JH, Nakib A, Edwards JE. Infarction of papillary muscles and mitral insufficiency associated with congenital aortic stenosis. *Circulation* 34:87, 1966.

66. Driscoll DJ, Glicklich LB, Gallen WJ. Chest pain in children: A prospective study. *Pediatrics* 67:648–651, 1975.

67. Fyfe DA, Moodie DS. Chest pain in pediatric patients presenting to a cardiac clinic. *Clin Pediatr* 23:321, 1984.

68. Rowley AH, Gonzalez Crussi F, Shulman ST. Kawasaki syndrome. *Rev Infect Dis* 10:1–15, 1988.

69. Gersony WM. Diagnosis and management of Kawasaki disease. *JAMA* 265:2699–2703, 1991.

70. Burns JC et al. Clinical and epidemiologic characteristics of patients referred for evaluation of possible Kawasaki disease. *J Pediatr* 118:680–686, 1991.

71. Burns JC et al. Clinical and epidemiologic characteristics of patients referred for evaluation of possible Kawasaki disease. United States Multicenter Kawasaki Disease Study Group. *J Pediatr* 118:680–686, 1991.

72. Newburger JW, Burns JC. Kawasaki syndrome. *Cardiol Clin* 7:453–465, 1989.

73. Dajani AS et al. Guidelines for long-term management of patients with Kawasaki disease. *Circulation* 89:916–922, 1994.

74. Corrigan JJ Jr. Neonatal thrombosis and the thrombolytic system: Pathophysiology and therapy. *Am J Pediatr Hematol Oncol* 10:83–91, 1988.

75. Fyfe DA et al. Transesophageal echocardiography detects thrombus formation not identified by transthoracic echocardiography after the Fontan operation. *J Am Coll Cardiol* 18:1733–1737, 1991.

76. Williams EC. Catheter-related thrombosis. *Clin Cardiol* 13:VI34–VI36, 1990.

77. Goetzman BW et al. Thrombolytic complications of umbilical artery catheters: A clinical and radiographic study. *Pediatrics* 56:374, 1975.

78. Neal WA et al. Umbilical artery catheterization: Demonstration of arterial thrombosis by aortography. *Pediatrics* 50:6, 1972.

79. Gupta JM, Robertson NRC, Wigglesworth JS. Umbilical artery catheterization in the newborn. *Arch Dis Child* 43:382, 1968.

80. Lam D, Emilson B, Rapaport E. Septic pulmonary embolic secondary to an infected right atrial thrombus. *Am Heart J* 114:178–180, 1987.

81. Corrigan JJ Jr. Coagulation disorders. In Miller DR, Baehner RL (eds): *Blood Diseases of Infancy and Childhood* (6th ed). St. Louis: Mosby, 1989. Pp 885–887.

82. Strife JL et al. Arterial occlusions in neonates: Use of fibrinolytic therapy. *Radiology* 166:395–400, 1988.

83. Corrigan JJ Jr. *Hemorrhagic and Thrombotic Diseases in Childhood and Adolescence.* New York: Churchill Livingstone, 1985.

84. Meister FL et al. Urokinase: A cost-effective alternative treatment of superior vena cava thrombosis and obstruction. *Arch Intern Med* 149:1209–1210, 1989.

85. Pritchard SL, Culham JAG, Rogers PCJ. Low-dose fibrinolytic therapy in infants. *J Pediatr* 106:594–598, 1985.

86. Bagnall HA, Gomperts E, Atkinson JB. Continuous infusion of low-dose urokinase in the treatment of central venous catheter thrombosis in infants and children. *Pediatrics* 83:963–966, 1989.

87. Chesebro JH, Adams PG, Fuster U. Antithrombotic therapy in patients with valular heart disease and prosthetic heart valves. *J Am Coll Cardiol* 8:41B, 1986.

88. Schaffer M et al. The St. Jude Medical cardiac valve in infants and children: Role of anticoagulant therapy. *J Am Coll Cardiol* 9:235, 1987.

89. Makhlous A et al. Prosthetic heart valve replacement in children. *J Thorac Cardiovasc Surg* 93:80, 1987.

90. Chesebro J, Fuster V, Elveback L. Trial of combined Warfarin pulus dipyridamole or aspirin therapy in prosthetic heart valve replacement. *Am J Cardiol* 51:1537, 1983.

91. Dreyer WJ. Congestive heart failure. In Garson A Jr, Bricker JT, McNamara DG (eds): *The Science and Practice of Pediatric Cardiology.* Philadelphia: Lea & Febiger, 1990. Pp. 2007–2023.

92. Fukushige J, Nihill MR. Kawasaki disease. In Garson A Jr, Bricker JT, McNamara DG (eds): *The Science and Practice of Pediatric Cardiology.* Philadelphia: Lea & Febiger, 1990. Pp 1542–1560.

93. Moller JH, Neal WA. *Fetal, Neonatal, and Infant Cardiac Disease.* East Norwalk, CT: Appleton-Lange, 1990.

Mary Etta E. King

23 ▶ Noninvasive Cardiovascular System Assessment and Monitoring

Over the past decade, two-dimensional imaging and Doppler ultrasound have emerged as key investigative tools for the noninvasive assessment of the cardiovascular system. They provide extensive information about the structure of the heart and great vessels as well as important data regarding cardiac function and intravascular blood flow. Cardiac ultrasound has tremendous advantage as a diagnostic and monitoring technique in the acute care environment by virtue of its portability, safety, and patient acceptance.

Technical Issues

Performance of a cardiac ultrasound study involves the placement of a transducer on the anterior chest wall and upper abdomen, coupled with an acoustic ultrasound gel to prevent air from interfering with the transducer-skin interface. Optimal insonation of the cardiac structures depends on passage of the interrogating ultrasound beam through the anterior chest wall or abdominal wall to the underlying heart without interference by air-containing lung or bony structures. Thus, the best echocardiographic windows are along the parasternal border between ribs, at the cardiac apex, and through solid organs (e.g., the liver) from the subcostal approach. In infants and small children, the cartilaginous nature of the ribs allows freer access to the heart without limitation to the intercostal spaces. In the older child, left lateral positioning may be required to move the heart closer to the chest wall and out from beneath the sternum.

A cursory ultrasound study can provide initial diagnosis and allow the physician caring for the patient to make appropriate changes in management. However, a complete anatomic study may require 45 minutes or longer of uninterrupted time to fully evaluate all aspects of the heart and great vessels. Nursing staff and sonographer should work together to ensure that the best echocardiographic data are obtained without harm or undue stress to the infant or child. It is impossible to acquire diagnostic images from a moving target. While the newborn infant or critically ill child may be easily examined, an agitated infant or child must be calmed or sedated to allow accurate echo-Doppler study.

Scanning can be performed on an open warming table, within an isolette or in a bassinet under warming lights. Attention to the infant's temperature is important. It should be noted that the usual position of an automatic temperature sensing probe for an open warming table lies directly beneath the sonographer's hand for much of the examination, and thus proper temperature sensing is impaired. The sensing probe should be readjusted before beginning the examination.

In infants and postoperative patients, the subxyphoid or subcostal region often provides the optimal window to image cardiac structures. However, this necessitates constant pressure of the transducer on the abdomen, which limits diaphragmatic excursion and may alter respiratory dynamics during this part of the study. Changes in patient position to left lateral decubitus or with shoulder elevation are sometimes required during scanning. Assistance of the nursing staff is important to ensure that intravenous or arterial lines, chest tubes, and endotracheal tubes are not compromised. Lastly, where issues of sterility are concerned (such as postoperative scanning near a fresh incision or posttransplant), sterile scanning gel and sterile transducer covers are available.

Structural Heart Disease

One of the primary applications of echocardiography is the diagnosis of structural heart disease in the neonatal intensive care unit (ICU). Suspicion of primary cardiac anomalies in an acutely ill newborn can be confirmed rapidly, allowing for immediate alteration in management. With the detailed structural and functional information provided by an experienced echocardiographer, many infants can be managed either medically or surgically without need for cardiac catheterization,[1,2] or if still needed, catheterization can be performed under more controlled circumstances for specific diagnostic or therapeutic purposes (e.g., balloon septostomy, balloon valvuloplasty).

The approach to a child with suspected congenital heart disease should be thorough and systematic, including analysis of all the major cardiac segments—abdominal and atrial situs, ventricular identification and location, great artery size and position, relationship between ventricles and great arteries, coronary artery origins and course, systemic and pulmonary veins, and associated valvular or septal defects.

Abdominal and Atrial Situs

Identifying the abdominal aorta and inferior vena cava can be done with a cross-sectional image at the level of the diaphragm where both vessels are seen in cross-section—the aorta lying just anterior to the spine and the inferior vena cava anteriorly and toward the patient's right when abdominal situs is normal. The aorta pulsates visibly, and Doppler sampling demonstrates pulsatile systolic flow. Imaging both vessels in their long axis allows the examiner to trace them cephalad and note the inferior caval entry into the right atrium joined by the hepatic veins, and the pulsatile aorta coursing behind the heart. With situs inversus, the right-to-left orientation of the inferior vena cava and aorta is reversed. The inferior cava can still be traced upwards into the right atrium, but the latter will then lie toward the patient's left.

Identifying anatomic right versus anatomic left atria is facilitated by several factors. The Eustachian valve is often a prominent feature crossing the floor of the right atrium and parenthetically should not be mistaken for a vegetation, tumor, or intravenous catheter. Caval and coronary sinus entry usually defines the functional right atrium; and pulmonary venous entry, the left atrium. (This would not pertain in those lesions with anomalous systemic or pulmonary venous connections, such as the heterotaxy syndromes where situs is frequently ambiguous.) The septum primum generally overlaps the septum secundum on the anatomic left atrial side. The right and left atrial appendages also have slightly different shapes, and when both can be visualized, they may assist in differentiating anatomic right and left atrial chambers.[3]

Atrioventricular Connection and Ventricular Chambers

The next major portion of the segmental evaluation of congenital heart disease requires evaluation of the atrioventricular connections and ventricular identification. The atria can connect to the ventricles via two distinct atrioventricular valves, a single A-V valve with atresia of the other inlet, or a common A-V orifice. The presence of only one ventricular chamber denotes a univentricular heart or severe hypoplasia of one of the ventricles (Fig. 23-1). When two ventricles are present, the anatomic right ventricle can be discerned by noting the moderator band crossing near the apex, three papillary muscles, a trabeculated septal surface, and a tri-

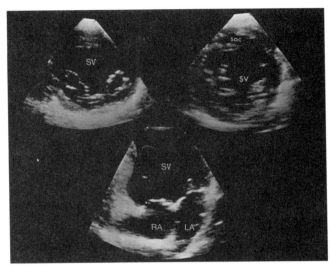

Figure 23-1. Echocardiographic views from a patient with univentricular heart. In the upper left panel, a single ventricular chamber is seen with two atrioventricular valves and no interventricular septum. In the upper right panel, a small outlet chamber is visible along the anterior aspect of the ventricle. The bottom panel demonstrates the image obtained from the apex, with both atrioventricular valves entering the single ventricle. LA, left atrium; RA, right atrium; soc, small outlet chamber; SV, single ventricle. (Prepared by M.E. King, MD, and reproduced with permission from Liberthson RR. Congenital heart disease in the child, adolescent, and adult. In Eagle KA, Haber E, DeSanctis RW, Austen WG (eds): *The Practice of Cardiology,* Boston, Little, Brown and Company, 1989.)

leaflet atrioventricular valve which inserts more apically along the interventricular septum than does the mitral valve. The anatomic left ventricle is characteristically less trabeculated, with a smooth septal surface, two papillary muscles, and a bileaflet atrioventricular valve.[4] With these distinguishing features, the echocardiographer can then identify the number of ventricular chambers, which ventricle is anatomically right and left, where the ventricles lie in anteroposterior and right-to-left orientation, and their relative size and wall thickness (Fig. 23-2).

Great Arteries

The aorta and pulmonary artery in the normal heart wrap around each other as they exit from their respective ventricles. This creates a so-called circle and sausage appearance when imaged echocardiographically in a cross-sectional plane (Fig. 23-3).[5] The semilunar aortic and pulmonic valves can be seen opening at the base of the great vessels, and by following the distal course of each vessel, the pulmonary artery can be distinguished by an early bifurcation into right and left branches, and the aorta by its arch and brachiocephalic vessels. The coronary arteries can also be seen with current high-frequency transducers, and their origins and proximal course should be sought to exclude anomalous course or origin.

When the great vessels are transposed, they arise in parallel from the base of the heart. This creates an image of both vessels running in parallel when viewed in their long axis, and both vessels in cross-section when viewed in the short axis plane (Fig. 23-4). The relationship of aorta to pulmonary artery in the transposition complexes can be described by noting the anteroposterior and right-to-left orientation in the cross-sectional plane—the aorta anterior and to the right in D-transposition, the aorta anterior and to the left in L-transposition, and side-by-side or direct anteroposterior orientation in double-outlet right ventricle or other types of malpositions. With aortic or pulmonary atresia, there is only one large semilunar valve and a small satellite vessel containing no moving valve tissue. Truncus arteriosus will demonstrate a large semilunar root (frequently with an abnormal valve), which gives off branch pulmonary vessels after exiting from the heart[6] (Fig. 23-5).

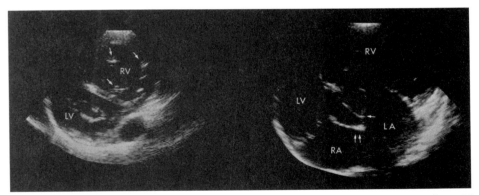

Figure 23-2. Images from a patient with physiologically corrected transposition with ventricular inversion to illustrate the echocardiographic features that distinguish anatomic right and left ventricles. The panel on the left is a cross-sectional view of the ventricles showing three papillary muscles *(arrows)* in the anterior left-sided ventricle and a smooth septal surface in the posterior right-sided ventricle. The panel on the right demonstrates the more apical origin of the tricuspid valve *(single arrow)* when compared with the origin of the mitral valve *(double arrow)* with respect to the atrioventricular septum. LA, left atrium; LV, left ventricle; RA, right atrium; RV, right ventricle. (Prepared by M.E. King, MD, and reproduced with permission from Liberthson RR. Congenital heart disease in the child, adolescent, and adult. In Eagle KA, Haber E, DeSanctis RW, Austen WG (eds): *The Practice of Cardiology,* Boston, Little, Brown and Company, 1989.)

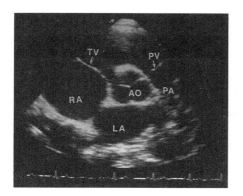

Figure 23-3. Cross-sectional echocardiographic view at the base of the heart depicting the normal wrapping of the right ventricular outflow tract over the aorta, creating the so-called circle (aorta) and sausage (RV outflow tract and PA) pattern. Ao, aorta; LA, left atrium; PA, pulmonary artery; PV, pulmonic valve; RA, right atrium; TV, tricuspid valve.

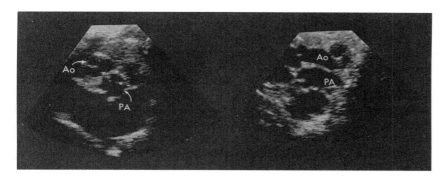

Figure 23-4. Parasternal echocardiographic images in a patient with complete transposition of the great arteries. In the panel on the left, the semilunar valves are both seen in cross-section with the aorta lying anterior and to the patient's right (D-transposition). In the panel on the right, the long axis of the great vessels demonstrates their parallel origin from the heart, with the aorta anterior to the pulmonary artery. Ao, aorta; PA, pulmonary artery. (Prepared by M.E. King, MD, and reproduced with permission from Levine RA et al. Echocardiography, principles of clinical applications. In Eagle KA, Haber E, DeSanctis RW, Austen WG (eds): *The Practice of Cardiology*, Boston, Little, Brown and Company, 1989.)

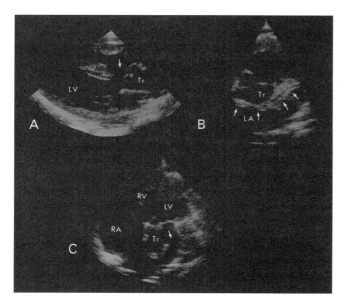

Figure 23-5. Echocardiographic images of a patient with truncus arteriosus Type I. **(A)** The large truncal root overrides the interventricular septum with a large outlet ventricular septal defect *(arrow)*. **(B)** The cross-sectional view at the level of the truncal valve demonstrates the anomalous origin of the left coronary artery from the noncoronary sinus. From the apical five-chamber view **(C)**, the origin of the main pulmonary artery can be seen from the lateral aspect of the truncus *(arrow)* as well as its proximal branching. LA, left atrium; LV, left ventricle; RA, right atrium; RV, right ventricle; TR, truncus arteriosus. (Reproduced by permission from King ME, Complex congenital heart disease II: A pathologic approach. In Weyman AE: *Principles and Practice of Echocardiography*, Lea and Febiger, 1994.)

Ventriculoarterial Relationship

Having established the number and orientation of the ventricular chambers and the number and orientation of the great arteries, it is necessary to define the relationship between ventricles and great vessels. In any of the long-axis views, these structures can be imaged in the same plane, and the origin of the aorta and pulmonary artery can be delineated. In this way, simple transposition can be diagnosed by the origin of the pulmonary artery from the left ventricle and the aorta from the right ventricle. Noting the relation-

ship of the great arteries to the ventricular septum allows detection of an overriding vessel, such as in tetralogy of Fallot or Taussig-Bing type of double-outlet right ventricle (Fig. 23-6).

Systemic and Pulmonary Venous Drainage

Systemic and pulmonary venous anatomy may have been noted earlier in the course of identifying the atrial situs. However, careful identification of all four pulmonary vein entries should be per-

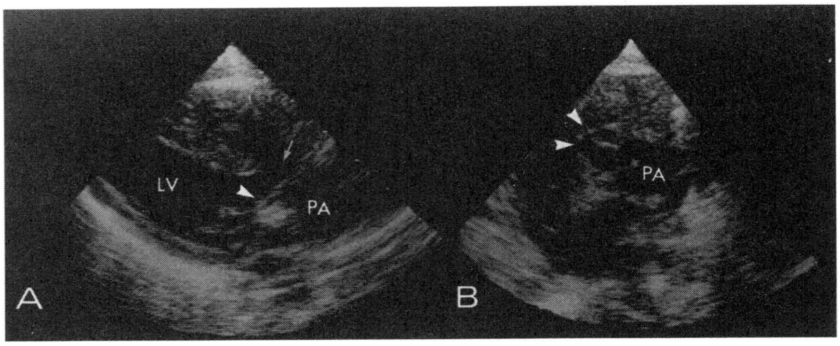

Figure 23-6. Parasternal echocardiographic views from a patient with Taussig-Bing type of double-outlet right ventricle. **(A)** The pulmonary artery overrides the interventricular septum above a large ventricular septal defect *(small arrow)*. The dense material *(caret)* beneath the pulmonic valve leaflets is subpulmonary conal tissue. **(B)** The cross-sectional view of the great vessels shows a side-by-side relationship with a hypoplastic aorta (carets) to the right of a larger pulmonary artery. (Prepared by M.E. King, MD, and reproduced by permission from Liberthson RR. Congenital heart disease in the child, adolescent, and adult. In Eagle KA, Haber E, DeSanctis RW, Austen WG (eds): *The Practice of Cardiology*, Boston, Little, Brown and Company, 1989.)

Figure 23-7. In the panel on the left, the parasternal long axis echocardiographic view of the left ventricular outflow tract shows doming of the aortic valve leaflets in systole *(arrows)*. The continuous wave Doppler spectral tracing on the right shows flow across the aortic valve obtained from the suprasternal notch. The peak systolic velocity of just under 3 m/sec predicts a peak instantaneous gradient of about 36 mm Hg. LA, left atrium; LV, left ventricle; m/s, meters/second (Prepared by M.E. King, MD, and reproduced with permission from Liberthson RR. Congenital heart disease in the child, adolescent, and adult. In Eagle KA, Haber E, DeSanctis RW, Austen WG (eds): *The Practice of Cardiology*, Boston, Little, Brown and Company, 1989.)

formed methodically. This can usually be done by imaging the left atrium from the suprasternal notch where the "crab-like" appearance denotes the four veins entering the body of the left atrium. Pulsed Doppler sampling or color flow mapping will confirm pulmonary venous flow from each vein (Color Plate 1). Marked aberration from this pattern is seen in total anomalous pulmonary venous drainage (TAPVD). The pulmonary veins return to a separate venous chamber in most forms of TAPVD, which must then be followed to its site of entry into the systemic venous system.

The course of the normal caval structures should be confirmed by tracing the vessels with two-dimensional imaging and noting venous flow patterns by pulsed or color flow Doppler. Abnormalities of systemic venous return may include persistence of a left superior vena cava with or without a connecting innominate vein, absence of a right-sided superior vena cava, and interruption of the inferior vena cava with azygos or hemiazygous continuation.

Valvular Stenosis and Regurgitation

The next aspect of evaluation of structural heart disease includes delineation of associated valvular lesions. Valvular stenosis is defined as doming of valve leaflets on opening. This is readily ascertained by two-dimensional imaging (Fig. 23-7). More important to clinical management, however, is the degree of obstruction across the stenotic valve. Doppler echocardiography provides an accurate estimate of transvalvular pressure gradients by measuring the peak velocity across the stenotic orifice.[7] Borrowing from the field of fluid dynamics, the modified Bernoulli equation relates

changes in pressure across a stenotic orifice to changes in velocity of the blood flowing across the valve:

$$P_1 - P_2 = 4(V_2^2 - V_1^2)$$

where P_1 is pressure proximal to the stenosis, P_2 is pressure distal to the stenosis, V_2 is velocity distal to the valve, and V_1 is velocity proximal to the valve (Fig. 23-8).

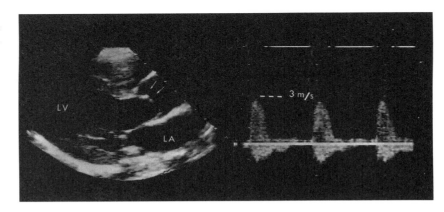

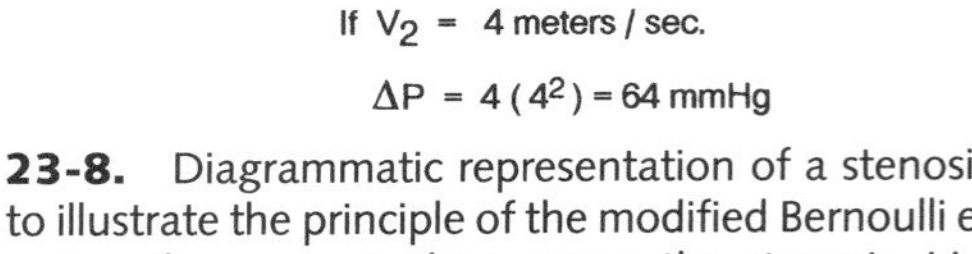

$$P_1 - P_2 = 4(V_2^2 - V_1^2)$$

$$\Delta P = 4V_2^2$$

If $V_2 = 4$ meters / sec.

$$\Delta P = 4(4^2) = 64 \text{ mmHg}$$

Figure 23-8. Diagrammatic representation of a stenosis within a vessel to illustrate the principle of the modified Bernoulli equation for estimating the pressure drop across the stenosis. V_2 and P_2 represent the velocity and pressure distal to the stenosis. V_1 and P_1 represent the velocity and pressure proximal to the stenosis. The equation states that the pressure drop across the obstruction (ΔP) varies as the square of the change in velocity across the stenosis.

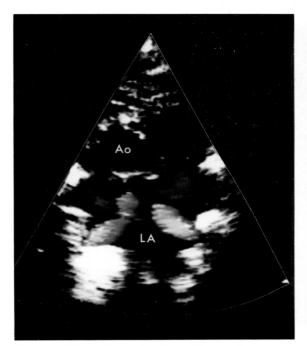

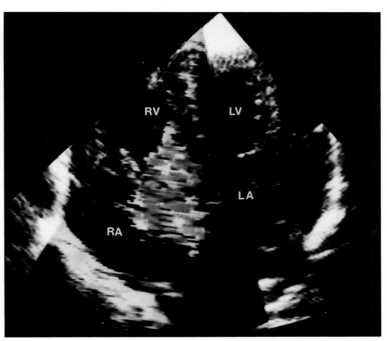

Plate 1. Echocardiographic view with color flow Doppler from the suprasternal notch, demonstrating flow entering the left atrium from four pulmonary veins. Flow from the left and right upper pulmonary veins is shown in blue, and the left and right lower veins in red. Ao, aorta; LA, left atrium.

Plate 2. Apical view of the heart in a child with severe tricuspid insufficiency. The regurgitant jet (shown in blue) begins at the coaptation point of the tricuspid leaflets and fills most of the right atrium. LA, left atrium; LV, left ventricle; RA, right atrium; RV, right ventricle.

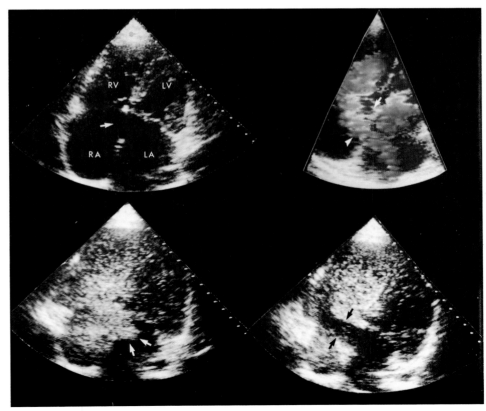

Plate 3. Series of apical four-chamber echocardiographic views in a patient with an ostium primum atrial septal defect. In the upper left panel, the dropout in the lower atrial septum (*arrow*) delineates the defect. Doppler color flow mapping (*upper right*) demonstrates a wide band of flow crossing from left atrium to right atrium (*arrows*). Following intravenous injection of agitated saline, microbubbles are detected as contrast within the cardiac chambers. In the lower left panel, right-to-left shunting can be seen across the defect (*arrows*), and left-to-right negative contrast is shown in the lower right panel as unopacified blood crosses the atrial defect. LA, left atrium; LV, left ventricle; RA, right atrium; RV, right ventricle. (Prepared by M. E. King, MD; and reproduced with permission from Levine RA, et al. Echocardiography: principles and clinical applications. In Eagle KA, Haber E, DeSanctis RW, Austen WG (eds): *The Practice of Cardiology*. Boston, Little, Brown and Company, 1989.)

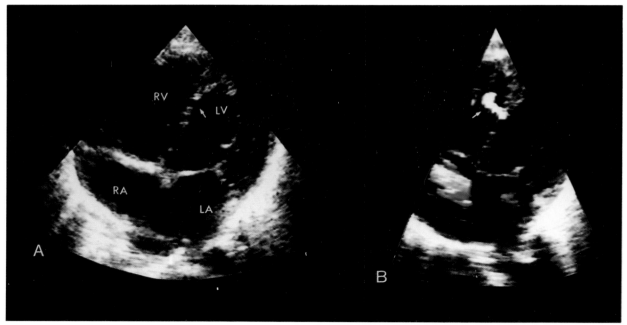

Plate 4. Apical four-chamber echocardiographic views of the heart, demonstrating a muscular ventricular septal defect in panel A with tissue dropout in the lower third of the interventricular septum (*arrow*) and in panel B the color flow Doppler signals crossing the defect (*arrow*). LA, left atrium; LV, left ventricle; RA, right atrium; RV, right ventricle.

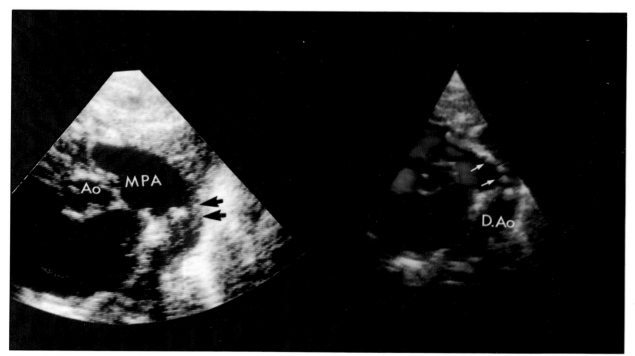

Plate 5. Parasternal short axis images at the base of the heart depicting a patent ductus arteriosus (*black arrows*) on the left, and the color Doppler appearance of the shunt flow from the descending aorta into the pulmonary artery (*white arrows*) on the right. Ao, aorta; DAo, descending aorta; MPA, main pulmonary artery. (Reproduced with permission from Nidorf SM, King ME. Echocardiography. In Thrall JH. *Cardiac Radiology: The Requisites*. St. Louis, C.V. Mosby Co., 1994.)

A

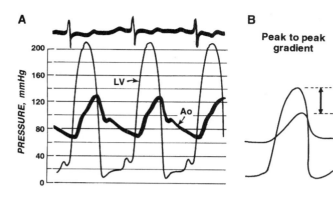

B

Peak to peak gradient

C

Peak instantaneous gradient

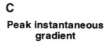

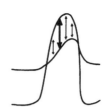

Figure 23-9. Pressure tracings in a patient with aortic stenosis obtained at cardiac catheterization, demonstrating the time course of pressure development within the left ventricle and aorta. **(A)** The left ventricular pressure tracing reaches a peak of over 200 mm Hg in systole. The aortic tracing reaches a peak systolic pressure of 120 mmHg. **(B)** Demonstrates the catheterization method of reporting the pressure gradient across the valve by determining the difference between the peak pressure of each tracing. **(C)** The dense arrow demonstrates the highest pressure difference between left ventricle and aorta at any point during systole, which is the peak instantaneous gradient measured by Doppler. The mean pressure difference integrates the area between the two curves and should be nearly identical for either method. Ao, aorta; LV, left ventricle.

For most clinical settings, V_1 can be neglected because it is less than 1, thus simplifying the equation to

$$\Delta P = 4V^2$$

Thus, the pressure gradient (ΔP) in millimeters of mercury can be estimated by detecting the peak velocity across the stenotic valve (V) in meters per second, squaring this velocity, and multiplying it by four.[8] Most current echocardiographic equipment calculates peak and mean gradients automatically from manually traced spectral Doppler velocity profiles. The correlation of mean gradients with catheterization-determined mean gradients is excellent. The Doppler peak gradient often overestimates the catheterization peak-to-peak gradient, because the Doppler measures the highest velocity at any point during transvalvular flow and gives a peak instantaneous gradient[9] (Fig. 23-9).

Valvular regurgitation can be detected readily by pulsed or color flow Doppler as flow occurring behind the closed valve leaflets into the proximal chamber (Color Plate 2). Indeed, with the availability of color flow Doppler, even tiny amounts of regurgitation are detected, which are probably physiologic and not indicative of valvular pathology. Trace regurgitation by Doppler is rarely audible by clinical examination. Its presence in children with structurally normal hearts is common for the tricuspid (75%) and pulmonic valves (84%), somewhat less frequent for the mitral valve (2%), and unusual for the aortic valve (0.3%).[10–12]

The Doppler color flow map provides a spatial picture of flow velocities that correlates roughly, but not precisely, with the volume of regurgitant flow.[13,14] Thus, the severity of valvular regurgitation is often graded visually as trace, mild, moderate or severe, based on the width of the regurgitant jet at the valve leaflets and the depth of its penetration into the receiving chamber. Chamber enlargement and increased forward flow velocities across the regurgitant valve also help to quantitate severity of regurgitation. The regurgitant fraction can be more specifically quantified by comparing pulsed Doppler estimates of forward stroke volume across a valve unaffected by the regurgitant flow with forward flow across the regurgitant valve (see section on Myocardial Function)[15] (Fig. 23-10). This requires meticulous attention to acquiring the imaging

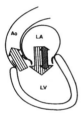

$$\text{REGURGITANT FRACTION} = \frac{\text{MITRAL FLOW} - \text{FORWARD FLOW}}{\text{MITRAL FLOW}}$$

Figure 23-10. Diagrammatic representation of the method for estimating mitral regurgitant fraction. The large arrow indicates forward flow across the mitral valve, which includes the forward cardiac output plus the volume of flow which has leaked across the valve during the previous beat. The flow across the aortic valve is the forward cardiac output. The regurgitant fraction can then be calculated by subtracting aortic flow from mitral flow and dividing by mitral flow. Ao, aorta; LA, left atrium; LV, left ventricle. (Reproduced by permission from Marshall SA, Weyman AE. Doppler estimation of volumetric flow. In Weyman AE: *Principles and Practice of Echocardiography*, Philadelphia, Lea and Febiger, 1994.)

and Doppler data and is somewhat time consuming to calculate, making it more often a research tool than a practical clinical method.

Septal Defects

Atrial and ventricular septal defects are found as isolated abnormalities but are also commonly associated with more complex congenital malformations, and thus should be sought as part of the complete evaluation of the infant or child with suspected congenital heart disease. The interatrial septum can be clearly recorded from the subcostal window.[16] Primum, secundum, or sinus venosus defects are apparent as defects in the septum in their respective locations (Fig. 23-11). Patency of the foramen ovale is noted by

Figure 23-11. Subcostal echocardiographic views of the heart focusing on the interatrial septum. On the left, a defect in the mid-atrial septum *(caret)* represents a secundum atrial septal defect. The central panel demonstrates a large area of dropout from the mid-septum to the atrioventricular groove, indicative of an ostium primum defect. In the panel on the right, a defect is present high in the atrial septum near the roof of the atrium, consistent with a sinus venosus defect. RA, right atrium. (Prepared by M.E. King, MD, and reproduced with permission from Liberthson RR. Congenital heart disease in the child, adolescent, and adult. In Eagle KA, Haber E, DeSanctis RW, Austen WG (eds): *The Practice of Cardiology*, Boston, Little, Brown and Company, 1989.)

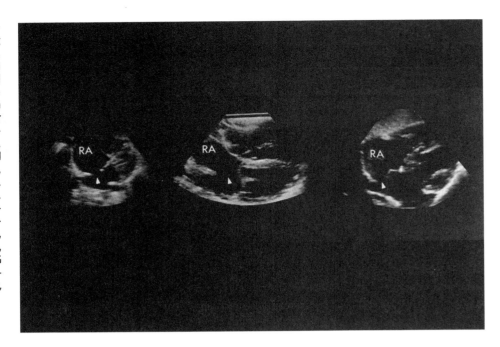

bowing or flapping of the septum primum covering the fossa ovalis away from the plane of the remainder of the septum. Color flow mapping can detect shunt flow across these defects either left to right or right to left (Color Plate 3, upper right). When atrial pressures are nearly equal, the velocity of shunt flow is quite low and may be difficult to detect by color Doppler. In this situation, if a suspected atrial defect must be confirmed, saline contrast echocardiography is helpful.[17] By rapidly injecting a small volume of agitated saline intravenously, a contrast effect is achieved by ultrasound reflection from the tiny microbubbles in the injectate. As the saline enters the right atrium, it passes right to left across the atrial septal defect, and contrast can be seen entering the left atrium (Color Plate 3, lower panels).

The ventricular septum is a more complex structure than the interatrial septum. It must be examined in all its segments to exclude ventricular communications. Large defects are easily apparent as dropout of the septal wall (Fig. 23-12). Smaller communications may be noted only by color flow Doppler as the shunt flow passes across the defect (Color Plate 4). As with atrial shunts, the pressure difference between the left and right heart will determine the velocity of shunt flow and the ease with which that shunt can be seen by color Doppler. In an infant with elevated right-sided pressures, small muscular defects may not be detected, as they are not large enough to see directly on imaging, and shunt flow velocities are too low to be detected unambiguously by pulsed or color Doppler. When the pulmonary vascular resistance falls, the left-to-right shunt flow across even the smallest defects will then be easily detected.

An atrial or ventricular shunt can be semiquantified by the size of the defect on two-dimensional imaging and the size of the color flow stream within the defect.[18] More precise estimates of shunt ratio (Q_p:Q_s) are possible using pulsed Doppler measurements of cardiac output across the aortic and pulmonic valves (see section on Myocardial Function).

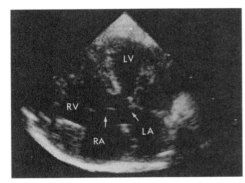

Figure 23-12. Apical four-chamber echocardiographic view of a large atrioventricular septal defect. The central fibrous crux of the heart is absent and the common atrioventricular valve passes through the defect *(arrows)*. LA, left atrium; LV, left ventricle; RA, right atrium; RV, right ventricle.

Distal Aorta, Pulmonary Artery, and Ductus Arteriosus

To complete the assessment of structural heart disease, the distal aspects of the aorta and pulmonary artery must be evaluated. Supravalvular aortic stenosis, coarctation of the aorta, aortic arch interruption, double aortic arch, and aberrant origins of the brachiocephalic vessels should be considered when imaging the aorta. From the suprasternal notch or high right parasternal approach, the long axis of the ascending aorta, aortic arch, and proximal descending thoracic aorta can be demonstrated. In a suprasternal cross-sectional plane, the relationship of the ascending and descending aorta can be shown to determine if the arch is to the left or to the right. Tracing the origin and course of the brachiocephalic vessels will also indicate a right or left arch pattern. In infants and small children, the aortic arch may also be well visualized from

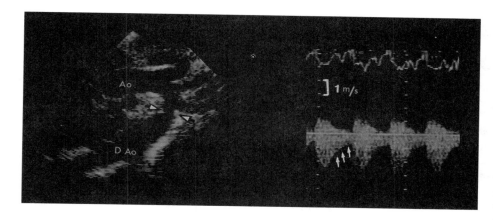

Figure 23-13. In the left panel, a suprasternal echocardiographic view depicts an aortic coarctation at the isthmus *(arrows)*. Mild tubular narrowing of the transverse arch is present, as well as poststenotic dilatation of the descending aorta. In the panel on the right, the continuous wave Doppler spectral tracing of flow in the descending aorta is high in velocity (3 m/sec), with a characteristic pattern of continued gradient into early diastole *(arrows)*. Ao, aorta; DAo, descending aorta; m/s, meters/second. (Prepared by M.E. King, MD, and reproduced with permission from Liberthson RR. Congenital heart disease in the child, adolescent, and adult. In Eagle KA, Haber E, DeSanctis RW, Austen WG (eds): *The Practice of Cardiology*, Boston, Little, Brown and Company, 1989.)

the subxyphoid approach. Doppler sampling assists in detecting discrete obstruction and in quantifying the gradient at the site of coarctation (Fig. 23-13).

The distal pulmonary artery should also be interrogated for the presence of branch stenoses or the rare case of absence of one of the pulmonary branches. In this portion of the examination, the patent ductus arteriosus should also be sought. Its course from the inner curvature of the aortic arch to the posterior aspect of the pulmonary artery bifurcation allows visualization from either the pulmonary artery bifurcation or the views of the aortic arch. Color flow mapping quickly detects left-to-right shunt flow into the main pulmonary artery as a stream of retrograde flow entering at the bifurcation in diastole (Color Plate 5). When pulmonary arterial pressures and resistance are high, ductal shunt flow will be low in velocity, reflecting the small differential in pressures between aorta and pulmonary artery. In this instance, shunting may be right to left and more difficult to detect by Doppler. When the ductus is large and imaged clearly, flow within it can be detected by either pulsed or color flow Doppler.

Monitoring Surgical and Nonsurgical Therapies for Structural Heart Disease

Following diagnosis of a congenital heart defect, cardiac ultrasound can be used to evaluate the effect of medical and/or surgical therapy of that lesion.

Patent Ductus Arteriosus

In newborn ICUs, the premature infant who develops a murmur, bounding pulses, and/or becomes difficult to wean successfully from mechanical ventilation is often suspected of having a patent ductus arteriosus with left-to-right shunt as a contributing factor. Echocardiography can image the ductus and show its size and direction of shunting.[19–21] Quantification of ductal shunt flow relies on evidence of left atrial and left ventricular chamber enlargement, width and extent of the color flow jet into the pulmonary artery, degree of retrograde flow in the aorta near the ductal origin, and

pulsed Doppler estimates of the ratio of pulmonary and systemic flow (see section on Myocardial Function).[22,23] Following administration of indomethacin, echo-Doppler study may be repeated to confirm clinical evidence of ductal closure or document continued shunt flow, which may require further intervention.

In the converse clinical setting, infants with critical obstruction to pulmonary blood flow or severe aortic coarctation must maintain patency of the ductus to provide pulmonary blood flow or peripheral arterial circulation until surgical repair can be accomplished. Usually, this occupies only a few hours of initial stabilization of the infant, but occasionally, longer delays are required. Echocardiographic monitoring of ductal patency may be helpful in these cases.

Balloon Septostomy

Infants with complete transposition of the great arteries or other complex lesions, which require free mixing of atrial blood, may need urgent balloon septostomy. Although in many instances this is done under fluoroscopic guidance in the catheterization laboratory, it can also be accomplished under echocardiographic guidance in the neonatal ICU.[24,25] This method allows rapid improvement in the cyanotic infant's hemodynamics without having to transport the child outside the neonatal unit. Catheter passage can be tracked with ultrasound imaging of the inferior vena cava and right atrium. Confirmation of catheter position is done by directly imaging the catheter within the chamber and by agitated saline injection if necessary. With the balloon inflated, echocardiography allows proper positioning in the left atrium, away from left atrial appendage, mitral valve, or pulmonary veins. Following septostomy, a freely mobile flap of septal tissue and a broad stream of shunt flow constitute a successful septostomy (Fig. 23-14).

Postoperative Evaluation of Structural Heart Disease

Echocardiographic study following surgery for congenital heart defects is important in order to establish the adequacy of the repair

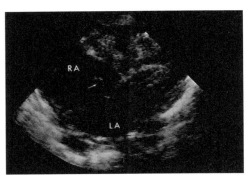

Figure 23-14. Subcostal echocardiographic view of the interatrial septum following balloon septostomy. A mobile flap of septal tissue can be seen moving into the right atrium *(arrow)*, indicating an adequate tear of the septum primum. LA, left atrium; RA, right atrium. (Prepared by M.E. King, MD, and reproduced with permission from Liberthson RR. Congenital heart disease in the child, adolescent, and adult. In Eagle KA, Haber E, DeSanctis RW, Austen WG (eds): *The Practice of Cardiology,* Boston, Little, Brown and Company, 1989.)

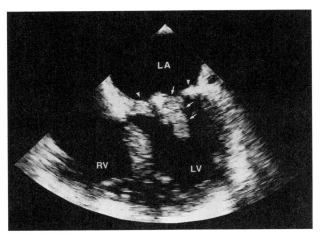

Figure 23-15. Transesophageal echocardiographic view of the heart in a patient with a Carpentier ring *(carets)* and endocarditis. A large prolapsing vegetation on the mitral valve *(small arrows)* was clearly visualized from the transesophageal window. LA, left atrium; LV, left ventricle; RV, right ventricle.

and detect residual lesions, ventricular dysfunction, or pericardial effusions. Early knowledge of these factors may make the difference between an uneventful recovery and a prolonged or unsuccessful postoperative course. Valvular regurgitation, residual atrial or ventricular shunts, outflow obstruction, and function of prosthetic valves or conduits are all readily performed in the postoperative recovery period.

Intraoperative ultrasound monitoring is now being increasingly used so that major problems can be corrected before leaving the operating room.[26–28] Once the patient has returned to the ICU, transthoracic echocardiographic access is often limited by surgical dressings and chest tubes. However, the subxyphoid approach or periapical windows in infants and smaller children may be sufficient to evaluate most anatomic and functional questions acutely.

Transesophageal echocardiography may be needed in the older child or the infant in whom adequate transthoracic echo is not possible. This relatively new application of cardiac ultrasound involves the use of a gastroscope that has been modified to include ultrasonic crystals on the tip. The standard probe is 10 to 14 mm in diameter at its widest point and can be used in children 15 kg or larger. Special pediatric probes should be used for children and infants smaller than 15 kg. Probe passage requires a well-sedated and carefully monitored patient. Cardiac structures can be visualized with excellent resolution by transmitting and receiving sound from within the nearby esophagus. The technique is particularly suited to evaluate pathology within the left atrium (thrombi, mitral regurgitation, interatrial baffles) or the mitral valve, and to assess prosthetic aortic and mitral valves (Fig. 23-15). It has also been utilized for evaluating anomalous pulmonary venous return, ventricular function, atrial and ventricular septal defects, and abnormalities of the pulmonary artery and valve. The aortic arch and thoracic aorta are also accessible by the transesophageal approach.

Hemodynamic Assessment

In addition to structural anatomic detail, echocardiography provides an accurate estimate of physiology and hemodynamics. Myocardial systolic and diastolic performance, intracardiac shunting,

and pulmonary artery pressures can all be derived from a combination of imaging and Doppler data.

Myocardial Function

Systolic performance of right and left ventricles can be made qualitatively with a fair degree of accuracy by an experienced observer by simply observing the contractility of the myocardium and change in ventricular size from diastole to systole.[29] Using this method, either ventricle can be described as normal, hyperkinetic, globally or segmentally hypokinetic, or akinetic.

More quantitative measures can be employed to give an estimated left ventricular **ejection fraction** by measuring left ventricular volume in diastole and systole and calculating the change in volume relative to the initial end-diastolic volume:

$$EF\ (\%) = \frac{EDV - ESV}{EDV} \times 100$$

where EF = ejection fraction

EDV = end-diastolic volume

ESV = end-systolic volume

Quantitative assessment of left ventricular volume generally requires an assumption of a geometric shape that resembles the left ventricle. The appropriate combination of linear dimensions and cavity areas which fit the equation for the volume of the assumed geometric shape can then be obtained from the two-dimensional echocardiographic images (Fig. 23-16). Good correlation has been demonstrated between left ventricular volumes and ejection fraction measured in this way when compared to angiographically determined volumes.[30,31] One of the simplest methods involves measuring a diameter of the left ventricle at the base of the heart (D) and cubing that dimension (D^3), assuming the ventricle to be spherical in shape. This method, of course, excludes the contribution to ventricular function provided by the apex. A practical method that involves a minimum of measurements is an area

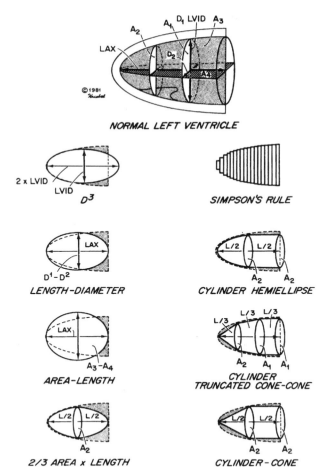

Figure 23-16. Diagrammatic representation of the left ventricle, showing the geometric models that have been used to calculate left ventricular volume. The shaded figures indicate the true chamber volume, with the superimposed solid figures demonstrating the geometric shape described by the formula. Simpson's rule comes closest to approximating the true shape of the ventricle. A, aorta; D, diameter; L, length; LAX, long axis length; LVID, left ventricular internal dimension. (Reproduced with permission from Weyman AE. *Cross-Sectional Echocardiography*, Philadelphia, Lea and Febiger, 1982.)

change at the base, with a percentage added or subtracted to account for apical function:

$$\text{EF (\%)} = \frac{D_d^2 - D_s^2}{D_d^2} \times 100 + \begin{cases} 10\% \text{ normal apex} \\ 5\% \text{ hypokinetic apex} \\ 0\% \text{ akinetic apex} \end{cases}$$

$$- [5\% \text{ to } 10\% \text{ dyskinetic apex}$$

where EF = ejection fraction

D_d = diastolic dimension at the base

D_s = systolic dimension at the base

These methods, which rely on a single dimension obtained at the base of the heart, are not accurate if there is segmental dysfunction affecting other portions of the myocardium. If other complex geometric figures are chosen to represent left ventricular shape (cylinder, truncated cone, cylinder hemi-ellipse), this necessitates more

complex formulae for calculating LV volume (see Fig. 23-16). These require careful attention to detail in obtaining the proper echocardiographic planes through the LV and more time to make the measurements needed. The use of Simpson's rule removes the need for an assumed geometric shape. With this method, the ventricle is cut into many stacked, parallel "slices," and the volume of each slice is summed to compute the total volume (see Fig. 23-16). This method requires measurement of a ventricular length and tracing of the cavity area from two orthogonal apical views of the left ventricle. Most current echocardiographic equipment has automated analysis to compute volumes from preprogrammed formulae using the dimensions or areas, which are entered by the sonographer.

Quantitative estimates of right ventricular function have been more problematic because the shape of this chamber is irregular, and obtaining reproducible echocardiographic planes is difficult.[32] A combination of apical and subcostal views provides the best assessment of both inflow and outflow portions of the right ventricle.[33]

Doppler echocardiography has introduced the capability to estimate **cardiac output** by measuring volumetric flow through the heart. Stroke volume can be calculated by measuring the cross-sectional area of a vessel or valve and integrating the flow velocities across a specific point in that vessel or valve throughout the period of transvalvular flow. The product of stroke volume and heart rate gives cardiac output (Fig. 23-17):

Stroke Volume (ml/beat) = **CSA** (cm²)
× **Flow Velocity Integral** (cm/beat)

Cardiac Output (ml/min) = **Stroke Volume** (ml/beat)
× **Heart Rate** (beats/min)

While cardiac output can be determined using the pulmonary, mitral, or tricuspid valve diameters and transvalvular flows, the aortic valve diameters and flow velocities have proven most accurate for reproducible measurement.[34,35] Experimentally, excellent correlations have been shown between Doppler cardiac outputs and cardiac outputs controlled by roller pumps ($r = 0.93–0.98$).[36] In the clinical setting, the absolute accuracy of Doppler cardiac outputs has been less encouraging. However, repetitive measurement of cardiac output in the same individual to follow relative changes with physiologic interventions has been useful.[37]

An additional application of Doppler-estimated cardiac output is the determination of **shunt ratios**. By comparing the cardiac output across the pulmonic and aortic valves, the $Q_p{:}Q_s$ can be calculated:

$$\frac{Q_p}{Q_s} = \frac{\text{CSA}_p \times \text{FVI}_p}{\text{CSA}_{ao} \times \text{FVI}_{ao}} = \frac{\pi \, [d_p/_2]^2 \times \text{FVI}_p}{\pi \, [d_{ao}/_2]^2 \times \text{FVI}_{ao}} = \frac{d_p^2 \times \text{FVI}_p}{d_{ao}^2 \times \text{FVI}_{ao}}$$

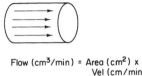

Flow (cm³/min) = Area (cm²) ×
Vel (cm/min)

Figure 23-17. Diagrammatic depiction of the principle of pulsed Doppler measurement of intracardiac blood flow. By measuring the cross-sectional area through which blood flow passes and the integral of pulsed Doppler peak flow velocity at that point, volumetric flow in cm³/min is the product of area (cm²) times the velocity integral (cm/min).

where Q_p = pulmonic flow

Q_s = systemic flow

CSA_p = cross-sectional area of the pulmonary annulus

CSA_{ao} = cross-sectional area of the aortic annulus

FVI_p = Doppler flow velocity integral across the pulmonic valve

FVI_{ao} = Doppler flow velocity integral across the aortic valve

d_p = diameter of the pulmonary annulus

d_{ao} = diameter of the aortic annulus

Thus, by simply measuring the aortic and pulmonic annuli and the flow velocity integrals across each of these valves, the size of atrial or ventricular shunts can be estimated. Ductal shunts require the reverse of the usual designation of systemic and pulmonary flow, because the pulmonic valve sees the preshunt systemic flow and the shunt flow passes subsequently across the aortic valve.[23] Thus, Q_p is measured from the trans**aortic** flow and Q_s from trans**pulmonic** flow. Any factor that may influence the velocity of flow across the aortic or pulmonic valves other than the volume of shunt flow (e.g., significant valvular regurgitation or stenosis) will interfere with the accuracy of this method and negate its use.[38]

Pulmonary Pressure Estimation

Several methods have been described to assess the degree of pulmonary hypertension noninvasively. By two-dimensional imaging, enlargement of the pulmonary artery and right ventricle and a mid-systolic notch of the pulmonic valve are suggestive of elevation of right-sided systolic pressures. The configuration of the interventricular septum is also helpful. When right ventricular systolic pressures are at least half of left ventricular pressure, the interventricular septum visibly flattens in systole when viewed in cross-section[39] (Fig. 23-18).

Doppler echocardiography has added more specific quantitative potential. The pulsed Doppler flow profile of pulmonary arterial flow can be analyzed both qualitatively and quantitatively. When pulmonary hypertension is present, the pulmonary flow profile demonstrates a rapid rise to peak velocity within the first third of systole, and often shows a mid-systolic notch (Fig. 23-19). Measurement of systolic time intervals from the pulmonary flow profile has also been used to predict pulmonary artery systolic and mean pressures.[40,41] The ratio of pre-ejection period (PEP) to acceleration time (AT), and acceleration time (AT) to right ventricular ejection time (RVET), have shown the best correlation with direct measurements of systolic and mean pressures.[40] Because many factors other than pulmonary artery pressure affect the systolic time intervals, however, the specificity of any of these ratios is limited in an individual patient and thus does not practically allow for quantitative estimation of pulmonary arterial pressure.

The most useful method for determining pulmonary artery pressure is the measurement of the peak velocity of the tricuspid regurgitation jet. Because most patients with significant pulmonary hypertension have right ventricular enlargement and dilatation of the tricuspid annulus, tricuspid regurgitation occurs frequently. Again making use of the Bernoulli equation, the pressure difference between right ventricle and right atrium can be predicted by measuring the peak velocity of the tricuspid regurgitant jet, squaring it and multiplying it by 4 [42] (Fig. 23-20). By adding the right atrial pressure to the pressure difference, the absolute right ventricular systolic pressure can be calculated:

$$\textbf{RVSP} \text{ (mm Hg)} = \textbf{Pressure gradient } (\Delta P)\text{(mm Hg)} + \textbf{Right Atrial Pressure (mm Hg)}$$

Right atrial pressure can be measured either directly from indwelling catheters, estimated from the jugular venous pressure, or simply assumed arbitrarily. Standard practice assumes a right atrial pressure of 10 mm Hg in the absence of a known figure for that chamber. The pulmonary artery systolic pressures are the same as right ventricular systolic pressures unless pulmonic stenosis is present.

If tricuspid regurgitation is not present, it is possible to determine pulmonary artery diastolic pressure from the pulmonic valve regurgitant jet. The peak velocity of the regurgitant flow reflects the

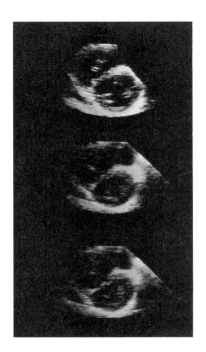 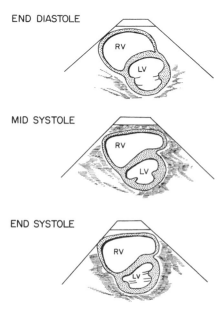

Figure 23-18. Series of parasternal short axis images of the left ventricle from end-diastole to end-systole, showing systolic flattening of the interventricular septum in a patient with pulmonary hypertension. In the normal heart, the interventricular septal configuration remains rounded and convex toward the right ventricle throughout the cardiac cycle. LV, left ventricle; RV, right ventricle. (Reproduced with permission of the American Heart Association, from King ME, et al. Interventricular septal configuration as a predictor of right ventricular systolic hypertension in children: A cross-sectional echocardiographic study. *Circulation* 1983;68:68.)

END DIASTOLE

MID SYSTOLE

END SYSTOLE

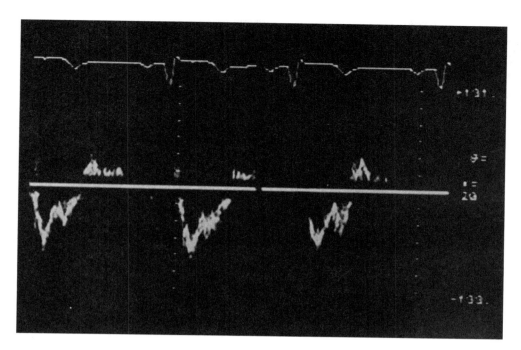

Figure 23-19. Pulsed Doppler spectral tracing of flow across the pulmonic valve in a patient with significant pulmonary hypertension. The spectral pattern shows a rapid rise to peak velocity and a mid-systolic notch (the "flying W"), which is characteristic of elevated pulmonary artery pressure.

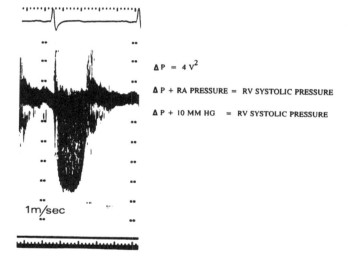

$$\Delta P = 4 \, V^2$$

$$\Delta P + RA \ PRESSURE = RV \ SYSTOLIC \ PRESSURE$$

$$\Delta P + 10 \ MM \ HG = RV \ SYSTOLIC \ PRESSURE$$

Figure 23-20. Continuous wave Doppler spectral tracing of tricuspid regurgitation illustrating a Doppler method for estimating right ventricular and pulmonary arterial systolic pressure. The peak velocity of the TR jet is 4.6 m/s. Using the formulae on the right, the pressure gradient between RV and RA is 4 × (4.6)² or 85 mm Hg. By adding an estimated RA pressure of 10 mm Hg, the estimated RV systolic pressure is 95 mm Hg. In the absence of pulmonic valve obstruction, the PA systolic pressure is also 95 mm Hg. m/sec, meters/second; mm Hg, millimeters of mercury; PA, pulmonary artery; RA, right atrium; RV, right ventricle. (Prepared by M.E. King, MD, and reproduced with permission from Liberthson RR. Congenital heart disease in the child, adolescent, and adult. In Eagle KA, Haber E, DeSanctis RW, Austen WG (eds): *The Practice of Cardiology,* Boston, Little, Brown and Company, 1989.)

pressure gradient between pulmonary artery diastolic pressure and right ventricular diastolic pressure. By assuming a value for right ventricular diastolic pressure (e.g., 5 mm Hg) and adding this to the diastolic pressure gradient obtained by Doppler, an estimate of pulmonary artery diastolic pressure can be made.

One of the clinical settings in which pulmonary hypertension is the predominant feature is **persistent fetal circulation** (PFC). The echo-Doppler findings in this situation are those detailed earlier as indicators of pulmonary artery hypertension, namely dilated right ventricle and pulmonary artery, systolic flattening of the interventricular septum, tricuspid and pulmonary regurgitation, and elevated pressures estimated from the regurgitant tricuspid jet. In addition, the reason for the infant's desaturation can be shown by color flow Doppler study of the patent foramen ovale (PFO) and the patent ductus arteriosus (PDA). With persistence of fetal levels of pulmonary arteriolar resistance, the elevation of right-sided pressures will cause right-to-left shunting at the atrial and ductal levels. If cyanosis is from major intrapulmonary shunting due to interstitial or alveolar processes, the findings of pulmonary artery hypertension will still be present, but the PFO and PDA shunts may be left to right. Evaluation of these infants must always consider the possibility of cyanotic structural congenital heart disease, particularly total anomalous pulmonary venous return, which closely mimics the physiology of PFC.

Echocardiography can be helpful in monitoring those infants requiring **extracorporeal membrane oxygenation** (ECMO). In venoarterial ECMO, substantial intracardiac volume is diverted to the membrane oxygenator, and the intracardiac flow velocities are quite low, decreasing 30% to 50% from pre-ECMO levels.[43] The aortic, left atrial, and left ventricular chamber dimensions show little change but the left and right ventricular stroke volumes fall, consistent with the drop in pre-load. The increase in afterload that occurs on ECMO may result in a decrease in ventricular contractility and an increase in myocardial wall stress. These findings return to normal as the ECMO flow rates are decreased. Doppler study frequently shows continued ductal patency during ECMO, with reversal of right-to-left shunting as the pulmonary resistance falls. The PDA will close spontaneously in the majority of infants following discontinuation of extracorporeal circulation.[43] It should be noted that the continuous inflow from the carotid arterial input line on venoarterial ECMO is detected by color flow Doppler as continuous turbulent flow in the transverse aortic arch. Care must be taken not to mistake this flow for ductal shunt flow. Decisions regarding the time and rate of weaning of ECMO can be assisted by following the echo-Doppler indices of pulmonary hypertension and the direction of intracardiac shunting.

Pericardial Effusion

Another clinical setting in which echocardiography is immensely valuable is in the evaluation of pericardial disease. Whether this occurs in the setting of bacterial sepsis, viral or rheumatic carditis, malignancy, chest trauma, or following cardiac surgery, echo-Doppler study can detect the presence of pericardial effusion, its distribution, and its hemodynamic effects. Fluid in the pericardial space is seen echocardiographically as an echo-lucent space adjacent to the heart between the visceral and parietal pericardium (Fig. 23-21). This may be seen only posteriorly where a small effusion will layer out in the supine patient, or in larger volume may surround the heart circumferentially. Determination of the volume of fluid is usually a qualitative process, with small effusions located posteriorly only, moderate effusions surrounding the heart anteriorly and posteriorly, and large effusions allowing swinging or free movement of the heart within the pericardial sac. If the fluid is roughly symmetrical in distribution, a quantitative estimate of fluid can be made by cubing the measurement of the anteroposterior dimension of the heart and subtracting this from the cube of an anteroposterior dimension of the heart plus pericardial fluid. This is not often accurate, however, because a larger volume of fluid accumulates around the apex that is not included in the anteroposterior dimension.[44]

Cardiac Tamponade

More important than the absolute volume of fluid is the hemodynamic effect of the effusion on cardiac function. In this regard, echo-Doppler study has added greatly to the assessment of cardiac tamponade. Although the diagnosis of cardiac tamponade is still a clinical determination, several features of the echo-Doppler exam are correlated strongly with tamponade physiology. When the intrapericardial pressure exceeds that of the right atrium and right ventricle, the free walls of the right atrium and right ventricle can be seen to buckle inward on two-dimensional echocardiographic study (see Fig. 23-21). The timing of this compression follows the time at which the intracardiac pressure within each of these chambers is at its lowest. The length of time during which the chamber remains compressed is indicative of the degree of elevation of intrapericardial pressure. Hence, if the right atrial free wall inverts for more than one third of the cardiac cycle, good correlation is seen with clinical evidence of cardiac tamponade. Inversion of the right ventricular outflow tract is less sensitive to small increases in intrapericardial pressure but more specific for tamponade physiology when it occurs. If right atrial and right ventricular inversion are both present, the likelihood of tamponade is very high.[45-47]

Pulsed Doppler flow velocities across the right- and left-sided valves also demonstrate alterations with large pericardial effusions. Inflow across the tricuspid valve normally shows a slight increase in velocity with inspiration, while transmitral and transaortic flows show no change or a minimal decrease in velocity. With cardiac tamponade, the Doppler equivalent of pulsus paradoxus can be demonstrated. The transmitral and transaortic flow velocities drop significantly with inspiration, while the transtricuspid flows show an exaggerated increase in flow velocity[48] (Fig. 23-22).

The nature of a pericardial process can often be ascertained by echocardiography as well. Serous pericardial effusions do not reflect the transmitted ultrasound and appear sonolucent. Organizing serous fluid, hematogenous or purulent fluid will produce ultrasonic reflectors that create an echodensity to the pericardial fluid. Solid tissue within the fluid, such as fibrin strands, inflammatory fibrinous deposits on the visceral pericardial surface, or metastatic tumor nodules, are readily displayed (Fig. 23-23).

Pericardiocentesis

When a pericardial effusion must be tapped emergently, echocardiography is often helpful at the bedside to localize the most direct access to the largest accumulation of fluid. After locating the

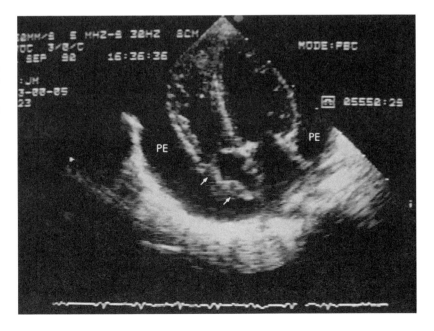

Figure 23-21. Apical four-chamber echocardiographic view of the heart in a patient with a large circumferential pericardial effusion. The echo-free space created by the fluid around the right atrial free wall allows easy visualization of the motion of this wall during the cardiac cycle. Indentation of the free wall *(arrows)* occurs when the pressure in the pericardial space exceeds that within the right atrium. PE, pericardial effusion.

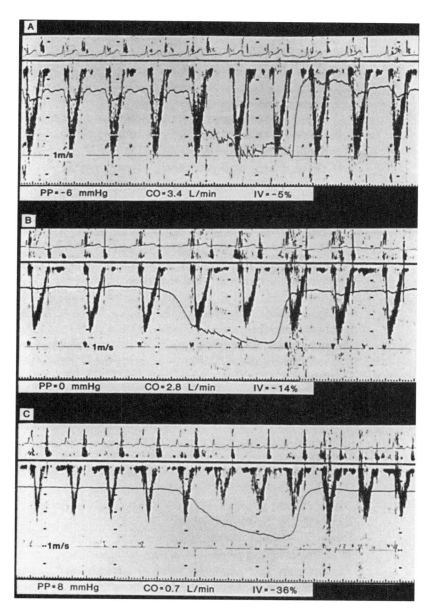

Figure 23-22. Pulsed Doppler spectral tracings of flow velocity across the aortic valve and intrapleural pressure tracing in an experimental model of pericardial effusion and increasing degrees of intrapericardial pressure. The top panel demonstrates the normal degree of variation in aortic flow velocity with respiration and normal intrapericardial pressure. The middle and lower panels show progressively more marked respiratory variation in flow velocity when intrapericardial pressure is raised. CO, cardiac output; IV, inspiratory variation; m/s, meters/second; PP, pericardial pressure. (Reprinted with permission from the American College of Cardiology, Picard MH et al. Quantitative relation between increased intrapericardial pressure and Doppler flow velocities during experimental cardiac tamponade. *J Am Coll Cardiol* 18:238, 1991.)

optimal site for the pericardial needle, the ultrasound transducer can be placed at a nearby position on the chest to follow the needle as it enters the pericardial space. Penetration of myocardium or ventricular chamber can be detected echocardiographically, and needle position can be verified by saline injection if necessary. Following pericardiocentesis, ultrasound study can assess the adequacy of fluid removal and document the improvement in hemodynamic parameters.

Pericardial Constriction

Pericardial constriction can be seen following pericardial inflammation from multiple causes: tuberculosis, viral pericarditis, radiation, or postoperative effusions. Echocardiographic signs of this hemodynamic state are subtle, but when present can pinpoint what is often an elusive problem. Pericardial thickening with separation of the visceral and parietal pericardial layers by echodense material can be noted by M-mode or two-dimensional imaging.

The impairment of ventricular filling, which occurs in pericardial constriction, can be qualitatively observed on real-time imaging of ventricular filling as a rapid early filling with no further late diastolic relaxation of the ventricular chambers. The interventricular septum has a characteristic "jiggle" in diastole as the augmentation of right ventricular filling with inspiration shifts the septum to the left, and left ventricular filling into a constricting pericardial sac quickly shifts it back toward the right. Pulsed Doppler sampling of the transmitral and transtricuspid flow demonstrates rapid early filling with a small or absent atrial filling wave.[49]

Infective Endocarditis

Infective endocarditis is often seen in the intensive care setting due to prolonged instrumentation, thermal burns, or infection in the immunocompromised host. Intravenous drug abuse also leads to serious manifestations of endocarditis, which may require an intensive care level of management.

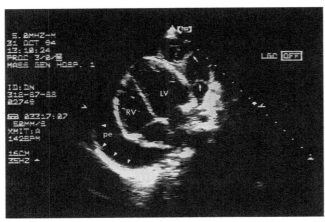

Figure 23-23. Apical four-chamber echocardiographic image in a patient with a large circumferential pericardial effusion from a viral pericarditis. The marked inflammatory reaction produced abundant fibrin strands *(arrows)* between the visceral and parietal layers of the pericardium. LV, left ventricle; RV right ventricle; pe, pericardial effusion.

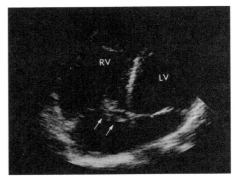

Figure 23-24. Apical four-chamber echocardiographic image in a patient with endocarditis, demonstrating a large prolapsing vegetation on the tricuspid septal leaflet *(arrows)*. LV, left ventricle; RV right ventricle. (Prepared by M.E. King, MD, and reproduced with permission from Levine RA et al. Echocardiography. In Eagle KA, Haber E, DeSanctis RW, Austen WG (eds): *The Practice of Cardiology*, Boston, Little, Brown and Company, 1989.)

Valvular Vegetations

The hallmark lesion of endocarditis is the vegetation that is most often found on the valvular apparatus but also occurs at sites of jet lesions (the wall of the right ventricular outflow tract opposite a ventricular septal defect) and on prosthetic materials within the heart. Echocardiography detects vegetations as localized echo-dense regions along the valve margins or supporting valve structures. Ultrasound is quite sensitive to very small vegetations, particularly if they are moving beyond the plane of motion of the underlying valve leaflet and can thus be recognized as a separate entity from the valve leaflet (Fig. 23-24). Sensitivity and specificity of ultrasound detection of vegetations varies from 35% to 65% in clinical series with a suspicion of endocarditis and up to 90% to 100% in patients undergoing surgical treatment for known infective endocarditis.[50,51] If the ultrasound images are suboptimal or if there is preexisting valve thickening, it may not be possible to distinguish valvular vegetations from the underlying pathology. Transesopha-

geal study may be needed when transthoracic access is limited in order to obtain the clarity of image necessary for making a definite diagnosis.

Significant infection usually results in destruction of valvular tissue and supporting elements, causing valvular regurgitation. The presence and severity of regurgitant flow can be assessed with Doppler techniques, as previously discussed (see section on Valvular Stenosis and Regurgitation).

Soft Tissue Extension

Extension of the infectious process into surrounding tissue leads to annular or root abscesses, fistulae, and purulent pericardial effusions. Echocardiography can serially monitor an infected valve for changes in the valve annulus or the aortic root. These generally appear as increased thickness and reflectivity that progresses to central clearing as cavitation and abscess formation occurs (Fig. 23-25). With aortic root abscesses, involvement of the proximal

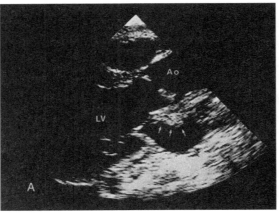
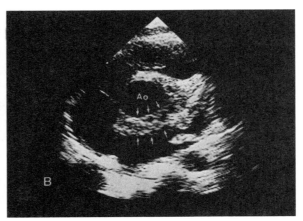

Figure 23-25. Parasternal echocardiographic images of the aortic root from a patient with aortic valve endocarditis and a root abscess. **(A)** The aortic leaflets are thickened and dome in systole. The posterior aortic root wall is markedly thickened *(arrows)*. **(B)** The aorta is seen in cross-section, with extensive thickening of the posterior aortic root wall *(arrows)*. Small lucent areas of liquefied material can be seen within the abscess. Ao, aorta; LV, left ventricle.

coronary orifices may occur, with resultant myocardial ischemia. Erosion through the root wall produces fistulous tracts into surrounding structures such as the left atrium, right ventricle, or right atrium. Pulsed and color flow Doppler readily demonstrate these fistulous shunts. The appearance of conduction disturbances by electrocardiogram suggests extension of infection into the atrial or ventricular septae. This can also be detected echocardiographically as thickening and increased density of the basilar interatrial septum or ventricular septal crest.

Blunt Chest Trauma

The child who has suffered major trauma from an automobile or bicycle accident is at obvious risk of injury to the chest wall and underlying cardiac structures. Echocardiography can quickly evaluate the pericardial and cardiac structures most likely to be affected. Pericardial contusion or laceration most frequently presents as an effusion. Myocardial contusion may also occur, which, if extensive enough, will be detectible as a segmental wall motion abnormality involving the anterior right ventricular free wall or anterior apex. The myocardium has increased echo reflectivity and decreased systolic thickening.[52] Traumatic injury to the aortic or mitral valve leaflets results in acute valvular regurgitation and partially flail valve apparatus. This is easily diagnosed by two-dimensional and Doppler assessment of valve function. The presence of a dissection flap within the aorta, with both false and true lumen by echo-Doppler study, may result from blunt injury to the aortic root.

Intracardiac Catheters

Indwelling central vascular catheters are used routinely in the management of infants and children in the ICU. If questions arise as to catheter position, ultrasound examination may be able to answer them. Catheters with a central lumen appear as two densely reflective parallel borders with a small central clearing. Scanning the abdominal aorta, inferior vena cava, or subclavian veins will often detect the catheter position. Problems are created, however, when the catheter bends out of the plane of the interrogating ultrasound beam. When the catheter is no longer perpendicular to the sound beam, strong reflections do not return from its surface and it will not be perceived by the ultrasound beam. Hence, localizing the catheter tip within the cardiac chambers when it loops on itself has not been reliable.

Pacing wires appear as a singular linear echodensity within the chamber involved. The tip is usually embedded in the myocardium, and perforation through the wall is often detected by the presence of a pericardial effusion rather than by direct visualization. Passage of the wire through the interventricular septum into the left ventricle is demonstrated clearly by following the linear echodensity through the myocardium and into the cavity of the left ventricle.

Intravascular catheters are often the site for bacterial vegetative material and thrombus formation. Echocardiography can evaluate the catheter terminus for mobile material that may be obstructing catheter function or providing septic or thrombotic emboli into the circulation (Fig. 23-26). In small infants, catheters may induce thrombosis of the large veins wherein they chronically reside. Edema of the head and neck or superior vena caval syndrome suggest major obstruction of the great veins. Two-dimensional imaging may visualize echogenic material within the lumen of the innominate vein and superior vena cava. Pulsed and color

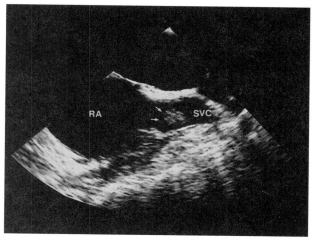

Figure 23-26. Transesophageal echocardiographic view of the superior vena cava and right atrium, demonstrating a fungal vegetation *(arrows)* that formed on a central venous line used for hyperalimentation. RA, right atrium; SVC, superior vena cava.

Doppler can determine whether normal venous return is present. If ambiguity remains, agitated saline can be injected through a vein distal to the obstruction and its passage traced into the heart. When serious superior vena caval obstruction occurs, collateral vessels are conscripted to carry some of the venous flow into the inferior cava. In this instance, agitated saline will be noted entering the right atrium via the inferior vena cava.[53]

References

1. Sharma S et al. The usefulness of echo in the surgical management of infants with congenital heart disease. *Clin Cardiol* 15:891–897, 1992.
2. Huhta JC et al. Two dimensional echocardiographic assessment of the aorta in infants and children with congenital heart disease. *Circulation* 70:417, 1984.
3. Chin AJ, Williams RG. Determination of atrial situs by two-dimensional echocardiographic imaging of atrial appendage morphology. In EE Doyle et al (eds): *Pediatric Cardiology: Proceedings of the Second World Congress.* New York: Springer, 1986. Pp 170–171.
4. Foale R et al. Left and right ventricular morphology in complex congenital heart disease defined by two-dimensional echocardiography. *Am J Cardiol* 49:93, 1982.
5. Henry WL et al. Differential diagnosis of anomalies of the great arteries with real-time two-dimensional echocardiography. *Circulation* 51:283, 1975.
6. Sanders SP, Bierman FZ, Williams RG. Conotruncal malformations: Diagnosis in infancy using subzyphoid 2-dimensional echocardiography. *Am J Cardiol* 50:1361–1367, 1982.
7. Snider AR et al. Comparison of high pulse repetition frequency and continuous-wave Doppler for velocity measurement and gradient prediction in children with valvular and congenital heart disease. *J Am Coll Cardiol* 7:873–879, 1986.
8. Hatle L, Angelsen B. *Doppler Ultrasound in Cardiology* (2nd ed). Philadelphia: Lea & Febiger, 1985.
9. Currie PH et al. Instantaneous pressure gradient: A simultaneous Doppler and dual catheter correlative study. *J Am Coll Cardiol* 7:800–806, 1986.
10. Choong CY et al. Prevalency of valvular regurgitation by Doppler echocardiography in patients with structurally normal hearts by two-dimensional echocardiography. *Am Heart J* 117:636–642, 1989.
11. VanDijk AP, VanOort AM, Daniels O. Right-sided valvular regurgita-

tion in normal children determined by combined colour-coded and continuous wave Doppler. *Acta Paediatr* 83(2):200–203, 1994.

12. Brand A et al. The prevalence of valvular regurgitation in children with structurally normal hearts: A color Doppler echocardiographic study. *Am Heart J* 123(1):177–180, 1992.

13. Miyatake K et al. Semiquantitative grading of severity of mitral regurgitation by real-time two-dimensional Doppler flow imaging technique. *J Am Coll Cardiol* 7:82, 1986.

14. Perry GJ et al. Evaluation of aortic insufficiency by Doppler color flow mapping. *J Am Coll Cardiol* 9:952, 1987.

15. Ascah KJ et al. A Doppler two-dimensional echocardiographic method for quantitation of mitral regurgitation. *Circulation* 72:377, 1985.

16. Shub C et al. Sensitivity of two-dimensional echocardiography in the direct visualization of atrial septal defects utilizing a subcostal approach: Experience with 154 patients. *J Am Coll Cardiol* 4:127–135, 1983.

17. Fraker TD et al. Detection and exclusion of interatrial shunts by two-dimensional echocardiography and peripheral vein injections. *Circulation* 54:558–562, 1976.

18. Pollick C et al. Doppler color-flow imaging assessment of shunt size in atrial septal defect. *Circulation* 78:522–528, 1988.

19. Sahn DJ, Allen HD. Real-time cross-sectional echocardiographic imaging and measurement of the patent ductus arteriosus in infants and children. *Circulation* 58:343–354, 1978.

20. Stevenson JG, Kawabori I, Guntheroth WG. Pulsed Doppler echocardiographic diagnosis of patent ductus arteriosus: Sensitivity, specificity, limitations, and technical features. *Cathet Cardiovasc Diagn* 6:255–263, 1980.

21. Liao P-K, Su W-J, Hung J-S. Doppler echocardiographic flow characteristics of isolated patent ductus arteriosus: Better delineation by Doppler color flow mapping. *J Am Coll Cardiol* 12:1285–1291, 1988.

22. Halliday HL, Hirata T, Brady JP. Echocardiographic findings of large patent ductus arteriosus in the very low birthweight infant before and after treatment with indomethacin. *Arch Dis Child* 54:744–749, 1979.

23. Stevenson JG. The use of Doppler echocardiography for detection and estimation of severity of patent ductus arteriosus, ventricular septal defect, and atrial septal defect. *Echocardiography* 4:321–346, 1987.

24. Allan LD et al. Balloon septostomy under two-dimensional echocardiographic control. *Br Heart J* 47:41–43, 1982.

25. Perry LW et al. Echocardiographically assisted balloon atrial septostomy. *Pediatrics* 70:403–408, 1982.

26. Cyran SE et al. Efficacy of intraoperative transesophageal echocardiography in children with congenital heart disease. *Am J Cardiol* 63:594–598, 1989.

27. Ritter SB. Transesophageal echocardiography in children: New peephole to the heart. *J Am Coll Cardiol* 16:447, 1990.

28. Fyfe DA, Kline CH. Transesophageal echocardiography for congenital heart disease. *Echocardiography* 8:573–585, 1991.

29. Wong M et al. Estimating left ventricular ejection fraction from two-dimensional echocardiograms: Visual and computer-processed interpretations. *Echocardiography* 8:1–7, 1991.

30. Silverman HN et al. Determination of left ventricular volume in children: Echocardiographic and angiographic comparisons. *Circulation* 62:548–557, 1980.

31. Mercier JC et al. Two-dimensional echocardiographic assessment of left ventricular volumes and ejection fraction in children. *Circulation* 65:962–969, 1982.

32. Hiraishi S et al. Two-dimensional echocardiographic assessment of right ventricular volume in children with congenital heart disease. *Am J Cardiol* 50:1368–1375, 1982.

33. Levine RA et al. Echocardiographic measurement of right ventricular volume. *Circulation* 69:497–505, 1984.

34. Rein MJ et al. Cardiac output estimates in the pediatric intensive care unit using a continuous-wave Doppler computer: Validation and limitations of the technique. *Am Heart J* 112:97–103, 1986.

35. Mellander M et al. Doppler determination of cardiac output in infants and children: Comparison with simultaneous thermodilution. *Pediatr Cardiol* 8:241–246, 1987.

36. Stewart WJ et al. Variable effects of changes in flow rate through the aortic, pulmonary and mitral valves on valve area and flow velocity: Impact on quantitative Doppler flow calculations. *J Am Coll Cardiol* 6:653–662, 1985.

37. Ihlen H et al. Changes in left ventricular stroke volume measured by Doppler echocardiography. *Br Heart J* 54:378–383, 1985.

38. Sanders SP et al. Measurement of systemic and pulmonary blood flow and Qp/Qs ratio using Doppler and two-dimensional echocardiography. *Am J Cardiol* 51:952, 1983.

39. King ME et al. Interventricular septal configuration as a predictor of right ventricular systolic hypertension in children: A cross-sectional echocardiographic study. *Circulation* 68:68, 1983.

40. Kitabatake A et al. Noninvasive evaluation of pulmonary hypertension by a pulsed Doppler technique. *Circulation* 68:302–309, 1983.

41. Isobe M et al. Prediction of pulmonary artery pressure in adults by pulsed Doppler echocardiography. *Am J Cardiol* 57:316–321, 1986.

42. Berger M et al. Quantitative assessment of pulmonary hypertension in patients with tricuspid regurgitation using continuous wave Doppler ultrasound. *J Am Coll Cardiol* 6:359–365, 1985.

43. Martin GR, Short BL. Doppler echocardiographic evaluation of cardiac performance in infants on prolonged extracorporeal membrane oxygenation. *Am J Cardiol* 62:929–934, 1988.

44. Horowitz MS et al. Sensitivity and specificity of echocardiographic diagnosis of pericardial effusion. *Circulation* 50:239–245, 1974.

45. Gillam LD et al. Hydrodynamic compression of the right atrium: A new echocardiographic sign of cardiac tamponade. *Circulation* 68:294, 1983.

46. Armstrong WF et al. Diastolic collapse of the right ventricle with cardiac tamponade: An echocardiographic study. *Circulation* 65:1491, 1982.

47. Leimgruber PP et al. The hemodynamic derangement associated with right ventricular diastolic collapse in cardiac tamponade: An experimental echocardiographic study. *Circulation* 68:612–620, 1983.

48. Picard MH et al. Quantitative relation between increased intrapericardial pressure and Doppler flow velocities during experimental cardiac tamponade. *J Am Coll Cardiol* 18:234–242, 1991.

49. King SW, Pandian NG, Gardin JM. Doppler echocardiographic findings in pericardial tamponade and constriction. *Echocardiography* 5:361–372, 1988.

50. King ME, Weyman AE. Echocardiographic findings in infective endocarditis. In Fowler NO (ed): *Non-Invasive Diagnostic Methods in Cardiology*. Philadelphia, Davis, 1983.

51. Martin RP et al. Clinical utility of two-dimensional echocardiography in infective endocarditis. *Am J Cardiol* 46:379–385, 1980.

52. Miller FA Jr et al. Two-dimensional echocardiographic findings in cardiac trauma. *Am J Cardiol* 50:1022–1027, 1982.

53. Silverman NH et al. Superior vena caval obstruction after Mustard's operation: Detection by two-dimensional contrast echocardiography. *Circulation* 64:392–396, 1981.

Edward P. Walsh

Richard R. Liberthson

24 ▸ Cardiac Arrhythmias in the Intensive Care Setting

In recent years, the incidence of cardiac arrhythmias in the pediatric intensive care unit (PICU) has risen dramatically. This rise can be attributed to several factors, including (1) improved monitoring and detection methods, (2) increased awareness of rhythm disorders among practitioners, and (3) a larger number of surviving postoperative cardiac patients with complex lesions who develop arrhythmias as a consequence of their disease. Associated with this increased recognition of arrhythmias has been an impressive expansion of available pharmacologic and nonpharmacologic treatment modalities. It has thus become necessary for pediatric intensivists to develop an improved understanding of the etiologies, mechanisms, and management of these entities. Our aim in this chapter is to provide a practical "front line" approach to the deductive diagnosis of specific arrhythmias' mechanisms and to outline suggestions for acute management of such disorders in the intensive care setting. For a more general discussion of pediatric arrhythmias, readers are referred to several comprehensive reviews.[1,2]

Pathophysiology of Cardiac Arrhythmias

Rhythm disorders may be separated into the broad categories of tachycardias and bradycardia, either of which may result from disorders of impulse formation or impulse conduction. Although our understanding of the cellular genesis of arrhythmias is still rudimentary, active basic science work is rapidly closing some major gaps in this knowledge.[3]

Based largely on study of in vitro heart tissue preparations, tachyarrhythmias are presently thought to develop from one of three cellular mechanisms (Fig. 24-1). The first is **abnormal automaticity,** which is due to early spontaneous depolarization of a cell outside the sinus node. This phenomenon can be caused by any change in a cell's membrane condition that lowers the threshold for depolarization or promotes a higher resting potential, thereby allowing the cell to prematurely activate.[4] Abnormal automaticity has been implicated as the possible cause of some atypical tachyarrhythmias in children, such as ectopic atrial tachycardia and junctional ectopic tachycardia, although the leap from this cellular model to the intact heart still involves considerable conjecture.

The second cellular model for tachycardia is **triggered activity** from "afterdepolarizations." Afterdepolarizations are small oscillations in the terminal portions of the cellular action potential[5] that occur under pathologic conditions. When these oscillations are of sufficient amplitude, the cell can be triggered to undergo one or more repetitive discharges. Although it is difficult to verify this model in vivo, triggered activity may be operative in some tachyarrhythmias seen with digoxin toxicity or certain atypical ventricular arrhythmias.[6]

The final model for tachyarrhythmias is the familiar concept of **reentry,** which is the best understood cause of clinical tachycardia. Reentry involves circular conduction or "circus movement" between two discrete cardiac pathways. The pathways must be functionally separated and must satisfy strict requirements in terms of conduction velocity and refractoriness.[7] When the proper conditions are met, an appropriately timed impulse can circle the loop

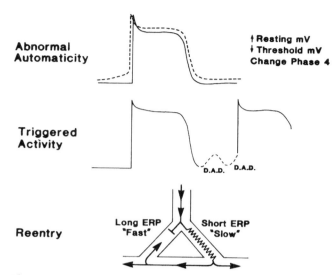

Figure 24-1. Cellular mechanisms for tachycardias. Abnormal automaticity may occur with deviations in either the resting membrane potential (mv), the threshold potential, or by spontaneous upward drift of the resting potential (phase 4 depolarization). Triggered activity results from small oscillations in the membrane potential during repolarization. One such type of oscillation is known as delayed afterdepolarizations (D.A.D.), which can reactivate the cell when they are at sufficient amplitude. Reentry involves circular conduction over two discrete pathways that are properly balanced in terms of their effective refractory periods (ERP) and conduction velocity (fast vs. slow). See text for further discussion.

to generate either single "echo beats" or sustained reentry tachycardia. Reentry is a well-verified phenomenon in the intact heart and is responsible for the majority of tachyarrhythmias discussed in this chapter.

Bradycardia may result from either depression of intrinsic pacemaker cell activity or block of the excitation process. Block can occur at multiple levels within the heart, including "exit block" from a pacemaker cell, or "conduction block" of an established depolarization wavefront.

Diagnostic Tools

Accurate diagnosis of arrhythmia mechanism is the cornerstone of successful therapy. The tools for this purpose are varied and sometimes complex, but the fact remains that a careful review of the standard electrocardiogram (ECG) is usually quite sufficient for arriving at a working diagnosis. The diagnostic clues available from the surface ECG will be outlined in detail later in this chapter during discussion of individual rhythm disorders.

The ECG does have some limitations, however, that relate primarily to occasions when the P wave is indistinct or obscured by the QRS. In the emergency setting, it is often essential to establish the precise timing of atrial electrical activity for rhythm diagnosis. The solution is placement of a recording electrode closer

Figure 24-2. Example of atrial ECGs obtained from temporary postoperative wires, showing an atrial signal (A), which is large and discrete. A bipolar recording from **two** atrial wires produces a signal with predominately atrial activity, and a small ventricular component (V). A unipolar recording from a **single** atrial wire reveals a sharp (but smaller) atrial signal, with an easily recognized ventricular component. When P waves are difficult to see on the standard ECG, such recordings will clarify atrial timing.

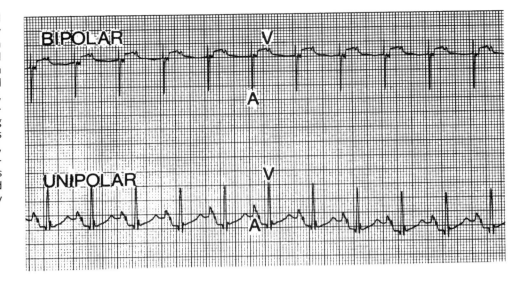

Figure 24-3. Sample recording from an esophageal (ESO) lead during normal sinus rhythm, shown with simultaneous surface ECG recordings. Note high-quality resolution of the atrial electrogram.

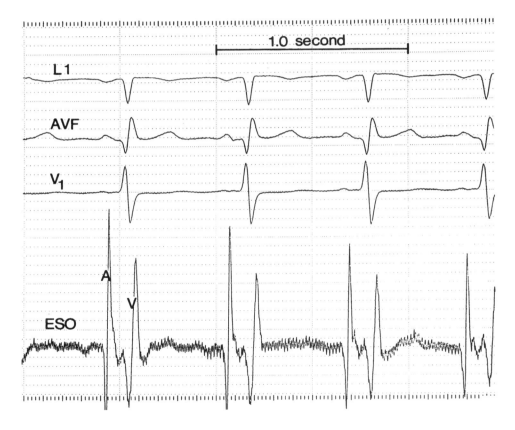

to atrial muscle. In postoperative cardiac patients, a convenient tool for this purpose is temporary atrial pacing wires, which are frequently left in place for several days after surgery.[8] When these wires are connected to standard recording equipment, high-quality atrial electrograms can be obtained (Fig. 24-2). If epicardial wires are not available, a small flexible electrode catheter can be inserted through the nose or mouth and positioned in the midesophagus[9] for recording of similar signals (Fig. 24-3). Both epicardial wires and the esophageal electrode can additionally be used for atrial pacing, including electrical stimulation to stop and start reentry supraventricular tachycardia (SVT) for diagnosis and/or therapy.

In some situations, it may be necessary to record cardiac electrical activity directly from intracardiac electrodes[10] (Fig. 24-4). The added data obtained with this technique include (1) recording of the His bundle depolarization, (2) pacing maneuvers to study functional characteristics and mechanism of abnormal rhythms, and (3) precise mapping of abnormal pathways or tachycardia foci. The His bundle electrogram is useful for determining levels of atrioventricular conduction disturbances and for distinguishing ventricular arrhythmias from some atypical SVTs. Careful intracardiac mapping also permits consideration of surgical or catheter ablation techniques for treatment of medically refractory disorders.

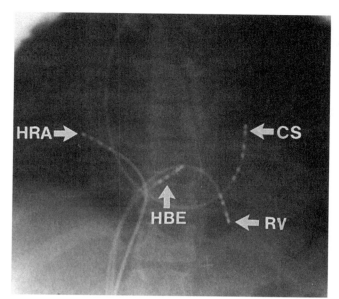

Figure 24-4. AP fluoroscopic image showing four electrode catheters in position for comprehensive electrophysiologic testing. HRA, high right atrium; HBE, His bundle electrogram; RV, right ventricular apex; CS, coronary sinus.

Tachycardias

Tachyarrhythmias can be separated into the general classes of SVTs and ventricular tachycardia (VT). The term *SVT* describes any inappropriately fast rhythm arising from the sinus node, atrial muscle, the proximal atrioventricular (AV) conducting system, or accessory pathways. The term *VT* describes any tachycardia arising below the bifurcation of the common His bundle. A proposed classification scheme that incorporates tachyarrhythmia location and probable cellular mechanisms are shown in Table 24-1 and will be used throughout this chapter.

When attempting to diagnosis a tachycardia from the surface ECG, the first step is to examine a full 12-lead trace for the width of the QRS complex. When the QRS is "narrow" (0.08 seconds or less), it is a safe assumption that the tachycardia is due to one of the supraventricular mechanisms. If a "wide" (0.10 seconds or more) QRS is seen, the disorder can be either VT or an atypical

SVT involving disturbance of bundle branch conduction or an accessory pathway. In practice, it is often quite difficult to distinguish VT from an atypical SVT on the basis of surface ECG alone. Hence, a wide QRS tachycardia should always be managed as VT in the acute setting until definitely proven otherwise.

Supraventricular Tachycardia

SVT is rarely life-threatening in the short run. On occasion, more damage may be done with inappropriate and hasty therapy than would have been caused by the tachycardia itself. The first rule in managing an SVT is to relax and attempt to pinpoint the arrhythmia mechanism and underlying cause before embarking on therapy. On the other hand, long-standing SVT leading to depressed ventricular function, or some atypical rapid forms of SVT in the Wolff-Parkinson-White syndrome, can cause hemodynamic collapse. Thus, one must rely on good clinical judgement and act aggressively to terminate SVT if the patient is severely compromised.

Although rational therapy of an SVT demands some knowledge of the specific mechanism for the disorder, some very general steps can be recommended in the acute setting (Table 24-2). These begin with physical assessment and a 12-lead ECG. The utility of a full 12-lead recording cannot be over emphasized, as it is far superior to a single-lead rhythm strip in providing clues to the exact arrhythmia mechanism (such as P wave timing and axis). When equipment is available, an atrial electrogram may also be obtained to uncover additional clues.

Once diagnostic data have been collected, attempts at terminating SVT may be initiated. First-line therapy usually begins with vagal stimulation, using techniques such as the Valsalva maneuver or application of ice to the face. If this is unsuccessful, intravenous (IV) adenosine is probably the safest and most generally effective drug option. If, at any time, the patient shows evidence of hemodynamic compromise, an emergency DC cardioversion should be performed.

Second- and third-line therapy, as outlined in Table 24-2, can be employed if SVT persists, but it is usually advisable to obtain the input of a cardiologist at this point in treatment. Several of the drugs listed in these latter two categories can have untoward effects and are best employed under direction of an individual experienced with their use. More importantly, the further one proceeds along this therapeutic scheme, the more crucial it is to

Table 24-1. Classification of tachyarrhythmias

	Proposed mechanism	
Site of origin	*Automaticity*	*Reentry*
Sinus node	Sinus tachycardia	?SA node reentry (rare)
Atrium	Ectopic atrial tachycardia Multifocal atrial tachycardia	Atrial flutter Atrial fibrillation
AV junction	Junctional ectopic tachycardia	AV node reentry
Accessory AV pathway	XXX	Orthodromic reentry Antidromic reentry Preexcited atrial Fl/Fib
Ventricle	Incessant VT (infants)	Monomorphic reentry VT Polymorphic reentry VT Torsade de pointes

Table 24-2. General guidelines for management of "narrow-QRS" tachycardia

Review history and evaluate condition

12-lead ECG

Atrial electrogram, if equipment available

First-line therapy
  Vagal stimulation
  IV adenosine
  If unstable, DC cardioversion

Second-line therapy
  Overdrive pacing, if equipment available
  IV esmolol or IV verapamil

Third-line therapy
  IV procainamide
  Elective DC cardioversion

know the exact tachycardia mechanism (both in terms of site of origin and whether it involves reentry or automaticity). Specific therapy for the individual forms of SVT is discussed next.

Sinus Tachycardia

Although not strictly pathologic, sinus tachycardia in the intensive care setting can sometimes become so pronounced that it may be confused with a primary rhythm disorder. Sinus tachycardia is due to enhancement of the normal automaticity of the sinus node and usually occurs under conditions of high-circulating catecholamines. The ECG features are typical for an "automatic" focus in that the rate will gradually accelerate and decelerate (warm up and cool down) in relation to sympathetic tone. This contrasts with reentry tachycardias, which tend to start and stop abruptly and exhibit minimal rate variation. The P wave axis on a 12-lead ECG during sinus tachycardia is always normal (+60 degrees), and the A:V conduction ratio is typically 1:1. These ECG features, combined with knowledge of the patient's clinical condition, should eliminate confusion with pathologic rhythms. Obviously, sinus tachycardia does not require therapy other than correction of the underlying cause. Additional etiologies for sinus tachycardia include fever, anemia, shock, heart failure, pain, and hyperthyroidism.

Ectopic Atrial Tachycardia and Multifocal Atrial Tachycardia

These two disorders are thought to be caused by **abnormal** automaticity arising from atrial cells outside the sinus node. Ectopic atrial tachycardia (EAT) describes a single abnormal focus, while multifocal atrial tachycardia (MAT) classically involves three or more such foci. Both conditions are rare, but they can cause severe hemodynamic compromise in children and are often difficult to control. They may arise spontaneously as a primary rhythm disorder or may be seen as a complication of cardiac surgery, cardiomyopathy, or multiorgan disease (e.g., respiratory failure). The ECG in ectopic atrial tachycardia[11] shows a rapid atrial rate with a single abnormal P wave axis. The rates tend to warm up and cool down in the pattern typical for automatic foci. The ventricular rate during EAT is independently determined by the AV node and His Purkinje system. First- and second-degree AV block, as well as intermittent bundle branch aberration, are common (Fig. 24-5). Multifocal atrial tachycardia presents a similar ECG pattern, although in this case multiple P wave morphologies are present.[12]

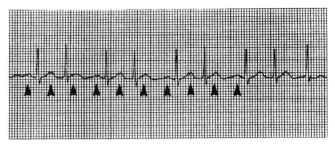

Figure 24-5. Surface ECG (lead II) from a patient with EAT. Note rapid atrial rate with variable AV conduction.

Control of these two tachycardias is difficult. Because they are due to automaticity rather than reentry, neither electrical cardioversion nor overdrive pacing techniques will terminate these disorders. Indeed, the diagnosis of an automatic tachycardia is often made retrospectively after these techniques have failed. Treatment is thus limited to pharmacologic trials or, whenever possible, removal of underlying cause. First line drug therapy in the PICU should begin with agents that primarily slow AV node conduction, such as digoxin. Although digoxin rarely has a primary effect on the atrial rhythm, it can slow a rapid ventricular response and provide some improvement in hemodynamics. Beta-blockers and verapamil may also be used to titrate the AV node response, and quite often they will suppress the abnormal atrial rhythm directly. Note that both of these drugs carry the potential risk of negative inotropic effects on a myocardium that may already be compromised. Beta-blockers or verapamil need to be used with caution; however, their efficacy in EAT and MAT is sometimes dramatic. Chronic therapy for these conditions should be chosen after consultation with a cardiologist.

Junctional Ectopic Tachycardia

Junctional ectopic tachycardia (JET) is an uncommon rhythm disorder caused by automaticity arising from the AV node or proximal His Purkinje system.[13] The typical clinical presentation is in the early postoperative period for an infant who has undergone cardiac surgery with procedures in the vicinity of the AV junction (e.g., ventricular septal defect closure). It may also be seen in myocarditis and severe central nervous system injury, and is occasionally reported as an idiopathic congenital rhythm disorder. JET has a very distinctive ECG appearance. The QRS is rapid and narrow and tends to exhibit warm up and cool down. Because the automatic focus is located below atrial muscle, however, one can often observe AV dissociation (Fig. 24-6). JET is the only narrow QRS tachycardia wherein the ventricular rate can be greater than the atrial rate. When there is uncertainty regarding P wave activity,

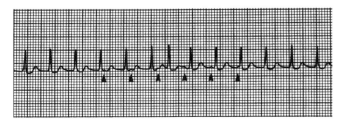

Figure 24-6. Surface ECG from a patient with rapid JET. Note that the QRS is narrow and rapid, at a rate faster than the P wave *(arrows)*.

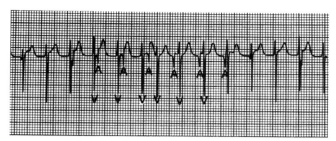

Figure 24-7. Atrial electrogram obtained from temporary post-operative wires in a patient with JET. Note how atrial activity (A) is clearly slower and dissociated from ventricular activity (V).

an esophageal recording or an atrial wire electrogram will provide clarification (Fig. 24-7).

JET at rates much over 170/min can cause critical hemodynamic compromise and, similar to EAT and MAT, will not respond to conventional therapy with cardioversion or overdrive atrial pacing. Treatment is difficult and begins with attempts to remove any underlying cause such as hypoxia, acidosis, or fever. If this is unsuccessful, one must institute aggressive efforts to both restore AV synchrony and lower the rate. Synchrony is achieved by pacing the atrium at a rate slightly faster than that of junctional discharge. At the same time, therapy is begun to lower the junctional rate to a more physiologic range. Conventional drugs are usually ineffective for this purpose, although occasional success has been reported with digoxin[14] and investigational trials of IV propafenone.[15] More commonly, the quickest and safest therapy for slowing JET is to drop the patient's body temperature to 34°C to 35°C by using a cooling blanket. The patient must be intubated and paralyzed to prevent shivering during this therapy. Induced hypothermia of this sort is usually effective in slowing JET.[16] In refractory cases, the addition of IV procainamide during hypothermia has been found to be highly effective,[17] even though procainamide exerts minimal influence on JET at normal body temperatures.

JET is usually a transient disorder lasting 24 to 72 hours after surgery, or for the first few days during the acute phase of myocarditis. This therapy should be weaned at intervals of 12 to 24 hours to determine if the transient arrhythmia has abated, so that therapy can be relaxed.

Atrial Fibrillation and Atrial Flutter

Atrial fibrillation and atrial flutter are caused by reentry within atrial muscle. Flutter represents a single reentry circuit, and fibrillation appears to represent multiple small and constantly changing reentry circuits. The potential etiologies include any process that promotes atrial enlargement or inflammation, such as congenital

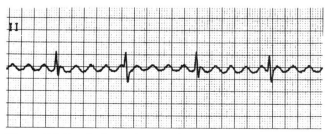

Figure 24-8. Surface ECG recording from a patient with atrial flutter and a slow ventricular response rate. The classical sawtooth pattern is clearly shown.

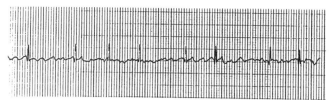

Figure 24-9. Surface ECG (lead II) from a patient with atrial fibrillation.

heart lesions or cardiomyopathy. Hyperthyroidism may cause atrial fibrillation in older patients.

The ECG features are fairly distinctive. Atrial flutter classically presents a sawtooth pattern best seen in leads II, III, and aVf at a very regular rate of 300 bpm (Fig. 24-8). However, many other P wave patterns can be observed, including rates as slow as 150 bpm in very dilated hearts, or rates as fast as 400 bpm in infants. The ECG in atrial fibrillation shows irregular and low-amplitude rapid atrial activity (Fig. 24-9).

The ventricular response rate in these two conditions is determined independently by the conduction properties of the AV junction, and often involves first-degree and second-degree AV block and occasional bundle branch aberration. The diagnosis may be confusing when AV conduction is rapid. Vagal stimulation can usually induce temporary slowing of conduction at the AV node to expose atrial activity. Alternatively, an esophageal lead or atrial pacing wires can be used (Fig. 24-10) to clarify atrial timing.

Acute termination of both conditions is fairly easy once the proper diagnosis has been made. Because the underlying mechanism is reentry, a synchronized DC cardioversion is virtually always successful in terminating these disorders. Cardioversion carries a small disadvantage of requiring an anesthetic, but is a quick and generally safe procedure. If cardioversion is not used, or is unsuccessful, one may consider attempts at pharmacologic conversion. Drug therapy must always begin with digoxin. Digoxin will increase the degree of AV block to lower the ventricular response rate and protects against the enhancement of AV conduction that can occur with second-line drugs used for these conditions. Once digitalization is complete, second-line therapy with an agent drug such as procainamide can be considered. Drugs of this type have direct effect on the conduction properties of atrial muscle, and in about 10% to 20% of cases will terminate the primary atrial disorder.

An attractive alternative therapy for atrial flutter is the use of overdrive atrial pacing, which can be performed via atrial wires, an esophageal lead, or an intracardiac electrode. The reentry circuit of atrial flutter can be broken in about 75% of patients[18] by using a short burst of atrial stimulation at rates slightly faster than the flutter. Overdrive pacing is not effective for atrial fibrillation, due to the presence of multiple rapid reentry circuits.

Atrioventricular Node Reentry

A rather common cause of SVT in older children and young adults is reentry within the AV node itself. The underlying substrate is the presence of dual AV-node conduction pathways, which can be a benign phenomenon in up to 35% of normal children.[19] In a small subset of these patients, however, it appears that refractoriness and conduction characteristics of the two pathways are balanced in a precise fashion that allows reentry to occur in response to appropriately timed premature beats.

The ECG pattern in AV node reentry is that of a rapid, regular, narrow QRS, with abrupt onset and termination. Atrial tissue is

Figure 24-10. Transesophageal atrial electrogram from a patient with atrial flutter. Note how this recording clarifies atrial timing, which may be indistinct on a surface ECG.

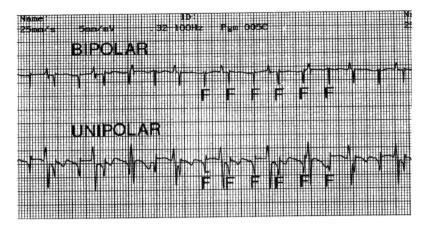

depolarized from below by retrograde conduction from the AV node, and the ventricle is depolarized nearly simultaneously in the anterograde fashion.[20] This results in the P wave occurring during (or just slightly after) the QRS. P waves are thus difficult to see in many instances, but an atrial wire or esophageal electrogram will clarify their timing when necessary (Fig. 24-11).

AV node reentry is generally quite easy to terminate. Any form of intense vagal stimulation can potentially slow AV node conduction and terminate the arrhythmia. Atrial overdrive pacing can also be used and is almost always successful. Drug therapy is also quite effective and involves agents such as adenosine, verapamil, and beta-blocker, all of which directly affect AV node conduction. Electrical cardioversion is also an effective technique, but is rarely necessary unless a patient is acutely compromised and other options are not readily available.

Accessory Atrioventricular Connections: (Wolff-Parkinson-White Syndrome and Concealed Pathways)

The presence of an abnormal conduction pathway is the most common cause of SVT in children. These connections can be of several types: (1) classical atrioventricular "Kent bundles" of the Wolff-Parkinson-White syndrome (WPW), which can conduct in both the anterograde and retrograde direction; (2) "concealed accessory pathways," which are capable of only unidirectional retrograde conduction; (3) "Mahaim fibers," which are thought to run between the AV junction and right ventricle[21]; and (4) "James fibers," which are postulated to run between the atrium and His Purkinje system.[22] The latter two fibers are rare and are beyond the scope of this chapter. The first two pathways, however, are responsible for more than 50% of cases of SVT in the first few years of life.

Figure 24-11. SVT due to AV nodal reentry, spontaneously converting to sinus rhythm in the later part of the tracing. Shown are three surface ECG leads with a simultaneous esophageal electrogram (ESO). The P wave timing (A) is nearly simultaneous with the QRS (V) during SVT and is not clearly visible on the surface ECG recordings. The esophageal electrogram demonstrates the superimposed A and V signals during SVT, which separate in the normal fashion when sinus rhythm resumes.

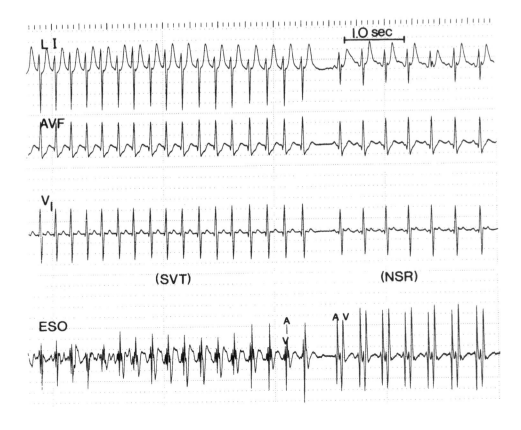

WPW syndrome presents a wide variety of ECG appearances during sinus rhythm and is capable of supporting several different varieties of tachycardia. During sinus rhythm, the pathognomonic observation is a short PR interval and a delta wave on the ECG (Fig. 24-12). This finding corresponds to early activation of a segment of ventricular muscle via the accessory pathway, which is ahead of schedule for the normal His Purkinje system (hence the term *preexcitation*). Ventricular activation during sinus rhythm is essentially a fusion beat of depolarization over the normal and abnormal pathways. The QRS morphologies can vary widely, depending on accessory pathway location[23] and the relative speed of conduction through the abnormal pathway versus the AV node. The preexcitation syndromes usually occur in patients with otherwise normal hearts, although the incidence is increased in patients with Ebstein's anomaly.

The most common reentry tachycardia of WPW occurs when all conduction proceeds over the normal AV node and is able to return retrograde to the atrium over the accessory pathway (so-called orthodromic reciprocating tachycardia). The ECG in this instance shows a regular **narrow** QRS complex with a fixed 1:1 A:V ratio and a P wave that usually does not occur until 70 to 150 msec after the QRS (Fig. 24-13). A less common arrhythmia in the WPW syndrome is the reverse reentry circuit, which proceeds anterograde over the accessory pathway and returns retrograde over the normal pathway (so-called antidromic reciprocating tachycardia). The QRS complex is **wide** in this instance because the ventricles are being activated exclusively by the accessory pathway (Fig. 24-14). The final and most serious arrhythmia in WPW syndrome is atrial fibrillation or atrial flutter in which the rapid atrial rhythm is capable of conducting anterograde over both the AV node and the accessory pathway. Depending on the conduction potential of the accessory pathway, this can occasionally result in a disastrously rapid ventricular response that may precipitate cardiac arrest.[24] The QRS during preexcited atrial fibrillation or flutter is rapid, irregular, and **wide** (Fig. 24-15). The QRS morphology may vary due to competition between normal and abnormal anterograde conduction.

Each SVT mechanism in WPW syndrome requires an individual approach to therapy. Orthodromic SVT is the easiest of the three to manage. One may begin with vagal stimulation, which may potentially slow the AV node and break the reentry circuit, although in the authors' experience this is effective less than one third of the time. There are numerous acute pharmacologic options. These include drugs that are aimed at acutely slowing AV

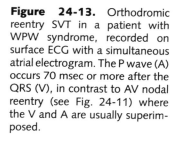

Figure 24-12. ECG recorded during sinus rhythms in a patient with WPW syndrome showing a short PR interval and delta wave.

Figure 24-13. Orthodromic reentry SVT in a patient with WPW syndrome, recorded on surface ECG with a simultaneous atrial electrogram. The P wave (A) occurs 70 msec or more after the QRS (V), in contrast to AV nodal reentry (see Fig. 24-11) where the V and A are usually superimposed.

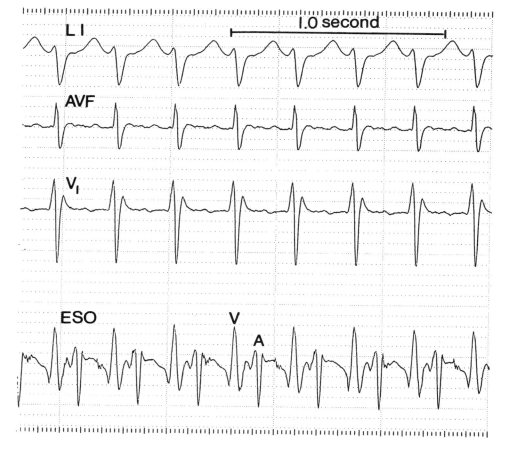

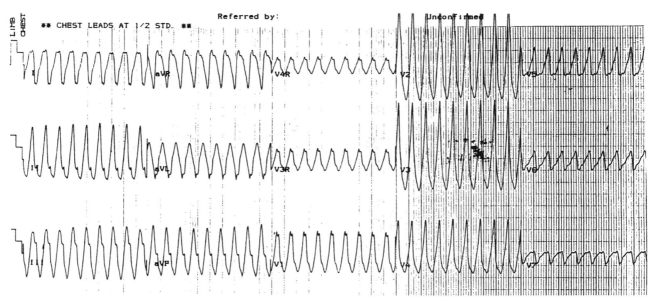

Figure 24-14. Surface ECG recorded from a patient with WPW syndrome during an episode of antidromic reciprocating tachycardia. Note the **regular wide** QRS.

Figure 24-15. Three simultaneous surface ECG leads recorded from a patient with WPW syndrome during atrial fibrillation. Note the **irregular wide** QRS at rapid rates.

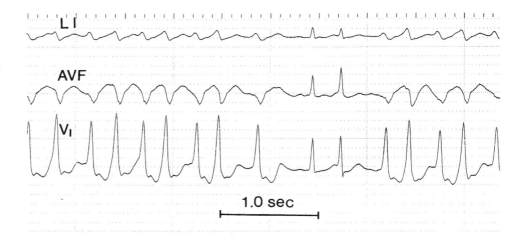

node conduction (adenosine, verapamil, beta-blocker) or drugs that act more specifically on the accessory pathway (e.g., as procainamide). Overdrive atrial pacing and elective cardioversion are also very effective for orthodromic tachycardia.

Antidromic tachycardia and preexcited atrial fibrillation/flutter require much more cautious management. Of central concern, they may present a diagnostic dilemma because their ECG appearance is very difficult to differentiate from ventricular tachycardia, and at first presentation, they may need to be managed as such. In a patient with a known history of WPW in whom the diagnosis of antidromic reentry or preexcited atrial fibrillation/flutter is firm, the specific treatment may involve elective cardioversion, intravenous procainamide, or trials of atrial overdrive pacing. It is essential to avoid the use of both digoxin[25] and verapamil[26] for acute therapy of any wide QRS tachycardia in the WPW syndrome. Both of these agents are known to shorten refractoriness of the accessory pathway and may thus increase the rate for anterograde conduction of fibrillation or flutter, resulting in acceleration of the ventricular

response and possible ventricular fibrillation. For this same reason, digoxin and verapamil are also generally avoided for chronic outpatient therapy of WPW, because one cannot accurately predict the occurrence of atrial fibrillation/flutter, even in patients who have never previously demonstrated the arrhythmia. In rare instances, when digoxin or verapamil are the only possible treatment options, they can be used if comprehensive electrophysiology testing has confirmed their safety.

"Concealed" accessory pathways are another common cause of orthodromic SVT in children. Although the ECG pattern during orthodromic reentry is identical to that seen with WPW, these patients lack the delta wave and short PR interval during sinus rhythm, due to the absence of anterograde conduction over the abnormal fiber. The treatment of orthodromic SVT in this case does not differ at all from WPW, but because concealed pathways cannot participate in antidromic reentry nor in preexcited atrial fibrillation/flutter, the warnings regarding digoxin and verapamil for chronic therapy do not apply.

Ventricular Tachycardia

Ventricular arrhythmias, although uncommon in pediatric patients, are the most malignant of the rhythm disorders—and the most challenging to treat. VT typically occurs in patients with abnormal myocardium who may already be compromised by poor ventricular function and may be at risk for abrupt degeneration to ventricular fibrillation. Most forms of VT are due to reentry mechanisms, although some atypical forms are thought to be due to automaticity or triggered activity.

Sustained wide QRS tachycardias should be treated as an emergency. If one is able to identify a treatable cause or toxic exposure, it should be reversed as soon as possible. Basic airway management and CPR measures should be instituted when necessary, and prompt attempts at converting the rhythm disturbance should be undertaken (discussion follows). Although some atypical SVT's are included in the differential diagnosis of wide QRS tachycardia, one should not risk delay in treatment when unsure of the exact diagnosis. To reiterate a prior caution, unless there is convincing evidence to the contrary, all wide QRS tachycardias should be managed acutely as VT.

The general therapeutic measures for VT are listed in the Table 24-3. Rapid physical assessment is performed, and if the situation permits, a formal 12-lead ECG should be recorded. In any unresponsive or hypotensive patient, the first therapeutic step should be an attempt at DC cardioversion. If the patient is awake and well perfused, or if DC cardioversion is not successful, pharmacologic therapy with lidocaine should be commenced.

Beyond lidocaine, treatment options vary depending on the etiology and type of the arrhythmia. One can recognize several distinct subcategories of VT based on ECG appearance. For purposes of this chapter, we will concentrate on three types: (1) common form of VT due to reentry within damaged ventricular muscle; (2) incessant VT, which does not respond to cardioversion or pacing and may be thought to arise from a discrete automatic focus; and (3) a specific form of VT known as "torsade de pointes," which typically occurs in the setting of QT interval prolongation.

Reentry Ventricular Tachycardia

Reentry at the ventricular level usually occurs within diseased or injured regions of muscle. The possible causes of this pathology are diverse, including long-standing pressure/volume loads and surgical scars from complex congenital heart defects,[27] coronary artery anomalies,[28] myocarditis, and various forms of cardiomyopathy or toxic exposure. The potential for reentry to occur at these sites is enhanced by many extrinsic factors, such as hypotension, electrolyte disturbances, acidosis, hypoxemia, and exposure to cer-

Table 24-3. General guidelines for management of "wide QRS" tachycardia

Review history and evaluate condition (basic CPR if needed)

12-lead ECG, if possible

If unresponsive or markedly hypotensive, DC cardioversion

IV lidocaine

Specific second-line therapy based on QRS morphology
   Monomorphic reentry VT—IV procainamide
   Torsade de pointes—Magnesium sulfate
   Any VT—DC cardioversion

Specific third-line therapy (see text)

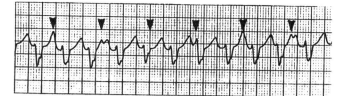

Figure 24-16. Surface ECG recorded from a patient with sustained monomorphic VT. The P waves *(arrows)* are clearly slower and dissociated from the wide QRS.

tain drugs (including the potential for "proarrhythmia" from antiarrhythmic agents).

The ECG appearance of reentry VT is a rapid, wide QRS rhythm, which may involve a single QRS morphology (monomorphic) or variable QRS shapes (polymorphic). On occasion, one may be able to demonstrate AV dissociation on the surface cardiogram (Fig. 24-16), but passive retrograde VA conduction may occur with VT, and in many instances the P wave may be difficult to see at all (Fig. 24-17). Atrial recordings from pacing wires or an esophageal lead may help demonstrate AV dissociation when the diagnosis is unclear.

The acute therapeutic response to sustained reentry VT in any hypotensive or unresponsive patient should be an immediate DC cardioversion using an energy of 1 to 2 joules/kg. If unsuccessful, the shock may be repeated for one or two additional trials, with doubling of the output at each new attempt. If the shock is unsuccessful, or VT recurs, pharmacologic therapy should begin with a bolus of lidocaine, followed by a continuous infusion. If additional drug therapy is still needed, procainamide is a reasonable second agent for reentry VT. Possible third-line agents include bretylium, esmolol, and phenytoin. If reentry VT remains resistant to this protocol, a transvenous pacing wire can be positioned in the ventricle to allow repeated overdrive pacing to terminate the tachycardia. The major caveat regarding pacing maneuvers is the potential to accelerate the tachycardia or precipitate ventricular fibrillation; this technique should thus be used cautiously by experienced individuals, with defibrillation equipment at the bedside. If the patient is stable, or the ventricular tachycardia is nonsustained, the treatment sequence can begin with pharmacologic trials, reserving DC shock or ventricular pacing as elective procedures under appropriate sedation.

Incessant VT from an Automatic Focus

This variety of VT is a rare condition that typically occurs during infancy and is rather unique in its resistance to cardioversion or overdrive pacing, suggesting automaticity as the possible cellular mechanism. Primary tumors of Purkinje-cell origin have been found at surgery in some afflicted infants.[29] This form of VT is usually monomorphic and moderate in rate (Figure 24-18), but so protracted in its duration that severe ventricular dysfunction may ensue. For ill patients, trials of cardioversion should be attempted as a matter of course, but they are often more diagnostic than therapeutic. When this proves ineffective, one should proceed to pharmacologic trials. Beta-blockers may be effective in cases where the ventricular function is still well preserved. Lidocaine, although safe, has minimal effect in most of these patients. Procainamide seems to be effective for terminating VT in some cases, or at least provides some slowing of the rate. Additional empiric trials with various intravenous and oral antiarrhythmic drugs may be tried if the child is sufficiently stable. In extreme cases, when pharmaco-

Figure 24-17. Recordings from a patient with rapid monomorphic VT. Atrial activity is poorly seen on surface ECG recording **(panel A)**, such that AV dissociation is difficult to verify. An esophageal recording **(panel B)** clearly demonstrates slower atrial rates (A), which confirms the diagnosis of VT. Of interest, the atria in this case are being activated by retrograde conduction, which occurs in a 6:5 Wenckebach pattern.

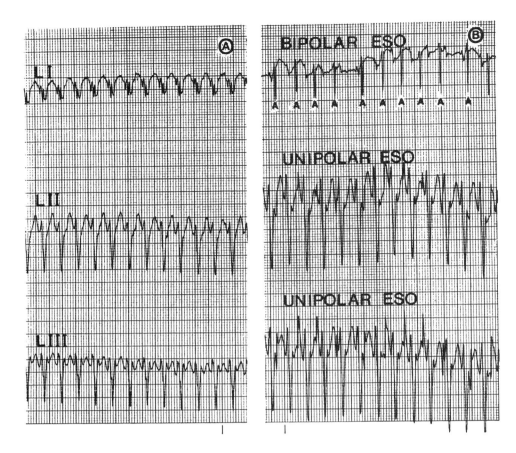

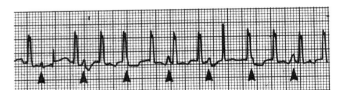

Figure 24-18. Surface ECG showing incessant VT from a 2-week-old girl. The VT is monomorphic, and P waves *(arrows)* are clearly dissociated. Occasional sinus capture beats and fusion beats are seen.

logic therapy is of no benefit, emergency intracardiac mapping followed by surgical or catheter ablation of the VT focus can be considered.

Torsade de Pointes

The phrase *torsade de pointes* refers to a specific pattern of polymorphic VT in which the direction of the QRS complex gradually twists around the isoelectric line of the ECG (Figure 24-19). Torsade is classically seen under conditions of abnormal QT prolongation, such as the congenital long QT disorders (Romano-Ward and the Jervell and Lange-Nielsen syndromes), toxicity from certain class I and class III antiarrhythmic drugs, electrolyte disturbance, and others.[30] The VT typically occurs at times of stress and will often start and stop of its own accord, causing transient dizziness, hypotension, or episodes of syncope with possible seizure-like activity. Sustained torsade de pointes can ultimately lead to ventricular fibrillation and death.

The management of this disorder is distinct from other forms of VT. In particular, one must avoid use of any drugs that could further prolong the QT interval (e.g., procainamide or quinidine).

Figure 24-19. Surface ECG showing torsade de pointes, which developed in a patient being treated with quinidine.

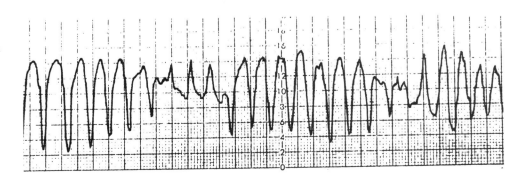

Sustained torsade de pointes should be treated with immediate DC shock of 1 to 2 joules/kg followed by medications to prevent recurrence. Patients with nonsustained episodes should be treated initially with drugs alone. The most useful agents are those that potentially shorten the QT interval, such as lidocaine or phenytoin. IV magnesium sulfate (25 mg/kg over 15–30 minutes) is also remarkably effective in stabilizing this disorder.[31] Although rapid overdrive ventricular pacing rarely corrects torsade, ventricular pacing per se at a physiologic rate seems to exert a stabilizing influence on ventricular muscle and is helpful in many cases. Alternatively, the induction of sinus tachycardia with an isoproterenol infusion or atrial pacing may be of benefit in difficult cases. Naturally, if an offending drug can be found, it should be stopped immediately, and any electrolyte disturbance (particularly hypokalemia, hypocalcemia, or hypomagnesemia) should be corrected promptly. Following acute stabilization, the administration of beta-blockers and/or chronic pacing may prevent recurrence of torsade de pointes.

Bradycardias

Bradycardia management is more straightforward than the treatment of tachycardia. If the disorder involves depression of natural pacemaker cells (e.g., sinus bradycardia), one needs to simply correct the underlying cause or consider pharmacologic therapy. Conduction block is generally easy to treat with artificial pacing in a cardiac chamber below the level of the block.

Sinus Bradycardia

Except for "sick sinus syndrome,"[32] which most often results from direct injury to sinus node tissue, most cases of sinus bradycardia are secondary to extrinsic factors. Any serious metabolic disturbance (e.g., acidosis, hypoglycemia, hypoxia) will depress sinus node automaticity, and the correction of these parameters will ultimately restore the heart rate. As a temporizing measure, one can enhance sinus node automaticity with infusions of catecholamines, and often with atropine if there is any significant vagal component to the slowing. In postoperative cardiac patients, one may also pace the heart via atrial or ventricular wires to increase the rate. An esophageal lead can be used for atrial pacing if epicardial wires are unavailable.

Atrioventricular Block

Disturbances of AV conduction may be divided into three major categories: (1) first-degree block (prolonged AV conduction time), (2) second-degree block (intermittent failure of conduction for an isolated atrial impulse), and (3) third-degree block (complete interruption of AV conduction).

First-degree block is typically due to delayed conduction at the level of the AV node, although the site of delay can be at the common His bundle on occasion. The ECG shows a PR interval that is prolonged for age (Figure 24-20A). First-degree block is generally well tolerated and does not require therapy. It may be caused by enhanced vagal tone, trauma or inflammation at the AV junction, and certain antiarrhythmic drugs.

Second-degree block is subdivided as either the Mobitz I or Mobitz II type. Mobitz I block classically results from delay at the level of the AV node and presents a stereotypic ECG sequence of gradual and progressive PR prolongation before the blocked atrial beat, known as Wenckebach periodicity (Figure 24-20B). The

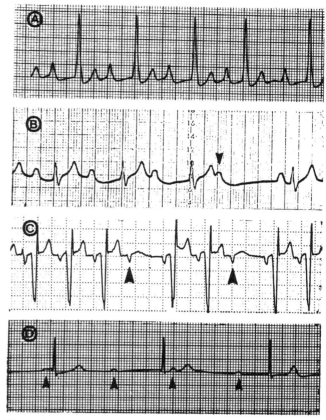

Figure 24-20. Varieties of AV block: **(A)** first-degree block with a prolonged PR interval, **(B)** second-degree block (Mobitz I type) with progressive PR prolongation culminating in a single nonconducted P wave *(arrow)*, **(C)** second-degree block (Mobitz II type) showing abrupt nonconducted P waves *(arrows)* without prior PR prolongation, **(D)** third-degree block with complete failure of atrial conduction.

causes of Mobitz I block are similar to those of first-degree block, and treatment is rarely needed. In a critically ill patient, however, Mobitz I block can complicate hemodynamic status and may require therapy on occasion. Atropine and/or isoproterenol will frequently improve conduction through the AV node.

Mobitz II block is a less predictable disorder that classically involves a conduction disturbance at the level of the common His bundle. It is usually caused by direct trauma or inflammation at this site, and in most all cases it is accompanied by more diffuse disturbances of His Purkinje conduction, such as bundle branch block. The ECG pattern is one of an abrupt, nonconducted P wave without preceding PR prolongation (Figure 24-20C). Unlike Mobitz I block, there exists a real potential for sudden progression to higher-grade block when the His Purkinje system is involved. Patients with Mobitz II block require very careful monitoring, and postoperative cardiac patients with Mobitz II should have the temporary-demand pacemaker wires for standby ventricular pacing. Isoproterenol may improve Mobitz II block in some instances, although atropine typically has no effect.

In third-degree block, there is complete electrical discontinuity between atrium and ventricle due to a disturbance of the AV node and/or His Purkinje system. The ECG shows normal atrial rates, with the slower ventricular rhythm generated independently from a junctional or ventricular escape focus (Figure 24-20D). The "congenital" forms of third-degree block (associated with maternal lupus or certain anatomic cardiac defects) are well tolerated, at least in the short run.[33] Third-degree block in the PICU setting is more likely to be the acquired variety, due to surgical trauma,[34] inflammatory processes, or myopathy. Acquired complete heart block generally leads to symptoms of low cardiac output and increased cardiac filling pressures, and thus requires therapy. Isoproterenol or atropine may increase the escape rate slightly, but pacing is the most reliable treatment option in this setting. As an acute measure, it is often sufficient to pace the ventricle alone, although optimal hemodynamic support is achieved when the atrium and ventricle can be paced in synchrony. Ventricular pacing can be performed from either transvenous catheters or epicardial wires when they are available. During an acute resuscitation, transcutaneous ventricular pacing is also possible using specialized electrode pads on the thorax and a specialized high-output generator. Such a device can cause serious skin burns in small infants and should be used only until more secure pacing electrodes are in place.

Antiarrhythmic Pharmacology

Antiarrhythmic drugs are semiselective cell poisons that have been adapted for clinical therapeutics based on their desirable "side effects" on cardiac tissue. Most of these agents have the potential for serious toxicity, including negative inotropic properties and paradoxical worsening of the rhythm disorder they were meant to treat (proarrhythmia). They should be used with extreme caution under appropriate monitoring and only when simple nonpharmacologic options have failed. Antiarrhythmic agents are classified according to their in vitro cellular effects,[35] as shown in Table 24-4. This discussion is limited to agents that are available for acute IV administration in the PICU setting. The interested reader is referred to in-depth reviews of pediatric electropharmacology[36] for a more general discussion of these agents.

Procainamide (Class IA)

As a sodium channel blocker, procainamide acts primarily on the so-called fast-response cardiac cells, which are highly dependent on sodium influx for their depolarization. Such cells occur in atrial muscle, ventricular muscle, His Purkinje tissue, and accessory pathways. Procainamide causes slowing of conduction and prolongation of refractoriness at these sites, and is thus suited to treatment of both atrial and ventricular reentry tachycardias (including atrial fibrillation and atrial flutter, VT, and tachycardia from WPW

Table 24-4. Classification of antiarrhythmic drugs

Class I	(IA)—**Procainamide**, quinidine, disopyramide
	(IB)—**Lidocaine**, mexiletine, tocainide, **phenytoin**, ethmozine
	(IC)—Flecainide, encainide, **propafenone***
Class II	(Nonselective)—**Propranolol**, nadolol
	(Cardioselective)—Atenolol, **esmolol**
Class III	**Amiodarone***, NAPA, **breytylium**, sotalol*
Class IV	**Verapamil**, diltiazem
Misc	Digoxin, **adenosine**

Bold print identifies agents available for IV administration.
*Investigational agents.

syndrome). Procainamide is occasionally effective in suppressing automatic foci at these sites as well.

IV procainamide administration begins with a slow loading dose of 5 to 15 mg/kg over 30 minutes, followed by a constant infusion of 20 to 60 µg/kg/min. In rare instances, hypotension secondary to vasodilation may occur during loading, but this is generally easy to correct with crystalloid administration. Serum levels should be checked periodically and should be maintained between 4 to 10 µg/ml. Potentially serious adverse effects include hypotension, widening of the QRS, QT prolongation, and proarrhythmia.

Lidocaine (Class IB)

IB drugs have subtle effects on sodium channels, which are most pronounced in damaged ventricular cells. Lidocaine use is thus restricted largely to suppression of ventricular arrhythmias. Unlike the class IA and class IC agents, lidocaine does not prolong the QT but, in fact, may shorten it slightly. It is therefore a reasonable treatment option for torsade de pointes.

IV lidocaine administration begins with a bolus of 1.0 mg/kg, which can be repeated for one or two additional trials at 10-minute intervals if needed. Loading is followed by constant infusion of 20 to 60 µg/kg/min. Serum levels should be maintained between 2 and 5 µg/ml. Higher levels may cause neurologic side effects such as vomiting, lethargy, and seizure. In the therapeutic range, lidocaine has minimal adverse effects and is a generally safe agent.

Phenytoin (Class IB)

Phenytoin is a weak IB agent that is useful for suppression of select ventricular arrhythmias but may also have occasional dramatic effect in treatment of ectopic atrial foci. IV administration of phenytoin involves a dosage of about 5 to 10 mg/kg given by slow IV infusion over 1 hour. Rapid administration can cause hypotension and bradycardia. Maintenance doses are begun 24 hours after loading, using a schedule of 5 mg/kg/d, divided in two doses 12 hours apart. The therapeutic serum level for antiarrhythmic therapy is similar to the anticonvulsant range (7–20 µg/ml). Acute adverse effects are mostly restricted to the central nervous system (lethargy, ataxia) and appear to be dose-related.

Propafenone (Class IC)

The IC drugs are very potent blockers of sodium channels and can cause profound decrease in conduction and automaticity in atrial muscle, ventricular muscle, His Purkinje system, and accessory pathways. Although they are often dramatically effective in suppressing arrhythmias, they have a high proarrhythmic potential, and use is restricted to life-threatening rhythm disorders.[37]

Propafenone is the only IV form of a IC agent currently available, and it is still restricted to select centers by investigational protocol. Efficacy has been reported for treatment of JET in children,[15] but experience is quite limited in other pediatric rhythm disorders.

Propranolol (Class II)

Propranolol is a nonselective beta-blocker that effects beta-1 and beta-2 receptors. Blockade at cardiac receptors results in a decrease in sinus node automaticity and slowing of conduction at the AV node. Beta-blockade may also decrease abnormal automaticity from atrial or ventricular foci and can stabilize ventricular cell membranes to increase the threshold for fibrillation. Beta-blockers are thus used for treatment of a wide variety of atrial and ventricular rhythm disorders.

Propranolol is the prototype beta-blocker and is available for IV use. The dose is 0.05 to 0.1 mg/kg by slow IV infusion over 10 to 15 minutes. The same dose can then be repeated at 6-hour intervals as needed.

The major cardiac side effects of IV propranolol are bradycardia, AV block, and hypotension. Because beta-2 blockade can affect bronchial smooth muscle, it may also aggravate reactive airway disease in some patients. Hypoglycemia can also occur because of its effects on hepatic glycogenolysis.

Because newer IV beta-blockers with cardioselectivity and shorter half-lives have now become available, propranolol is being used less often in the acute setting.

Esmolol (Class II)

Esmolol is a beta-1 selective agent possessing a short half-life of approximately 10 minutes, which is an effective and perhaps preferred alternative to propranolol in the acute setting. It is administered as an IV loading dose of 0.5 mg/kg, followed, if needed, by an infusion of 50 to 100 μg/kg/min. Cardiac side effects are similar to those of propranolol, but they can be reversed quickly by discontinuing the drug.

Bretylium (Class III)

All class III agents have complex action on both cardiac cells and the autonomic nervous system. Their hallmark antiarrhythmic action is prolongation of cellular action potential duration, which results in increased refractoriness and prolonged conduction time in the fast-response cells of atrial muscle, ventricular muscle, and the His Purkinje system.

Bretylium has a biphasic cardiac response. After initial administration, it causes release of norepinephrine from sympathetic nerve endings, leading to sinus tachycardia, hypertension, and occasional aggravation of the abnormal rhythm. This is gradually followed by onset of its class III antiarrhythmic activity and a block of norepinephrine release, which can result in bradycardia and hypotension.

The primary indication for bretylium is treatment of recurrent or refractory ventricular fibrillation during difficult resuscitation.[38] It is also used for some cases of VT that have not responded to standard therapy.

Bretylium is administered as an IV load of 5 mg/kg over 15 minutes, followed if necessary by an infusion of 20 to 50 μg/kg/min, with careful monitoring for both proarrhythmia and hypotension.

Verapamil (Class IV)

As a calcium channel blocker, verapamil acts primarily on the so-called slow-response cardiac cells, which are highly dependent on calcium influx for their depolarization. Such cells occur primarily in the sinus and AV nodes. Verapamil will slow automaticity and depress conduction at these areas and is thus suited to termination of reentry SVT, which involves the AV node as part of its circuit, or for temporary slowing of the ventricular response rate in other forms of SVT. With rare exception,[39] verapamil is not useful for treatment of VT (or any wide QRS tachycardia wherein the mechanism is uncertain).

Verapamil should not be administered to infants under age 12 months because of an exaggerated hypotensive and bradycardic response in this age group.[40] Likewise, it should not be administered to patients of any age who are receiving beta-blocker, because of synergistic myocardial suppression. As discussed earlier in this chapter, verapamil is also a generally poor choice of therapy in WPW syndrome, except for acute termination of orthodromic reentry in which the QRS is narrow.

The dosage for administration of verapamil is 0.05 to 0.1 mg/kg by rapid IV push. This dose may be repeated at 15-minute intervals for two additional trials if needed. Hypotension and bradycardia are occasionally observed that can be treated with IV calcium and/or isoproterenol.

Digoxin

The antiarrhythmic actions of digoxin are mediated primarily by enhancement of vagal tone, which causes mild depression of sinus node automaticity and some slowing of AV node conduction. The major disadvantage of this agent is delayed onset of action, requiring 12 to 24 hours until digitalization is complete. Although the cardiac glycosides were, for many years, the mainstay of acute therapy for SVT in children, use is declining as alternate, faster-acting options are introduced.

Although not ideal for acute therapy, digoxin is often an effective agent for maintenance therapy in SVT due to AV node reentry, concealed accessory pathways, or for controlling a rapid ventricular response in atrial fibrillation and atrial flutter. Whenever possible, digoxin should be avoided in WPW syndrome for reasons previously discussed.

The dosage of digoxin for antiarrhythmic therapy is similar to the standard digitalization and maintenance schedules used in the treatment of congestive heart failure.

Adenosine

Adenosine is a new and very promising treatment option for reentry SVT.[41] It is rapidly replacing digoxin, verapamil, and beta-blocker for acute termination of these disorders. Adenosine is an endogenous nucleoside that will cause transient but profound sinus node slowing and AV block when administered as a large, rapid bolus. It is removed quickly from the circulation by endothelial cells and blood cells, resulting in a half-life of less than 15 seconds. The dosage in children is 0.05 to 0.25 mg/kg by rapid IV push. Attempts should be made to administer this drug as close to the central circulation as possible to prevent rapid metabolism before the bolus reaches the heart. When this drug is effective, the result is almost immediate.

Transient bradycardia and AV block can be observed after administration, but they resolve within a few seconds. Although experience is still limited, serious cardiac side effects have been decidedly uncommon when using this drug in children and adults.

Nonpharmacologic Therapy

For an acutely ill child in a PICU setting, it is desirable, whenever possible, to avoid lingering exposure to potential side effects of antiarrhythmic drugs. With the exception of adenosine, esmolol, and lidocaine, one must usually contend with elimination half-lives lasting up to several hours for these agents, which is particularly disadvantageous if the drug is ineffective or proarrhythmic. Treatment of arrhythmias should thus involve initial attempts to reverse any underlying cause, or consideration of nonpharmaco-logic options.

Vagal Stimulation

The principal sites of vagal influence in the heart occur at the levels of the sinus and AV nodes. By enhancing vagal tone, reentry SVT involving the AV node can often be terminated. Vagal stimulation can also be used for temporary depression of AV node conduction to assist in the diagnosis of other forms of SVT (e.g., atrial flutter).

Several techniques can be used for this purpose.[42] The most common is the Valsalva maneuver, which results in a complex series of vasomotor reflexes that ultimately enhances vagal tone. A proper Valsalva maneuver requires considerable patient cooperation and must involve an intense effort for 10 to 15 seconds before release. It is usually only successful in older children.

The application of an ice bag to the face, or facial immersion in very cold water, is also an effective form of vagal stimuli and is less dependent on patient performance. Alternatively, carotid massage or elicitation of the gag reflex with a tongue blade or passage of a nasogastric tube can be used. Ocular compression, perhaps the most intense of the vagal stimuli, is contraindicated because of the risk of retinal detachment.

Cardioversion and Defibrillation

A DC shock of proper intensity and timing will terminate most all reentry tachycardias at the atrial and ventricular levels.[43] The procedure is termed a *cardioversion* when this energy is applied for treatment of SVT or an organized VT. *Defibrillation* refers to a larger shock used for termination of rapid polymorphic VT or ventricular fibrillation.

A DC shock is painful, and patients must be fully sedated prior to the procedure, unless they already have altered consciousness from their abnormal rhythms or other underlying disease processes. Electrode paddles must be positioned to optimize the flow of current through the heart. If paddles are positioned too closely together, the energy may arc between them, causing skin burn

and poor energy delivery to the cardiac tissue. Anterior-posterior paddle positioning is thus usually preferred in small children over the standard apex-upper-chest position.

When cardioversion is performed for SVT or an organized VT, the shock should be "synchronized" to cause discharge at the same time as the QRS complex. Energy delivery during this precise moment prevents random discharge, which could potentially coincide with the T wave and precipitate ventricular fibrillation. For polymorphic VT or ventricular fibrillation when there is no suitable QRS for sensing, the energy must be delivered in a unsynchronized random fashion.

For most forms of SVT, a starting energy of 0.25 to 0.5 joules/kg is used, and it can be doubled for one or two additional attempts when needed. For an organized VT, a starting energy of 1.0 joules/kg is employed, and for VF, 2.0 joules/kg is the proper starting dose. Excess energy delivery or multiple repeated DC shocks can cause depression of myocardial function and should be avoided.

Overdrive Pacing

Reentry tachycardias can often be interrupted with pacing maneuvers if some of the involved tissue can be depolarized faster than the conduction capacity of the reentry circuit.[10] Overdrive pacing is often effective for atrial flutter, AV node reentry, many tachycardias involving accessory pathways, and some forms of VT (Fig. 24-21). It is not effective for atrial fibrillation or rapid VT, nor will it terminate tachycardia due to automatic foci.

The potential danger with overdrive pacing relates to a small but real risk of accelerating the rate of reentry or causing degeneration to fibrillation in either the atrium or ventricle. These problems are most likely to occur when very prolonged and/or rapid bursts of pacing are used. Overdrive pacing should be employed only by those familiar with the technique and with defibrillation equipment on standby at the bedside.

The key to successful overdrive pacing and avoidance of the aforementioned complications is to use the minimum number of paced beats, delivered at the slowest effective rate. Thus, one typically begins with only three or four paced beats chosen at a rate just slightly faster than the tachycardia. In a sequential fashion,

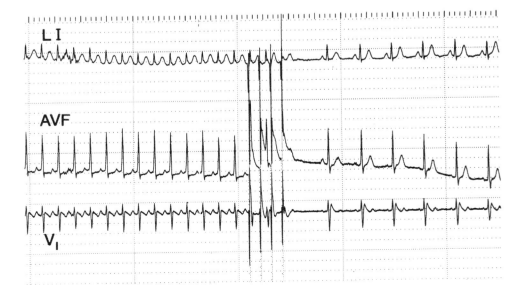

Figure 24-21. An example of overdrive atrial pacing (performed with an esophageal lead), using a train of four premature beats to terminate reentry SVT.

both the rate and duration of pacing may be gradually increased on each additional attempt. In general, the slower the original reentry circuit, the higher the chance of success.

Prognosis

Cardiac arrhythmias in a PICU setting can usually be stabilized with the techniques described in this chapter, and quite often will relent as the child's general condition improves. When endogenous and exogenous catecholamines are lowered, automatic foci tends to slow or become quiescent, and the number of premature atrial or ventricular beats that serve as triggers for reentry tachycardias tends to decrease.

The long-term risk of arrhythmia recurrence is highly dependent on the cause and mechanism of the disorder. Before a child leaves the PICU, these data must be determined to avoid an unpredictable relapse under conditions of reduced surveillance. Thus, proper diagnosis of the arrhythmia mechanism is essential, not only for acute stabilization in the PICU, but also for determining prognosis and long-term management when the child moves to an unmonitored ward or is discharged home.

Formal cardiac evaluation is recommended prior to PICU dismissal for any patient in whom an arrhythmia was not clearly related to a reversible cause, or is otherwise thought to result from a primary cardiac abnormality. This evaluation may include 24-hour Holter monitoring, echocardiography, cardiac catheterization, exercise testing, and electrophysiology testing with transesophageal or intracardiac pacing maneuvers. Depending on etiology, long-term prevention of arrhythmia may include chronic oral drug therapy, pacing, or even surgical[44] or catheter ablation techniques[45] for abnormal foci or pathways.

References

1. Gillette PC, Garson A. *Pediatric Arrhythmias: Electrophysiology and Pacing.* Philadelphia: Saunders, 1990.
2. Walsh EP, Saul JP. Cardiac arrhythmias. In Fyler DC (ed): *Nadas' Pediatric Cardiology.* Philadelphia: Hanley & Belfus, 1991. Pp 377–434.
3. Gilmore RF, Zipes DP. Cellular basis for cardiac arrhythmias. *Cardiol Clinics* 1:3–11, 1983.
4. Akhatar M, Tchou PJ, Jazayeri M. Mechanism of clinical tachycardias. *Am J Cardiol* 61:9A–19A, 1988.
5. Gorgels AP et al. The clinical relevance of abnormal automaticity and triggered activity. In Brugada P, Wellens HJ (eds): *Cardiac Arrhythmias: Where to Go from Here?* Mount Kisco, NY: Futura, 1987.
6. Walsh EP, Rhodes LA, Saul JP. Triggered activity as the possible mechanism for exercise induced ventricular tachycardia in young patients (abstract). *PACE* 13:541, 1990.
7. Cranefield PF, Hoffman BF. Reentry: Slow conduction, summation, and inhibition. *Circulation* 44:309–316, 1971.
8. Humes RA et al. Utility of temporary atrial epicardial electrodes in postoperative pediatric patients. *Mayo Clin Proc* 64:516–521, 1989.
9. Benson DW et al. Transesophageal cardiac pacing: History, application, technique. *Clin Prog Pace Electrophysiol* 2:360–327, 1984.
10. Walsh EP, Keane JF. Electrophysiologic studies in congenital heart disease. In Lock JE, Keane JF, Fellows KE (eds): *Diagnostic and Interventional Catheterization in Congenital Heart Disease.* Boston: Martinus Nijhoff, 1987. Pp 161–181.
11. Gillette PC, Garson A. Electrophysiologic and pharmacologic characteristics of automatic ectopic atrial tachycardia. *Circulation* 56:571–575, 1977.
12. Scher DL, Arsura EL. Multifocal atrial tachycardia: Mechanisms, clinical correlates, and treatment. *Am Heart J* 118:574–580, 1989.
13. Gillette PC. Diagnosis and management of postoperative junctional ectopic tachycardia. *Am Heart J* 118:192–194, 1989.
14. Grant JW et al. Junctional tachycardia in infants and children after open heart surgery for congenital heart disease. *Am J Cardiol* 59:1216–1218, 1987.
15. Garson A, Moak J, Smith RT. Control of postoperative junctional ectopic tachycardia with propafenone. *Am J Cardiol* 59:1422–1424, 1987.
16. Bash SE et al. Hypothermia for the treatment of postoperative greatly accelerated junctional ectopic tachycardia. *J Am Coll Cardiol* 10:1095–1099, 1987.
17. Sholler GF et al. Evaluation of a staged treatment protocol for postoperative rapid junctional tachycardia (abstract). *Circulation* 78(II):597, 1988.
18. Campbell RM et al. Atrial overdrive pacing for conversion of atrial flutter in children. *Pediatrics* 75:730–736, 1985.
19. Casta A, Wolff GS, Mehta AV. Dual atrioventricular nodal pathways: A benign finding in arrhythmia-free children with heart disease. *Am J Cardiol* 46:1013–1018, 1980.
20. Akhtar M et al. Anterograde and retrograde conduction characteristics in three patterns of paroxysmal reentrant tachycardia. *Am Heart J* 95:22–42, 1978.
21. Gallagher JJ et al. Role of mahaim fibers in cardiac arrhythmias in man. *Circulation* 64:176–189, 1981.
22. Brechenmacher C. Atrio-His bundle tracts. *Br Heart J* 37:853–857, 1975.
23. Gallagher JJ et al. The preexcitation syndromes. *Prog Cardiovasc Dis* 20:285–327, 1978.
24. Klein GJ et al. Ventricular fibrillation in the Wolff-Parkinson-White syndrome. *N Engl J Med* 301:1080–1085, 1979.
25. Sellers TD, Bashore TM, Gallagher JJ. Digitalis in the preexcitation syndrome: Analysis during atrial fibrillation. *Circulation* 56:260–267, 1977.
26. McGovern B, Garan H, Ruskin JN. Precipitation of cardiac arrest by verapamil in patients with Wolff-Parkinson-White Syndrome. *Ann Intern Med* 104:791–794, 1986.
27. Walsh EP et al. Late results in patients with tetralogy of Fallot repaired during infancy. *Circulation* 77:1062–1067, 1988.
28. Liberthson RR, Dinsmore RE, Fallon JT. Aberrant coronary artery origin from the aorta. *Circulation* 59:748–754, 1979.
29. Garson A et al. Incessant ventricular tachycardias in infants: Myocardial hamartomas and surgical cure. *J Am Coll Cardiol* 10:619–626, 1987.
30. Jackman WM et al. The long QT syndromes: A critical review, new clinical observations, and a unifying hypothesis. *Prog Cardiovas Dis* 31:115–172, 1988.
31. Tzivoni D et al. Treatment of Torsade de Pointes with magnesium sulfate. *Circulation* 77:392–397, 1988.
32. Greenwood RD et al. Sick sinus syndrome after surgery for congenital heart disease. *Circulation* 52:208–213, 1975.
33. Sholler GF, Walsh EP. Congenital complete heart block in patients without anatomic cardiac defects. *Am Heart J* 118:1193–1198, 1989.
34. Hofschire PJ, Nicoloff DM, Moller JH. Postoperative complete heart block in 64 children treated with and without cardiac pacing. *Am J Cardiol* 39:559–562, 1977.
35. Vaughan Willams EM. Classification of antiarrhythmic drugs. In Sandoe E, Flenshted-Jansen E, Olesen KH (eds): *Symposium on Cardiac Arrhythmias.* Sodertalje, Sweden: AB Astra, 1970. Pp 449–472.
36. Moak JP. Pharmacology and electrophysiology of antiarrhythmic drugs. In Gillette PC, Garson A (eds): *Pediatric Arrhythmias: Electrophysiology and Pacing.* Philadelphia: Saunders, 1990. Pp 37–117.
37. Zipes DP. Proarrhythmic events. *Am J Cardiol* 61:70A–76A, 1988.
38. Lucchesi BR. Rationale of therapy in the patient with acute myocardial infraction and life-threatening arrhythmias: A focus on bretylium. *Am J Cardiol* 54:14A–19A, 1984.
39. Ohe T et al. Idiopathic sustained left ventricular tachycardia: Clinical and electrophysiologic characteristics. *Circulation* 77:560–568, 1988.
40. Epstein ML, Kiel EA, Victoria BE. Cardiac decompensation following

verapamil therapy in infants with supraventricular tachycardia. *Pediatrics* 75:737–740, 1985.

41. Lerman BB, Belardinelli L. Cardiac electrophysiology of adenosine. *Circulation* 83:1499–1509, 1991.
42. Waxman MB et al. Vagal techniques for termination of paroxysmal supraventricular tachycardia. *Am J Cardiol* 46:655–664, 1980.
43. Kerber RE et al. Energy, current, and success in defibrillation and cardioversion. *Circulation* 77:1038–1046, 1988.
44. Garson A et al. Surgical treatment of arrhythmias in children. *Cardiol Clinics* 7:319–329, 1989.
45. Walsh EP, Saul JP. Transcatheter ablation for pediatric tachyarrhythmias using radiofrequency electrical energy. *Pediatr Ann* 20:386–392, 1991.

James W. Ziegler
Robert Englander
John H. Fugate

25 Pharmacologic Support of the Circulation

The top priority in managing the critically ill patient is maximizing the delivery of oxygen to the vital organs of the body. To accomplish this, one must understand the concept of **oxygen delivery,** which is represented by the following equation:

$$DO_2 = CaO_2 \times CO \qquad (1)$$

where DO_2 equals oxygen delivery, CaO_2 equals the arterial oxygen content of blood, and CO equals the cardiac output. This equation states that the delivery of oxygen in the bloodstream is equal to the concentration of oxygen in blood (in milliliters of oxygen per 100 ml of blood) times the flow of blood (in milliliters of blood per minute). The arterial oxygen content is further described by the equation:

$$CaO_2 = (\text{hemoglobin concentration} \times 1.34 \qquad (2)$$
$$\times \,\%\text{saturation}) + (0.003 \times PaO_2)$$

The majority of oxygen carried in blood is combined with hemoglobin, and the first part of Eq. 2 represents this fraction. The constant 1.34 represents the amount of oxygen (in milliliters) that can maximally combine with 1 g of hemoglobin; %saturation represents the oxygen-hemoglobin saturation. The second half of Eq. 2 represents the dissolved portion of oxygen in the blood: 0.003 ml of oxygen will dissolve in 100 ml of blood for every millimeter mercury of pressure. It is easily seen that only at very high PaO_2s, or at very low hemoglobin concentrations, will the dissolved fraction of oxygen contribute significantly to the overall arterial oxygen content. If one cancels the units in Eq. 2, one is left with milliliters of oxygen per 100 ml of blood.

$$CaO_2 = \frac{\text{grams Hg}}{100 \text{ ml blood}} \times \frac{1.34 \text{ ml O}_2}{\text{gram Hg}} \times \%\text{saturation} \qquad (3)$$
$$+ \frac{0.003 \text{ ml O}_2 \times \text{mm Hg}}{100 \text{ ml blood} \times \text{mm Hg}}$$

CaO_2 can be maximized by optimizing oxygenation (either with supplemental oxygen or with mechanical ventilatory support and the use of positive end-expiratory pressure [PEEP]) in concert with maintaining an adequate RBC mass. Although the remainder of this chapter deals with the second component of oxygen delivery, the cardiac output, it is important to remember that arterial oxygen content must be maintained if one is to accomplish the overall goal of therapy—maximizing oxygen delivery! Also, the optimal oxygen delivery is that which maintains the oxygen consumption required by the cells of the body. In addition to maximizing oxygen delivery, simple measures to reduce unnecessary oxygen consumption (Table 25-1) should be initiated to ensure that an adequate supply-demand ratio is maintained.

Cardiac output is the amount of blood pumped by the heart per unit time. It is represented by the following:

$$CO = \text{heart rate} \times \text{stroke volume} \qquad (4)$$

Stroke volume depends on three variables: (1) the preload, (2) the afterload, and (3) the contractile state of the myocardium. Thus, there are four factors that determine cardiac output.

Heart Rate

Table 25-2 shows the range of normal heart rates for given age groups. An abnormally low heart rate directly impairs cardiac output and may necessitate the use of a **chronotrope,** an agent that increases heart rate. An excessively rapid heart rate adversely affects cardiac output by providing insufficient time for ventricular filling during diastole, causing stroke volume and ultimately cardiac output to fall.

Preload

The importance of preload on cardiac output was first described by Starling in 1914. Preload is equivalent to the diastolic "load" placed on the myocardium; by increasing this load, one increases resting myocardial fiber length, which optimizes the overlapping of action and myosin filaments within sarcomeres.[1] The end result is an increased force of contraction and improved performance by the heart. Figure 25-1 shows Starling curves for a normal and a failing heart. Note that preload improves cardiac performance to a certain point, beyond which further stretching of the myocar-

Table 25-1. Reducing unnecessary caloric expenditure in patients with compromised hemodynamics

Maintain neutral thermal environment

Aggressively treat fever

Avoid unnecessary muscle activity
   Phenothiazines/benzodiazepines for shivering or muscle spasms
   Aggressive anticonvulsant therapy for seizures

Early endotracheal intubation with controlled ventilation if increased work of breathing
   Muscle relaxants if patient "fighting" ventilator

Provide adequate sedation and analgesia

Mild hypothermia in noninfants

Table 25-2. Age-specific heart rates

Age	2%	Mean	98%
<1 d/o	93	123	154
1–2 d/o	91	123	159
3–6 d/o	91	129	166
1–3 w/o	107	148	182
1–2 w/o	121	149	179
3–5 m/o	106	141	186
6–11 m/o	109	134	169
1–2 y/o	89	119	151
3–4 y/o	73	108	137
5–7 y/o	65	100	133
8–11 y/o	62	91	130
12–15 y/o	60	85	119

From H Cole. *The Harriet Lane Handbook* (13th ed). St. Louis: Mosby, 1993. P 101. With permission.

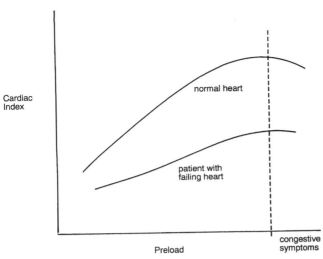

Figure 25-1. Starling curves reflecting the effect of increasing preload on cardiac output in the normal and failing heart.

dium depresses function and leads to circulatory congestion. The failing heart, with depressed contractility, has less preload reserve; that is, the increase in cardiac output for a given increase in preload is less than in the normal heart.

In clinical practice, preload is estimated by directly or indirectly measuring right or left atrial filling pressures with a central venous or pulmonary artery catheter, respectively. Preload is manipulated by giving fluid to increase venous return or, if signs of congestion are present, by removing fluid (with diuretics or hemofiltration). The type of fluid needed to increase preload will depend on the clinical situation.

Changes in heart rate, contractility, and afterload may indirectly affect preload. For example, increasing the inotropic state of the myocardium or decreasing afterload will improve systolic function, increase the ejection fraction, and decrease end-systolic volume. This ultimately decreases end-diastolic volume and leads to a drop in filling pressures.

Afterload

Afterload represents the impedance against which the heart must pump. Increasing afterload impairs ventricular emptying and cardiac output; conversely, decreasing afterload improves cardiac performance and augments stroke volume and cardiac output. In a practical sense, afterload is represented by vascular resistance. In a patient with a failing heart and a high peripheral vascular resistance, vasodilation may be a rational therapeutic goal. Two conditions, however, must be met before attempting vasodilation. First, venous return and filling pressures must be adequate. Vasodilation in the face of hypovolemia will further reduce filling pressures, and the effect of decreasing preload will negate any benefit of decreasing afterload. Second, the patient must be normotensive. Because BP is a reflection of both cardiac output and systemic vascular resistance (SVR), a drop in vascular resistance in a hypotensive patient exacerbates the hypotension, impairs coronary perfusion, and negatively influences myocardial performance. In the hypotensive patient who does not respond to fluids and agents that improve contractility, it may be necessary to use a **vasopressor,** a drug that increases vascular resistance. Although this will increase afterload, the improvement in diastolic pressure and coronary perfusion will enhance cardiac performance and end-organ perfusion.

Contractility

The contractile state of the myocardium represents the intrinsic ability of the heart to perform work (i.e., to effectively pump blood). It is dependent on preload and afterload, but contractility is also dependent on several other factors, including serum pH and PaO_2, glucose and calcium concentrations, body temperature, and circulating levels of inotropic substances.[2-4]

An inotrope is an agent that increases the stroke work of the heart at a given preload and afterload; it improves the contractile state of the myocardium. The use of an inotrope in a failing heart will improve performance and increase cardiac output. It will shift myocardial contractility to a new Starling curve (Fig. 25-2).

In the pediatric population there are many systemic and cardiac conditions that result in circulatory failure (Table 25-3). The guiding principle in the therapy of these diseases is the optimization of oxygen delivery and preservation of vital organ function. A rational approach includes initiating therapy for underlying disease

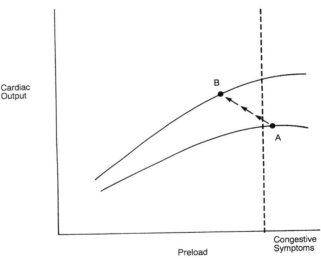

Figure 25-2. The use of intropes in the falling heart will shift the failing heart (point A) to a new curve (point B) and increase cardiac output while improving congestive symptoms.

Table 25-3. Causes of circulatory failure in the pediatric patient

Hypovolemic
    Hemorrhage
    Gastroenteritis and dehydration
    Diabetic ketoacidosis
Cardiogenic
    Congenital heart disease (left to right shunts, left-sided obstructive processes, valvular disease)
    Acquired heart disease (myocarditis, cardiomyopathy, ischemia, trauma, vasculitis)
    Postoperative open-heart surgery and cardiopulmonary bypass
    Arrhythmias
Distributive
    Sepsis
    Anaphylaxis
    Spinal shock

states and optimizing the arterial oxygen content, the metabolic milieu, and ventricular filling pressures. If the BP and/or perfusion remain inadequate despite these measures, the use of pharmacologic agents to improve hemodynamics is indicated.

The Sympathetic Nervous System

An understanding of the pharmacologic effects of agents used to support the cardiovascular system in pediatric intensive care requires a working knowledge of the sympathetic nervous system. The authors provide, therefore, a review of the anatomy, physiology, and neurotransmitters of the "involuntary," or autonomic, nervous system.

Anatomy

The central and peripheral nervous systems comprise the nervous system connections of humans. The peripheral nervous system is further subdivided into the somatic and autonomic nervous systems. The latter, also known as the involuntary, visceral, or vegetative nervous system, provides innervation to the heart, blood vessels, glands, viscera, and smooth muscles. It is separated into two often antagonistic divisions: the sympathetic and parasympathetic nervous systems. Pharmacologic manipulation of the **sympathetic nervous system** provides the primary basis for pharmacologic support of the circulation in pediatric critical care.

The preganglionic fibers of the sympathetic nervous system originate primarily in the intermediolateral and intermediomedial columns of the spinal cord from the first thoracic to the second lumbar segment, although some preganglionic fibers have been demonstrated as high as the seventh cervical segment and as low as the fourth lumbar segment. Preganglionic pathways may remain intraspinal for up to 12 segments before exiting the spinal cord via ventral roots.[5]

The preganglionic axons traverse to the sympathetic chain where they may synapse within sympathetic chain ganglia, or pass through these ganglia to synapse in collateral ganglia near viscera. After synapsing in the sympathetic ganglia, the postganglionic fibers traverse to target organs via peripheral nerves or may alone form visceral nerves. Each preganglionic nerve fiber may synapse with a single neuron or many postganglionic neurons. There are three groups of sympathetic ganglia: the paravertebral, prevertebral, and terminal.

The postganglionic neurons enter the effector organs, where they branch several times. At intervals along the terminal axons, "bulges" occur in the cell membrane; these are referred to as varicosities. Vesicles in these varicosities store a neurotransmitter. In the postganglionic sympathetic neurons, this neurotransmitter is generally noradrenaline, thus the term *adrenergic neurons*. Stimulation of these sympathetic nerves results in the release of noradrenaline (norepinephrine), which crosses the synaptic space and binds to adrenoceptors in the cell membrane of the cells of the target organ. Norepinephrine is then taken up by the cells of effector organs and metabolized to inactive by-products. Of note, postganglionic sympathetic neurons that innervate sweat glands and some blood vessels are cholinergic; that is, they release acetylcholine at the nerve terminal, which acts on cholinoceptors in the cell membrane of cells in those effector organs.

For the primary purpose of this chapter, one needs to focus on the sympathetic innervation of the heart and blood vessels. However, a working knowledge of the anatomy and physiology of the entire sympathetic nervous system is mandatory in order to understand and anticipate the side effects of pharmacologic agents used

to support the circulation in pediatric intensive care patients. With this general background of the anatomy of the sympathetic nervous system, we now turn to a discussion of its receptor physiology.

Adrenergic Receptor Physiology

Adrenergic receptors are glycoproteins that exist within the cell membrane and have highly specific binding affinity for catecholamines. Stimulation of these receptors activates the sympathetic response in those organs where the receptors exist. In 1948, Ahlquist first described two distinct populations of adrenergic receptors, which he labeled alpha and beta.[6] In 1967, Lands et al. found experimental evidence of at least two subtypes of beta receptors — now referred to as beta-1 and beta-2.[7] In 1977, Bethelsen and Pettinger found similar experimental evidence suggesting subdivision of the alpha receptors, resulting in presynaptic alpha receptors classified as alpha-2 and postsynaptic receptors as alpha-1.[8] Finally, receptors highly specific for dopamine, which had been recognized for more than 15 years, were subdivided into DA-1 and DA-2 receptors as a result of experiments conducted by Kebabian and Calne in 1979.[9]

Beta-Adrenergic Receptors

On a molecular level, beta receptor activation by catecholamines circulating or released at nerve terminals results in an intracellular increase in cyclic AMP (cAMP) concentration. Experimental evidence suggests that sympathetic nerves terminate at beta-1 receptors, whereas circulating catecholamines have enhanced binding at beta-2 receptors.[10] The specific result of increased intracellular cAMP depends on the target organ whose cell membranes house the beta receptor.

Because the focus of this chapter is the pharmacologic support of the circulation, we will begin with the effects of beta receptor activation in the heart and blood vessels. Beta receptors mainly affect cardiac function. Stimulation of beta-1 receptors in the myocardium results in positive chronotropy, positive inotropy, and positive dromotropy (increased conduction velocity). Beta receptors also exist in coronary artery smooth muscle, where their stimulation results in vasodilation.

Beta receptors are found primarily in the vascular smooth muscle of skeletal muscles, and their stimulation results in vasodilation. Some evidence exists also to suggest that beta-2 receptors enhance catecholamine-induced inotropy, although the vast majority of beta receptor effects on the heart are beta-1-mediated.[11]

Beta receptors exist in other organs, and administration of beta agonists can thus have far-reaching, and often untoward, side effects. Beta-1 receptors can be found in the gastrointestinal tract, where stimulation results in decreased tone, motility, and secretory activity. Stimulation of beta-1 receptors present in lipocytes results in lipolysis and an increase in circulating free fatty acids. In skeletal muscle, beta-2 stimulation, in addition to causing vasodilation, results in glycogenolysis. On lymphocytes, beta-2 receptors mediate mitogenesis, and on polymorphonuclear leukocytes and mast cells, their stimulation results in inhibition of granule release. In the kidney, beta-2 receptors mediate renin release.

Alpha-Adrenergic Receptors

The alpha-adrenergic receptors, as noted, have also been subdivided into alpha-1 and alpha-2. Alpha-1 receptors are found in the membranes of effector organ cells and are excitatory. Alpha-2 receptors are found in the neuronal cell membrane at the adrenergic nerve terminal where their stimulation results in inhibition of further norepinephrine release.

Alpha receptors are not present in the myocardium. The use of alpha agonists in intensive care, therefore, is aimed primarily at changing afterload, as alpha receptors are abundant in vascular smooth muscle. Alpha receptors are present in the vascular smooth muscle of cutaneous, visceral, pulmonary, coronary, cerebral, and skeletal muscle arteries and arterioles. Excitation results in vasoconstriction with a resultant increase in systemic vascular resistance and BP. Alpha receptors are present diffusely in veins, where stimulation results in venoconstriction.

Alpha receptors are abundant in many other organs. In the eye, stimulation of alpha receptors results in constriction of the radial muscle, producing pupillary dilation. In the gastrointestinal tract, alpha receptor excitation results in decreased tone, motility, and secretory activity, as well as contraction of gastrointestinal sphincters. Likewise, alpha receptors mediate trigone-sphincter muscle contraction of the urinary bladder, as well as contraction of the splenic capsule. Finally, insulin secretion decreases as a result of stimulation of alpha receptors located in the cell membranes of beta islet cells of the pancreas.

Dopaminergic Receptors

Receptors that have a higher affinity for dopamine than other catecholamines, and that are not inhibited by alpha-blockers and beta-blockers, have been recognized as dopaminergic receptors. Dopaminergic receptors are found in specific vascular beds as well as in the CNS. Like the beta adrenoceptors, dopamine receptors found in vascular beds work primarily through increasing cAMP concentration in the target organ cell.

The DA-1 receptor is found postsynaptically in renal, splanchnic, coronary, and cerebral vascular beds. Stimulation results in smooth muscle relaxation and, thus, vasodilation in these organs.[12] The DA-1 receptor is also found in the adrenal cortex, and evidence suggests that its stimulation results in suppression of aldosterone secretion.[13] As a result, although dopamine's renal vasodilatory effect may increase renal blood flow by up to 50%, renal sodium excretion may be increased by up to 500% during the administration of dopamine.

The DA-2 receptors are found in the carotid body, gastrointestinal tract, and anterior pituitary gland. In the carotid body, stimulation of DA-2 receptors results in decreased afferent input to the CNS, with a resultant diminishing of the hypoxic ventilatory drive.[14] In the anterior pituitary gland, stimulation of DA-2 receptors results in inhibition of thyroid-stimulating hormone (TSH) and prolactin release.[15] Of note, thyroid function studies will not be accurate in a pediatric or neonatal intensive care patient receiving a dopamine infusion.

The Catecholamines

With this background of the anatomy of the sympathetic nervous system and the physiology of its receptors, one can examine the endogenous and exogenous agents utilized by the intensivist to stimulate or replicate the action of the sympathetic nervous system, the catecholamines.

Endogenous catecholamines include norepinephrine, epinephrine, and dopamine. These substances are synthesized in the adrenal medulla and share a common pathway, which begins with tyrosine. Tyrosine is converted to dopa by the enzyme tyrosine hydroxylase, and dopa is converted to dopamine through a decar-

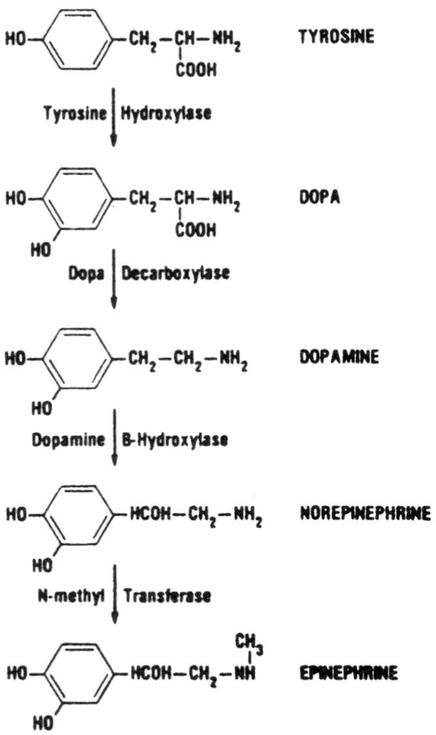

Figure 25-3. The endogenous catecholamines

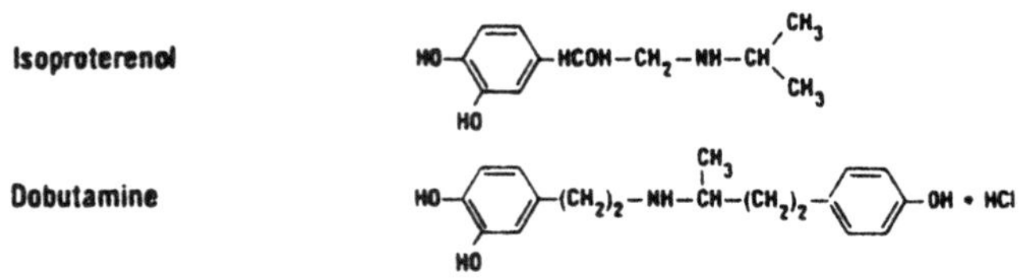

Figure 25-4. Isoproterenol and dobutamine

boxylase. Dopamine serves as the precursor to norepinephrine, which is then converted to epinephrine (Fig. 25-3).

In adrenergic neurons, tyrosine is actively transported into the cytosol. In the cytosol, it is converted to dopa by the same pathway as in the adrenal medulla. Dopa is then converted to dopamine, which is actively transported into storage vesicles. Within the vesicles, dopamine is converted to norepinephrine. The final conversion to epinephrine, which occurs in the adrenal medulla, does not occur in sympathetic neurons secondary to a lack of the converting enzyme, phenylethanolamine N-methyltransferase, in the neuronal storage vesicles.

Figure 25-4 illustrates the chemical structure of the two major synthetic catecholamines, isoproterenol and dobutamine. These agents share the skeletal structure of the catecholamines, varying in their substitutions at the alpha and beta carbons of the catechol ring, as well as at the terminal amino group. All of the catecholamines exert their effects by interacting with end-organ adrenoceptors. Their sites and amplitudes of action depend on their relative selectivity for alpha-1, alpha-2, beta-1, beta-2, DA-1, or DA-2 adrenoceptors.

Before discussing the individual catecholamines, it is worthwhile to explore some of the developmental changes that occur in the cardiovascular system of the growing human. The response to pharmacologic interventions is dictated, at least to some degree, by the developmental stage of the patient.

Developmental Changes

Several dramatic functional changes occur in the neonatal circulation after birth as it changes from the fetal circulation to the adult "circuits in series." Aside from these functional changes, there are important structural and physiologic differences between the immature and mature heart and circulation. These differences affect all of the factors that determine cardiac output, and the response of the neonate or young infant to pharmacologic and other therapeutic interventions may be different than that of the adult. Although most of the following information has been derived from animal studies, it probably applies to the immature human subject as well.

Preload

The chambers of the immature heart are less compliant than those of the mature heart. In addition, although the Starling mechanism is operational, the increase in contractility for a given preload is less in the fetal heart when compared with the adult (Fig. 25-5).[2,16] Further, it takes a smaller increase in ventricular filling to reach the point of myocardial decompensation.[17-19] Thus, the preload, or diastolic "reserve," of the fetal and neonatal heart is limited and increases with age.

Contractility

The myocardium of the immature heart contains a greater proportion of noncontractile elements and fewer myofilaments (the myofilaments that are present are capable of generating the same force as adult myofilaments).[2] This may explain, at least in part, the suboptimal response to digoxin and other inotropes that has been noted by several authors.[20,21] Incomplete sympathetic innervation of the myocardium with decreased myocardial norepinephrine stores and disproportionate cholinergic innervation may also contribute.[2,22-24] Because augmentation of stroke volume as a means of increasing cardiac output is attenuated, the "systolic reserve" of the immature myocardium is limited.[25]

Limited diastolic and systolic reserve translates into greater ventricular interdependence in the immature heart.[2] Clinically, this manifests as a more rapid progression to biventricular failure in neonates and young infants with disease processes that primarily affect one ventricle. Ventricular interdependence decreases with age.[26]

Afterload

The distribution and functional integrity of adrenergic receptors in the peripheral vasculature of the fetus and neonate have not been fully elucidated. Diminished vascular sensitivity to different catecholamines has been observed in immature animals by several authors, although this has been an inconsistent finding.[27,28]

Heart Rate

As mentioned earlier, cardiac output is related directly to heart rate to a certain limit. An increase in heart rate beyond this limit compromises ventricular filling by decreasing diastolic filling time, and cardiac output falls. The neonate functions close to this maximal limit of heart rate, even at rest, and thus "heart rate reserve" is limited as a means of increasing cardiac output. In addition, because diastolic and systolic reserve are both limited in the immature heart, cardiac output is dependent on heart rate, and bradycardia is not tolerated well by the neonate.

From these data, it can be seen that at rest the young heart functions at nearly peak performance and possesses a limited capacity to respond to stress. This limited "total cardiac reserve" is offset to some degree by two features unique to the immature circulation.[29] First, coronary artery disease is not prevalent in the young, and thus coronary underperfusion and disruption of the myocardial oxygen supply-demand ratio are lesser concerns than in adult patients. Second, the young heart is better able to handle hypoxic stress. This probably reflects age-related differences in mitochondrial oxidative phosphorylation along with an increased anaerobic capacity of the immature heart.[2,30]

Having discussed the concept of oxygen delivery, the determinants of cardiac output, the anatomy, physiology, and chemistry of the sympathetic nervous system, and the developmental peculiarities of the pediatric circulation, we may now proceed to a discussion of the specific agents used to support the circulation in pediatric intensive care patients. Much of the following information has been generated from adult trials. Whenever possible, we will attempt to emphasize responses which are unique to the pediatric population.

Dobutamine

Pharmacology

Dobutamine was developed in the early 1970s. Investigators at that time were interested in finding a pure inotrope, one that lacked the chronotropic, arrhythmogenic, and vasoactive properties of isoproterenol, dopamine, and norepinephrine. Dobutamine came close to filling this requirement.

Dobutamine exists as a racemic mixture of ($-$) and ($+$) isomers.[31] Both stereoisomers have a high affinity for beta-1 receptors. The ($-$) isomer also maintains some activity on alpha-1 receptors of blood vessels, while the ($+$) isomer has weak affinity for beta-2 receptors. These effects are minimal when compared with the beta-1 effect. In addition, because the commercial mixture contains equal concentrations of both isomers, the alpha-1 and beta-2 effects on the peripheral vasculature are balanced. Most patients treated with dobutamine do have a slight drop in systemic vascular

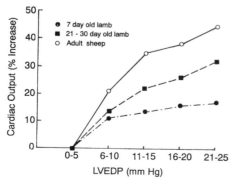

Figure 25-5. Starling curves in sheep of different ages. (From WF Friedman, BF George. New concepts and drugs in the treatment of congestive heart failure. *Pediatr Clin North Am* 30:1207, 1984. With permission.)

resistance, reflected as a slight drop in diastolic BP. This effect most likely represents reflex withdrawal of vascular tone resulting from the improved cardiac output associated with the use of dobutamine, rather than a direct effect of dobutamine on the peripheral vasculature.

Like other catecholamines, dobutamine has a very short half-life of 2.37 minutes, necessitating administration via a continuous intravenous (IV) infusion.[32] There is a linear relationship between the infusion rate and the plasma dobutamine concentration and also between the plasma concentration and hemodynamic effect.[33,34] Dobutamine's short half-life is primarily a reflection of rapid redistribution and metabolism by the liver, with excretion of inactive metabolites in the urine and stool.

Actions

Dobutamine is a potent inotropic agent that acts directly on beta-1 receptors within the heart. It does not cause the endogenous release of norepinephrine from sympathetic nerve terminals in the heart, nor does it have any effect on dopaminergic receptors.

Figure 25-6 illustrates the systemic hemodynamic effects of dopamine and dobutamine in anesthetized dogs. Although both agents increase cardiac output, dobutamine does so to a greater degree than dopamine and has less of an effect on BP (actually causing a slight fall in mean arterial pressure at higher doses) and vascular resistance. As illustrated in Fig. 25-7, the increased cardiac output associated with dobutamine is preferentially diverted to muscle beds, with an actual decrease in the percentage of cardiac output perfusing mesenteric and renal vascular beds. Despite this "relative" decrease in renal blood flow noted in the dog model, the experience with adult humans in congestive heart failure is that the overall increase in cardiac output associated with the administration of dobutamine promotes improved renal blood flow and increased urine flow and urine sodium excretion.[35-37]

In adults with low-output heart failure, dobutamine in the dose range of 5 to 15 µg/kg/min augments cardiac output primarily by increasing stroke volume.[33,37-39] The increased stroke volume is associated with a drop in right- and left-sided filling pressures and a slight drop in SVR and mean BP. Heart rate is minimally affected relative to the increase in inotropy, and myocardial oxygen balance is not influenced adversely, even in patients with underlying coronary artery disease.[40-42] When compared with dopamine in the treatment of heart failure, for a given increase in cardiac output, dobutamine causes filling pressures to fall, while dopamine may

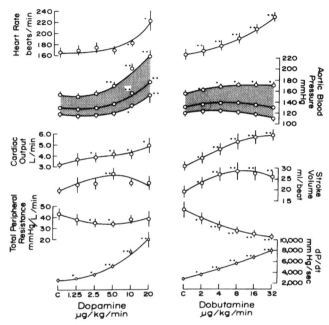

Figure 25-6. The hemodynamic effects of dopamine and dobutamine in anesthetized dogs. (From NW Robie, LI Goldberg. Comparative systemic and regional hemodynamic effects of dopamine and dobutamine. *Am Heart J* 90:340–345, 1975. With permission.)

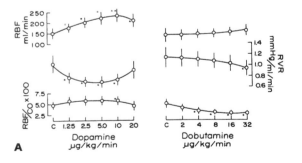

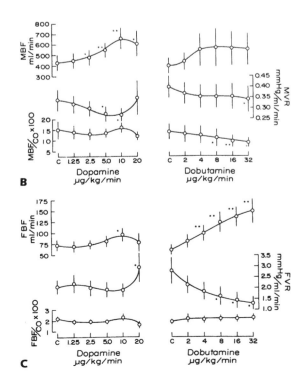

Figure 25-7. **(A)** Renal, **(B)** mesenteric, and **(C)** femoral artery hemodynamic responses to dobutamine infusion. RBF, renal artery blood flow; RVR, renal vascular resistance; RBF/CO, % of cardiac output (CO) perfusing renal artery; MBF, mesenteric artery blood flow; MVR, mesenteric artery; FBF, femoral blood flow; FVR, femoral vascular resistance; FBF/CO, % cardiac output perfusing femoral artery. From NW Robie, LI Goldberg. Comparative systemic and regional hemodynamic effects of dopamine and dobutamine. *Am Heart J* 90:340–345, 1975. With permission.)

increase left-sided filling pressures and worsen pulmonary vascular congestion and pulmonary edema.[43,44] Also, dopamine tends to have more chronotropic effect than dobutamine when used in this setting.

Figure 25-8 compares the effect of dobutamine with isoproterenol and norepinephrine on measured hemodynamic indices in dogs with experimentally induced low cardiac output. It can be seen that dobutamine has greater inotropic activity and less of an effect on heart rate, BP, and vascular resistance than either isoproterenol or norepinephrine.[45]

Table 25-4 summarizes the published experience with dobutam-

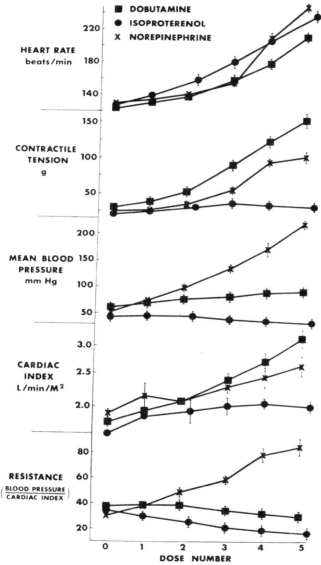

Figure 25-8. Mean hemodynamic values in response to dobutamine, isoproterenol, and norepinephrine after coronary artery ligation and ganglionic blockade in the perfused canine heart. Dose numbers 0–5 represent (in mcg/kg/min): dobutamine 0, 1.0, 2.0, 5.0, 10.0, and 20.0, isoproterenol 0, 0.02, 0.05, 0.1, 0.2, and 0.5, and norepinephrine 0, 0.1, 0.2, 0.5, 1.0, and 2.0. As shown, dobutamine increases cardiac index and contractile tension while exerting little effect on heart rate, blood pressure, and systemic resistance. (From RR Tuttle, J Mills. Dobutamine, development of a new catecholamine to selectively increase cardiac contractility. *Circ Res* 36:185–195, 1975. With permission.)

ine in the pediatric population. In general, dobutamine maintains its inotropic activity in younger patients, although this activity is attenuated when compared with adults. Also, dobutamine tends to be more chronotropic in pediatric patients. One potentially deleterious effect noted in infants is a stepwise increase in pulmonary capillary wedge pressure with increasing dobutamine dosage, similar to the effect seen with dopamine in older patients.[21] The reason for this is unclear.

Indications

The ideal candidate for dobutamine therapy is the patient with low-output congestive heart failure associated with elevated filling pressures and **normal or only slightly reduced BP.** In this type of patient, the use of dobutamine enhances cardiac performance and improves clinical status. In adults, it has proven beneficial in disease states such as cardiomyopathy, ischemic heart disease, and postmyocardial infarction.[33–42] In patients with septic shock who are typically vasodilated with low filling pressures, it is less efficacious, but in the subset of septic patients with elevated filling pressures, dobutamine improves cardiac output and systemic perfusion.[46]

In the pediatric population, dobutamine has been used successfully in a variety of disease states associated with myocardial failures, including asphyxia and myocarditis, and after open-heart surgery.[21,47–55] Response may be less predictable than in adults, and higher doses may be required to achieve the desired hemodynamic affect. In some patients, tachycardia may be problematic. Because dobutamine does not affect PVR, it may be the agent of choice in conditions associated with pulmonary hypertension, such as adult respiratory distress syndrome and persistent pulmonary hypertension, if inotropic support is required.[56]

In patients who remain hypotensive after volume expansion, a vasopressor rather than dobutamine is the agent of choice. In this setting, dobutamine may be used as adjunctive therapy. In combination with dopamine, dobutamine additionally improves cardiac output and BP, allowing the use of smaller dopamine doses and off-setting the rise in pulmonary capillary wedge pressure and increase in myocardial oxygen consumption encountered with high-dose dopamine. Renal blood flow may also be better preserved with combined therapy.

Dose

The usual dose range for dobutamine varies between 5 and 15 μg/kg/min. At rates greater than 15 μg/kg/min, the incidence of untoward side effects, including tachycardia, arrhythmias, and symptomatic complaints, increases. In addition, hemodynamic benefit seems to be maximal in the 5 to 15 μg/kg/min range, although higher infusion rates may be needed in infants and neonates. Tolerance to the inotropic action of dobutamine may develop over time. In an adult study, cardiac output at 72 hours into an infusion was 66% of what it was at 2 hours into the infusion. In this instance, increasing the dose to the desired effect eliminated the problem.[57]

Side Effects

Dobutamine shares most of the adverse effects that are common to all catecholamines, but in general, the propensity to develop complications from dobutamine is less than with these other agents. It tends to be less arrhythmogenic, though it does increase arterioventricular (AV) conduction and may increase the ventricu-

Table 25-4. The use of dobutamine in pediatric patients

Ref. no.	Population	Dosage (μg/kg/min)	Hemodynamic effects (sign Δ from baseline)	Comments
48	10 children (2–11 years old) following open-heart surgery and cardiopulmonary bypass	2.5–15	↑ CI, ↑ HR at ≥10 μg/kg/min No Δ in MAP, PAP, LAP, CVP, SI, SVR, PVR	↑ CI mostly 2° to ↑ HR
47	18 neonates with clinically diagnosed heart failure	7.5–10	↑ inotropy by echocardiographic criteria; ↑ HR, ↑ MAP (4/9)	Echocardiographic evidence of improved LV function but also sign. ↑ in HR
49	12 children (2.3–16.7 yrs) with congenital heart disease evaluated during diagnostic cardiac catheterization	2.0 and 7.75	↑ CI, ↑ SI, ↑ MAP, ↓ PCWP No Δ HR, CVP, SVR, PVR	Only 2 patients with CHF at time of catheterization
37	13 critically ill neonates requiring inotropic support	2.5–7.5	↑ CI by pulsed Doppler No Δ MAP, HR	No Δ in plasma catecholamine [] during infusion
51	4 pediatric patients with acute myocarditis	Not described	↑ CI by echocardiographic criteria, ↑ systolic BP No Δ HR	No significant arrhythmias observed
52	17 hemodynamically unstable premature infants	10.0	↑ HR, ↑ inotropy by echocardiographic data (systolic time intervals), ↑ MAP	Echocardiographic evidence of improved LV function but sign. ↑ HR
21	33 infants and children with cardiogenic or septic shock	2.5–10.0	↑ CI; no Δ in HR, MAP, PAP, CVP, PVR, ↓ SVR	Best response with cardiogenic shock. ↑ PCWP seen in infants
54	11 children after open-heart surgery	1.0–10.0	↑ CI, ↑ HR, ↑ MAP No Δ SVR	Increase in CI predominantly a chronotropic effect
55	12 infants and children with clinical shock	7.5–10.0	↑ CI, ↑ HR, ↑ MAP, ↑ SVR with no Δ in PVR	Increase CI at least partly 2° to ↑'d chronotropy

lar response to atrial tachyarrhythmias. In addition, some patients may develop an exaggerated chronotropic or hypertensive or hypotensive response, prohibiting its use even at low doses. Increases in heart rate of more than 10% may induce or exacerbate myocardial ischemia.[59] Infiltration into subcutaneous tissues is less likely to cause tissue necrosis, but this complication has been described.[61] All of these effects are dose-related.

As mentioned, infants tend to have a rise in pulmonary capillary wedge pressure with the administration of dobutamine. This effect may potentiate the development of pulmonary edema causing hypoxemia.

With long-term usage, the inhibition of platelet function has been described with dobutamine. This is in contrast to other catecholamines, which promote platelet aggregation.

Dopamine

Pharmacology

Dopamine is an endogenous catecholamine that serves as a precursor to norepinephrine in the adrenal medulla and sympathetic neurons. It is pharmaceutically supplied as dopamine hydrochloride (Intropin), which has a pH of 2.5 to 4.5. It is destabilized at a pH of greater than 5, and thus should not be given in an IV line with sodium—bicarbonate or acetate.

Dopamine is metabolized rapidly after oral or IV administration and must be given as a continuous IV infusion. Steady-state concentrations are reached rapidly after starting an IV infusion, usually within 30 minutes. The steady-state concentrations are dose-dependent. Dopamine's elimination follows a biphasic pattern.

The rapid early phase has a half-life of 2 minutes. The elimination phase is also rapid, with a half-life of 9 minutes.[60] Clearance of dopamine is achieved through extraneuronal uptake, methylation in the liver, and secretion into urine by the kidney. In patients with hepatic or renal dysfunction, clearance may be prolonged, suggesting a need for caution in the use of dopamine in critically ill patients with renal or hepatic failure.[61] Neonates represent another subpopulation warranting special caution; response may be unpredictable, and often hemodynamic effects are obtained at infusion rates lower than expected.

Actions

Since the early 1900s, dopamine has been recognized to have vasoactive effects on specific vascular beds. Its vasodilatory action in the renovascular bed, unique among catecholamines, led to the hypothesis that a dopamine-specific receptor was located in the renal vasculature.[62–66] Identification of specific dopaminergic receptors occurred in the 1970s. Further, dopamine is singular in its ability to stimulate dopaminergic, beta-adrenergic, and alpha-adrenergic receptors in a dose-dependent fashion. This ability is thought to be the result of flexibility of the dopamine molecule, which allows alteration in its configuration to fit different receptors.[66]

At low doses, 0.5 to 2.0 μg/kg/min, dopamine selectively stimulates dopaminergic receptors, resulting in vasodilation in the renal, mesenteric, coronary, and cerebral vascular beds. This vasodilatory effect of dopamine is blocked by haloperidol, a specific dopamine-receptor antagonist, but not by alpha- and beta-adrenergic blocking agents. At these low doses, dopamine also acts on dopaminergic receptors in the adrenal cortex to inhibit aldosterone secretion, resulting in a natriuresis that acts synergistically with renal vasodilatation to increase free-water clearance via increased urine output.[67]

At doses between 2 and 5 μg/kg/min, dopamine acts on both DA and beta receptors. At doses between 5 and 10 μg/kg/min, dopamine's effects are primarily beta-adrenergic-mediated. In the peripheral vasculature, dopamine is a weak beta-adrenergic agonist, approximately one thousandth as potent as isoproterenol.[68] Its primary utility as a beta agonist, therefore, is in its effects on the heart. Dopamine in the beta-agonist range is both an inotrope and a chronotrope. Positive inotropy probably occurs at all doses between 2 and 10 μg/kg/min, whereas positive chronotropy generally requires doses greater than 5 μg/kg/min. Dopamine's beta effect reflects direct stimulation of the beta-adrenoceptor and also norepinephrine release at the terminal axon. This latter mechanism is probably primary to dopamine's inotropic effect, while the former is likely primary to dopamine's chronotropic effect.[68] In patients with chronic heart failure and depleted myocardial norepinephrine stores, the inotropic response to dopamine may be blunted. The increased inotropy and chronotropy from dopamine result in a slight increase in myocardial oxygen consumption, which is paralleled by an increase in coronary blood flow, the latter thought to be a dopaminergic rather than a beta-adrenergic effect.[66] The positive chronotropy and inotropy result in a moderate increase in cardiac output.

At doses greater than 10 μg/kg/min, dopamine exerts an increasing alpha-adrenergic effect. Its effects between 10 and 20 μg/kg/min vary in vascular beds, depending on relative alpha- and beta-adrenoceptor stimulation. Positive chronotropy and positive inotropy persist with an increased heart rate, BP, and, often, an alpha-adrenergic-mediated increase in SVR. Alpha-adrenergic-mediated vasoconstriction occurs virtually unopposed in all sympathetically innervated vascular beds at doses over 20 μg/kg/min, with a resultant increase in SVR and myocardial work.[69] Dopamine has several other vascular actions. It causes venoconstriction in all venous beds. Its actions on the pulmonary vasculature are less clear. In some animal models, dopamine causes alpha-adrenergic-mediated pulmonary vasoconstriction, with a resultant increase in PVR.[70] In human studies with adults, dopamine causes pulmonary vasoconstriction in patients with preexisting pulmonary hypertension, thus exacerbating elevation in PVR.[71] For this reason, higher-dose dopamine should be used cautiously in disease states associated with elevated pulmonary artery pressure (i.e., adult respiratory distress syndrome, persistent pulmonary hypertension).

Dopamine has noncardiovascular actions worthy of note. Dopamine acts on receptors on beta-islet cells in the pancreas to inhibit insulin release, causing hyperglycemia.[72] It also acts on the anterior pituitary to inhibit TSH and prolactin release via stimulation of DA-2 receptors. Finally, dopamine stimulates DA-2 receptors found in the carotid body, resulting in a decrease in the hypoxic drive to breathe.[14]

Indications

Dopamine is perhaps the best studied of the agents used to support the circulation of pediatric intensive care patients. Specifically, clinical studies have investigated dopamine's effectiveness in (1) shock states of all etiologies, (2) patients following open-heart surgery and cardiac bypass, (3) hypoxic or asphyxiated states, (4) adjunctive therapy for congestive heart failure, and (5) hemodynamic support following liver transplant.

Dopamine Treatment in Shock/Oliguric States

In 1966 MacCannell et al. provided the first clinical study of the use of dopamine in treating shock of all etiologies in adult patients; they found improvement in cardiac output and urine output.[73] Several studies over the next decade confirmed the beneficial effects of dopamine in shock, specifically, improved cardiac output and urine flow.[74–77] These studies also suggested that dopamine was superior to the prior mainstays of pressor therapy in shock, especially isoproterenol and norepinephrine. Isoproterenol often causes a drop in BP, whereas dopamine either improves arterial BP or has no significant effect.[74] Norepinephrine improves BP but at the expense of cardiac output and urine flow, while dopamine improves BP, cardiac output, and urine flow. Of note, the doses of dopamine used in all of these adult studies were between 1.0 and 10.0 μg/kg/min, the dosage range at which one would expect primarily dopaminergic and beta-adrenergic effects, with little alpha-adrenergic stimulation.

Driscoll et al. provided the first study of dopamine therapy in infants and children with shock.[78] They examined 24 patients with clinical shock defined as hypotension (BP <2 SDs below normal for age) or oliguria (<1 ml/kg/hr of urine output), or both, associated with tachycardia, and/or elevated central venous pressure, and/or compromised peripheral circulation. Dopamine infusion resulted in a significant increase in systolic BP and urine flow, with no significant effect on central venous pressure or heart rate. The infusions used ranged from 0.3 to 25.0 μg/kg/min. No significant adverse reactions were directly attributable to the dopamine infusion. No significant effect on outcome was reported, and the study had no control group.

Cuevas et al. examined the effects of low-dose dopamine in premature infants with respiratory distress syndrome.[79] A control group received no dopamine, a second group received 1.0 μg/kg/min for 72 hours, and a third group received 2.5 μg/kg/min for 72 hours. They found a significant effect on hemodynamics only in newborns with preexisting hypotension. No effect on outcome was noted.

In summary, dopamine appears to be effective in improving hemodynamics in shock and oliguric states. It provides clinical improvement without the untoward side effects of isoproterenol and norepinephrine. It also maintains renal perfusion and urine output. It is for these reasons that dopamine has become the first-line agent for providing hemodynamic support to the failing circulation in pediatric patients.

Dopamine Treatment following Bypass for Cardiac Surgery

Myocardial dysfunction and low cardiac output have been well described following cardiac bypass for open-heart surgery. Several studies have investigated the use of dopamine in the early postoperative period. Daenen et al., in a discussion published by the proceedings of the Royal Society of Medicine, elucidated the theoretical benefits of dopamine use following cardiac surgery: (1) Dopamine has a positive inotropic effect that exceeds its chronotropic effect at low doses (e.g., <10 μg/kg/min). (2) Dopamine causes coronary vasodilation, resulting in an improved supply-demand ratio for myocardial oxygen utilization. This effect is especially important when compared with other agents commonly used after bypass surgery, such as epinephrine and isoproterenol. (3) Dopamine causes increased renal blood flow, increased sodium excretion, and increased free-water clearance, effectively maximizing urine output.[80]

Studies in the early 1970s provided strong evidence for dopamine's advantageous effect on hemodynamic indices (specifically, cardiac index, mean arterial BP, and urine output) following bypass surgery in adults.[81,82] Lang et al. examined dopamine's effects on infants with low cardiac output following corrective cardiac surgery and found that heart rate, BP, and cardiac index increased significantly at doses of 15 μg/kg/min or greater, without significant changes in right atrial pressure, SVR, PVR, or stroke volume.[20] Their population size was small and no controls or comparisons to other pressor agents were used. No data were presented on changes in urine output, free-water clearance, or sodium clearance. The authors noted that to achieve hemodynamic changes similar to those found in adult patients, higher doses of dopamine were required in infants.

Outwater et al. reproduced the findings of Lang's group in a study of dopamine's effects in six infants after cardiac surgery.[83] They found improved cardiac index at an infusion rate of 15 μg/kg/min, without changes in right atrial pressure, left atrial pressure, systemic arterial pressure, SVR, or PVR. They also measured urine output and glomerular filtration rate and found a significant increase in both parameters at doses of 5 and 10 μg/kg/min, with a return to baseline at doses of 15 μg/kg/min. The authors concluded that higher doses of dopamine were required in infants, compared with adults, to achieve similar changes in hemodynamic indices.

Stephenson et al. found statistically significant increases in cardiac index and heart rate in 28 children treated with dopamine after cardiac surgery.[84] They also examined combination therapy with dopamine and nitroprusside and found consistent inotropic and chronotropic improvement from dopamine augmented by a decrease in pulmonary and systemic vascular resistances resulting from coadministration of nitroprusside.

In summary, the research to date supports the use of dopamine for correcting low-output states following bypass and open-heart surgery in infants and children. Some evidence suggests a need for higher doses for infants than children to achieve a significant increase in cardiac index. One should exercise caution, however, as some young infants will manifest increased sensitivity to dopamine; thus, dopamine should be started at low infusion rates and titrated to the desired hemodynamic effect.[85]

Dopamine Therapy in Hypoxic or Anoxic States

Studies examining dopamine's effects in hypoxic or asphyxiated states have focused primarily on neonates. Fiddler et al. published four case reports of infants with persistent fetal circulation following hypoxic perinatal insults who had clinical evidence of myocardial dysfunction.[86] All four received dopamine in doses of 2 to 5 μg/kg/min, and all were noted to have "marked" clinical improvement. No objective data were obtained regarding cardiac output, and no controls were used. DiSessa et al. performed a randomized, blinded study comparing dopamine infusion with placebo in 14 asphyxiated neonates.[87] The dopamine-treated patients had significant improvement in echocardiographic measurements of shortening fraction and mean velocity of circumferential fiber shortening, as well as in systolic BP. The dopamine dosage used in this study was only 2.5 μg/kg/min, a dose usually considered within the "renal" or dopaminergic range, yet the findings suggested significant stimulation of myocardial beta-1 adrenoceptors. Walther et al. examined 22 newborn infants with myocardial dysfunction, 11 of whom had suffered severe perinatal asphyxia.[88] Echocardiographic and hemodynamic data were used to demonstrate myocardial dysfunction (hypotension in eight; low cardiac output and low

stroke volume in 20) in their study infants. Six of the 11 infants with perinatal asphyxia were then treated with dopamine in doses of 4 to 10 μg/kg/min. Within 1 hour, myocardial contractility normalized in all of the treated infants.

None of these studies examining the use of dopamine in hypoxia- or anoxia-induced myocardial dysfunction reports significant adverse reactions to the drug infusion. All suggest that myocardial dysfunction is significantly improved by dopamine infusion. Conclusions regarding an effect on outcome cannot be made, because long-term outcome was not examined in these studies.

Dopamine as Adjunctive Therapy for Congestive Heart Failure

In both adult and pediatric medicine, digitalis in combination with diuretics remains the mainstay of treatment for congestive heart failure. In the adult literature, several studies have demonstrated dopamine's efficacy in improving cardiac index, glomerular filtration rate, and sodium clearance in patients who are refractory to treatment with digitalis and diuretics.[66,89] The pediatric literature is scant regarding this indication for dopamine use. Artman et al. published a review of the recognition and management of congestive heart failure in children and adolescents.[90] They mention dopamine as "another inotropic agent which can be useful for acute parenteral therapy," noting its advantage of dilating the renal vasculature at low-to-moderate doses. The major limiting factor to the use of dopamine in congestive heart failure is its requirement for continuous IV infusion necessitating close hemodynamic monitoring, restricting its use to the intensive care unit (ICU). Also, caution needs to be used when dosing dopamine for the treatment of congestive heart failure in order to avoid alpha-adrenergic doses, which increase afterload and may exacerbate the congestive heart failure.

Dopamine Use Following Liver Transplant

Postoperative renal insufficiency is a well-described complication of liver transplantation. This is a result of hemorrhagic renal vasoconstriction intraoperatively as well as the use of nephrotoxic immunosuppressant drugs such as cyclosporin A. Polson et al. performed a randomized study of prophylactic low-dose dopamine in 34 patients undergoing orthotopic liver transplantation.[91] They found that only 9.5% of patients receiving prophylactic dopamine developed renal impairment, whereas 67% of patients in the control group developed renal impairment, with 40% of them progressing to acute renal failure. The authors concluded that orthotopic liver transplant is an indication for prophylactic renal doses of dopamine.

Dose

Dosing of dopamine is titrated to desired effect. As noted in the Actions section, at doses of 0.5 to 2.0 μg/kg/min, dopamine acts on dopaminergic receptors. At doses of 2.0 to 5.0 μg/kg/min, dopamine exerts its effects on both dopaminergic and beta-adrenergic receptors. At doses of 5 to 10 μg/kg/min, dopamine is primarily a beta-adrenergic stimulant, with some residual dopaminergic effects. At doses between 10 and 20 μg/kg/min, dopamine exerts an increasing alpha-adrenergic effect and a decreasing beta-adrenergic effect. Finally, at doses above 20 μg/kg/min, dopamine acts mostly as an alpha-adrenergic agonist. These are **general guide-**

lines with large interpatient variability, especially in neonates and infants.

It is the authors' practice to institute, as a minimum, continuous monitoring of ECG, respiratory rate, BP, and urine output in all patients receiving dopamine. Because infiltration of dopamine into subcutaneous tissues causes potent local effects, we recommend it be given through a central venous line whenever possible. If only peripheral access is available, the line must be monitored closely for local blanching and changed immediately if any evidence of infiltration develops. Dopamine is generally mixed in a dextrose solution. In our units, we use the "Rule of Sixes" to prepare the mixture for patients under 50 kg:

$$6 \times \text{patient's weight (kg)}$$
$$= \text{mg of dopamine to be added to 100 mol solvent}$$

With this mixture, each 1 ml/hr provides 1 μg/kg/min. This solution can be further concentrated to a 2×, 4×, 8×, or 10× mix, so that each 1 ml/hr provides 2 μg/kg/min, 4 μg/kg/min, 8 μg/kg/min, or 10 μg/kg/min, respectively. If only peripheral access is available, we recommend using dilute solutions, with a maximum concentration of a 2× mix.

Adverse Reactions

Adverse effects of dopamine are related to its physiologic actions, most of which have already been discussed. Its primary toxicity is on the cardiovascular system. In the beta-adrenergic range, dopamine increases myocardial oxygen demand, and there are several reports in adults of myocardial ischemia exacerbated by the use of dopamine. This adverse effect is rare in most children due to their preserved coronary arteries. Dopamine has also been implicated in tachyarrhythmias as a direct result of its beta-1 receptor stimulation. This latter effect has been well described in children.[92] In the pulmonary vascular bed, dopamine may worsen V/Q mismatch and increase intrapulmonary shunting of blood, especially in patients with preexisting pulmonary hypertension.

Dopamine's effects on the CNS and endocrine system have already been addressed. Probably the most commonly encountered adverse effect noted with dopamine is IV infiltration with resulting tissue ischemia or necrosis. Many cases have been reported of infiltrates causing necrosis severe enough to require amputation.[93–95] Treatment of a dopamine infiltrate includes prompt, local administration of a solution of phentolamine (2 mg phentolamine mixed in 5 ml of 0.9% saline) directly into the infiltrated tissues. This therapy should also be provided for IV infiltration of other agents with alpha-adrenergic activity, such as norepinephrine, epinephrine, and phenylephrine. Because of this complication, as noted, alpha-adrenergic agents should be infused centrally whenever possible.

Epinephrine

Mechanism of Action and Pharmacology

Epinephrine (adrenaline) is an endogenous catecholamine synthesized in the adrenal medulla. Norepinephrine is converted to epinephrine by N-methyl transferase (see Fig. 25-5) through the addition of a methyl group to the N-terminus. (The term Nor-*epinephrine* is derived from "N ohne radical," that is, epinephrine minus the CH_3 group.)

Epinephrine is synthesized and stored in the chromaffin granules in the adrenal medulla, and it constitutes 80% of the catechola-

mines of the chromaffin granules. It is released rapidly after stimulation by nerve impulses from the sympathetic nervous system, and an influx of calcium is necessary for this process to occur. Epinephrine then acts on adrenergic receptor sites, causing increased levels of cAMP and an increase of calcium infusion intracellularly.

As epinephrine is released from the adrenal medulla, it acts like a circulating hormone, with only small changes in concentration affecting cardiovascular hemodynamics. Normal resting levels of epinephrine are between 24 and 74 pg/ml, while concentrations of 75 to 125 pg/ml will produce increases in heart rate and systemic BP.[90,96] In a study of critically ill children, however, mean levels of 508 pg/ml were measured.[93]

Epinephrine is the most potent endogenous alpha and beta catecholamine activating receptors of alpha-1, alpha-2, beta-1, and beta-2. Low concentrations of epinephrine stimulate beta-1 receptors in the myocardium and conducting systems, resulting in increased heart rate and shortened systolic time intervals. An increase in myocardial contraction occurs (inotropic effect), while myocardial oxygen consumption increases. Epinephrine also stimulates beta-2 receptors, leading to relaxation of arterioles, resulting in a significant decrease in SVR and diastolic BP. The concentration of beta-2 adrenergic receptors varies in different vascular beds. Skeletal muscle vascular beds are rich in beta-2 receptors, while renal vascular beds have a low concentration of beta-2 receptors. The latter fact is responsible for reduced blood flow to the kidneys with epinephrine infusions because of the unopposed alpha-1 vasoconstriction activity in renal blood vessels. Epinephrine also reduces cutaneous blood flow, and it increases coronary blood flow. Thus, with low-dose epinephrine infusions, the hemodynamic effects include increased stroke volume, increased heart rate, increased ventricular stroke work, and increased cardiac output (as long as intravascular volume is adequate) along with widened pulse pressure and decreased SVR and PVR.[97]

Increased concentrations of epinephrine, however, activate alpha-1 receptors, leading to an increase in SVR. With BP increase, slowing of the heart may occur through the baroreceptor reflex. Cardiovascular effects of epinephrine are a balance between the opposing actions of alpha-1 vascular receptors, which lead to vasoconstriction, and beta-2 vascular receptors, which lead to vasodilation. The positive inotropic effect is maintained, however, although cardiac output may vary, dependent on the balance of increased SVR versus increased inotropy.

Epinephrine produces marked bronchodilation by activating bronchial smooth muscle beta-2 receptors. In high doses, epinephrine increases respiratory rate and tidal volume. It also causes restlessness, apprehension, and muscle tremors. Metabolically, it causes increases in plasma concentrations of glucose, lactate, and free fatty acids.[90,98]

Epinephrine also induces a fall in plasma potassium and phosphorus.[99,100] The hypokalemia is through beta-2 mechanisms, and flattening of T waves and QTc prolongation may occur.[99] These electrophysiologic changes along with the hypokalemia may predispose the patient to life-threatening dysrhythmias.

Metabolism

The metabolism of epinephrine is by two enzyme systems, monamine oxidase and catechol-o-methyl transferase (COMT). The metabolic pathways are similar to those of norepinephrine and are discussed in that section.

Indications and Dosage

Epinephrine is a potent adrenergic agonist that improves myocardial dysfunction in a number of different settings. Postoperative cardiac surgical patients may require continuous epinephrine infusion for up to 12 to 24 hours to augment myocardial contractility. Patients in cardiogenic shock may also benefit from epinephrine infusions, with usual infusion rates being 0.05 to 0.3 μg/kg/min.[12] Plasma concentrations are linearly related to infusion rates and in one study ranged from 670 to 9430 pg/ml for rates of 0.05 to 0.2 μg/kg/min, with clearance rates similar to those for dopamine and dobutamine.[101]

In the treatment of septic shock in children, intravascular volume expansion and inotropic support to the myocardium are key parts of the patient's management. Epinephrine may play a helpful role in these patients by improving the myocardial dysfunction, should it progress to a low cardiac-output state. Its alpha-1 adrenergic action is helpful in increasing vascular tone, increasing BP and thus coronary artery perfusion pressure. Infusion rates of approximately 0.1 to 0.3 μg/kg/min will achieve this effect. With high infusion concentrations of 1 to 2 μg/kg/min, marked vasoconstriction through alpha-1 adrenergic effects may lead to reduced blood flow to some organs and produce a marked increase in afterload that could compromise myocardial contractile force.

For the treatment of asystole and electromechanical dissociation (EMD), bolus injections of epinephrine is the therapy of choice. The recommended standard dose of 0.01 mg/kg is given intravenously or by intraosseous infusion. However, animal studies have shown that higher doses of epinephrine (0.4–0.2 mg/kg) produce better responses.[102–105] In recent years, clinical studies have demonstrated that these higher doses of epinephrine do increase return of spontaneous circulation but have no statistically significant improvement in survival rates.[106–108] It is recommended in the recent guidelines of Pediatric Advanced Life Support that if no effect is achieved in 3 to 5 minutes, then high-dose epinephrine (0.1–0.2 mg/kg) may be given and repeated within 3 to 5 minutes if necessary.[109] For administration of the drug via the endotracheal tube, the high dose is administered from the beginning.[110,111]

Interactions

Anesthetic agents, especially the fluorinated hydrocarbons, may sensitize the heart to the effects of epinephrine, leading to serious arrhythmia. Epinephrine administered to a patient receiving a beta-blocker (e.g., propranolol) may cause an exaggeration of the alpha effects (e.g., hypertension) because of unopposed beta effects.

Norepinephrine

Mechanism of Action and Pharmacology

Norepinephrine is an endogenous catecholamine that is synthesized in the body from L-tyrosine (see Fig. 25-3). Its chemical structure is a dehydroxylated phenyl-B-ethanolamine and as such, exhibits properties of phenols, alcohols, and amines. Norepinephrine is produced in the brain, chromaffin cells of the adrenal medulla, and the sympathetic neurons of the sympathetic nervous system.

Norepinephrine is released from its storage in vesicles at the nerve cell endings after nerve stimulation. The release from vesicles is by the process of exocytosis, is aided by the contraction of the neurofibrils of the cells, and is an energy-dependent process requiring the production of ATP.[112]

Once released, norepinephrine acts on effector sites by binding to the adrenergic receptors, and by stimulating these, there is intracellular release of AMP. Beta-adrenergic stimulation in the heart causes increased inotropy, dromotropy, and to a lesser extent, chronotropy. Alpha-1 adrenergic stimulation, especially in the peripheral vasculature, causes vasoconstriction, mediated by increased cAMP and increased calcium infusion intracellularly. Alpha-2 stimulation on the terminal nerve endings actually will inhibit further norepinephrine release from the storage vesicles. Once norepinephrine is excreted from adrenergic nerve endings or the adrenal medulla, it generally has a short plasma half-life. It is inactivated rapidly, mostly through re-uptake of storage granules, but also through conversion to metabolites and excretion. There are two significant enzymatic events that may occur in either order, but which finally result in production of vanillylmandelic acid (VMA) or, to a lesser extent, methoxyhydroxyphenylglycol (MHPG), which are then excreted in the urine. COMT is an important enzyme for metabolism and is found in the cytoplasm of most tissues, especially kidney, liver, and RBC. Oxidative deamination via monamine oxidase (MAO) is the other metabolic enzyme, and it works at the adrenergic nerve endings.

Actions

In the brain, norepinephrine-containing neurons are found in the cerebellum, the cerebral cortex, and the hypothalamus, and these neurons help control alertness, mood, balance, coordination, thirst, hunger, temperature, and BP.

Peripherally, norepinephrine is the predominant neurotransmitter in the sympathetic nervous system, including the adrenergic nerve endings, and it has generalized effects because of the receptor sites. It also travels via the circulation as a neurohumor secondary to spillover from the sympathetic system and via synthesis and secretion from the chromaffin cells in the adrenal medulla.

The actions of norepinephrine are many throughout the body, but this discussion deals mainly with its effects on the peripheral and central circulation. Norepinephrine has both beta-1 and beta-2 adrenergic effects and alpha-1 and alpha-2 adrenergic effects. Its alpha effects are some of the most potent of any of the endogenous catecholamines, but it still has significant beta effects, although not as potent as epinephrine. Some sympathetic nerve fibers branch and terminate in the heart muscle, sinus node, and AV junction. When norepinephrine is released from these fibers, heart rate is increased by increased pacemaker firing and facilitated conduction, and force of muscular contraction is increased in the atria and the ventricles. With increased levels of norepinephrine, the peak velocity of blood flow increases and the duration of contraction shortens as dP/dT (first derivative of pressure) rises.

Sympathetic nerve fibers branch and supply all arteries throughout the body with norepinephrine-containing adrenergic nerve endings. These nerve endings reach all blood vessels except true capillaries and cause intense vasoconstriction, especially in the small arteries and arterioles, which are richly innervated. Thus, peripherally norepinephrine may significantly elevate systemic BP, and the vasoconstriction may significantly impair regional blood flow. Venule and venous vasoconstriction (not as richly innervated) by norepinephrine does increase blood return to the heart. Adrenal medulla stimulation following stimulation of the lateral columns of the spinal cord, splanchnic nerves, vasomotor center of the medulla oblongata or the lateral hypothalamus also exhibits neurohumoral control by releasing epinephrine and lesser quantities of norepinephrine.

Also, the secretion atrial natriuretic factor (ANF) is increased by stimulation of norepinephrine and thus promotes saluresis. This is probably secondary to receptor stimulation by norepinephrine.[113]

Indications

The use of norepinephrine as a therapeutic agent became limited in the late 1970s, especially after studies showed renal vasoconstriction and decreased renal blood flow with use in humans and the development of acute renal failure with use in animals.[114–116] Because of concerns of excessive vasoconstriction, it became a little-used inotropic agent. Recently, however, norepinephrine has again found use in septic shock patients and in those patients with ventricular failure, especially after bypass during cardiac surgery. Also, norepinephrine has been used in tricyclic antidepressant overdose, and there are some animal data on the use of norepinephrine as a cardiopulmonary resuscitation medication. These situations will now be reviewed.

The hemodynamic management of patients with septic shock includes volume loading and inotropic agents. Usually, dopamine and dobutamine are the initial agents, but some patients continue to remain hypotensive in spite of these efforts. It has been shown that even in patients who die from septic shock, many of them have a normal or above-normal cardiac index and have a very low SVR.[117] Several studies have shown that norepinephrine improves the clinical course of patients with septic shock, including improvement of hypotension, improved renal output, decreased heart rate, and increased SVR, without decreasing cardiac output.[118–121] It seems that a reasonable therapeutic goal in patients with septic shock is to raise their cardiac indices to greater than 4.5 liters/min/m^2, their SVR indices to greater than 700 to 800 dyne-sec/cm^5, and to substantially increase their oxygen delivery by using norepinephrine, fluid loading, and dobutamine. There have been several studies indicating that use of norepinephrine in septic shock patients actually improves urine output and creatinine, osmolar, and free-water clearances, although one study noted that these improvements did not occur in patients with high lactate levels.[122–124]

It is not surprising that norepinephrine improves urine flow and renal blood flow in patients with septic shock, as opposed to excessive vasoconstriction and decreased renal blood flow in normal hosts. It is known that the adrenergic effects of norepinephrine are significantly down-regulated in sepsis, and the use of norepinephrine as catechol in this situation may help overcome these down-regulatory effects, thus returning to more normal flow.[125] Thus, norepinephrine seems a reasonable therapy in hyperdynamic septic shock with low SVR and especially after no clinical improvement has occurred with volume loading and other inotropic agents.

Norepinephrine is also frequently used in the treatment of tricyclic antidepressant (TCA) overdose. TCA overdose compromises the endogenous stores of norepinephrine, and thus norepinephrine is usually a first- or second-line drug to be used in the treatment of hypotension unresponsive to volume loading or dopamine.[126]

There have been several reports of using norepinephrine in combination with other inotropes in ventricular failure in adults. In patients with low cardiac output or difficulty in coming off cardiopulmonary bypass, norepinephrine and amrinone have been found to be a good combination in improving the clinical course.[127–130]

Finally, there are some data from animal studies showing that norepinephrine may be equal or superior to epinephrine in cardiopulmonary resuscitation models.[131,132] One potential reason for this is the decreased cardiac oxygen consumption with norepinephrine (not as strong beta effects as epinephrine), thus improving the balance between increased oxygen delivery and oxygen consumption.[133]

Dose

Norepinephrine is presently used as an infusion rather than bolus medication. Because of its potent vasoconstrictor effects, it should be administered through secure venous access, preferably in a central venous catheter.

The publicized infusion rates are quite variable, ranging from high levels of 0.5 to 1.5 μg/kg/min to more moderate ranges of 0.03 to 0.89 μg/kg/min.[118,122,123] Most infusions are started in the 0.05- to 0.10-μg/kg/min ranges and then titrated until the desired effects are attained, such as improved BP, perfusion, urine output, or SVR. If untoward effects of excessive vasoconstriction occur, the dosage should be lowered.

Side Effects

The major concern with norepinephrine is excessive vasoconstriction, thus impairing regional blood flow. Also, increased PVR may occur, increasing right ventricular workload, although this is usually offset by increased inotropy and oxygen delivery.[129] Finally, all catechols including norepinephrine may cause an increase in dysrhythmias.

Isoproterenol

Pharmacology

Isoproterenol is a beta-specific synthetic catecholamine that was developed and first studied in the 1940s. It exists as a racemic mixture of stereoisomers with the L isomer being more potent than the D isomer.[134] Its affinity for beta-1 and beta-2 receptors is equal, and it has virtually no activity at alpha receptors.

Isoproterenol has a very short half-life of approximately 2 minutes and must be given as a continuous infusion when used as a parenteral medication. There exist linear relationships between the rate of infusion of isoproterenol and the measured serum concentration and also between the serum concentration of isoproterenol and the hemodynamic effect.[135] Its short half-life can be attributed to rapid clearance and metabolism by the liver and other effector organs throughout the body, with minimal to no reuptake by sympathetic neurons.[134]

Effects

Isoproterenol is the most potent beta agonist employed in clinical practice. It directly stimulates beta-1 and beta-2 receptors and thus possesses inotropic, chronotropic, and vasodilatory properties. The combination of these properties accounts for its effects on the cardiovascular system. In general, the administration of isoproterenol causes an increase in stroke volume reflected as an increase in cardiac output and systolic BP. Its afterload-reducing beta-2 effect results in a fall in SVR and PVR and a drop in diastolic BP. The net effect on BP is an increase in pulse pressure with essentially no change or a slight decrease in mean BP.[134] Isoproterenol also markedly affects heart rate. It increases conduction velocity, shortens AV conduction time, and directly stimulates the SA node.

This direct chronotropic effect is accentuated by the reflex tachycardia that accompanies vasodilation. In animal as well as human studies, the use of isoproterenol results in a relatively greater chronotropic than inotropic response.[134,136–138] This may be problematic for two reasons. First, the incidence of trachyarrhythmias is increased, and isoproterenol is the most arrhythmogenic of the catecholamines. Second, isoproterenol significantly increases myocardial oxygen consumption. At the same time, by decreasing diastolic BP and diastolic filling time, it limits coronary perfusion and myocardial oxygen delivery. This resultant imbalance between oxygen delivery and oxygen consumption may promote myocardial ischemia, and clinically this has been noted, especially in the setting of ischemic heart disease in adults.[139–141] Myocardial ischemia, manifested as elevated isoenzymes and fatal myocardial infarction, has also been encountered in asthmatic children without underlying heart disease who were treated with IV isoproterenol.[29,142–146]

In addition to its additive effect on increasing chronotropy, the vasodilation encountered with isoproterenol may lead to other unwanted physiologic side effects. Vasodilation occurs primarily in skeletal muscle vascular beds (because of the high density of beta-2 receptors in these beds), which can cause a vascular "steal" phenomenon from vital organs.[29,147] In neonates, a decrease in renal blood flow has been documented during the administration of isoproterenol.[137] Also, isoproterenol's effect on the pulmonary vasculature abolishes hypoxic pulmonary vasoconstriction, and in patients with parenchymal lung disease, increases V/Q mismatch and hypoxemia.[148–151]

Isoproterenol has other end-organ beta-1 and beta-2 effects. When administered as a nebulized aerosol or continuous IV infusion, it is a potent bronchodilator. It also affects intermediary metabolism, acting as an insulin antagonist; lipolysis and, rarely, hyperglycemia may result.[134]

Indications

Isoproterenol's usefulness is limited by its deleterious side effects. In the treatment of shock, other more selective agents have replaced it as first-line therapy. In selected instances, however, isoproterenol still has clinical utility.

Isoproterenol is most commonly utilized in the setting of severe asthma refractory to conventional therapy.[152–154] A continuous infusion starting at 0.05 μg/kg/min and titrated upward is employed. The endpoint in therapy is determined by either a therapeutic response or the development of untoward side effects, including excessive tachycardia (a heart rate greater than 180 bpm), dysrhythmia, or evidence of myocardial ischemia. In one series of asthmatics, a mean infusion rate of 0.36 μg/kg/min was necessary to elicit the desired therapeutic response.[152] Usually, clinical improvement occurs at doses that push the limit of tachycardia. In treating severe asthmatics, the use of isoproterenol should be restricted to the ICU where continuous monitoring of heart rate, ECG, and arterial BP is available. An arterial line should be placed and arterial blood gases checked after each change in infusion rate. The presence of high-flow supplemental oxygen is mandatory to compensate for the initial drop in oxygenation that results from increased V/Q mismatch secondary to pulmonary vasodilation. Abrupt discontinuation of the infusion should be avoided by always keeping a second functional IV line in place. As the arterial PCO$_2$ normalizes, the infusion rate should be slowly weaned over 24 to 36 hours. More rapid withdrawal of isoproterenol may lead to rebound bronchospasm.[153,154] Isoproterenol enhances the metabolism of theophylline, resulting in a drop in serum theophylline levels.[155,156] Because theophylline potentiates the toxic effects of isoproterenol on the myocardium, it is prudent not to "chase" theophylline levels.[156,157] A level in the 10- to 15-μg/ml range is acceptable. The complications associated with the use of isoproterenol in asthmatics can be life-threatening. If dysrhythmias or clinical evidence of myocardial ischemia develop, the infusion should be discontinued. The use of IV isoproterenol has declined in recent years because of the development of such less cardiotoxic medications as continuous bronchodilation, either as nebulizers or IV therapy.

Isoproterenol is useful in the treatment of hemodynamically significant bradycardia.[158] It may provide temporary improvement in the patient with complete heart block awaiting placement of a pacemaker. It may also normalize the heart rate (and thus the cardiac output) in cardiac surgery patients who have undergone procedures involving the atria or AV node and have postoperative bradycardia associated with poor perfusion.

There are other settings in which isoproterenol may have clinical efficacy. In the patient in shock who has high filling pressures and high SVR and PVR, isoproterenol may augment cardiac output.[74,159,160] In this setting, it is often used as an adjunct to other catecholamines. In children with pulmonary hypertension (and excessive pulmonary vascular lability) secondary to large left-to-right shunts, isoproterenol may lessen PVR and unload the right ventricle in the postoperative period.[151,161] Finally, the administration of isoproterenol during the tilt test is a standardized method of evaluating and diagnosing vasodepressor syncope.[162]

Dose

Isoproterenol is initiated as a continuous infusion starting at 0.05 μg/kg/min. The dose is increased by 0.05 to 0.1 μg/kg/min until the desired therapeutic effect is achieved or until excessive tachycardia or other side effects become limiting. The usual IV dose range is between 0.05 and 1.0 μg/kg/min. Higher doses result in an unacceptable incidence of side effects.

In the treatment of asthma, isoproterenol can be delivered via nebulization. A dose of 0.1 ml/kg (to a maximum of 0.3 ml) of a 1:200 preparation is mixed with 2 to 3 ml of 0.9% saline and given as an aerosol. Unwanted side effects may also be encountered with this mode of therapy.

Side Effects

Most of the adverse effects associated with isoproterenol are as described earlier. Isoproterenol also commonly causes minor symptoms, including headache, palpitations, flushing, nausea, vomiting, and dizziness. It is essential that practitioners who utilize this drug are well aware of its toxicities so that complications can be **anticipated and rapidly addressed**. Because isoproterenol possesses no alpha activity, extravasation from an infiltrated IV does not produce tissue necrosis. It can be safely given through a peripheral IV, even at high doses.

Amrinone

Mechanism of Action and Pharmacology

The bipyridines, amrinone, milrinone, and related agents, have inotropic and vasoactive properties that are independent of adrenergic stimulation (nonsympathomimetic) or inhibition of sodium-potassium ATPase (nonglycosidic).[163] Amrinone, which was approved by the Food and Drug Administration in 1984 for the short-term therapy of severe congestive heart failure, is the major bipyridine that presently has clinical utility in the intensive care setting.

Amrinone inhibits the enzyme phosphodiesterase, resulting in an increased intracellular concentration of cAMP in target organs (primarily the myocardium and the smooth muscle of blood vessels).[164–167] The increase in intracellular cAMP affects cellular calcium metabolism, probably at several levels, ultimately increasing intracellular availability of calcium.[168–171] That intracellular cAMP and calcium are both pivotal in mediating the effects of amrinone is supported by in vitro evidence that demonstrates that carbachol[3] (an inhibitor of adenyl cyclase and thus cAMP formation), calcium channel blockers, and hypocalcemia all attenuate amrinone's effects.[159,160] Exactly how cAMP affects calcium's intracellular availability has not been fully elucidated. An effect on the sarcolemmal slow, inward calcium channel along with an alteration in the sarcoplasmic reticulum's sequestration and release of calcium have both been implicated.[163,168,170–172] It is interesting that the increase in intracellular cAMP does not correlate temporally with the hemodynamic effects noted with amrinone.[168–172] Thus, amrinone has additional, as yet undefined, mechanisms of action.

Amrinone's hemodynamic effects are dependent on both the dose administered and the resulting serum concentration.[172–177] Its half-life is variable, depending on age as well as disease state. It averages approximately 3.0 hours in healthy adults, 5.8 hours in adults with congestive heart failure, 6.8 hours in infants, and 22.2 hours in neonates after open-heart surgery.[178–180] Metabolism via acetylation and glucuronidation occurs in the liver, although approximately 40% of the drug is excreted unchanged in the urine.[174,178]

Actions

In the laboratory, experimental models using isolated myocardium and vascular smooth muscle demonstrate that amrinone has both inotropic and vasodilatory properties. There are important interspecies as well as age-dependent variations in the end-organ response to this drug. Of particular concern has been the finding that in myocardium isolated from newborn puppies, amrinone acts as a negative inotrope for the first 3 days of life, with positive inotropy of increasing magnitude demonstrated with advancing age beyond 4 days.[181–183] The reason for this negative inotropic response is unclear, possibly explained by developmental immaturity of the sarcoplasmic-tubular system in myocytes in the first few days of life. This effect is not related to phosphodiesterase activity, as cAMP concentrations rise in a dose-dependent manner, as expected.[181]

In humans, controversy exists as to whether amrinone's hemodynamic effects are due primarily to improved contractility or to afterload reduction via vasodilation. Some studies suggest that amrinone possesses no inotropic activity and that it acts purely as a vasodilator.[184–186] Other studies demonstrate increased contractility associated with reduced filling pressures, implying a direct inotropic effect.[187,188] Taken as a whole, available data suggest amrinone's hemodynamic effects involve both improved inotropy and increased afterload reduction, with afterload reduction probably assuming greater importance.

In adult patients with congestive heart failure, usual therapeutic doses of amrinone result in improved cardiac output associated with decreased filling pressures and decreased SVR and PVR. BP and heart rate are minimally affected.[175,177,187,189–192] Coronary artery vasodilation and decreased ventricular wall tension improve myo-

cardial oxygen balance, and a decrease in myocardial lactate production along with a diminished coronary artery-coronary sinus oxygen difference have been demonstrated.[184,187–189] Although AV nodal conduction is enhanced, dysrhythmias are not encountered in clinical practice with usual therapeutic doses.[193]

Indications

Amrinone's prolonged half-life and potential for causing hypotension limit its usefulness in treating critically ill patients. In adults, it has proven efficacy in the short-term treatment of severe, refractory congestive heart failure associated with high filling pressures and high peripheral vascular resistance.[177,187,189–194] In this setting, it is often used as a second-line agent in the patient with a diminished stroke volume despite the administration of dobutamine and other first-line agents such as dopamine and epinephrine. Its hemodynamic effects appear to be additive to those of these other agents with no increase in the incidence of toxic side effects such as tachycardia, myocardial ischemia, or arrhythmias. Disease states in which amrinone has been used with satisfactory results include congestive cardiomyopathy, severe congestive heart failure secondary to coronary artery disease, and low-output states after open-heart surgery and cardiopulmonary bypass. Amrinone's role in the therapy of septic shock and other forms of shock needs further assessment.

In the pediatric age range, experience with amrinone is limited to a few small series, case reports, and anecdotal experience. In one series of pediatric patients with severe congestive heart failure after cardiac surgery, the administration of amrinone resulted in an increased ejection fraction and decreased vascular resistance with no change in heart rate or BP.[195] In another series of postoperative cardiac patients, the use of amrinone resulted in a decrease in vascular resistance and BP, but no change in stroke volume or cardiac output.[196] These somewhat contradictory results require further clinical evaluation. It is the authors' opinion that amrinone possesses clinical efficacy in pediatric patients with low-output states associated with high filling pressures. It should be considered adjunctive therapy to conventional first-line agents.

Dose

Amrinone is approved only for IV administration. The usual adult dose is 0.75 to 3.0 mg/kg, given as a loading dose over 3 to 5 minutes followed by a continuous infusion of 5 to 15 µg/kg/min. Because amrinone is a potent vasodilator of both arterial and venous beds, it is preferable to monitor left-sided filling pressures prior to its administration. Too rapid infusion of the loading dose, and continuous infusions greater than 10 µg/kg/min, may cause hypotension necessitating fluid administration to restore filling pressures.

In the pediatric age range, a dose for amrinone has not been established. One study of 18 postsurgical infants assessed the pharmacokinetic and safety profiles of amrinone.[180] The conclusion reached was that to achieve and maintain steady-state serum levels of 2 to 7 µg/ml (the therapeutic range for adults), neonates require a loading dose of 3.0 to 4.5 mg/kg followed by a continuous infusion of 3 to 5 µg/kg/min. Infants greater than 1 month of age require a loading dose of 3.0 to 4.5 mg/kg followed by a continuous infusion of 10 µg/kg/min. If these larger loading doses are utilized, they should be broken into repeated smaller doses, each given as a slow push.

Amrinone is incompatible with glucose and should be prepared in a glucose-free solution such as 0.9% saline. In patients with renal failure, there is a real risk of drug accumulation, and when used in this setting, low-dose infusions should be employed.

Side Effects

Initial trials of long-term, oral amrinone revealed a high incidence of gastrointestinal symptomatology, elevation of liver enzymes, and thrombocytopenia. The oral preparation was subsequently taken off the market.

IV amrinone has been well tolerated by most patients in both the adult and pediatric age ranges. The most commonly reported adverse side effect is hypotension, usually associated with too rapid administration of the loading dose; it is easily reversed with restoration of filling pressures. Reversible liver enzyme elevation and thrombocytopenia may also occur. If prolonged infusions are used, liver function tests and platelet counts should be followed.

Phenylephrine

Pharmacology

Phenylephrine is a noncatecholamine sympathomimetic agent first studied in 1910 by Barger and Dale.[197] It differs in structure from epinephrine by lacking a hydroxyl group in the fourth position of the benzene ring.

In the ICU, phenylephrine hydrochloride is given in the IV form. After IV administration, phenylephrine levels in the serum show a biphasic decline. Response to phenylephrine lasts up to 20 minutes following IV administration. Phenylephrine is excreted in the urine. Deamination accounts for approximately two thirds of metabolism, with conjugated phenylephrine accounting for less than 10% of the metabolism. The remainder is excreted as the free amine.[198] Studies of phenylephrine metabolism in patients with renal insufficiency have not been done; however, because the drug is excreted renally, caution should be exercised in these patients.

Actions

Phenylephrine is a direct-acting alpha-adrenoceptor agonist with little beta-adrenoceptor effects. As such, its primary effect is in vascular beds where it acts as a potent vasoconstrictor. As a result, systolic and diastolic BPs increase as does SVR. As an exception, coronary blood flow may be increased slightly following phenylephrine administration.[199] Pulmonary vasoconstriction occurs with phenylephrine use, with an increase in pulmonary artery systolic pressure and PVR. A reflex bradycardia may occur secondary to baroreceptor stimulation. This latter action may be blocked by atropine. Otherwise, phenylephrine is a unique sympathomimetic in its lack of direct cardiac effects.

Additional potential actions of phenylephrine result from its alpha-adrenergic properties. These include contraction of GI sphincters; decreased tone, motility, and secretion in the GI tract; decreased insulin secretion; constriction of the radial muscle of the eye; contraction of the urinary bladder trigone-sphincter muscle; and contraction of the splenic capsule. Venoconstriction from phenylephrine is minimal.

Indications

A dearth of literature has been written regarding the uses of phenylephrine. Reports in humans are limited to case studies, while the available clinical studies have been done in animal models. A review of this literature suggests four indications for phenylephrine use: (1) in shock states, (2) resuscitation of cardiac arrest, (3) tetralogy of Fallot hypoxemic spells, and (4) supraventricular tachycardia (SVT).

Perhaps the most common use of phenylephrine is in the treatment of hypotension and shock. As a potent vasoconstrictor, phenylephrine increases the BP and SVR. The goal of therapy is to provide adequate perfusion pressure to vital organs. Phenylephrine may provide a benefit over traditional mainstays of pressor therapy for shock—dopamine, epinephrine, and norepinephrine—in its lack of direct cardiac effects. This is especially important in patients who develop tachyarrhythmias from administration of other pressors.[200] In our unit, we have used phenylephrine successfully in the treatment of spinal shock following cervical spine injuries. This specific use may be especially appropriate due to the major contribution of lack of vascular tone in spinal shock, with relatively less contribution from cardiac depression. Bonfiglio et al. provide a case report of the successful use of phenylephrine in a patient with septic shock.[200] Caution should be used in cardiogenic shock, however, as phenylephrine will increase the afterload burden on the heart.

Epinephrine has been the mainstay of therapy for cardiac arrest. Academic disagreement existed as to whether its success in resuscitation was a result of elevation of diastolic pressure, thereby reestablishing coronary blood flow, or beta-adrenergic-mediated increased chronotropy and inotropy. Using a dog model, Yakaitis et al. found 100% resuscitation in dogs treated with phenylephrine who had been beta-blocked prior to the arrest. Alpha-blocked dogs treated with isoproterenol had only 27% successful resuscitation. The authors concluded that alpha-receptor stimulation was more important to successful resuscitation than beta-stimulation.[201] Several studies since that time, all in dog models, have corroborated the data on phenylephrine's efficacy in resuscitation from cardiac arrest.[202–205] Some authors suggest that pure alpha-agonists may be preferable to mixed agonists. Pure alpha-agonists avoid the increased myocardial oxygen consumption caused by beta-adrenergic stimulation.[206] One study examined neurologic outcome following resuscitation with phenylephrine or epinephrine, and found no difference in dogs examined 24 hours following arrest.[203] The body of literature certainly suggests that phenylephrine can be a useful therapy in cardiac arrest; however, its benefit over traditional mainstays of therapy remains unclear, and human studies have not been performed.

A third indication for phenylephrine use is in the treatment of refractory cyanotic spells in patients with tetralogy of Fallot. The final common pathway for these spells is life-threatening reduction in pulmonary blood flow. Traditional treatment aimed at increasing pulmonary blood flow has included knee-to-chest positioning and the administration of oxygen, morphine, and beta-blockers. Use of alpha-adrenergic agents has been advocated as well, to increase SVR, and thereby decrease right-to-left shunting at the ventricular level.[207] Shaddy et al. reported three infants with tetralogy of Fallot with refractory hypoxemic spells, unresponsive to the traditional therapeutic interventions.[208] All three had reversal of hypoxemia following administration of phenylephrine and successfully underwent palliative surgery while on a continuous phenylephrine IV infusion. The authors have also found that phenylephrine can be a life-saving intervention in pediatric patients with tetralogy of Fallot who have hypoxemic spells refractory to traditional treatment.

Finally, phenylephrine has been used to convert SVT. Vagal maneuvers generally are the primary intervention for SVT, such as administration of ice to the face or performance of the Valsalva maneuver. Alpha-adrenergic stimulation is perhaps the most potent vagal maneuver, as it stimulates arterial baroreceptors with a reflex augmentation of vagal discharge. Jacobson et al. reported the successful use of phenylephrine in SVT refractory to vagal maneuvers, calcium channel blockers, and procainamide.[209] This use of phenylephrine should be reserved for the intensive care setting where continuous BP monitoring can be provided and cardioversion is available should it fail.

Adverse Reactions

Adverse reactions are related primarily to phenylephrine's physiologic effects on the cardiovascular system. These include hypertension and reflex bradycardia. The former can be reversed by alpha-blockers, and the latter can be blocked by atropine. Exacerbation of ventricular tachycardias can occur, and caution should be exercised in using phenylephrine in patients who have exhibited such arrhythmias. Phenylephrine can also cause adverse reactions in the CNS. These include headache, excitability, and restlessness. Finally, phenylephrine hydrochloride contains sodium metabisulfite. This sulfite has been reported to cause allergic reactions, including anaphylaxis, in susceptible individuals. Sulfite sensitivity is more common in patients with asthma, although the overall incidence, even in these patients, is probably quite low.

Dose

For the treatment of hypotension, phenylephrine is given as a continuous IV infusion. It is compatible with dextrose or saline solutions. In our unit, we begin at a dose of 0.1 μg/kg/min and titrate to the desired effect on BP.

For use in cardiac arrest, tetralogy of Fallot cyanotic spells, and SVT, phenylephrine is given as a single IV dose. The initial dose is usually 0.1 mg, but up to 0.5 mg may be used safely if the desired effect is not attained at the lower dose. This bolus dose can then be followed by a continuous infusion to maintain alpha blockade.

Sodium Nitroprusside

Mechanism of Action and Pharmacology

In acute and chronic circulatory failure associated with a low cardiac output, the body's main compensatory mechanism for preserving BP is vasoconstriction. This increase in SVR increases the afterload of the heart and adversely affects cardiac output. In providing pharmacologic support to the failing circulation, vasodilation is a rational therapeutic goal if fluid administration and the use of inotropes do not improve cardiac output.[210] As mentioned in an earlier section, BP should be normal or near normal, and filling pressures must be maintained if vasodilation is to be effective. There are many vasodilating agents available for clinical use. The one that is utilized most frequently in the intensive care setting is sodium nitroprusside.

Nitroprusside exists as an unstable, iron-coordination complex molecule (Fig. 25-9) that decomposes on contact with sulfhydryl groups present in RBC.[211,212] Nitric oxide is liberated during this reaction and activates quanylate cyclase present in vascular smooth muscle, resulting in vasodilation.[213] Nitroprusside relaxes arterial and venous smooth muscle equally.

Nitroprusside (and its metabolic end product nitric oxide) is

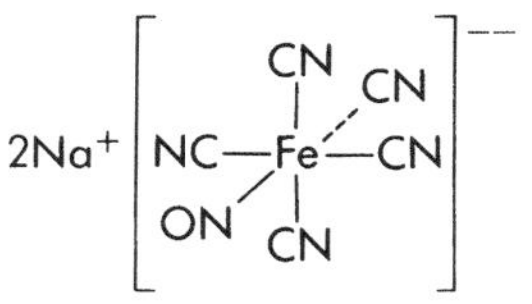

Sodium Nitroprusside

Figure 25-9. The structure of nitroprusside.

very rapidly inactivated and must be given as a continuous IV infusion. Its onset of action is rapid, within seconds of initiating an infusion. In addition, its effect is short-lived, dissipating within minutes of terminating an infusion. Because of these characteristics, it is an ideal agent for use in the ICU, titrating the infusion to the desired hemodynamic effect.[212,213]

During the in vivo decomposition of nitroprusside, free cyanide is formed. Cyanide is metabolized by the liver to thiocyanate, which is then slowly excreted by the kidneys. With prolonged infusions and with renal insufficiency, thiocyanate toxicity may occur.

Effects

Nitroprusside is a potent vasodilator of both venous and arterial vascular beds, and its hemodynamic effects are secondary to venous pooling (decreased preload) and arterial vasodilation (decreased afterload). The effect of nitroprusside on cardiac performance depends on the existing state of the myocardium.[211] With normal left ventricular function, the decrease in preload outweighs the decrease in afterload, and cardiac output and BP fall. In contrast, with a failing heart, a decrease in afterload "unloads" the left ventricle, and cardiac output rises. In general, in the critically ill patient, nitroprusside decreases filling pressures, decreases SVR and PVR, and increases cardiac output. BP falls unless filling pressures are maintained, and heart rate increases slightly.

All of nitroprusside's hemodynamic effects result from its activity on vascular smooth muscle; there is no direct effect on the heart itself. Nitroprusside also has no direct effect on the autonomic or central nervous system nor on smooth muscle in other organs of the body.[214] Because it acts on all blood vessels of the body equally, it does not alter the regional distribution of blood flow. One potentially adverse effect of this generalized vasodilation is the overriding of hypoxic pulmonary vasoconstriction (also seen with catecholamines with beta-2 activity), and patients with chronic pulmonary disease may become hypoxemic during the administration of nitroprusside if supplemental oxygen is not provided.[213]

Indications

Because of its potent vasodilating properties, nitroprusside is a very effective antihypertensive medication. It is a first-line agent for the treatment of severe hypertension, especially if rapid lowering of BP is crucial, as with hypertensive encephalopathy. It is also used to induce "controlled hypotension" during surgery to minimize intraoperative bleeding. Peak antihypertensive response occurs within 2 minutes of initiating an infusion; thus, an infusion should be titrated upward every few minutes until BP is controlled.[213] In a series of 20 children with severe hypertension, nitroprusside controlled BP in all 20 patients at a mean infusion rate of 1.4 μg/kg/min.[215] No tachyphylaxis was observed. When used in this setting, abrupt withdrawal of the infusion should be avoided, as rebound hypertension may occur.

Nitroprusside augments cardiac output in disease states associated with acute and chronic heart failure, such as cardiomyopathy, ischemic heart disease, valvular heart disease, and in the early postoperative period after intracardiac surgery.[216–227] In most of these disease states, nitroprusside is used in conjunction with inotropic agents, volume expansion, and diuretics. After acute stabilization, nitroprusside can be switched to longer-acting oral agents if prolonged afterload reduction is deemed necessary.

Dose

Nitroprusside is diluted in 5% dextrose water. It should be initiated at a starting dose of 0.5 µg/kg/min and titrated upward until the desired clinical effect is achieved. In most series, average infusion rates range between 1 and 3 µg/kg/min.

Nitroprusside is inactivated by alkaline solutions and should not be given with bicarbonate. It is also light-sensitive, undergoing photochemical degradation over time with exposure to light. It should be protected from light by wrapping the IV container and tubing with foil.

Side Effects

Acute toxicity includes hypotension and tachycardia. Continuous monitoring of BP and pulse is thus mandatory. Monitoring of central venous or pulmonary capillary wedge pressure is also desirable. The hypotensive effect is rapidly reversed by stopping the infusion and administering fluids to restore filling pressures.

Because cyanide is liberated during the degradation of nitroprusside, cyanide toxicity (marked by metabolic acidosis, tachycardia, tachypnea, headache, vomiting, and depressed mentation) is at least a theoretical consideration. The liver handles the amount of cyanide generated during the usual course of nitroprusside efficiently, and unless hepatic failure is present, cyanide toxicity is not encountered.

Thiocyanate, the end product of the metabolism of cyanide, may accumulate with prolonged, high-dose (>5 µg/kg/min) infusions.[211,214] Toxicity manifests as fatigue, nausea, tinnitus, disorientation, and muscle spasms.[228] Thyroid function can also be depressed with prolonged infusions, presumably the result of a direct toxic effect of thiocyanate on the thyroid gland.[229] By convention, thiocyanate levels are usually followed every 24 hours if infusions are greater than 48 hours, if doses are greater than 5 µg/kg/min, or if renal insufficiency is present. A serum level greater than 5 µg/dl necessitates termination of the infusion. In practice, thiocyanate toxicity is rare, and nitroprusside maintains a good safety profile in all age groups, including neonates.[230]

References

1. Sonnenblick EH, Spiro D, Spotnitz HM. The ultrastructural basis of Starling's law of the heart. The role of the sarcomere in determining ventricular size and stroke volume. *Am Heart J* 68:336–346, 1964.
2. Friedman WF. The intrinsic physiologic properties of the developing heart. *Prog Cardiovasc Dis* 15:87–111, 1972.
3. Downing SE, Talner NS, Gardner TH. Influences of arterial oxygen tension and pH on cardiac function in the newborn lamb. *Am J Physiol* 211:1203–1208, 1966.
4. Lee JC, Downing SE. Developmental aspects of the myocardial staircase phenomenon: Effects of insulin. *J Mol Cell Cardiol* 10:953–966, 1978.
5. Appenzeller O. *The Autonomic Nervous System.* New York: Elsevier, 1990. Pp 2–8.
6. Ahlquist RP. A study of the adrenotropic receptors. *Am J Physiol* 153:586–600, 1948.
7. Lands AM et al. Differentiation of receptor systems activated by sympathomimetic amines. *Nature* 214:597–598, 1967.
8. Bethelsen S, Pettinger WA. A functional basis for classification of α-adrenergic receptors. *Life Sci* 21:595–606, 1977.
9. Kebabian JW, Calne DB. Multiple receptors for dopamine. *Nature* 277:93–96, 1979.
10. Bryan LJ et al. A study designed to explore the hypothesis that Beta-1 adrenoceptors are 'innervated' receptors and Beta-2 adrenoceptors are 'hormonal' receptors. *J Pharmacol Exp Ther* 216:395–400, 1981.
11. Anderson KE. Aspects of the pharmacology of B-adrenoceptor agonists and antagonists. *Acta Anaesthesiol Scand* 76(Suppl):12–19, 1982.
12. Zaritsky A, Chernow B. Use of catecholamines in pediatrics. *J Pediatr* 105:341–350, 1984.
13. Carey RM, Thorner MD, Ortt EM. Dopaminergic inhibition of metoclopramide-induced aldosterone secretion in man. *J Clin Invest* 66:10–18, 1980.
14. Ward DS, Bellville JW. Reduction of hypoxic ventilatory drive by dopamine. *Anesth Analg* 61:333–337, 1982.
15. Kaptein EM et al. Effects of prolonged dopamine infusion on anterior pituitary function in normal males. *J Clin Endocrinol Metab* 51:488–491, 1980.
16. Downing SE, Talner NS, Gardner TH. Ventricular function in the newborn lamb. *Am J Physiol* 208:931–937, 1965.
17. Kirkpatrick SE et al. Frank-Starling relationship as an important determinant of fetal cardiac output. *Am J Physiol* 231:495–500, 1976.
18. Klopfenstein HS, Rudolph AM. Postnatal changes in the circulation and responses to volume loading in sheep. *Circ Res* 42:839–845, 1978.
19. Romero TE, Friedman WF. Limited left ventricular response to volume overload in the neonatal period: A comparative study with the adult animal. *Pediatr Res* 13:910–915, 1979.
20. Lang P et al. The hemodynamic effects of dopamine in infants after corrective cardiac surgery. *J Pediatr* 96:630–634, 1980.
21. Perkin RM et al. Dobutamine: A hemodynamic evaluation in children with shock. *J Pediatr* 100:977–983, 1982.
22. Holbrook PR, Schaible DH. Pediatric pharmacotherapy. In Chernow B (ed): *The Pharmacologic Approach to the Critically Ill Patient.* Baltimore: Williams & Wilkins, 1983. Pp 50–64.
23. Sinha SN, Armour JA, Randall WC. Development of autonomic innervation of the heart (abstract). *Circulation* Supp IV:37, 1973.
24. Roan Y, Galant SP. Decreased neutrophil beta adrenergic receptors in the neonate. *Pediatr Res* 16:591–593, 1982.
25. Rudolph AM, Heymann MA. Cardiac output in the fetal lamb: The effects of spontaneous and induced changes of heart rate on right and left ventricular output. *Am J Obstet Gynecol* 124:183–192, 1976.
26. Romero T, Covell J, Friedman WF. A comparison of pressure volume relations of the fetal, newborn, and adult heart. *Am J Physiol* 222:1285–1290, 1972.
27. Buckly NM, Brazeau P, Gootman PM. Maturation of circulatory responses to adrenergic stimuli. *Fed Proc* 42:1643–1647, 1983.
28. Duckles SP, Banner W Jr. Changes in vascular smooth muscle reactivity during development. *Annu Rev Pharmacol Toxicol* 24:65–83, 1984.
29. Friedman WF, George BL. New concepts and drugs in the treatment of congestive heart failure. *Pediatr Clin North Am* 31:1197–1227, 1984.
30. Jolley RL, Cheldelin VH, Newburgh RW. Glucose catabolism in fetal and adult heart. J Biol Chem 233:1289–1294, 1958.
31. Ruffolo RR Jr et al. Alpha and beta adrenergic effects of the stereoisomers of dobutamine. *J Pharmacol Exp Ther* 219:447–452, 1981.
32. Kates RE, Leier CV. Dobutamine pharmacokinetics in severe heart failure. *Clin Pharmacol Ther* 24:537–540, 1978.

33. Leier CV, Unverforth DV, Kates RE. The relationship between plasma dobutamine concentrations and cardiovascular responses in cardiac failure. *Am J Med* 66:238–242, 1979.

34. Martinez AM, Padbury JF, Thio S. Dobutamine pharmacokinetics and cardiovascular responses in critically ill neonates. *Pediatrics* 89:47–51, 1992.

35. Robie NW, Goldberg LI. Comparative systemic and regional hemodynamic effects of dopamine and dobutamine. *Am Heart J* 90:340–345, 1975.

36. Vatner SF, McRitchie RJ, Braunwald E. Effects of dobutamine on left ventricular performance, coronary dynamics, and distribution of cardiac output in conscious dogs. *J Clin Invest* 53:1265–1273, 1974.

37. Leier CV, Webel J, Bush CA. The cardiovascular effects of the continuous infusion of dobutamine in patients with severe cardiac failure. *Circulation* 56:468–472, 1977.

38. Beregovich J et al. Hemodynamic effects of a new inotropic agent (dobutamine) in chronic cardiac failure. *Br Heart J* 37:629–634, 1975.

39. Andy JJ et al. Cardiovascular effects of dobutamine in severe congestive heart failure. *Am Heart J* 94:175–182, 1977.

40. Bendersky R et al. Dobutamine in chronic ischemic heart failure: Alterations in left ventricular function and coronary hemodynamics. *Am J Cardiol* 48:554–558, 1981.

41. Gillespie TA et al. Effects of dobutamine in patients with acute myocardial infarction. *Am J Cardiol* 39:588–594, 1977.

42. Pozen RG et al. Myocardial metabolic and hemodynamic effects of dobutamine in heart failure complicating coronary artery disease. *Circulation* 63:1279–1284, 1981.

43. Loeb HS, Bredakis J, Gunna RM. Superiority of dobutamine over dopamine for augmentation of cardiac output in patients with chronic low output cardiac failure. *Circulation* 55:375–381, 1977.

44. Stoner JD III, Bolen JL, Harrison DC. Comparison of dobutamine and dopamine in treatment of severe heart failure. *Br Heart J* 39:536–539, 1977.

45. Tuttle RR, Mills J. Development of a new catecholamine to selectively increase cardiac contractility. *Circ Res* 36:185–195, 1975.

46. Jardin F et al. Dobutamine: A hemodynamic evaluation in human septic shock. *Crit Care Med* 9:329–332, 1981.

47. Stopfkuchen H et al. Effects of dobutamine on left ventricular performance in newborns as determined by systolic time intervals. *Eur J Pediatr* 146:135–139, 1987.

48. José AB et al. Hemodynamic effects of dobutamine in children. *Anesthesiology* 55:A61, 1981.

49. Driscoll DJ et al. Hemodynamic effects of dobutamine in children. *Am J Cardiol* 43:581–585, 1979.

50. Berner M, Rouge JL, Friedli B. The hemodynamic effect of phentolamine and dobutamine after open-heart operations in children: Influence of the underlying heart defect. *Ann Thorac Surg* 35:643–650, 1983.

51. Rees AH et al. The use of dobutamine in the treatment of infants and children with acute myocarditis (abstract). *Clin Res* 29:876A, 1981.

52. Stopfkuchen H, Queisser-Luft A, Vogel K. Cardiovascular responses to dobutamine determined by systolic time intervals in preterm infants. *Crit Care Med* 18:722–724, 1990.

53. Miall-Allen VM, Whitelaw AGL. Response to dopamine and dobutamine in the preterm infant less than 30 weeks gestation. *Crit Care Med* 17;1166–1169, 1989.

54. Bohn DJ et al. Hemodynamic effects of dobutamine after cardiopulmonary bypass in children. *Crit Care Med* 8:367–371, 1980.

55. Schranz D et al. Hemodynamic effects of dobutamine in children with cardiovascular failure. *Eur J Pediatr* 139:4–7, 1982.

56. Gnidec AG, Finley RR, Sibbald WJ. Effect of dobutamine on lung microvascular fluid flux in sheep with "sepsis syndrome." *Chest* 93:180–186, 1988.

57. Unverferth AV, Blanford M. Tolerance to dobutamine after a 72 hour continuous infusion. *Am J Med* 69:262–266, 1980.

58. Rude RE et al. Effects of inotropic and chronotropic stimuli on acute myocardial ischemic injury, I: Studies with dobutamine in the anesthetized dog. *Circulation* 65:1321–1328, 1982.

59. Hoff JV, Beatty PA, Wade JL. Dermal necrosis from dobutamine (letter). *N Engl J Med* 300:1280, 1979.

60. Jarnberg PO et al. Dopamine infusion in man. Plasma catecholamine levels and pharmacokinetics. *Acta Anaesth Scand* 25:328–231, 1981.

61. Zaritsky A et al. Steady-state dopamine clearance in critically ill infants and children. *Crit Care Med* 16:217–220, 1988.

62. McDonald RH Jr et al. Augmentation of sodium excretion and blood flow by dopamine in man. *Clin Res* 11:248, 1963.

63. McDonald RH Jr et al. Effect of dopamine in man. Augmentation of sodium excretion, glomerular filtration rare and renal plasma flow. *J Clin Invest* 43:1116–1124, 1964.

64. McNay JL, McDonald RH Jr, Goldberg LI. Comparative effects of dopamine on renal and femoral blood flow. *Pharmacology* 5:269, 1963.

65. McNay JL, McDonald RH Jr, Goldberg LI. Direct renal vasodilatation produced by dopamine in the dog. *Circ Res* 16:510–517, 1965.

66. Goldberg LI, Hsich YY, Resnekov L. Newer catecholamines for treatment of heart failure and shock: An update on dopamine and a first look at dobutamine. *Prog Cardiovasc Dis* 19:327–340, 1977.

67. Noth RH et al. Tonic dopaminergic suppression of plasma aldosterone. *J Clin Endocrinol Metab* 51:64–69, 1980.

68. Goldberg LI. Cardiovascular and renal applications of dopamine: Potential clinical applications. *Pharmacol Rev* 24:1–29, 1972.

69. Chernow B, Rainey TG, Lake CR. Endogenous and exogenous catecholamines in critical care medicine. *Crit Care Med* 10(6):409–416, 1982.

70. Drummond WH, Webb IB, Percell KA. Cardiopulmonary response to dopamine in chronically catheterized neonatal lambs. *Pediatr Pharmacol* 1:347–355, 1981.

71. Holloway EL, Polumbo RA, Hamson DC. Acute circulatory effects of dopamine in patients with pulmonary hypertension. *Br Heart J* 37:482–485, 1975.

72. Zern RT et al. Characteristics of the dopaminergic and noradrenergic systems of the pancreatic islets. *Diabetes* 28:185–189, 1979.

73. MacCannell KL et al. Dopamine in the treatment of hypotension and shock. *N Engl J Med* 275:1389–1398, 1966.

74. Talley RC et al. A hemodynamic comparison of dopamine and isoproterenol in patients in shock. *Circulation* 39:361–378, 1969.

75. Loeb HS et al. Acute hemodynamic effects of dopamine in patients with shock. *Circulation* 44:163–173, 1971.

76. Jardin F et al. Effect of dopamine on intrapulmonary shunt fraction and oxygen transport in severe sepsis with circulatory and respiratory failure. *Crit Care Med* 7:273–277, 1979.

77. De la Cal MA et al. Dose-related hemodynamic and renal effects of dopamine in septic shock. *Crit Care Med* 12:22–25, 1984.

78. Driscoll DT, Gillette PC, McNamara DG. The use of dopamine in children. *J Pediatr* 92:309–314, 1978.

79. Cuevas L et al. The effect of low-dose dopamine infusion on cardiopulmonary and renal status in premature newborns with respiratory distress syndrome. *Am J Dis Child* 145:799–803, 1991.

80. Daenen W, LeVal M, Stark J. Dopamine in open heart surgery for congenital heart disease. *Proc R Soc Med* 70:48–50, 1977.

81. Steen PA et al. Efficacy of dopamine, dobutamine, and epinephrine during emergence from cardiopulmonary bypass in man. *Circulation* 57:378–384, 1978.

82. Stephenson LW, Blackstone EH, Kouchoukos NT. Dopamine vs. epinephrine in patients following cardiac surgery: Randomized study. *Surg Forum* 22:272–275, 1976.

83. Outwater KM et al. Renal and hemodynamic effects of dopamine in infants following cardiac surgery. *J Clin Anesth* 2:253–257, 1990.

84. Stephenson LW et al. Effects of nitroprusside and dopamine on pulmonary arterial vasculature in children after cardiac surgery. *Circulation* 60(Suppl):I-104–I-110, 1979.

85. Padbury JF et al. Dopamine pharmacokinetics in critically ill newborn infants. *J Pediatr* 110:293–298, 1987.

86. Fiddler GI et al. Dopamine infusion for the treatment of myocardial dysfunction associated with a persistent transitional circulation. *Arch Dis Child* 55:194–198, 1980.

87. DiSessa TG et al. The cardiovascular effects of dopamine in the severely asphyxiated neonate. *J Pediatr* 99:772–776, 1981.

88. Walther FT et al. Cardiac output in infants with transient myocardial dysfunction. *J Pediatr* 107:781–785, 1985.

89. Goldberg LI. Dopamine—Clinical uses of an endogenous catecholamine. *N Engl J Med* 291:707–710, 1974.

90. Artman M, Parrish MD, Graham TP. Congestive heart failure in childhood and adolescence: Recognition and management. *Am Heart J* 105:471–480, 1983.

91. Polson RJ et al. The prevention of renal impairment in patients undergoing orthotopic liver grafting by infusion of low dose dopamine. *Anesthesia* 42:15–19, 1987.

92. Guller B et al. Changes in cardiac rhythm in children treated with dopamine. *Crit Care Med* 6:151–154, 1978.

93. Notterman DA. Inotropic agents: Catecholamines, digoxin, amrinone. *Crit Care Clin* 7:583–613, 1991.

94. Maggi JC, Angelats J, Scott JP. Gangrene in a neonate following dopamine therapy. *J Pediatr* 100:323–325, 1982.

95. Koerber RK et al. Peripheral gangrene associated with dopamine infusion in a child. *Clin Pediatr* 23:106–107, 1984.

96. Clutter WE et al. Epinephrine plasma metabolic clearance rates and physiologic thresholds for metabolic and hemodynamic actions in man. *J Clin Invest* 66:94, 1980.

97. Chernow B (ed). *The Pharmacologic Approach to the Critically Ill Patient* (2nd ed). Baltimore: Williams & Wilkins, 1988. P 586.

98. Soman VR, Shamoon H, Sherwin RS. Effects of physiologic infusion of epinephrine in normal humans: Relationship between the metabolic response and β-adrenergic binding. *J Clin Endocrinol Metab* 50:294, 1980.

99. Struthers AD, Whitesmith R, Reid JL. Metabolic and haemodynamic effects of increased circulating adrenaline in man. *Br Heart J* 50:277, 1983.

100. Body J-J et al. Epinephrine is a hypophosphatemic hormone in man. *J Clin Invest* 71:572, 1983.

101. Fisher D, Schwartz P, Davis A. Pharmacokinetics of exogenous epinephrine in critically ill children. *Crit Care Med* 21:111–117, 1993.

102. Lindner KH, Ahnefeld FW, Bowdler IM. Comparison of different doses of epinephrine on myocardial perfusion and resuscitation success during cardiopulmonary resuscitation in a pig model. *Am J Emerg Med* 9:27–31, 1991.

103. Brown CG et al. Effect of standard doses of epinephrine on myocardial oxygen delivery and utilization during cardiopulmonary resuscitation. *Crit Care Med* 16:536–539, 1988.

104. Brown CG et al. Comparative effect of graded doses of epinephrine on regional brain blood flow during COR in a swine mode. *Ann Emerg Med* 15:1138–1144, 1986.

105. Kosnik JW et al. Dose-related response of centrally administered epinephrine on the change in aortic diastolic pressure during closed-chest massage in dogs. *Ann Emerg Med* 14:204–208, 1985.

106. Lindner KH, Ahnefeld FW, Prengel AW. Comparison of standard and high-dose adrenaline in the resuscitation of asystole and electromechanical dissociation. *Acta Anaesthesiol Scand* 35:253–256, 1991.

107. Stiell IG et al. A study of high-dose epinephrine in human COR. *Ann Emerg Med* 21:206, 1992.

108. Callahan M et al. A randomized clinical trial of high-dose epinephrine and norepinephrine versus standard-dose epinephrine in prehospital cardiac arrest. *Ann Emerg Med* 21:606–607, 1992.

109. Pediatric advanced life support. *JAMA* 268:2262–2274, 1992.

110. Roberts JR et al. Blood levels following intravenous and endotracheal epinephrine administration. *JACEP* 8:53–56, 1979.

111. Aitkenhead AR. Drug administration during CPR: What route? *Resuscitation* 22:191–195, 1991.

112. Guyton AC. The autonomic nervous system: The adrenal medulla. In Guyton AC (ed): *Textbook of Medical Physiology*. Philadelphia: Saunders, 1991. P 670.

113. Wildey GM, Kunio SM, Graham RM. Atrial natriuretic factor: Biosynthesis and mechanism of action. In Fozzard HA (ed): *The Heart and Cardiovascular System* (2nd ed). New York: Raven, 1992. P 1783.

114. Gombos EA et al. Reactivity of renal and systematic circulation to vasoconstrictor agents in normotensive and hypertensive subjects. *J Clin Invest* 41:203, 1962.

115. Cronin RE et al. Pathogenic mechanisms in early norepinephrine-induced acute renal failure: Functional and histologic correlates of protection. *Kidney Int* 14:115, 1978.

116. Patak RV et al. Study of factors which modify the development of norepinephrine-induced acute renal failure in the dog. *Kidney Int* 15:227, 1979.

117. Parker MM et al. Serial hemodynamic patterns in survivors and nonsurvivors of septic shock in humans. *Crit Care Med* 12:311, 1984.

118. Desjars P et al. A reappraisal of norepinephrine therapy in human septic shock. *Crit Care Med* 15:134, 1987.

119. Dasta JF. Norepinephrine in septic shock: Renewed interest in an old drug. *Drug Intell Clin Pharm* 24(2):153, 1990.

120. Martin C et al. Septic shock: A goal-directed therapy using volume loading, dobutamine and/or norepinephrine. *Acta Anaesthesiol Scand* 34:413, 1990.

121. Schreuder WO et al. Effect of dopamine vs norepinephrine on hemodynamics in septic shock. Emphasis on right ventricular performance. *Chest* 95:1282, 1989.

122. Desjars P et al. Norepinephrine therapy has no deleterious renal effects in human septic shock. *Crit Care Med* 17:426, 1989.

123. Hesselvik J, Brodin B. Low dose norepinephrine in patients with septic shock and oliguria: Effects of afterload, urine flow, and oxygen transport. *Crit Care Med* 17:179, 1989.

124. Fukuoka T et al. Effects of norepinephrine on renal function in septic patients with normal and elevated serum lactate levels. *Crit Care Med* 17:1104, 1989.

125. Zaritsky A, Chernow B. Catecholamines and other inotropes. In Chernow B (ed): *The Pharmacologic Approach to the Critically Ill Patient* (2nd ed). Baltimore: Williams & Wilkins, 1988. P 585.

126. Teba L et al. Beneficial effect of norepinephrine in the treatment of circulatory shock caused by tricyclic antidepressant overdose. *Am J Emerg Med* 6:566, 1988.

127. Robinson RJ, Tchervenkov C. Treatment of low cardiac output after aortocoronary artery bypass surgery using a combination of norepinephrine and amrinone. *J Cardiothorac Anesth* 1:229, 1987.

128. Lathi KG et al. The use of amrinone and norepinephrine for inotropic support during emergence from cardiopulmonary bypass. *J Cardiothorac Vasc Anesth* 5:250, 1991.

129. Coyle JP et al. Left atrial infusing of norepinephrine in the management of right ventricular failure. *J Cardiothorac Anesth* 4:80, 1990.

130. Nakatsuka M, Mobley K. The combined use of noradrenaline, amrinone and nitroglycerin in the management of severe low cardiac output after coronary artery surgery. *Anaesth Int Care* 16:485, 1988.

131. Lindner KH, Ahnefeld FW, Schuermann W. Epinephrine and norepinephrine in cardiopulmonary resuscitation. Effects on myocardial oxygen delivery and consumption. *Chest* 97:1458, 1990.

132. Lindner KH et al. Epinephrine versus norepinephrine in prehospital ventricular fibrillation. *Am J Cardiol* 67:427, 1991.

133. Lindner KH, Ahnefeld FW. Comparison of epinephrine and norepinephrine in the treatment of asphyxial or fibrillatory cardiac arrest in a porcine model. *Crit Care Med* 17:437, 1989.

134. Hoffman BB, Lefkowitz RJ. Catecholamines and sympathomimetic drugs. In Gilman AG et al (eds): *Goodman and Gilman's The Pharmacological Basis of Therapeutics*. New York: Pergamon, 1990. Pp 201–202.

135. Goldstein DS et al. Plasma catecholamine and hemodynamic responses during isoproterenol infusions in humans. *Clin Pharmacol Ther* 40:233–238, 1986.

136. Crone RK. The cardiovascular effects of isoproterenol in the preterm newborn lamb. *Crit Care Med* 12:33–35, 1984.

137. Driscoll DJ. Use of inotropic and chronotropic agents in neonates. *Clin Perinatol* 14:931–949, 1987.

138. Driscoll DJ et al. Comparative hemodynamic effects of isoproterenol, dopamine, and dobutamine in the newborn dog. *Pediatr Res* 13:1006–1009, 1979.

139. Gunnar RM et al. Ineffectiveness of isoproterenol in shock due to acute myocardial infarction. *JAMA* 202:64–68, 1967.

140. Mueller H et al. Hemodynamics, coronary blood flow, and myocardial metabolism in coronary shock; response to 1-norepinephrine and isoproterenol. *J Clin Invest* 49:1885–1900, 1970.

141. Lekven J, Kjekshus JK, Mjos OD. Cardiac effects of isoproterenol during graded myocardial ischemia. *Scand J Clin Lab Invest* 33:161–171, 1974.

142. Maguire JF, Geha RS, Umetsu DT. Myocardial specific creatinine phosphokinase isoenzyme elevation in children with asthma treated with intravenous isoproterenol. *J Allergy Clin Immunol* 78:631–636, 1986.

143. Mikhail MS et al. Myocardial ischemia complicating therapy of status asthmaticus. *Clin Pediatr* 26:419–421, 1987.

144. Matson JR, Loughlin GM, Strunk RC. Myocardial ischemia complicating the use of isoproterenol in asthmatic children. *J Pediatr* 92:776–778, 1978.

145. Kurland G, Williams J, Lewiston NJ. Fatal myocardial toxicity during continuous infusion intravenous isoproterenol therapy of asthma. *J Allergy Clin Immunol* 63:407–411, 1979.

146. Maguire JF et al. Cardiotoxicity during treatment of severe childhood asthma. *Pediatrics* 88:1180–1186, 1991.

147. Rosenblum R, Berkowitz WD, Lawson D. Effect of acute intravenous administration of isoproterenol on cardiorenal hemodynamics in man. *Circulation* 38:158–168, 1968.

148. Furman WR et al. Comparison of the effects of dobutamine, dopamine, and isoproterenol on hypoxic pulmonary vasoconstriction in the pig. *Crit Care Med* 10:371–374, 1982.

149. Crowley MR, Fineman JR, Soifer SJ. Effects of vasoactive drugs on thromboxane A₂ mimetic-induced pulmonary hypertension in newborn lambs. *Pediatr Res* 29:167–172, 1991.

150. Gazioglu K et al. Effect of isoproterenol on gas exchange during air and oxygen breathing in patients with asthma. *Am J Med* 50:185–190, 1971.

151. Mentzer RM, Alegre CA, Nolan SP. The effects of dopamine and isoproterenol on the pulmonary circulation. *J Thorac Cardiovasc Surg* 71:807–814, 1976.

152. Parry WH, Martorano F, Cotton EK. Management of life-threatening asthma with intravenous isoproterenol infusions. *Am J Dis Child* 130:39–42, 1976.

153. Herman JJ, Noah ZL, Moody RP. Use of intravenous isoproterenol for status asthmaticus in children. *Crit Care Med* 11:716–720, 1983.

154. Klaustermeyer WB, DiBernardo RL, Hale FC. Intravenous isoproterenol: Rationale for bronchial asthma. *J Allergy Clin Immunol* 55:325–333, 1975.

155. O'Rourke PP, Crone RK. Effect of isoproterenol on measured theophylline levels. *Crit Care Med* 12:373–375, 1984.

156. Horowitz LN et al. Effects of aminophylline on the threshold for initiating ventricular fibrillation during respiratory failure. *Am J Cardiol* 35:376–379, 1975.

157. Urthaler F, James TN. Both direct and neurally mediated components of the chronotropic actions of aminophylline. *Chest* 70:24–32, 1976.

158. Notterman DA. Pharmacologic support of the failing circulation: An approach for infants and children. *Probl Anesth* 3:288–309, 1989.

159. Eichna LW. The treatment of cardiogenic shock, the use of isoproterenol in cardiogenic shock. *Am Heart J* 74:848–852, 1967.

160. Carey JS et al. Cardiovascular function in shock, responses to volume loading and isoproterenol infusion. *Circulation* 35:327–338, 1967.

161. Lupi-Herrera E et al. The role of isoproterenol in the preoperative

162. evaluation of high-pressure, high-resistance ventricular septal defect. *Chest* 81:42–46, 1982.

163. Waxman MB et al. Isoproterenol induction of vasodepressor-type reaction in vasodepressor-prone persons. *Am J Cardiol* 63:58–65, 1989.

164. Colucci WS, Wright RF, Braunwald E. New positive inotropic agents in the treatment of congestive heart failure. *N Engl J Med* 314:349–357, 1986.

165. Endoh M et al. Effects of new inotropic agents on cyclic nucleotide metabolism and calcium transients in canine ventricular muscle. *Circulation* 73(Suppl III):117–131, 1986.

166. Endoh M, Yamashita S, Taira N. Positive inotropic effect of amrinone in relation to cyclic nucleotide metabolism in the canine ventricular muscle. *J Pharmacol Exp Ther* 221:775–783, 1982.

167. Levine SD et al. The effects of amrinone on transport and cyclic AMP metabolism in toad urinary bladder. *J Pharmacol Exp Ther* 216:220–224, 1981.

168. Gaide MS et al. Effects of amrinone on contraction and K⁺-induced contracture of normal and subacutely failed cat ventricular muscle. *Circulation* 73(Suppl III):36–43, 1986.

169. Sys SU et al. Inotropic effects of amrinone and milrinone on contraction and relaxation of isolated cardiac muscle. *Circulation* 73(Suppl III):25–34, 1986.

170. Alousi AA, Johnson DC. Pharmacology of the bypyridines: Amrinone and milrinone. *Circulation* 73(Suppl III):10–23, 1986.

171. Rapundalo ST et al. Myocardial actions of milrinone: Characterization of its mechanism of action. *Circulation* 73(Suppl III):134–141, 1986.

172. Sutko JL, Kenyon JL, Reeves JP. Effects of amrinone and milrinone on calcium influx into the myocardium. *Circulation* 73(Suppl III):52–57, 1986.

173. Adams HR, Rhody J, Sutko JL. Amrinone activates K⁺-depolarized atrial and ventricular myocardium of guinea pigs. *Cir Res* 51:662–665, 1982.

174. Kondo N et al. Electrical and mechanical effects of amrinone on isolated guinea pig ventricular muscle. *J Cardiovasc Pharmacol* 5:903–912, 1983.

175. Hoffman BF, Bigger JT. Digitalis and allied cardiac glycosides. In Gilman AG et al (eds): *Goodman and Gilman's The Pharmacological Basis of Therapeutics.* New York: Pergamon, 1990. Pp 836–837.

176. Edelson J et al. Relationship between amrinone plasma concentration and cardiac index. *Clin Pharmacol Ther* 29:723–728, 1981.

177. Alousi AA et al. Cardiotonic activity of amrinone. *Circ Res* 45:666–677, 1979.

178. Goldstein RA. Clinical effects of intravenous amrinone in patients with congestive heart failure. *Circulation* 73(Suppl III):191–194, 1986.

179. Kullberg MP et al. Amrinone metabolism. *Clin Pharmacol Ther* 29:394–401, 1981.

180. Edelson J et al. Pharmacokinetics of the bypyridines amrinone and milrinone. *Circulation* 73(Suppl III):145–150, 1986.

181. Lawless S et al. Amrinone in neonates and infants after cardiac surgery. *Crit Care Med* 17:751–754, 1989.

182. Binah O et al. The inotropic effects of amrinone and milrinone on neonatal and young canine cardiac muscle. *Circulation* 73(Suppl III):46–50, 1986.

183. Binah O et al. Developmental changes in the cardiac effects of amrinone in the dog. *Circ Res* 52:747–752, 1983.

184. Binah O, Danilo P, Rosen MR. Developmental changes in the effects of amrinone on cardiac contraction. *Am J Cardiol* 49:993, 1982.

185. Wilmshurst PT et al. Comparison of the effects of amrinone and sodium nitroprusside on hemodynamics, contractility, and myocardial metabolism in patients with cardiac failure due to coronary artery disease and dilated cardiomyopathy. *Br Heart J* 52:38–48, 1984.

186. Firth BG et al. Assessment of the inotropic and vasodilator effects of amrinone versus isoproterenol. *Am J Cardiol* 54:1331–1336, 1984.

187. Wilmshurst PT et al. Haemodynamic effects of intravenous amrinone

in patients with impaired left ventricular function. *Br Heart J* 49:77–82, 1983.

187. Benotti JR, Grossman W, Braunwald E. Hemodynamic assessment of amrinone. *N Engl J Med* 299:1373–1377, 1978.

188. Jentzer JH et al. Beneficial effect of amrinone on myocardial oxygen consumption during acute left ventricular failure in dogs. *Am J Cardiol* 48:75–83, 1981.

189. Benotti JR et al. Effects of amrinone on myocardial energy metabolism and hemodynamics in patients with severe congestive heart failure due to coronary artery disease. *Circulation* 62:28–34, 1980.

190. Likoff MJ et al. Amrinone in the treatment of chronic cardiac failure. *J Am Coll Cardiol* 3:1282–1290, 1984.

191. Weber KT et al. Amrinone and exercise performance in patients with chronic heart failure. *Am J Cardiol* 48:164–169, 1981.

192. Klein NA et al. Hemodynamic comparison of intravenous amrinone and dobutamine in patients with chronic congestive heart failure. *Am J Cardiol* 48:170–175, 1981.

193. Naccarelli GV et al. Amrinone: Acute electrophysiologic and hemodynamic effects in patients with congestive heart failure. *Am J Cardiol* 54:600–604, 1984.

194. Siskind SJ et al. Acute substantial benefit of inotropic therapy with amrinone on exercise hemodynamics and metabolism in severe congestive heart failure. *Circulation* 64:966–973, 1981.

195. Wessel A, Seiffert P. Amrinone in the treatment of congestive heart failure after cardiac surgery in infants and children. *Monatsschr Kinderheilkd* 137:712–715, 1989.

196. Berner M et al. Hemodynamic effects of amrinone in children after cardiac surgery. *Intensive Care Med* 16:85–88, 1990.

197. Barger G, Dale HH. Chemical structure and sympathomimetic action of amines. *J Physiol* 41:19–59, 1910.

198. Hengstmann JH, Goronzy J. Pharmacokinetics of ³H-phenylephrine in man. *Eur J Clin Pharmacol* 21:335–341, 1982.

199. Weiner N. Norepinephrine, epinephrine, and the sympathomimetic amines. In Goodman AG, Gillman LS, Gilman A (eds): *The Pharmacological Basis of Therapeutics*. New York: Macmillan, 1980. Pp 138–175.

200. Bonfiglio MF et al. High-dose phenylephrine infusion in the hemodynamic support of septic shock. *Ann Pharmacother* 24:936–939, 1990.

201. Yakaitis RW, Otto CW, Blitt CD. Relative importance of α and β adrenergic receptors during resuscitation. *Crit Care Med* 7:293–296, 1979.

202. Joyce SM, Barsan WG, Doan LA. Use of phenylephrine in resuscitation from asphyxial arrest. *Ann Emerg Med* 12:418–421, 1983.

203. Brillman JA et al. Outcome of resuscitation from fibrillatory arrest using epinephrine and phenylephrine in dogs. *Crit Care Med* 13:912–913, 1985.

204. Brillman J et al. Comparison of epinephrine and phenylephrine for resuscitation and neurologic outcome of cardiac arrest in dogs. *Ann Emerg Med* 16:27–33, 1987.

205. Midei MG et al. Preservation of ventricular function by treatment of ventricular fibrillation with phenylephrine. *J Am Coll Cardiol* 16:489–494, 1990.

206. Otto CW, Yakaitis RW. The role of epinephrine in CPR: A reappraisal. *Ann Emerg Med* 13:840–843, 1984.

207. Nudel DB, Berman MA, Talner NS. Effects of acutely increasing systemic vascular resistance on oxygen tension in tetralogy of Fallot. *Pediatrics* 58:248–251, 1976.

208. Shaddy RE et al. Continuous intravenous phenylephrine infusion for treatment of hypoxemic spells in tetralogy of Fallot. *Pediatrics* 114:468–470, 1989.

209. Jacobson L, Turnquist K, Masley S. Wolff-Parkinson-White syndrome: Termination of paroxysmal supraventricular tachycardia with phenylephrine. *Anaesthesia* 40:657–660, 1985.

210. Friedman WF, George BL. Treatment of congestive heart failure by altering loading conditions of the heart. *J Pediatr* 106:697–706, 1985.

211. Palmer RF, Lasseter KC. Sodium nitroprusside. *N Engl J Med* 292:294–297, 1975.

212. Artman M, Graham TP. Guidelines for vasodilator therapy of congestive heart failure in infants and children. *Am Heart J* 113:994–1005, 1987.

213. Gerber JG, Nies AS. Antihypertensive agents and the drug therapy of hypertension. In Gilman AG et al (eds): *Goodman and Gilman's The Pharmacological Basis of Therapeutics*. New York: Pergamon, 1990. Pp 803–804.

214. Page IH et al. Cardiovascular actions of sodium nitroprusside in animals and hypertensive patients. *Circulation* 11:188–198, 1955.

215. Gordillo-Paniagua G et al. Sodium nitroprusside treatment of severe arterial hypertension in children. *J Pediatr* 87:799–802, 1975.

216. Guiha NH et al. Treatment of refractory heart failure with infusion of nitroprusside. *N Engl J Med* 291:587–592, 1974.

217. Dillon TR et al. Vasolidator therapy for congestive heart failure. *J Pediatr* 96:623–629, 1980.

218. Beekman RH et al. Vasodilator therapy in children: Acute and chronic effects in children with left ventricular dysfunction or mitral regurgitation. *Pediatrics* 73:43–51, 1984.

219. Franciosa JA et al. Improved left ventricular function during nitroprusside infusion in acute myocardial infarction. *Lancet* i:650–654, 1972.

220. Chatterjee K et al. Hemodynamic and metabolic responses to vasodilator therapy in acute myocardial infarction. *Circulation* 48:1183–1193, 1973.

221. Nakano H, Ueda K, Saito A. Acute hemodynamic effects of nitroprusside in children with isolated mitral regurgitation. *Am J Cardiol* 56:351–355, 1985.

222. Chatterjee K et al. Beneficial effects of vasodilator agents in severe mitral regurgitation due to dysfunction of subvalvar apparatus. *Circulation* 48:684–690, 1973.

223. Goodman DJ et al. Effect of nitroprusside on left ventricular dynamics in mitral regurgitation. *Circulation* 50:1025–1032, 1974.

224. Bolen JL, Alderman EL. Hemodynamic consequences of afterload reduction in patients with chronic aortic regurgitation. *Circulation* 53:879–883, 1976.

225. Appelbaum A et al. Afterload reduction and cardiac output in infants early after intracardiac surgery. *Am J Cardiol* 39:445–451, 1977.

226. Benzing G et al. Nitroprusside after open-heart surgery. *Circulation* 54:467–471, 1976.

227. Rubis LJ et al. Comparison of effects of prostaglandin E₁ and nitroprusside on pulmonary vascular resistance in children after open-heart surgery. *Ann Thorac Surg* 32:563–570, 1981.

228. Deichmann WB, Gerarde HW. *Toxicology of Drugs and Chemicals*. New York: Academic, 1969.

229. Nourok DS et al. Hypothyroidism following prolonged sodium nitroprusside therapy. *Am J Med Sci* 248:129–138, 1964.

230. Benitz WE et al. Use of sodium nitroprusside in neonates: Efficacy and safety. *J Pediatr* 106:102–110, 1985.

IV ⬥ Central Nervous System

Thomas V. Brogan

Jeremy M. Geiduschek

Harry J. Kallas

Elliot J. Krane

26 Pathophysiology of Intracranial Emergencies

Intracranial emergencies may be precipitated by a number of diverse etiologies, including trauma, central nervous system (CNS) infections, malignancies, and systemic illness. Unfortunately, neuronal damage usually continues after patients are admitted to the hospital, and secondary insults often impair CNS healing, adding to primary damage. Often, little can be done to reverse primary CNS damage attendant on intracranial emergencies. The primary goal, then, of neurologic intensive care is to limit secondary injury. A basic understanding of the physiology of cerebral blood flow (CBF), cerebral ischemia, and the mechanics of the intracranial vault establishes the groundwork for treating patients with intracranial pathology.

Recent advances in research have provided the basis for an understanding of the events that occur at the cellular and molecular levels during and after brain injury. Many of the methods used in studying brain injury are applicable only in animal models, and extrapolation of the data to humans often remains difficult. In addition, therapies that were thought to have potential benefit in providing protection to brain-injured patients because of promising results in animal experiments have either been disproved (e.g., the use of barbiturates following cardiac arrest) or have yet to be proven helpful in the clinical setting (e.g., use of calcium channel blockers to prevent the "no reflow" phenomenon).[1,2] On the other hand, certain positive results obtained in adult series, such as the use of calcium channel blockers to prevent vasospasm following subarachnoid hemorrhage from ruptured cerebral aneurysms, and the use of hypovolemic hemodilution with dextran to improve CBF following a stroke, should lead to advances in treatment of children with brain injuries.[3,4] In this chapter we present a review of the physiology of the intracranial contents that can be used for selecting currently available and accepted treatments for children with intracranial emergencies.

Cerebral Blood Flow

A normal adult brain receives 15% of the cardiac output and has a total CBF of 50 ml/100 g tissue/min.[5] Relatively few studies have measured CBF during childhood. These studies have generally demonstrated that both cerebral oxygen consumption ($CMRO_2$) and CBF are 10% to 50% greater in the developing brain.[6,7] The major energy requirements in the brain result from the establishment and maintenance of ionic gradients, from the maintenance of cellular membranes, and from the molecular transport of various substances.[8]

CBF is not distributed uniformly throughout the brain. Areas with higher metabolic activity, such as the cortical gray matter, receive greater blood flow than areas with less activity, such as the subcortical white matter.[9] The blood flow to a **region** of the brain (rCBF) is regulated by that **region's** demand for oxygen (rCMRO$_2$). The brain has no oxygen reserve, and because the brain extracts most of the oxygen contained in its perfusing blood, the only mechanism possible to increase regional utilization of oxygen and of other metabolic substrates is to increase blood flow to that region.

The cerebral circulation possesses a number of unique features that distinguish it from the remainder of the systemic blood supply and that appear to be designed to assure delivery of adequate metabolic substrates in the face of a variety of physiologic challenges. The cerebral vasculature intrinsically regulates cerebral blood supply in response to three major physiologic parameters: cerebral metabolic rate (also $CMRO_2$), cerebral perfusion pressure (CPP), and the viscosity of the blood perfusing the brain. The mechanisms that alter blood flow as a result of changes in these three parameters have been called metabolic, pressure, and blood viscosity autoregulation, respectively.

Metabolic Autoregulation

Cerebral vessels are able to couple CBF to $CMRO_2$ in an exquisitely precise fashion. The exact mechanism of this metabolic autoregulation, which appears to occur on a localized level, remains obscure.[10] This coupling remains intact in normal individuals and usually under certain physiologic and pathologic conditions, such as seizures, changes in temperature, and anesthesia.[11] Neuronal release of vasodilator metabolites couples blood flow to metabolic rate. The identity of these metabolites has not been firmly established, although adenosine and its phosphorylated derivatives may play a critical role in regulating rCBF.[8]

Adenosine and its derivatives have been shown to relax cerebral vessels both *in vitro* and *in vivo* in animal preparations.[12–14] Adenosine acts on cerebral vessels in an endothelium-independent fashion.[15] Adenosine levels rise rapidly in the brain, and cerebral vascular resistance (CVR) decreases concomitantly after cerebral hypoxia, hypotension, ischemia, and seizures.[16] As adenosine triphosphate (ATP) is consumed for energy utilization, and high-energy phosphate bonds are broken, adenosine is released into the regional extracellular fluid (ECF). It is proposed that adenosine works by interacting with intracellular calcium-sequestering mechanisms decreasing the smooth muscle, free calcium concentration, which is needed to form actin-myosin complexes necessary for muscle contraction, ultimately resulting in vasodilatation.[17] Although initial work has demonstrated that adenosine may be responsible for control of metabolic autoregulation, more recent discoveries support a role for nitric oxide.

Nitric oxide (NO), recently discovered to be the first gas that serves as a biologic messenger molecule in mammalian physiologic systems, has also been implicated in the coupling of CBF to metabolic rate. NO is derived from the terminal guanidine group of L-arginine as it is converted to L-citrulline by nitric oxide synthase (NOS).[18] NO exerts its effect by diffusing into target cells, including vascular smooth muscle cells, and stimulating the enzyme, guanyl cyclase. This leads to increases in intracellular cGMP production, which promotes smooth muscle cell relaxation. NO has been shown to cause vasodilatation of a number of vascular beds, including cerebral blood vessels.[19] This vasodilatation requires the presence of the vascular endothelium.

NO is produced by the endothelium of large cerebral arteries in response to a variety of stimuli, including receptor agonists such as acetylcholine, ADP, and substance P.[20,21] NO concentrations increase acutely in the brain after middle cerebral artery occlusion, as do brain nitrites and cGMP levels.[22–24] These increases in NO are effectively blocked by prior administration of NOS inhibitors.[24]

Furthermore, inhibitors of NOS, when administered locally, produce profound changes in CBF, including constriction of cerebral blood vessels, diminution of the hypercapneic increases in CBF, and an inhibition of the hypercapneic increase in $CMRO_2$.[25,26] These studies suggest that NO contributes to the maintenance of basal CBF under a variety of physiologic circumstances.

Metabolic autoregulation may suffer disturbances after severe brain trauma. In such cases, CBF exceeds metabolic demands, and frequently this hyperemia may ensue because damaged neurons cannot utilize the oxygen delivered to them.[27,28]

Pressure Autoregulation

Another extremely important physiologic property intrinsic to the cerebral circulation is the ability to maintain a constant CBF over a broad range of perfusion pressures when metabolism remains fixed. This pressure autoregulation was first confirmed experimentally by direct visualization of pial vessels in the cat during fluctuations in arterial pressure.[29,30] Vasoconstriction and vasodilatation occur in response to increases or decreases in BP, respectively, preserving a normal CBF. Resistance changes begin to occur within seconds of a change in perfusion pressure. A return to baseline blood flow occurs within 2 minutes.[31] Again, the precise mechanism of pressure autoregulation remains unknown. Adenosine probably does not play a key role in pressure autoregulation, nor do changes in extracellular H^+ and K^+ appear to be involved.[32,33] Currently, pressure autoregulation is considered to be the result of an interplay between intrinsic myogenic reflexes of the smooth muscle in cerebral arterioles and metabolic mechanisms.[34]

In adult humans, autoregulation is intact when the mean arterial pressure (MAP) is between 50 and 150 mm Hg.[5] When the MAP is less than 50 mm Hg, cerebral vessels will dilate maximally and CBF will decline passively with any further decrease in MAP. When the MAP exceeds 150 mm Hg, CBF will increase with further increments of MAP because the cerebral resistance vessels are maximally constricted (Fig. 26-1). Ultimately, if the MAP becomes high enough, damage to the blood-brain barrier occurs, with resultant vasogenic cerebral edema or acute intracranial hemorrhage due to the exposure of the cerebral capillary beds to excessively high hydrostatic pressure or shearing forces.[35,36] Conse-

quently, extremes in BP often compound any existing neurologic damage.

Physiologic changes can reset autoregulation. For instance, when there is high sympathetic nervous output, as in hemorrhagic arterial hypotension, the lower limit of autoregulation is increased and with it, the threshold BP for the onset of cerebral ischemia.[37] If sympatholytics are used to lower BP, the mean BP can drop as low as 40 mm Hg without cerebral ischemia.[38] When chronic hypertension is present, autoregulatory curves are shifted to the right of normal. When the hypertension is treated, the curve may gradually shift back to its normal position. This has been demonstrated in animal models as well as in humans[39,40] (Fig. 26-2). If BP is rapidly lowered in patients with chronic hypertension, however, CBF may decrease below the reset ischemic threshold, at a level that would ordinarily be tolerated by normal individuals. In contrast, infants normally have a MAP less than 60 mm Hg, and, therefore, it is assumed that the autoregulatory limits are probably lower than in adults, although this has not been confirmed experimentally. The upper limit of autoregulation in infants is not known.

CNS injury may alter pressure autoregulation. Pressure autoregulation is impaired in the vicinity of focal abnormalities caused by trauma, ischemia, or hypoxemia.[41-43] This disturbance may occur shortly after the injury or may be delayed up to a week after the initial insult.[44-49] In these cases, CBF passively follows changes in MAP (Fig. 26-3). In the absence of physical injury, pressure autoregulation can be overridden when vasodilatation is induced by hypercarbia, hypoxia, seizure activity, and administration of volatile anesthetic agents or opiate antagonists[50] (Figs. 26-4, 26-5, 26-6).

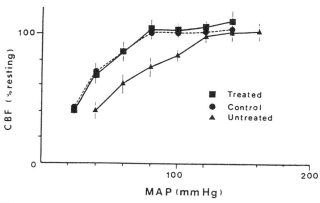

Figure 26-2. Lower part of the CBF autoregulation curve in renal hypertensive rats after 8 weeks of antihypertensive treatment with reserpine, dihydralazine, and hydrochlorothiazide. Also shown are untreated renal hypertensive and normotensive control rats. CBF measurements were made at approximately 10-mm Hg MAP intervals during angiotensin II–induced elevations of MAP and during controlled hemorrhagic hypotension. Results are expressed as percent baseline CBF and grouped at 20-mm Hg MAP intervals. The lower limit of autoregulation was in the MAP range of 50 to 69 mm Hg in control rats. In the untreated renal hypertensive rats, the lower limit was shifted to the MAP range of 90 to 109 mm Hg, whereas in the treated rats it was restored to normal (i.e., 50–69 mm Hg). Values are mean ± SEM. (From S Vorstrup et al. Chronic antihypertensive treatment reverses the hypertension-induced changes in cerebral blood flow autoregulation. *Stroke* 15:312–318, 1984. Reproduced with permission. *Stroke.* Copyright © 1984 American Heart Association.)

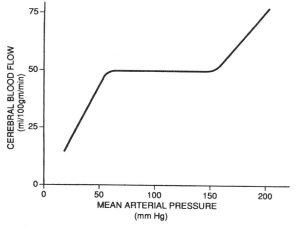

Figure 26-1. The normal pressure autoregulation curve for cerebral blood flow in humans. The lower limits of pressure autoregulation in newborns and infants is not known. See text for details.

Figure 26-3. Mean values of cerebrovascular resistance (CVR) in control, low-trauma, and severe-trauma groups of cats during progressive hemorrhagic hypotension. Injury was induced by fluid percussion. In control animals there is a progressive fall in CVR as MAP is reduced from 140 to 60 mm Hg. This signifies that progressive cerebrovascular dilation is occurring to maintain normal CBF. Below 60 mm Hg, CVR increases and CBF decreases (not shown), implying that vascular dilation from this point was inadequate to maintain CBF. The CVR curves in the trauma groups demonstrate that some autoregulatory activity is preserved, but the threshold below which CBF falls (associated with a rise in CVR) is increased by 20 to 30 mm Hg from control levels. MAP, mean arterial pressure. (From W Lewelt, LW Jenkins, JD Miller. Autoregulation of cerebral blood flow after experimental fluid percussion injury of the brain. *J Neurosurg* 53:500–511, 1980. With permission.)

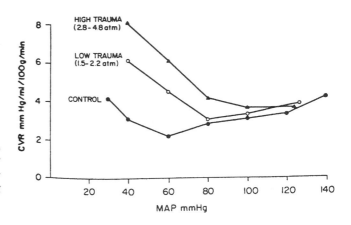

Figure 26-4. Loss of autoregulation due to reduction in arterial pressure during prolonged hypoxia (6% inspired oxygen) in a dog model. Changes in BP are induced by withdrawing and reinfusing blood. Arterial blood gasses were measured 1 minute before and during pressure reduction. Cort. B.F., cortical blood flow. (From K Kogure et al. Effects of hypoxia on cerebral autoregulation. *Am J Physiol* 219:1393–1396, 1970. With permission.)

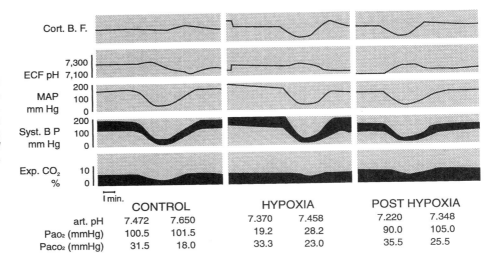

	CONTROL		HYPOXIA		POST HYPOXIA	
art. pH	7.472	7.650	7.370	7.458	7.220	7.348
Pao₂ (mmHg)	100.5	101.5	19.2	28.2	90.0	105.0
Paco₂ (mmHg)	31.5	18.0	33.3	23.0	35.5	25.5

Figure 26-5. Response of cortical blood flow to changes in mean arterial blood pressure in normocapnic dogs. (From AM Harper. Autoregulation of cerebral blood flow: Influence of the arterial blood pressure on the blood flow through the cerebral cortex. *J Neurol Neurosurg Psychiatry* 29:398–403, 1966. With permission.)

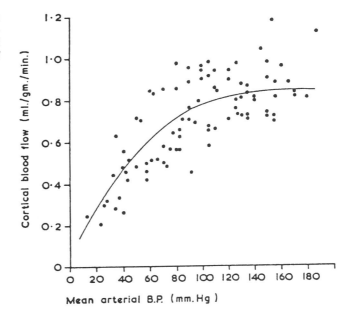

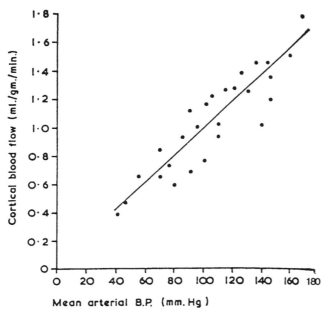

Figure 26-6. Response of cortical blood flow to changes in MAP in hypercapnic ($PaCO_2$ 66–91 mm Hg) dogs. Autoregulation is abolished during hypercapnia. This may be due to maximal dilation of vessels that cannot dilate further in response to a decrease in BP. Line is calculated linear regression. (From AM Harper. Autoregulation of cerebral blood flow: Influence of the arterial blood pressure on the blood flow through the cerebral cortex. *J Neurol Neurosurg Psychiatry* 29:398–403, 1966. With permission.)

Blood Viscosity Autoregulation

Blood viscosity serves as the final trigger for autoregulatory control of CBF. Cranial window experiments in cats demonstrated that a bolus infusion of 1 g/kg of mannitol, which decreased blood viscosity by 23%, resulted in cerebral arteriolar constriction 10 minutes later.[51,52] One hour after the mannitol infusion, viscosity increased 10%, with an accompanying 12% increase in vessel diameter. Cerebral blood viscosity autoregulation occurs with hemodilution to approximately 70% of baseline hematocrit.[53]

Carbon Dioxide and Oxygen as Chemical Mediators of Cerebral Blood Flow

Among the most important chemical mediators of CBF are arterial carbon dioxide and oxygen tensions. Increases in $PaCO_2$ between approximately 20 and 80 mm Hg augment CBF, while reductions of $PaCO_2$ cause vasoconstriction and decreased CBF.[5,54] A change 2znin $PaCO_2$ by 1 mm Hg results in a change of approximately 2% to 3% in CBF (Fig. 26-7). Carbon dioxide readily diffuses across the blood-brain barrier and enters the cerebral spinal fluid (CSF); a rise of CSF carbon dioxide tension lowers CSF pH, which in turn produces vessel smooth-muscle relaxation.[55] At a $PaCO_2$ of 80 mm Hg, the cerebral vasculature essentially reaches maximal dilatation, and further incremental increases in $PaCO_2$ result in smaller changes in CBF. Also, as $PaCO_2$ drops below 20 mm Hg, vasoconstriction may produce cerebral ischemia[56] (Figs. 26-8,26-9).

$PaCO_2$-induced changes in CBF occur rapidly and reach full equilibrium within 12 minutes. However, if the $PaCO_2$ is reduced

for prolonged periods (i.e., >36 hours), CSF bicarbonate will increase and CSF pH will return toward normal.[57] This has important implications for therapy, as control of CBF by hyperventilation becomes progressively less effective over time as pH changes are buffered.[58] Molecular carbon dioxide and bicarbonate ions have no intrinsic effect on cerebral vessels but rather produce their effect via changes in pH. Furthermore, intravascular pH does not affect pH in the CSF because H^+ and HCO_3^- do not penetrate the blood-brain barrier; hence, a metabolic acidosis or alkalosis will not cause rapid changes in CBF.[59]

Reactivity to carbon dioxide may be altered by a number of insults, including trauma, surgery, arterial hypotension, focal ischemia, and hemorrhage.[43,60,61] In focal cerebral ischemia, vascular reactivity to changes in $PaCO_2$ is impaired locally and blood vessels become maximally dilated. If the $PaCO_2$ is allowed to rise in such patients, blood vessels in the uninjured portion of the brain will dilate, and blood flow will be diverted from the injured areas to other areas of the brain because of the loss of vasomotor reactivity.

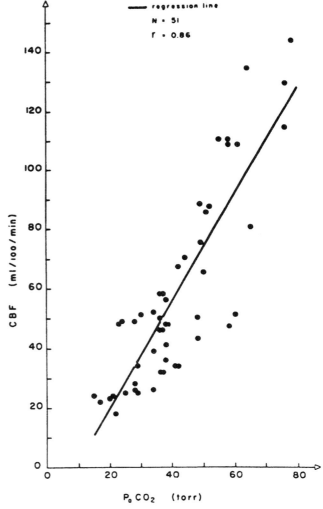

Figure 26-7. CBF versus $PaCO_2$ in rhesus monkeys. (From RL Grubb Jr et al. The effects of changes in $PaCO_2$ on cerebral blood volume, blood flow, and vascular mean transit time. *Stroke* 5:630–639, 1974. Reproduced with permission. *Stroke.* Copyright © 1974 American Heart Association.)

Figure 26-8. The effect of arterial hypocapnia on mean regional cerebral blood flow (rCBF) and mean cerebral metabolic rate for oxygen consumption (rCMRO$_2$) in the brain cortex of cats. (From J Grote, K Zimmer, R Schubert. Effects of severe arterial hypocapnia on regional blood flow regulation, tissue PO$_2$ and metabolism in the brain cortex of cats. *Eur J Physiol [Pflugers Arch]* 391:195–199, 1981. With permission.)

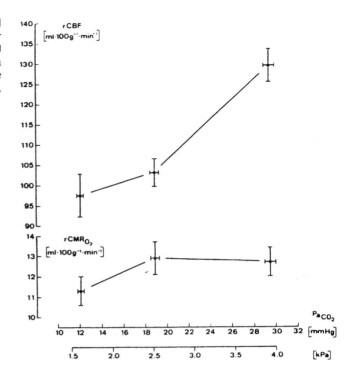

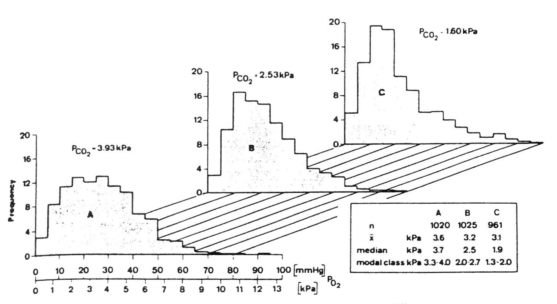

Figure 26-9. Tissue PO$_2$ frequency histograms in the brain cortex of cats determined at different levels of arterial carbon dioxide tension. **(A)** Conditions of normocapnia (PaCO$_2$ = 30 mm Hg) and normoxia. Tissue PO$_2$ ranges from less than 10 to 95 mm Hg. **(B)** Moderate PaCO$_2$ reduction (PaCO$_2$ = 19 mm Hg) results in a shift of PO$_2$ histograms to lower values. **(C)** Severe hypocapnia (PaCO$_2$ = 12 mm Hg) generates a significant increase in the number of tissue PaO$_2$ measurements less than 10 mm Hg. (From J Grote, K Zimmer, R Schubert. Effects of severe arterial hypocapnia on regional blood flow regulation, tissue PO$_2$ and metabolism in the brain cortex of cats. *Eur J Physiol [Pflugers Arch]* 391:195–199, 1981. With permission.)

This diversion of blood flow can result in extension of infarction or worsening of ischemia and is known as "intracerebral steal."[62] Conversely, if PaCO$_2$ is lowered, blood flow to the ischemic area will be promoted. This is known as "inverse steal" or "Robin Hood steal" (Figs. 26-10, 26-11).

At first glance, CBF appears to respond less dramatically to changes in PaO$_2$. This is true to a limit and results from the variable affinity of oxygen for hemoglobin as dictated by the hemoglobin oxygen-dissociation curve. Thus, significant decreases in oxygen delivery, whether due to anemia, hypoxemia, or carbon monoxide

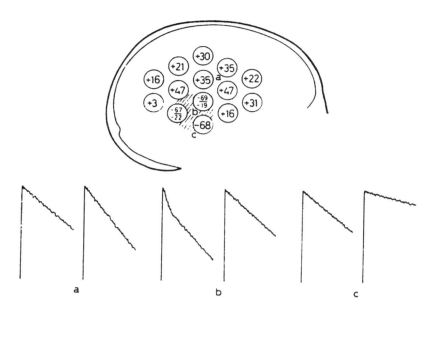

Figure 26-10. The steal syndrome. The diagram depicts a patient with a malignant glioma *(shaded area)* and the position of multiple scintillation detectors. Pairs of clearance curves from the counters, labeled a, b, and c, are shown at the bottom. The speed with which counts disappear is proportional to the blood flow to the underlying area of brain. The left clearance curve of each pair is at a $PaCO_2$ of 40 mm Hg and the right, at 55 mm Hg. An increase in blood flow at the higher $PaCO_2$ is indicated by an greater slope in the right-hand clearance curve. A decrease in blood flow at a $PaCO_2$ of 55 mm Hg would result in a lesser slope in the right curve. Numbers in circles represent the percentage change from control blood flow at $PaCO_2$ 40 mm Hg. When two percentages are contained in the circle, they represent the change from each phase of the control clearance curve (e.g., the left curve registered from counter (b) has two distinct phases. When the $PaCO_2$ is increased to 55, blood flow decreases 69% from the initial portion of the clearance curve (approx. 1 minute in duration) and 19% for the remainder of the time that clearance was calculated. (From L Symon. The concept of intracerebral steal. *Int Anesthesiol Clin* 7:597–615, 1969. With permission.)

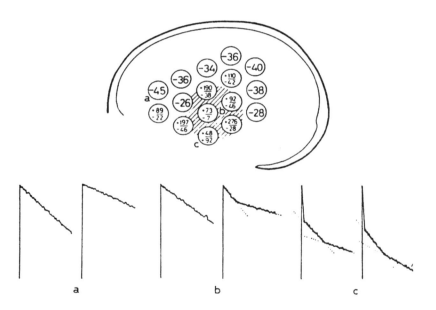

Figure 26-11. Inverse steal syndrome. Parameters are the same as in Fig 26-10, but here the right-hand members of the pairs were taken at a $PaCO_2$ of 29 mm Hg. Hyperventilation has caused a decreased flow in normal brain and an increased flow in the tumor zone. (From L Symon. The concept of intracerebral steal. *Int Anesthesiol Clin* 7:597–615, 1969. With permission.)

poisoning, produce increases in CBF. Hence, when PaO_2 drops below 50 mm Hg, CBF rapidly increases[63] (Fig. 26-12). The coupling mechanism between hypoxemia and cerebral vasodilatation may be related to a fall in extracellular fluid pH or to a rise in ECF adenosine. The latter is supported by experiments in which administration of theophylline, an adenosine antagonist, results in attenuated CBF responses to hypoxemia.[64,65] Oxygen reactivity may also be altered in the face of CNS injury, which impairs carbon dioxide reactivity.[63]

Neurologic Input and Autonomic Innervation

Cerebral blood vessels are innervated by a generous array of autonomic nerves. Sympathetic nerves supplying cerebral vessels originate predominantly from the ipsilateral superior cervical gan-

glia.[66,67] Sympathetic nerves appear to have only minimal effect on resting CBF, although there has been a great deal of debate about the extent of this influence.[66,68] However, sympathetic stimulation during arterial hypertension decreases the augmentation of CBF, especially when MAP exceeds autoregulatory limits, and this sympathetic activation attenuates disturbances in the blood-brain barrier.[69,70] During systemic hypercapnia and hypoxia, sympathetic input produces vasoconstriction of large cerebral arteries, reducing the augmentation of CBF in response to these stimuli.[63–71] Although innervation is less dense in cerebral veins than in arteries, pial veins appear to be more sensitive to sympathetic stimulation than are pial arteries, producing constriction in these capacitance vessels, with resultant decreases in CBV.[72]

Cerebral vessels are also supplied with a rich network of cholinergic parasympathetic nerves.[73] In contrast to sympathetic nerves, parasympathetic nerves appear to have no influence on cerebral

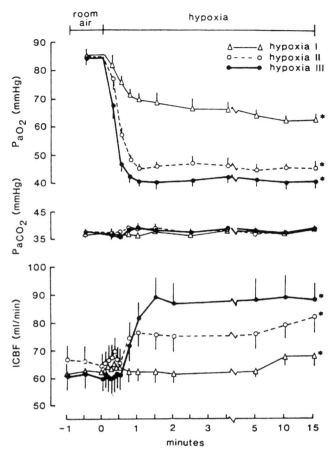

Figure 26-12. The effect of isocapnic hypoxia in unanesthetized ponies. Time course of changes in partial pressure of arterial oxygen and carbon dioxide, and internal carotid artery blood flow (ICBF). Hypoxia I, II, and III correspond to an FiO_2 of 16%, 11%, and 8%, respectively. *15-min value significantly different from prehypoxia value ($p < 0.05$). (From LC Wagerle et al. Cerebrovascular response to acute decreases in arterial PO_2. *J Cereb Blood Flow Metab* 3:507–515, 1983. With permission.)

veins and do not innervate intraparenchymal arteries.[67] The origin of cholinergic nerves is not well understood, although the greater superficial petrosal nerve and cranial nerves III, VII, IX, and X have been implicated.[66,73] Cholinergic stimulation principally produces increases in CBF via vasodilatation, although this effect does not appear to be significant during hypercapnia.[74] A significant effect of these cholinergic nerves may be to modulate the effects of sympathetic nerve stimulation.[66]

Cerebral arteries also appear to be supplied by autonomic nerves containing the neurotransmitters' vasoactive intestinal peptide (VIP) and substance P.[66,73] Both neurotransmitters relax cerebral arteries, and the vasodilation caused by VIP is blocked by cyclooxygenase inhibitors, suggesting a possible involvement of prostaglandins in this response.[75] Like cholinergic fibers, VIP-containing fibers do not appear to mediate vasodilatation during hypercapnia.[43]

Cerebral Blood Flow Measurement

Alterations in CBF and autoregulatory mechanisms profoundly affect the potential for secondary cerebral injury and ultimate

recovery in children with severe neurologic injuries. In a study of traumatic brain injury, CBF was the second most consistent predictor of patient outcome after $CMRO_2$.[76] When the hyperperfusion state of the acute posttraumatic phase receded, the predictive value equaled that of $CMRO_2$. Consequently, a great deal of effort has been invested in establishing convenient and accurate methods of measuring CBF. However, the only methods available for direct measurement of CBF remain cumbersome and do not allow for repeated measurements in the clinical setting. A number of indirect methods have been developed and have now achieved a wider spectrum of application. The following section details some of the more important direct and indirect means of CBF assessment.

Several inert substances and isotope clearance techniques exist to measure CBF. The Kety-Schmidt method relies on the Fick principle to measure the washout of inhaled nitrous oxide (N_2O) from the brain. N_2O is not metabolized by the brain, so as the brain becomes saturated with N_2O, the venous content approximates the arterial content. CBF is calculated based on the rate at which the venous content approaches the arterial content according to the equation:

$$CBF \ (ml/100 \ g/min) = \frac{(100 \times Vt \times S)}{\int (AV)dt}$$

where Vt is the cerebral venous content of N_2O at equilibrium, S is the blood-brain partition coefficient, and (AV)dt is the arteriovenous difference of N_2O from the beginning of inhalation to the time of equilibrium.

This method requires both jugular bulb venous and arterial blood sampling and provides measurement of mean hemispheric blood flow.[77] The venous sample cannot be contaminated with extracerebral blood.

Measurement of rCBF can be accomplished with external scintillation counters following intracarotid injections or inhalational administration of [133]Xe.[78–80]

Positron emission tomography (PET) evaluates rCBF and metabolism in a noninvasive fashion. Radioisotopes, which emit positrons, are either injected intravenously or inhaled. The positrons collide with electrons in the surrounding tissue, releasing gamma rays, which are measured by external scanners.[81] Anatomic distribution of blood flow is determined by measuring the local radiotracer concentration over the time of the scan, the concentration of the radiotracer in the arterial blood over the same period, and the blood-brain barrier partition coefficient for the tracer. Newer scanners have a resolution of 5 mm, with excellent uniformity of resolution throughout the field of view.

In addition to blood flow, PET provides measurements of physiologic and metabolic function as it detects small changes in the concentration of radioactively labeled tracer in tissues over time. PET scanners measure $rCMRO_2$, regional oxygen extraction fraction, regional cerebral metabolic rate for glucose, rCBV, pH, and blood-brain barrier permeability. PET can follow the evolution of an area of brain from ischemia to infarction and distinguishes areas of ischemia from areas of infarction.[82,83]

The half-life of positron-emitting compounds is very short so that an on-site or nearby cyclotron and radiochemistry facility are often required for their production, although some PET scanners may use rubidium scanners.[84] Unfortunately, these requirements make the cost of PET scanning prohibitive for most medical centers. Another nuclear medicine technique, single photon emission computed tomography (SPECT) also utilizes radiolabeled compounds such as Technetium 99 or Iodine 123 to provide tomographic images. SPECT provides images with poorer spatial resolution than does PET.[85]

Transcranial Doppler (TCD) provides a noninvasive estimation of intracranial CBF by utilizing ultrasound technology to measure blood velocity in cerebral arteries at the base of the brain. The low-frequency signals (1–2 MHz) introduced by Aaslid and colleagues contrasts with earlier probe signals (4–10 MHz) by their superior penetration of bony tissues and ability to insonate the arteries of the circle of Willis, which reside deep within the brain.[86] The TCD equipment employs a pulsed, range-gated design and the depth of insonation can be adjusted by changing the time between the emission and the reception of the signal by the probe.[87] This also differs from the continuous wave Doppler ultrasound, which samples everything in the ultrasound path.

Views of intracranial vessels are commonly limited to only three transcranial windows with this technique. The transtemporal window is located just above the zygomatic arches. Here, the Doppler signal passes through the thin temporal bone to visualize the middle cerebral artery and its proximal branches, the distal intracranial carotid artery, and the proximal portions of the anterior and posterior cerebral arteries. The ophthalmic artery and the siphon (genu) of the internal carotid artery can be insonated through the transorbital window. The suboccipital window is located by placing the Doppler probe at the inion and directing the signal through the foramen magnum, allowing for visualization of the distal intracranial vertebral and basilar arteries.

Common measurements obtained using TCD include peak systolic, peak diastolic, and mean blood flow velocities. TCD can evaluate only relative changes in blood flow through inflow channels when the arterial diameter at the recording site does not change significantly during the period of insonation. Current Doppler equipment can also estimate the pulsatility index (PI) where

$$PI = \frac{(Vs - Vd)}{Vm}$$

where Vs is peak systolic velocity, Vd is end-diastolic velocity, and Vm is mean velocity.[88] PI is an attempt to use waveform analysis to evaluate the resistance in the distal vasculature. The value of PI, unlike absolute blood velocity, does not vary with the angle of incidence between the blood flow and the ultrasound beam axis. Generally, the PI is decreased in conditions that result in diminished intracranial vascular resistance and increased in conditions that result in augmented intracranial vascular resistance. Changes in cardiac contractility, however, will also affect PI, which may make repeated measurements difficult to compare in critically ill patients.

Blood velocity measurements can vary with age, sex, $PaCO_2$, hematocrit, cardiac output, BP, intracranial pressure (ICP), vessel anatomy, and brain activation. The reliability of this method of measuring CBF depends to a large degree on the knowledge and experience of the technician and interpreter. Anatomic variations and even obscure positioning may be difficult to distinguish from disease.

In those patients with vascular anomalies, identification of vessels and interpretation of TCD studies can be problematic. For these individuals, a flow mapping technique has been developed that utilizes a computerized three-dimensional image of the cerebral vasculature reconstructed from angiographic data. This image can then be used in guiding proper placement of the TCD probe.[89]

TCD has the advantages of being noninvasive, portable, and easily reproducible. It may be employed in monitoring brain-injured patients, diagnosing vasospasm in patients with subarachnoid hemorrhage, identifying vascular stensosis, establishing the presence of feeding arteries of AV malformations and monitoring the hemodynamic effects of their treatment, confirming the clinical diagnosis of brain death, and postoperative monitoring of neurosurgical patients. TCD may also provide a noninvasive method to study the CBF response to various medications, such as anesthetics and vasoactive compounds.

Laser Doppler flowmetry (LDF) utilizes the Doppler shift of laser waves to measure the movement of RBCs within the microcirculation. LDF has a small sample volume, approximately 1 μL, imparting a high spatial resolution and is therefore better suited for the monitoring of local CBF rather than rCBF.[90] LDF can be applied to vessels with a diameter of 5 to 500 μm, which would include arterioles, capillaries, and venules.[91–93] Blood flow to various cerebral tissues may be measured by using a variety of different probes, including straight standard, surface angular, needle, microneedle, endoscopic, integrated, and implantable.[94,95] Probe movement during LDF measurements will degrade image resolution and may result in moderate changes in the measurement of CBF.[96–98]

CBF measurements obtained by LDF are not expressed in absolute flow units (ml/100 g/min) but rather are measured in arbitrary units (mV). The conversion of LDF measurements to absolute flow units has been shown to be unreliable.[92,93,99] However, LDF-measured changes in CBF during continuous measurement correlate linearly with values obtained by other, established techniques.[92,93,99,100]

LDF was used initially to measure CBF in a continuous fashion during surgical treatment of AV malformations and tumors.[91,101,102] These studies demonstrate the ability to evaluate microcirculatory hemodynamic changes produced during surgery. Multimodal probes that continuously measure LDF, NADH redox state, and concentrations of K^+, Ca^{2+}, and Na^+ simultaneously in cerebral tissue of patients have also been employed during surgery.[103] The first postoperative measurements were performed by Hashimoto and colleagues on patients with ruptured cerebral aneurysms.[104] Probes were placed on the cortex intraoperatively, and measurements of CBF were continued after the patients were transferred to the intensive care unit (ICU). Since then, probes have been placed in various fashions to assure stability for long-term monitoring (up to several weeks). These placement methods include tunneling under the scalp and then securing in a subdural position and insertion through a burr hole that had previously served as the site of an intraventricular cannula.[98,105]

LDF has proved useful in combination with TCD. The LDF probe may be positioned near the suspected area of brain injury or pathology to obtain continuous monitoring of microvascular blood flow.[90] TCD complements LDF measurements by providing CBF data on a wider surrounding region of the brain.[90] The clinical value of LDF data increases when the information is compared with other routinely monitored hemodynamic parameters. Recurrent CBF patterns may indicate physiologic events, changes in the clinical status of the patient, or iatrogenic manipulations. Bolognese and colleagues demonstrated an increase in pulmonary artery pressure coincident with the onset and resolution of cerebral hyperemia over a 48-hour interval following removal of a large sphenoid wing meningioma. There were no pathologic changes in ICP.[90]

The electroencephalogram (EEG) directly reflects neuronal electrical activity and, consequently, cerebral metabolism. Changes in CBF are reflected in the EEG, and electrical changes consistent with ischemia have been well established. The EEG can be used to establish the threshold and reversibility of impaired function in ischemia.[106] As CBF drops below 25 ml/100 g of cerebral tissue/min, EEG voltage decreases. Below 15 ml/100 g/min, transmembrane ionic gradients can no longer be maintained, indicated by increases in slow frequencies and loss of postsynaptic evoked responses. Cellular edema and neuronal death occur when CBF is below 10 ml/100 g/min with an isoelectric (flat) EEG.[107] On recovery from certain injuries, however, CBF and metabolism may be partially dissociated, and in these situations, EEG better reflects cerebral metabolism than CBF.

Continuous monitoring of a 16-lead EEG is cumbersome and requires trained technical personnel. More recently, bedside computerized compressed spectral array (CSA) analysis of the EEG has become commercially available. The CSA is relatively easy to apply in the clinical setting and may be used to follow minute-to-minute changes in brain function of the patient, particularly in situations when the clinical examination has been obscured by pharmacologic agents.

Mechanisms of Secondary Brain Injury

Brain injury occurs by two main processes: primary processes, such as trauma, infection, or degeneration; and secondary processes. Primary brain injury directly produces death of a group of neurons. Secondary brain injury results in the death of neurons in other portions of the brain that remain viable after the primary event; for instance, the cerebral edema surrounding an infarction may result in ischemia adjacent to the area of brain immediately killed by the infarction process itself. Hypoxemia and ischemia are among the most common events leading to brain injury. When present, hypoxemia is usually a global phenomena; ischemia, however, may be either global or focal. Many biochemical events occur as a result of these injuries.

The events that result in secondary neuronal injury, despite numerous, disparate etiologies, seem to share similar, final, common pathways. Studies of ischemia and hypoxemia have provided invaluable insight into these injuries. As mentioned earlier, the vulnerability of various cerebral tissues to ischemic injury depends on the anatomy of the tissue in addition to the quality and duration of the ischemia and the effectiveness of reperfusion.[108,109] Furthermore, the area immediately surrounding ischemic injury initially remains viable, and the fate of these cells rests with the events following the initial insult. This area, known as the "ischemic penumbra," places an important onus on the practitioners of neurologic intensive care to act in a timely and effective manner in the face of ischemic damage.

The most significant metabolic disturbances resulting from ischemia include acidosis, energy failure, free radical production, and disruption of ion gradients, especially for calcium. These pathophysiologic processes are mutually reinforcing (Fig. 26-13). Because the brain has no oxygen or glucose reserves and very limited glycogen stores, rapid and extensive energy failure begins within seconds of complete global brain ischemia and is maximal within 3 to 5 minutes.[8] As blood supply becomes limited, anaerobic glycolysis is stimulated. Lactate is produced instead of carbon dioxide, and less ATP is created per molecule of glucose consumed. This occurs at arterial oxygen tensions or mean arterial BPs greater than those that would lead to gross energy failure.[110–113] Unless circulation and oxygenation are rapidly restored, gross energy failure ensues, followed by cytotoxic edema and cell death.

Coincident with this acidosis, ischemic energy failure dissipates

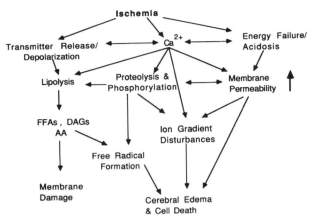

Figure 26-13. The progression from cerebral ischemia to cerebral edema and neuronal necrosis. Ischemia leads to excitotoxic neurotransmitter release, energy failure and acidosis, and a nonphysiologic rise in intracellular calcium. These in turn lead to other major adverse effects, including proteolysis, lipolysis, and membrane destruction. The result is cellular edema and necrosis. FFA, free fatty acid; DAG, diacylglyceride; AA, arachidonic acid.

neuronal ion gradients. Disturbances of ionic homeostasis and gross cellular energy failure occur at similar CBF values.[113,114] Neurons contain a number of ATP-dependent ion pumps to maintain cellular ion gradients. Such pumps include the Na+-K+ ATPase and the Ca2+-H+-antiporter. Furthermore, the energy stored in the transmembrane chemical gradients established by these two ATP-dependent pumps is utilized in the maintenance of other ionic gradients created by the Ca2+-Na+ and H+-Na+ exchangers (Fig. 26-14). As ATP and phosphocreatine are depleted, ionic homeostasis cannot be maintained because of failure of ionic pumps and increased membrane permeability.[115] Intracellular [Na+], [Ca2+], and [Cl−] rise. Osmotically obligated water follows the influx of Na+ and Cl−, leading to cerebral edema. Extracellular [K+] increases,

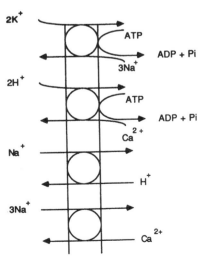

Figure 26-14. Four of the common ion channels used in maintaining neuronal ionic homeostasis. Left is extracellular and right is intracellular. From top to bottom, the pumps are (1) sodium-potassium ATPase, (2) calcium-hydrogen ion antiporter (also an ATPase), (3) hydrogen-sodium exchange pump, and (4) calcium-sodium exchange pump.

leading to membrane depolarization, often in waves that propagate into the ischemic penumbra.[116] This depolarization resembles "spreading depression," which is a propagated disturbance of membrane function that extends over the cortical surface, and may trigger or exacerbate energy failure by activating ion fluxes.[117–119] Waves of depolarization may recruit damaged cells, and infarction size has been found to correlate strongly with the number of depolarizations.[120]

Free-radical formation represents another important consequence of ischemia and contributes to neuronal injury.[121–124] Free-radical species—superoxide ($\cdot O_2^-$), hydrogen peroxide (H_2O_2), and hydroxyl ($\cdot OH$)—may be produced by the accumulation of reduced compounds in ischemic areas at low oxygen tensions. Although reperfusion of ischemic areas is required for cell survival, improved blood flow may paradoxically promote increased cellular injury by resulting in the generation of more of the harmful oxygen free radicals.[125] During ischemia, proteases will convert xanthine dehydrogenase to xanthine oxidase. Hypoxanthine and xanthine accumulate and are the purine substrates for the xanthine oxidase–mediated formation of uric acid. Superoxide anions are generated as a by-product of this reaction. These are usually scavenged by superoxide dismutase, but in ischemic states, the free radicals may overwhelm clearance systems. Left in excess, superoxide species are very reactive with cellular molecules and may be involved in the destruction of cell membranes and the development of cerebral edema. Free radicals appear to have their most significant destructive effects during prolonged periods of ischemia, with or without reperfusion.[126] The cerebral microvasculature appears to be one of the most sensitive areas to free-radical damage.[127]

Metabolic disturbances caused by ischemia, including the formation of free-radical species, are exacerbated by profound disturbances in calcium regulation. Intracellular calcium is an important second messenger involved in the regulation of many basic cellular functions. Elevations of calcium concentrations activate a series of enzymes, including protein kinase C, phospholipases, proteases (calpains), protein phosphatases, and nitric oxide synthase.[128–130] The activation of protein kinase C may result in phosphorylation of membrane receptors or ionic channels, helping to establish the sustained rise of intracellular calcium. Stimulation of phospholipase A2 and phospholipase C causes hydrolysis of membrane phospholipids and an increase of lysophospholipids diacylglycerides (DAGs) free fatty acids (FFAs), and arachidonic acid (AA).[131,132] Lysophospholipids and FFAs may act as membrane detergents and ionophores.[126] AA serves as the precursor for prostaglandins, thromboxane, platelet activating factor (PAF), and leukotrienes, all of which mediate numerous elements of the inflammatory response and play a significant role in normal and pathologic vascular functions.[132–135] Additionally, AA metabolism may produce oxygen free radicals, leading to further stimulation of phospholipases, creating a positive feedback loop for inducing cellular injury.[136] AA also potentiates N-methyl-D-aspartate (NMDA)-evoked currents.[137] Elevated calcium ultimately activates endonucleases that produce condensation of nuclear chromatin, DNA fragmentation, and nuclear breakdown. This processes is known as apoptosis.[138]

Excitotoxic Hypothesis of Cell Death

Disturbances in calcium balance appear to play a primary role in neuronal cytotoxicity, but the augmentation of intracellular $[Ca^{2+}]_i$ is probably mediated by a certain group of neurotransmitters known as "excitotoxins."[139] These amino acid neurotransmitters, including glutamate, aspartate, and others, result in excitatory activation of neurons. In high concentrations, these neurotransmitters may actually destroy neurons. The excitotoxic hypothesis is based on several observations. First, the sensitivity of neurons to injury in the face of global ischemia varies considerably but does not appear to correlate well with the level of blood flow.[140] As described earlier, ischemia-induced cytotoxic reactions coincide with elevations of $[Ca^{2+}]_i$.[141] Second, excitatory neurotransmitters produce a pattern of brain injury closely resembling that of ischemia.[139] Third, extracellular glutamate levels increase significantly following global and focal ischemia.[139] Furthermore, brain regions vulnerable to ischemia are protected when their glutamatergic afferents are removed prior to the insult.[142,143] Finally, postsynaptic glutamate receptors activate calcium channels.[144] Thus, the excitotoxic hypothesis states that when excitatory neurotransmitters reach abnormally high concentrations in the synaptic cleft, excessive Ca^{2+} influx occurs, leading to cellular injury and necrosis. This hypothesis has been expanded to include neuronal injury due to hypoglycemia, seizures, and trauma as well as in certain neurodegenerative diseases, such as Alzheimer's.[138]

Glutamate is the most closely studied excitotoxin. Excitotoxins and ischemia damage the soma and dendrites preferentially, usually sparing the axons.[139,145] Myelinated axons lack glutamate receptors and synapses but may be injured by other mechanisms, such as direct trauma, hypoxia, or free radical–mediated injury.[121,139,145] The initial event of glutamate toxicity is neuronal swelling, which results from excessive entry of sodium and chloride together with water into the cell.[139] If the insult continues, swelling is followed by degeneration of intracellular organelles and nuclear pyknosis, then finally neuronal necrosis. The latter phase appears to be related to calcium entry through specific glutamate-activated channels, resulting in the biochemical cascade described earlier.[139]

The differential vulnerability of individual neurons to glutamate depends on their particular array of receptors and ionic channels.[146] The areas that are most vulnerable to glutamate toxicity include the CA1 region of the hippocampus, the hilus of the dentate nucleus, the ventromedial portion of the caudoputamen, as well as the middle and lower cortical layers of the neocortex.[117] Postsynaptically, glutamate acts primarily at two major receptor subtypes: ionotropic (receptors linked directly to membrane ion channels) and metabotropic (receptors coupled to G proteins, resulting in alterations of intracellular second messengers). There are five types of glutamate receptors, the characterization of which is based on the specificity of agonist binding: NMDA, high- and low-affinity kainate, alpha-amino-3-hydroxyl-5-methyl-4-isoxazole propionate (AMPA), and quisqualate. Only the first four receptors types are ionotropic. Many neurons, which are most susceptible to ischemic degeneration, have a high density of NMDA receptors. NMDA channels allow the influx of both calcium and sodium but are normally blocked by Mg^{2+} in physiologic concentrations.[147] This block is relieved when the membrane depolarizes. The AMPA/kainate receptors also lead to influxes of Na^+ and Ca^{2+} after glutamate stimulation.[148] These receptors mediate fast excitatory responses in the CNS, but it has yet to be determined whether this is mediated via distinct AMPA or kainate receptors[148] (Fig. 26-15).

Influx of calcium through these receptor channels depolarizes cellular membranes and activates voltage-sensitive calcium channels (VSCC). The four types of VSCC described thus far include the N-type (found in neurons), T-type (transient current), L-type (long-duration current, large conductance channels), and P (Purkinje cells of the cerebellum).[149] The stimulation of these channels by cellular depolarization further increases intracellular calcium

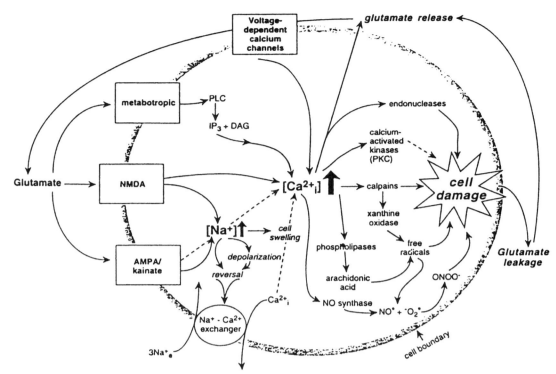

Figure 26-15. The possible mechanisms by which intracellular calcium may be increased in neurons during ischemia and the putative intracellular targets that may mediate cell damage and eventually cell death. Glutamate acts on NMDA, AMPA/kainate, and metabotropic receptors to produce an increase in cytosolic free Ca²⁺. The cytosolic Ca²⁺ interacts with diacylglyceride (DAG) to activate protein kinase C (PKC), which acts via a number of mechanisms (primarily by altering membrane ion channels) to increase neuronal excitability and further increase cytosolic Ca²⁺. Elevated cytosolic Ca²⁺ also activates several enzymes (calpains, endonucleases, and phospholipases) capable of either directly or indirectly (through free-radical formation) destroying cellular structure. The increased levels of intracellular Ca²⁺ may also activate the nitric oxide pathway and thus produce cell damage through free-radical formation. The cytosolic Ca²⁺ levels are normally maintained via the Na⁺-Ca²⁺ exchanger. The activation of AMPA receptors may also be involved in reversal of the Na⁺-Ca²⁺ exchanger. Therefore, all these mechanisms contribute to cell death. Furthermore, the glutamate released from the synaptic terminals or leaking nonspecifically from ruptured neurons may contribute to additional injury propagation. (From R Gill. The pharmacology of α-amino-3-hydroxy-5-methyl-4-isoxazole propionate (AMPA)/kainate antagonists and their role in cerebral ischaemia. *Cerebrovasc Brain Metab Rev* 6:225–256, 1994. With permission.)

concentrations and leads to the release of glutamate into the synaptic cleft. These cationic fluxes are normally terminated and inhibited by receptors and channels controlling K⁺ and Cl⁻ permeability: Increased K⁺ conductance hyperpolarizes membranes, and increased Cl⁻ conductance tends to "clamp" the membrane potential near the resting potential. Calcium homeostasis is normally restored by ATP-dependent transport of Ca²⁺ out of the cell and by an electrogenic 3Na⁺/Ca²⁺ antiporter, which is driven by the Na⁺ gradient and the membrane potential. [Ca²⁺]ᵢ depends therefore on a balance between leakage of calcium into the cell, plasma membrane calcium pumps, intracellular calcium binding, and mitochondrial sequestration (Fig. 26-16).[141]

Energy failure is also responsible for activation of glutamate-receptor–dependent mechanisms. Energy depletion leads to failure or even reversal of glutamate transport in both neurons and astrocytes that depend on a Na⁺/K⁺ ATPase.[150] Furthermore, energy failure reduces the conversion of glutamate to glutamine in astrocytes, increasing intracellular accumulation of glutamate. This may reduce the capacity of inward glutamate transport. The net result is a prolongation of exposure time of glutamate receptors to glutamate in the synaptic cleft.

Neurons and astroglia release NO in response to activation by glutamate, kainate, and quisqualate, and serve as an important mediator of normal glutamatergic signal transduction. NOS is stimulated by the calcium influx that occurs with glutamate binding its receptors[24,151,151a] (Fig. 26-17). NO is released by nonadrenergic, noncholinergic vasodilator nerves and has also been implicated in neurogenic vasodilation of cerebral vessels.[152–154] NMDA-induced neurotoxicity has been shown to be attenuated in a dose-dependent fashion with the use of NOS inhibitors. Further studies with mutant mice that lack neuronal NOS activity in the brain show reduced ischemic damage after permanent and transient cerebral vessel occlusion, despite similar cardiovascular parameters before and after the insult.[155] This neuroprotective effect does not appear to be related to vascular factors but may actually be due to either reduced free-radical formation or depressed release of excitotoxins.[146]

Studies of the effects of NO in the brain have been complicated

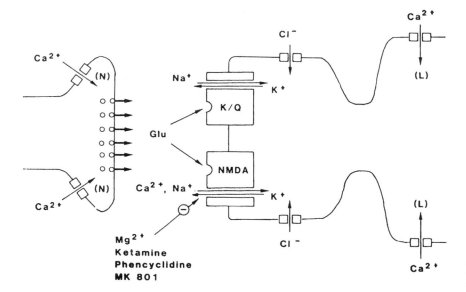

Figure 26-16. Presynaptic voltage-sensitive calcium channels (VSCCs) and post-synaptic agonist–operated calcium channels. Presynaptically, VSCCs involved in transmitter release are assumed to be of the N-type (N), which is not sensitive to calcium antagonists. At the postsynaptic site, kainate/quisqualate-operated channels (K/Q) are assumed to allow Na+ influx and thereby to cause depolarization, while NMDA-operated channels are assumed to allow calcium influx. The ionic shifts at the K/Q- and NMDA-gated channels occur when the K/Q and NMDA receptors are activated by glutamate (Glu). When Na+ enters the cell postsynaptically, electrostatic forces are assumed to cause Cl- influx along voltage-sensitive or agonist-operated anion channels. Na+ and Cl- entry is accompanied by osmotically obligated water that can result in swelling of apical dendrites. On the central dendrite or cell-soma, VSCCs of the L-type (L) are assumed to be located to allow Ca^{2+} entry. (From BK Siesjö, F Bengtsson. Calcium fluxes, calcium antagonists, and calcium-related pathology of brain ischemia, hypoglycemia and spreading depression: A unifying hypothesis. *J Cereb Blood Flow Metab* 9:127–140, 1989. With permission.)

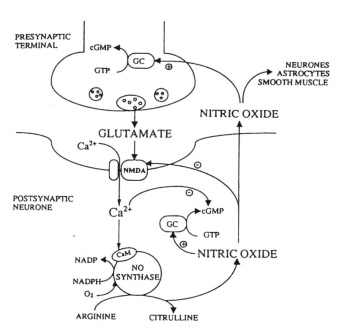

Figure 26-17. Nitric oxide–mediated signal transduction at the glutamate NMDA receptor. Glutamate released from the presynaptic terminal activates the NMDA receptor–gated ion channel resulting in Ca^{2+} influx into the postsynaptic neuron. The increase in free intracellular Ca^{2+} then activates the calmodulin-dependent NO synthase that releases NO in the conversion of L-arginine to L-citrulline. The freely diffusible NO can then pass into neighboring target cells (neurons, glia, or vascular smooth muscle) or back into the presynaptic neuron to activate guanylate cyclase (GC) and increase cGMP production. Two negative feedback systems operate to prevent over-activation of the NMDA receptor and limit accumulation of cGMP in the NO generator neuron itself: (1) NO reduces Ca^{2+} influx by interacting with the redox modulatory site on the NMDA receptor to reduce the frequency of channel opening, and (2) the increase in intracellular Ca^{2+} also activates a calmodulin-dependent cGMP phosphodiesterase that rapidly hydrolyses cGMP. (From DA Dawson. Nitric oxide and focal cerebral ischemia: Multiplicity of actions and diverse outcome. *Cerebrovasc Brain Metab Rev* 6:299–324, 1994. With permission.)

by the multiplicity of actions, cell types, and tissues that can produce NO. Other studies have belied the neuroprotective effect of NOS inhibitors.[156] These disparate results may stem from varying experimental conditions, such as the redox state of the NO species. Superoxide anions can terminate NO-mediated vasodilatation by reacting with NO to form peroxynitrite (ONOO-) and other free-radical species that are toxic to neurons.[157] Nitrosium, on the other hand, is the oxidized form of NO that binds to a regulatory site on the NMDA

receptor and produces a decrease in activity of the receptor. This serves as a cellular protective mechanism in conditions in which there is excessive stimulation by glutamate.[150] The vasodilatory action of NO may also counteract excitotoxic damage.

$$Arginine + O_2 + NADPH ———\rightarrow Citruline + NO\cdot + NADP$$
$$NO\cdot + \cdot O_2^- ———\rightarrow ONOO^- + H^+ ———\rightarrow ONOOH$$
$$ONOOH ———\rightarrow \cdot OH + NO_2\cdot$$

Calcium and Glutamate Antagonists

Elucidation of the role of cellular calcium flux in promoting neuronal injury has led to attempts to use calcium and glutamate antagonists to improve outcome. A number of discrepant results have been achieved in various models, but, in general, medications that reduce the intracellular increase in calcium do not diminish neuronal damage when there is either global ischemia or transient forebrain ischemia.[158–162] The calcium channel blockers nimodipine and isradipine, both dihydropyridine antagonists, have been shown to decrease infarction size in models of focal ischemia when given before, but not after, vessel occlusion.[118,158,159] These agents may only block the L-type VSCC.[163] Isradipine is a vasodilator and may act by increasing blood flow in the perifocal areas. Nimodipine reduces the rise in intracellular calcium that occurs during ischemia and will also reduce the severity of acidosis, possibly by improving mitochondrial function.[160–162]

In contrast, the calcium channel blockers flunarizine and nicardipine demonstrated some effect in separate models of global and forebrain ischemia, but isradipine was ineffective in forebrain ischemia models.[164] Both flunarizine and nicardipine have effects on T-type VSCCs that may be involved in fast excitation, reducing postsynaptic excitation and depolarization during recovery from transient ischemia.[165] Their protective action resembles that of AMPA receptor antagonists.

Antagonists to glutamate receptors have been employed in a number of animal models in an attempt to limit damage promoted by excitotoxins. NMDA receptor antagonists, both competitive and noncompetitive, do not appear to be protective in animal models of global or severe forebrain ischemia.[148] This may be because massive depolarization and severe energy depletion in dense ischemia leads to cellular injury via a multitude of chemical pathways, and antagonism of the NDMA receptors alone cannot reduce the rise in $[Ca^{2+}]_i$. In models of focal cerebral ischemia, however, both competitive and noncompetitive NMDA receptor antagonists were effective, reducing infarction size.[166,167] The mechanism of protection provided by NMDA antagonists in focal ischemia may be through the blocking of cortical-spreading, depression-like activity that can be recorded in the ischemic penumbra.[166]

AMPA receptors mediate fast excitatory responses and depolarization in the CNS, a necessary step for the triggering calcium influx.[148] 2,3-dihydroxy-6-nitro-7-sulfamoyl-benzo(F)quinoxaline (NBQX), a competitive AMPA antagonist, and 1-(aminophenyl)-4-methyl-7,8-methylenedioxy-5H-2,3-benzodiazepine (GYKI 52446), a noncompetive AMPA antagonist, were protective in animal models of focal ischemia.[168,169] These AMPA antagonists may also act by blocking cortical-spreading depression in the penumbra following focal ischemia by preventing glutamate-induced neuronal depolarization.[148] These AMPA antagonists also appear to possess greater neuroprotective effects in the face of global ischemia than do NMDA antagonists.[170] Combinations of NDMA and AMPA receptor antagonists did not prove additive in their neuroprotective effects and, in fact, resulted in profound neurologic depression in animals.[169,171]

Finally, attempts at regulating the effects of NO in models of cerebral ischemia are being tested. Preliminary data have shown that 7-nitroindazole, an inhibitor of NOS with somewhat greater selectivity for the neuronal isoform, decreases infarction size after vessel occlusion.[172]

Recently, high-affinity free-radical scavengers, including allopurinol, alpha-tocopherol, dimethylurea, and 21-aminosteroids, have been employed in models of CNS injury. Beneficial effects were observed with free-radical scavengers used in models of ischemia, trauma, intracranial hemorrhage, and circulatory shock. Allopurinol and dimethylurea decreased neurologic damage, edema, H_2O_2 production, and infarction size in models of long-term ischemia.[125,173] Models of focal ischemia in transgenic mice that overexpressed superoxide dismutase demonstrated less edema and smaller infarctions than in controls. Inhibition of lipid peroxidation by a 21-aminosteroid improved somatosensory evoked potential recovery and accelerated normalization of pH and inorganic phosphate concentration when given prior to the ischemic insult.[174]

No-Reflow Phenomena

When global cerebral ischemia occurs, followed by restoration of blood flow (e.g., following cardiac arrest and resuscitation), CBF initially increases above baseline, but within 30 minutes decreases to less than 20% of baseline values. This is known as the postreperfusion no-flow phenomenon, or postreperfusion vasospasm.[175] This phenomenon has also been observed with less severe focal ischemia, although the resuscitation times are longer.[119] This intense vasoconstriction is associated with increased levels of thromboxane A_2 (TxA_2).

Laboratory research has naturally focused on the prevention of the no-reflow phenomenon. Unfortunately, inhibition of cerebral synthesis of TxA_2 in the dog ischemia model does not prevent the no-reflow phenomenon, nor has the later increase in vascular resistance been found to be due to platelet plug formation.[176,177]

Principles of Neurointensive Care

Intracranial Pressure

By the age of 1 year, the anterior and posterior fontanels are closed, and by the age of 10 years, the cranial sutures are fused. At this point, the volume of the intracranial contents is fixed, and any increase in volume of one of the tissue components results in an increment of ICP, unless it is compensated for by a decrease in volume of another component. This concept is the Monro-Kellie doctrine. The intracranial vault contains three substances: neural tissue and supporting structures (approximately 70% by volume), blood (10%), and extracellular fluid plus CSF (20%).

Normally, ICP is less than 15 mm Hg. If there is a gradual increase in volume of one of the brain's components (e.g., a slow-growing hemispheric tumor), compensatory mechanisms can occur until a critical tumor volume is reached, at which time the ICP rises precipitously. Early compensation can be due to a decrease in CSF volume by translocation of CSF through the foramen magnum to the area surrounding the spinal cord, an increase in CSF fluid resorption rate secondary to increased CSF pressure, and a decrease in cerebral blood volume by compression of cerebral venous sinuses. If a change in volume occurs rapidly, such as with an intracranial hemorrhage, compensatory mechanisms are inadequate and ICP acutely increases (Fig. 26-18).

When ICP is not elevated, the normal CPP is equal to the difference between the MAP and the jugular venous pressure (JVP):

$$CPP = MAP - JVP$$

When the ICP is greater than JVP,

$$CPP = MAP - ICP$$

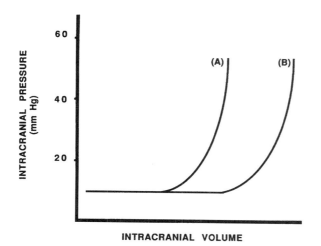

Figure 26-18. The effects of changes in volume of intracranial contents on intracranial pressure. **(Curve A)** A rapid increase in the volume of an intracranial component will not allow adequate time for compensation, and ICP increases at a volume less than if the change occurred over a longer period **(Curve B).**

As ICP approaches the MAP, CPP approaches zero. Clinically this represents no cerebral blood flow. Also,

$$CPP = CBF \times CVR$$

where CVR is cerebral vascular resistance. As ICP rises, CPP falls, unless there is a concurrent rise in BP. A decrease in CPP stimulates cerebral vasodilatation as a means of increasing CBF. However, cerebral vasodilatation will also increase cerebral blood volume (CBV), although CBV may not be directly proportional to CBF. The net effect may be a further rise in ICP and a decrease in CBF and CPP[178] (Fig. 26-19). In seriously injured patients this self-sustaining cycle is often initiated by a fall in MAP and will persist until the cerebral resistance vessels are maximally dilated or until appropriate therapy is instituted.

Intracranial Pressure Monitoring

ICP monitoring is a well-established clinical tool in neurologic intensive care, and therapeutic strategies are often based on controlling ICP and optimizing CPP. A word of caution is appropriate at this point. The efficacy of ICP monitoring in improving outcome has been proven only in patients in two clinical situations: (1) stage III Reye's syndrome in children and (2) following head trauma.[179–181] Extrapolation of this therapy to other clinical situations, such as near-drowning, may not always be appropriate or effective. Current recommendations for using ICP monitors are (1) history or physical examination consistent with severe brain injury; (2) when treatment is used to lower ICP, especially in situations in which neurologic examination is not obtainable (e.g., the patient receiving neuromuscular junction blocking agents); and (3) to detect acute changes in ICP, such as obstructive hydrocephalus or hemorrhage.

ICP can be measured by several means, each with its distinct advantages and disadvantages. A catheter placed in the lateral ventricle via a burr hole, for direct measurement of CSF pressure using a pressure transducer, is the original and probably most accurate method of measuring ICP. Intraventricular catheters remain the standard against which other devices are compared. With this technique, the pressure transducer can be calibrated after catheter placement so that a drift in pressure baseline is avoided. Furthermore, small (<1 ml) volumes of normal saline can be injected into the catheter to measure cerebral compliance, although this is an uncommon and potentially dangerous procedure that is not used often at this time. In addition to their monitoring capabilities, intraventricular catheters also serve as potential therapy for elevated ICP, as CSF can be aspirated from the intraventricular catheters.

The disadvantages of this system are significant and have limited the routine use of this monitor. Because the monitor is placed through the brain substance into the lateral ventricles, there is a risk of hemorrhage (approximately 1%–2% of cases) or direct neuronal damage.[182] If cerebral edema becomes severe enough, the ventricles may be compressed, making catheter placement technically difficult. Cerebral edema may accumulate after placement of the catheter, resulting in compression of the ventricles around the catheter and obfuscation of the pressure signal. The catheter holes may also plug with particulate matter. Finally, these invasive catheters carry a rate of infection higher than the rates of other methods of 6% to 21%, and infections involving the ventricle are often severe.[182,183] In light of the progress made in the sensitivity of less invasive monitors, intraventricular catheters are rarely indicated and should probably be reserved for those patients who may require CSF withdrawal during therapy.

Subarachnoid catheters are devices commonly used for measuring ICP. A burr hole is made in the skull, and a small cruciate incision of the dura is made under direct vision. A bolt is screwed into the burr hole. The bolt is hollow and contains a fluid-filled column that contacts CSF. A continuous fluid column from CSF to a pressure transducer allows for CSF pressure to be measured. Interruptions of this fluid column by air bubbles will dampen or distort this signal. The advantages of this system include facility and rapidity of placement. Additionally, there is lower risk of hemorrhage and infection, and such infection generally remains superficial. Subarachnoid catheters can also be periodically zeroed to baseline. The disadvantages include underestimation of ICP, as compared with intraventricular pressure measurements, due to the problem of surface tension.[184] Subarachnoid monitors do not allow for withdrawal of CSF as a therapeutic modality. There is significant difficulty in placement through the thin friable skulls of neonates and infants. Like the intraventricular catheter, subarachnoid bolts may become occluded by edematous brain or by debris, making pressure measurements unreliable.

Camino monitors, like subarachnoid bolts, are inserted by placing a screw through a burr hole. The monitor contains a fiberoptic tip that may be placed in a number of locations, including the subdural space, within the brain parenchyma, or within the lateral ventricle. These monitors can be calibrated after their placement. The Camino monitor is also easily placed, contains a closed system, does not require recalibration after initial placement, and can monitor intraparenchymal pressures. This device has been shown

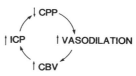

Figure 26-19. A fall in CPP can initiate a vicious cycle, generating a rise in ICP and further falls in CPP.

to be accurate, although when placed in a subdural position, its accuracy becomes less precise at higher ICPs.[185] Disadvantages include the requirement of a burr hole and measurement drift over long periods of monitoring (>5 days).[185,186]

Epidural discs (Ladd monitors) are solid-state devices that use fiberoptic transducers, which require no fluid column. Their distinct advantage resides in the need for no dural incision during placement.[187] The major disadvantage is that the catheter cannot be calibrated or zeroed after placement.

ICP Interpretation

Continuous real-time stripchart recording of ICP should be done for all patients receiving ICP monitoring. Three types of ICP waveforms can be seen on the record, and events associated with their occurrence (e.g., seizures, endotracheal suctioning, position changes, etc.) should be noted on the stripchart. C waves are rapid oscillations of ICP associated with changes in arterial pressure or intrapleural pressure. These are not pathogenic waveforms. B waves have an amplitude of 10 to 50 mm Hg and occur approximately every 2 minutes. They are self-limited and indicate a poor or marginal cerebral compliance. B waves may herald the onset of A waves (plateau waves), which have a similar amplitude as B waves but of much longer duration. A waves are associated with global ischemia and herniation[187] (Figs. 26-20, 26-21, 26-22).

Retrograde Jugular Bulb Catheterization

As the name implies, a jugular venous catheter is passed superiorly through the internal jugular vein into the jugular bulb where venous oxygenation can be monitored. Standard central venous catheters allow intermittent monitoring of blood gas values, while fiberoptic oximetry catheters can be used to obtain continuous measurement of jugular venous hemoglobin saturation ($SjvO_2$)[188] The catheters must be accurately placed in the jugular bulb, a few millimeters away from the superior wall. Failure to advance the catheter completely into the bulb will lead to sample contamination with blood from the pharyngeal veins and common facial vein, creating false measurements. Also, head movement following placement may lead to catheter tip migration.[189]

Jugular venous bulb monitors allow an estimation of global

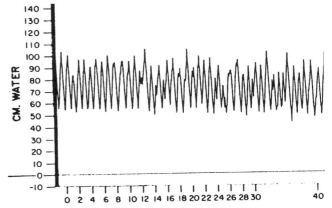

Figure 26-20.   Series of B waves recorded with a fiberoptic ICP monitoring system. (From AB Levin. The use of a fiberoptic intracranial pressure monitor in clinical practice. *Neurosurgery* 1:266–271, 1977. With permission.)

cerebral metabolism by providing data on global cerebral oxygen extraction (CEO_2), but they cannot distinguish areas of heterogeneous metabolism or blood flow. This technique, because of its global nature, is insensitive to detection of even large areas of infarction or ischemia.[190] Cerebral venous oxygen content can be calculated by multiplying the $SjvO_2$ by the hemoglobin content. The AV oxygen content difference can also be calculated to assess the effect on therapeutic maneuvers on CEO_2. Cruz has relied on CEO_2, which he defined as the difference in hemoglobin saturations between SaO_2 and $SjvO_2$. The CEO_2 reflects the global ratio of $CMRO_2$ to CBF without measuring either of those two variables.[190]

When patients are hyperventilated, differential tissue flow patterns in various cerebral regions tend to decrease. That is, areas in which autoregulation is compromised and normal areas will both receive decreased blood flow due to contraction of resistance arterioles. Hyperventilation is believed to improve the accuracy of the jugular bulb technique.[189,191,192] Generally, there is an inverse relationship between rCBF and CEO_2, except when patients pres-

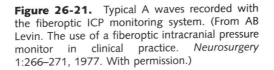

Figure 26-21.   Typical A waves recorded with the fiberoptic ICP monitoring system. (From AB Levin. The use of a fiberoptic intracranial pressure monitor in clinical practice. *Neurosurgery* 1:266–271, 1977. With permission.)

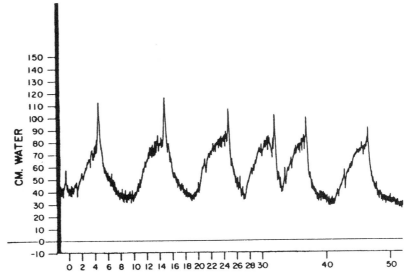

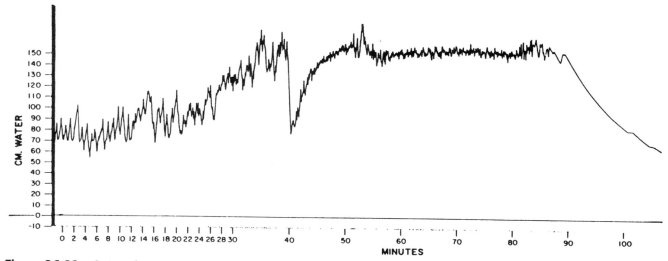

Figure 26-22. Series of progressive A waves ending in a terminal plateau wave followed by decompensation. (From AB Levin. The use of a fiberoptic intracranial pressure monitor in clinical practice. *Neurosurgery* 1:266–271, 1977. With permission.)

ent with clinical signs of impending or actual brain death.[191] Under these circumstances, a low CBF is associated with a significant decrease in CEO_2. This pathologic decrease in oxygen extraction with respect to CBF is known as "cerebral luxury perfusion."

The AV difference in oxygen content ($AVDO_2$) is a highly dynamic parameter that responds to extracranial factors, such as changes in BP or hemoglobin oxygen saturation, as well as to intracranial events, such as changes in ICP.[193] Increases in ICP most commonly result in increases in the $AVDO_2$, because increases in MAP are transmitted to the intracranial compartment in patients in whom autoregulation has been severely impaired. Patients with the largest $AVDO_2$ fluctuations appear to have the poorest outcome.[193]

Therapy for Intracranial Emergencies

The primary goal of therapy in the face of CNS emergencies is to prevent any further injury. To accomplish this, the demands of cellular metabolism must match the nutrient supply. Many creative therapies have been employed that aim either to decrease neuronal cellular metabolic rate or to increase cerebral blood supply. A substantial quantity of work has been performed to define the efficacy of these therapies. For instance, hyperventilation has commonly been used to decrease ICP and thus improve CBF. However, studies suggest that prolonged hyperventilation does not improve outcome and may actually add to secondary injury by decreasing blood supply to the ischemic penumbra.[191,194] Consequently, application of therapeutic maneuvers affecting cerebral homeostasis must be applied on an individualized basis, rendering frequent, careful clinical observation indispensable.

Preventing or minimizing secondary brain injury is the central goal of neurointensive care; this end will presumably lead to improved patient outcome. An abundance of research into the basic mechanisms of brain injury was produced during the past two decades. No doubt, a better understanding of these mechanisms will result in improved care of the brain-injured patient. Already, insights gained from these investigations have led to novel therapeutic strategies. However, the underlying foundation of neurointensive care still must center on basic physiologic principles,

including the restoration of oxygenation, ventilation, and perfusion, with special attention to maintaining normoglycemia, normal electrolytes, and controlling intracranial pressure, seizures, and fever. The emergence of new therapies should not obscure the need for providing this basic and fundamental care.

The initial priority in all intracranial emergencies is to follow basic resuscitation paradigms. All patients with a Glasgow Coma Scale of 8 or less should have a secured airway (Table 26-1). Otherwise, the normal criteria for endotracheal intubation should be applied. It cannot be overemphasized that even mild hypotension or hypoxemia does not benefit the patient with neurologic injury, and meticulous concern for hemodynamic stability must precede all other maneuvers.

Decreased oxygen delivery will result in cerebral vasoconstriction and consequent increases in ICP. Adequate oxygenation has been shown to improve quality of life in pediatric head-trauma victims.[195] In one study of pediatric patients with severe brain injury, outcome was worse in patients who demonstrated poor

Table 26-1. Glasgow Coma Scale

Activity	Best response	Score
Eye opening	Spontaneous	4
	To verbal stimuli	3
	To pain	2
	None	1
Best verbal response	Oriented	5
	Confused	4
	Inappropriate	3
	Nonspecific sounds	2
	None	1
Best motor response	Follows commands	6
	Localizes pain	5
	Withdraws to pain	4
	Flexion response to pain	3
	Extension response to pain	2
	None	1

oxygenation by arterial blood gas.[196] The improved oxygenation correlated with the absence of chest trauma.

CBV and thus ICP may be reduced by head elevation and by placing the head in a neutral, midline position. Rotation of the head causes jugular venous obstruction, which increases JVP, CBV, and ICP. Doubts have been cast on the common practice of routine head elevation by showing that head elevation of any degree is associated with ICP plateau waves and with a decrease in CPP[197] (Figs. 26-23, 26-24). However, head elevation to 15 to 30 degrees has been shown to significantly reduce ICP while having no untoward effect on CPP or on $SjvO_2$.[198] Head elevation to 60 degrees does result in reduced cardiac index and CPP, and variable ICP response, with some patients having an ICP above values recorded at 0 degrees.[199] Other authors found that optimal brain compliance (measured by injecting saline into an intraventricular catheter and recording pressure changes) varied between

patients; some patients have improved compliance with head lowering[200] (Figs. 26-25, 26-26). We recommend individualizing the degree of head elevation to provide the lowest ICP, while maintaining CPP above 50 mm Hg.

Fluid restriction is another cornerstone of tissue volume reduction and control of cerebral edema formation. Again, the primary concern is resuscitation to an adequate circulating volume. Once this is attained, fluid can be administered at a rate of 60% to 80% of daily maintenance requirements. We recommend using lactated Ringer's or D_5 ½ NS, with close attention to urine output and serum electrolytes. Because patients with brain injury are prone to develop the syndrome of inappropriate antidiuretic hormone secretion (SIADH) or even diabetes inspidus (DI), fluid balance must be assiduously monitored. Hypotonic fluid administration should be avoided because decreases in serum osmolarity will promote brain swelling. Prudence dictates monitoring of right

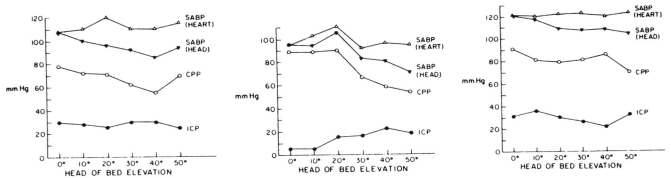

Figure 26-23. Three different effects from head elevation in three separate patients. **(Left)** 19-year-old with acute subdural hematoma. Head elevation had little effect on ICP, but systemic arterial blood pressure (SABP) decreased and CPP declined. **(Center)** 62-year-old with glioblastoma multiforme. CPP maintained with head elevation up to 20 degrees, beyond which systolic BP could not be maintained, CPP fell, and ICP rose, probably as a result of the fall in CPP. **(Right)** 52-year-old with cerebellar and frontal hemorrhage. The ICP increased slightly at 10 degrees' elevation, but ultimately fell to 22 mm Hg before rising again. The SABP at heart level changed little and declined by 18 mm Hg at head level. The CPP never improved over that at 0 degrees' elevation. (From MJ Rosner, IB Coley. Cerebral perfusion pressure, intracranial pressure, and head elevation. *J Neurosurg* 65:636–641, 1986. With permission.)

Figure 26-24. Composite graph from 18 patients with ICP monitoring. ICP declines as head elevation progresses, but the decrement in systemic arterial blood pressure (SABP) at head level is greater. Therefore, cerebral perfusion pressure (CPP) declines. Only the tendency for SABP to increase when the head is elevated beyond 40 degrees prevents a greater CPP decrement. CVP, central venous pressure; NS not significant. Values are means ± SEM. (From MJ Rosner, IB Coley. Cerebral perfusion pressure, intracranial pressure, and head elevation. *J Neurosurg* 65:636–641, 1986. With permission.)

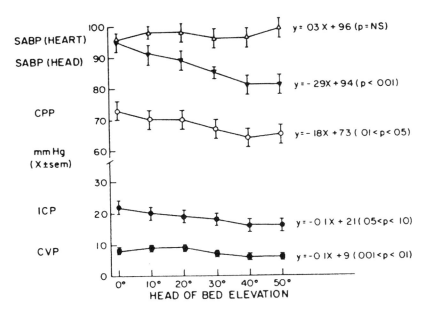

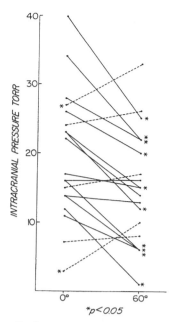

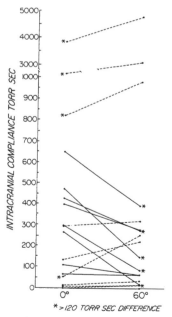

Figure 26-25. Resting mean ICP over 40 seconds at 0 degrees and 60 degrees in 19 patients. Solid lines indicate patients with lower ICPs at 60 degrees (10) or no significant difference (7), and interrupted lines indicate patients with lower ICPs at 0 degrees (2). (From AH Ropper, D O'Rourke, SK Kennedy. Head position, intracranial pressure, and compliance. *Neurology* 32:1288–1291, 1982. With permission.)

Figure 26-26. Volume tolerance in torr-sec at 0 and 60 degrees of head elevation in 19 patients, following injection of 0.1 ml of fluid into a subarachnoid screw. Measures were obtained by integrating the area under the ICP curve above baseline for 60 seconds. Solid lines indicate patients with better volume tolerance at 60 degrees (5) or no significant difference (10), and interrupted lines indicate patients with better volume tolerance at 0 degrees (4). (From AH Ropper, D O'Rourke, SK Kennedy. Head position, intracranial pressure, and compliance. *Neurology* 32:1288–1291, 1982. With permission.)

atrial filling pressures and possibly cardiac output in patients who have associated myocardial dysfunction.

During cerebral ischemia, the degree of intra- and extracellular acidosis depends in part on glucose concentration. Hyperglycemic subjects have worse intracellular acidosis, compared with subjects with normoglycemia.[201,202] Several retrospective studies in humans have demonstrated a poorer neurologic outcome when cerebral ischemia, either from a stroke or a cardiac arrest, coincided with hyperglycemia.[201,203,204] Subsequently, it has been strongly recommended that hyperglycemia be avoided in conditions associated with cerebral ischemia or other insults.[205]

In animal models, neurologic outcome (as measured by EEG and sensory evoked potentials) was worse in animals that had glucose administered prior to complete or incomplete cerebral ischemia, when compared with a group of animals that had been fasted.[206] During ischemia, partial CBF may provide inadequate oxygen for aerobic metabolism, while supplying enough glucose to be incompletely oxidized to lactate. This results in a greater intracellular acidosis and worse cellular injury than in animals who were fasted or had complete cerebral ischemia (Fig. 26-27).

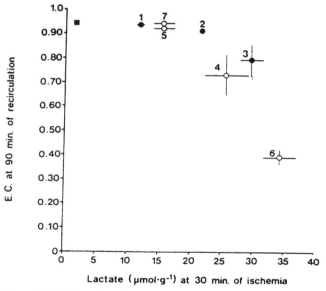

Figure 26-27. The adenylate energy charge: E.C. = [(ATP) + 0.5(ADP)]/[(ATP) + (ADP) + (AMP)] of rat cortical tissue at 90 min of recirculation following 30 min of cerebral ischemia as a function of the cortical lactate concentration at the end of ischemia. Experimental groups: *Shaded square*, nonischemic controls. *Shaded circles*, reversible complete ischemia. (Infusion of artificial CSF into cisterna magna to pressure > systolic BP, reversed with discontinuation of CSF infusion): *1*, normally fed; *2*, fasted, infused with glucose prior to ischemia; *3*, fasted, hypercapnic, and infused with glucose prior to ischemia. *Open circles*, reversible incomplete ischemia (created by ligating both carotid arteries and lowering mean arterial BP to 50 mm Hg by hemorrhage. Reversed by removal of carotid clamps and reinfusion of blood); *4*, normally fed; *5*, fasted, infused with Krebs-Hensleit solution prior to ischemia; *6*, fasted, infused with glucose prior to ischemia; *7*, fasted, infused with glucose during recirculation. There were 6 or 8 animals in each group. The symbols represent mean ± SE. Postischemic E.C. differed significantly from controls in groups with ischemic lactate concentrations exceeding 20 μmol/g of tissue. (From S Rhencrona, I Rosen, BK Siesjö. Excessive cellular acidosis: An important mechanism of neuronal damage in the brain? *Acta Physiol Scand* 110:435–437, 1980. With permission.)

Hyperthermia increases cerebral metabolic and oxygen demands, which can increase CBF, CBV, and ICP. "Neurogenic" fever commonly accompanies cerebrovascular pathology when the hypothalamus is involved.[207] Cerebral hyperthermia may also occur after global ischemic events, such as cardiac arrest. Even small increases in body temperature may jeopardize the brain's resistance to periods of ischemia.[208–210] Fever should be controlled with acetaminophen and/or cooling blankets. Shivering should be prevented with either neuromuscular blocking agents, meperidine, or phenothiazines.

Seizures should be prevented whenever possible and aggressively treated when they occur. Seizures cause an increase in $CMRO_2$ and often increase ICP. Approximately 10% of head-injury patients develop posttraumatic seizures, which usually occur within the first 24 hours following injury.[211,212] Phenytoin (10 mg/kg loading dose, followed by a maintenance of 5 mg/kg/d) has been shown to decrease the risk of posttraumatic seizures during the first week after severe head injury, but it does not prevent late seizures.[196,212] For patients receiving neuromuscular blockade, seizures cannot be detected clinically and may manifest themselves only as ICP spikes or plateau waves. The use of continuous EEG or CSA monitoring in these patients is therefore helpful. Subclinical seizures should be suspected when there is an abrupt, otherwise unexplainable, rise in ICP in patients with CNS trauma.

Anxiety and nociception must be assessed and appropriately treated in all patients, especially those who are comatose or receiving neuromuscular blocking agents. Painful and uncomfortable procedures (e.g., arterial line catheterization or endotracheal tube suctioning) can be associated with dramatic spikes in ICP. Local anesthesia should be used for all painful procedures, and sedatives (e.g., benzodiazepines, barbiturates, etc.) should be administered routinely to patients who receive neuromuscular blockers. For example, 0.5 to 3.0 mg/kg of IV sodium thiopental will blunt the ICP response to endotracheal intubation or suctioning. Because barbiturates can cause myocardial depression, BP should be followed closely, adequate fluid resuscitation must be assured, and doses should be titrated slowly. Barbiturates should not be used for this purpose in a patient who is hemodynamically unstable.

Sustained elevations of ICP negatively affect outcome in head-injured patients.[213] Consequently, much effort should be directed at reducing intracranial hypertension. The most rapid method of decreasing ICP involves reducing CBF, and probably CBV, via hyperventilation. Many references recommend that once a patient is hemodynamically stable, she should have initial treatment with controlled hyperventilation to lower the $PaCO_2$ to approximately 25 mm Hg. It has also been suggested that hyperventilation may produce its beneficial effect by compensating for CSF acidosis, which also is associated with poor outcome.[214,215] While hyperventilation has been shown to restore autoregulation in certain pathologic states (i.e., postictal animals), the decline in CBF with hyperventilation may tip a compromised but viable area of the brain into the abyss of frank ischemia in the patient with increased ICP.[119,194] Furthermore, arteriolar constriction in response to hyperventilation appears to be short-lived, and thus the duration of decreased ICP may be quite brief.[216]

In one review, it was concluded that hyperventilation was ineffective in the treatment of intracranial hypertension, cerebral edema, and stroke.[213] Since then, others have prospectively found that the prophylactic use of sustained hyperventilation for a period of 5 days was found to delay recovery from severe head injury.[215]

A possible mechanism is that there is a reduction in buffer capacity with lower bicarbonate concentrations, rendering the cerebral vessels more sensitive to changes in $PaCO_2$, and this could lead to more pronounced ICP elevations during transient increases in $PaCO_2$. Hyperventilation alone may increase lactate levels in the CSF and serum and produce intracellular hypoxia. The hypoxia results from two possible mechanisms. First, the decrease in CBF may limit oxygen supply to damaged tissue, resulting in ischemia. Second, the alkalosis that occurs with hyperventilation leads to a shift in the oxygen-hemoglobin dissociation curve to the left, further decreasing oxygen delivery to the tissues. However, brief episodes of hypocapnea are effective in the treatment of acute elevations of intracranial pressure.[213]

Hyperventilation to a $PaCO_2$ level between 25 and 30 mm Hg in the face of acute intracranial injuries should help minimize spikes of ICP and normalize CBF. Hyperventilation to this level has been shown to decrease CBV and prevent excessive CBF, which can worsen vasogenic cerebral edema.[217] Lowering $PaCO_2$ below 25 mm Hg should be reserved for the acute setting when there is an imminent risk of cerebral herniation. Maintenance of the $PaCO_2$ below 25 mm Hg should be avoided because this may exacerbate cerebral ischemia and result in decrease efficacy of this modality.[56,218]

Mannitol also serves as an important treatment for elevated intracranial pressure, as it produces acute cerebral vasoconstriction and delayed brain dehydration. IV mannitol decreases blood viscosity, resulting in vascular contraction by autoregulation. Additionally, it increases intravascular osmolality, creating an osmotic gradient across the blood-brain barrier. This leads to free water movement into the intravascular space, with eventual clearance through diuresis. The subsequent diuresis can lead to hypovolemia (and possibly shock) and hyponatremia. A dose of 1 g/kg may be associated with a rise in systolic arterial pressure and ICP. If other measures are not also being incorporated to lower ICP when this occurs, the results can be deleterious. Lower doses (0.25–0.5 g/kg) are as effective in reducing ICP and are associated with a smaller increase in serum osmolarity.[219] Repeated use of mannitol can cause rebound increases in ICP. This may be due to the influx of mannitol into damaged brain in areas where the blood-brain barrier is not intact.[220,221] The duration of action for lowering ICP from a single dose of mannitol is approximately 6 hours. When the duration becomes less than 4 hours, the likelihood of improving brain compliance with further doses is diminished and alternative means of therapy should be employed.

When tachyphylaxis to mannitol occurs, furosemide (0.5–1.0 mg/kg IV) decreases ICP by further intracellular dehydration and has the added benefit of decreasing CSF production. The onset of action of furosemide is 30 minutes, compared with 5 to 10 minutes for mannitol. Long-term use can result in hypovolemia and a hypochloremic alkalosis.

In patients receiving positive pressure ventilation and positive end-expiratory pressure (PEEP), concern often exists that PEEP may increase right atrial pressure and JVP. If PEEP is high enough, cerebral venous drainage is decreased, and an increase in CBV and ICP can occur. In addition, PEEP may reduce left atrial filling pressures and cardiac output. In the mechanically ventilated patient with no PEEP, however, atelectasis may occur, resulting in augmented intrathoracic pressure. Consequently, in patients with intracranial emergencies, minimal PEEP to assure optimal oxygenation and pulmonary compliance should be used, as this will decrease both ICP and intrathoracic pressure.

Areas of Controversy

Barbiturates

Barbiturates decrease $CMRO_2$, CBV, CBF, and ICP even in patients in deep coma.[222,223] Barbiturates also increase intracellular pH through diminished production of lactate.[223] Results from study protocols wherein ICP was measured have consistently shown that high-dose barbiturate therapy can control elevated ICP that has been refractory to other conventional measures.[179,224–227] Some authors argue that elevated ICP correlates with poorer outcome in head-trauma patients. Studies that have evaluated outcome, however, have not shown that high-dose barbiturate administration improves survival.[228–230]

Barbiturates decrease CBF and CBV by increasing CVR.[231] As with hyperventilation, this decrease in CBF could actually result in local ischemia. Due to the abysmal results in patients with persistent elevations in ICP, however, the appeal of this approach of lowering ICP and $CMRO_2$ remains high.[232–234] The most commonly used agent for barbiturate therapy is pentobarbital. An initial loading dose of 5 to 10 mg/kg is administered over 1 to 2 hours. A maintenance infusion is started at 3 to 4 mg/kg/hr and is titrated according to the response of ICP, while maintaining the CPP with cardiovascular support, often necessitating the use of a continuous IV catecholamine infusion (e.g., dobutamine at 5–15 μg/kg/min). The physiologic end point of high-dose barbiturates is suppression of the EEG to a burst-suppression or isoelectric pattern.

Hypothermia

Induced hypothermia decreases $CMRO_2$, and therefore ICP. Hypothermia has been shown to reduce infarction size after transient, but not after permanent, middle cerebral artery occlusion in animal models.[210,235] Animal studies have shown that hypothermia improves both functional and histopathologic outcome, but only if applied shortly after the ischemic insult.[236] Additionally, hypothermia improves EEG potentials in permanent focal ischemia despite diminished residual flow to the ischemic territory.[237] Temperature is lowered to 32°C by using a cooling blanket. Neuromuscular blockade is used to prevent shivering. Routine surveillance cultures are necessary, because hypothermia inhibits neutrophil function, increasing the patient's risk for infection.[238] Also, the patient is incapable of manifesting infection by a fever. Rewarming should be attempted every 24 to 48 hours and hypothermia reinduced if ICP control is unsuccessful at warmer temperatures. As with barbiturate coma, hypothermia has not been shown to improve outcome in clinical trials. Use of this therapy should be reserved only for severe ICP that is refractory to standard therapeutic measures.

Steroids

Steroids can reduce vasogenic cerebral edema surrounding brain tumors and will decrease ICP associated with mass lesions and brain abscesses.[239,240] Extrapolation of steroid therapy to patients with traumatic head injury and coma, or local or global cerebral ischemia, has proven to be ineffective in reducing cerebral edema.[241–247] Complications from steroid use include hyperglycemia, gastrointestinal hemorrhage, and immunosuppression.[243,244] The current recommendation is that steroid use to control ICP be limited to patients suspected of having vasogenic cerebral edema surrounding mass lesions. Co-administration of an H-2 blocker (e.g., ranitidine) should be considered for anyone receiving chronic steroid therapy.

Sodium Bicarbonate

The acidosis that accompanies CNS insults often leads to secondary neuronal damage and exacerbates other injurious molecular and cellular processes. Consequently, it appears logical to treat that acidosis. However, reducing acidosis would probably require large doses of bases, and the bicarbonate ion does not penetrate the normal blood-brain barrier. Furthermore, bicarbonate has been shown to have deleterious effects that may be a result of paradoxical intracellular acidosis, hyperosmolarity, hypernatremia, and shifting of the oxyhemoglobin saturation curve to the left, inhibiting the release of oxygen in the tissues. Bicarbonate has been shown to cause irreversible damage to otherwise potentially viable cells.[248]

Tromethamine

Tromethamine (THAM) is a weak base and buffering agent that crosses the blood-brain barrier, and in its non-ionized form traverses the plasma membrane. It is not metabolized to any significant extent and is excreted via the kidneys in equimolar amounts of bicarbonate, and so acts as an osmotic diuretic.

Patients with severe head injury have abnormal energy metabolism, which is manifested by elevated levels of lactate in the CSF. In an experimentally traumatized cat brain, postinjury treatment with THAM reduced lactate production, brain edema, and mortality.[249,250] THAM has been demonstrated to be more effective than bicarbonate in resolving CSF acidosis. Additionally, THAM returned oxidative stores (phosphocreatine/inorganic phosphate ratios) to normal after they had fallen with sustained hyperventilation. When combined with prolonged, prophylactic hyperventilation, THAM reversed the delayed recovery produced by hyperventilation in head-injury patients. When THAM was employed with conventional treatment, however, there was no difference between the THAM group and the controls.[251] THAM has been shown to be effective in producing sustained control of elevated ICP.[251,252] The mechanism of ICP control by THAM is unclear, but THAM does buffer pH changes with $PaCO_2$ alterations in the CSF, which may translate to improved intracerebral compliance with dampened ICP fluctuations.

Presently, it would seem appropriate to consider THAM in the face of persistently increased ICP, especially if long-term hyperventilation is employed to control ICP.

Conclusion

The recent discoveries regarding the deleterious effects of energy failure, calcium fluxes, excitotoxin release, and NO and free radical production have engendered a veritable industry directed at limiting the CNS damage mediated by these various processes. Many agents remain in the animal-model stage of testing. However, research continually moves into the area of clinical trials. Agents that have been shown to be effective in humans include the following:

1. The NMDA antagonists dextrophan and CNS 1102 are currently in phase 2 trials among patients with strokes.[253]

2. Nimodipine, the calcium channel antagonist, has been shown to be effective in reducing the incidence of arterial spasm following subarachnoid hemorrhage from cerebral aneurysms.[3] It has also been employed in a study of AIDS dementia complex, which is felt to be partially mediated by excitotoxic action.[138]

3. Riluzole, which inhibits glutamate release from presynaptic neurons, possibly by blocking sodium channels, appears to slow

the rate of progression of amyotrophic lateral sclerosis. Such a medication may be found to be effective in more acute excitotoxic CNS injury.[254]

The mediators of CNS injury are manifold, and treatment options rest squarely on sound physiologic principles. Although a number of clinical studies have examined important therapeutic modalities, such as hyperventilation or the use of bicarbonate, and found their application to be limited, individual variation appears to exist, and frequent, careful clinical reassessment remains the mainstay of neurologic intensive care. Secondary neurologic injuries appear to have a shared common biochemical pathway. Investigation into therapeutic strategies to limit this excitotoxic damage may provide efficacious future therapies.

References

1. Brain Resuscitation Clinical Trial I Study Group. Randomized clinical study of thiopental loading in comatose survivors of cardiac arrest. *N Engl J Med* 314:397–403, 1986.
2. Steen P et al. Nimodipine improves cerebral blood flow and neurologic recovery after complete cerebral ischemia in the dog. *J Cereb Blood Flow Metab* 3:38–43, 1983.
3. Allen G et al. Cerebral arterial spasm: A controlled trial of nimodipine in patients with subarachoid hemorrhage. *N Engl J Med* 308:619–624, 1983.
4. Strand T et al. A randomized controlled trial of hemodilution therapy in acute ischemic stroke. *Stroke* 15:980–989, 1984.
5. Lassen N, Christensen M. Physiology of cerebral blood flow. *Br J Anaesth* 48:719–734, 1976.
6. Kennedy C, Sokoloff L. An adaptation of the nitrous oxide method to the study of the cerebral circulation in children; normal values for cerebral blood flow and cerebral metabolic rate in childhood. *J Clin Invest* 36:1130–1137, 1957.
7. Settergren G, Lindblad B, Persson B. Cerebral blood flow and exchange of oxygen, glucose, ketone bodies, lactate, pyruvate, and amino acids in anesthetized children. *Acta Pediatr Scand* 69:457–465, 1980.
8. Siesjö BK. Cerebral circulation and metabolism. *J Neurosurg* 60:883–908, 1984.
9. Frackowiak RS et al. Regional cerebral oxygen utilization and blood flow in normal man using oxygen-15 and positron emission tomography. *Acta Neurol Scand* 62:336–344, 1980.
10. Sokoloff L. Localization of functional activity in the central nervous system by measurement of glucose utilization with radioactive deoxyglucose. *J Cereb Blood Flow Metab* 1:7–36, 1981.
11. Nilsson B, Rehncrona S, Siesjö BK. Coupling of cerebral metabolism and blood flow in epileptic seizures, hypoxia, and hypoglycemia. In Purves M (ed): *Cerebral Vascular Smooth Muscle and Its Control.* CIBA Foundation Symposium 56 (New Series). Amsterdam: Elsevier, 1978. Pp 199–214.
12. Wahl M, Kuschinsky W. The dilatory action of adenosine on pial arteries of cats and its inhibition by theophylline. *Pflügers Arch* 362:55–59, 1976.
13. Toda N et al. Responses to adenine nucleotides and related compounds of isolated dog cerebral, coronary, and mesenteric arteries. *Blood Vessels* 19:226–236, 1982.
14. Morii S, Ngai AC, Winn HR. Reactivity of rat pial arterioles and venules to adenosine and carbon dioxide: With detailed descriptions of the closed cranial window technique in rats. *J Cereb Blood Flow Metab* 6:34–41, 1986.
15. Hardebo JE et al. Endothelium-dependent relaxation in cerebral arteries. *J Cereb Blood Flow Metab* 5(Suppl 1):S533–S534, 1985.
16. Phillis JW. Adenosine in the control of the cerebral circulation. *Cerebrovasc Brain Metab Rev* 1:26–54, 1989.
17. Kovach AGB et al. Effect of the organic calcium antagonist D-600 on cerebrocortical vascular and redox responses evoked by adenosine, anoxia, and epilepsy. *J Cereb Blood Flow Metab* 3:51–61, 1983.
18. Palmer RM, Ashton DS, Moncada S. Vascular endothelial cells synthesize nitric oxide from L-arginine. *Nature* 333:664–666, 1988.
19. Marshall JJ, Wei EP, Kontos HA. Independent blockade of cerebral vasodilation from acetylcholine and nitric oxide. *Am J Physiol* 255:H847–H854, 1988.
20. Shimokawa H, Kim P, Vanhoutte PM. Endothelium-dependent relaxation to aggregating platelets in isolated basilar arteries of control and hypercholesterolemic pigs. *Circ Res* 63:604–612, 1988.
21. Murphy S et al. An astrocyte-derived lipoxygenase product evokes endothelium-dependent relaxation of the basilar artery. *J Neurosci Res* 38:314–318, 1994.
22. Stamler JS, Singel DJ, Loscalzo J. Biochemistry of nitric oxide and its redox-activated forms. *Science* 258:1898–1902, 1992.
23. Malinski T et al. Nitric oxide measured by a porphyrinic microsensor in rat brain after transient middle cerebral artery occlusion. *J Cereb Blood Flow Metab* 13:355–358, 1993.
24. Kadder A et al. Nitric oxide production during focal cerebral ischemia in rats. *Stroke* 24:1709–1716, 1993.
25. Garthwaite J, Southam E, Anderton M. A kainate receptor linked to nitric oxide synthesis from arginine. *J Neurochem* 53:1952–1954, 1989.
26. Niwa K et al. Blockade of nitric oxide synthesis in rats strongly attentuates the CBF response to extracellular acidosis. *J Cereb Blood Flow Metab* 13:535–539, 1993.
27. Muizelaar JP et al. Cerebral blood flow and metabolism in severely head-injured children. Part 2: Autoregulation. *J Neurosurg* 71:72–76, 1989.
28. Bouma GJ, Muizelaar JP. Cerebral blood flow, cerebral blood volume, cerebrovascular reactivity after severe head injury. *J Neurotrauma* 9(Suppl 1):S333–S348, 1992.
29. Fog M. Cerebral circulation: The reaction of the pial arteries to a fall in blood pressure. *Arch Neurol Psychiatry* 37:351–364, 1937.
30. Fog M. Cerebral circulation II: Reaction of pial arteries to increase in blood pressure. *Arch Neurol Psychiatry* 41:260–278, 1939.
31. Miller JD, Stanek A, Langfitt TW. Concepts of cerebral perfusion pressure and vascular compression during intracranial hypertension. *Prog Brain Res* 35:411–432, 1972.
32. Phillis JW, DeLong RE. The role of adenosine in cerebral vascular regulation during reductions in perfusion pressure. *J Pharm Pharmacol* 38:460–462, 1986.
33. Wahl M, Kuschinsky W. Unimportance of perivascular H^+ and K^+ activities for adjustment of pial arterial diameter during changes in arterial blood pressure in cats. *Pflugers Arch* 382:203–208, 1979.
34. Paulson OB, Strandgaard S, Edvinsson L. Cerebral autoregulation. *Cerebrovasc Brain Metab Rev* 2:161–192, 1990.
35. Lassen NA, Agnoli A. The upper limit of autoregulation of cerebral blood flow—On the pathogenesis of acute hypertensive encephalopathy [sic]. *J Clin Lab Invest* 30:113–116, 1973.
36. Johansson BB. The blood-brain barrier and cerebral blood flow in acute hypertension. *Acta Med Scand* (Suppl 1):107–112, 1983.
37. Heistad DD et al. Effect of sympathetic nerve stimulation on cerebral blood flow and on large cerebral arteries of dogs. *Circ Res* 41:342–350, 1977.
38. Fitch W, MacKenzie ET, Harper AM. Effects of decreasing arterial blood pressure on cerebral blood flow in the baboon: Influence of the sympathetic nervous system. *Circ Res* 37:550–557, 1975.
39. Strandgaard S. Autoregulation of cerebral blood flow in hypertensive patients: The modifying influence of prolonged antihypertensive treatment on the tolerance to acute drug-induced hypotension. *Circulation* 53:720–727, 1976.
40. Vorstrup S et al. Chronic antihypertensive treatment in the rat reverses hypertension-induced changes in cerebral blood flow autoregulation. *Stroke* 15:312–318, 1984.
41. Symon L, Branston NM, Strong AJ. Autoregulation in acute focal ischemia. An experimental study. *Stroke* 7:547–554, 1976.
42. Waltz AG. Effect of blood pressure on blood flow in ischemic and

in nonischemic cerebral cortex. The phenomena of autoregulation and luxury perfusion. *Neurology* 18:613–621, 1968.

43. Enevoldsen EM, Jensen FT. Autoregulation in CO_2 responses of cerebral blood flow in patients with acute severe head injury. *J Neurosurg* 48:689–703, 1978.

44. Harper AM. Autoregulation of cerebral blood flow: Influence of the arterial blood pressure on the blood flow through the cerebral cortex. *J Neurol Neurosurg Psychiatry* 29:398–403, 1966.

45. Fieschi C et al. Derangement of regional cerebral blood flow and of its regulatory mechanisms in acute cerebrovascular lesions. *Neurology* 18:1166–1179, 1968.

46. Kogure K et al. Effects of hypoxia on cerebral autoregulation. *Am J Physiol* 219:1393–1396, 1970.

47. Reilly PL, Farrar JK, Miller JD. Vascular reactivity in the primate after acute cryogenic injury. *J Neurol Neurosurg Psychiatry* 40:1092–1101, 1977.

48. Lewelt W, Jenkins LW, Miller JD. Autoregulation of cerebral blood flow after experimental fluid percussion injury of the brain. *J Neurosurg* 53:500–511, 1980.

49. Lewelt W, Jenkins LW, Miller JD. Effects of experimental fluid percussion injury of the brain in cerebrovascular reactivity to hypoxia and hypercapnia. *J Neurosurg* 56:332–338, 1982.

50. Walker JL Jr, Brown AM. Unified account of the variable effects of carbon dioxide on nerve cells. *Science* 167:1502–1504, 1970.

51. Muizelaar JP et al. Mannitol causes compensatory cerebral vasoconstriction and vasodilation in response to blood viscosity changes. *J Neurosurg* 59:822–828, 1983.

52. Muizelaar JP et al. Cerebral blood flow is regulated by changes in blood pressure and in blood viscosity alike. *Stroke* 17:44–48, 1986.

53. Hudak ML et al. Hemodilution causes size-dependent constriction of pial arterioles in the cat. *Am J Physiol* 257:H912–H917, 1989.

54. Grubb RL et al. The effects of changes in $PaCO_2$ on cerebral blood volume, blood flow, and vascular mean transit time. *Stroke* 5:630–639, 1974.

55. Wahl M et al. Micropuncture evaluation of the importance of perivascular pH for the arteriolar diameter on the brain surface. *Pflugers Arch* 316:152–163, 1970.

56. Grote J, Zimmer K, Schubert R. Effects of severe arterial hypocapnia on regional blood flow regulation, tissue PO_2 and metabolism in the brain cortex of cats. *Pflugers Arch* 391:195–199, 1981.

57. Severinghaus JW et al. Cerebral blood flow in man at high altitude: Role of cerebrospinal fluid pH in normalization of flow in chronic hypocapnia. *Circ Res* 19:274–282, 1966.

58. Plum F, Seisjö BK. Recent advances in CSF physiology. *Anesthesiology* 42:708–730, 1975.

59. Harper AM, Bell RA. The effect of metabolic acidosis and alkalosis on the blood flow through the cerebral cortex. *J Neurol Neurosurg Psychiatry* 26:341–344, 1963.

60. Ovegaard J, Tweed WA. Cerebral circulation after head injury. Part 1: Cerebral blood flow and its regulation after closed head injury with emphasis on clinical correlations. *J Neurosurg* 41:531–541, 1974.

61. Saunders ML et al. The effects of graded experimental trauma on cerebral blood flow and responsiveness to CO_2. *J Neurosurg* 51:18–26, 1979.

62. Symon L. The concept of intracerebral steal. *Int Anesthesiol Clin* 7:597–615, 1969.

63. Wagerie LC et al. Cerebrovascular response to acute decreases in arterial PO_2. *J Cereb Blood Flow Metab* 3:507–515, 1983.

64. Emerson TE, Raymond RM. Involvement of adenosine in cerebral hypoxic hyperemia in the dog. *Am J Physiol* 241:H134–H138, 1981.

65. Morii S, Winn HR, Berne RM. Effect of theophylline, an adenosine receptor blocker, on cerebral blood flow during rest and transient hypoxia. *J Cereb Blood Flow Metab* 3 (Suppl 1):S480–S481, 1983.

66. Busija DW, Heistad DD. Factors involved in the physiological regulation of the cerebral circulation. *Rev Physiol Biochem Pharmacol* 101:162–210, 1984.

67. Edvinsson L et al. Concentration of noradrenaline in pial vessels, choroid plexus, and iris during two weeks after sympathetic ganglionectomy or decentralization. *Acta Physiol Scand* 85:201–206, 1972.

68. Edvinsson L, MacKenzie ET. Amine mechanism in the cerebral circulation. *Pharmacol Rev* 28:275–348, 1977.

69. Heistad DD, Marcus ML. Effect of sympathetic stimulation on permeability of the blood-brain barrier to albumin during acute hypertension in cats. *Circ Res* 45:331–338, 1979.

70. Bill A, Linder J. Sympathetic control of cerebral blood flow in acute arterial hypertension. *Acta Physiol Scand* 96:114–121, 1976.

71. Busija DW, Heistad DD. Effects of activation of sympathetic nerves on cerebral blood flow during hypercapnia in cats and rabbits. *J Physiol (Lond)* 347:35–45, 1984.

72. Edvinsson L, McCullough J, Uddman R. Feline cerebral veins and arteries: Comparison of autonomic innervation and vasomotor responses. *J Physiol (Lond)* 318:161–173, 1982.

73. Edvinsson L et al. Concentration of noradrenaline in pial vessels, choroid plexus, and iris during two weeks after sympathetic ganglionectomy or decentralization. *Acta Physiol Scand* 85:201–209, 1972.

74. Busija DW, Heistad DD. Effects of indomethacin in cerebral blood flow during hypercapnia in cats. *Am J Physiol* 244:H519–H524, 1982.

75. Wei EP, Kontos HA, Said SI. Mechanism of action of vasoactive intestinal polypeptide on cerebral arterioles. *Am J Physiol* 239:H765–H768, 1980.

76. Jaggi JL et al. Relationship of early cerebral blood flow and metabolism to outcome. in acute head injury. *J Neurosurg* 72:176–182, 1990.

77. Kety SS, Schmidt CF. The determination of cerebral blood flow in man by the use of nitrous oxide in low concentrations. *Am J Physiol* 143:53–65, 1945.

78. Olesen J, Paulson OB, Lassen NA. Regional cerebral blood flow in man determined by the initial slope of the clearance of intra-arterially injected ^{133}Xe. *Stroke* 2:519–540, 1971.

79. Obrist WD et al. Regional cerebral blood flow estimated by ^{133}xenon inhalation. *Stroke* 6:245–256, 1975.

80. Risberg J et al. Regional cerebral blood flow by ^{133}xenon inhalation. *Stroke* 6:142–148, 1975.

81. Ter-Pogossian MM et al. A positron-emission transaxial tomograph for nuclear imaging (PETT). *Radiology* 114:89–98, 1975.

82. Lenzi GL, Frackowiak RS, Jones T. Cerebral oxygen metabolism and blood flow in human cerebral ischemic infarction. *J Cereb Blood Flow Metab* 2:321–335, 1982.

83. Wise RJS et al. Serial observations on the pathophysiology of acute stroke: The transition from ischaemia to infarction as reflected in regional oxygen extraction. *Brain* 106:197–222, 1983.

84. Gardner SF et al. Principles and clinical applications of positron emission tomography. *Am J Hosp Pharm* 49:1499–1506, 1992.

85. Wyper DJ. Functional neuroimaging with single photon emission computed tomography (SPECT). *Cerebrovasc Brain Metab Rev* 5:199–217, 1993.

86. Aaslid R, Markwalder T-M, Nornes H. Noninvasive transcranial Doppler ultrasound recording of flow velocity in basal cerebral arteries. *J Neurosurg* 57:769–774, 1982.

87. Petty GW, Wiebers DO, Meissner I. Transcranial Dopple ultrasonography: Clinical applications in cerebrovascular disease. *Mayo Clin Proc* 65:1350–1364, 1990.

88. Gosling RG, King DH. Arterial assessment by Doppler shift ultrasound. *Proc R Soc Med* 67:447–449, 1974.

89. Niderkorn K et al. Three-dimensional transcranial Doppler blood flow mapping in patients with cerebrovascular disorders. *Stroke* 19:1335–1344, 1988.

90. Bolognese P et al. Laser-Doppler flowmetry in neurosurgery. *J Neurosurg Anesthesiol* 5:151–158, 1993.

91. Rosenblum BR, Boner RF, Oldfield EH. Intraoperative measurement of cortical blood flow adjacent to cerebral AVM using laser Doppler velocimetry. *J Neurosurg* 66:396–399, 1987.

92. Haberl RL, Heizer ML, Ellis EF. Laser Doppler assessment of the brain microcirculation: Effect of local alterations. *Am J Physiol* 256:H1255–H1260, 1989.

93. Haberl RL et al. Laser-Doppler assessment of brain microcirculation: Effect of systemic alterations. *Am J Physiol* 256:H1247–H1254, 1989.

94. Salerud EG, Nilsson GE. Integrating probe for tissue laser Doppler flowmeters. *Med Biol Eng Comput* 24:415–419, 1986.

95. Salerud EG, Oberg PÅ. Single-fiber laser Doppler flowmetry. A method for deep tissue perfusion measurements. *Med Biol Eng Comput* 25:329–334, 1987.

96. Newson TP et al. Laser Doppler velocimetry: The problem of fibre movement artefact. *J Biomed Eng* 9:169–172, 1987.

97. Tenland T et al. Spatial and temporal variations in human skin blood flow. *Int J Microcirc Clin Exp* 2:81–90, 1983.

98. Meyerson BA et al. Bedside monitoring of regional cortical blood flow in comatose patients using laser Doppler flowmetry. *Neurosurgery* 29:750–755, 1991.

99. Dirnagl U et al. Continuous measurement of cerebral cortical blood flow by laser Doppler flowmetry in a rat stroke model. *J Cereb Blood Flow Metab* 9:589–596, 1989.

100. Lindsberg PJ et al. Validation of laser-Doppler flowmetry in measurement of spinal and blood flow. *Am J Physiol* 257:H674–H680, 1989.

101. Arbit E et al. Intraoperative measurement of cerebral and tumor blood flow with laser-Doppler flowmetry. *Neurosurgery* 24:166–170, 1989.

102. Fasano VA et al. Intraoperative use of laser Doppler in the study of cerebral microvascular circulation. *Acta Neurochir (Wien)* 95:40–48, 1988.

103. Mayevsky A et al. A fiber optic based multiprobe system for intraoperative monitoring of brain function. In Chance B, Katzir A (eds): *Time-resound Spectroscopy and Imaging of Tissues.* Los Angeles: SPIE, 1991. Pp 303–313.

104. Hashimoto T et al. Monitoring of hemodynamics in subarachnoid hemorrhage using transcranial Doppler and laser Doppler. In Frowen RA, Brock M, Klinger M (eds): *Advances in Neurosurgery.* Vol 17. Berlin: Springer, 1989. Pp 337–343.

105. Haberl RL, Villringer A, Dirnagl U. Applicability of laser-Doppler flowmetry for cerebral blood flow monitoring in neurological intensive care. *Acta Neurochir (Wien)* 59(Suppl):64–68, 1993.

106. Astrup J, Siesjö BK, Symon L. Thresholds in cerebral ischemia: The ischemic penumbra. *Stroke* 12:723–725, 1981.

107. Shapiro H. Monitoring in neurosurgical anesthesia. In Saidman L, Smith N, (eds): *Monitoring in Anesthesia* (2nd ed). Boston: Butterworths, 1984. Pp 269–309.

108. Heiss W-D. Experimental evidence for ischemic thresholds and functional recovery. *Stroke* 23:1668–1672, 1992.

109. Inoue T et al. Emphasized selective vulnerability after repeated nonlethal cerebral ischemic insults in rats. *Stroke* 23:739–745, 1992.

110. Siesjö BK, Zwetnow NN. The effect of hypovolemic hypotension on extra- and intracellular acid-base parameters and energy metabolites in the rat brain. *Acta Physiol Scand* 79:114–124, 1970.

111. Siesjö BK, Nilsson L. The influence of arterial hypoxemia upon labile phosphates and upon extracellular and intracellular lactate and pyruvate concentrations in the rat brain. *Scand J Clin Lab Invest* 27:83–96, 1971.

112. Meyer FB et al. Intracellular brain pH, indicator tissue perfusion, electroencephalography, and histology in severe and moderate focal cortical ischemia in the rabbit. *J Cereb Blood Flow Metab* 6:71–78, 1986.

113. Naritomi H et al. Flow thresholds for cerebral energy disturbance and Na^+ pump failure as studied by in vivo ^{31}P and ^{23}Na nuclear magnetic resonance spectroscopy. *J Cereb Blood Flow Metab* 8:16–23, 1988.

114. Obrenovitch TP et al. Brain tissue concentrations of ATP, phosphocreatine, lactate and tissue pH in relation to reduced cerebral blood flow following experimental acute middle cerebral artery occlusion. *J Cereb Blood Flow Metab* 8:866–874, 1988.

115. Wieloch T et al. Influence of severe hypoglycemia on brain extracellular calcium and potassium activities, energy, and phospholipid metabolism. *J Neurochem* 43:160–168, 1984.

116. Hansen AJ. Effect of anoxia on ion distribution in the brain. *Physiol Rev* 65:101–148, 1985.

117. Nedergaard M. Mechanisms of brain damage in focal cerebral ischemia. *Acta Neurol Scand* 77:81–101, 1988.

118. Sauter A, Rudin M. Prevention of stroke and brain damage with calcium antagonist in animals. *Am J Hypertens* 4:121s–127s, 1991.

119. Siesjö BK. Pathophysiology and treatment on focal ischemia. Part I: Pathophysiology. *J Neurosurg* 77:169–184, 1992.

120. Mies G, Iijima T, Hosman KA. Correlation between peri-infarct DC shifts and ischaemic neuronal damage in the rat. *Neuroreport* 4:709–711, 1993.

121. Porlishock JT et al. Axonal change in minor head injury. *J Neuropath Exp Neurol* 42:225–242, 1983.

122. Kontos HA. Oxygen radicals in CNS damage. *Chem Biol Interact* 72:229–255, 1989.

123. Kontos HA. Oxygen radicals in cerebral vascular injury. *Circ Res* 57:508–516, 1985.

124. Garthwaite J. Glutamate, nitric oxide and cell-cell signaling in the nervous system. *TINS* 14:60–67, 1991.

125. Patt A et al. Xanthine oxidase-derived hydrogen peroxide contributes to ischemia reperfusion-induced edema in gerbil brains. *J Clin Invest* 81:1556–1562, 1988.

126. Siesjö BK. Pathophysiology and treatment of focal ischemia. Part II: Mechanisms of damage and treatment. *J Neurosurg* 77:337–354, 1992.

127. Chan PH et al. Brain injury, edema, and vascular permeability changes induced by oxygen-derived free radicals. *Neurology* 34:315–320, 1984.

128. Choi DW. Glutamate neurotoxicity and diseases of the nervous system. *Neuron* 1:623–634, 1988.

129. Dawson TM, Dawson VL, Snyder SH. A novel neuronal messenger in the brain: The free radical nitric oxide. *Ann Neurol* 32:297–311, 1992.

130. Trout JJ et al. N-methyl-D-aspartate receptor excitotoxicity involves activation of polyamine synthesis: Protection by alpha difluoromethylornithine. *J Neurochem* 60:352–355, 1993.

131. Prough DS, DeWitt DS. Cerebral protection. In Chernow B (ed): *The Pharmacologic Approach to the Critically Ill Patient* (2nd ed). Baltimore: Williams & Wilkins, 1988. Pp 198–218.

132. Bazán NG. Free arachidonic acid and other lipids in the nervous system during early ischemia and after electroshock. *Adv Exp Med Biol* 72:317–335, 1976.

133. Bevan S, Wood JN. Arachidonic-acid metabolites as second messengers. *Nature* 328:20, 1987.

134. Moskowitz MA et al. Synthesis of compounds with properties of leukotrienes C_4 and D_4 in gerbil brains after ischemia and reperfusion. *Science* 224:886–889, 1984.

135. Bhakoo KK, Crockard HA, Lascelles PT. Regional studies of changes in brain fatty acids following experimental ischaemia and reperfusion in the gerbil. *J Neurochem* 43:1025–1031, 1984.

136. Lafon-Cazal M et al. NMDA-dependent superoxide production and neurotoxicity. *Nature* 364:535–537, 1993.

137. Miller B et al. Potentiation of NMDA receptor currents by arachidonic acid. *Nature* 355:722–725, 1992.

138. Lipton SA, Rosenberg PA. Excitatory amino acids as a final common pathway for neurologic disorders. *N Engl J Med* 330:613–622, 1994.

139. Rothman SM, Olney JW. Glutamate and the pathophysiology of hypoxic-ischemic brain damage. *Ann Neurol* 19:105–111, 1986.

140. Pulsinelli WA, Levy DE, Duffy TE. Regional cerebral blood flow and glucose metabolism following transient forebrain ischemia. *Ann Neurol* 11:499–509, 1982.

141. Siesjö BK, Bengtsson F. Calcium fluxes, calcium antagonists, and calcium-related pathology in brain ischemia, hypoglycemia and spreading depression: A unifying hypothesis. *J Cereb Blood Flow Metab* 9:127–140, 1989.

142. Johansen FF, Jørgensen MB, Diemer NH. Ischemic CA-1 pyramidal cell loss is prevented by preischemic colchicine destruction of dentate gyrus granule cells. *Brain Res* 377:344–347, 1986.

143. Jørgensen MB, Johansen FF, Diemer NH. Removal of the entorhinal cortex protects hippocampal CA-1 neurons from ischemic damage. *Acta Neuropathol (Berl)* 73:189–194, 1987.

144. Benveniste H et al. Calcium accumulation by glutamate receptor activation is involved in hippocampal cell damage after ischemia. *Acta Neurol Scand* 78:529–536, 1988.

145. Albers GW, Goldberg MP, Choi DW. N-methyl-D-aspartate antagonists: Ready for a clinical trial in brain ischemia? *Ann Neurol* 25:398–403, 1989.

146. Phillis JW et al. Characterization of glutamate, aspartate, and GABA release from ischemic rat cerebral cortex. *Brain Res Bull* 34:457–466, 1994.

147. Siesjö BK. Cell damage in the brain: A speculative synthesis. *J Cereb Blood Flow Metab* 1:155–185, 1981.

148. Gill R. The pharmacology of α-amino-3-hydroxy-5-methyl-4-isoxazole propionate (AMPA)/kainate antagonists and their role in cerebral ischaemia. *Cerebrovasc Brain Metab Rev* 6:225–256, 1994.

149. Bean BP. Classes of calcium channels in vertebrate cells. *Annu Rev Physiol* 51:367–384, 1989.

150. Lipton SA et al. A redox-based mechanism for the neuroprotective and neurodestructive effects of nitric oxide and related nitroso-compounds. *Nature* 364:626–632, 1993.

151. Dawson VL et al. Nitric oxide mediates glutamate neurotoxicity in primary cortical cultures. *Proc Natl Acad Sci USA* 88:6368–6371, 1991.

151a. Dawson DA. Nitric oxide and focal cerebral ischemia: Multiplicity of actions and diverse outcome. *Cerebrovasc Brain Metab Rev* 6:229–324, 1994.

152. Toda N, Okamura T. Possible role of nitric oxide in transmitting information from vasodilator nerve to cerebroarterial muscle. *Biochem Biophys Res Commun* 170:308–313, 1990.

153. Toda N, Okamura T. Role of nitric oxide in neurally induced cerebroarterial relaxation. *J Pharmacol Exp Ther* 258:1027–1032, 1991.

154. Lee TJF, Sarwinski SJ. Nitric oxidergic neurogenic vasodilation in the porcine basilar artery. *Blood Vessels* 28:407–412, 1991.

155. Huang Z et al. Effects of cerebral ischemia in mice deficient in neuronal nitric oxide synthase. *Science* 265:1883–1885, 1994.

156. Demerlé-Pallardy C et al. Absence of implication of L-arginine/nitric oxide pathway on neuronal cell injury induced by L-glutamate or hypoxia. *Biochem Biophys Res Commun* 181:456–464, 1991.

157. Vigé X et al. Antagonism by NG-nitro-L-arginine of L-glutamate-induced neurotoxicity in cultured neonatal rat cortical neurons. Prolonged application enhances neuroprotective efficacy. *Neuroscience* 55:893–901, 1993.

158. Mohamed AA et al. Effect of pretreatment with the calcium antagonist nimodipine on local cerebral blood flow and histopathology after middle cerebral artery occlusion. *Ann Neurol* 18:705–711, 1985.

159. Gotoh O et al. Nimodipine and the haemodynamic and histopathological consequences of middle cerebral artery occlusion in the rat. *J Cereb Blood Flow Metab* 6:321–331, 1986.

160. Uematsu D et al. Cytosolic free calcium, NAD/NADH redox state and hemodynamic changes in the cat cortex during severe hypoglycemia. *J Cereb Blood Flow Metab* 9:149–155, 1989.

161. Hakim AM. Cerebral acidosis in focal ischemia: II. Nimodipine and verapamil normalize cerebral pH following middle cerebral artery occlusion in the rat. *J Cereb Blood Flow Metab* 6:676–683, 1986.

162. Meyer FB et al. Effect of nimodipine on intracellular brain pH, cortical blood flow, and EEG in experimental focal ischemia. *J Neurosurg* 64:617–626, 1986.

163. Nowycky MC, Fox AP, Tsien RW. Three types of neuronal calcium channel with different calcium agonist sensitivity. *Nature* 316:440–443, 1985.

164. Ohta S, Smith M-L, Siesjö BK. The effect of a dihyropyridine calcium antagonist (isradipine) on selective neuronal necrosis. *J Neurol Sci* 103:109–115, 1991.

165. Akaike N, Kostyuk PG, Osipchuk YV. Dihydropyridine-sensitive low-threshold calcium channels in isolated rat hypothalamic neurones. *J Physiol (Lond)* 412:181–195, 1989.

166. Gill R et al. The effect of MK-801 on cortical spreading depression in the penumbral zone following focal ischaemia in the rat. *J Cereb Blood Flow Metab* 12:371–379, 1992.

167. Minematsu K et al. Effects of a novel NMDA antagonist on experimental stroke rapidly and quantitatively assessed by diffusion-weighted MRI. *Neurology* 43:397–403, 1993.

168. Gill R, Nordholm L, Lodge D. The neuroprotective action of 2,3-dihydroxy-6-nitro-7-sulfamoyl-benzo (F) quinoxaline (NBQX) in a rat focal ischaemia model. *Brain Res* 580:35–43, 1992.

169. Xue D et al. Delayed treatment with AMPA, but not NDMA, antagonists reduces neocortical infarction. *J Cereb Blood Flow Metab* 14:251–261, 1994.

170. Meldrum B. Protection against ischaemic neuronal damage by drugs acting on excitatory neurotransmission. *Cerebrovasc Brain Metab Rev* 2:27–57, 1990.

171. Foutz AS, Pierrefiche O, Denavit-Saubie M. Combined blockade of NMDA and non-NMDA receptors produces respiratory arrest in the adult cat. *Neuroreport* 5:481–484, 1994.

172. Yoshida T et al. The NOS inhibitor, 7-nitroindazole, decreases focal infarct volume but not the response to topical acetylcholine in pial vessels. *J Cereb Blood Flow Metab* 14:924–929, 1994.

173. Martz D et al. Allopurinol and dimethylthiourea reduce brain infarction following middle cerebral artery occlusion in rats. *Stroke* 20:488–494, 1989.

174. Maruki Y et al. Effect of the 21-aminosteroid trilizad on cerebral pH and somatosensory evoked potential recovery after incomplete ischemia. *Stroke* 24:724–730, 1993.

175. Ames A III et al. Cerebral ischemia: II. The no-reflow phenomenon. *Am J Pathol* 52:437–453, 1968.

176. Prough DS et al. Inhibition of thromboxane A_2 production does not improve post-ischemic brain hypoperfusion in the dog. *Stroke* 17:1272–1276, 1986.

177. Little JR, Kerr FW, Sundt TM. Microcirculatory obstruction in focal cerebral ischemia: Relationship to neuronal alterations. *Mayo Clin Proc* 50:264–270, 1975.

178. Rosner M. Cerebral perfusion pressure: Link between intracranial pressure and systemic circulation. In Wood J (ed): *Cerebral Blood Flow: Physiologic and Clinical Aspects*. New York: McGraw-Hill, 1987. Pp 425–448.

179. Shaywitz BA, Rothstein P, Venes JL. Monitoring and management of increased intracranial pressure in Reye's syndrome: Results in 29 children. *Pediatrics* 66:198–204, 1980.

180. Bruce DA et al. Outcome following severe head injuries in children. *J Neurosurg* 48:679–688, 1978.

181. Saul TG, Ducker TB. Effect of intracranial pressure monitoring and aggressive treatment on mortality in severe head injury. *J Neurosurg* 56:498–503, 1982.

182. Aucoin JP et al. Intracranial pressure monitors. Epidemiologic study of risk factors and infections. *Am J Med* 80:369–376, 1986.

183. Narayan RK et al. Intracranial pressure: To monitor or not to monitor? A review of our experience with severe head injury. *J Neurosurg* 56:650–659, 1982.

184. Mendelow AD et al. A clinical comparison of subdural screw pressure measurements with ventricular pressure. *J Neurosurg* 58:45–50, 1983.

185. Chambers IR et al. A clinical evaluation of the Camino subdural screw and ventricular monitoring kits. *Neurosurgery* 26:421–423, 1990.

186. Crutchfield JS et al. Evaluation of a fiberoptic intracranial pressure monitor. *J Neurosurg* 72:482–487, 1990.

187. Levin AB. The use of a fiberoptic intracranial pressure monitor in clinical practice. *Neurosurgery* 1:266–271, 1977.

188. Cruz J et al. Cerebral oxygenation monitoring. *Crit Care Med* 21:1242–1246, 1993.

189. Cruz J et al. Continuous monitoring of cerebral oxygenation in

acute brain injury: Assessment of cerebral hemodynamic reserve. *Neurosurgery* 29:743–749, 1991.

190. Cruz J. Continuous monitoring of cerebral oxygenation in acute brain injury: Assessment of cerebral hemometabolic regulation. *Minerva Anestesiol* 59:555–562, 1993.

191. Obrist WD et al. Cerebral blood flow and metabolism in comatose patients with acute head injury. Relationship to intracranial hypertension. *J Neurosurg* 61:241–253, 1984.

192. Cruz J, Gennarelli TA, Hoffstad OJ. Lack of relevance of the Bohr effect in optimally ventilated patients with acute brain trauma. *J Trauma* 33:304–311, 1992.

193. Bullock R et al. Continuous monitoring of jugular bulb oxygen saturation and the effect on drugs acting on cerebral metabolism. *Acta Neurochir (Wien)* Suppl 59:113–118, 1993.

194. Cold GE. Does acute hyperventilation provoke cerebral oligaemia in comatose patients after acute head injury? *Acta Neurochir (Wien)* 96:100–106, 1989.

195. Mayer T, Walker ML. Emergency intracranial pressure monitoring in pediatrics: Management of the acute coma of brain insult. *Clin Pediatr* 21:391–396, 1982.

196. Michaud LJ et al. Predictors of survival and severity of disability after severe brain injury in children. *Neurosurgery* 31:254–264, 1992.

197. Rosner M, Coley IB. Cerebral perfusion pressure, intracranial pressure, and head elevation. *J Neurosurg* 65:636–641, 1986.

198. Schneider GH et al. Influence of body position on jugular venous oxygen saturation intracranial pressure and cerebral perfusion pressure. *Acta Neurochir (Wien)* 59(Suppl):107–112, 1993.

199. Durward Q et al. Cerebral and cardiovascular responses to changes in head elevation in patients with intracranial hypertension. *J Neurosurg* 59:938–944, 1983.

200. Ropper AH, O'Rourke D, Kennedy SK. Head position, intracranial pressure and compliance. *Neurology* 32:1288–1291, 1982.

201. Longstreth WT Jr, Inui TS. High blood glucose level on hospital admission and poor neurological recovery after cardiac arrest. *Ann Neurol* 15:59–63, 1984.

202. Sutherland GR et al. Forebrain ischemia in diabetic and non-diabetic BB rats studied with ^{31}P magnetic resonance spectroscopy. *Diabetes* 41:1328–1334, 1992.

203. Pulsinelli WA et al. Increased damage after ischemic stroke in patients with hyperglycemia with or without established diabetes mellitus. *Am J Med* 74:540–544, 1983.

204. Longstreth WT Jr et al. Neurologic outcome and blood glucose levels during out-of-hospital cardiopulmonary resuscitation. *Neurology* 36:1186–1191, 1986.

205. Yatsu FM, McKenzie JD, Lockwood AH. Cardiopulmonary arrest and intravenous glucose. *J Crit Care* 2:1–3, 1987.

206. Rhencrona S, Rosen I, Seisjö BK. Excessive cellular acidosis: An important mechanism of neuronal damage in the brain? *Acta Physiol Scand* 110:435–437, 1980.

207. Massonnet B, Ont M, Cibanc M. Hypothalamic fever in a human. In Lipton JM (ed): *Fever.* New York: Raven, 1980. Pp 243–248.

208. Kuroiwa T, Bonnekoh P, Hossman K-A. Prevention of postischemic hyperthermia prevents ischemic injury of CA1 neurons in gerbils. *J Cereb Blood Flow Metab* 10:550–556, 1990.

209. Dietrich WD et al. Effects of normothermic versus mild hypothermic forebrain ischemia in rats. *Stroke* 21:1318–1325, 1990.

210. Morikawa E et al. The significance of brain temperature in focal cerebral ischemia: Histopathological consequences of middle cerebral artery occlusion in the rat. *J Cereb Blood Flow Metab* 12:380–389, 1992.

211. Hahn YS et al. Factors influencing posttraumatic seizures in children. *Neurosurgery* 22:864–867, 1988.

212. North JB et al. Phenytoin and postoperative epilepsy: A double-blind study. *J Neurosurg* 58:672–677, 1983.

213. Raichle ME, Plum F. Hyperventilation and cerebral blood flow. *Stroke* 3:566–575, 1972.

214. Gordon E, Rossanda M. Further studies on cerebrospinal fluid acid-base status in patients with brain lesions. *Acta Anaesthesiol Scand* 14:97–109, 1970.

215. Muizelaar JP et al. Adverse effects of prolonged hyperventilation in patients with severe head injury. A randomized clinical trial. *J Neurosurg* 75:731–739, 1991.

216. Muizelaar JP et al. Pial arteriolar vessel diameter and CO_2 reactivity during prolonged hyperventilation in the rabbit. *J Neurosurg* 69:923–927, 1988.

217. Greenberg JH et al. Local cerebral blood volume response to carbon dioxide in man. *Circ Res* 43:324–331, 1978.

218. Kennealy JA et al. Hyperventilation-induced cerebral hypoxia. *Am Rev Respir Dis* 122:407–412, 1980.

219. Marshall LF et al. Mannitol dose requirements in brain-injured patients. *J Neurosurg* 48:169–172, 1978.

220. Stuart FP et al. Effects of single, repeated and massive mannitol infusion in the dog: Structural and functional changes in kidney and brain. *Ann Surg* 172:190–204, 1970.

221. Wise BL et al. Penetration of C^{14}-labeled mannitol from serum into cerebral spinal fluid and brain. *Exp Neurol* 10:264–270, 1964.

222. Michenfelder JD. The interdependency of cerebral functional and metabolic effects following massive doses of thiopental in the dog. *Anesthesiology* 41:231–236, 1974.

223. Nordström C-H et al. Cerebral blood flow, vasoreactivity, and oxygen consumption during barbiturate therapy in severe traumatic brain lesions. *J Neurosurg* 68:424–431, 1988.

224. Rockoff MA, Marshall LF, Shapiro HM. High-dose barbiturate therapy in humans: A clinical review of 60 patients. *Ann Neurol* 6:194–199, 1979.

225. Marshall LF, Smith RW, Shapiro HM. The outcome with aggressive treatment in severe head injuries: Part II: Acute and chronic barbiturate administration in the management of head injury. *J Neurosurg* 50:26–30, 1979.

226. Conn AW, Edmonds JF, Barker GA. Cerebral resuscitation in near-drowning. *Pediatr Clin North Am* 26:691–701, 1979.

227. Eisenberg HM et al., Comprehensive Central Nervous System Trauma Centers. High-dose barbiturate control of elevated intracranial pressure in patients with severe head injury. *J Neurosurg* 69:15–23, 1988.

228. Consensus Conference: Diagnosis and treatment of Reye's syndrome. *JAMA* 246:2441–2444, 1981.

229. Ward JD et al. Failure of prophylactic barbiturate coma in the treatment of severe head trauma. *J Neurosurg* 62:383–388, 1985.

230. Bohn DJ et al. Influence of hypothermia, barbiturate therapy, and intracranial pressure monitoring on morbidity and mortality after near-drowning. *Crit Care Med* 14:529–534, 1986.

231. Louis PT et al. Barbiturates and hyperventilation during intracranial hypertension. *Crit Care Med* 21:1200–1206, 1993.

232. Berger MS et al. Outcome from severe head injury in children and adolescents. *J Neurosurg* 62:194–199, 1985.

233. Miller JD et al. Significance of intracranial hypertension in severe head injury. *J Neurosurg* 47:503–516, 1977.

234. Pittman T, Bucholz R, Williams D. Efficacy of barbiturates in the treatment of resistant intracranial hypertension in severely head-injured children. *Pediatr Neurosci* 15:13–17, 1989.

235. Ridendour TR et al. Mild hypothermia reduces infarct size resulting from temporary but not permanent focal ischemia in rats. *Stroke* 23:733–738, 1992.

236. Kuboyama K et al. Delay in cooling negates the beneficial effect of mild resuscitative cerebral hypothermia after cardiac arrest in dogs: A prospective, randomized study. *Crit Care Med* 21:1348–1358, 1993.

237. Lo EH, Steinberg GK. Effects of hypothermia on evoked potentials, magnetic resonance imaging, and blood flow in focal ischemia in rabbits. *Stroke* 23:889–893, 1992.

238. Bohn D, Kent G, Beggar WD. Changes in polymorphonuclear leukocyte function in vivo and in vitro with anesthesia and hypothermia. *Anesthesiology* 57(Suppl):A133, 1982.

239. Galicich JH, French LA, Melby JC. Use of dexamethasone in treat-

ment of cerebral edema associated with brain tumors. *Lancet* 81:46–53, 1961.

240. Reulen HJ. Vasogenic brain oedema: New aspects in its formation, resolution, and therapy. *Br J Anaesth* 48:741–752, 1976.

241. Dearden NM et al. Effects of high-dose dexamethasone on outcome from severe head injury. *J Neurosurg* 64:81–88, 1986.

242. Saul TG et al. Steroids in severe head injury. A prospective randomized clinical trial. *J Neurosurg* 54:596–600, 1981.

243. Cooper PL et al. Dexamethasone and severe head injury: A prospective double-blind study. *J Neurosurg* 51:307–316, 1979.

244. Gudeman SK, Miller JD, Becker DP. Failure of high-dose steroid therapy to influence intracranial pressure in patients with severe head injury. *J Neurosurg* 51:301–306, 1979.

245. Donley RF, Sundt TM Jr. The effect of dexamethasone on the edema of focal cerebral ischemia. *Stroke* 4:148–155, 1974.

246. Lee MC et al. Ineffectiveness of dexamethasone for treatment of experimental cerebral infarction. *Stroke* 5:216–218, 1974.

247. Plum F, Alvord EC Jr, Posner JB. Effect of steroids on experimental cerebral infarction. *Arch Neurol* 9:571–573, 1963.

248. Jefferson LS, Mayes TC. Cardiopulmonary resuscitation. In Garson A Jr, Bricker T, McNamara DG (eds): *The Science and Practice of Pediatric Cardiology.* Malvern: Lea & Febiger, 1990. Pp 401–427.

249. Yoshida K, Marmarou A. Effects of tromethamine and hyperventilation on brain injury in the cat. *J Neurosurg* 74:87–96, 1991.

250. Rosner MJ, Becker DP. Experimental brain injury: Successful therapy with the weak base, tromethamine. With an overview of CNS acidosis. *J Neurosurg* 60:961–971, 1984.

251. Wolf AL et al. Effect of THAM upon outcome in severe head injury: A randomized prospective clinical trial. *J Neurosurg* 78:54–59, 1993.

252. Gaab MR, Seegers K, Goetz C. THAM (tromethamine, "tris-buffer"): Effective therapy of traumatic brain swelling. In Hoff JT, Betz AL (eds): *Intracranial Pressure VII.* Berlin: Springer, 1989. Pp 616–619.

253. Albers GW et al. Safety, tolerability, and pharmacokinetics of the N-methyl-D-aspartate antagonist dextrorphan in patients with acute stroke. Dextrorphan study group. *Stroke* 26:254–258, 1995.

254. Bensimon G et al., Riluzole Study Group. A controlled trial of Riluzole in amyotrophic lateral sclerosis. *N Engl J Med* 330:585–591, 1994.

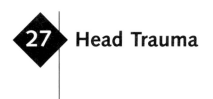

27 Head Trauma

Despite efforts at prevention, head injury remains a significant source of mortality and neurologic morbidity in the pediatric population. There are an estimated 12,000 deaths per year from head injury in the U.S. population aged 19 or less.[1] Five times as many children aged 0 to 14 die of head injuries as from leukemia, the next leading killer. Although brain tumors are a significant source of neurologic morbidity, head trauma causes more deaths than all other neurologic diagnoses combined. Ongoing neuroprotection studies notwithstanding, little can currently be done to actively repair neuronal damage occurring at the time of injury; the goal of intensive care unit (ICU) management in head trauma should be to prevent secondary injury while attempting to minimize neurologic and systemic complications.

Pathophysiology

The underlying pathophysiology varies with both the mechanism of injury and the age of the child.[2] Although neuronal division and migration are completed by about the twentieth fetal week, glial proliferation, dendritic maturation, and myelination begin in midgestation and continue for years after birth. Glial mitosis begins about fetal week 15 and continues to age 2 years; astrocytes apparently retain their ability to divide throughout life.[3] Neurons undergo progressive dendritic maturation, with the number of dendritic spines increasing until about age 7 years.[4] Oligodendroglia begin myelination of the vestibular system in late gestation, optic tracts myelinate for 6 months postnatally, pyramidal tracts for 2 years, and the reticular formation and cortical association areas continue myelination into adulthood.[1] Although significant brain development occurs postnatally, it matures rapidly in comparison with other organ systems. At birth, the brain is 25% of adult weight, 50% by 6 months, and 90% by 5 years; skeletal growth is 5% of adult weight at birth and 50% at 10 years.[5] Head injury in infancy and childhood thus both acts on an immature substrate with an altered response to injury and impairs the ability of the maturing brain to proceed with normal differentiation and development. Although experimental evidence suggests that the developing nervous system exhibits considerable plasticity after injury, it remains unclear whether this plasticity is truly functional or only aborted normal development.[6]

Cellular Response to Injury

Direct CNS trauma sets off a cascade of events involving both the brain parenchyma and vasculature, which can result in local and diffuse edema, ischemia, and widespread cell death.[7,8] The immediate impact causes membrane disruption and release of intracellular contents, with formation of free radicals,[9] arachidonic acid metabolites, and release of lysosomal enzymes. Loss of membrane integrity leads to loss of ionic gradients, with an increase in intracellular Ca^{++}, membrane depolarization, and increased extracellular K^+. Transmitter release, especially glutamate, has been implicated in the excitotoxicity mechanism of cell death, where the uncontrolled excitatory action of glutamate leads to neuronal destruction.[10] Loss of membrane integrity also leads to breakdown of osmotic gradients, with cytogenic edema. Trauma to the microcirculation causes opening of the blood-brain barrier, with influx of prostaglandins, activation of the kallikrein-kinin system, and development of vasogenic edema. Platelet activation from vascular injury causes release of serotonin and histamine, two potent vasodilators, with loss of vasomotor tone and autoregulation. The result of this complicated and poorly understood system is focal and diffuse edema, with elevated intracranial pressure (ICP), and decreased cerebral perfusion, with ongoing cerebral ischemia and neuronal damage. The ongoing cerebral injury, separate from the initial injury, is known as the secondary injury cascade, and much current research is directed at preventing its progression.[11]

Pathophysiology of Intracranial Pressure and Blood Flow

In a child with fused sutures, the skull acts as a fixed container that must accommodate noncompressible brain, cerebral spinal fluid (CSF), and the intravascular volume. This three-compartment model has been developed to account for the relationship between ICP and intracranial volume—cerebral compliance.[12,13] A hemorrhagic mass lesion and focal or diffuse edema cause distortion of the surrounding brain; this mass effect is initially compensated by movement of CSF into the lumbar subarachnoid space. With progressive edema or mass effect, ICP will rise as compensatory mechanisms fail, and one moves into the more vertical portion of the exponential ICP compliance curve. At this point, even small changes in intracranial volume result in large increases in ICP. Cerebral perfusion pressure (CPP), defined as the difference between arterial blood pressure (MAP) and ICP, will fall as ICP rises.[14] As CPP falls, cerebral ischemia progresses, with further activation of the injury cascade. Clinical and experimental evidence in normal adults suggests that a CPP below about 40 torr is associated with cerebral ischemia, and this corresponds to a MAP of 80 torr and ICP of 30 to 40 torr.[15] The ischemic threshold appears to be lowered after trauma, and perfusion pressures of 70–80 torr may be required to maintain adequate tissue oxygenation.

Local factors may also be significant. ICP near an area of damaged brain may be higher than that obtained at the site of an epidural or subarachnoid pressure sensor, and local changes in autoregulation may lead to altered flow despite presumably adequate perfusion pressure. Focal expansion at the tentorial hiatus or posterior fossa may lead to devastating brainstem compression, despite normal or marginally elevated ICP at the site of pressure measurement. In general, diffuse elevation of ICP can be well tolerated for long periods (e.g., pseudotumor cerebri), if not associated with shifts in brainstem structures.

Although perfusion pressure is a useful concept, the therapeutic goal is to maintain cerebral blood flow (CBF) at a level adequate to prevent ongoing ischemia, and perfusion pressure simply represents one related measurable parameter. Cell death occurs with CBF less than 12 ml/100 g/min[16] and loss of electrical activity below about 18 ml/100 g/min.[17] The intact cerebral vasculature is able to maintain—autoregulate—CBF over a range of perfusion pressures.[18] Between a MAP of about 60 to 120 torr, CBF is held relatively constant; pressures outside this range lead to a parallel change in CBF with MAP. Autoregulation can be impaired in injured brain tissue, with increasing BP leading directly to increased intravascular volume and increased ICP. The significance of ischemia (inadequate tissue perfusion to meet metabolic needs) in head injury has received increasing attention. CBF measurements shortly after severe head injury (within the first 6–8 hours) show ischemic levels in 20% to 30% of patients.[19–21] The routine use of therapeutic manuevers that may conceivably lower perfusion pressure (dehydration, induced hypotension) or lead to vasoconstriction and decreased CBF (hyperventilation) has therefore come into question.[22]

Management

Control of Elevated Intracranial Pressure

Although it is clear that raised ICP is associated with poor outcome in the severely head injured patient, it is more difficult to show cause and effect.[23,24] Raised ICP may be the result of severe irreversible trauma occurring at the time of injury, and control of ICP may not necessarily improve outcome in these cases. A significant number of patients, however, appear to deteriorate in association with elevation in ICP as a secondary event, and control of ICP in this setting may be reasonably expected to have a beneficial effect on outcome.[25] It is difficult, however, to show conclusively that monitored patients have improved outcome when compared with unmonitored patients receiving empiric therapy.[23] Most large trauma centers place ICP monitors in those patients who have a Glasgow Coma Score (GCS) of 7 or less, in those patients undergoing prolonged anesthetics for other surgical procedures, or in those requiring neuromuscular paralysis for respiratory management.

A variety of ICP monitors are available. Ventricular catheters allow direct measurement of CSF pressure and withdrawal of fluid for ICP control; but small ventricles shifted from mass effect are difficult to cannulate, and fluid-coupled systems are prone to drift and damping. Intraparenchymal fiberoptic transducers are commonly used, and miniature parenchymal strain gauges have been recently introduced. (See Pathophysiology of Intracranial Emergencies by Brogan, Geiduschek, and Kane, this volume.)

The goal of medical management is to maintain cerebral perfusion and blood flow within acceptable limits. In the three-compartment model, control of ICP can be achieved either by removal of the offending mass, if possible, or by decreasing the volume of edematous and normal brain, removing CSF, or decreasing intravascular volume (which, if associated with decreased CBF, may worsen ischemia).

Cerebral Spinal Fluid Removal

If a ventriculostomy has been placed for ICP monitoring, it also serves as a means of withdrawing CSF. Although only small amounts of CSF can be drained from collapsed ventricles, in some cases this may be useful in controlling ICP.

Osmotherapy

Osmotherapy remains one of the most effective means of controlling ICP. Its mechanism of action is multifactorial: its major effect may be to improve microvascular flow by decreasing blood viscosity.[26] It may also establish an osmotic gradient between brain and blood across an intact blood-brain barrier[27] and improve cerebral perfusion.[28] Its action is not due to systemic dehydration; intravascular volume must be maintained to avoid reduction of CPP and worsening ischemia. The osmotic gradient required for its effectiveness may not be present if the blood-brain barrier is exten-

sively disrupted, and mannitol is theoretically less effective in withdrawing water from areas of brain injury. Because it may eventually equilibrate across the blood-brain barrier, a rebound rise in ICP after withdrawal has been reported; this is of uncertain clinical importance.[29] A transient increase in CBF may be seen with bolus injection.[30] Dosing regimens of 0.5 to 1.0 g/kg as a loading dose will raise serum osmolality 10 to 20 mosm/liter and reduce ICP. Maintenance doses of 0.25 g/kg every 2 to 4 hours appear to be as effective as larger doses given less frequently, and are associated with fewer metabolic complications.[31] Maximum serum osmolality should not exceed 315 to 320 mosm/liter, as renal damage may occur, and frequent monitoring of electrolytes is required. The dehydration associated with diuretic use may lead to hypovolemia, hypotension, and decreased CPP; therefore adequate intravascular volume must be maintained. This may require central venous pressure monitoring for accurate replacement. Loop diuretics (furosemide) will decrease intravascular volume and CBF, as well as decrease CSF production,[32] but may also lead to dehydration and reduced CPP.

Cerebral Perfusion Pressure

In many cases, cerebral blood flow after severe head injury appears to follow a phasic pattern: There is an initial fall to sometimes ischemic levels within the first eight hours, followed by an increased hyperemic flow, followed by normalization. Therapeutic maneuvers designed to control ICP may also influence CBF, as when hyperventilation results in vasoconstriction, or osmotherapy leads to dehydration. Our goal in general is to maintain adequate perfusion (CPP > 70–80 torr in adults), with pressors if needed, while avoiding luxury perfusion and increased intravascular volume. Some have suggested that induced hypertension may in fact be beneficial, as it may allow autoregulatory mechanisms to lower ICP through reflex vasoconstriction.[33]

Hyperventilation

Both carbon dioxide and oxygen appear to have a direct effect on the cerebral vasculature, although the effect of carbon dioxide usually predominates. Cerebral vasoconstriction occurs in response to CSF alkalosis. A change in pCO_2 to 30 torr will lower CBF by 25 to 30%; hypoventilation to a pCO_2 of 80 will double CBF.[33] The effect is almost immediate, but resolves over hours as the alkalosis equilibrates across the blood-brain barrier.[34] Additional hypocarbia is effective down to a pCO_2 of about 20 torr but will be associated with extreme alkalosis and decreased CBF. Significant hypoxia results in vasodilation, with resultant increased CBF and elevated ICP, although CBF remains relatively constant until the pO_2 is less than 50 torr.[35] An arterial pO_2 of 90 to 100 torr should be maintained if possible.

The routine use of hyperventilation after head trauma is now in question, as the resulting vasoconstriction may worsen cerebral ischemia and lead to potentially worse outcome. It has been suggested that hyperventilation (to a $PCO_2 < 33$–35 torr) be instituted after other measures, including withdrawal of CSF via ventriculostomy, optimizing perfusion pressure to greater than 70–80 torr, and osmotherapy, have proved inadequate. The concomitant use of bedside measures of tissue oxygenation, especially jugular venous oxygen saturation, may allow the degree of hyperventilation to be optimized, depending upon the relative extraction of oxygen by the brain as evidenced by the arteriovenous difference of oxygen ($AVDO_2$).[37]

Respiratory mechanics can influence ICP through the apparent effect of positive end-expiratory pressure (PEEP) and mean airway pressures on intravascular volume. In those patients with poor pulmonary compliance—stiff lungs—increased airway pressure can impede cerebral venous drainage to the extent that ICP may be elevated.[36,37] This can often be relieved by elevating the patient's head to improve venous drainage, and low PEEP pressures are usually well tolerated. Because of the risk of ICP elevation, however, its use must be individualized.

Head position itself may influence ICP. Lowering venous pressure by raising the head to 30 degrees will usually lower ICP,[38] as will maintaining the head in a laterally neutral position to prevent venous congestion. In a hypovolemic patient, however, head elevation may cause hypotension with a decrease in CPP, and this should be avoided.[39]

Steroids

The use of steroids is clearly effective in treating edema associated with brain tumors, but their beneficial effect in head trauma has not been well established. Literature can be cited to support either view. Early reports, although favorable, have now been supplanted by more recent studies that suggest minimal, if any, beneficial effect on outcome.[40–44] There is, however, reasonable experimental evidence to suggest that extremely high doses of methyl prednisolone (30 mg/kg) in head-injured mice lead to an improved outcome,[45] and another study has shown some benefit with such high-dose regimens after acute spinal cord trauma.[46] Current practice at many institutions is to minimize the use of steroids in head trauma, while following study protocol for spinal cord injury. The presumed mechanism of action of high-dose steroids in experimental head trauma—free-radical scavenging—remains under intense investigation, and a number of new agents are under development.[47]

Barbiturates

Anesthetic doses of barbiturates, usually thiopental or pentobarbital, will reproducibly lower ICP, but whether they significantly affect outcome has been more difficult to prove.[48,49] They may act by lowering CBF and decreasing brain water content, and perhaps as free-radical scavengers.[50] Complications from their use are related to hypotension and decreased cardiac output,[51] and perhaps predisposition to infection.[52] They should obviously not be used without an accurate ICP monitor in place. Maximal reduction in ICP and cerebral metabolism can be gauged by the development of electrocerebral silence or burst suppression on EEG. The most commonly used agent is pentobarbital, with a serum half-life of about 30 hours. It is given as a loading dose of 3 to 5 mg/kg, followed by a maintenance dose of 0.5 to 1.0 mg/kg/hr. Dosage can be increased until ICP begins to respond or until EEG evidence of electrocerebral silence or burst suppression occurs. Hypotension may require inotropic support. It has been suggested that a therapeutic trial of thiopental may give an empiric indication of the usefulness of inducing barbiturate coma: If there is no ICP drop after bolus thiopental administration, large doses of pentobarbital are unlikely to be of benefit.[34] Although original studies suggested that barbiturate therapy may improve outcome, these studies were open to criticism in their use of historical controls and in their definition of failure of conventional therapy. A multicenter trial from 1988 suggested, however, that barbiturate therapy does indeed improve survival in a small proportion of patients, although this increase occurred in the most severely injured groups.[53] These studies also showed that aggressive conventional therapy is often effective in controlling ICP in most situations, making routine use unnecessary. The prophylactic use of barbiturates has been shown to be of no benefit.[54]

Hypothermia

Mild hypothermia (34°C), instituted immediately after injury, is receiving increasing attention as a means of controlling ICP and minimizing secondary injury.[57,58] Although not yet universally recommended, the results of clinical trials are awaited.

Head Injury in Children

After the perinatal period, falls become the leading cause of head injury, followed by motor vehicle accidents and child abuse. These may be falls from highchairs, changing tables, windows, or stairs. Walkers have been implicated in a significant number of falling injuries. With closure of sutures and progressive myelination, injuries pathologically begin to follow a more adult pattern, as true *contre coup* injuries appear and contusions replace subcortical tears. Injuries may include fractures, meningeal hemorrhages, or direct parenchymal injuries.

Skull Fractures

Linear nondepressed fractures, unassociated with any underlying injury, usually only require observation. Open scalp injuries can be sutured in the emergency room or operating room and ICU management is seldom required. Depressed fractures, if closed, will require operative elevation if there is significant underlying contusion, dural laceration, or a need for cosmetic refigurement. Open depressed fractures require surgical exploration and debridement. Basilar fractures present with hemotympanum or CSF oto- and rhinorrhea. Acute CSF leaks often stop spontaneously, but persistent leaks require surgical repair. Meningitis is a potential risk; the benefit of prophylactic antibiotic is debatable. Entrapment of the facial nerve from petrous fracture, or hearing loss from dislocation of the ossicles, requires otolaryngology evaluations and consideration for surgical intervention.

Meningeal Hemorrhage

Epidural hemorrhage in the young child may be associated with bleeding from bony fracture lines rather than from the more characteristic tear of the middle meningeal artery. In the infant with open sutures, a significant amount of blood can accumulate and lead to acute anemia. Although classically a lucid interval is described, this is present in only about 50% of patients. These lesions usually require surgical evacuation. Although fatal brainstem compression may result if not treated in time, the prognosis is otherwise good, as underlying brain injury is often not severe. The reverse is true in subdural hematomas, as there is often underlying cortical injury. The hematoma is the result of tearing a bridging vein or dural laceration, although occasionally a cortical artery is torn. Clinical presentation may include lethargy, focal neurologic findings, or seizures; there is an association with retinal hemorrhage. In infants with an open fontanelle, subdural taps can be performed, especially if the clot has liquefied. With acute clots and closed sutures, surgical evacuation is required. Edema associated with underlying brain injury may necessitate aggressive ICP management.

Cerebral Injury

The spectrum of parenchymal injury ranges from minor concussion to focal contusion to diffuse axonal injury. Aggressive ICU management is required in children with significant focal contusions. Depending on the extent of the hemorrhage and its location, medical control of ICP can be attempted before proceeding to surgical debridement. With progressive edema unresponsive to medical therapy, surgical treatment will be required. Diffuse axonal injury (DAI) occurs with a generalized shearing injury to the deep white matter. The patients are deeply comatose at presentation, but computed tomography (CT) will show only diffuse edema with small focal hemorrhages in the deep white matter and corpus callosum. ICP may be low initially. Prognosis is poor, with usual outcomes of either death or a persistent vegetative state. Pathologic findings at autopsy show axonal retraction balls in corpus callosum and white matter tracts.

Young children may occasionally present with progressive obtundation after a lucid interval, even after relatively minor trauma.[55] CT scanning will show severe generalized edema, with little evidence of parenchymal injury. This "malignant brain edema" appears to be secondary to a generalized loss of vasomotor tone with hyperemia of unclear etiology. These children will require aggressive ICP monitoring and treatment, but prognosis may be good if underlying parenchymal injury is slight and ICP can be controlled.

Head Injury from Child Abuse

A significant proportion of childhood head injuries is unfortunately caused by child abuse. Intentional injury results in damage from either direct impact—throwing or hitting the child—or from what Caffey has described as the "whiplash–shaken infant syndrome."[56] Direct impact will cause skull fractures with underlying contusions, white matter shearing, and subdural hematomas—both acute and chronic—often with associated signs of external trauma. The whiplash–shaken infant syndrome occurs when the child is shaken without direct impact. External signs of trauma are not seen, but the rapid acceleration-deceleration imparts shearing forces that lead to parenchymal tearing and vascular injury, with retinal hemorrhages as well as subdural or intraparenchymal bleeding.

Medical Problems in the Head-Injured Child

Seizures

Seizures occurring in the setting of severe head injury require aggressive management, because increased metabolic requirements lead to elevated CBF and ICP, even in patients under neuromuscular paralysis. Initial control can usually be achieved with diazepam or lorazepam, and maintenance therapy using phenytoin or phenobarbital. The prophylactic use of anticonvulsants to prevent late-onset epilepsy has been debated; the risk of late epilepsy increases with compound fractures, dural lacerations, and parenchymal injury. Prophylactic treatment has been reported to decrease the risk of late epilepsy from 30% to 40% to 5% to 10% in some series,[57] although data suggest that the beneficial effect is significant only during the first week, with similar incidence of late epilepsy in both treated and untreated adults.[58] Seizure management is discussed in detail in Status Epilepticus by Krishnamoorthy, this volume.

Metabolic Abnormalities

Many of the metabolic abnormalities associated with head injury are iatrogenic, as ICP control measures (hyperventilation, osmotherapy) have metabolic consequences and their use requires careful monitoring. Abnormalities in antidiuretic hormone secretion are seen with elevated ICP, and the syndrome of inappropriate

diuretic hormone (SIADH) has been described with basilar skull fractures. Severe injury may result in trauma to the pituitary stalk, with diabetes insipidus and endocrine insufficiency.

Neurogenic Pulmonary Edema

Life-threatening pulmonary edema has been described in association with severe head injury, presumably as the result of an overwhelming sympathetic discharge.[59] This may lead to peripheral vasoconstriction with shift of intravascular volume to the lung, high pulmonary venous resistance, and perhaps a direct effect on the permeability of the pulmonary vasculature.

Gastrointestinal Complications and Nutrition

Cushing described the relationship between hypothalamic damage and "stress" ulceration in 1932,[60] and erosive gastritis and stress ulceration remain clinically significant problems after head injury. Prophylactic antacids, H-2 blockers, or enteric coating agents (sucralfate) are administered routinely in cases of severe injury. Nutritional requirements may increase after severe trauma, especially in cases of persistent seizures or posturing. Enteral feeding should begin as soon as tolerated, based on appropriate nutritional assessment; in multiply injured patients, total parenteral feeding may be required.

Outcome

Given the variability in mechanism of injury, age of patient population, and different methodologies of study, it has proven difficult to determine average mortality and morbidity after severe pediatric head injury. In children with a GCS of 3 to 7 (or 8), mortality varies from 6% to 60%, with most reports in the range of 25% to 35%.[61] In more moderate injures (GCS of 7–8) mortality should approach 0%. Morbidity has proven even harder to assess, because there are neurobehavioral sequelae after even minor head injury and quantifying long-term morbidity in a developing nervous system after major trauma has proven difficult.

Although ICU management is directed toward the acute care of the head-injured child, the physicians providing this care—neurosurgeon, neurologist, intensivist—need to work for prevention of these devastating injuries. Public education efforts directed toward increasing infant safety (e.g., seat belt and infant restraint systems) require especially vigorous support.

References

1. Amacher AL. Pediatric head injury: A national tragedy. In *Concepts in Pediatric Neurosurgy* Basel: Karger, 1985. P 76.
2. Peacock WJ. The postnatal development of the brain and its coverings. In Raimondi AJ, Choux M, DiRocco C (eds): *Head Injuries in the Newborn and Infant.* New York: Springer, 1986. P 53.
3. Yakovlev PI, Lecours AP. The myelogenetic cycle of regional maturation of the brain. In Minkowski A (ed): *Regional Development of the Brain in Early Life.* Oxford: Blackwell, 1967. Pp 3–70.
4. Purpura DP. Dendritic differentiation in human cerebral cortex: Normal and aberrant developmental patterns. In GW Kreuteberg (ed): *Advances in Neurology.* New York: Raven Press, 1975.
5. Cheek DB. *Fetal and Postnatal Cellular Growth.* New York: Wiley, 1975.
6. Lenin NJ. Neuroplasticity and the developing brain: Implications for therapy. *Pediatr Neurosci* 13:176–183, 1987.
7. Bakay RAE, Sweeney KM, Wood JH. Pathophysiology of cerebrospinal fluid in head injury: Part I. *Neurosurgery* 18:234–243, 1986.

8. Choi D. Cerebral hypoxia: Some new approaches and unanswered questions. *J Neurosci* 10:2493–2501, 1990.

9. Hall ED, Braughler JM. Free radicals in CNS injury. In Waxman SG (ed): *Molecular and Cellular Approaches to the Treatment of Neurological Disease.* New York: Raven, 1993. Pp 81–105.

10. Rothman SM. Synaptic release of excitatory amino acid neurotransmitter mediates anoxic neuronal death. *J Neurosci* 4:1884–1891, 1984.

11. Mattson MP, Scheff SW. Endogenous neuroprotection factors and traumatic brain injury: Mechanisms of action and implications for therapy. *J Neurotrauma* 11:3–33, 1994.

12. Shapiro HM. Intracranial hypertension: Therapeutic and anesthetic considerations. *Anesthesiology* 43:445–471, 1975.

13. Leech P, Miller JD. Intracranial volume pressure relationships during experimental brain compression in primates. *J Neurol Neurosurg Psychiatry* 37:1099–1104, 1974.

14. Marsh ML, Marshall LF, Shapiro HM. Neurosurgical intensive care. *Anesthesiology* 47:149–163, 1977.

15. Jennet WB et al. Relation between cerebral blood flow and cerebral perfusion pressure. *Br J Surg* 57:390–397, 1970.

16. Astrup J, Siesjo BK, Symon J. Thresholds in cerebral ischemia—The ischemic penumbra. *Stroke* 12:723–725, 1981.

17. Sharbrough FW, Messick JM, Sundt TF. Correlation of continuous electroencephalograms with cerebral blood flow measurements during carotid endarterectomy. *Stroke* 4:674–683, 1974.

18. Lassen NA. Control of cerebral circulation in health and disease. *Circ Res* 34:749–760, 1974.

19. Bouma GJ et al. Cerebral circulation and metabolism after severe traumatic brain injury: The elusive role of ischemia. *J Neurosurg* 75:685–693, 1991.

20. Bouma GJ et al. Ultra early evaluation of regional cerebral blood flow in severely head injured patients using xenon enhanced computed tomography. *J Neurosurg* 77:360–368, 1992.

21. Muizelaar JP et al. Cerebral blood flow and metabolism in severely head-injured children. Part 1: Relationship with GCS score, outcome, ICP, and PVI. *J Neurosurg* 71:63–71, 1989.

22. Muizelaar JP et al. Adverse effects of prolonged hyperventilation in patients with severe head injury: A randomized clinical trial. *J Neurosurg* 75:731–739, 1991.

23. Miller JD et al. Significance of intracranial hypertension in severe head injury. *J Neurosurg* 47:503–516, 1977.

24. Stuart CG et al. Severe head injury managed without intracranial pressure monitoring. *J Neurosurg* 59:601–605, 1983.

25. Marshall LM, Smith RW, Shapiro HM. The outcome with aggressive treatment in severe head injuries. Part I: The significance of intracranial pressure monitoring. *J Neurosurg* 50:20–25, 1979.

26. Nath F, Galbraith S. The effect of mannitol on cerebral white matter water content. *J Neurosurg* 65:41–43, 1986.

27. Mendelow AD et al. Effect of mannitol on cerebral blood flow and cerebral perfusion pressure in human head injury. *J Neurosurg* 63:43–48, 1985.

28. Muizelaar JP et al. Mannitol causes compensatory cerebral vasoconstriction and vasodilation in response to blood viscosity changes. *J Neurosurg* 59:822, 1983.

29. Goluboff B, Shankin A, Haft H. The effects of mannitol and urea on cerebral hemodynamics and cerebrospinal fluid pressure. *Neurology* 14:891–898, 1964.

30. Jafar JJ, Johns LM, Mullan SF. The effect of mannitol on cerebral blood flow. *J Neurosurg* 64:754–759, 1986.

31. Marshall LF et al. Mannitol dose requirements in brain-injured patients. *J Neurosurg* 48:169–172, 1978.

32. Cottrell JE et al. Furosemide and mannitol induced changes in intracranial pressure and serum osmolality and electrolytes. *Anaesthesia* 47:642–648, 1977.

33. Rosner MJ. Pathophysiology and management of increased intracranial pressure. In Andrews BT (ed) *Neurosurgical Intensive Care.* New York: McGraw-Hill, 1993. Pp. 57–112.

34. Ropper AH, Rockoff MA. Treatment of intracranial hypertension. In Ropper AH, Kennedy SF (eds): *Neurological and Neurosurgical Intensive Care.* Rockville, MD: Aspen, 1988. Pp 23–42.

35. Siesjo BK et al. Brain metabolism in the critically ill. *Crit Care Med* 28:1465–1471, 1970.

36. Aidinis SJ, Lafferty J, Shapiro HM. Intracranial responses to PEEP. *Anesthesiology* 45:275–286, 1976.

37. Gopinath SP et al. Jugular venous desaturation and outcome after head injury. *J Neurol Neurosurg Psychiatry* 57:717–23, 1994.

38. Feldman Z et al. Effect of head elevation on intracranial pressure, cerebral perfusion pressure, and cerebral blood flow in head-injured patients. *J Neurosurg* 76:207–211, 1992.

39. Rosner MJ, Coley IB. Cerebral perfusion pressure, intracranial pressure, and head elevation. *J Neurosurg* 65:636–641, 1986.

40. French LA. The use of steroids in the treatment of cerebral edema. *Bull NY Acad Med* 42:301–311, 1977.

41. Cooper PR et al. Dexamethasone and severe head injury. A prospective double-blind study. *J Neurosurg* 58:307–316, 1979.

42. Gudeman SK, Mulla JD, Becker DP. Failure of high dose steroid therapy to influence intracranial pressure in patients with severe head injury. *J Neurosurg* 51:301–306, 1979.

43. Saul TG et al. Steroids in severe injury: A prospective randomized clinical trial. *J Neurosurg* 54:596–600, 1981.

44. Giannotta SL. High dose glucocorticoids in the management of severe head injury. *Neurosurgery* 15:497–501, 1984.

45. Hall ED. High-dose glucocorticoid treatment improves neurological recovery in head injured mice. *J Neurosurg* 62:882–887, 1985.

46. Bracken MB et al. A randomized, controlled trial of methylprednisolone or naloxone in the treatment of acute spinal cord injury. *N Engl J Med* 322:1405–1411, 1990.

47. Hall ED, Braughler JM. Free radicals in CNS injury. In Waxman SG (ed): *Molecular and Cellular Approaches in the Treatment of Neurological Disease.* New York: Raven, 1993. Pp 81–105.

48. Marshall LF, Smith RW, Shapiro HM. The outcome with aggressive treatment in severe head injuries. Part II: Acute and chronic barbiturate administration in the management of head injury. *Neurosurgery* 50:26–30, 1979.

49. Rockoff MA, Marshall LM, Shapiro HM. High dose barbiturate therapy in humans. A clinical review of 60 patients. *Ann Neurol* 6:194–199, 1979.

50. Piatt J, Schiff SJ. High dose barbiturate therapy in neurosurgery and intensive care. *Neurosurgery* 15:427–444, 1984.

51. Etsen B, Li TH. Hemodynamic changes during thiopental anesthesia in humans: Cardiac output, stroke volume, peripheral resistance, and intrathoracic blood volume. *J Clin Invest* 34:500–510, 1955.

52. Neuwelt EA et al. Barbiturate inhibition of lymphocyte function. *J Neurosurg* 56:254–259, 1982.

53. Eisenberg HM et al. High-dose barbiturate control of elevated intracranial pressure in patients with severe head injury. *J Neurosurg* 69:15–23, 1988.

54. Ward JD et al. Failure of prophylactic barbiturate coma in the treatment of severe head injury. *J Neurosurg* 62:383–388, 1985.

55. Marion DW et al. The use of moderate therapeutic hypothermia for patients with severe head injuries: a preliminary report *J Neurosurg.* 79:354–62, 1993.

56. Shiozaki T et al. Effects of mild hypothermia on uncontrollable intracranial hypertension after severe head injury. *J. Neurosurg.* 79:363–8, 1993.

57. Chiofalo N, Madsen J, Basauri L. Perinatal and posttraumatic seizures. In Raimondi AJ, Choux M, DiRocco C (eds): *Head Injuries in the Newborn and Infant.* New York: Springer, 1986. Pp 217–232.

58. Temkin NR, Dikmen SS, Wilensky AJ. A randomized double-blind study of phenytoin for the prevention of post-traumatic seizures. *N Engl J Med* 323:497–501, 1990.

59. Ducker TB. Increased intracranial pressure and pulmonary edema. *J Neurosurg* 28:112–117, 1968.

60. Cushing HC. Peptic ulcers and the interbrain. *Surg Gynecol Obstet* 55:1–34, 1932.

61. Luerssen TG, Klauber MR. Outcome from pediatric head injury: On the nature of prospective and retrospective studies. In Marlin AE (ed): *Concepts of Pediatric Neurosurgery.* Basel: Karger, 1989. Pp 198–210.

Kalpathy S.
Krishnamoorthy

28 Status Epilepticus

Status epilepticus is a dramatic clinical disorder that may be life-threatening. It is one of the common emergencies encountered in the pediatric emergency rooms and pediatric intensive care units (PICUs).

Frequently, status epilepticus is thought to be synonymous with generalized tonic-clonic seizures (convulsive type). Other types of status epilepticus encountered in the setting of PICUs include complex partial status epilepticus (psychomotor), absence status (petit mal), and focal tonic-clonic status (epilepsia partialis continua). Thus, status epilepticus, is classified as **convulsive** (generalized tonic-clonic and focal tonic-clonic) and **nonconvulsive** (complex partial and absence status). In this chapter, we specifically deal with these four types of status epilepticus (Table 28-1).

Generalized Tonic-Clonic Status Epilepticus

By definition, tonic-clonic status epilepticus implies a state of repetitive tonic-clonic seizures lasting 30 to 60 minutes or longer, and between seizures the consciousness is impaired. Approximately 5% of children with tonic-clonic seizure disorder will experience status epilepticus some time in their lives. In children, 75% of tonic-clonic status occurs below 3 years of age.[1] Frequently, it may be the initial presentation of an epileptic disorder in the setting of elevated temperature in a child with preexisting brain disorder. Some of the causes of generalized tonic-clonic status include congenital disorders of the brain development (congenital encephalopathy), epileptic disorders, poor compliance with anticonvulsant therapy, abrupt cessation of anticonvulsant therapy in the setting of chronic epileptic disorder, hypoxic-ischemic encephalopathy (following cardiorespiratory arrest), viral encephalitis, acute metabolic derangements (hyponatremia and hypernatremia), severe head trauma, and intoxications.

Pathophysiology

Animal studies indicate that prolonged seizure activity, even in paralyzed and ventilated animals, may result in irreversible neuronal damage.[2,3] There are several biochemical and pathophysiologic changes that follow acute tonic-clonic convulsions. They relate both to systemic changes and local events that set in at the cellular level. It is the perpetuation of these changes that ultimately leads to irreversible damage to the nervous system.

Table 28-1.   Classification of status epilepticus

Convulsive status epilepticus
  Generalized tonic-clonic
  Myoclonic
  Infantile spasms with status epilepticus
  Focal convulsive status epilepticus
Nonconvulsive status epilepticus
  Complex partial status epilepticus
  Absence status epilepticus
  Atonic; akinetic; myoclonic status epilepticus (related to myoclonic epilepsy; infantile spasms; Lennox-Gastaut syndrome)

The onset of tonic-clonic seizures is accompanied by an abrupt alteration in cardiovascular dynamics, leading to tachycardia, elevation of systemic BP, an increase in cerebral blood flow, and elevation of central venous pressure. These changes occur during the first 20 minutes, accompanied at the cellular level by an increased cerebral metabolic rate ($CMRO_2$). Arterial oxygen desaturation, elevation of carbon dioxide, and metabolic acidosis set in. Blood lactic acid is elevated within 15 to 30 minutes, while blood glucose is initially mildly elevated. The changes that occur beyond 30 minutes are even more severe. The pulse becomes weak, accompanied by hypotension. Severe metabolic acidosis (pH 6.7–7.1) develops, associated with hypoglycemia and lactic acidosis. Hyperpyrexia may occur at late stages of tonic-clonic status in nonparalyzed animals and, by itself, may have deleterious effects on the brain, especially the cerebellum. The summation of these events leads to a severe disparity between the available sources of cerebral energy substrate and depletion of the substrate. Thus, cellular death follows because of oxygen debt.

The neuropathologic changes that occur in the brain, even in paralyzed and ventilated animals, following tonic-clonic status epilepticus resemble those of severe hypoxic-ischemic injury. Thus, the topographic distribution of brain injury includes most structures of the neocortex, hippocampus, brain stem, and cerebellum. Microscopic changes typically resemble ischemic cell death of the neurons.[2] Further, neuropathologic changes and extent of brain injury depend on the underlying etiology of status epilepticus. Thus, for example, severe cortical neuronal necrosis and brain swelling following profound hypoxic-ischemic injury, or severe inflammatory changes following encephalitis, may contribute to further brain injury. Animal studies suggest, however, that even in uncomplicated tonic-clonic status epilepticus, prolonged seizure activity longer than 30 to 60 minutes may be deleterious to the integrity of the nervous system.

Management of Generalized Tonic-Clonic Status Epilepticus

The principles of management include

1. Maintenance of vital functions
2. Identification and treatment of underlying etiologic factors
3. Prevention or correction of secondary medical complications
4. Initiation of anticonvulsant drug therapy

Maintenance of Vital Functions

Careful monitoring and maintenance of vital signs, and careful positioning to avoid aspiration, asphyxia, or physical injury are important. An oral airway should be taped in place, but forcible opening of the mouth to insert an airway through clenched teeth should be avoided. Intubation may become necessary if there is prolonged apnea, cyanosis, aspiration, or significant respiratory compromise. An intravenous (IV) catheter should be promptly placed for administration of fluids and drugs. As soon as the IV line is placed, it is prudent to draw blood samples for routine laboratory determinations, including anticonvulsant levels. An IV bolus of dextrose 50% should be administered in patients who are seizing and unconscious without prior history of seizures. Fluid restriction to two-thirds maintenance and avoidance of hypotonic fluids are important.

Identification and Treatment of Underlying Etiologic Factors

Frequently, there is an underlying etiology for a patient with a history of epilepsy to develop status epilepticus. Included are fever, sleep deprivation, drug withdrawal, or poor compliance with anticonvulsant drug therapy. The source of fever should be investigated, and prompt control of fever and infection is necessary. An acute CNS process, such as meningitis, encephalitis, trauma, or a cerebrovascular event, should be considered. Drug intoxications (e.g., tricyclics, isoniazid) should be suspected in those with no previous CNS disorder. Substance abuse (e.g., cocaine) should be investigated in suspected cases by a toxic screen test. A massive lesion in the brain rarely may present as clonic tonic status.

Studies that need to be performed after stabilizing the patient include a lumbar puncture, a CT brain scan or a magnetic resonance imaging (MRI) of the brain. The decision to perform these studies should be dictated by a high index of clinical suspicion and a careful review of the risks versus benefits to the patient. Before performing lumbar puncture, a careful examination of the fundi for increased intracranial pressure should be done. Therefore, a CT scan is particularly important prior to a lumbar puncture in those cases of suspected massive cerebral swelling, hematoma, tumors, or focal inflammatory CNS conditions. MRI is often performed later in the evaluation and is especially useful to diagnose major and minor structural changes, tuberous sclerosis, neurofibromatosis, brain tumors, focal encephalitis, and posttraumatic white matter changes.

In summary, most cases of generalized tonic-clonic status occur due to an underlying precipitating factor which should be vigorously sought.

Prevention or Correction of Secondary Medical Complications

Arterial blood gas determination should be performed early in the management of status epilepticus. Severe metabolic acidosis and a profound deficit of base reserve often complicate status epilepticus and may prevent satisfactory seizure control with antiepileptic drugs by increasing the amount of extracellular potassium. This may contribute to irreversible cerebral damage during status epilepticus. Fluid overload should be avoided by careful titration of isotonic fluids. Determinations of electrolytes in blood and urine and urine specific gravity should be done to detect the syndrome of inappropriate ADH (SIADH). Other medical complications include pneumonia, myoglobinuria, pulmonary edema, hyperthermia, orthopedic injuries, disseminated intravascular coagulation, and hypertension.

Initiation of Anticonvulsant Therapy

The mainstay of treatment of status epilepticus is stabilizing the patient with anticonvulsant drugs.

Principles of Drug Therapy

In the management of status epilepticus, it is imperative to administer drugs by an IV route. There is no role for intramuscular administration of anticonvulsant drugs because the absorption is erratic and there is thus a delay in control of seizures. One should follow the recommended dose and route for drug therapy, because undertreatment may delay the seizure control and cause further damage. It is important to use one drug at a time to the maximum loading dose before administering a second drug. This is especially applicable to the long-acting drugs used in status epilepticus. It is very helpful to be familiar with all commonly used anticonvulsant drug preparations, their basic pharmacokinetics, and drug combinations. Monitoring drug levels is very important, and one should check the drug levels 2 hours after an IV loading dose of long-acting anticonvulsants (e.g., phenytoin and phenobarbital). Further measurement of drug levels will be dictated by the frequency of dose, type of drug, and the seizure control. Although it may become necessary to measure and monitor frequent drug levels of most anticonvulsants, note that it takes approximately five half-lives' duration for most anticonvulsants to reach a steady state and maintain a therapeutic level. This is important to keep in mind during the adjustment of maintenance drug dosage. After the initial seizure control with a long-acting IV drug or drugs, it is important to initiate maintenance drug therapy. Improper attention to adequate maintenance therapy may result in recurrence of seizures. In choosing a long-acting anticonvulsant drug, the ideal one should be safe, rapidly control seizures, and be able to be used as the maintenance drug for continued seizure control. Only phenobarbital and phenytoin fulfill most of these criteria. The adverse side effects of various drugs on respiration, hemodynamics, and sensorium should be constantly kept in mind while using the anticonvulsants. Neither overtreatment nor undertreatment with anticonvulsants is advisable, although in the ICU setting, it may become necessary to exceed the usually recommended doses if seizure control is difficult and life-threatening. In this situation, a neurologic consultation, frequent neurologic evaluations, and possibly continuous electroencephalographic studies will be important.

In emergent situations if establishing IV access in the child becomes difficult or the child has been seizing for more than 30 minutes, vascular access through intraosseous (IO) route should be obtained. All fluids and medications that are given IV may be administered by IO infusion.

Medications for Treatment of Generalized Tonic-Clonic Status Epilepticus

The three initial main drugs used to treat generalized tonic-clonic status epilepticus have been benzodiazepines, phenytoin, and phenobarbital. Paraldehyde is not often used but is useful in the patient who does not respond to conventional drug therapy.

Lorazepam

Reports on the use of lorazepam in status epilepticus have demonstrated that it is a very effective and safe anticonvulsant.[4-7] It has the benefit of rapid onset of action, stopping seizure activity within 3 to 10 minutes after an IV bolus. Unlike diazepam, the duration of seizure control is longer with lorazepam, lasting for 4 to 24 hours in 50% to 80% of cases. Serious complications are less common, although the danger of respiratory depression should not be underestimated. Lorazepam is highly efficacious in treating generalized tonic-clonic status.

Lorazepam is given intravenously and may be repeated at 10- to 20-minute intervals. However, its anticonvulsant property diminishes with successive doses. It is frequently possible to fully control the tonic-clonic seizures with a single dose of lorazepam combined with a loading dose of phenytoin. The usual dose is 0.05 to 0.1 mg/kg (maximal dose 4 mg), given over 1 to 2 minutes.

Diazepam

The use of diazepam as the first drug to control generalized tonic-clonic convulsions is widely practiced. After IV infusion of diazepam, maximal brain concentrations in humans is reached within 1 to 12 minutes. This rapid anticonvulsant effect is a great advantage in acute emergencies. However, diazepam brain parenchyma concentration falls rapidly at a rate that closely follows the fall in serum concentration. This rapid clearance of diazepam makes the duration of anticonvulsant effect short-lived (as short as 15 minutes) and probably accounts for the frequent recurrence of seizure activity when diazepam alone is used to control status epilepticus.[4,8]

A judicious use of diazepam is especially indicated in generalized tonic-clonic status if the seizure activity is compromising vital functions. Typical situations for the use of diazepam include status epilepticus associated with structural lesions and viral encephalitis. To avoid cardiorespiratory depression, care must be exercised when diazepam is used in conjunction with phenobarbital or other depressant drugs. A frequently recommended therapeutic strategy is the initial use of IV diazepam to achieve immediate seizure control, followed by prompt administration of an appropriate loading dose of phenytoin to maintain seizure control. The use of repeated doses of diazepam should be avoided because toxic concentrations of diazepam and its metabolites will accumulate and result in overdosage.

The recommended dose is 0.25 to 0.40 mg/kg, given intravenously (maximum dose, 5–10 mg/dose). It may be repeated in 15 to 20 minutes, up to a maximum of 3 doses. In children older than 5 years of age, the recommended dose is 1 mg every 2 to 5 minutes, and in children younger than 5 years, 0.2 to to 0.5 mg slowly every 2 to 5 minutes, to a maximum of 5 mg. For the treatment of status epilepticus, diazepam is not effective by intramuscular route.

Midazolam

Recent reports have indicated midazolam to be an effective anticonvulsant.[9–11] It seems highly efficacious as an intramuscular (IM) anticonvulsant in emergent situations where IV access becomes difficult.[9] It causes little irritation as an IV or IM injection. It has a rapid onset of action (1.5–5.0 minutes) and a short duration of action (1–5 hours). The initial IV or IM dose is 0.05 to 0.20 mg/kg, with a maximum dose of 5 mg.

Even though midazolam is not used routinely to control generalized tonic-clonic status in children, it has been used successfully in adults and, therefore, can be also used in children in the form of a continuous infusion in selected cases of refractory status.[10,11]

Phenytoin

Phenytoin is an effective drug for treatment of tonic-clonic status epilepticus when administered intravenously. It is safe and does not depress respiration or alter the sensorium, all of which are distinct advantages, especially in a patient who is comatose without an obvious cause. Phenytoin is also an excellent anticonvulsant for long-term maintenance treatment of tonic-clonic seizures. The typical clinical settings for the use of phenytoin include craniocerebral trauma, encephalitis, and anticonvulsant withdrawal seizures.

Peak brain concentrations of phenytoin occur between 20 and 60 minutes after IV infusion. It is slower in onset of action than lorazepam or diazepam. Therefore, one of these latter two drugs is often used as the first agent to control tonic-clonic status epilepticus, followed by IV phenytoin to achieve adequate serum and brain concentrations. The use of IM or oral loading dose of phenytoin to control tonic-clonic status epilepticus is ineffective.[4,12,13]

A dose of 10 to 20 mg/kg IV achieves and maintains therapeutic levels for 24 hours. It is recommended that the maintenance dose be commenced 24 hours after the loading dose. The maximum recommended rate for IV infusion is 50 mg/min in older children and 0.5 to 1.0 mg/kg/min in younger children.

The toxicity of IV phenytoin depends chiefly on the rate of administration rather than the dose administered. The threat of bradycardia, hypotension, and cardiac arrhythmia would dictate careful and slow IV administration of phenytoin. It is important to frequently monitor pulse, BP, and ECG during the IV loading dose of phenytoin. Because phenytoin is an irritative substance, precaution should be taken to avoid extravasation by using a large infusion catheter and flushing with sterile saline solution following the drug's infusion.[4]

Phenobarbital

The use of phenobarbital as the first drug to control tonic-clonic status in children is widely practiced. It is a well-known drug with considerably less acute side effects and as a maintenance drug for tonic-clonic seizures, phenobarbital is a good anticonvulsant for infants and children. Peak brain concentrations of phenobarbital do not occur for about 60 minutes, although seizure control generally occurs within 20 minutes after IV infusion. Because of its long half-life (up to 120 hours) and its sedative effects, patients treated with large doses of phenobarbital may remain heavily sedated for several days.

IM phenobarbital is not recommended for treatment of tonic-clonic status epilepticus because peak serum concentrations are not achieved rapidly. Respiratory depression is a serious risk when large doses are administered, and especially when used in combination with diazepam. The typical clinical settings for the use of phenobarbital include febrile status epilepticus and young children and infants. Large doses should be infused slowly to avoid hypotension and cardiac irregularities.

Loading doses of 15 to 20 mg/kg are required to achieve therapeutic levels in serum and adequate seizure control. If seizures persist for 20 to 30 minutes after the first dose, a second, and even a third dose, can be given at 3 to 5 mg/kg/dose at 20- to 30-minute intervals (maximal dose, 360 mg). The rate of infusion recommended is 100 mg/min. The maintenance dose of phenobarbital is started 12 to 24 hours following the loading dose.

Paraldehyde

When phenytoin, phenobarbital, diazepam, or lorazepam fail to control tonic-clonic status epilepticus, paraldehyde may then be useful as a second-line drug. Paraldehyde is very effective intramuscularly, but due to its local irritative effects, this route is no longer used. Even though it is effective intravenously, the safety of paraldehyde by IV route is controversial and is no longer recommended. Absorption by oral route is slower and best avoided for status epilepticus due to the risk of aspiration. Thus, rectal paraldehyde is most commonly used, and its ease of administration by this route accounts for its popularity. Peak concentrations by rectal route occur in 20 to 30 minutes. To obtain a serum concentration high enough to control seizures, administration of large doses of paraldehyde will be necessary, and toxic concentrations might occur.[4,14]

The dose of 0.3 ml/kg of paraldehyde for rectal administration is diluted 2:1 in oil (olive or cottonseed). The doses can be repeated every 2 to 4 hours, if necessary, up to a maximum of 4 to 6 doses in a 24-hour period.

In summary, the three drugs commonly used to treat generalized tonic-clonic status epilepticus are benzodiazepines, phenytoin, and phenobarbital. The use of high and frequent doses of benzodiazepines is limited by the functional tolerance to anticonvulsant effect and progressive resistance (tachyphylaxis) to increasing doses. Phenobarbital offers the beneficial property of having a relatively linear and predictable volume of distribution and elimination kinetics. Phenytoin offers the advantage of being a nonsedative drug with fairly rapid action, and in most cases is able to control seizures within 10 minutes after the full loading dose. It is important to emphasize, however, that only a few comparative studies have been conducted in a prospective randomized manner, and there are therefore virtually no solid data on which to base one's choice of diazepam, lorazepam, phenytoin, or phenobarbital in the initial management of generalized tonic-clonic status epilepticus.

Refractory Tonic-Clonic Status Epilepticus

By definition, when tonic-clonic status epilepticus continues beyond 60 minutes, it is usually considered **refractory**. Some of the factors that contribute to refractory status include inadequate drug treatment, medical and metabolic complications, improper management of the precipitating factors, presence of a large cerebral lesion (tumor, encephalitis), or an intractable epileptic disorder.

Management

The first principle is to reevaluate and attend to the medical and metabolic complications that might prevent adequate seizure control. Particular attention should be paid to metabolic acidosis, electrolyte imbalance, hypoglycemia, infections, hyperthermia, and fluid therapy. Neuroimaging studies, such as CT scan or MRI, are helpful in detecting cerebral edema, hemorrhage, encephalitis, or tumor. At all times, adequate ventilation should be maintained by tracheal intubation and, if necessary, by assisted ventilation and neuromuscular blockade (e.g., pancuronium).

Drug Therapy

A round of phenytoin and phenobarbital is reasonable as the initial step. If this fails, rectal paraldehyde may be tried.

A variety of drug treatments for refractory status epilepticus have been attempted in both adults and children. None of them is entirely satisfactory in children. Among the extraordinary measures used are continuous IV diazepam infusion, general anesthesia with inhalational agents, neuromuscular blockade, and short-acting barbiturates (e.g., pentobarbital).

Continuous midazolam IV infusion has been used in generalized tonic-clonic status epilepticus with good response.[10,11] When maximal doses of first-line drugs fail, the use of IV continuous infusion of midazolam appears to be a reasonable step: 0.1 mg/kg/hr, to be titrated and increased as needed to 0.2 to 0.4 mg/kg/hr.

Continuous IV diazepam has been used in the treatment of refractory status epilepticus.[4,15] There are several problems associated with this mode of therapy. Definitive efficacy data are not available because none of the studies performed was randomized or controlled. Certain types of IV bottle and tubing material (polyvinyl chloride) could cause adsorption of the lipid-soluble drug to the organic tubing material. In solution, diazepam is unstable in higher concentrations, and the safety margin is narrow during continuous IV administration. Tolerance occurs in some patients when infused continuously for more than 24 hours. Thus, continu-

ous diazepam infusion should be used judiciously in cases of refractory status when other conventional methods have failed.

General Anesthesia (Pentobarbital, Isoflurane)

The use of general anesthetics is the last resort in an attempt to stop generalized tonic-clonic seizures. These agents reduce tonic and clonic activity, allow control of respirations, diminish seizure discharges, and reduce cerebral metabolic requirements. However, the duration of action and efficacy are somewhat limited. There are dangers in the use of these agents because they may cause severe cardiorespiratory depression, especially when very high doses are required in the management of refractory status epilepticus.

In those cases resistant to the first- and second-line drugs, the use of either pentobarbital or thiopental should be the next mode of therapy.[16-18] Some of the benefits of these agents include the ease of administration in the ICU, their ameliorating effects on the intracranial pressure, the ability to monitor the dosage, and the ease of reversibility of treatment. It is necessary to monitor EEG continuously when general anesthesia is used in the management of refractory status epilepticus. The use of pentobarbital coma is one of the standard therapies for refractory status epilepticus in children. The dose of pentobarbital recommended is 2 to 8 mg/kg loading dose and a maintenance dose of 1 to 3 mg/kg/hr to achieve a level of 3 to 5 μg/ml, which usually produces burst supression pattern on the EEG.

The guidelines used for adjustment of dosage include the EEG monitoring, clinical seizure control, and vital functions. Ideally, blood level should be monitored frequently. These short-acting barbiturates may produce significant cardiac and respiratory depression. Therefore, patients should be intubated and mechanically ventilated during treatment. Continuous hemodynamic monitoring is necessary. Hypotension may require the use of vasopressor agents. High-dose pentobarbital therapy may cause pulmonary edema and ileus.

Isoflurane is the inhalational anesthetic that is administered in resistant cases of status epilepticus. Its use requires special equipment and experienced personnel (e.g., an anesthesiologist) to administer the agent and monitor therapy. The advantages of isoflurane over halothane include its ability to suppress EEG and clinical seizure activity at hemodynamically tolerated concentrations, ease of dose adjustment based on clinical and EEG monitoring, and its relative lack of adverse effects on intracranial pressure.[4,19] The experience of its use in children is limited. A major disadvantage of general anesthetics in the management of refractory status epilepticus is that the duration of action of these agents is temporary and relapse of seizures may therefore occur once the agent is discontinued.

Lidocaine

Lidocaine may be effective against refractory tonic-clonic status epilepticus, given intravenously either in boluses or by continuous infusion.[20] The antiepileptic effect of IV lidocaine is rapid, with a decrease in seizures noted in 20 to 30 seconds. The effects may be transient, however, lasting 20 to 30 minutes. In **high** doses, lidocaine may cause convulsions, hypotension, and cardiac arrhythmias.

A single initial dose of 1 to 2 mg/kg is administered intravenously. If seizures recur, lidocaine infusion is run at a rate of 3 to 10 mg/kg/hr, with close titration of the rate of infusion depending on the clinical response, frequency of seizures, and side effects. Rate of infusion should not exceed 2.5 to 5.0 mg/kg/hr. There is limited experience with lidocaine use in pediatric cases of status epilepticus.

Muscle Relaxants

Neuromuscular blockade will abolish tonic-clonic muscle movements, but this form of treatment does not prevent ongoing electrical seizure discharges. Studies on paralyzed and ventilated animals indicate that prolonged and repetitive electrical seizure activity alone may cause irreversible neuronal injury.[2] In some cases of refractory status epilepticus, however, pharmacologic paralysis will be necessary to allow one to adequately ventilate the patient.

Sodium Valproate (Valproic Acid)

Valproic acid may be helpful in refractory tonic-clonic status epilepticus.[21–24] Because there is no parenteral form of valproic acid available, nasogastric or rectal administration is used. Rectally, sodium valproate is reasonably well absorbed, reaching peak levels at 2 to 4 hours after administration. It is an effective and practical route in situations when the oral route is not feasible. There is some concern that liver enzyme elevations may be higher after rectal administration of sodium valproate, so liver functions must be followed carefully. In selected cases of refractory status, the nasogastric route may be used.

A dose of 20 mg/kg of sodium valproate syrup (250 mg/5 ml) is diluted 1:1 with tap water and administered as a tap water retention enema. A similar dose of sodium valproate may be used through the nasogastric route.

Several studies indicate that a variety of newer approaches may be used in the treatment of recurrent generalized tonic-clonic seizures and refractory status epilepticus. The use of oral or rectal loading of valproate[24] and oral loading of carbamazepine[25] may be effective. Rectal diazepam may be effective against recurrent febrile seizures.[26,27] The use of a very high dose of phenobarbital without a predetermined upper limit (median level, 114 μg/ml) was found to be effective in a large series of children in controlling refractory tonic-clonic status.[28] Crawford et al. administered 15- to 20-mg/kg IV boluses of phenobarbital every 30 to 60 minutes until cessation of clinical seizures or burst supression. Phenobarbital levels in the range of 60 mg/ml (range, 30–120 mg/ml) achieved good seizure control.[28] Treatment must be handled on an individual-patient basis when following any of these newer approaches. Tables 28-2 and 28-3 summarize the management of tonic-clonic status epilepticus.

Focal Motor Status Epilepticus (Simple Partial Seizures)

The management of focal motor status epilepticus can be a challenge to the intensivist. The motor seizures may remain localized, or there may be impairment of consciousness or generalization of seizure activity. The EEG abnormalities are often focal, localized in frontal, temporal, or central regions. Among the etiologic factors, vascular, tumor, and focal encephalitic lesions are most important. Although most focal motor seizures come under prompt control with the use of IV diazepam, phenytoin, or phenobarbital, a small group of children with epilepsia partialis continua can continue to seize for hours, days, and even months.

Drug Therapy

Drug therapy for focal motor status epilepticus is similar to that for generalized tonic-clonic status epilepticus. In intractable cases, one should endeavor to optimize the use of IV phenytoin and phenobarbital. If these fail, rectal paraldehyde, rectal or nasogastric

Table 28-2. Management of tonic-clonic status epilepticus

Assess neurologic, general physical, and cardiorespiratory status; elicit quick history and obtain samples of blood for laboratory studies. Insert IV catheter, oral airway, and administer oxygen if needed.

Begin IV infusion with dextrose 5% and 0.45% saline solution. Administer dextrose 50% if no cause is obvious.

If seizures continue, give a benzodiazepine (lorazepam or diazepam). Infuse a long-acting anticonvulsant (phenytoin or phenobarbital). Be prepared to intubate the trachea.

If seizures persist, repeat at least three times, giving maximal doses of each drug, one at a time, until seizures are controlled. Protect airway by intubation. Consult neurologist.

If seizures still continue, one might be dealing with refractory status. Look for a cause, metabolic complications, and review therapy. Give a round of all drugs previously tried. If seizures persist, try rectal paraldehyde or, in selected cases, nasogastric valproic acid or carbamazepine. Consider the use of continuous midazolam or diazepam infusion. Anticipate the need for general anesthesia and, therefore, consult anesthesia and neurology. Review all laboratory data.

Use pentobarbital therapy or other anesthetics as per availability of resources of personnel and monitoring facilities.

---

sodium valproate, and carbamazepine should be considered. On rare occasions, IV lidocaine or pentobarbital therapy is helpful.

Complex Partial Status Epilepticus (Psychomotor/Temporal Lobe Status)

Children with complex partial status epilepticus may have diverse clinical manifestations. These include prolonged twilight state, speech arrests, automatisms, staring, eyelid fluttering, eye rolling, oral buccal-lingual involuntary movements, autonomic changes (dilated pupils, sweating, tachycardia, and elevated BP), and generalized seizures. The EEG is characteristic during the seizures, showing continuous high-voltage, slow electroencephalographic changes, or is associated with spike and slow-wave activity from the temporal leads. A rare form of prolonged complex partial status epilepticus in children may present predominantly with psychiatric symptoms and generalized seizures, all of which may be resistant to the conventional drug therapy.[29]

Drug Therapy

Most cases of complex partial status epilepticus will respond to doses of IV diazepam, lorazepam, phenytoin, or phenobarbital. A common and successful strategy is to use one of the benzodiazepines intravenously, followed by a loading dose of phenytoin to maintain adequate seizure control. A methodical use of all major anticonvulsants will become necessary. There are intractable cases that may not respond easily and may take several days to weeks to be seizure-free. In such cases, a trial of both carbamazepine and sodium valproate (rectally or by nasogastric tube) should be attempted,[24,25] and successful seizure control can be expected.

Absence Status Epilepticus (Petit Mal Status)

Typically, absence status epilepticus is characterized by altered consciousness and clonic movements of the eyelids and hands

Table 28-3. Drug dosage in the treatment of status epilepticus

Drug	Route of administration	Dose	Onset of action	Duration of action
Diazepam	IV, IO PR	0.25–0.40 mg/kg 0.05 mg/kg Max. 10 mg/dose 40 mg/24 hr May repeat Q 10–15 min	1–3 min	5–15 min
Lorazepam	IV, IO	0.05–0.10 mg/kg Max. 4.0 mg/dose May repeat Q 10–15 min	2–3 min	24–48 hr
Midazolam	IV, IO IM	0.05–0.20 mg/kg 0.20 mg/kg Max. 5 mg/dose	2–5 min	1–5 hr
Phenytoin	IV, IO	18–20 mg/kg initial bolus Max. 1000 mg Infusion rate must be <0.5–1.0 mg/kg/min to a max. rate <50 mg/kg	10–30 min	12–24 hr
Phenobarbital	IV, IO	20 mg/kg initial bolus Max. 400 mg/dose Infusion rate <100 mg/min	10–20 min	1–3 d
Paraldehyde	PR	0.3 ml/kg May repeat 4–6 hourly/24 hr	10–15 min	
Valproic acid	NG, PR	20 mg/kg Maintenance 10–50 mg/kg		
Carbamazepine	NG, PR	10–30 mg/kg Maintenance 10–30 mg/kg		
Pentobarbital	IV	2–8 mg/kg initial bolus Maintenance 3–5 mg/kg/hr continuous infusion		
Lidocaine	IV	2–3 mg/kg initial bolus		
Thiopental	IV	5 mg/kg IV bolus 5 mg/kg/hr continuous infusion		
Inhalation anesthesia (isoflurane)		0.5%–3.0%		

IV, intravenous; IM, intramuscular; PR, per rectum; IO, intraosseous; NG, nasogastric.
Data from Tunik and Young.[9]

with automatisms of face and hands. Some children may become stuporous. Absence seizure status should be distinguished from drug intoxication, complex partial status, psychosis, metabolic encephalopathy, and hysteria.

Differentiation of petit mal status from complex partial status may be difficult but is important therapeutically. The first attack of petit mal seizure may start as petit mal status. Medical history is very important to uncover the seizure type. Another useful diagnostic point is the manner in which the attacks end. Petit mal status usually ends abruptly without postictal behavior, whereas complex partial status is associated with postictal depression, confusion, or malaise. The EEG is often decisive. Petit mal status shows generalized continuous epileptiform (spike and wave) activity, while complex partial status is associated with focal abnormalities and generalized or focal runs of high-voltage slow waves.

Drug Therapy

A common strategy employed to control absence seizure status is to give IV diazepam or acetazolamide (diamox), followed by oral

administration of ethosuximide or sodium valproate. Because it takes several days for oral ethosuximide to reach steady-state serum concentration, a higher than usual recommended dose (750 mg/d) may be started. Diazepam may be used intermittently while one of the long-acting drugs is slowly titrated to a therapeutic level. A combination of sodium valproate and ethosuximide may be necessary in difficult cases.

Doses for the three primary agents are as follows:

1. Acetazolamide: 250 to 500 mg intravenously
2. Ethosuximide: Orally, 20 mg/kg in 2 to 3 divided doses, with maximum starting dose of 750 mg/d
3. Sodium valproate: Orally, 10 to 50 mg/kg in 2 to 3 divided doses, with a starting dose of 10 mg/kg and gradual increments up to 50 mg/kg

Surgical Treatment

A small number of patients who are refractory to medication may be evaluated for epilepsy surgery. Most children who are identified as candidates for epilepsy surgery are referred to specialized centers for further presurgical evaluation. Types of surgery currently performed include temporal lobectomy, focal cortical resection of the lesion, hemispherectomy, and corpus callosotomy.[30]

Prognosis

In children, the presence of any underlying neurologic abnormality is associated with an increased risk of status epilepticus, especially during a febrile illness. The 1% to 2% mortality reported is often related to the underlying neurologic condition or treatment complications.[31] There is an increased risk of recurrent seizures and intellectual dysfunction following an episode of status epilepticus.[32] The causal association is not clear, but it appears that the outcome of tonic-clonic status epilepticus in children is related to the underlying cause rather than to the duration of seizure or the response to treatment.[31–33]

The outcome of epilepsia partialis continua is almost always guarded because it is related to a serious focal neuropathologic process. The outcome of prolonged nonconvulsive status may be associated with undesirable sequelae, such as memory disorders, intellectual deterioration, and behavior problems.[34,35]

References

1. Aicardi J, Chervie JJ. Convulsive status epilepticus in infants and children. A study of 239 cases. *Epilepsia* II:187, 1970.
2. Meldrum B. Metabolic factors during prolonged seizures and their relation to nerve cell death. *Adv Neurol* 34:261–275, 1983.
3. Lothman E. The biochemical basis and pathophysiology of status epilepticus. *Neurology* 40:13, 1990.
4. Browne TR, Mikati M. Status epilepticus. In Ropper AH, SF Kennedy (eds): *Neurological and Neurosurgical Intensive Care* (2nd ed). Rockville, MD: Aspen, 1988. Pp 269–288.
5. Lacey DJ et al. Lorazepam therapy for status epilepticus in children and adolescents. *J Pediatr* 108:771, 1986.
6. Leppik IE et al. Double blind study of lorazepam and diazepam in status epilepticus. *JAMA* 249:1452, 1983.
7. Crawford TO, Mitchell WG, Snodgrass SR. Lorazepam in childhood status epilepticus and serial seizures. *Neurology* 37:190, 1987.
8. Smith BT, Masotti E. Intravenous diazepam in the treatment of prolonged seizure activity in neonates and infants. *Dev Med Child Neurol* 13:630, 1981.
9. Tunik MA, Young GM. Status epilepticus in children. The acute management. *Pediatr Clin North Am* 39:1007, 1992.
10. Galvin GM, Jelinke GA. Midazolam: An effective intravenous agent for seizure control. *Arch Emerg Med* 4:169–172, 1987.
11. Kumar A, Bleck TP. Intravenous midazolam for the treatment of refractory status epilepticus. *Crit Care Med* 20:483, 1992.
12. Cranford RE et al. Intravenous phenytoin in acute treatment of seizures. *Neurology* 29:1474, 1979.
13. Albani M. Phenytoin in infancy and childhood. *Adv Neurol* 34:457, 1983.
14. Curless RH, Holzman BH, Ramsay RE. Paraldehyde therapy in childhood status epilepticus. *Arch Neurol* 40:477, 1983.
15. Bell HE, Bertino JS Jr. Constant infusion of diazepam in the treatment of continuous seizure activity. *Drug Intell Clin Pharm* 18:963, 1984.
16. Young RSK et al. Pentobarbital in refractory status epilepticus. *Pediatr Pharmacol* 3:63, 1983.
17. Rashkin MC, Young C, Penovich P. Pentobarbital treatment of refractory status epilepticus. *Neurology* 37:500, 1987.
18. Tasker RC et al. EEG monitoring of prolonged thiopentone administration for intractable seizures and status epilepticus in infants and young children. *Neuropediatrics* 20:147, 1989.
19. Kofke WA et al. Isoflurane anesthesia for status epilepticus. *Neurology* 37:103, 1987.
20. Leppik IK. Status epilepticus. *Neurology* 30:4, 1990.
21. Thorpy MJ. Rectal valproate syrup and status epilepticus. *Neurology* 30:1113, 1980.
22. Viani F et al. Rectal administration of sodium valproate for neonatal and infantile status epilepticus. *Dev Med Child Neurol* 26:277, 1984.
23. Rosenfield WE et al. Valproic and loading during intensive monitoring. *Arch Neurol* 44:709, 1987.
24. Snead OC, Miles MV. Treatment of status epilepticus in children with rectal sodium valproate. *J Pediatr* 106:323, 1985.
25. Miles MV et al. Rapid loading of critically ill patients with carbamazepine suspension. *Pediatrics* 86:263, 1990.
26. Knudsen FU. Rectal administration of diazepam in solution in the acute treatment of convulsions in infants and children. *Arch Dis Child* 54:855, 1979.
27. Camfield CS et al. Home use of rectal diazepam to prevent status epilepticus in children with convulsive disorders. *J Child Neurol* 4:125, 1989.
28. Crawford TO et al. Very high dose phenobarbital for refractory status epilepticus in children. 38:1035, 1988.
29. Mikati MA et al. Protracted epileptiform encephalopathy: An unusual form of partial complex status epilepticus. *Epilepsia* 26:563, 1985.
30. Wyllie E, Rothner DA, Luders H. Partial seizures in children; clinical features, medical treatment and surgical considerations. *Pediatr Clin North Am* 36:343–364, 1989.
31. Hauser WA. Status epilepticus: Epidemiologic considerations. *Neurology* 40:9, 1990.
32. Lockman LA. Treatment of status epilepticus in children. *Neurology* 40:43, 1990.
33. Dodrill CB, Wilensky AJ. Intellectual impairment on outcome of status epilepticus. *Neurology* 40:28, 1990.
34. Manning DJ, Rosenbloom L. Nonconvulsive status epilepticus. *Arch Dis Child* 62:37, 1987.
35. Doose H, Volzke E. Petit mal status in early childhood and early dementia. *Neuropaediatrie* 10:10, 1979.

29 Coma

Comatose infants and children require aggressive management after initial evaluation and stabilization of their respiratory function and circulation. Coma results from an alteration in level of consciousness and has been classified as **light** coma, a state in which arousal responses may be elicited with mild stimuli, and **deep** coma, a state in which only limited, if any, reflex reactions are obtained with strong stimuli. The pediatric modification of the Glasgow Coma Scale[1] may be useful in making prognostications about the outcome of comatose infants and children, once the basis for coma, a symptom of an underlying disease, has been identified. The availability of neuroimaging and monitoring equipment has been beneficial in the management of comatose patients, but these advances are no substitute for preventive measures.

Pathophysiology

Coma occurs where there is bilateral disease of the cerebral hemispheres or dysfunction of the reticular activating system of the upper pons and mesencephalon. Neurophysiologic studies have shown that structural or metabolic lesions induce states of prolonged unresponsiveness and cause the cortical waves of an EEG to be slow and usually synchronous. Strong sensory stimulation does not reverse the unresponsiveness. The reticular formation of the upper brain stem is interspersed among the paramedian tegmentum, the septal region, and the hypothalamus, and includes certain thalamic nuclei. Nuclei of the reticular formation in the brain stem receive collaterals from spinothalamic tracts and project to the parietal sensory cortex and other parts of the cerebral cortex, which have corticofugal connections back to the reticular formation.[2] Experimental studies of acceleration injuries in monkeys by Denny-Brown and Russell[3] led them to conclude that coma resulted from immediate disruption of respiratory and vasomotor responses. Ommaya and Gennarelli[4] have postulated that coma supervenes because of disconnection of the reticular system of the upper brain stem due to shear strain. Shear or diffuse axonal injuries causing disconnection of supratentorial and infratentorial structures occur more often in areas of bony protrusion and rough surfaces, such as the orbitofrontotemporal regions. Neuropathologic studies, by Adams and Victor[2] and others, of patients who had been comatose before death, showed the following two results: (1) **Discrete** lesions of cortex and subcortical white matter, including tumors, abscesses, and hemorrhages (epidural, subdural, intracerebral, and subarachnoid), rarely primarily involving the thalamus or midbrain, but causing temporal lobe–tentorial herniation syndromes with consequent compression, ischemia, and secondary (Duret) hemorrhages in the midbrain and subthalamic regions—or, infrequently, **massive**, diffuse, bilateral damage of the cortex and underlying white matter with apparent sparing of the thalamus and midbrain; (2) more often, no gross anatomic lesion, thus suggesting that coma was due to subcellular or metabolic dysfunction. Those lesions that displace the brain stem may do so by downward central displacement and bilateral compression or by unilateral displacement with uncal herniation. The major difference between the two processes is that in the latter, there is early drowsiness that may be accompanied by unilateral pupillary changes, usually ipsilateral dilatation.

Alteration of normal functioning of mesencephalic-diencephalic-cortical systems may result from metabolic disturbances that include hypoxia, hyperglycemia, hypoglycemia, hyperthermia, hypothermia, acidosis, alkalosis, hypokalemia, hypernatremia, hyperammonemia, lactic acidosis, and deficiency of thiamine, nicotinic acid, vitamins B_{12} and B_6. Such derangements affect cellular function but have little effect on cerebral blood flow (CBF). In hypoglycemia, there is insufficient glucose to support cellular needs. In hyperglycemia, ketone bodies and acidosis may have a toxic effect on cellular metabolism. In hyponatremia, the intraneuronal influx of water leads to cellular swelling and diffusion of chloride from the cells. Drugs such as alcohol, anticonvulsants, and phenothiazines may have a direct toxic effect on neuronal membranes. Other drugs may produce a metabolic acidosis or alter CBF. Hypotension also will cause decreased CBF and adversely affect the metabolic rate. Excessive neuronal discharge during status epilepticus often produces coma.

In head trauma, significant increased intracranial pressure (ICP) up to 200 to 700 lb/sq in. may occur in a few milliseconds. The resulting vibrations in the skull may be transmitted to the brain, or a sudden, marked increase in ICP may cause abrupt paralysis of neurologic function. Easily deformed by blunt injury, the skull of a young child may absorb the energy of impact and severe acceleration-deceleration forces, but underlying blood vessels may be torn, and shear or diffuse axonal injury may occur.[5] High-velocity injuries such as misaimed baseballs and free falls are more likely to cause depressed fractures and cerebral contusions than simple linear fractures. A blow to the unfixed head causes a shifting of the brain, which is only loosely secured by dura and piaarachnoid, within the cranium and torsion of the upper brain stem, and causes more severe damage than a similar blow to a head fixed in place. Contrecoup injuries may occur when there is an impact injury to one side of an older child's head and force is distributed directly across or diagonally to the opposite cerebral hemisphere to cause cortical or subcortical contusions.

Clinical Presentation

The patient must be examined carefully after the airway, respirations, and circulation are evaluated and stabilized. The general physical examination may disclose signs of a metabolic or infectious disease to explain the origin of coma or offer clues to a predisposing neurologic condition to account for coma (Table 29-1). The neurologic examination is performed to define the deficits, focal or generalized, and so attempt to localize the intracranial anatomic site of the disease process.

The skin, nailbeds, and lips may provide information about underlying disease conditions, such as the hyperpigmented, hypopigmented, hemangiomatous, or telangiectatic lesions of the phakomatoses; clubbing of the fingers and toes because of pulmonary or cyanotic heart disease; cherry-red lips resulting from carbon monoxide exposure; systemic illnesses reflected by petechiae, purpura, rashes, or burns; child abuse indicated by new and old scars; or evidence of self-mutilation associated with purine metabolism or psychiatric disorders. The scalp should be examined for abrasions and lacerations and ticks. The texture of the hair should be

Table 29-1. Diseases causing coma in infants and children

Trauma
    Motor vehicle accidents
    Falls
    Abuse
    Blows during fights or sports
    Drowning
    Hanging
    Electrocution

Infection
    Meningitis
    Encephalitis
    Brain abscess
    Sepsis

Vascular
    Epidural hematoma
    Subdural hematoma
    Subarachnoid hemorrhage
    Arteriovascular malformation
    Congenital aneurysm
    Mycotic aneurysm
    Arterial dissection
    Cerebral infarction
    Hemolytic-uremic syndrome
    Leukemia
    Idiopathic thrombocytopenia
    Sickle-cell disease
    Thalassemia
    Blood dyscrasias
    Moya-moya

Status epilepticus
    Idiopathic
    Complex febrile
    Withdrawal
    Subtherapeutic drug levels
    Noncompliance

Metabolic-toxic
    Ingestion, overdose
    Inborn error of metabolism
    Diabetes
    Reye's syndrome
    Hypoglycemia
    Carbon monoxide poisoning
    Lead poisoning
    Hypothyroidism
    Adrenal insufficiency

Acute hydrocephalus
    Shunt malfunction
    Tumor
    Herniation

noted; steely or kinky hair may be indicative of disorders of copper metabolism, such as Menkes disease. A bulging fontanel in an infant reflects increased ICP and may be associated with persistent downward deviation or "sunsetting" of the eyes. Blood or cerebrospinal fluid drainage from the nose or ears or periorbital ecchymoses ("raccoon eyes") occur with basilar skull or an orbital fracture or an underlying bony deformity associated with a meningocele or encephalocele. Lymphadenopathy should be recorded because of streptococcal, viral, and tubercular infections; mononucleosis and cat scratch fever; lymphoma; and other malignancies. The excursions of the chest should be observed for symmetry and depth. Guarding of the abdomen and the size of the liver and spleen should be assessed. In infants, certain urine odors are typical of metabolic diseases: mousy with phenylketonuria, maple syrup with branched-chain amino acids, and rancid with organic acidurias. Patients with diabetic ketoacidosis often have a sweet or fruity odor to their breaths.

Observation of the eye movements and resting posture of the comatose patient may yield important information. Calling the patient's name in a loud voice may provoke an arousal or a motoric response. If the patient shows no reaction and does not follow simple commands, such as when asked to squeeze the examiner's hand or move a body part, stronger stimuli should be used. A response to pain may be elicited by sternal or supraorbital rubbing, pinching of the inner aspects of the upper arms and thighs, or pressure applied to the nailbeds. Grimacing, avoidance of, or withdrawal from pain indicates light coma, and there may be incoherent vocalizations. The pupillary size and reactions (direct and consensual) should be noted and the ocular movements assessed. If there are no spontaneous movements of the eyes, and if there is no cervical spine injury, the oculocephalic responses should be checked by rotating the head quickly to either side and in the vertical plane to produce conjugate eye movements in the opposite direction, thus assessing the intactness of the tegmental structures of the pons and midbrain regulating these movements. In the absence of eye movements with the so-called doll's head maneuver, the oculovestibular responses can be evaluated by instilling ice water into the intact ear canal. If the eyes move rapidly in a nystagmoid manner to the side opposite of the side of irrigation, the patient is in light coma. When a lesion of the brain stem causes loss of the fast component of gaze, the eyes will be deflected from the midline to the side of irrigation. Disconjugate eye movements indicate that the pathologic process is infratentorial. The gag reflex and cough should be evaluated. During the aforementioned testing, the patient may move all or none of the extremities. If there is consistent lack of movement of the ipsilateral arm and leg, and the tone in these limbs is flaccid, the patient may be hemiplegic on the basis of a structural lesion or a postictal paralysis. Reflex asymmetry may confirm the impression of unilateral weakness. Recognizable patterns of motor response to painful stimuli are seen. Extension and inward rotation of the arms and extension of the legs are typical of **decerebrate** posturing and usually indicate more severe dysfunction than the flexion of the arms and extension of the legs that is characteristic of **decorticate** posturing.

In newborns who become comatose within hours or days after birth, congenital infections, inborn errors of metabolism, and serious congenital malformations must be considered. TORCH studies of the baby and mother should be obtained if there are lesions such as jaundice, rashes, petechiae, chorioretinitis, hepatosplenomegaly, macro- or microcephaly, and seizures. If the mother is immunocompromised because of substance abuse or other risk factors, HIV testing should be performed. If the baby is found to have severe lactic acidosis, errors of the electron transport system and short-, medium-, long-, and very long chain fatty acid disorders must be assessed. A specific diagnosis may require analysis of skin fibroblasts or samples of muscle or liver. Acute-phase serum and blood for amino acids, urine for organic acids, and serum for ammonia and carnitine should be obtained. Intracranial malformations such as congenital hydrocephalus may be apparent on bedside examination, but further studies, such as cranial ultrasound, computed tomography (CT), or magnetic resonance imaging (MRI) scans, may disclose the presence of aqueductal stenosis (Chiari 1, resulting in cerebellar tonsillar herniation and medullary compression), periventricular or diffuse calcifications, a teratoma, choroid plexus papilloma, or poorly differentiated malignancy. In older infants, a febrile illness or exposure to anesthesia for a routine procedure may be the provocation for exposure of a previously unrecognized metabolic disorder. Toddlers who become comatose must be evaluated for unwitnessed falls, child abuse, accidental ingestions of toxins or household medications, and infrequent idiosyncratic reactions to medications or vaccinations. A detailed history will be most helpful in these instances. Shaken-baby syndrome or Trauma X must always be considered in comatose children who have no apparent precipitating illness. Older children who play contact sports or have access to bicycles, roller skates or blades, or skateboards, or are unsupervised in a playground, are at greater risk for coma resulting from head injury, especially because of peer pressure, which often includes teasing of the children who wear protective helmets.

Special Investigations

At this time, a CT scan of the head, providing more information than skull x-rays, is so readily obtained in most community hospitals that it may not be considered a special investigation. When hemorrhage is suspected, contrast material should not be used, because the high attenutation of hemorrhagic lesions may be obscured by areas of contrast enhancement. Should a brain tumor be under consideration, it is useful to review the plain scan to look for areas of calcification or hemorrhage before contrast is injected. Shear or diffuse axonal injuries are best imaged with MRI. If subdural hematomas are suspected because of focal seizures, anemia, and retinal hemorrhages, but are not seen on CT scanning, an MRI with axial and coronal images should be obtained. Processes involving the basal structures of the brain are better visualized on MRI scans, but many scanners cannot accommodate a patient who requires ventilation, unless special arrangements are made. Noncontrast MR angiography (MRA) using phase contrast or time-of-flight sequences can demonstrate aneurysms or arterial dissections and allows serial examinations of such abnormalities without subjecting an infant or small child to invasive arteriography. Transfemoral arteriography is performed in patients whose sudden decline in level of consciousness results from an intracranial hemorrhage from an arteriovenous malformation or, less commonly, a ruptured congenital or mycotic aneurysm. The risk-benefits of MRA and conventional angiography are being delineated. At this time, some vascular lesions may not be visualized as readily and accurately on MRA. Bedside telemetry or video-EEG monitoring is useful in determining whether the altered consciousness is caused by ongoing electrical status epilepticus, with or without overt clinical seizures. The value of testing evoked responses in comatose patients remains to be clarified. Radionuclide CBF studies are useful in infants or small children when the clinical criteria for brain death are present and there has been one isoelectric EEG. An apnea test is used in conjunction with the assessment of brain death.

Management

General Principles

Because a comatose patient is unable to provide any history or complaints, an immediate brief but thorough evaluation of the patient is necessary. Any person who was present when the patient became comatose or found the patient in coma must be sought to answer questions. This is especially important for comatose older children and adolescents. The adequacy of the patient's airway and respirations must be assessed immediately, and the vital signs must be checked for evidence of circulatory shock. If there is external trauma, bleeding should be stopped. While an endotracheal tube or oral airway is inserted, intravenous (IV) access should be established after obtaining blood samples for hematologic and coagulation studies, type and crossmatching, glucose, creatinine, BUN, electrolytes, liver function tests, toxic screen, and blood gases. Anticonvulsant levels should always be checked in a patient known to have seizures. A bladder catheter should be inserted, and urine should be sent for analysis and toxic screen. In a patient with a known or suspected head injury, in which there may be concomitant injury of the cervical vertebrae, the patient's neck should be immobilized in a cervical collar until x-rays of the cervical spine are obtained and interpreted. As soon as the patient is stabilized, if there is suspected head injury or no obvious cause for coma, a CT scan without contrast should be obtained and glucose administered intravenously. It may be feasible to obtain a CT scan of the cervical spine also, if there are any questions about the plain x-rays of the cervical spine. If seizures occur, they should be controlled. Medication-induced respiratory depression by anticonvulsants is of less concern when there are an adequate airway, controlled ventilation, and a nasogastric tube in place. If a patient has been partly responsive but required sedation or paralysis for intubation and does not return to the previous level of arousal within an appropriate time, a portable EEG should be obtained to exclude subclinical status epilepticus. Administering flumazenil, a short-acting benzodiazepine antagonist, can be useful in assessing whether ingestion of a benzodiazepine is the basis of coma or altered consciousness. In patients who are dependent on benzodiazepines, there is risk of inducing seizures with flumazenil.

Specifics

Patients with intracranial lesions such as epidural, subdural, or intracerebral hematomas may require emergency neurosurgical evacuation of the hematoma. Any patient with findings of increased ICP, suggested by slow or irregular respirations, high BP, and slow pulse, should be fluid-restricted to two-thirds or three-fourths maintenance with isoosmolar fluids for the first 72 to 96 hours to reduce the incidence of cerebral edema, unless there is an electrolyte imbalance or circulatory shock. The serum osmolality should be kept at 295 to 305 until the period of maximal hyperemia has passed. If changing vital signs suggest an increase in ICP, additional measures, such as hyperventilation to keep the arterial pCO_2 between 25 and 30 torr, and administration of furosemide, 0.5 to 1.0 mg/kg every 4 to 6 hours, or mannitol, 0.25 to 1.0 g/kg (of a 20% solution), may be used. Urine output should be measured. ICP monitors may be useful in selected cases, but the bolt must be checked for accuracy of readings, so the aforementioned measures can be instituted for bolt reading of ICP over 20 torr. Placement of a bolt is not a substitute for careful bedside monitoring of the child's temperature, BP, respirations, and heart rate. Correction of alkalosis or acidosis is important. If the patient is febrile and has evidence of meningismus, a lumbar puncture should be performed after the CT scan is obtained. If the patient is in septic shock, antibiotics should be given as soon as possible, even if the lumbar puncture is deferred. Naloxone should be administered if there may have been ingestion of narcotics. Gastric lavage and instillation of charcoal should be performed in instances of toxic ingestion. Although steroids are extremely effective in decreasing tumor-related edema in patients with brain tumors, there is controversy about their usefulness in patients with head trauma or meningitis.[6] One study has shown, however, that very high dose steroids are beneficial if given within the first 8 hours in patients with spinal cord injuries.[7]

Prognosis and Outcomes

The tempo of the child's recovery of consciousness is a reliable indicator of the likely outcome when it is combined with the score on the Glasgow Coma Scale or modified Pediatric Coma Scale (Table 29-2). Patients with initial scores less than 5 usually have sequelae. About 75% of children who remain comatose for 3 weeks or more are incapable of independent living. In the absence of a structural lesion or focal deficit, a child who regains alertness within 12 to 24 hours and has a Coma score of 8 or higher will not have significant neurologic problems superimposed on any that may have contributed to the onset of coma. A prospective study by Levy et al.[8] of the outcome of 210 older patients who had cardiac arrests showed that 92 of 93 patients were accurately identified as being in a poor outcome category because of abnormal motor responses and the absence of orienting or roving eye movements. Sacco et al.[9] performed a prospective study of outcome of 169 patients older than 10 years who had nontraumatic coma and determinations of Glasgow Coma Scale scores within 72 hours of hospitalization. They found that 61% of the patients were dead or in persistent coma by 2 weeks after onset of coma, regardless of age, sex, or ethnicity. Patients who lack pupillary reactions, oculovestibular responses, or corneal reflexes within a few hours of coma rarely regain independent function. The Multi-Society Task Force on Persistent Vegetative State (PVS)[10] stated that recovery of consciousness after 12 months of PVS is unlikely in children with traumatic injuries; recovery of consciousness after 3 months

is rare in children with nontraumatic injuries. Emerman et al.[11] found that patients with drug-induced coma had a better outcome than those with coma due to hypoxia or ischemia. The initial level of consciousness in 92 patients who were hospitalized because of tricyclic overdose was a better predictor of outcome than the patients' QRS intervals on the ECG. They stated that fewer complications occurred in the 55 patients who did not require emergency intubation because of obtundation. In their study of the outcome of near-drowning in 142 children who ranged in age from 8 months to 14 years, Brezner et al.[12] found that 43 of the 69 comatose children died during the first week; of the 26 who survived, 15 remained in PVS for 1 to 8 years. Fields et al.[13] evaluated the long-term outcome of 20 children in PVS who were cared for at home after hospitalization. Eight children died; only minimal awareness in the other children was reported by their caretakers after an average of 4.5 years' home care. A prospective study by Kaufmann et al.[14] of children 6 months after they sustained severe closed-head injury showed that the patients had attentional disturbances.

As soon as the patient's respiratory and circulatory functions have become stable and the basis for coma has been identified and remedied, it is important to involve rehabilitative therapists from physical therapy, occupational therapy, and speech and language therapy in the daily management of the patient. Early intervention may prevent contractures and other disabilities that occur in comatose patients. Social service and child psychiatry will play important roles in support and after-hospital care.

References

1. Simpson D, Reilly P. Paediatric coma scale. *Lancet* 2:450, 1982.
2. Adams RD, Victor M. Coma and related disorder of consciousness. In Adams RD, Victor M (eds): *Principles of Neurology* (5th ed). New York: McGraw-Hill, 1993. Pp 300–318.
3. Denny-Brown D, Russell WR. Experimental brain concussion. *Brain* 64:7–164, 1941.
4. Ommaya AK, Gennarelli TA. Cerebral concussion and traumatic unconsciousness: Correlation of experimental and clinical observations on blunt head injuries. *Brain* 97:633–654, 1974.
5. Menkes JH, Till K. Postnatal trauma and injuries by physical agents. In JH Menkes (ed): *Textbook of Child Neurology* (5th ed). Baltimore: Williams & Wilkins, 1995. Pp. 557–597.
6. Prober CG. The role of steroids in the management of children with bacterial meningitis. *Pediatrics* 95:29–31, 1995.
7. Bracken MB, Holford TR. Effects of timing of methyl-prednisolone or naloxone administration on recovery of segmental and long-tract neurological function in NASCIS 2. *J Neurosurg* 79:500–507, 1993.
8. Levy DE et al. Predicting outcome from hypoxic-ischemic coma. *JAMA* 253:1420–1426, 1985.
9. Sacco RL et al. Glasgow coma scale and coma etiology as predictors of 2-week outcome. Nontraumatic coma. *Arch Neurol* 47:1181–1184, 1990.
10. The Multi-Society Task Force on PVS. Medical aspects of the persistent vegetative state (in two parts). *N Engl J Med* 330:1499, 1572, 1994.
11. Emerman CL, Connors AR, Burma GM. Level of consciousness as a predictor of complications following tricyclic overdose. *Ann Emerg Med* 16:326–330, 1987.
12. Brezner A, Molnar GE, Aoki BY. Long-term outcome of near-drowning in children. *Arch Phys Med Rehabil* 71:770, 1990.
13. Fields AI et al. Outcomes of children in a persistent vegetative state. *Crit Care Med* 21:1890–1894, 1993.
14. Kaufmann PM et al. Attentional disturbance after pediatric closed head injury. *J Child Neurol* 8:348–353, 1993.

Table 29-2. Pediatric Coma Scale

Eyes	Open spontaneously	4
	Open to speech	3
	Open to pain	2
	Not open	1
Motor	Obeys commands	6
	Localizes pain	5
	Flexion to pain	4
	Decorticate posturing	3
	Decerebrate posturing	2
	No reaction	1
Verbal	Obeys commands	5
	Says words	4
	Vocalizes	3
	Cries	2
	No sounds	1
"Normal" score for age:	0–6 mo	9
	6–12 mo	11
	1–2 yr	12
	2–5 yr	13
	>5 yr	14

Brooke Swearingen

30 Perioperative Management of the Neurosurgical Patient

Improvements in operative mortality after neurosurgery in the pediatric population have resulted both from changes in surgical technique and from major advances in pediatric neuroanesthesia and perioperative critical care. The goal of intensive care unit (ICU) management should be to maintain a physiologic homeostasis while preventing potential complications arising from the operative procedure. This requires attention to each organ system as it impacts on the underlying neurologic condition.

Neurologic Observation

Probably the most common reason for neurosurgic admission to the ICU is for intensive surveillance of possible postoperative neurologic deterioration. This could occur from raised intracranial pressure (ICP) as a result of postoperative hemorrhage or edema, and obviously requires immediate neurosurgical consultation and possible computed tomography (CT) imaging. Specific neurologic complications can be anticipated based on the location of the previous surgery. Deficits from posterior fossa surgery might include acute hydrocephalus with early ocular motility problems, persistent vomiting, or apnea, or perisellar surgery may lead to visual deficits or endocrine abnormalities, especially diabetes insipidus. Close cooperation and communication between the intensivist and the neurosurgeon is of paramount importance. To minimize the risk of such complications, routine postoperative care should include measures for control of ICP, respiratory support, control of BP, and appropriate fluid and nutritional management.

Control of Raised Intracranial Pressure

The pathophysiology of elevated ICP is discussed in detail in Head Trauma, by Swearingen, in this volume. In the postoperative period, increased ICP can result from unresolved peritumoral edema, edema from the original injury or surgical intervention itself, or the development of a postoperative hemorrhage or infarct. If significant postoperative edema is expected, an ICP measuring device will have been placed intraoperatively. Routine postoperative measures to control ICP, even without an ICP monitor, include fluid restriction and steroid administration, with hyperventilation and osmotherapy sometimes required. Cerebral spinal fluid (CSF) drainage through a ventriculostomy can be employed to both monitor ICP and control ICP by decreasing the volume of the CSF compartment. Cerebral ischemia has been recognized as an increasingly important factor after head injury and as a complication of vasospasm following subarachnoid hemorrhage. The balance required in ICU management requires

1. Maintaining sufficient tissue perfusion to prevent ischemia while preventing hemorrhagic complications
2. Minimizing cerebral edema while avoiding the ischemia induced by ICP reduction techniques (hyperventilation, osmotherapy, fluid restriction)

The goal of such therapy is to maintain adequate brain-blood flow and oxygenation, as measured by the cerebral perfusion pressure (CPP). This is defined as the difference between the mean arterial pressure (MAP) and the ICP (CPP = MAP − ICP). In adults, an adequate CPP is felt to be above 50 torr,[1,2] although in the case of head trauma or a subarachnoid hemorrhage patient with vasospasm, significantly higher CPPs can be required to maintain adequate CBF.[3-5] The interaction between CBF, ICP, and systemic BP is complex. In the intact brain, CBF is maintained (autoregulated) over a range of systemic arterial pressures, but this autoregulation is impaired after head trauma or intracranial surgery.[6] Under these circumstances, it is important to control both the ICP and the systemic arterial pressure to maintain adequate cerebral perfusion. Although relatively rare in the pediatric population, vasospasm after subarachnoid hemorrhage further complicates postoperative management. This delayed arterial constriction, occurring 3 to 10 days after subarachnoid hemorrhage, can lead to severe ischemia, neurologic deficit, and infarction. Especially in cases in which early surgery for aneurysm clipping has minimized the risk of rebleeding, vasospasm is best managed by induced hypertension, volume expansion, and hemodilution,[4,5,7] and with administration of prophylactic nimodipine, a calcium channel blocker.[8,9]

Fluid Management

Routine postoperative fluid administration should provide two-thirds maintenance, usually as dextrose 5% and ½ normal saline or dextrose 5% and normal saline, unless euvolemia is required to maintain adequate perfusion. Use of hypotonic glucose solutions should be avoided, as excess free water in the setting of postoperative blood-brain barrier disruption can exacerbate intracranial edema. Blood glucose should be maintained within the normal range, as both hypo- and hyperglycemia have been associated with neuronal injury. Electrolyte abnormalities are common after head injury and may be seen in the postoperative patient; they are often iatrogenic as a result of fluid restriction and osmotherapy. Serum sodium often rises above 140 mEq/liter, but levels above 150 mEq/liter are to be avoided. Diabetes insipidus, with a rising serum sodium in association with an increasing urine output, can be seen after pituitary or hypothalamic surgery or severe head trauma. It is effectively treated with vasopressin (Pitressin) or DDAVP.[10] Mild hyponatremia may result from stress-induced release of antidiuretic hormone (ADH), but progressive hyponatremia with an inappropriate urine hyperosmolality (SIADH) is sometimes seen after head trauma or surgery in the perisellar region.[11] Although it usually responds to fluid restriction, severe hyponatremia (<120 mEq/liter) requires the use of a loop diuretic and sodium chloride administration.[12]

Osmotherapy

Use of osmotherapy in the postoperative patient is based on the likelihood of persistent ICP elevation, and is usually unnecessary for the routine craniotomy. In cases of diffuse postoperative edema, maintaining the elevation of serum osmolality achieved intraoperatively is sometimes required, and this is best obtained by small (0.25 g/kg) frequent doses of mannitol.[13] Because most patients (even uncomplicated craniotomies) are loaded with mannitol intraoperatively, a loading dose is usually not necessary. The dose frequency needs to be tailored to maintain a serum osmolality of not greater than 320 mosm/liter, as higher osmolalities are associated with renal damage. Small doses of a loop diuretic can also be used to maintain an elevated serum osmolality.

Steroids

Although the use of steroids in head injury is controversial, they unequivocally decrease peritumor edema and are routinely used in the perioperative period.[14] Dexamethasone in doses of 0.25 to 0.5 mg/kg/d is commonly given. Its use may be associated with gastrointestinal complications, including stress ulceration or gastritis, as well as hyperglycemia, poor wound healing, and immunosuppression.

Respiratory Management

The need for postoperative intubation depends on the neurologic status of the patient as well as the risk of persistent elevation in ICP. Extubation of the patient postoperatively requires that the child be awake and able to protect its airway and handle secretions appropriately. These functions may be altered, especially after posterior fossa surgery, and prophylactic intubation for airway protection is sometimes indicated. Hyperventilation is effective in the acute lowering of elevated ICP by decreasing CBF through cerebral vasoconstriction.[15] Postoperative elevation in ICP can be controlled in the short term by ventilating to a pCO_2 of 30 torr, although the vasoconstrictive effect wears off after a few hours, and more prolonged measures (removal of any mass lesion, osmotherapy, barbiturates) are then required. Aggressive hyperventilation (pCO_2 25 to 30 or less) may worsen cerebral ischemia by decreasing CBF, and caution has been suggested regarding its routine use,[16] although it remains necessary in cases of refractory intracranial hypertension. Hypercarbia results in cerebral vasodilation with a resultant increase in ICP, and therefore oversedation or excessive analgesia with hypoventilation is to be avoided. Hypoxemia will also increase ICP through vasodilation and increased CBF, and maintenance of adequate oxygenation ($pO_2 > 80$ torr) is essential. The use of positive end-expiratory pressure (PEEP) to decrease atelectasis and improve ventilation is usually well tolerated. Theoretically, PEEP may result in elevated venous pressures, which may in turn elevate ICP.[17,18]

Barbiturate Therapy

Chronic administration of barbiturates (pentobarbital) to control ICP is reserved for those cases refractory to all, more conservative measures, usually after severe head trauma, and is of questionable long-term benefit. (See Head Trauma, by Swearingen, this volume.) Small doses of a short-acting barbiturate (thiopental) are useful in the intubated postoperative patient with elevated ICP who requires transient sedation for a brief procedure (e.g., endotracheal suctioning).

Medical Management of the Postoperative Patient

Cardiovascular Management

Control of BP in the postoperative period is necessary to ensure adequate cerebral perfusion, as well as to decrease the risk of hemorrhagic complications and minimize elevations in ICP. A MAP of 60 to 100 torr is optimal, although this will vary with the age of the child, and data directly relating CBF to perfusion pressure are not available in children. BP support is often best achieved by small volumes of fluid or colloid, followed by peripheral vasoconstrictors (phenylephrine) or inotropes (dopamine), if needed. Antihypertensives are commonly needed postoperatively, although often mild hypertension will resolve with adequate analgesia. Most agents that lower systemic arterial pressure also act as cerebral vasodilators, and thus their use is a compromise between the need to lower MAP and the risk of elevating ICP by cerebral vasodilation.[1] IV labetolol, with both anti-alpha- and anti-beta-adrenergic activity, appears useful as a first-line drug to control systemic hypertension without reflex tachycardia and with minimal increase in ICP. If unsuccessful, nitroprusside, nitroglycerine, or trimethophan may be required. Nitroprusside is a potent vasodilator, but use may be complicated by cyanide toxicity. Trimethophan (Arfonad), as a ganglionic blocker, causes little increase in ICP but leads to pupillary dilation, and its use is limited by rapid tachyphylaxis.

Gastrointestinal Complications

Stress ulceration was originally described in association with hypothalamic damage by Cushing in 1932,[19] and the common use of steroids may have exacerbated the incidence of ulceration or gastritis in neurosurgical patients. Prophylaxis for gastrointestinal hemorrhage is given to all patients perioperatively and is maintained as long as steroids are administered. Lowering gastric acidity appears to be effective in decreasing the risk of hemorrhage, either with H-2 antagonists[20] or frequent antacid use.[21] Because gastric acidity may serve as a barrier to nosocomial infection, sucralfate prophylaxis has been suggested as an alternative that does not lower gastric pH and may therefore decrease the risk of nosocomial infection.[22]

Nutritional support is required in those patients whose neurologic condition prevents their obtaining adequate independent caloric intake. Because gastrointestinal motility often returns quickly after neurosurgical procedures, enteric feeding through a flexible, small-bore feeding tube can usually meet caloric needs, and it is well-tolerated over long periods. With associated abdominal trauma or prolonged gut immotility (often seen with barbiturate use), total parenteral nutrition is required. Some have suggested that, in the hypercatabolic state associated with severe head injury, total parenteral nutrition may in fact be more effective than enteral feedings in providing optimal nutrition.[23]

Hematologic Complications

Hemorrhagic hypovolemia is uncommon in the postoperative period, except in infants, who may lose a significant amount of their intravascular volume into large subgaleal collections. This is an important consideration in those procedures requiring extensive bone work, as in craniofacial reconstructions, in which the volume status and postoperative hematocrit should be closely monitored. Head trauma with severe scalp injuries can also lead to large external blood losses. In general, however, falling hematocrits in the postoperative period should prompt a search for causes other than neurosurgical. Clotting abnormalities are described after severe head trauma, especially disseminated intravascular coagulation.[24]

References

1. Marsh ML, Marshall LF, Shapiro HM. Neurosurgical intensive care. *Anesthesiology* 47:149–163, 1977.

2. Jennet WB et al. Relation between cerebral blood flow and cerebral perfusion pressure. *Br J Surg* 57:390–97, 1970.

3. Rosner MJ. Pathophysiology and management of increased intracranial pressure. In Andrews BT (ed): *Neurosurgical Intensive Care*. New York, McGraw-Hill, 1993.

4. Awad IA et al. Clinical vasospasm after subarachnoid hemorrhage: Response to hypervolemic hemodilution and arterial hypertension. *Stroke* 18:365, 1987.

5. Kassell NF et al. Treatment of ischemic deficits from vasospasm with intravascular expansion and induced arterial hypertension. *Neurosurgery* 11:337, 1982.

6. Lassen NA. Control of cerebral circulation in health and disease. *Circ Res* 34:749–760, 1974.

7. Levy ML, Giannotta SL. Induced hypertension and hypervolemia for treatment of cerebral vasospasm. *Neurosurg Clin North Am* 1:357, 1990.

8. Ljunggren B et al. Outcome in 60 consecutive patients treated with early aneurysm operation and intravenous nimodipine. *J Neurosurg* 61:864, 1984.

9. Pickard JG et al. Effect of oral nimodipine on cerebral infarction and outcome after subarachnoid hemorrhage: British aneurysm nimodipine trial. *Br J Med* 298:636, 1989.

10. Robinson AG. DDAVP in the treatment of central diabetes insipidus. *N Engl J Med* 312:1121–1122, 1985.

11. Bartter FC, Schwartz WB. The syndrome of inappropriate secretion of antidiuretic hormone. *Am J Med* 42:790–806, 1967.

12. Hantman D et al. Rapid correction of hyponatremia in the syndrome of inappropriate secretion of antidiuretic hormone. *Ann Intern Med* 78:870–875, 1973.

13. Marshall LF et al. Mannitol dose requirements in brain-injured patients. *J Neurosurg* 48:169–172, 1978.

14. Shapiro HM. Intracranial hypertension: Therapeutic and anesthetic considerations. *Anaesthesia* 56:53–54, 1982.

15. Crockard HA, Coppel DL, Morrow WFK. Evaluation of hyperventilation in the treatment of head injuries. *Br J Med* 4:634–664, 1973.

16. Muizelaar JP et al. Adverse effects of prolonged hyperventilation in patients with severe head injury: A randomized clinical trial. *J Neurosurg* 75:731–739, 1991.

17. Aidinis SJ, Lafferty J, Shapiro HM. Intracranial responses to PEEP. *Anesthesiology* 45:275–286, 1976.

18. Apuzzo MLJ et al. Effect of positive end-expiratory pressure ventilation on intracranial pressure in man. *J Neurosurg* 46:227–232, 1977.

19. Cushing HC. Peptic ulcers and the midbrain. *Surg Gynecol Obstet* 55:1–34, 1932.

20. Strauss RJ, Stern TA, Wise L. Prevention of stress ulcerations using H2 receptor antagonists. *Am J Surg* 135:120–126, 1978.

21. Priebe HJ et al. Antacid versus cimetidine in preventing acute gastrointestinal bleeding. A randomized trial in 75 critically ill patients. *N Engl J Med* 302:426–430, 1980.

22. Driks MR et al. Rates of ventilator-associated pneumonia in patients randomized to treatment with sucralfate versus antacids or H2 blockers. *Am Rev Respir Dis* 135:212, 1987.

23. Rapp RP et al. The favorable effect of early parenteral feeding on survival in head-injured patients. *J Neurosurg* 58:906–912, 1983.

24. Van der Sande JJ et al. Head injury and coagulation disorders. *J Neurosurg* 49:357–365, 1978.

Paul H. Chapman

31 Pediatric Hydrocephalus

Neurosurgical patients in a pediatric intensive care unit (PICU) tend to fall into relatively few categories. Aside from children requiring perioperative care for intracranial surgery, one typically sees patients with head injury or those requiring control of elevated intracranial pressure (ICP) from some other condition, such as hepatic encephalopathy. More often than not, there is also a child with some form of hydrocephalus. This may be associated with neonatal intracranial hemorrhage, a congenital neural tube defect such as myelomeningocele, or brain tumor. The child may also represent a critical management problem because of malfunction or infection of a previously placed shunt. The hydrocephalus may or may not be the primary focus of attention at the moment but when present, seems to always lurk in the background as a complicating factor in the patient's care. For this reason, it is appropriate that physicians caring for children in the ICU have more than a passing grasp of the subject and its ramifications. Detailed discussions of the topic are available for the interested reader.[1]

Pathophysiology

Cerebral Spinal Fluid Formation and Absorption

To put the discussion into proper context, it is useful to consider a few relevant facts regarding the physiology of the cerebrospinal fluid (CSF). The rate of formation of CSF is approximately 20 ml/hr.[2] This figure is valid for any individual from late infancy to adulthood. In younger infants, the rate is not known, although it is probably not much below that figure. The choroid plexus accounts for at least 80% to 90% of CSF production. Before shunts were available to treat hydrocephalus, surgical removal of the choroid plexus was occasionally used in an effort to control the problem. This was generally unsuccessful, for reasons not entirely clear. In fact, virtually normal rates of CSF production have been measured after ablation of the entire choroid plexus of the lateral ventricles. CSF production by the choroid plexus is an energy-requiring process with involvement of the enzymes carbonic anhydrase and Na-K ATPase. Efforts have been made to take advantage of this and treat hydrocephalus by pharmacologic reduction of CSF production. The most commonly used drug is acetazolamide, which acts as a carbonic anhydrase inhibitor. In doses up to 100 mg/kg/d, it may decrease the rate of CSF production by 50% to 60%. Furosemide, which probably interferes with chloride transport, also affects CSF production adversely. It is generally used with acetazolamide in doses up to 1 mg/kg/d.[3]

Cause of Hydrocephalus

Brain Tumor

In the pediatric population, brain tumors are the most common cause of noncommunicating hydrocephalus. Cerebellar tumors such as benign astrocytomas and medulloblastomas represent about half of all childhood brain tumors. These obstruct CSF circulation within the fourth ventricle, resulting in acute hydrocephalus. With the advent of computed tomography (CT) and magnetic resonance imaging (MRI) scanning, earlier diagnosis of such tumors is now the rule, thus avoiding extreme life-threatening hydrocephalus before the situation is detected. Because of this, precraniotomy emergency shunting or external ventricular drainage is usually no longer required; nonetheless, tumor surgery should be performed in a timely fashion to relieve the CSF obstruction. If CSF flow cannot be restored, shunting at the time of craniotomy will be necessary.

In spite of what seems to be adequate surgical decompression of a posterior fossa tumor, as many as 20% of such children will have persistent hydrocephalus and require shunting before discharge from hospital. It is of particular importance that ICU personnel caring for these patients postoperatively appreciate the potential for acute hydrocephalus and be alert for its clinical signs, which include deteriorating level of consciousness, bradycardia, and respiratory depression. Depressed breathing with carbon dioxide retention will exacerbate already elevated ICP and lead to eventual respiratory arrest.

Pineal and third ventricular tumors are also relatively common in childhood and may typically manifest themselves by producing hydrocephalus at those sites. Suprasellar tumors such as craniopharyngiomas and optic gliomas can cause hydrocephalus, but do so less commonly. When this occurs, it is because the tumor has grown to a large size and extends upward to obstruct the foramen of Monro. This prevents CSF from exiting either lateral ventricle into the third ventricle. The result is so-called biventricular hydrocephalus, which is important to identify because each ventricle will need to be drained independently to effectively relieve the problem.

Congenital Hydrocephalus

The intensive care pediatrician can expect to encounter hydrocephalus resulting from a variety of conditions other than brain tumor. In an adult population, the hydrocephalus is often acquired as a consequence of head injury, aneurysmal subarachnoid hemorrhage, or meningitis. By contrast, during infancy and childhood, congenital causes are common. An intrauterine catastrophe such as toxoplasmosis infection or a cerebrovascular accident may be responsible. More often, there is a structural anomaly of the brain resulting from abnormal central nervous system (CNS) morphogenesis. The best examples of this include myelodysplasia, encephalocele, and the Dandy-Walker cyst of the posterior fossa. The importance of this fact to the treating physician is that he or she understands the way in which hydrocephalus may manifest itself in relation to the child's other CNS problems. Myelodysplasia is the most common of the congenital conditions. It also best illustrates this point. Ninety percent of infants with spina bifida can be expected to require shunting for hydrocephalus. This incidence is due to the presence of a posterior fossa Chiari malformation, which obstructs the outflow of CSF from the fourth ventricle. The malformation itself includes a small posterior fossa with caudal herniation of cerebellum and brain stem through the foramen magnum into the cervical spinal canal.[4] The brain stem is distorted and kinked with abnormal cytoarchitecture. Active hydrocephalus can cause symptoms of brain stem dysfunction in such children, the most common manifestations being apnea/bradycardia, dysphagia, and stridor. When such symptoms require ICU management, the physician should be alert to the possibility that hydrocephalus is the immediate cause of the problem. If the child already has a shunt, malfunction of this device should be ruled out before considering direct surgical decompression of the malformation.

The Dandy-Walker malformation is a less frequent but important cause of congenital hydrocephalus.[5] It is also an anomaly that illustrates the way in which hydrocephalus can interact with its anatomic substrate to cause an atypical or potentially confusing diagnostic problem. Like the Chiari malformation, it is a hindbrain anomaly with obstruction of CSF outflow from the fourth ventricle. In this instance, however, there is cystic enlargement of the fourth ventricle with associated agenesis of the cerebellar vermis and expansion of the posterior fossa. Shunting the dilated lateral ventricular system alone may initially control the hydrocephalus problem. At a later time, the posterior fossa cyst can become isolated from the rest of the ventricular system. This results in a pressure gradient across the tentorial hiatus with consequent upward herniation and signs that reflect brain stem dysfunction. Shunting of the posterior fossa cyst is necessary to correct the problem.

Monitoring Techniques and Temporizing Measures in the Intensive Care Unit

Although shunting is the definitive treatment for most hydrocephalus, there may be a period during a child's ICU management when this is undesirable or inappropriate. In this circumstance, monitoring of the hydrocephalus and ICP will be necessary. In addition, one may require a means of controlling CSF accumulation and elevated ICP until shunting can be done. There is a variety of methods available for monitoring ICP.[6] Most are invasive and include the subarachnoid bolt, subdural catheter, and fiberoptic probe. A completely implantable telemetric system can also be used.[7] These methods all have the disadvantage of not providing a means of removing CSF. For this reason, direct ventricular cannulation is preferred. The ventricular catheter is usually then attached to a closed external ventricular drainage (EVD) system for either constant or intermittent venting of CSF. Alternatively, it may be connected to a plastic reservoir that has been implanted beneath the scalp. This can then be tapped percutaneously as necessary[8] (Fig. 31-1). A principal concern with any method that has tubes or wires leading through the scalp externally is, of course, infection, which can be minimized by using a closed system with strict aseptic technique. Equally important is the need for physicians and nurses to be completely familiar with the mechanics of the system to avoid accidental obstruction, inappropriate pressure settings, or retrograde contamination.

The means chosen to monitor and control ICP elevation may vary, depending on the underlying cause of the hydrocephalus. In the case of tumors, one ideally treats hydrocephalus by removing the mass that blocks CSF circulation. Even when this is done, approximately 20% of children will have persistent hydrocephalus.[9] This may be due to residual tumor or communicating hydrocephalus related to aseptic meningitis. External ventricular drainage may be helpful to monitor and control hydrocephalus in the immediate postoperative period. Its disadvantage is that the hydrocephalus often persists beyond the period when use of an EVD is advisable. For this reason, we prefer to implant a telemetric pressure sensor and subcutaneous reservoir attached to a ventricular catheter when there is concern about postoperative hydrocephalus.[8] This can be converted to a conventional shunt system at any time, as necessary.

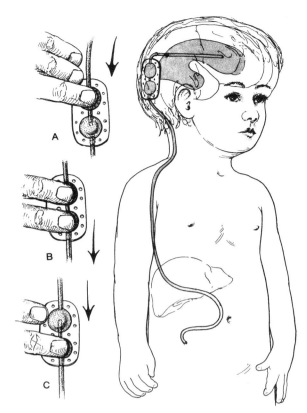

Figure 31.1.   Ames design "double bubble" ventricular peritoneal shunt. To evaluate patency, **(A)** compress proximal bubble, which ensures filling of distal bubble; **(B)** compress both bubbles, and fluid should easily pass distally into abdomen if there is no obstruction; and **(C)** remove compression of proximal bubble, and it should fill within 1 second if there is no obstruction.

A common source of concern in the neonatal ICU is hydrocephalus that complicates intracranial hemorrhage associated with prematurity. Temporizing measures to control fluid buildup are usually necessary. Early hydrocephalus will eventually compensate or resolve without shunting in a significant percentage of these infants. Even in those cases in which it is clear that a shunt will be required, one prefers to delay until the ventricles are clear of blood products and proteinaceous debris; otherwise, the new shunt may obstruct repeatedly. Serial lumbar punctures may suffice to control pressure, although if the hydrocephalus is not communicating, direct ventricular decompression is necessary. Percutaneous ventricular taps are effective but risk further brain injury or bleeding if done repeatedly.[10] An indwelling ventricular catheter is appropriate when one anticipates a long period of temporizing treatment. This may be used with either external drainage or a subgaleal reservoir, which can be tapped through the scalp as necessary.[11,12] The chief concern with either technique is infection with resulting bacterial ventriculitis, which may seriously complicate the hydrocephalus problem.

Another common hydrocephalus-related problem encountered in the PICU is management of shunt infection.[13] Such cases may require close monitoring of ICP and neurologic status while the infection is brought under control. Because the typical hydrocephalic child is shunt-dependent, it is important to continue to provide adequate CSF drainage during the interval of treatment before a new shunt can be placed. This is usually achieved by using an EVD, which also allows one to instill antibiotics into the ventricle, monitor CSF antibiotic levels, and culture CSF from day to day.

Shunt Types

Shunts typically divert CSF from the cerebral ventricles to an extracranial body site, from which the fluid is then reabsorbed. The usual elements of a shunt system are (1) a proximal catheter, which is inserted into the ventricle through a burr hole; (2) a valve, which controls pressure and assures unidirectional flow of CSF; (3) a reservoir beneath the scalp that allows percutaneous tapping of the system; and (4) a distal catheter, which is placed in the body cavity to which CSF is being diverted. The peritoneal cavity is the most common site used today. Ventriculoperitoneal (VP) shunts are easily inserted. They have the advantage of being relatively unaffected by the child's growth, because a considerable length of distal tubing can be inserted into the abdominal cavity when the shunt is first placed. Occasionally, ventriculoatrial (VA) shunts are used. These devices divert CSF into the venous system (ideally the right atrium of the heart) via the internal jugular vein and superior vena cava. Siting of the distal catheter is technically more difficult than with peritoneal shunting, and excess distal tubing cannot be used to compensate for the child's future growth. VA shunts are now used only as an alternative when VP shunting is not feasible. Ventriculopleural shunting is also an accepted procedure for children.[14] It is rarely used and is reserved for cases in which neither VP nor VA shunting can be employed. Pleural effusion with respiratory distress can occur, particularly below 5 years of age.

Shunt Complications

There are a variety of shunt complications with which the pediatric intensive care specialist should be familiar. The most common complication is obstruction of the device by tissue or organic debris. Because of the close relationship of the ventricular catheter tip to choroid plexus and the walls of the ventricle, proximal obstruction is more common than distal. In either case, the typical symptoms of headache, vomiting, and lethargy are related to increased ICP. Atypical symptoms and signs may also occur, particularly those referrable to brain stem dysfunction in cases of Arnold-Chiari or Dandy-Walker malformation. Shunt patency can be assessed by various means, although the clinical course alone may cause one to proceed directly with surgery. The presence of papilledema is also compelling. Plain x-rays of the shunt may show a disconnection or kink in the tubing. CT scanning allows one to assess ventricular size, although this may be helpful only if a prior study is available for comparison. Ventricular size cannot be expected to change dramatically immediately following shunt obstruction, even in the presence of elevated ICP. If one taps the shunt reservoir percutaneously with a small-gauge needle, pressures and run-off can be measured in the system. An alternative noninvasive technique that gives the same information utilizes a telemetric pressure measuring device in the shunt.[15] Figures 31-1 and 31-2 and Table 31-1 provide details for evaluation of shunt malfunction.

Shunt infection is a troublesome complication that occurs in 2% to 5% of cases. Although details of this problem are beyond the scope of this chapter, aspects of its treatment do relate to the PICU. Usually, this involves monitoring for signs of increased ICP and management of an external ventricular drainage device.

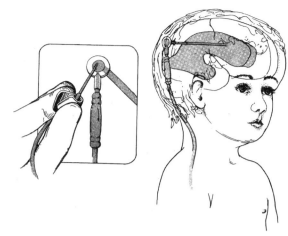

Figure 31.2. Single-reservoir Holter shunt, a common shunt type presently used. Circular chamber *(inset)* is used to obtain specimens and assess pressure. Distal compressible pump may be checked for refill and patency.

Some complications are related to the specific type of shunt used. For example, the presence of a peritoneal catheter can lead to delayed perforation of a viscus such as bowel or bladder. The tube may even extrude spontaneously through the umbilicus. If the shunt becomes infected for this or other reasons, peritonitis can result. One must consider this possibility in the differential diagnosis of the acute abdomen in shunted children. VP shunts are associated with abdominal pseudocyst formation as well as CSF ascites. In either case, the possibility of indolent shunt infection exists.

The complications of VA shunting are more troublesome. The tip of the distal catheter must be located within a short segment of the venous system to remain patent; therefore, growth of the young child will usually require multiple shunt revisions to maintain an adequate length of distal tubing. Complications of VA shunts are of greater consequence because they involve the cardiovascular system. Problems include cardiac arrhythmias, valvular damage, catheter migration into the pulmonary artery, and cardiac perforation with tamponade. Thrombus formation with chronic embolization can lead to pulmonary hypertension and cor pulmonale.[16] Incidental bacteremia may contaminate the distal catheter, leading to a shunt infection. Conversely, an infected shunt may cause septicemia or even nephritis.[17]

Problems Associated with Normal Shunt Function

Although shunts are effective in treating hydrocephalus, they do not restore the physiologic mechanisms that normally control intracranial volume, and hence pressure, relationships. Specifically, all

Table 31-1. Signs and symptoms of shunt malfunction

Vomiting	Bradycardia
Drowsiness	Coma
Headaches	Focal neurologic findings
Seizures	Swelling around shunt site

of the commonly used valves are activated by the pressure difference across the device. This "opening pressure" is built into the design to regulate CSF flow and prevent overdrainage with resultant low ICP. This is only effective with the child in a horizontal position. Once an upright posture is assumed, the valve cannot prevent abnormally low pressures because of the hydrostatic column between the proximal and distal ends of the shunt.[18] This is the so-called siphoning phenomenon. It can result in a variety of clinical problems, from postural headache to subdural hematoma. The latter is a particular concern in children whose skulls have become oversized due to chronic hydrocephalus with marked ventriculomegaly prior to shunting.

The most common clinical problem associated with siphoning is the slit ventricle syndrome.[19] As the name implies, the ventricles have become unusually small due to chronic shunting since early infancy. This may cause repeated ventricular catheter obstruction, and such children are commonly managed in the ICU because of concern about shunt malfunction. Operative treatment consists of replacing the ventricular catheter and inserting devices into the shunt system that are designed to increase resistance to flow. Occasionally, the signs of shunt malfunction are transient and will resolve without operative intervention. In either situation, the ICU physician may be called on to assist in the management of this difficult problem.

References

1. Chapman PH. Hydrocephalus in childhood. In Youmans JR (ed): *Neurological Surgery* (3rd ed). Philadelphia: Saunders, 1990. Pp 1236–1276.
2. McComb JG. Recent research into the nature of cerebrospinal fluid formation and absorption. *J Neurosurg* 59:369–383, 1983.
3. Shinnar S et al. Management of hydrocephalus in infancy: Use of acetazolamide and furosemide to avoid cerebrospinal fluid shunts. *J Pediatr* 107:31–37, 1985.
4. Naidich TP, McLone DG, Fulling KH. The Chiari II malformation: Part IV. The hindbrain deformity. *Neuroradiology* 25:179–197, 1983.
5. Hirsch J et al. The Dandy-Walker malformation. *J Neurosurg* 61: 515–522, 1984.
6. Barnett GH, Chapman PH. Insertion and care of intracranial pressure monitoring devices. In Ropper AH, Kennedy SF (eds): *Neurological and Neurosurgical Intensive Care* (2nd ed). Rockville, MD: Aspen, 1988. Pp 43–56.
7. Zervas NT, Cosman ER, Cosman BJ. A pressure-balanced radio-telemetry system for the measurement of intracranial pressure. *J Neurosurg* 47:899–911, 1977.
8. Chapman PH, Cosman E, Arnold M. Telemetric ICP monitoring after surgery for posterior fossa and third ventricular tumors. Technical note. *J Neurosurg* 60:649–651, 1984.
9. Papo I, Caruselli G, Luongo A. External ventricular drainage in the management of posterior fossa tumors in children and adolescents. *Neurosurgery* 10:13–15, 1982.
10. Fleischer AC et al. Sonographic depiction of changes in ventricular size associated with repeated ventricular aspirations. *J Ultrasound Med* 2:499–504, 1983.
11. Harbaugh RE, Saunders RL, Edwards WH. External ventricular drainage for control of posthemorrhagic hydrocephalus in premature infants. *J Neurosurg* 55:766–770, 1981.
12. Marlin AE. Protection of the cortical mantle in premature infants with post hemorrhagic hydrocephalus. *Neurosurgery* 7:464–468, 1980.
13. Chapman PH, Borges LF. Shunt infections: Prevention and treatment. *Clin Neurosurg* 32:652–664, 1984.
14. Hossman HJ, Hendrick EB, Humphreys RP. Experience with ventriculo-pleural shunts. *Childs Brain* 10:404–413, 1983.
15. Cosman ER et al. A telemetric pressure sensor for ventricular shunt systems. *Surg Neurol* 11:287–294, 1979.
16. Roa PS, Molthan ME, Lipow HW. Cor pulmonale as a complication of ventriculoatrial shunts. Case report. *J Neurosurg* 33:221–225, 1970.
17. Wyatt RJ, Walsh JW, Holland NH. Shunt nephritis. Role of the complement system in its pathogenesis and management. *J Neurosurg* 55:99–107, 1981.
18. Chapman PH, Cosman ER, Arnold MA. The relationship between ventricular fluid pressure and body position in normal subjects and subjects with shunts: A telemetric study. *Neurosurgery* 26:181–189, 1990.
19. Epstein F, Lapras C, Wisoff JH. Slit-ventricle syndrome: Etiology and treatment. *Pediatr Neurosci* 14:5–10, 1988.

32 ▸ Infections of the Central Nervous System

Infections of the central nervous system (CNS) pose a special challenge to the intensive care physician because of the unique anatomic features of the neuraxis. Since the brain and spinal cord are enclosed within rigid containers, inflammatory edema or mass lesions may increase intracranial pressure (ICP) and lead to ischemic infarction and/or herniation of supratentorial structures. Thus, CNS infections may lead rapidly to death or catastrophic brain injury in addition to any systemic toxicity (e.g., shock, disseminated intravascular coagulation, etc.) or metastatic infection that may be present. In addition, the limited phagocytic function of granulocytes in cerebrospinal fluid (CSF), a medium poor in opsonizing antibodies and complement, results in the need for potent bactericidal therapy. However, the so-called blood-brain barrier provides a special impediment to antibiotic therapy, since penetration of most antibiotics into the CSF is significantly impaired in comparison with achievable blood levels.

CNS infections are readily classified into a limited number of discrete syndromes: meningitis, meningoencephalitis, brain abscess, and parameningeal infections. The spectrum of pathogens responsible in each of these syndromes may be approached systematically by detailed analysis of the CSF, since different classes of pathogens evoke characteristic changes. These abnormalities can be organized into a diagnostic matrix, as shown in Table 32-1, based on the glucose, protein, and cellular formula. In addition, consideration of each patient's unique clinical features (age, underlying diseases, trauma, surgery, exposure history, travel, immunosuppression, etc.) will help determine whether opportunistic or exotic agents must be considered seriously in addition to conventional pathogens. Bacterial meningitis is the most commonly encountered treatable infection of the CNS and must always be considered in the differential diagnosis. A comprehensive review on this subject is available for the interested reader.[1]

Bacterial Meningitis

Bacterial meningitis generally develops as a consequence of transient or sustained bacteremia. Meningitis may arise after a brief prodrome of fever without an apparent focus of infection, or may complicate a focal suppurative process such as otitis media. The presenting clinical features and usual etiologic agents are dependent on the age of the child. Neonatal meningitis is usually due to the dominant neonatal bacterial pathogens (i.e., group B streptococci [*Streptococcus agalactiae*] and enteric Gram-negative bacilli), although *Listeria monocytogenes* remains an important consideration and is responsible for up to 10% of cases. **Early-onset neonatal meningitis** is defined as occurring within the first week of life and is more frequently observed in high-risk infants (prematurity, prolonged prepartum rupture of membranes, invasive fetal monitoring, etc.). Early-onset infection is often fulminant, with the clinical picture usually dominated by hypotension and shock and/or group B streptococcal pneumonia rather than the signs or symptoms of meningitis per se. **Late-onset meningitis** is defined as occurring after the first week of life and may develop at any time during the first 3 months of life. Many of these infections develop in otherwise normal infants with uncomplicated perinatal courses, and in these patients the meningitic process dominates the clinical picture.

The signs and symptoms of meningitis in neonates are usually nonspecific and entirely nonlocalizing. Fever is usually present, although in neonates fever over 102°F is infrequent. Neurologic signs may be limited to poor feeding, hypotonia, and lethargy or, conversely, to increased motor tone and irritability. Although the fontanelles may be full, this is not entirely reliable, and classic signs of meningismus, such as stiff neck or positive Kernig and Brudzinski signs, are rare. Consequently, all neonates with fever require careful neurologic assessment and lumbar puncture as part of their initial evaluation.

Table 32-1. CSF findings in intracranial infections

	Pressure (mm H$_2$O)	Cell count (WBCs/μL)	Glucose (mg/dl)	Protein (mg/dl)
Normal values	90–180	0–5 lymphs	50–75	15–40
Bacterial meningitis	200–300	100–5,000; neutrophils usually > 80%	Reduced (<40)	100–1,000
Brain abscess	180–300	10–200; lymphocytes predominate	Normal	70–400
Subdural empyema	200–300	10–2,000; usually lymphocytes predominate; PMNs dominate after surgery or if accompanying meningitis	Normal (<40 if meningitis)	50–500
Cerebral epidural abscess	180–250	10–300; lymphocytes predominate	Normal	50–200
Tuberculous meningitis	180–300	<500 lymphocytes	Reduced (<50)	100–200 (increased if CSF block)
Cryptococcal meningitis	180–300	10–200 lymphocytes	Reduced (<40)	50–200
Viral meningitis	90–200	10–300 lymphocytes; early echovirus disease may have up to 80% PMN predominate	Normal (may be reduced in mumps and LCM)	50–100

In older infants and children, during the first few years of life, bacterial meningitis is caused almost exclusively by the encapsulated pathogens *Haemophilus influenzae*, *S. pneumoniae*, and *Neisseria meningitidis*. The polysaccharide capsules of these bacteria are poor immunogens during the first 2 years of life, and consequently, pharyngeal colonization (or even invasive infection) fails to elicit protective opsonizing antibodies. Although *H. influenzae* meningities formerly predominated in this age group, a dramatic fall in invasive *H. influenzae* infections, including meningitis, has been observed since conjugate *H. influenzae* vaccines have become widely used in the first six months of life. In children 6 to 24 months of age, with acute nonlocalizing febrile illnesses, with fever exceeding 103°F, there is a significant incidence of bacteremia due to *S. pneumoniae* approximately 2% of these cases are complicated by the development of meningitis.[2] In some children, primary foci of infection such as otitis media, pneumonia, cellulitis, or septic arthritis may be present, but frequently no primary focus is identifiable. Typically, children with meningitis present with a prodromal febrile illness of 1 or a few days' duration which progresses to develop high fever, vomiting, headache (in older children), lethargy progressing to obtundation, and stiff neck (often with positive Kernig and Brudzinski signs). Grand mal seizures may be present in approximately 20% of cases, which may simply represent febrile seizures or reflect cortical inflammation and/or cortical venous thrombosis. Sixth cranial neuropathy is associated with increased intracranial pressure, but facial paresis or hemiparesis may be present and reflect parenchymal injury.[3] A petechial exanthem usually indicates meningococcemia, but meningococcal infection may be associated with maculopapular eruptions or occur without cutaneous involvement. *H. influenzae* may occasionally produce significant thrombocytopenia and petechial lesions, and petechial eruptions may occasionally be seen with enteroviral disease as well.[4] Papilledema is generally absent in patients with acute bacterial meningitis because of the rapid course of their illness.

Diagnostic efforts should be focused, expedited, and dovetailed with the institution of supportive measures. The necessity for the rapid initiation of therapy cannot be overstated. In addition to the risk of metastatic infection or cardiovascular collapse, particularly with meningococcal or *H. influenzae* infection, the development of sensorineural hearing loss is generally an early sign of complication of meningitis due to cochlear inflammation.[5–7] In principle, the risk of this complication may be reduced by the prompt administration of appropriate antibiotic therapy and dexamethasone (discussion follows).

Immediate laboratory studies may be limited to a complete blood count, with differential white cell count and platelet count, blood culture, electrolytes, BUN, and creatinine. A lumbar puncture should be performed promptly, and if turbid CSF is present, antibiotics may be administered by rapid intravenous (IV) bolus infusion. The CSF evaluation should include Gram stain and culture (typically on blood agar plate, chocolate agar slant, and in thioglycollate broth; the latter two media should receive generous inocula >0.5 ml); cell count and differential white cell count; and determination of glucose, protein, and xanthochromia. Multiple rapid diagnostic tests for polysaccharide antigens are generally reserved for those specimens in which no organisms are present by Gram stain, especially if the child has received antibiotics prior to presentation. If the Gram stain of CSF suggests a single morphology (e.g., gram-positive lancet-shaped diplococci for *S. pneumoniae*, kidney-bean-shaped gram-negative diplococci for *N. meningitidis* or pleomorphic gram-negative rods for *H. influenzae*),

an antigen detection test for that organism may confirm the presumptive diagnosis. The utility of antigen detection tests is hampered by the absence of reagents for certain pneumococcal serotypes and group B meningococcus, as well as by the presence of false-negative and false-positive results, particularly with the polyspecific pneumococcal reagents. After the lumbar puncture is performed and therapy initiated, a chest X-ray should be obtained to assess a possible primary focus of infection or a secondary complication such as aspiration pneumonitis.

In the occasional instance when initial attempts at lumbar puncture are unsuccessful or confounded by a traumatic tap, initial antibiotic therapy should not be delayed unnecessarily. Although current therapeutic regimens are highly efficacious at sterilizing the CSF, a lumbar puncture performed 1 to 2 hours after initial antibiotic therapy is given is still likely to yield an organism. Even if sterile, the characteristic CSF pleocytosis and chemistries will confirm the diagnosis of pyogenic meningitis,[8] and rapid antigen detection techniques may still identify the responsible pathogen. In a small number of patients with focal neurologic deficits at the time of presentation, the diagnostic consideration of brain abscess would require a cranial imaging procedure (computed axial tomography [CAT] or magnetic resonance imaging [MRI]) prior to lumbar puncture to minimize the chance of post-lumbar puncture transtentorial herniation. In such instances, empiric antibiotic therapy should be administered after blood cultures are obtained, prior to imaging and lumbar puncture.

Routine laboratory data suggest a severe acute inflammatory insult with marked leukocytosis (or leukopenia) with the presence of band forms. Mild anemia is often present. The platelet count may be depressed, especially with gram-negative infections, and if disseminated intravascular coagulation (DIC) has developed, the prothrombin time (PT) and partial thromboplastin time (PTT) will be prolonged. The serum sodium may be depressed if the child has received hypotonic fluids prior to admission. This may be a consequence of inappropriate ADH secretion in euvolemic children, or appropriate ADH secretion if poor intake and vomiting produce significant dehydration prior to admission.[9]

The CSF in acute bacterial meningitis almost always reveals a significant pleocytosis with the predominance of granulocytes, hypoglycorrachia (commonly below 30 mg/dl), and elevated protein. This is true even in the patient who received prior antibiotics (e.g., for otitis media[8]). These findings pose little difficulty in interpretation, except for the occasional patient with early viral meningitis who demonstrates an exuberant cellular response.[10] In such cases, clinical features of illness and epidemiologic considerations may readily identify those children with viral meningitis, but when the patient is very young (e.g., less than 1 year of age) or ill-appearing, it is appropriate to initiate empiric antibiotic therapy for the first 72 hours. During summertime epidemics of viral meningitis, older nontoxic patients with presumed viral meningitis, who have granulocyte-predominant formulae with normal CSF protein may undergo repeat lumbar puncture after 4–6 hours of observation. A more typical mononuclear cell pleocytosis with normal chemistries may obviate the need for antibiotic therapy.[10]

Patients with bacterial meningitis are admitted to the ICU for close observation, sequential neurologic evaluation, and therapy. Those patients with meningitis due to *H. influenzae* or *N. meningitidis*, and those patients with purulent meningitis due to an as yet unknown pathogen are housed under respiratory precautions for the first 24 hours of therapy to prevent nosocomial spread of these organisms. Fluid management is an important aspect of supportive care. Although concerns over the syndrome of inappropriate secretion of antidiuretic hormone (SIADH) and cerebral edema traditionally led to routine fluid restriction, decreased extracellular volume in fluid-restricted patients may reduce cerebral perfusion and exacerbate cerebral injury (11). Patients who are hypotensive or clinically dehydrated should not undergo fluid restriction. Euvolemic patients with a normal initial serum sodium concentration should receive maintenance fluids, with careful monitoring of serum electrolytes, urine output and specific gravity, urine and serum osmolality, and body weight for the first 48 hours of hospitalization. A minority of patients will have hyponatremia and inappropriately concentrated urine and an increase in body weight, indicating inappropriate ADH secretion; in these patients fluid intake should be restricted to roughly 1000 ml/m²/day.[11] Patients are generally not able to ingest fluids initially due to obtundation, and so for the first 48 to 72 hours, required fluids are administered parenterally to minimize the risk of aspiration. The head circumference of infants should be carefully measured daily to monitor the development of subdural effusions or hydrocephalus. Since meningococcal and *H. influenzae* meningitis have a significant risk of secondary spread within households, rifampin prophylaxis (10 mg/kg bid up to 600 mg bid for 2 days for the former, and 20/mg/kg qid up to 600 mg/d for 4 days for the latter) should be administered to siblings and other pediatric household contacts at the time of diagnosis.[12] Adult contacts should receive 600 mg rifampin bid for 2 days for meningococcal prophylaxis, and 600 mg qid for 4 days for *H. influenzae* prophylaxis. The index patient should receive prophylaxis at the completion of parenteral therapy because pharyngeal carriage of these pathogens is not reliably eradicated during therapy, and invasive disease does not reliably evoke protective immunity in children less than 2 years old.

Initial antibiotic therapy for bacterial meningitis is based on the patient's age and the expected spectrum of pathogens. In neonatal meningitis, ampicillin and gentamicin provide synergistic bactericidal therapy against group B streptococci and *L. monocytogenes*, and would be optimal therapy in those infants whose CSF Gram stain and/or antigen detection test suggested these organisms. When the initial CSF Gram stain demonstrates enteric gram-negative bacilli, ampicillin and a third-generation cephalosporin such as cefotaxime may be considered because the spectrum of activity of these agents is broad, their potency is great, their penetration into CSF is favorable, and their ease of use exceeds gentamicin, which requires careful drug-level monitoring. Ceftriaxone generally is not used in neonates because it competes with bilirubin for conjugation and secretion into bile. If the initial Gram stain fails to disclose a pathogen, either combination would represent reasonable empiric coverage. The antibiotic regimen may then be revised once initial culture data are available and the infant has responded to therapy. Therapy is usually continued for 3 weeks, since relapse may occur with shorter regimens. Such prolonged antibiotic therapy may mandate the placement of a central venous catheter for antibiotic administration. After initial synergistic therapy has led to clear-cut clinical improvement, prolonged therapy for group B streptococcal and listerial meningitis may be achieved with penicillin as monotherapy. If possible, the minimal inhibitory concentration (MIC) and minimal bactericidal concentration (MBC) of group B streptococci against penicillin should be determined in the laboratory, because occasional isolates are "tolerant," with a low MIC (<1 U/ml) but a high MBC (>100 U/ml), and in this setting some authors recommend prolonged therapy with penicillin together with gentamicin.[13] Repeat lumbar puncture is recommended at 3 to 4 days in the management of neonatal meningitis, particularly when treating enteric gram-negative bacilli

and tolerant group B streptococcus. If the CSF culture remains positive, the addition of gentamicin to a third-generation cephalosporin in the case of *Escherichia coli* meningitis should be considered. Rarely, in refractory cases, intrathecal or intraventricular aminoglycoside therapy (e.g., 1 mg qi.d.-qod.) administered via a ventriculostomy drain may be necessary to achieve CSF sterilization.

Recommendations for initial empiric antibiotic therapy for older infants and children with bacterial meningitis are presently undergoing significant change. In addition to the dramatic decline in *H. influenzae* disease, there has been a rising worldwide incidence of pneumococci which are relatively or highly resistant to penicillin (with MICs 0.1–1 µg/ml and > 1 µg/ml, respectively) due to altered penicillin-binding proteins. These isolates are often multiply resistant to a variety of other antibiotics, including chloramphenicol, erythromycin, and trimethoprim-sulfamethoxazole, and frequently are relatively or highly resistant to third-generation cephalosporins as well (e.g., ceftriaxone or cefotaxime MIC ≤ 0.5 µg/ml and ≥ 1 µg/ml, respectively). Thus, routine initial empiric therapy with third-generation cephalosporins is hazardous, particularly when an initial CSF Gram stain demonstrates pneumococcal infection. The routine use of vancomycin in this setting has raised concern regarding its efficacy, since its penetration into the CSF may result in subtherapeutic levels, especially if administered together with dexamethasone (see below).[14]

At present, initial therapy for bacterial meningitis must provide coverage for resistant pneumococci, the rare *H. influenzae* isolate (which may be ampicillin-resistant), as well as meningococci. The combination of high dose vancomycin (60 mg/kg/d in 4 divided doses) together with ceftriaxone (100 mg/kg/d in 2 divided doses) or cefotaxime (200 mg/kg/d in 4 divided doses) has been recommended.[15] Antibiotic susceptibility testing of pneumococci is crucial: all CSF isolates should undergo MIC testing against penicillin and a third-generation cephalosporin by E-test or broth dilution testing. In addition, early assessment of response to initial therapy by repeat lumbar puncture at 24 to 36 h after starting therapy is important in patients with meningitis due to resistant pneumococci. In patients who fail to respond to initial vancomycin/ceftriaxone therapy by clinical and/or microbiologic criteria, the addition or substitution of rifampin (20 mg/kg/d in 2 divided doses) for vancomycin should be considered. Children with a history of late-onset morbilliform drug eruption to penicillin who have meningococcal, *H. influenzae*, or cephalosporin-susceptible pneumococcal meningitis may be treated with cefotaxime or ceftriaxone. If there is a history of beta-lactam associated immediate hypersensitivity, pneumococcal infection should be treated with chloramphenicol or high dose vancomycin based on susceptibilities, and the alternate encapsulated pathogens may be treated with chloramphenicol. Occasionally, desensitization to a beta-lactam agent followed by intravenous therapy may be necessary.

In selected clinical situations, a broader spectrum of bacterial pathogens may be encountered, and initial therapy must provide broader coverage. For example, patients who have sustained head injury with disruption of the dura (e.g., after basilar skull fracture) or who have undergone neurosurgical exploration are at risk of developing meningitis due to a CSF leak. It is important to remember that the diagnosis of meningitis in an obtunded patient may be a difficult one and that the effects of postoperative dexamethasone therapy may dampen the clinical features of meningitis in these patients. Hence, lumbar puncture should be considered as part of an evaluation for unexplained fever in these patients. Although pneumococci once were the most commonly encountered pathogens in this situation,[16] meningitis developing in the head trauma or postoperative neurosurgical patient who has received numerous antibiotics during a protracted stay in the ICU may be due to staphylococci, resistant nosocomially acquired gram-negative bacilli, or even mixed infection. The importance of CSF Gram stain and culture in this setting must be underscored, and initial therapy may include an antistaphylococcal penicillin such as nafcillin, oxacillin, or vancomycin, given together with an antipseudomonal agent such as ceftazidime. If gram-negative infection is confirmed, dual therapy with a third-generation cephalosporin together with an aminoglycoside may be considered. In patients with ventriculostomy drains or other prosthetic materials, coagulase-negative staphylococcal infection and corynebacteria are frequently encountered, mandating the initial use of IV vancomycin therapy and, if possible, removal of the contaminated prosthetic materials with CSF pressure controlled by serial lumbar punctures or the placement of a temporary ventriculostomy drain.

Certain clinical settings require early structural or physiologic investigations, because meningitis may serve as the clue for a significant underlying host defect. Acute meningitis due to organisms other than the more commonly encountered encapsulated pathogens raises the possibility of infection developing from a contiguous focus of infection, such as sinusitis or mastoiditis, or from an anatomic defect (e.g., dermal sinus). Although initial medical therapy is directed against the recovered pathogen, failure to improve after a limited trial of therapy (e.g., 48 hours) may lead to consideration of surgical intervention, such as sinus exploration or mastoidectomy, to drain the "feeding focus" of infection.[17] These considerations also apply to older children with pneumococcal meningitis, which is often associated with a parameningeal suppurative focus. Patients with recurrent meningitis due to respiratory tract flora and/or encapsulated pathogens frequently possess an occult breach of the dural barrier, typically in relation to the cribriform plate, sinus walls, or cochlea, and should be evaluated by audiometric testing, cranial imaging studies, and fluorescein study of the CSF in an attempt to localize the defect.[18,19] In such patients, appropriate surgical intervention to obliterate the defect is necessary. Patients with recurrent neisserial meningitis, either *N. meningitidis* or *N. gonorrheae*, should undergo complement function tests at the termination of therapy, because a significant fraction of such patients will be shown to have defects in the terminal components of the complement cascade.[20] Recurrent meningitis due to enterococci or enteric gram-negative bacilli may have an unrecognized sinus tract in the sacral region.

Guidelines for the duration of antibiotic therapy must be individualized, based on each child's pathogen and clinical course. Neonatal meningitis is usually treated for 3 weeks. Ceftriaxone therapy of meningococcal or *H. influenzae* meningitis with ceftriaxone is usually administered for seven days.[21] Pneumococcal infection is usually treated for 10 to 14 days to reduce the risk of relapse and to treat any parameningeal focus (e.g., sinusitis or mastoiditis) that may be present. Traditionally, antibiotic therapy is continued until the patient is afebrile for at least 5 days.

Despite the efficacy of current antibiotic regimens, the course of therapy is often complicated by continuing fever.[22] Persistent fever (lasting as long as 1 week) occurs in approximately 15% of patients, but is particularly associated with *H. influenzae* infection. Greatly prolonged fever, exceeding 10 days of therapy, occurs in perhaps 10% of patients. These protracted fevers may reflect metastatic foci of infection (e.g., septic arthritis), other nosocomial infections (e.g., urinary tract infection or pneumonia), or noninfec-

tious conditions such as phlebitis or drug allergy. Secondary fever (return of fever after 1 or more afebrile days) is rarely a harbinger of relapse and is associated with similar causes as the continuing fevers. In approximately 25% of patients with continuing fever, cranial imaging studies will demonstrate the presence of subdural effusions. These collections are usually sterile but may contribute to an ongoing inflammatory response. A reasonable approach includes careful evaluation for a secondary focus of infection, careful repeated neurologic examination, replacement of IV cannulae, and possible switch in therapy to chloramphenicol (if supported by susceptibility data) to exclude possible drug allergy as a cause of fever. In children who are not thriving, repeat lumbar puncture to document improvement of the CSF formula, sterilization of the CSF, and cranial imaging to look for subdural effusions is indicated. Although these collections are not routinely sampled, in occasional patients who experience persistent systemic toxicity, or significant neurologic dysfunction, or whose effusions enhance with contrast CT scanning, it is prudent to obtain a fluid sample to exclude the possibility that the protracted fever is due to an infected subdural effusion (i.e., a subdural empyema).

Experimental investigations of the pathophysiology of bacterial meningitis have shown that the characteristic pleocytosis is a response to proinflammatory cytokines (e.g., tumor necrosis factor, interleukin-1, etc.) elicited by certain bacterial products (grampositive cell wall proteoglycan, gram-negative lipopolysaccharide).[23] The polymorphonuclear pleocytosis is not effective at eradicating infection (which is accomplished by the bactericidal antibiotics employed in therapy) but rather is responsible for the disruption of the blood-brain barrier and inflammatory sequellae that result in intracranial hypertension, hypoperfusion, and vascular injury. Such considerations have led to experimental and clinical trials of dexamethasone therapy, (0.15 mg/kg administered every 6 hours for the first 4 days of therapy) begun just prior to antibiotic administration as an adjunctive measure in the therapy of acute bacterial meningitis. Several clinical trials have now shown that the risk of neurosensory hearing loss is moderately reduced in children treated with dexamethasone.[24,25] Additional randomized, multicenter trials are in progress, and the use of dexamethasone (or other antiinflammatory agents) has become somewhat routine in the initial treatment of bacterial meningitis.

In one recent multicenter trial, no benefit was observed.[26] In these trials, the vast majority of children had *H. influenzae* meningitis, and data regarding the use of dexamethasone in pneumococcal meningitis (which has the highest rate of audiologic sequellae) is limited. Experimental studies, retrospective clinical analysis [27] and limited prospective study[28] seem to support its use in pneumococcal meningitis as well, but this decision should be individualized. Although the 4-day regimen has been used most widely, two-day courses of dexamethasone (using either 0.6 mg/kg/d in 4 divided doses or 0.8 mg/kg/d in 2 divided doses) have been used at some centers[29,30] with the hope of decreasing the hemorrhagic risks associated with dexamethosone. Considerable controversy persists as to whether dexamethasone therapy will have a significant impact in reducing the substatial neurologic[31] and audiologic[32] sequellae of bacterial meningitis.[33]

It is important to reconsider the differential diagnosis of bacterial meningitis in children with initially sterile CSF and poor responses to initial therapy. Brain abscess, subdural empyema, tuberculous or fungal meningitis, viral encephalitis, and rare instances of neoplastic or amebic meningoencephalitis may be responsible for a child's neurologic illness, and the nonspecific anti-inflammatory effects of dexamethasone may suggest an initial response to therapy.[34] Clinical deterioration should prompt an early reinvestigation and modification of the initial empiric therapy.

Tuberculous and Fungal Meningitis

These meningitides are considered together because they share a progressive subacute or chronic course and evoke a characteristic CSF formula (i.e., lymphocytic pleocytosis with hypoglycorrhachia and elevated protein).

The clinical features of tuberculous meningitis differ somewhat, depending on the age of the child. In infants and young children, tuberculous meningitis is usually a complication of progressive primary infection. Replication of *Mycobacterium tuberculosis* at the initial pulmonary focus of infection results in the spread of mycobacteria to the draining hilar lymph nodes. Inadequate cell-mediated immunity fails to contain the infection at this site, and large numbers of tubercle bacilli are disseminated hematogenously. The meninges and/or cerebral cortex are readily seeded, and infection spreads directly to the CSF. From a clinical perspective, these children may have evidence of an active pulmonary focus, with a focal pulmonary infiltrate and hilar adenopathy apparent on chest x-ray. Other evidence of hematogenous dissemination may be present as well, such as miliary pulmonary infiltrates or evidence of hepatic, renal, or marrow involvement, with obstructive chemistries, abnormal urinanalysis, or cytopenia(s), respectively. The absence of these ancillary findings, however, never excludes the diagnosis of tuberculous meningitis. PPD testing in these patients frequently is nonreactive, a common finding in life-threatening tuberculous disease at any age and consistent with the impaired cell-mediated immunity observed in this population. In older children, a previously established cortical granuloma (Rich focus) breaks down and releases viable tubercle bacilli into the CSF. Thus, tuberculous infection is limited to a single extrapulmonary focus, and the chest film is either normal or shows evidence of past granulomatous disease with discrete parenchymal and/or nodal calcification.

Untreated tuberculous meningitis progresses through three classic stages, defined by the severity of neurologic dysfunction. In stage I disease, the sensorium is normal and symptoms reflect the meningitic process with headache, fever, meningismus, and so on. CSF examination usually already displays a classic lymphocytic pleocytosis with low sugar and elevated protein, but rarely, CSF abnormalities are so modest that the picture closely resembles viral aseptic meningitis. In contrast to this benign entity, symptoms persist and sequential lumbar punctures demonstrate disease progression. In stage II disease, there is obtundation and other focal neurologic defects, and the progression to coma defines stage III disease. Progressive tuberculous infection elicits a thick basilar meningitic exudate, which can entrap cranial nerves and produce discrete cranial nerve palsies. In addition, the inflammatory reaction produces vasculitis with focal parenchymal ischemic injury and damages the arachnoid villi with resultant (communicating) hydrocephalus. In some instances, the presence of hydrocephalus may be largely responsible for the observed neurologic deterioration. The prognosis of tuberculous meningitis depends on the state of consciousness when therapy is initiated, so that routine consideration of tuberculous meningitis must become part of the clinician's diagnostic approach in this setting.

The diagnosis of tuberculous meningitis is largely **clinical** because the tuberculin reaction is frequently nonreactive (up to 50%), the chest x-ray is frequently normal, the acid-fast smear of CSF is generally nondiagnostic, and the results of CSF culture (which are positive in only 50%–70% of cases) are unknown for 4 to 6 weeks when conventional culture techniques are employed. When tuberculous meningitis is part of a syndrome of disseminated (miliary) tuberculosis, cultures of urine, bone marrow, respiratory tract secretions (via gastric aspirates or bronchoscopy), or liver biopsy may improve the chances of recovering an isolate, and the strategy for obtaining these specimens is based on pursuing those specimens in which the chances of tuberculous infection are highest, based on laboratory or radiologic abnormalities. Nevertheless, it is not unusual for all cultures to be unrevealing, and for these children, a clinical and laboratory response to empiric antituberculous chemotherapy confirms the presumptive diagnosis. Epidemiologic considerations are important in considering this diagnosis, because most cases of childhood tuberculosis result from close contact with immediate family members, relatives, or friends with (often unrecognized) pulmonary tuberculosis. If a member of the child's household has recently been diagnosed as having tuberculosis, the likelihood that a child with "aseptic meningitis" in fact has tuberculous meningitis is much increased. Conversely, the confirmation of the diagnosis of tuberculosis mandates a search within the family for the index case.

Antituberculous chemotherapy with isoniazid and rifampin has become the mainstay of treatment. Current approaches (Table 32-2) utilize intensive multidrug "induction" therapy with isoniazid (INH), rifampin, and pyrazinamide for 2 months, followed by INH and rifampin to complete 12 months of therapy.[35,36] The use of supervised, twice weekly therapy during the "maintenance" phase has proven valuable in managing poorly compliant patients. Although most cases of tuberculosis acquired in the United States are caused by highly susceptible isolates, in many urban areas and among the homeless and immigrant populations, the incidence of drug-resistant disease is increased. Thus, in high-risk children, initial therapy must be broadened to include four agents by adding ethambutol or streptomycin to ensure that at least two effective agents are administered concurrently at all times. An additional benefit of recovering an isolate of *M. tuberculosis* is to confirm drug susceptibilities prior to embarking on prolonged therapy. Although corticosteroids are not believed to alter the ultimate mortality rate of tuberculous meningitis, corticosteroid therapy has been advocated in the setting of severe intracranial hypertension to reduce acute mortality from cerebral edema and transtentorial herniation.[37] If imaging studies document hydrocephalus, ventriculoperitoneal shunting may be performed without delay.

Fungal meningitis generally follows the same path of pulmonary infection with subsequent lymphohematogenous dissemination as that observed with mycobacterial infection, but occurs in two diverse patient populations. The endemic dimorphous soil fungi (*Coccidioides immitis*, *Histoplasma capsulatum*, and *Blastomyces dermatitidis*) infect only those individuals who are exposed to these agents in rather well defined geographic areas (southwestern United States; the central great river basins; and the southeastern United States, respectively). On rare occasions, meningitis may develop in apparently normal children, as well as in those children with recognizable cellular immunodeficiency. The course of illness is more indolent than tuberculosis, with headache, obtundation, and meningismus, with a waxing and waning course, but nevertheless there is a high ultimate mortality rate.[38–40] Meningitis usually develops in association with or subsequent to other foci of invasive disease (pulmonary, skeletal, cutaneous, lymphadenitis,

Table 32-2.   Chemotherapeutic regimens for tuberculous meningitis

	Dose	*Route*	*Toxicity*
Agents			
Isoniazid	10 mg/kg/d (300 mg/d max.)	PO, IM	Hepatotoxicity, peripheral neuropathy (give pyridoxine 10 mg/d)
Rifampin	10 mg/kg/d (600 mg/d max.)	PO, IV	Hepatotoxicity, drug fever, thrombocytopenia
Pyrazinamide	25 mg/kg/d (2.5 g/d max.)	PO	Hepatotoxicity
Ethambutol	25 mg/kg/d × 8 weeks, then 15 mg/kg/d	PO	Optic neuritis (requires monthly visual acuity and red/green testing)
Streptomycin	15 mg/kg/d × 8 weeks (1 g/d max.); then 15 mg/kg/d twice weekly	IM	Vertigo, sensorineural hearing loss
Clinical-setting			

Low suspicion of drug resistance
  Isoniazid + rifampin + (pyrazinamide or ethambutol) for first 2 months; isoniazid + rifampin to complete 9 months of therapy
High suspicion of drug resistance
  Isoniazid + rifampin + pyrazinamide + ethambutol for first 3 months
    Isoniazid + rifampin to complete 9 months of therapy if isolate is sensitive
    Isoniazid + rifampin + pyrazinamide and/or ethambutol to maintain at least two effective agents to complete 9 months of therapy if resistance
      pattern of isolate is available
Six-month, supervised therapy (low suspicion of drug resistance)
  Isoniazid + rifampin + pyrazinamide + (ethambutol or streptomycin) for first 2 months

osteomyelitis, etc.). CSF cultures have a variable yield in recovering organisms, but may be enhanced by large-volume cultures of CSF or, on occasion, by meningeal biopsy. As with tuberculosis, the diagnosis of fungal meningitis is usually based on the clinical picture, together with recovery of the pathogen at distant sites of infection and compatible serologic findings. Amphotericin B administered intravenously (discussion follows) (with coccidioidomycosis, intrathecally) is the mainstay of therapy, but requires prolonged treatment because of the high risk of relapse. Hydrocephalus due to basilar meningitis or arachnoiditis requiring shunting is a frequent complication. The newer imidazole antifungal agents fluconazole and infraconazole may play a role in the long-term control of these infections.

Cryptococcus neoformans meningitis is observed almost exclusively in patients with defects in cell-mediated immunity as a result of intrinsic disease processes or as a consequence of immunosuppressive therapy. The course is usually indolent, with progressive headache, low-grade fever, and eventual signs of increased ICP (vomiting, sixth-nerve palsies) and alteration in mentation. CSF examination reveals the typical lymphocytic pleocytosis with decreased glucose and elevated protein. Microscopic examination of CSF in India ink demonstrates yeast forms approximately the size of lymphocytes with a large clear cell wall in a minority of cases, but direct rapid analysis for cryptococcal antigen is almost always diagnostic, as is fungal culture. A minority of patients may demonstrate a primary pulmonary focus of infection on chest x-ray. In patients with evidence of increased ICP or focal neurologic deficits, imaging studies should be performed prior to lumbar puncture, because this compromised patient population may have a variety of focal parenchymal lesions (toxoplasmosis, nocardiosis, or cryptococcosis).

Amphotericin B has been the traditional mainstay of therapy. Patients are routinely premedicated with acetaminophen and diphenhydramine to minimize typical febrile reactions and may require infusion with hydrocortisone (0.25 mg/kg) or narcotic analgesics to control immediate toxicity. After the administration of a test dose of 1 mg or 0.1 mg/kg, whichever is less, over 1 to 2 hours and observation for possible anaphylaxis, therapy is continued

immediately thereafter with a second dose (0.1–0.2 mg/kg) and escalated over 3 days to 0.7 mg/kg/d, administered as a single dose over approximately 4 hours. Amphotericin readily produces phlebitis when administered via peripheral sites, and therapeutic courses of this drug frequently require placement of a central venous catheter. If rigors or febrile reactions persist despite routine premedication, the drug can be diluted, infused more slowly, or the patient can be retreated with acetaminophen during infusion. The use of 5-fluocytosine (5-FC) in the treatment of cryptococcal meningitis (150 mg/kg/d divided q6h), together with amphotericin B, has facilitated reduction in the dose of amphotericin B in adult patients, which reduces its toxicity.[41] However, 5-FC has significant myelosuppressive potential, which may be limiting in neutropenic hosts, and is excreted by renal mechanisms, which may be compromised by concurrent amphotericin therapy. It is important to monitor 5-FC levels and adjust dosage based on optimal peak levels of 50–100 μg/ml 2 hours after an ingested dose. Although extended therapy is generally effective in truly curing many patients with cryptococcal meningitis, severely immunocompromised patients, such as those with AIDS, often experience relapses after the completion of therapy. In such cases, long-term suppressive therapy with an oral imidazole antifungal agent that achieves therapeutic levels in CSF, such as fluconazole, appears promising in controlling symptomatic disease.[42]

Aseptic Meningitis

Aseptic meningitis defines a **syndrome** of meningeal inflammation associated with bacteriologically sterile CSF. The presence of meningeal inflammation with minimal cerebral dysfunction comprises one pole in the spectrum of nonbacterial meningoencephalitis, with the encephalitis syndrome representing the opposite pole of progressive cerebral dysfunction. In contrast to the hypoglycorrhachia, elevated protein, and granulocyte-predominant CSF pleocytosis observed in patients with bacterial meningitis, patients with aseptic meningitis are generally recognized by the presence of lymphocytic pleocytosis associated with essentially normal CSF glucose and protein levels. In the vast majority of cases, aseptic meningitis is due to a viral pathogen, and in fact, most of these are due to enteroviruses. Nevertheless, the differential diagnosis of aseptic meningitis includes a wide variety of viral pathogens as well as selected nonviral agents. A list of possible etiologic agents for the syndrome of aseptic meningitis is provided in Table 32-3. Direct recovery of an etiologic agent from CSF is generally difficult, and an etiologic diagnosis must often be made by indirect means, such as recovery of a viral agent from another body site (pharynx, stool), by antigen or nucleic acid detection, or by serologic methods.[45] Presumptive diagnoses are often invoked on the basis of clinical features and epidemiologic considerations.

The clinical features of a patient with aseptic meningitis depend in part on the extraneurologic symptoms and signs evoked by the specific etiologic agent; nevertheless, certain generalizations can be made regarding the neurologic features seen in this syndrome. In infants and toddlers, fever and irritability predominate as presenting features, while in older children, discrete complaints of headache, stiff neck, and photophobia may be present. Systemic toxicity is almost always less striking than that seen in bacterial meningitis.

Enteroviral infections are responsible for most cases of aseptic meningitis treated during the warmer months (e.g., May through September in temperate climates). Such illnesses may be accompanied by symptoms of diarrhea or rash. The cutaneous involvement may be a typical maculopapular (morbilliform) eruption or may have a prominent petechial appearance mimicking meningococcal disease.[4] Vesicular lesions of the hands and feet (hand-foot-mouth syndrome, typically due to Coxsackie virus 5) or small ulcerative lesions of the posterior oropharynx (herpangina) may be present. Infection in other household members may be frequent and supports the diagnosis. Summertime arboviral infection, especially that due to St. Louis encephalitis virus, may present with aseptic meningitis, but more frequently is responsible for meningo-

encephalitis. Leptospirosis may produce aseptic meningitis at this time of year as well, but requires epidemiologic linkage to rodents or dogs in the environment, such as bathing in a pond or other stagnant water in a rural environment.[44,45] Lyme disease may produce aseptic meningitis or even meningoencephalitis during the subacute stage of infection, and may be difficult to diagnose in the absence of the pathognomonic erythema chronicum migrans.[46–48]

In autumn, when field rodents seek refuge in warm shelters, children may develop aseptic meningitis due to lymphocytic choriomeningitis virus (LCM). LCM may also be seen when children acquire commercially raised rodents as pets. During winter months, aseptic meningitis in older children may be a feature of mycoplasma infection.[49] In occasional cases, virtually no signs of pulmonary disease are present, and the diagnosis may be elusive. Older children may also develop aseptic meningitis from Epstein-Barr virus infection, which displays little seasonal preference.[50,51] The diagnosis will be apparent in children with typical infectious mononucleosis, but may be a difficult one in those children with few extraneurologic symptoms. Acute infection with HIV may be associated with an acute retroviral syndrome, a mononucleosis-like illness with fever, pharyngitis, lymphadenopathy, maculopapular eruption, and aseptic meningitis.[52,53] With the decline in mumps, aseptic meningitis due to this virus has become rare. It is important to consider that in its very earliest stages, tuberculous meningitis may mimic aseptic meningitis, with minimal alterations in CSF chemistry, but will evolve to life-threatening infection if undiagnosed (discussion follows).

The management of children with aseptic meningitis is supportive. The major emphasis is placed on appropriate fluid management, especially when vomiting and diarrhea are prominent features of illness, and on excluding treatable causes of infection. In all young infants (e.g., those under 12 months of age), appropriate empiric antibacterial therapy should be administered, after the initial lumbar puncture is performed, for a period of 48 to 72 hours, until the CSF cultures are confirmed as sterile. In occasional instances, particularly when oral antibiotics have been administered prior to lumbar puncture and the CSF examination demonstrates a granulocytic pleocytosis, a full course of antibacterial therapy is administered despite negative CSF cultures. In older patients, initial empiric therapy may be restricted to those patients with disturbing systemic toxicity, nonclassical CSF formulae (most often a disturbingly high polymorphonuclear pleocytosis observed early in the course of enteroviral, mumps, and lymphocytic choriomeningitis virus disease), and those patients receiving prior antibiotic therapy in whom partially treated bacterial meningitis may be an important consideration. Diagnostic studies, such as viral culture of CSF, pharynx, or stool, and/or serologic analyses, must be individualized based on clinical and epidemiologic features of illness, because the results of such studies are often uninformative and, in any case, unavailable until after the child recovers. The prognosis of viral aseptic meningitis depends largely on the etiologic agent and the age of the patient. In general, the prognosis is favorable,[54,55] but long-term sequellae have been observed more frequently in some series of young infants with enteroviral disease.[56,57]

Table 32-3. Infectious causes of aseptic meningitis syndrome

Viruses
  Picornaviruses:
    poliovirus
    coxsackievirus
    echovirus
    newer enteroviruses
  Mumps
  Epstein-Barr virus
  Lymphocytic choriomeningitis virus
  Varicella
  Herpes simplex
  Human immunodeficiency virus (HIV)
  California equine encephalitis
  St. Louis encephalitis

Bacteria
  Syphilis (*T. pallidum*)
  Lyme Disease (*B. bergdorferi*)
  Leptospirosis
  Mycoplasma pneumoniae

Mycobacteria (earliest stage)
  M. tuberculosis

Fungi (early stages)
  C. neoformans
  C. immitis
  B. dermatidis

Encephalitis

Encephalitis is distinguished clinically from aseptic meningitis by the prominence of cerebral dysfunction (i.e., alterations in mentation, seizures, and focal neurologic deficits, rather than isolated meningeal irritation). Although a syndrome of encephalitis is occasionally encountered with certain bacterial infections, such as *Staphylococcus aureus* cerebritis associated with high-grade bacteremia, or *Listeria* meningitis, the etiology of encephalitis is almost always due to a viral pathogen. As with aseptic meningitis, limitations of viral diagnostic techniques may make precise etiologic diagnoses difficult, and a variety of clinical and epidemiologic considerations may be utilized to make a presumptive diagnosis. The need for a precise diagnosis has grown in order to direct specific antiviral therapy for herpes group viruses and to minimize the chance that a treatable infection (such as tuberculosis) is mistaken for a viral process.

Children often manifest encephalitic symptoms following a brief febrile flu-like illness, which is sometimes associated with gastrointestinal complaints. Headache and/or stiff neck are often present. Neuropsychiatric symptoms may subsequently become apparent, with confusion, hallucinations, agitation, or delirium, and progress over hours or a few days to obtundation or even coma. Seizures may be present and may be focal or generalized. A variety of focal neurologic deficits may be present as well. In some instances, initial neuropsychiatric complaints may precede the development of a toxic, febrile illness. In the case of rabies, autonomic dysfunction with relative preservation of cognition (rhombdencephalitis) may precede progressive obtundation and coma.

Initial physical examination documents the extent of neurologic dysfunction and may provide clues regarding an etiologic diagnosis. Cutaneous examination may reveal a viral exanthem suggestive of enteroviral infection, measles, or varicella. Parotitis may be seen in mumps, while pharyngitis, adenopathy, and splenomegaly may suggest infectious mononucleosis. Pulmonary findings may suggest mycoplasma infection, although secondary aspiration pneumonia must always be considered. The presence of labial *H. simplex* may merely reflect recurrent "fever blisters" and is not diagnostic of *H. simplex* encephalitis. The epidemiologic considerations that were discussed previously in relation to aseptic meningitis must be considered in this situation as well. Additional queries must be raised regarding exposure to animals, particularly unprovoked attacks by pets as well as any attack by animals at risk of harboring rabies (e.g., foxes, raccoons, skunks, etc.).[58] Mosquitoes serve as the vector for the transmission of arborviral encephalitis viruses (Eastern equine, Western equine, California, St. Louis) in endemic areas, but because mosquito bites are ubiquitous and sometimes unrecognized, this provides less useful information than a history of prolonged outdoor exposure in high-risk areas. HIV infection is commonly associated with progressive encephalopathy, but acute neurologic deterioration is far more likely to result from superimposed opportunistic infection or intracranial neoplasm rather than from HIV encephalitis per se.

Most routine laboratory studies provide important baseline information but fail to help elucidate an etiologic diagnosis. Leukocytosis, often with a mild left shift, may be present. Renal and electrolyte studies help to define the patient's fluid balance and possible inappropriate ADH secretion. Hepatic chemistries are usually normal, although anicteric hepatitis occurs frequently with Epstein-Barr virus infection. In the absence of focal neurologic signs, prompt lumbar puncture should be performed and the pressure measured (if possible), in addition to the routine CSF diagnostic studies. Cerebrospinal fluid examination usually reveals a moderate mononuclear cell pleocytosis, with relative preservation of CSF glucose and mild elevation of CSF protein. In several encephalitides (e.g., mumps, enterovirus, or lymphocytic choriomeningitis virus), polymorphonuclear pleocytosis as well as hypoglycorrhachia may be seen, especially early in the disease, and thus mimic bacterial meningitis. CSF should be cultured for bacterial pathogens. CSF viral culture may be considered, but the yield of recovering viral pathogens is quite low. CSF antigen detection and nucleic acid tests (based on polymerase chain reaction technology) for specific etiologic agents appear promising, but are not yet available for routine clinical use. When focal findings are prominent, CT scanning should precede lumbar puncture, because mass lesions such as abscess or tumor may produce similar clinical findings. Imaging studies are usually nondiagnostic and at most reveal diffuse cerebral edema. Hypodense areas of cerebral cortex are late findings and are usually seen only after 4 or more days of illness in necrotizing encephalitides, such as *H. simplex* or arboviral disease. Electroencephalography can be useful in diagnosis because a discordance between mild or moderate symptomatology and severely disorganized EEG suggests *H. simplex* disease, especially when seizure activity localizes to the temporal region. In those rare instances when rabies is suspected on a clinical or epidemiologic basis, skin biopsy and immunofluorescence testing for rabies antigen serves as a rapid diagnostic test. Repeat lumbar puncture after 48 to 72 hours of illness usually shows stable or improved parameters, except in herpetic or arboviral disease, in which there is rising pleocytosis, rising protein, and stable or falling glucose.

Antibacterial therapy for the presumptive therapy of meningitis is indicated for the first 72 hours of observation if the initial CSF formula has a predominance of polymorphonuclear leukocytes or if prior antibiotic therapy has been administered. Specific antiviral therapy is limited to the use of acyclovir in the treatment of *H. simplex* and varicella encephalitis, or to appropriate antibiotics in those rare situations in which encephalitic symptoms reflect underlying bacterial infection. Because *H. simplex* encephalitis occurs sporadically throughout the year, its diagnosis must be entertained in any sporadic case of encephalitis. Ultimate prognosis depends in part on the severity of clinical disease at the start of therapy, so early initiation of acyclovir is crucial. Rapid confirmation of this diagnosis requires brain biopsy for histologic, immunologic, and virologic study. In many centers, the logistical difficulties and morbidity associated with prompt brain biopsy lead to routine empiric use of acyclovir in this setting. Acyclovir therapy (30 mg/kg/d divided q8h)[59] must be maintained for at least 2 weeks of therapy because of the possibility of relapse occasionally reported after shorter courses of therapy. The diagnosis of *H. simplex* encephalitis can sometimes be made retrospectively in some patients by serologic testing of acute and convalescent sera.

Supportive measures involve control of fever by antipyretics and careful fluid management to control hyponatremia as well as ICP. In this situation, it is occasionally necessary to monitor ICP technically. The airway needs to be protected in obtunded patients to prevent aspiration, and in patients who are not intubated, care must be taken to avoid restraining the patient in the supine position. Oral feeding should be avoided in obtunded or agitated patients. Anticonvulsant therapy is indicated if seizures are present, and adequate control of seizures may require the concurrent administration of two or three different agents. In children who have survived the acute phase of illness with persisting obtundation or coma, efforts to place tracheostomy and gastrostomy tubes should be made to reduce the hazards of nosocomial infection complicating long-term parenteral nutrition. Persistent fever in these patients may be due to nosocomial infections such as pneumonia, nasotracheal tube-associated sinusitis or otitis media, catheter-related urinary tract infection, or IV catheter-related bacteremia. Drug-induced fever or hepatitis may develop due to concurrently administered antibiotics, anticonvulsants, etc. Additional noninfectious sources of fever may include IV catheter-associated thrombophlebitis or, rarely, deep venous thrombosis in older children.

Parameningeal Infections

A number of different focal disease processes, including brain abscess and subdural and epidural empyema, are classified together as parameningeal infections because they exist in close proximity to the meninges and evoke a characteristic CSF formula (including a moderate lymphocytic pleocytosis, often with a modestly elevated protein but normal glucose) but do not directly infect the CSF.

Brain Abscess

Brain parenchyma can become the site of progressive suppurative infection in three different ways: direct inoculation, either by penetrating head trauma or neurosurgery, by contiguous spread of infection from adjacent structures, and by hematogenous seeding. In the first case, the historical features of the patient's illness provide a high index of suspicion, and the diagnosis is usually straightforward. In the latter two instances, the patient's history may offer evidence of important predisposing factors, but at times the history is remarkably benign and the diagnosis overlooked.

The extension of parameningeal infection to produce brain abscess in immunologically competent children was a relatively common event in the preantibiotic era, but the routine early and effective treatment of sinusitis, otitis media, and mastoiditis has made progressive infection from these foci rare. Brain abscesses generally developed in close proximity to these primary foci, with infection spreading via venous or lymphatic channels or occasionally extending directly across a bony barrier to invade the brain. Thus, frontal sinusitis led to frontal lobe abscesses, and mastoiditis led to cerebellar and/or temporal lesions. In contrast, brain abscesses developing as a result of hematogenous spread of infection may occur in a variety of intracerebral locations. Such lesions are almost never seen in association with the commonly encountered bacteremias, but instead occur in situations in which there is chronic suppurative disease, such as with advanced intraoral infection, or chronic pulmonary infection due to lung abscess or bronchiectasis. In these situations, there appears to be an element of right-to-left shunting (e.g., due to fistulae between the pulmonary and bronchial arterial systems). Patients with cyanotic heart disease have significant shunting from the pulmonary to the systemic circulation and are at risk of developing brain abscess even without a recognized primary focus of infection. Brain abscesses are also occasionally seen in infective endocarditis, whereby the brain may be seeded by septic embolic material. This occurs more frequently in acute endocarditis, in which metastatic abscesses are frequent, than in subacute infective endocarditis, in which emboli usually result in bland cerebral infarction rather than in abscess formation.

Patients with brain abscess may present with predominant features of a slowly progressive, focal space-occupying lesion, with focal neurologic deficits, or seizures (focal or generalized), without findings such as fever, leukocytosis, or elevated erythrocyte sedimentation rate to indicate the presence of an infectious process. Other patients may have greater inflammatory features and fewer prominent neurologic complaints. In many of the latter children, empiric antibiotic therapy has often been administered prior to hospitalization.

The management of brain abscess must be individualized, depending on each child's clinical features. Traditionally, neurosurgi-

cal exploration for drainage and/or excision provided material for microbiologic analysis and removed the bulk of infected tissue,[60] particularly for abscesses associated with contiguous sinusitis.[61] Parenteral antibiotic therapy aimed at the pathogens recovered at surgery was then administered for 6 weeks. However, relative contraindications to surgical excision include the presence of technically difficult and rather inaccessible, deep lesions, the presence of very large or multiple abscesses, and location in the dominant hemisphere or in other sensitive regions, although in older children, stereotactic needle biopsy for bacterial culture may be considered. Experience in defining the spectrum of pathogens recovered from brain abscesses has shown that these lesions are usually polymicrobial in nature, with a predominance of streptococci and anaerobic flora. In addition, CT and MRI scanning have facilitated frequent sequential monitoring of brain abscesses during therapy. Consequently, medical therapy of these lesions may be considered in selected cases with the long-term administration of a broad-spectrum regimen, including metronidazole, penicillin, and a third-generation cephalosporin, and with careful interval monitoring by scanning techniques.[62,63] The initial extended period of parenteral therapy may be followed by protracted oral administration of metronidazole and amoxicillin or penicillin (e.g., for 6 months). Scans usually show interval improvement of these lesions, with resolution of edema and diminution in abscess volume during therapy, but the final involution of the process occurs over months after the completion of antibiotic therapy.

Although conventional bacterial brain abscesses may develop in the absence of local or systemic anatomic risk factors, such lesions are infrequent. Focal tuberculous lesions (tuberculomas[64,65]) or parasitic lesions due to the larval stage of *T. solium* (cysticercosis[66]) may be present. These diseases have widely varying incidence rates, depending on the epidemiologic setting. In India, for example, tuberculomas are the most commonly encountered parenchymal lesion, while in many parts of Latin America, cysticercosis is far more common. The latter diagnosis may be straightforward when multiple and/or calcified cystic lesions are present, particularly if discrete larvae are visualized along the surface of the lesions. In children, single noncalcified lesions are the rule and thus may provoke diagnostic uncertainty. The diagnosis may be confirmed by the detection of anticysticercal antibodies in serum and CSF, which together offer a high degree of sensitivity in confirming the diagnosis. Therapy with praziquantel, 50 mg/kg/d divided into 3 doses daily for 2 weeks,[67] may be initiated empirically in the proper clinical setting while awaiting the results of the serologic tests. Dexamethasone is often administered as an adjunctive antiinflammatory agent to prevent possible deterioration due to increased edema at the initiation of praziquantel therapy.[67,68] Follow-up cranial imaging generally shows involution of the cysts and resolution of inflammatory edema when performed weeks to months after the completion of therapy.

Patients with underlying congenital or acquired T cell immunodeficiency syndromes may develop focal brain abscesses due to opportunistic pathogens. These include *Nocardia asteroides, Cryptococcus neoformans, M. tuberculosis,* and *Toxoplasma gondii.* Serologic tests for cryptococcal antigen in serum and/or CSF and serum antibodies against *T. gondii* may facilitate rapid diagnosis of these processes, but skin test reactivity against mycobacteria is generally absent in these immunodeficient patients, and surgical exploration for diagnosis is frequently required in these selected patients. In selected HIV-infected patients, empiric therapy for toxoplasmosis may be initiated, with biopsy restricted to those patients who fail to improve.

Subdural Empyema

These focal infections usually develop as complications of contiguous infections, specifically sinusitis or mastoiditis, or bacterial meningitis.[69,70] Focal subdural empyema should be suspected when a child with significant sinusitis or mastoiditis presents with seizures, obtundation, focal neurologic signs, disproportionate systemic toxicity, or typical CSF findings despite appropriate medical or combined medical and surgical therapy of the primary infection. Cranial CT scanning demonstrates the presence of subdural fluid or, occasionally, a mixture of fluid and gas in the subdural space, generally accompanied by enhancement of the adjoining cerebral cortex and often associated with reactive cerebral edema and/or mass effect. The contiguous primary focus of infection, such as sinusitis, should be apparent as well. Subdural empyemas may sometimes localize to a falcine location between the hemispheres. Management requires immediate neurosurgical consultation and generally requires urgent surgical drainage. Collections located along the convexity of the cortex may be drained by the placement of burr holes, but collections in relation to the frontal tips may require bifrontal craniotomy in addition to sinus exenteration. Operative specimens should be Gram stained and cultured for anerobes as well as for routine pathogens. Initial empiric antibiotic management should cover anerobes, *S. aureus*, encapsulated pathogens, and possibly enteric gram-negative bacilli, depending on the clinical setting. Nafcillin and chloramphenicol represent a traditional antibiotic regimen used in this situation; less experience is available using the newer cephalosporin and other beta-lactam agents. Sequential cranial imaging is helpful for monitoring the efficacy of therapy.

Subdural empyemas may also occur with conventional bacterial meningitis in early infancy and childhood.[61] In this setting, it is presumed that (initally sterile) subdural effusions become secondarily infected by the offending pathogen, despite adequate initial therapy. Typically, the children demonstrate a persisting submaximal clinical response, with continuing fever and lethargy, and cranial imaging documents subdural fluid with the inflammatory features described earlier. Alternatively, there may be an initial interval of satisfactory response, perhaps complicated only by persistent fever or by recurrence of fever, in which case, cranial scanning is performed in pursuit of the source of fever. Although the subdural effusions typically seen in this setting are sterile and do not require diagnostic or therapeutic drainage, diagnostic aspiration is occasionally recommended because of worsening fever, deteriorating clinical status, or enlarging effusions. If the cultures of the drainage specimen are positive, more definitive drainage via additional burr holes, or even craniotomy, may be necessary.

References

1. Feigin RD, McCracken GH, and Klein JO. 1992. Diagnosis and management of meningitis. *Pediatr. Infect. Dis. J.* 11:785.
2. Teele DW, Marshall R, Klein JO. Unsuspected bacteremia in young children. *Pediatr Clin North Am* 26:773, 1979.
3. Kaplan, SL, and Woods CR. 1992. Neurologic complications of bacterial meningitis in children. *Current Clin. Topics in Infect. Dis.* 12:37.
4. Lerner AM. New viral exanthems. *Ann Intern Med* 60:703, 1964.
5. Kaplan SL et al. Onset of hearing loss in children with bacterial meningitis. *Pediatrics* 73:575, 1984.
6. Vienny H et al. Early diagnosis and evolution of deafness in childhood bacterial meningitis: A study using brainstem auditory evoked potentials. *Pediatrics* 73:579, 1984.
7. Dodge PR et al. Prospective evaluation of hearing impairment as a sequela of acute bacterial meningitis. *N Engl J Med* 311:869, 1984.
8. Converse GM et al. Alteration of cerebrospinal fluid findings by partial treatment of bacterial meningitis. *J Pediatr* 83:220, 1973.
9. Powell KR et al. Normalization of plasma arginine vasopressin concentrations when children with meningitis are given maintenance plus replacement fluid therapy. *Pediatrics* 117:515, 1990.
10. Feigin RD, Shackelford PG. Value of repeat lumbar puncture in the differential diagnosis of meningitis. *N Engl J Med* 289:571, 1973.
11. Singhi SC, Singhi PD, Srinivas B, Narakesri HP, Ganguli NK, Sialy R, and Walia BNS. 1995. Fluid restriction does not improve the outcome.
12. Shapiro ED. Prophylaxis for contacts of patients with meningococcal or *Haemophilus influenzae* type B disease. *Pediatr Infect Dis* 1:132, 1982.
13. Siegel SD, Shannon KM, DePasse BM. Recurrent infection associated with penicillin-tolerant group B streptococci: A report of two cases. *J Pediatr* 81:920, 1981.
14. Paris MM, Hickey SM, Uscher MI, Shelton S, Olsen KD, and McCracken GH. 1993. Effect of dexamethasone on therapy of experimental penicillin- and cephalosporin-resistant pneumococcal meningitis. *Antimicrob. Agents Chemother.* 38:1320.
15. Paris MM, Ramilo O, and McCracken GH. 1995. Management of meningitis caused by penicillin-resistant *Streptococcus pneumoniae*. *Antimicrob. Agents Chemother.* 39:2171.
16. Hand WL, Sanford JP. Posttraumatic bacterial meningitis. *Ann Intern Med* 72:869, 1970.
17. Swartz MN, Dodge PR. Bacterial meningitis—A review of selected aspects. I. General clinical features, special problems and unusual reactions mimicking bacterial meningitis. *N Engl J Med* 272:725–731, 779–787, 842–848, 898, 1965.
18. Pappas DG, Hammerschlag PE, and Hammerschlag M. 1993. Cerebrospinal fluid rhinorrhea and recurrent meningitis. *Clin. Infect. Dis.* 17:364.
19. Hyslop NE, Montgomery WW. Diagnosis and management of meningitis associated with cerebrospinal fluid leaks. In Remington JS, Swartz MN (eds): *Current Clinical Topics in Infectious Disease.* New York: McGraw-Hill, 1982. P 254.
20. Ellison RT et al. Prevalence of congenital or acquired complement deficiency in patients with sporadic meningococcal disease. *N Engl J Med* 308:913, 1983.
21. Lin T et al. Seven days of ceftriaxone therapy is as effective as ten days' treatment for bacterial meningitis. *JAMA* 253:3559, 1985.
22. Lin T, Nelson JD, McCracken GH Jr. Fever during treatment for bacterial meningitis. *Pediatr Infect Dis* 3:319, 1984.
23. Quagliarello VJ, and Scheld WM. 1993. New perspectives on bacterial meningitis. *Clin. Infect. Dis.* 17:603.
24. Lebel MH et al. Dexamethasone therapy for bacterial meningitis: Results of two double-blind, placebo-controlled trials. *N Engl J Med* 319:964, 1988.
25. Odio CM et al. The beneficial effects of early dexamethasone administration in infants and children with bacterial meningitis. *N Engl J Med* 324:1525, 1991.
26. Wald ER, Kaplan SL, Mason EO, Sabo D, Ross L, Arditi M, Wiedermann BL, Barson W, Kim KS, Yogev R, and Hofkosh D for the Meningitis Study Group. 1995. Dexamethasone therapy for children with bacterial meningitis. *Pediatrics* 95:21.
27. Kennedy WA, Hoyt MJ, and McCracken GH. 1991. The role of corticosteroid therapy in children with pneumococcal meningitis. *AJDC* 145:1374.
28. Kanra GY, Ozen H, Secmeer G, Ceyhan M, Ecevit Z, and Belgin E. 1995. Beneficial effects of dexamethasone in children with pneumococcal meningitis. *Pediatr. Infect. Dis. J.* 14:490.
29. Syrogiannopoulos GA, Lourida AN, Thodoridou MC, Pappas IG, Babilis GC, Economidis JJ, Zoumboulakis DJ, Beratis NG, and Matsaniotis NS. 1994. Dexamethasone therapy for bacterial meningitis in children: 2- versus 4-day regimen. *J. Infect. Dis.* 169:853.
30. Schaad UB, Gnehm HE, Blumberg A, Heinzer I, and Wedgwood J

for the Swiss Meningitis Study Group. 1993. Dexamethasone therapy for bacterial meningitis in children. *Lancet* 342:457.

31. Grimwood K, Anderson VA, Bond L, Catroppa C, Hore RL, Keir EH, Nolan T, and Roberton DM. 1995. Adverse outcomes of bacterial meningitis in school-age survivors. *Pediatrics* 95:646.

32. Fortnum HM. 1992 . Hearing impairment after bacterial meningitis: a review. *Arch. Dis. Child.* 67:1128.

33. Prober CG. 1995. The role of steroids in the management of children with bacterial meningitis. *Pediatrics* 95:29.

34. Bradley JS. 1994. Dexamethasone therapy in meningitis: potentially misleading antiinflammatory effects in central nervous system infections. *Pediatr. Infect. Dis. J.* 13:823.

35. Newton RW. 1994. Tuberculous meningitis. *Arch. Dis. Child.* 70:364.

36. Starke JR, and Correa AG. 1995. Management of mycobacterial infection and disease in children. *Pediatr. Infect. Dis. J.* 14:455.

37. Escobar HA et al. Mortality from tuberculous meningitis reduced by steroid therapy. *Pediatrics* 56:1050, 1975.

38. Gonyea EF. The spectrum of primary blastomycoticmeningitis: A review of central nervous system blastomycosis. *Arch Neurol* 3:26, 1978.

39. Bouza E et al. Coccidiodal meningitis: An analysis of thirty-one cases and review of the literature. *Medicine* 60:139, 1981.

40. Goodwin RA Jr et al. Disseminated histoplasmosis: Clinical and pathologic correlations. *Medicine* 59:1, 1959.

41. Dismukes WE et al. Treatment of cryptococcal meningitis with combination amphotericin B and flucytosine for four as compared with six weeks. *N Engl J Med* 317:334, 1987.

42. Bozzette SA et al. A placebo-controlled trial of maintenance therapy with fluconazole after treatment of cryptococcal meningitis in the acquired immunodeficiency syndrome. *N Engl J Med* 324:580, 1991.

43. Wildin S, Chonmaitree T. The importance of the virology laboratory in the diagnosis and management of viral meningitis. *Am J Dis Child* 141:454, 1987.

44. Peter G. Leptospirosis: A zoonosis of protean manifestations. *Pediatr Infect Dis* 1:282, 1982.

45. Pierce JF, Jabbari B, Shraberg D. Leptospirosis: A neglected cause of nonbacterial meningoencephalitis. *South Med J* 70:150, 1977.

46. Logigian EL, Kaplan RF, Steere AC. Chronic neurologic manifestations of Lyme disease. *N Engl J Med* 323:1438, 1990.

47. Reik L et al. Neurologic abnormalities of Lyme disease. *Medicine* 58:281, 1979.

48. Rahn DW, Malawista SE. Lyme disease: Recommendations for diagnosis and treatment. *Ann Intern Med* 114:472, 1991.

49. Ponka A. Central nervous system manifestations associated with serologically verified Mycoplasma pneumoniae infection. *Scand J Infect Dis* 12:175, 1980.

50. Grose C, Henle W, Henle G, and Feorino PM. 1975. Primary Epstein-Barr virus infections in acute neurologic diseases. *New Engl. J. Med.* 292:392.

51. Silverstein A, Steinberg G, Nathanson M. Nervous system involvement in infectious mononucleosis: The heralding and/or major manifestation. *Arch Neurol* 26:353, 1972.

52. Ho DD et al. Primary human T-lymphotropic virus type III infection. *Ann Intern Med* 103:880, 1985.

53. Hollander H, Stringari S. Human immunodeficiency virus-associated meningitis: Clinical course and correlations. *Am J Med* 83:813, 1987.

54. Bergman I et al. Outcome in children with enteroviral meningitis during the first year of life. *J Pediatr* 110:705, 1987.

55. Rorabaugh ML, Berlin LE, Heldrich F, Roberts K, Rosenberg LA, Doran T, and Modlin JF. 1993. Aseptic meningitis in infants younger than 2 years of age: acute illness and neurologic complications. *Pediatrics* 92:206.

56. Wilfert CM et al. Longitudinal assessment of children with enteroviral meningitis during the first three months of life. *Pediatrics* 67:811, 1981.

57. Wilfert CM, Lehrman SN, Katz SL. Enteroviruses and meningitis. *Pediatr Infect Dis* 2:333, 1983.

58. Anderson LJ et al. Human rabies in the United States, 1960–1979: Epidemiology, diagnosis and prevention. *Ann Intern Med* 100:728, 1984.

59. Whitley RJ et al. Vidarabine versus acyclovir therapy in Herpes simplex encephalitis. *N Engl J Med* 314:144, 1986.

60. Rosenblum ML, Mampalam TJ, Pons VG. Controversies in the management of brain abscesses. *Clin Neurosurg* 33:603, 1986.

61. Johnson DL et al. Treatment of intracranial abscesses associated with sinusitis in children and adolescents. *J Pediatr* 113:15, 1988.

62. Boom WH, Tuazon CU. Successful treatment of multiple brain abscesses with antibiotics alone. *Rev Infect Dis* 7:189, 1985.

63. Keren G, Tyrrell DLJ. Nonsurgical treatment of brain abscesses: Report of two cases. *Pediatr Infect Dis* 3:331, 1984.

64. Tyler B, Bennett H, Kim J. Intracranial tuberculomas in a child: Computed tomographic scan diagnosis and nonsurgical management. *Pediatrics* 71:952, 1983.

65. Harder E, Al-Kawi MZ, Carney P. Intracranial tuberculoma: Conservative management. *Am J Med* 74:570, 1983.

66. Earnest MP et al. Neurocysticercosis in the United States: 35 cases and a review. *Rev Infect Dis* 9:961, 1987.

67. Sotelo J et al. Therapy of parenchymal brain cysticercosis with praziquantel. *N Engl J Med* 310:1001, 1984.

68. Nash T, Neva FA. Recent advances in the diagnosis and treatment of cerebral cysticercosis. *N Engl J Med* 311:1492, 1984.

69. Jacobson PL, Farmer TW. Subdural empyema complicating meningitis in infants: Improved prognosis. *Neurology* 31:190, 1981.

70. Coonrod JD, Dans PE. Subdural empyema. *Am J Med* 53:85, 1972.

John H. Fugate

33 Metabolic Encephalopathy Including Reye's Syndrome

Metabolic encephalopathies are noninflammatory encephalopathies caused by toxic metabolites. These metabolites deleteriously affect the brain by direct neuronal injury, vascular damage, cerebral edema, neurotransmitter blockade, demyelination, or hypoxic-ischemic injury and may retard brain growth.[1] There are a wide variety of causes for these encephalopathies, but the two most common are Reye's syndrome and inborn errors of metabolism. Reye's Syndrome will be discussed in this chapter. Other metabolic encephalopathies and their treatment are discussed in Metabolic Disorders by Herrin, this volume.

Classically, Reye's syndrome is a biphasic illness with a prodrome of an acute viral illness followed 3 to 7 days later by the development of encephalopathy. Usually, other metabolic encephalopathies are precipitated by a number of factors, and the encephalopathy develops in conjunction with the precipitating factor. These factors may include starvation, infection, fever, hypoxemia, and exercise. Protein overload in the diet or certain vitamin deficiencies and specific toxins (e.g., valproate, aspirin, or copper) may precipitate the development of metabolic encephalopathies.[1] Frequently, these types of encephalopathies may be associated with hepatocellular injury and may be termed *Reye's-like illness*.

Table 33-1 lists the most common inherited metabolic disorders that mimic Reye's syndrome. Several features may be helpful in differentiating these from Reye's syndrome: absence of the biphasic illnesses, unusual odor, jaundice, and inadequately elevated serum ammonia and liver enzymes. Also, there may be a previous history of similar episodes, developmental delay, seizures, hypoglycemia, or unexplained infant deaths in the family.[2]

In general, the treatment for the metabolic encephalopathies is similar in that supportive care is given to the patient to ensure adequate circulation and normal oxygenation. The etiology of the encephalopathy is vigorously pursued and systematically treated if possible, and neurointensive care treatment principles are utilized to minimize secondary brain injury. These concepts are discussed further in this chapter and in Pathophysiology of Intracranial Emergencies by Brogan, Geiduschek, and Krane, this volume.

Reye's syndrome is a rare, acute disorder, primarily of children, causing encephalopathy with fatty infiltration of the liver and other organs. The disease is usually self-limiting, but survivors may have permanent neurologic injury. In 1963, Reye and his colleagues first described this syndrome, which occurred primarily in infants and young children less than 2 years of age and had distinctive clinical and biochemical characteristics.[3] Also in 1963, George Johnson and co-workers described patients in North Carolina that were older, mostly between 6 and 13 years of age.[4] These patients developed illness during an outbreak of influenza B in the community. The similarities between the two descriptions led to the common designation of this clinical pathologic entity as Reye's syndrome.

Over the past 30 years since these reports, there has been a great deal of effort in trying to find the etiology and pathogenesis of this disease, along with improving the methods of treatment. Incidence of the disease peaked in the late 1970s and early 1980s when the Centers for Disease Control estimated between 600 and 1200 cases each year in the United States.[5] Since that time there has been a dramatic decline in the cases of Reye's syndrome. Also, the overall mortality rate is significantly less than was originally described at 80%, with the overall mortality now between 20% and 30%.[6]

Epidemiology and Differential Diagnosis

The epidemiology of Reye's syndrome (or Reye's-like syndromes) seems to have two separate groups, which also coincides with the two initial reports. The type of patients described by Johnson includes older children who had the syndrome shortly after having a viral illness, usually with strains of influenza infection, either B or A, or chicken pox. They have the typical history of a viral prodrome illness, followed 3 to 5 days later by protracted vomiting, then progression of variable sensorial changes. There appears to be a few other diseases clinically mimicking this disorder in this age group, especially in the appropriate setting, either in winter influenza months or following chicken pox. The incidence of Reye's syndrome in this older group of children was much higher in the United States, especially in the 1970s and early 1980s, until the widespread use of aspirin in the United States dramatically declined. The other epidemiologic group appears to be in children less than 5 years of age, especially infants. Prior to 1981, approximately 20% of the cases reported each year were children less than 5 years of age, whereas in the past several years, as the older

Table 33-1. Inborn errors of metabolism that mimic Reye's syndrome

Disorder	Example
Fatty-acid oxidation disorders	MCAD—medium-chain fatty-acid acyl CoA dehydrogenase deficiency
Carnitine transport disorders	Carnitine palmitoyl transferase deficiency
Organic acidurias	Proprionic acidurea
Urea cycle disorders	Ornithine transcarbomylase deficiency
Pyruvate metabolism disorders	Respiratory-chain enzyme deficiency
Ketone utilization disorders	Acetoacetyl succinyl CoA transferase deficiency
Carbohydrate disorders	Fructose—1,6-diphosphatase deficiency

Table 33-2. Two epidemiologic groups of Reye's syndrome and Reye's-like syndromes

Older children	Younger children
Primarily children 5–12 yrs	Primarily infants <2 yrs
Aspirin-associated	Nonseasonal; nonepidemic
Viral epidemics (influenza A,B) or chicken pox	Usually no latent period if associated with viral illness
Latent period 3–5 days after viral illness	
Declining incidence	Unchanged incidence
Peaked in the United States in 1970s, early '80s	Inborn errors of metabolism likely

age group number of children has declined, the younger age group incidence has increased to greater than 50% of the total cases.[7] This group of children appears to have a mixture of metabolic and other disorders, including typical Reye's syndrome. The difference between these two groups is outlined in Table 33-2.

From an epidemiologic standpoint in the United States, the second group, which is a heterogenous group frequently made up of inborn errors in metabolism, is now the more common cause of Reye's (or Reye's-like) syndrome. Because of this increased number, it is important for any child, especially under 2 years of age, and occasionally even older children, to be considered for metabolic evaluation. When one looks for the criteria of the diagnosis of Reye's syndrome, as seen in Table 33-2, it is important

that no other explanation for cerebral or hepatic abnormalities can be found, which includes eliminating all of the inherited errors of metabolism.

The differential diagnosis of Reye's syndrome in the older child includes any disease that causes acute encephalopathy or acute severe hepatic injury. These include drug overdose, valproic acid toxicity, acute severe hepatitis, acetaminophen toxicity, connective tissue diseases with chronic salicylate ingestion, systemic carnitine deficiency, encephalitis, and occasionally late diagnoses of inborn errors of metabolism.

The differential diagnosis in the younger age group includes infections that cause acute encephalitis or acute severe hepatic injury, but most commonly includes metabolic disorders with a Reye's-like syndrome presentation. There have been a number of inherited metabolic disorders that have been reported to present with a Reye's-like syndrome. This most frequently occurs in children who present with hypoglycemia and hyperammonemia. These disorders may include organic acidemias, urea cycle defects, aminoacidurias, and disorders of carbohydrate metabolism. Metabolic studies should be done on any patient who presents with Reye's-like symptoms. It is also important to do these studies early in the clinical course, especially urine studies for organic acids and serum for amino acids. Once the patient has had no protein intake for a few days it may be difficult to interpret the studies. Investigations may also need to include liver tissue and sterile skin biopsy specimens for fibroblast culture. Figure 33-1 shows a flow tree of the different metabolic disorders associated with the Reye's-like symptoms. It is important to keep in mind that several of these syndromes will present with mixed symptoms. Further treatment

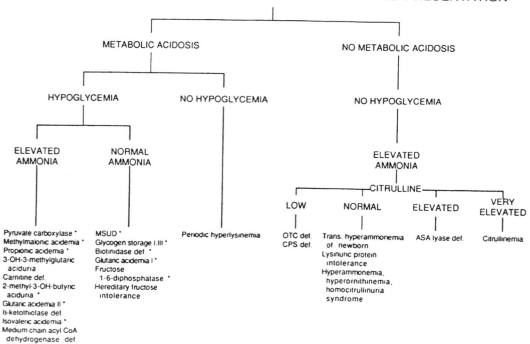

Figure 33-1. An approach to evaluation of metabolic disorders in which symptoms are similar to those of Reye's syndrome. In disorders with metabolic acidosis, the most useful diagnostic test is evaluation of organic acids. In the second group, plasma amino acids are most helpful. Asterisks, ketonuria; def., deficiency. (From Green CL, Blitzer MG, Shapira E. Inborn errors of metabolism and Reye syndrome: Differential diagnosis. *J Pediatr* 113:156–159, 1988. With permission.)

protocols and information regarding specific co-enzyme or vitamin therapy for some of the specific inborn errors of metabolism can be found in Metabolic Disorders by Herrin, this volume. It is important that a diagnosis be found for genetic counselling.

Finally, there has been much discussion about Reye's syndrome and aspirin use, from both an epidemiologic and differential diagnosis standpoint. Studies have pointed out a close relationship between aspirin usage and Reye's syndrome, and children on chronic salicylates have an increased incidence of the syndrome.[8–11] Intoxication with aspirin also causes encephalopathy and liver dysfunction, like Reye's syndrome. Since recommendations in 1982 warning of this association, there has been a significant decline in both aspirin usage and Reye's syndrome.

There is much speculation as to whether aspirin use and the development of Reye's syndrome is a proven correlation. This is because there are other reports of Reye's syndrome in children with no history of aspirin use, and there is some question as to the validity of the initial studies.[12–15] Most likely, salicylates are not the single causal agent in the development of Reye's syndrome, but probably contribute to its development, as will be discussed later.

Etiology and Pathogenesis

While the incidence of Reye's syndrome has continued to decrease, the etiology remains enigmatic. There has been significant progress in elucidating the pathophysiology of Reye's syndrome, however, and with the development of good animal models, further developments in both etiology and pathophysiology should come.

Clinically, after an initial viral prodrome, patients develop severe vomiting after a latent phase of 3 to 7 days. Vomiting and lethargy are usually the first signs of encephalopathy. Elevations of free fatty acids, hepatic enzymes (AST, ALT), and prolonged prothrombin time with or without hyperammonemia accompany the early findings. As increasing encephalopathy develops, associated with increasing intracranial pressure, hyperammonemia becomes markedly elevated as free fatty acids continue to rise.

At the cellular level there appears to be a primary injury to the mitochondria. It is uncertain whether the defect occurs in multiple organs, including the liver, brain, and muscle, or primarily affects liver cells with secondary injury to other sites through metabolic derangements. Most likely it is the latter.

The major defect in mitochondrial injury in Reye's syndrome appears to be disordered fatty-acid oxidation. This is evidenced by microvascular fat deposits in the liver of affected children and the presence of fatty-acid conjugates and partially degraded fats in urine and serum of these children—all indicating alternative pathways of fatty-acid metabolism.[16] Figure 33-2 depicts the interactions between the mitochondrial fatty-acid oxidation systems showing the abnormal sequelae. This figure demonstrates the various derangements that have been found in patients with Reye's syndrome and includes the following:

1. Decreased urine and serum ketone bodies, and decreased acetyl-CoA levels. A block in mitochondrial beta oxidation of fatty acids leads to decreased acetyl-CoA production and decreased production ketone bodies.

2. Increased medium-chain and mono- and dicarboxylic acids. Increased use of the omega oxidation pathway, as an alternative pathway, leads to increased medium-chain dicarboxylic acids after conversion from medium-chain acyl-CoA intermediates.

3. Increased urine losses of free and acetyl carnitine. Blocked

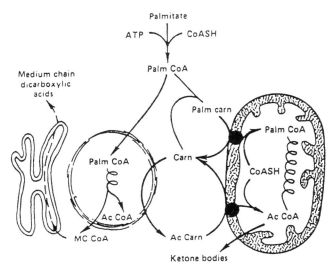

Figure 33-2. A model illustrating the actions between hepatic mitochondrial beta-oxidation, peroxisomal beta oxidation, and omega oxidation. This model shows oxidation of a long-chain fatty acid, as illustrated, as palmitoyl-CoA by both mitochondria and peroxisones. A block in mitochondrial beta oxidation (●) results in decreased production of ketone bodies and increased formation of acetyl carnitine (Ac Carn) and medium-chain acyl CoA (MC CoA) intermediates by beta-oxidation of the peroxisomes. The MC CoA intermediates are then converted to medium-chain dicarboxylic acids by omega oxidation in the endoplasmic reticulum. (From Kilpatrick-Smith L, Hale DE, Douglas SD. Progress in Reye syndrome: Epidemiology, biochemical mechanisms and animal models. *Dig Dis* 7:135–146, 1989. Copyright © 1989, Karger Basel. With permission.)

pathways of mitochondrial beta oxidation causes carnitine to be utilized in removal of toxic intermediates.

4. Accumulation of short- and medium-chained acyl-CoA compounds. Alternate pathway shunting increases these intermediate compounds as short- and medium-chained acyl-Co esters are used up.[16]

These cellular findings can explain the major clinical findings seen in Reye's syndrome, especially hyperammonemia and hypoglycemia. The intermediate products, especially acyl-CoA intermediates, now compete for the enzyme binding sites, profoundly altering normal pathways. These fatty-acid intermediates especially compete with acetyl-CoA and other acyl-CoA substrates, which then inhibits gluconeogenesis, ureagenesis, ketogenesis, the citric acid cycle, and metabolism through pyruvate dehydrogenase.[16] These alterations may produce the specific hepatocellular injury and the abnormal and histopathologic findings that comprise Reye's syndrome. The cause of the start of this mitochondrial injury in Reye's syndrome is uncertain, however.

As mentioned, Reye's syndrome frequently follows a viral infection and appears to be associated with aspirin use. A possible triggering agent is bacterial endotoxin, as elevated levels of endotoxin have been found in patients with Reye's syndrome.[17] A mechanism for the elevation could be the impairment of Kupffer cells which clear endotoxin. This impairment frequently follows viral infections.[18] Other hepatotoxins, such as pesticides and aflatoxin, may also impair Kupffer cells, but most children with Reye's syndrome do not have exposure to either of these chemicals.[19] Also,

Table 33-3. Differing characteristics of physical examination according to the stage of Reye's syndrome

Stage	Level of consciousness	Posture	Response to painful stimuli	Pupillary reaction to light	Oculocephalic reflex (doll's eye)	Glasgow Coma Scale
I	Lethargic but follows verbal commands	Normal	Purposeful	Brisk	Normal response	8+
II	Combative/stuporous, verbalizes inappropriately	Normal	Purposeful or nonpurposeful	Sluggish	Conjugate deviation of eyes	6–8
III	Coma	Decorticate	Decorticate	Sluggish	Conjugate deviation of eyes	5
IV	Coma	Decerebrate	Decerebrate	Sluggish	Inconsistent or absent response	4
V	Coma	Flaccid	No response	No response	No response	3

fibronectin, which is thought to have a significant role in clearing endotoxins, has been found in lower levels than normal in patients with Reye's syndrome.[20] An animal model has been developed in rats that shows much of the same biochemical, clinical, and histopathologic characteristics as seen in patients with Reye's syndrome.[21–23] Hepatic microvesicular fat deposition and mitochondrial swelling with cristae disruption without parenchymal inflammation or necrosis is seen in fasted rats given low doses of *Escherichia coli* endotoxin. Elevated ammonia levels, lactate, free fatty acids, and decreased hepatic ketones are also observed. These clinical and histopathologic changes are the same as those in patients with Reye's syndrome. The addition of aspirin to this model produces the same unusual pattern of hepatic acyl-CoA esters as seen in patients with Reye's syndrome. This unusual pattern is not seen when aspirin or endotoxin is given separately. This possibly supports the idea that aspirin is not a direct cause but may further contribute to its development.[8]

Increased levels of endotoxin stimulate macrophage production and secretion of endogenous monokines, especially interleukin-1 (IL-1) and tumor necrosis factor (TNF). Aspirin appears to augment the macrophage release of TNF in the presence of endotoxin, and these released mediators (TNF and IL-1) produce significant intracellular alterations at the effected target cells.[24] In the liver, this includes inhibiting mitochondrial fatty-acid oxidation with the previously described sequelae.

In conclusion, Reye's syndrome appears to be caused by disordered fatty-acid metabolism, which then effects significant disruption of multiple metabolic pathways. The intermediate products of fatty-acid metabolism compete with normal acyl-CoA substrates and inhibit gluconeogenesis, ureagenesis, ketogenesis, and the citric acid cycle, among others. These disruptions injure normal cellular function, especially hepatocytes effecting the histopathologic changes seen in Reye's syndrome. The triggering mechanism may be increased levels of endotoxin liberated from viral illnesses associated with Kupffer cell injury and decreased fibronectin levels, both of which help to clear endotoxin. Endogenous monokines stimulated by endotoxin appear to cause the injury. Aspirin seems to compound the metabolic derangement in these patients, by augmenting TNF (one of the endogenous monokines).

Clinical History and Physical Examination

The clinical history of Reye's syndrome generally starts with a viral illness, usually during influenza A and B epidemics, occasionally associated with varicella, mumps, Coxsackie, Epstein Barr, or echo

viruses. During the peak years of the syndrome, the incidence of disease was highest in January through March, which is generally when these epidemic viruses occur. Thirty percent of Reye's syndrome follows varicella with sporadic incidence, and 10% follows diarrhea illnesses, also with a sporadic incidence. After the prodromal illness of the viral infection, approximately 3 to 7 days later, protracted vomiting begins. Then the progression of variable neurologic changes may develop. The encephalopathy that occurs may rapidly progress to severe or lethal neurologic dysfunction or may remain stable. The peak incidence is between the ages of 4 and 16 years, although the incidence now is highest in children less than 2 years of age with Reye's-like illness. (The children with Reye's-like illness frequently have a viral prodrome but usually develop encephalopathy very early in their illness.) Physical examination usually shows that the preceding viral illness has faded. Generally, fever is absent, although occasionally it may be low-grade. Usually, there is no evidence of meningismus, but if it is present, it most likely represents encephalitis or meningitis. Hepatomegaly frequently occurs with peak liver size, usually about 3 to 5 days after the development of the vomiting. Focal neurologic signs are usually absent, but generalized neurologic dysfunction usually occurs and has been staged according to severity. Table 33-3 gives the staging currently followed by the National Institutes of Health, which indicates the different characteristics of physical examination according to the stage of Reye's syndrome.

The diagnosis of Reye's syndrome in a patient depends on meeting the defined criteria, as seen in Table 33-4. This includes the characteristic abnormal liver studies of a threefold or greater rise in either the AST, ALT, or ammonia, or more importantly, the

Table 33-4. Centers for Disease Control definition of Reye's syndrome

Acute noninflammatory encephalopathy documented clinically by an alteration in consciousness and, if available, a record of cerebrospinal fluid containing <8 leukocytes per millimeter, or by histological specimen demonstrating cerebral edema without perivascular of meningeal inflammation

Hepatopathy documented by results of either a liver biopsy or autopsy considered to be diagnostic of Reye's syndrome, or a threefold or greater rise in the levels of either the AST, ALT, or serum ammonia

No more reasonable explanation for cerebral or hepatic abnormalities

AST, aspartate aminotransferase; ALT, alanine aminotransferase.

histopathologic changes found on biopsy. The following is a list of laboratory tests that aid in the initial evaluation of possible Reye's syndrome and also therapeutic decisions:

1. Liver function tests
   a. AST, ALT, ammonia—threefold or greater rise should be seen
   b. Hepatitis screening, bilirubin, and alkaline phosphatase—should be normal
2. Coagulation studies—to assess liver function or coagulopathy
3. CNS imaging—to evaluate other causes of encephalopathy or the extent of cerebral edema
4. EEG—helpful in correlating staging
5. Arterial blood gas—to evaluate hyperventilation and amount of metabolic acidosis
6. Serum glucose—to evaluate hypoglycemia, especially common in infants
7. Routine studies—CBC, BUN, creatinine, electrolytes, osmolarity, and urinalysis, as baseline studies
8. Serum and urine organic and amino acids—to rule out inborn error of metabolism
9. Lumbar puncture—if there is a question of meningitis or encephalitis
10. Viral studies—to evaluate possible etiology
11. Routine cultures—blood, urine, tracheal, cerebrospinal fluid, if appropriate
12. Serum amylase and lipase—occasionally Reye's syndrome is associated with pancreatitis
13. Toxic screen—part of encephalopathy workup
14. Uncommon tests—lactate, fatty-acid intermediate metabolites, carnitine, fibronectin, and endotoxin levels

Treatment

The treatment of patients with Reye's syndrome is dependent on the stage of encephalopathy that the child develops. Any child with the presumptive diagnosis of Reye's syndrome should be transferred to a hospital with an intensive care unit (ICU) familiar with the management of critically ill children, especially those who have problems with intracranial hypertension.

The major thrust of therapy for Reye's syndrome has been supportive rather than specific, in that treatment has been directed at supporting the complications of liver injury (i.e., hypoglycemia, hyperammonemia) and at reducing intracranial hypertension. With these general supportive measures in a modern ICU setting, mortality in Reye's syndrome is generally less than 30%. Therapies at the cellular level specific for reversing or shortening of time of injury are only presently being developed as animal models are developed, and thus supportive guidelines comprise the major treatment modalities.

Routine care for all patients with Reye's syndrome includes the following general guidelines:

1. All patients should be closely monitored with frequent neurologic evaluations. Pulse oximetry is important, as are daily weights and strict input and output recording, and children should be kept NPO. Generally, patients are kept partially fluid-restricted to three-fourths maintenance rates, after correcting for dehydration. Nonhypotonic fluids should be used.
2. Elevated ammonia levels. Lactulose is given via a nasogastric tube with 0.5 g/kg given every hour until stooling occurs, then 0.25

mg every 6 hours. Neomycin is also frequently added. Exogenous protein sources are initially withheld.

3. Hypoglycemia. Treatment is based on giving enough IV dextrose to maintain serum glucose greater than 80 mg%. This may mean giving high dextrose solutions via a central line in patients who are volume-restricted.
4. Prolonged prothrombin time. Vitamin K is given as a slow IV dose of 0.1 mg/kg, usually daily or twice daily. For problems with clinical bleeding, fresh frozen plasma blood transfusions are needed, and cryoprecipitate as needed should be given.
5. Laboratory monitoring includes frequent assessment of glucose, serum electrolytes and osmolarity, serum ammonia, liver function studies, BUN, creatinine, CBC, and coagulation studies. Less frequent studies may include calcium, phosphorus, magnesium, amylase, cultures, and chest radiographs. Liver biopsy may be indicated in most patients because of the low incidence of Reye's syndrome.

As encephalopathy worsens, treatment becomes more directed at reducing intracranial hypertension and maintaining normal cerebral perfusion pressure (CPP), hopefully preserving neurologic function. Once a patient develops stage II encephalopathy (see Table 33-4), hyperosmolar therapy is usually instituted by giving mannitol, 0.25 to 0.5 g/kg intravenously every 4 to 6 hours, either as bolus therapy or as a continuous infusion. Serum osmolality is maintained at 300 to 315 mosm/liter. An arterial catheter and/or a central venous catheter is also recommended.

Once a patient has reached stage III or greater encephalopathy, she should be anesthetized (usually with thiopental and a muscle relaxant) and intubated. A CT scan should be performed, if not already done, and a mechanism for measuring intracranial pressure (ICP) should be employed. This can be done by using an intraventricular catheter, a subdural bolt, or fiberoptic transducer. It is important to keep cerebral perfusion (CPP = mean arterial BP − ICP) above 50 torr. One study has shown that outcome in children with Reye's syndrome did not correlate with ICP levels but did correlate to minimum CPP levels, with poor outcomes in children having a minimum CPP of 31.5.[25]

General therapy in these higher stages of encephalopathy includes the previously mentioned guidelines, along with therapy to control ICP, thus maintaining CPP in a normal range. The basics for controlling ICP include the following (This is discussed in detail in Pathophysiology of Intracranial Emergencies by Brogan, Geiduschek, and Krane, this volume.):

1. Positioning the patient midline, head elevated approximately 15 to 30 degrees
2. Hyperventilation to $PaCO_2$ of 25 to 30 mm Hg
3. Hyperosmolar therapy to maintain osmoles in the 310 to 315 mosm/liter range. This is done using mannitol, 0.25 to 0.5 g/kg every 4 to 6 hours as needed, and furosemide, 1 mg/kg to aid in restricting free water.
4. Maintain normothermia (avoid hyperthermia and significant hypothermia) and normovolemia, monitoring fluid balance closely.
5. Maintain sedation and avoid excessive stimulation. ET suctioning, venipuncture, NG tube placement, and so on, should be preceded by sedation, mannitol, and/or lidocaine (1 mg/kg).
6. Positive end-expiratory pressure should be kept at the minimal levels needed to ensure oxygenation without excessive FiO_2.
7. Vasodilators should be avoided.

8. Prophylactic anticonvulsant therapy should be considered, or if seizures do occur, they need to be treated aggressively.

9. Muscle relaxation helps reduce ICP, but precludes ongoing neurologic assessment. It is important for patients who are refractory to other therapeutic measures and for those with dyssynchronized breathing. When it is used, continuous EEG monitoring is advised, along with the use of sedation.

If CPP becomes less than 50 mm Hg, with normal ICP pressure levels (<15–20 mm Hg), crystalloid may be given to ensure normovolemia or an inotropic agent started to increase systemic BP. If ICP rises to greater than 20 mm Hg, mannitol and lasix should be given, after ensuring that the previously mentioned basics are being maintained. If mannitol has been maximized, or serum osmoles are greater than 320 mosm/liter, barbiturate therapy is advised for treating the increased ICP. Thiopentone as a 1- to 4-mg/kg bolus may be tried to evaluate for a beneficial response, and then thiopentone as a drip (2–10 mg/kg/hr) or pentobarbital (4–10 mg/kg load with 1–3-mg/kg/hour drip) may be used.

Barbiturate therapy may cause systemic hypotension, reducing systemic BP, and thus normovolemia should be maintained and inotropic support may be needed. Cardiac output monitoring may be helpful in these circumstances. Normal pentobarbital levels are 2.5 to 4.0 mg/dl, but occasionally higher levels are needed. Extreme caution is needed to maintain cardiovascular integrity at the higher levels.

Once the patient has maintained stability (normal CPP and ICP levels), the therapy can gradually be reduced, starting with the barbiturates, if used, and then progressing to reductions in mannitol, hyperventilation, and sedation.

Outcome

Mortality from Reye's syndrome is usually less than 20%, with fatalities most commonly occurring in children with stages IV and V encephalopathy.[25,26] Usually these patients have severe intracranial swelling and brain injury, even though the biochemical and pathologic abnormalities resolve quickly.

Arterial-venous difference of oxygen saturation (AVD$_{O_2}$), as measured by a catheter placed at the jugular bulb, appears to be of benefit in determining severe CNS insult and thus prognosis. In children with Reye's syndrome who do poorly, there is an ongoing decreased oxygen extraction as measured by AVD$_{O_2}$, despite normal or above-normal cerebral blood flow.[27,28] This decreased oxygen extraction is indicative of severe cellular CNS injury, both in Reye's syndrome and other widespread CNS injuries. Children who do improve neurologically have daily improvements in their arterial-jugular AVD$_{O_2}$, indicative of better cellular extraction of oxygen and thus better cellular integrity.

Although most children with Reye's syndrome survive, there may be ongoing morbidity. The majority of children appear to recover with relatively normal neurologic function, although a small number may have severe dysfunction. A study by Quart et al. indicated that there appears to be significant short- and long-term memory impairment in children recovered from Reye's syndrome.[29] An earlier study demonstrated deficits in measured intelligence, concept formation, visual-motor integration, and sequencing in children following Reye's syndrome.[30] All of these areas affect school performance, and there appears to be an association between the severity of encephalopathy and behavioral outcome.[31] Finally, there may be an increased incidence of vocal cord paralysis and absent laryngeal sensation as a sequelae to Reye's syndrome, thus putting these children at risk for aspiration.[32]

References

1. Brown JK, Imam H. Interrelationships of liver and brain with special reference to Reye Syndrome. *J Inherited Metab Dis* 14:436–458, 1991.
2. Glasgow JFT, Moore R. Current concepts in Reye's syndrome. *Br J Hosp Med* 50:599–604, 1993.
3. Reye RDK, Morgan G, Baral J. Encephalopathy and fatty degeneration of the viscera: A disease entity in childhood. *Lancet* 2:749–752, 1963.
4. Johnson GN, Scurletis TD, Carroll NG. A study of 16 fetal cases of encephalitis-like disease in North Carolina children. *NC Med J* 24:464–473, 1963
5. Hurwitz ES. The changing epidemiology of Reye's Syndrome in the United States: Further evidence for a public health success: *JAMA* 260:3178–3180, 1988.
6. Hurwitz ES et al. National surveillance for Reye syndrome: A five year review. *Pediatrics* 70:895–900, 1982.
7. Barrett MG et al. Changing epidemiology of Reye syndrome in the United States. *Pediatrics* 77:598–602, 1986.
8. Waldman RJ et al. Aspirin as a risk factor in Reye syndrome. *JAMA* 247:3089–3094, 1982.
9. Starko JM et al. Reye's syndrome and salicylate use. *Pediatrics* 66:859–864, 1980.
10. Young RSK et al. Reye's syndrome associated with long term aspirin therapy. *JAMA* 251:754–756, 1984.
11. Rennebohm RN et al. Reye's syndrome in children on salicylate therapy for connective tissue disease. *JAMA* 107:877–880, 1985.
12. White JM. Reye's syndrome and salicylates (letter). *N Engl J Med* 314:920, 1986.
13. Chu AB et al. Reye's syndrome: Salicylate metabolism, viral antibody level and other factors in surviving patients and unaffected family members. *Am J Dis Child* 140:1005–1012, 1986.
14. Partin JS et al. Serum salicylate concentration in Reye's disease. *Lancet* i:191–194, 1982.
15. Kang ES, Crocker JFS, Johnson GM. Reye's syndrome and salicylates (letter). *N Engl J Med* 314:920–921, 1986.
16. Kilpatrick-Smith L, Hale DE, Douglas SD. Progress in Reye syndrome: Epidemiology, biochemical mechanisms, and animal models. *Dig Dis Sci* 7:135–146, 1989.
17. Cooperstock MS, Tucker RP, Baubles JV. Possible pathogenic role of endotoxin in Reye's syndrome. *Lancet* i:1272–1274, 1975.
18. Kirn A, Gut J, Gendrault J. Interactions of viruses with sinusoidal cells. *Prog Liver Dis* 7:377–392, 1982.
19. Heubi JE et al. Reye's syndrome: Current concepts. *Hepatology* 7:155–164, 1987.
20. Yoder MC et al. Plasma fibronectin deficiency in Reye syndrome. *J Pediatr* 105:436–438, 1984.
21. Yoder MC et al. Metabolic and mitochondrial orphological changes that mimic Reye syndrome after endotoxin administration to rats. *Infect Immun* 47:329–331, 1985.
22. Kilpatrick-Smith L et al. Endotoxin-induced changes in nitrogen metabolism. *Res Commun Chem Pathol Pharmacol* 53:381–398, 1986.
23. Kilpatrick-Smith L et al. Effects of sublethal doses of endotoxin and aspirin on rat hepatic energy metabolism: An animal model of Reye syndrome. *Pediatr Res* 21:343A, 1987.
24. Larrick JW, Kunkel SL. Is Reye's syndrome caused by augmented release of tumor necrosis factor? *Lancet* ii:132–133, 1986.
25. Jenkins JG et al. Reye's syndrome: Assessment of intracranial monitoring. *Br Med J* 294:337–338, 1987.
26. Chi CS et al. Continuous monitoring of intracranial pressure in Reye's syndrome—5 year experience. *Acta Paediatr Jpn* 32:426–434, 1990.
27. Frewen TC, Kisson N. Cerebral blood flow and brain oxygen extraction in Reye syndrome. *J Pediatr* 110:903–905, 1987.
28. Swedland D et al. Cerebral oxygen extraction in Reye syndrome. *Crit Care Med* 10:205, 1982.

29. Quart EJ, Buchtel HA, Sarnaik AP. Long lasting memory deficits in children recovered from Reye's syndrome. *J Clin Exp Neuropsychol* 10:409–420, 1988.

30. Brunner RL et al. Neuropsychologic consequences of Reye's syndrome. *J Pediatr* 95:706, 1979.

31. Rockoff MA, Pascucci RC. Reye's syndrome. *Emerg Med Clin North Am* 1:87–101, 1983.

32. Thompson JW, Rosenthal P, Camilon FS Jr. Vocal cord paralysis and superior laryngeal nerve dysfunction in Reye's syndrome. *Arch Otolaryngol* 116:46–48, 1990.

I. David Todres

34 ◆ Brain Death

The first report of brain death appeared in 1959.[1] French physicians described a condition referred to as "coma dépassé"—a state beyond coma. In 1968, an ad hoc committee of the Harvard Medical School published a report that listed criteria that needed to be satisfied in the diagnosis of "brain death."[2] The term used by the committee to define the condition of brain death was *irreversible coma*, a potentially confusing term, as this state is usually applied to a patient in a vegetative condition. The Harvard criteria consisted of the following requirements: (1) unreceptivity and unresponsivity, (2) no movements, (3) no elicitable reflexes, (4) apnea, and (5) isoelectric electroencephalogram (EEG). All the tests needed to be repeated 24 hours later, with no changes noted. The committee proposed this clinical state to be one of death—a new concept in light of the technology now available to support respiration and circulation.

The Harvard criteria were incorrect in one diagnostic aspect, namely that spinal reflexes might still persist even in the presence of **whole brain** death. The Harvard criteria's recommendation for an electroencephalographic determination of electrocerebral

silence as being of great confirmatory value has been a subject of debate as to its necessity in the determination of whole brain death. In this regard it is noteworthy that Beecher, who chaired the ad hoc committee later, stated that the committee was unanimous in its belief that an EEG was not essential to a diagnosis of irreversible coma but could provide "valuable supporting data."[3] The Harvard Criteria, with the exception of spinal reflexes, were demonstrated to be accurate and were widely adopted. Over the following years, the criteria have stood the test of time. Support for this concept and the criteria in its establishment came from the President's Commission report in 1981 and 1982.[4,5] Minor changes have been introduced, particularly relating to the observation period, which has been reduced.[6–9] A task force has established guidelines for the determination of brain death in children, and this has assisted the pediatric intensivist in clarifying the criteria required for the determination of brain death at all ages.[10] (Table 34-1). Brain death in the pediatric patient can be seen from a number of perspectives. A recent paper by Farrell and Levin reviews well the historical, sociological, medical, religious, cultural, legal, and ethical considerations.[11]

Clinical Diagnosis

With the advent of artificial methods to support circulation and respiration, it became necessary to develop a new means of diagnosing death. Capron has stated that there is a "misperception that what is involved is a 'redefinition' of human death, when all that is actually involved is a reformulation of the standards for measuring death."[12] The extent of the problem may be gauged from a number of published reports, indicating an overall incidence of 2% of admissions to pediatric ICUs will be declared "brain dead."[13–15]

The first step in the diagnosis of brain death is to **identify a causative proximal agent** appropriately responsible for the clinical state the child presents. It should also be determined that this state is **not** reversible. The major cause of brain death is the result of a hypoxic insult to the brain.[16] This may arise from breathing a hypoxic mixture (e.g., near-drowning, smoke inhalation) or follow failure of the cerebral circulation to deliver required oxygen for metabolism (e.g., following cardiac arrest). Insults to the brain, such as infection (e.g., meningitis), may cause loss of brain stem reflexes but leave cortical function intact and be associated with complete recovery. Metabolic causes (e.g., overdose of barbiturates) may also be reversible. A clear history of the events leading to a state suggestive of brain death is critical in order to determine the proximate cause of the coma.

Interpretation of the clinical examination may be affected by drugs such as sedatives or neuromuscular blocking drugs employed to help control ventilation. Thus the presence of these drugs must be excluded. In the case of sedatives, laboratory testing will reveal their presence, and measurement of blood levels of these agents will assist in clarifying whether the drug is significantly contributing to the coma status noted on clinical examination.

For the diagnosis of brain death, the whole brain (i.e., cortical and brain stem) is evaluated. In examination for the presence or absence of brain stem reflexes, the absence of spontaneous

Table 34-1. Guidelines for the determination of brain death in children

History

Determination of proximate cause of coma to ensure absence of remediable or reversible conditions (exclude toxic and metabolic disorders, sedatives or hypnotic drugs, paralytic agents, hypothermia, hypotension, and surgically remediable conditions).

Physical examination criteria
1. Coma and apnea
2. Absence of brain stem function
   a. Midposition or fully dilated pupils (exclude drugs)
   b. Absence of spontaneous, oculocephalic ("doll's eye") and caloric (oculovestibular) indirect eye movements
   c. Absence of movement of bulbar musculature and corneal, gag, cough, sucking, and rooting reflexes
   d. Absence of spontaneous respiratory movements (apnea) with standardized testing
3. Patient must not be hypothermic or hypotensive
4. Flaccid tone and absence of spontaneous or induced movements, excluding spinal cord–medicated reflexes
5. Examination should remain consistent for brain death throughout observation period testing

Observation period according to age

7 d–2 mo: Two examinations and EEGs 48 hours apart

2 mo–1 yr: Two examinations and EEGs 24 hours apart. A repeat examination and EEG are unnecessary if a radionuclide angiogram shows no cerebral blood flow.

Over 1 yr: Two examinations 12–24 hours apart. Laboratory testing (EEG, cerebral blood flow studies) is not required. However, observation period may be reduced if EEG shows electrocerebral silence or radionuclide studies demonstrate no cerebral blood flow.

Adapted from Task Force for the Determination of Brain Death in Children. Guidelines for Determination of Brain Death in Children. *Ann Neurol* 21:616, 1987; *Arch Neurol* 44:587, 1987; *Neurology* 37:1077, 1987; *Pediatr Neurol* 3:242, 1987; *Pediatrics* 80:298; 1987. With permission.

respiratory movements (i.e., apnea) is probably the most critical. Testing for apnea should be carried out using standardized tests.[17,18] The patient is removed from the ventilator, with the arterial PCO_2 at normocarbic levels (i.e., 36–44 mm Hg), and carbon dioxide is allowed to accumulate while close observation is made for the appearance of any spontaneous ventilations. Blood gas samples are drawn, and the $PaCO_2$ is determined. When the $PaCO_2$ reaches 55 mm Hg (a rise of ± 2.5 mm Hg/min is expected) and no spontaneous respirations have resumed, apnea has been adequately demonstrated. To sustain vital functions during the test, the patient is preoxygenated for 5 minutes with 100% oxygen, and oxygen is then insufflated (8–12 liters/min) via a tracheal cannula through the endotracheal tube. This provides diffusion oxygenation and will generally maintain a stable hemodynamic state. Should there be significant changes in heart rate, BP, or oxygen desaturation (measured with a pulse oximeter), however, the apnea test procedure must be terminated. Diabetes insipidus due to insufficient antidiuretic hormone production and release was noted in 14 of 16 brain dead children.[19] However, a study by Fackler et al. noted that diabetes insipidus was not a useful clinical sign of brain death.[20]

Ancillary Tests

Ancillary laboratory tests are required to establish the presence of brain death when the clinical history is uncertain, in which case the clinical examination alone may not suffice. The tests that are considered the most dependable are the EEG and the cerebral blood flow (CBF) studies.

The Electroencephalogram

The appropriateness of the EEG in confirming the clinical diagnosis of brain death is generally accepted in the United States but is considered nonessential in Great Britain. The EEG must be considered with the criteria of establishing the proximate cause, to ensure the absence of reversible conditions, and the physical examination of the patient. The EEG must not be considered as a diagnostic tool on its own (i.e., the sole determinant of brain death).[21]

Interpretation of the EEG for a diagnosis of electrocerebral silence (ECS) or electrocerebral inactivity (ECI) is fraught with technical difficulties. There are no official guidelines for recording ECS in pediatric patients. Guidelines established for adults are difficult to apply to the young child. For example, interelectrode distance should be 10 cm or more—a situation that is impractical because of the infant's small head size. Artifacts may make the tracing unsatisfactory for diagnostic purposes, particularly those due to the respirator. The pediatric EEG requires greater technical and interpretive expertise than that required for the adult EEG.

Hypotension and hypothermia are two important clinical states that may affect the true interpretation of brain death, both from a clinical diagnostic point of view as well as the EEG. The core body temperature that produces ECS is unknown. Arbitrarily, a core temperature of 32.2°C must be reached to validate the EEG interpretation. The degree of hypotension that correlates with ECS is also unknown. Large doses of sedatives and hypnotics may cause ECS. Barbiturates are employed in the management of intracranial hypertension (increased intracranial pressure) and status epilepticus. The precise levels at which barbiturates cease to produce ECS is unknown—thus the practice of validating ECS only in

the presence of subtherapeutic levels of those agents or confirming suspected brain death with radionuclide brain blood flow studies.

Studies of brain death by Alvarez et al. and Moshé et al. in pediatric patients demonstrated that clinical criteria as used in adults could be applied to children above 3 months of age. In addition, it was stated that a single EEG demonstrating ECS was sufficient to confirm brain death.[22,23] The EEG may not correlate with the neurologic examination or CBF studies. Studies have confirmed the finding of clinically diagnosed brain death with persistence of some activity on the EEG.[24] Thus its limitations must be appreciated.

Cerebral Blood Flow Studies

Intravenous (IV) radionuclide cerebral angiography is now a well-established confirmatory test for brain death in children. Arrest of the carotid circulation at the base of the skull and unequivocal absence of intracranial arterial circulation imply death of the whole brain. Some authors have stated that this test is a valid diagnostic procedure for infants and even neonates. In the absence of CBF, Goodman and others have stated that no further testing is required.[25,26] Still others recommend an EEG, even when the radionuclide study shows no flow.

The advantage of radionuclide imaging studies is that the procedure may be performed at the bedside—a critical issue because the patient is usually in an ICU with maximal therapy to support the brain pending the diagnostic evaluation by the scan. Four-vessel angiography is an alternate method but is more complex to perform and has been superseded by IV radionuclide imaging studies. According to Schwartz and others, incorrect identification of brain death by radioimaging is not unknown.[27,28] Not infrequently, with this technique one may demonstrate no flow through the carotid arteries but some minimal flow through the vertebral arteries. The absence of cerebral perfusion using the technique of radionuclide angiography is valuable confirmatory evidence of cerebral death.

Observation Periods

The Task Force proposed three sets of guidelines for the observation period and the use of ancillary testing to confirm the state of brain death. These guidelines were set according to the child's age: (1) For children 7 days to 2 months, two EEGs are recommended 48 hours apart. The cut-off of 2 months is arbitrary, and Alvarez et al. have used 3 months as a cut-off period because the EEG generally acquires the characteristic childhood pattern at this age. Prior to this time the EEG closely resembles the neonate pattern. (2) For children 2 months to 1 year, an observation period of 24 hours was recommended, with a repeat EEG at the end of this period. (3) For children over 1 year, confirmatory ancillary testing was not required. The observation period recommended was 12 hours. A period of 24 hours was recommended when the child was thought to have suffered a hypoxemic-ischemic encephalopathy condition in which it is difficult to assess the extent and reversibility of brain damage.

Some commentators have pointed to what they consider shortcomings in the guidelines, particularly with reference to the observation periods recommended. Fackler et al. reviewed the findings in 47 brain dead children and found that the criteria (observation periods and laboratory data) to establish brain death were uniform in children aged 2 months to 5 years of age.[20] Freeman and Ferry have stated, "In view of the lack of supporting evidence, it is difficult to understand the rationale for these proposed time and ancillary testing requirements."[29] Shewmon has stated that "neither 24 to 48 hours of absent brainstem reflexes, nor electrocerebral silence, nor absence of supratentorial blood flow establishes irreversibility of brainstem nonfunction: thus, they do not establish brain death."[30]

Physicians' Attitudes toward the Concept of Brain Death

Lynch and Eldadah undertook a questionnaire survey of pediatric intensivists and explored the practice of clinical determination of brain death and the use of confirmatory studies of the physicians involved in the determination and the reevaluation intervals.[31] The survey revealed that all intensivists found a positive apnea test, absent corneal reflexes, fixed and dilated pupils, and no motor response to pain to be reliable signs of brain death. The confirmatory tests most routinely used were radionuclide cerebral flow scan and EEG. The majority surveyed (80%) considered it necessary to have more than one physician make the determination, and that a neurospecialist should be included. In addition, most physicians (77%) stated that a second clinical examination was required within 12 to 24 hours.

Although the medical and legal definitions of death based on brain determination measurements are identical, there remains much confusion in the minds of the health care profession. To illustrate this, we recently undertook a questionnaire study illustrated by a case in which a young child (9 years old) was struck by a motor vehicle and sustained severe head injuries.[32] The child presented with a Glasgow Coma Score of 3, fixed dilated pupils, and absent corneal, oculocephalic, oculovestibular, cough, and gag reflexes. A subdural bolt pressure of 60 cm H_2O, with cerebral perfusion pressure of 20, was recorded for four hours. The patient's clinical examination was consistent with whole brain death. Medical treatment included "pentobarbital coma." Because the pentobarbital therapy could potentially affect the clinical evaluation of brain death, however, a radionuclide scan was performed. The procedure demonstrated absent CBF.

The questionnaire was mailed to 45 pediatric ICUs. The response was 96%. When asked if they would diagnose brain death with the aforementioned findings, 82% of neurologists and 73% of pediatric intensivists indicated that they would. However, only 17% of neurologists and 56% of pediatric intensivists would declare the patient brain dead when specifically asked to consider the medicolegal aspects of the case. Thus, despite guidelines published in 1987 by a task force endorsed by both medical and legal societies, inconsistencies in the interpretation of brain death continue to exist among physicians. With this disparity among physicians in their comprehension of brain death, it is not surprising that this concept of death is confusing to the public. As noted by Annas, there is also no meaningful distinction between "medical death" and "legal death." A "brain death" pronouncement can be made in the absence of a statute because this practice has been accepted by the medical community and the courts.[33]

References

1. Mollaret P, Goulan M. Lé coma dépassé (mémoire préliminaire). *Rev Neurol (Paris)* 101:3, 1959.
2. Ad Hoc Committee of the Harvard Medical School to Examine the Definition of Brain Death. A definition of irreversible coma. *JAMA* 205:85, 1968.
3. Beecher HK. After the "definition of irreversible coma." *N Engl J Med* 281:1070, 1969.
4. President's Commission for the Study of Ethical Problems in Medicine and Biomedical and Behavioral Research. Defining death. Washington, DC: Government Printing Office, 1981.
5. President's Commission for the Study of Ethical Problems in Medicine and Biomedical and Behavioral Research. Guidelines for the determination of death. *Neurology* 32:395, 1982.
6. Ad Hoc Committee on Brain Death, The Children's Hospital, Boston. Determination of brain death. *J Pediatr* 110:15, 1987.
7. Ashwal S, Schneider S. Brain death in children: Part I. *Pediatr Neurol* 3:5, 1987.
8. Ashwal S, Schneider S. Brain death in children: Part II. *Pediatr Neurol* 3:69, 1987.
9. Ad Hoc Committee on Brain Death, The Children's Hospital, Boston. Determination of brain death. *J Pediatr* 110:15, 1987.
10. Task Force for the Determination of Brain Death in Children. Guidelines for the determination of brain death in children. *Ann Neurol* 21:616, 1987; *Arch Neurol* 44:587, 1987; *Neurology* 37:1077, 1987; *Pediatr Neurol* 3:242, 1987; *Pediatrics* 80:298, 1987.
11. Farrell MM, Levin DL. Brain death in the pediatric patient: Historical, sociological, medical, religious, cultural, legal and ethical consideration. *Crit Care Med* 21:1951, 1993.
12. Capron AM. The legal status of brain-based determination of death. In Kaufman HH (ed): *Pediatric Brain Death and Organ/Tissue Retrieval.* New York: Plenum, 1989.
13. Black P, Todres ID. Brain death in children. Guidelines and experiences at the Massachusetts General Hospital in pediatric brain death. In Kaufman HH (ed): *Pediatric Brain Death and Organ/Tissue Retrieval.* New York: Plenum, 1989.
14. Edmonds JF, Wong SN. Pediatric brain death and organ transplantation. In Kaufman HH (ed): *Pediatric Brain Death and Organ/Tissue Retrieval.* New York: Plenum, 1989.
15. Bruce D. Brain death in children: The Philadelphia experience. In Kaufman HH (ed): *Pediatric Brain Death and Organ/Tissue Retrieval.* New York: Plenum, 1989.
16. Edmonds JF, Wong SN. Pediatric brain death and organ transplantation. In Kaufman HH (ed): *Pediatric Brain Death and Organ/Tissue Retrieval.* New York: Plenum, 1989.
17. Outwater KM, Rockoff MA. Apnea testing to confirm brain death in children. *Crit Care Med* 12:357, 1984.
18. Rowland TW, Donnelly JH, Jackson AH. Documentation for determination of brain death in children. *Pediatrics* 74:505, 1984.
19. Outwater KM, Rockoff MA. Diabetes insipidus accompanying brain death in children. *Neurology* 34:1243, 1984.
20. Fackler JC, Troncoso JC, Bivoa FR. Age-specific characteristics of brain death in children. *Am J Dis Child* 142:999, 1988.
21. Schneider S. Usefulness of EEG in the evaluation of brain death in children: The cons. *Electroencephalog Clin Neurophysiol* 73:276, 1989.
22. Alvarez LA et al. EEG and brain death determination in children. *Neurology* 38:227, 1988.
23. Moshé SL, Alvarez LA, Davidoff BA. Role of EEG in brain death determination in children. In Kaufman HH (ed): *Pediatric Brain Death and Organ/Tissue Retrieval.* New York: Plenum, 1989.
24. Grigg MM et al. Electroencephalographic activity after brain death. *Arch Neurol* 44:948, 1987.
25. Goodman JM, Heck LL. Confirmation of brain death at bedside by isotope angiography. *JAMA* 238:966, 1977.
26. Goodman JM, Heck LL, Moore BD. Confirmation of brain death with portable isotope angiography: A review of 204 consecutive cases. *Neurosurgery* 16:492, 1985.
27. Schwartz JA, Baxter J, Brill DR. Diagnosis of brain death in children by radionuclide cerebral imaging. *Pediatrics* 73:14, 1984.
28. Schwartz JA, Brill D, Baxter J. Detection of blood flow to the brain

by radionuclide cerebral imaging. In Kaufman HH (ed): *Pediatric Brain Death and Organ/Tissue Retrieval*. New York: Plenum, 1989.

29. Freeman JM, Ferry PC. New brain death guidelines in children: Further confusion. *Pediatrics* 81:301, 1988.

30. Shewmon DA. Commentary on guidelines for the determination of brain death in children. *Ann Neurol* 24:789, 1988.

31. Lynch J, Eldadah MK. Brain-death criteria currently used by pediatric intensivists. *Clin Pediatr* 31:456, 1992.

32. Castillo L, Todres ID. Inconsistencies in the diagnosis of brain death in children (abstract). American Academy of Pediatrics (Section on Critical Care Medicine), San Francisco, CA, October, 1992.

33. Annas GJ. *Judging Medicine*. Clifton, NJ: Humana, 1988. P 368.

Brenda Stewart **34.1**   **Consideration of Organ and Tissue Donation**

It is essential that health care professionals give consideration to organ and tissue donation from every critically ill patient diagnosed with a fatal brain injury wherein the criteria for brain death could be fulfilled. Tissue donation should be considered following the death of all patients. Organs that may be donated for life-saving transplantation include the heart, lungs, liver, kidneys, pancreas, and small bowel. Tissues that provide life-enhancing benefit to their recipients include corneas, heart valves, bone, saphenous vein, and skin. The benefits of donation for potential transplant recipients are obvious. Equally significant is the value of offering the option of donation as a source of comfort to the dying patient's family. Families who have consented to donation have reported that their grief was eased by the donation.[1] The donation process can allow families to participate in their loved ones' end-of-life decisions, it helps them to acknowledge the death, and it provides a sense of peace and consolation through altruistic giving.

The success of organ transplantation for the treatment of end-organ failure has contributed to the steady increase in the number of patients awaiting this life-saving therapy. As of February 28, 1995, the number of patients waiting for organ transplant in the United States was 38,364. Pediatric candidates constitute 1,375 of the total number waiting, with a diverse breakdown according to age and organ needed (Table 34.1-1).[2] A new name is added to the national waiting list approximately every 20 minutes, while every day between eight to ten people die before an organ becomes available for them. This tragic reality is caused primarily by the insufficient availability of donor organs.

The 1993 Gallup poll, "The American Public's Attitudes toward Organ Donation and Transplantation," has shown overwhelming public support of this process. Donation of organs for transplantation was supported by 85% of the respondents, with 90% strongly agreeing that organ donation allowed something positive to come out of a person's death.[3] Given these results, it is surprising that organ recovery efforts in the United States are only between 37% to 59% efficient.[4] The number of organ donors has remained relatively constant, at approximately 4,500 per year, despite many efforts to increase this yield. To maximize the number of families comforted by donation and the number of recipients benefitted, it is essential to address limiting factors that are within our control.

It is important to establish a clear mechanism of identification and referral of potential donors by hospital staff; without this step the process cannot begin. Anyone on the health care team, including but not limited to physicians, nurses, social workers, or pastoral caregivers, is encouraged to consider donation when caring for a patient whose prognosis is terminal and irreversible. Often, the responsibility for contacting the local organ procurement organization (OPO) rests on the intensive care unit (ICU) intensivist or primary nurse due to their close association with the medical details of the case and the family. It is best to initiate contact with the OPO as early as possible, even in advance of the anticipated declaration of brain death, to discuss donor suitability and plan a coordinated team approach to donation.

The donor criteria are intentionally broad to prevent inappropriate exclusion of patients. They are also constantly evolving as management practices and surgical techniques are perfected. The OPO staff is aware of the most current donation policies, experienced in the process, and available 24 hours a day. This is why discussion on a case-by-case basis is encouraged. Early contact with the OPO does not initiate an immediate on-site visit by the donation coordinator (DC) or family contact with them unless it is warranted and requested by the hospital. This team approach allows for more effective management of any obstacles to donation, such as offering donation to families of patients who are not suitable donors and then having to withdraw the option from them, as well as excessive delays for families waiting to speak with the DC. Minimizing the family's distress is always the focus of care.[5]

Many cases referred for donation fall under the jurisdiction of the local medical examiner's office due to the circumstance of death. On these cases, permission for donation must be obtained from the medical examiner in order to proceed. A recent nationwide survey of OPOs indicated that from 1990 to 1992 there was a relative increase by 65% in the number of cases in which donation

Table 34.1-1. Pediatric candidates waiting, by age and organ, as of 2/28/95

Age	Kidney	Liver	Pancreas	Kidney/ pancreas	Intestine	Heart	Heart/lung	Lung	Total
0–5 yr	62	284	7	10	39	72	8	10	492
6–10 yr	97	104	2	1	6	18	12	17	257
11–17 yr	314	136	8	1	8	50	21	88	626
TOTAL	473	524	17	12	53	140	41	115	1375

Data from the United Network for Organ Sharing, research department.

was denied by the medical examiner or coroner. Denial for donation was reported highest in cases involving child abuse and gunshot wound to the head. There are, however, variations across the country, with some regions reporting few to no medical examiner denials and some reporting a high degree of restriction. The OPOs who report having favorable working relationships with their local medical examiner's office have the greatest likelihood of success surrounding these delicate negotiations. Their successful models include having protocols established that support the medical examiner's need for identification, preservation, collection, and documentation of evidence.[6] For these reasons, including the OPO staff in discussions with the medical examiner is recommended.

Sensitivity toward the needs of the donor family and their comfort with consent for donation are the highest priorities for the coordinator. Referrals that are determined to be suitable proceed to offering the option of donation to the family. Given each case's unique issues, the DC will collaborate with the physician and nurse regarding how best to proceed, often with their participation in the consent discussion. This discussion should occur only after brain death has been determined and the family has had adequate explanation and time to understand what this means. The donation discussion includes an informed consent of the entire process of donor evaluation and organ and tissue recovery and a detailed medical and social history of the donor. Families are encouraged to make the decision that is best for them after having a complete explanation with all of their questions answered. Following consent, most families say their good-byes and return home. This is their choice as well, and they decide whether to communicate by telephone or during the stay at the hospital.

A period of specific organ evaluation occurs next, with multiple tests and procedures to determine each organ's suitability for transplantation. The DC remains in the ICU during this time, managing the care of the donor in concert with the intensive care team. The organ recipients are determined according to the allocation process through discussion with individual transplant centers. A coordinated organ and tissue recovery in the operating room concludes this phase of the process. The OPO extends continued care to the family following the donation. One example of this is by sending a letter of acknowledgment to them several weeks after the recovery which shares information on the transplant outcomes. Organ and tissue donation is an opportunity for families to choose to give the gift of life for solace in their grief. The principle of giving in this way is based on altruism and generosity. Most families do not initiate the consideration of this voluntary process but are assisted in this by the hospital and OPO staff.[7] Our responsibility is to allow families this privilege.

References

1. National Kidney Foundation. *National Kidney Foundation Survey of Organ and Tissue Donor Families.* National Donor Family Council. October, 1993.
2. United Network for Organ Sharing. *UNOS Update.* March, 1995.
3. Gallup Organization. *The American Public's Attitudes toward Organ Donation and Transplantation.* Princeton, NJ: Gallup Organization, 1993.
4. Evans RW, Orians CE, Ascher NL. The potential supply of organ donors: An assessment of the efficiency of organ procurement efforts in the United States. *JAMA* 267:239, 1992.
5. Albert P. Overview of the donation process. *Crit Care Nurs Clin North Am* 6:553, 1994.
6. Shafer T et al. Impact of medical examiner/coroner practices on organ recovery in the United States. *JAMA* 272:1607, 1994.
7. Prottas J. *The Most Useful Gift: Altruism and the Public Policy of Organ Transplants.* San Francisco: Jossey-Bass, 1994.

V Renal Diseases

David Link

35 ▸ Fluids, Electrolytes, Acid-Base Disturbances, and Diuretics

Deranged fluid and electrolyte homeostasis commonly afflicts children in the intensive care unit (ICU). While sometimes resulting from a kidney disorder, the problems can also occur as primary derangements, as in hypernatremic dehydration or as disturbances further compounding nonrenal problems, as in the chemotherapy of solid tumors. A basis of pathophysiology is essential to applying the principles of practice and management. Extended pathophysiologic dissertation is available from standard textbooks.[1-7]

Fluid and Electrolytes

Effective circulating volume must be restored regardless of the underlying clinical insult or consequent pathophysiologic derangement so that normal cellular metabolism can proceed. Physicians must correctly interpret the laboratory results and gauge initial therapy according to volume requirements and specific metabolic needs. Mistakes can produce immediate, serious, and life-threatening complications that aggravate an already precarious condition. In the intensive care setting, a child with metabolic imbalance faces dangers ranging from seizures, renal impairment, permanent CNS insults to cardiac dysrhythmias, and shock. These events in turn threaten the cellular integrity of vital systems with temporary or irreversible injury or even death. Table 35-1 provides a classification of

Table 35-1. Classification of pediatric metabolic disturbances

Water imbalances
  Dehydration
  Water intoxication
  Hyperosmolar state

Electrolyte abnormalities
  Hypernatremia
  Hyponatremia
  Hyperkalemia
  Hypokalemia
  Hypercalcemia
  Hypocalcemia

Acid-base disturbances
  Acidosis
  Alkalosis

Disorders of carbohydrate metabolism
  Hyperglycemia
  Hypoglycemia
  Diabetic ketoacidosis
  Galactosemia

Inherited aminoacidopathy

Urea cycle abnormality

Reye's syndrome

Iatrogenic emergency
  Fluid overload (especially in renal failure)
  Hypernatremia due to sodium bicarbonate administration
  Parenteral nutrition without adequate laboratory monitoring
  Chemotheraphy with tumor lysis

common metabolic disturbances. However, especially in infants, many of these conditions present with generalized clinical findings, making differentiation difficult. These symptoms include poor feeding, failure to gain weight, persistent vomiting, weakness, lethargy, or seizures. In the absence of major trauma, the differential diagnosis of this constellation of findings includes overwhelming sepsis, circulatory failure, or metabolic crisis. Regardless of the ultimate diagnosis, initial management entails the following priorities: (1) Establish and maintain an adequate airway and ventilation, (2) restore circulatory volume, (3) draw appropriate blood samples for diagnosis of the underlying condition, (4) establish and sustain adequate urine output, and (5) correct fluid, electrolyte, and acid-base disturbances as guided by test results. Laboratory screening should include electrolytes, BUN, creatinine, pH, pCO$_2$, bicarbonate, calcium, glucose, ketones, ammonia, a complete blood count with differential, blood, and other cultures as indicated. Reserving a small sample of blood is useful in case further determinations are warranted. With intravenous (IV) access in place, BP, pulse, respiratory rate and **weight** are checked. **Change in weight is the best and most reliable indicator of volume status** (and subsequent acute changes) but is often overlooked.

The classification in Table 35-1 lists a variety of discrete disturbances. However, many clinical circumstances will combine several of those abnormalities. For example, acute renal failure due to illness (sepsis or postsurgical) often involves water intoxication, hyponatremia, hyperkalemia, hypocalcemia, or acidosis. This illustrates the complexity and interplay of metabolic disturbances arising from single-organ failure. Children with multiple-organ failure present even more complicated management challenges, necessitating very careful treatment of chemical disturbances, which may be additive in their effects (e.g., hypocalcemia and hyperkalemia) or even offset each other (e.g., severe vomiting with loss of acid and potassium in the face of severe renal failure, which generates acidosis and hyperkalemia).

The appendix at the end of the chapter summarizes the fluid and electrolyte needs in specific medical conditions.

Water Imbalances

Dehydration

The loss of water and electrolytes defines dehydration. Although gastroenteritis is a common childhood illness, patients with symptoms severe enough to be admitted to the ICU have 10% or greater weight loss from the disease. A number of other conditions, however, may mimic gastroenteritis. In the infant or young child, amino acid disturbances and other organic acid disorders commonly present as vomiting; measurement of acid-base status, glucose, ammonia, urea, and a check of the urine with a ferric chloride test may help identify the underlying problem. Formal assay of blood and urine for amino and organic acids will reveal an inborn error of metabolism.

Pathophysiology

Infants and children requiring admission to the ICU will have severe dehydration, circulatory instability, marked electrolyte im-

Table 35-2. Composition of body fluids

Source	Na^+ (mEq/liter)	K^+ (mEq/liter)	Cl^- (mEq/liter)	HCO_3 (mEq/liter)	pH	Osmolality (mosm/liter)
Gastric	50	10–15	150	0	1	300
Pancreas	140	5	50–100	100	9	300
Bile	130	5	100	40	8	300
Ileostomy	130	15–20	120	25–30	8	300
Diarrhea	50	35	40	50	Alk	
Sweat	50	5	55	0		
Blood	140	4–5	100	25	7.4	285–295
Urine	0–100*	20–100*	70–100*	0	4.5–8.5	50–1400

*Varies considerably with intake.

balance, and/or renal impairment. These children are not candidates for oral rehydration but require careful parenteral management.[8–11] Effective strategies for the management of these disorders must rest on a knowledge of normal fluid and electrolyte homeostasis.[12]

One needs to consider the normal chemical composition of body fluids that can be lost through disease or surgical manipulation in the ICU (Table 35-2). The composition of fluids should be considered when reviewing the pathophysiology of dehydration.

Water Anatomy and Distribution

There are important contrasts in water anatomy in the infant and the adult (Table 35-3). Note that extracellular fluid (ECF) constitutes a higher fraction of body weight in infants than in adults and highlights the higher (three times) body water turnover in infants, compared with adults.[13,14] Thus, dehydration is more common and more serious in children and continues to carry a higher mortality (especially in the developing world).

The net maintenance fluid requirement is approximately 1500 ml/m²/24 hr in the healthy, nonfebrile child.[15] A nomogram for calculating body surface area is shown in Fig. 35-1. The relationship between weight (kg) and body surface area is roughly linear up to about 10 kg, and one can simply estimate 100 ml/kg/24 hr as a normal fluid requirement for the first 10 kg (about the first year of life). By the time one reaches 30 kg, or roughly the weight of a 7- or 8-year-old child, body surface area is one square meter (1 m²), with a normal net maintenance requirement of 1500 ml/24 hr. The 70-kg individual has a body surface area of 1.73 m², which is the standard reference for renal functions such as glomerular filtration rate.

Table 35-3. Body water (as percentage of total body weight)

Water anatomy	Infant (%)	Adult (%)
Total body water	70–80	60
Extracellular fluid	35–45	15
Intravascular fluid	5	5
Intracellular fluid	30	40
Turnover rate Extracellular fluid	50 per 24 hr	15 per 24 hr

Clinical Cases

Clinical presentation of dehydration is best considered as isotonic (isonatremic), hypotonic (hyponatremic), and hypertonic (hypernatremic) dehydration. Three cases illustrate these different modes of presentation.

Case 1

Isotonic Dehydration, 10%. A 5-month-old girl has been ill for 3 days with diarrhea. On presentation, weight is 4.5 kg, down from 5.0 kg 1 week earlier. Laboratory results show Na 140, K 4.0, Cl 100, pH 7.10, and bicarbonate 9. Urinalysis reveals SG 1.029, pH 5, + ketones.

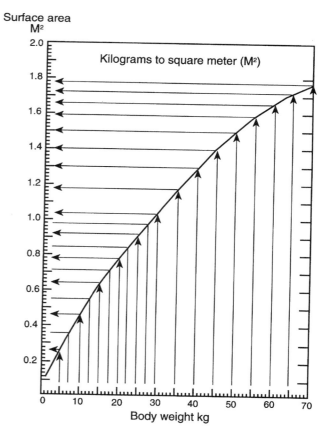

Figure 35-1. Nomogram for calculating body surface area.

Case 2

Hypertonic Dehydration, 10%. Similar clinical history as in Case 1, except the 5-month-old girl received boiled skim milk. On examination, skin turgor is reasonably good, with adequate perfusion and a temperature of 39°C. Laboratory results show Na 160, Cl 120, and K 4.5.

Case 3

Hypotonic Dehydration, 15%. A boy of the same age and weight as the girl in Case 1 is admitted for treatment of gastroenteritis. He now weighs 4.25 kg. No urine has been noted in the past 15 hours and explosive diarrhea persists. He received Kool-aid and water. BP is 40 mm Hg, skin is cool and clammy. Laboratory results include Na 125, Cl 85.

These three examples are typical of moderate-to-severe dehydration. Note that the hypotonic child has lost 15% of body weight, which accounts for the dramatic circulatory impairment (Table 35-4)

The first child, with isotonic dehydration, has experienced balanced loss of salt and water. The second child, with hypertonic dehydration, experiences principally intracellular fluid depletion with relative preservation of circulation. This allows for more severe and chronic dehydration before clinical signs are evident. The hypotonic child suffers ECF depletion with relative sparing of intracellular contents; hence, vascular compromise occurs early with signs of dehydration. In this circumstance, the intracellular environment is relatively higher in ion content than the surrounding fluid bathing cells, and water is drawn from the extracellular into the intracellular space. This imbalance further aggravates circulatory compromise, leading to the early presentation.

Although the precise quantitative losses need not be calculated, helpful general principles result from quantitative comparison of the losses. Usually, water loss in dehydration is roughly 60% extracellular and 40% intracellular. The child with hypotonic dehydration, however, has an exaggerated ECF loss, while the child with hypertonic dehydration has relative ECF sparing with much larger intracellular loss and contraction of cell volume. The child with isotonic dehydration will have nearly balanced losses of water and electrolytes, leading to a slight predominance of ECF water loss overall.

The clinical distinctions among the different forms of dehydration reflect pathophysiology and help predict clinical presentation. These presenting signs may be subtle or overt. The hypertonic child typically presents with neurologic signs. As the cells of the nervous system dehydrate, infants and children pass through stages of irritability and lethargy to coma or seizures over several days' time. Children may have a doughy skin turgor, sunken fontanel, and "neurologic" cry, and later in the illness they may be virtually unresponsive. By contrast, hypotonic dehydration presents earlier, with symptoms of circulatory impairment, incipient shock, or vascular collapse. Because the pathophysiologic derangements tend to exacerbate intravascular fluid loss, children often present sooner in the course of their illness. Their overall clinical condition is difficult to distinguish from sepsis, and workup proceeds along parallel lines for dehydration and infection. Quantitative assessment of dehydration by clinical findings is noted in Table 35-5.

Acute Fluid Resuscitation

In children who are seriously ill from dehydration, acute resuscitation proceeds in parallel with clinical and laboratory assessment. The management approach listed here is aimed at restoring circulation, minimizing the possibility of further harm to the patient from treatment, and rapidly extracting the basic qualitative and quantitative information necessary to determine which type of dehydration is occurring and how extensive the insult has become.[16]

Calculation of the patient's requirements should be carried out, and accurate intake and output flow charts must be maintained at the bedside for physicians and nurses to monitor fluid and electrolyte replacement, changes in mental status, and renal output and function. The management of the seriously dehydrated child includes the following (also Fig. 35-2):

Table 35-4. Dehydration—5-kg child: Comparison of losses

	Volume (ml)	Free H$_2$O (ml)	Na (mEq)	K (mEq)
Isotonic (10%)	500	Balanced	42	30
Hypertonic (10%)	500	300	18	12
Hypotonic 15%	750	−66	74	45

Table 35-5. Quantitative assessment of dehydration by clinical findings

	Mild	Moderate	Severe
Behavior	Normal	Irritable	Hyperirritable to lethargic
Thirst	Slight	Moderate	Intense
Mucous membrane	May be nl	Dry	Parched
Tears	Present	+/−	Absent
Ant. fontanelle	Flat	+/−	Sunken
Skin	Normal	+/−	Tenting (doughy with hyper-Na⁺)
Urinary specific gravity	Slight change	Increased	Greatly increased with oliguria

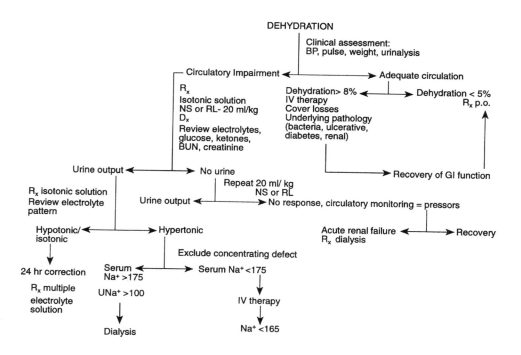

Figure 35-2. Algorithm for management of dehydration.

1. Weigh patient.

2. If shock is present or urine output is questionable, give 20 to 30 ml/kg lactated Ringers's or normal saline over 15 minutes and assess adequacy of perfusion. Repeat if circulation remains inadequate.

3. Continue to give 10 ml/kg/hr of D_5 lactated Ringer's until shock is alleviated and actual fluid and electrolyte profile can be accurately determined and appropriate replacement therapy planned.

4. Use multiple electrolyte solution with 5% dextrose for repair; rule of thumb for moderate dehydration, 2500 to 3000 ml/m²/24 hr (twice maintenance), and for severe dehydration 3500 to 4000 ml/m²/24 hr (three times maintenance).

5. If the patient is stable and dehydration is hypotonic or isotonic, give one half total calculated fluid deficit plus maintenance during the first 8 hours. The remaining half should be administered over the subsequent 16 hours.

6. If hypertonic dehydration is present, after restoring circulation, correct the deficit slowly and evenly over 48 hours while providing daily maintenance requirements.

7. Body temperature will affect fluid losses, and total maintenance needs require modification; with fever add 10% of maintenance per °C fever.

8. Ongoing fluid losses (i.e., diarrhea and vomiting) will increase fluid requirements and must be replaced.

9. Potassium supplement for the IV fluid should not occur until urine output is established or a normal serum creatinine is identified.

10. Ideally, circulation should improve promptly, BP should rise, and urine output should reach a value of at least 1.0 ml/kg/hr in response to resuscitation.

All children should be reassessed at 4 to 6 hours to ascertain that a therapeutic response has occurred. Circulation should be improved, with BP normal. Body weight may already start rising (in severely dehydrated infants and children, body weight should

be monitored twice daily), with urine output also starting to increase. For children with evident acute renal failure see Acute Renal Failure, by Herrin and Trompeter, this volume. Evidence of an endocrine cause for the electrolyte imbalance (i.e., congenital adrenal cortical hyperplasia or other adrenal abnormality) will require additional management, such as treatment with hydrocortisone or deoxycorticosterone (DOC). Proprietary multiple electrolyte solutions are generally satisfactory. However, they can cause serious complications in particular clinical settings, such as patients with renal or adrenal compromise who are at risk for potassium toxicity and life-threatening complications from the high potassium load (10 times the normal serum concentration) (Table 35-6).

Acid-base disturbance also may be ongoing and warrant treatment beyond the initial phase of resuscitation. However, aggressive treatment of acidosis with sodium bicarbonate may produce problems because of the excess sodium administered in concentrated solutions. If renal perfusion can be restored, acidosis will be far better treated by natural endogenous correction through kidney and lung rather than by treatment with alkaline solutions. Formal

Table 35-6. Instances in which multiple electrolyte solution cannot be used

Example	Reason
Infant	Excess load
Renal compromise	Excess K^+, PO_4
Acute resuscitation of dehydration	Hypotonic solution, excess K^+
Hypernatremic dehydration–acute management	Hypotonic solution, excess K^+
Hypoadrenal, Addison's disease, adrenogenital syndrome	Excess K^+
Volume expansion	Hypotonic solution

correction of metabolic acidosis is indicated only if serum bicarbonate falls below 15 mEq/liter, usually accompanied by a pH less than 7.20. Severe acidosis in an infant should trigger a search for underlying disease. Screening of blood and urine for amino and organic acid abnormalities and review for new onset ketoacidosis due to diabetes mellitus are appropriate if the anion gap is elevated.

Overhydration/Water Intoxication

Clinically important overhydration usually occurs acutely as an increase of total body water. While edema is often evident (e.g., nephrotic syndrome, congestive heart failure, acute glomerulonephritis), an increase in plasma volume may not be accompanied by evident ECF accumulation, such as in the syndrome of inappropriate antidiuretic hormone (SIADH), congenital adrenal cortical hyperplasia, or chronic renal failure.

Etiology

Circumstances leading to excess hydration, basically through too much salt intake, too much water intake, or a reduction in the excretion of either, are depicted in Table 35-7.[17] Water intoxication in a normal child is uncommon except in the setting of freshwater drowning. Normal renal function will usually cope with polydipsia and excessive IV infusion of fluids. With impaired renal function, however, the problem will be exacerbated. Furthermore, when tubular diluting function is impaired, as is seen with an ADH analog (DDAVP, as now used for the control of enuresis or hematologic disorders) or chlorpropamide, volume expansion results from the retained water.

Table 35-7. Causes of overhydration

Water excess
  Fresh water drowning
  SIADH secretion
  Psychogenic polydipsia
  Excessive intravenous infusion—D₅W

Sodium excess
  Increased intake
  Salt poisoning
  Saltwater drowning
  Undiluted infant formula concentrate
  Sodium bicarbonate, intravenous
  Intravenous albumin or plasma
  Salt tablets for athletics

Sodium retention/decreased excretion
  Acute glomerulonephritis
  Chronic renal failure
  Nephrotic syndrome
  Cirrhosis
  Congestive heart failure
  Drugs
  Vasodilators
  Nonsteroidal antiinflammatory drugs
  Mineralocorticoid

Steroid excess
  Congenital adrenal cortical hyperplasia
  Exogenous mineralocorticoids
  Cushing's syndrome
  Conn's syndrome
  Iatrogenic excess

Salt poisoning can occur when infants receive an undiluted formula concentrate or in malevolent circumstances when salt poisoning is deliberate.[18] Saltwater drowning with ingestion of large amounts of water can result in sodium intoxication. The use of large amounts of serum albumin (5% solution) or plasma causes a sodium load not immediately appreciated. In the setting of impaired renal plasma flow or tubular function, the retained sodium will obligate water retention.

Both endogenous and exogenous drugs containing steroids will lead to sodium and water retention. The most dramatic clinical circumstances are Cushing's syndrome, the variant congenital adrenal hyperplasia involving 11- or 17-hydroxylase deficiency, or hyperaldosteronism (Conn's syndrome).[19] Treatment of these patients requires measurement of a variety of glucocorticoid and mineralocorticoid hormones, and management rests ultimately on controlling and correcting the underlying disorder. Note that steroids also may be used to excess therapeutically, to the point that sodium retention develops. Obvious cases usually involve deliberate steroid abuse. However, long-term management of asthma with poor patient monitoring can result in protracted use of high-dose steroids and fluid retention.

Sodium retention due to diminished excretion occurs most commonly in children in the setting of impaired renal function, either glomerular or tubular. Overhydration results from the obligatory fluid retention, which accompanies retained sodium, and also from impaired tubular ability to excrete free water. When "effective circulating volume" is reduced, as in the nephrotic syndrome, cirrhosis, and congestive heart failure, the physiologic response is to stimulate increased production of ADH as well as angiotensin and aldosterone. All will lead to further reabsorption of sodium and water, which expand the ECF with edema formation. In acute glomerulonephritis, impaired renal plasma flow inhibits normal excretion of salt and water so that fluid retention results. The derangement of renal function in chronic renal failure impairs water balance with net fluid retention and potential volume overload. Because chronic renal failure evolves slowly, the problem usually does not present acutely. By contrast, in acute glomulonephritis, severe salt and water retention can occur very rapidly and lead to pulmonary edema requiring intensive care management.

Drugs that lead to sodium retention include the vasodilator class of antihypertensives. Minoxidil, diazoxide (usually used acutely), and nifedipine (calcium channel blocker) reduce BP sufficiently to impair sodium excretion. Nonsteroidal antiinflammatory drugs cause mild retention of sodium. When these drugs are used in patients with underlying nephrotic syndrome, cirrhosis, or congestive heart failure, the sodium retention can become sufficiently severe to augment edema substantially. Use of minoxidil for BP control in patients with renal impairment almost invariably requires the concomitant use of a loop diuretic to prevent severe fluid retention.[20] SIADH secretion is prominent as a cause of overhydration in the ICU setting.

Clinical Features

Overhydration manifests through the symptoms of an increase in total body water. Weight gain occurs by definition, but the location of the excess fluid will determine specific clinical findings. Acute fluid retention in the intravascular space will lead to pulmonary edema and hypertension, as is seen in acute glomerulonephritis. On the other hand, if the excess fluid accumulates primarily in the interstitial space, peripheral edema, ascites, and pleural effusion will become evident.

Management

The treatment for overhydration rests principally on acute measures to reduce local accumulations of fluid and, more importantly, measures aimed to curb the underlying disturbance. The general approach includes the use of diuretics, fluid restriction, and some form of dialysis (peritoneal or hemofiltration).

Immediate fluid restriction should be instituted by controlling intake at the level of insensible water loss plus urine output. Severe restriction entails a limit of 350 to 400 ml/m²/24 hr; in the anuric patient with fluid overload, this is appropriate. A more modest restriction would be set at half fluid requirement or 750 to 800 ml/m²/24 hr. If restoration of intravascular oncotic pressure is necessary to improve "effective circulating volume," infusion of albumin—either 5% or 25% as salt-poor solution—is appropriate. Great caution should be exercised not to infuse the albumin dose too rapidly, as this may mobilize fluid at an excessive pace, leading subsequently to refractory pulmonary edema. In general, 1 gm/kg of albumin is the maximum safe dose to be administered intravenously over no less than a 4-hour time span. The use of loop diuretics during the albumin infusion can be helpful in the nephrotic syndrome to promote excretion of the mobilized fluid. In patients with fluid overload due to acute renal failure or salt poisoning, dialysis helps both in fluid removal as well as in managing the metabolic disturbance. In addition to fluid restriction, sodium restriction becomes important in patients with congestive heart failure and, to a lesser extent, in those with nephrotic syndrome. In both of these groups, the addition of diuretics can help to reduce ongoing fluid retention and enhance excretion of water when mobilized by other therapies.

Sodium

Hypernatremia

Sodium acts to control and shape body water content and as such is a prime mover in body tonicity, hydration, and osmolarity. A variety of physiologic mechanisms work to maintain sodium in a normal range of 135 to 145 mEq/liter of ECF. When the sodium level exceeds 160 mEq/liter, the pathophysiologic consequences of this derangement become clinically evident. In most children, hypernatremia is due to excessive loss of free water rather than excess intake of salt[21] (Table 35-8). In infants and small children, however, excess salt may be the culprit. Neonates treated with liberal IV doses of sodium bicarbonate, infants inadvertently given salt as substitute for sugar in formula preparation (or given formula concentrate instead of a properly diluted mixture), and small children subject to malicious salt poisoning are exceptions to the generalization. It is important to note that hypernatremia does not necessarily indicate an excess of total body sodium.[22] Although the patient will be hypertonic, body weight, and therefore body water, may be decreased, resulting in hypernatremia without addition of exogenous salt. The effort to ascertain whether the patient with hypernatremia is overhydrated or dehydrated must be undertaken promptly. Management of the patient's condition hinges on whether one must add missing water (a dehydrated patient) or remove excess salt and water (overhydrated patient) to restore normal equilibrium.

With increased serum sodium, water shifts from the intracellular to the extracellular compartment, resulting in intracellular dehydration. In hypernatremic dehydration, the circulation and ECF are relatively preserved because the ionic gradient created by increased sodium draws water out of the cell into these spaces. As cells shrink, the vulnerable brain is at great risk for acute and

Table 35-8. Causes of hypernatremia in children

Loss of water in excess of sodium
  Gastroenteritis
  Inadequate fluid replacement
  Fever
  Burns
  Mechanical overventilation
  Primary CNS disease limiting water access
  Renal water loss
    Diabetic ketoacidosis
    Diabetes insipidus; central or nephrogenic
    Osmotic diuresis (glucose, mannitol, urea, x-ray contrast media)
    Postobstructive diuresis
    Concentrating defect
Excessive salt intake
  Improper mixing of infant formula
  Sodium bicarbonate therapy
  Boiled skim milk
  Salt poisoning (accidental, malicious)
  Salt tablets (for athletics, etc.)

sometimes permanent damage. If brain cell shrinkage is extensive, cerebral contents may pull away from the fixed cranial vault, resulting in tearing of blood vessels and CNS bleeding.[23] In hypernatremia with overhydration, the principal acute danger is pulmonary edema. The generalized hypervolemia also can result in increased intracranial pressure and seizures.

The diagnostic challenge of sorting out concomitant dehydration versus overhydration is important in the child's management. In the child newly admitted to the ICU, the distinction may be evident based on history and absence of underlying other diseases. This is certainly not the case in the long-term resident of the ICU who may have multisystem problems, including renal impairment and requiring mechanical ventilation, and who had received multiple medications with IV fluids running. Careful review of the patient's weight may establish volume status one way or the other. Obvious clinical findings, such as peripheral edema and ascites, will suggest overhydration, while decreased skin turgor, BP, and urine output may indicate dehydration.

Clinical Signs of Hypernatremic Dehydration

If dehydration reaches a level of 8% to 10% of body weight loss, predictable symptoms result. Shock is unusual because plasma water and circulation are relatively spared by the pathophysiology of hypernatremic dehydration. Skin turgor has a characteristic doughy feel, evident where the skin is loose over the abdomen or forehead.[22,24] The patient presents with irritability and high-pitched cry; there is unusual somnolence alternating with irritability.[25] With progression of the hypernatremia, the CNS disturbances become more evident, with increasing somnolence, seizures, and coma. As the serum sodium rises above 160 mEq/liter, irritability and tremulousness occur. With serum sodium in the range of 180 to 200 mEq/liter, the progression to coma and death is likely.

In approximately half of patients with a serum sodium above 155 mEq/liter, hyperglycemia occurs. This problem corrects spontaneously with resolution of the hypernatremia. The glucose elevation may be helpful by acting as an "osmotic umbrella" under whose protection ionic shifts can occur with gradual re-equilibration. The slow metabolism of the glucose provides a continuous release of free water and is helpful. Hypocalcemia also occurs commonly with hypernatremia and tends to resolve with treatment. Specific measures to increase serum calcium are rarely needed.

The presence of several free amino acids, the alcohol myoinositol, and other organic substances (idiogenic osmols) helps permit the equilibration of intracellular brain fluid in chronic hypernatremia. Brain water content is pulled toward normal by the presence of these osmotically active substances and is a vital neuronal adaptation. In acute hypernatremia, this corrective mechanism is impaired.

Treatment

Therapy for severe hypernatremia generally rests on one central principle: **Make haste slowly.** With the exception of acute salt poisoning, hypernatremia should be treated slowly to avoid rapid osmolar shifts. While the child with acute salt poisoning will benefit from rapid sodium removal through combined vigorous diuresis and peritoneal dialysis, infants and children who have had time to "equilibrate" at a hypernatremic level (i.e., those with dehydration, undiluted formula, diabetes insipidus) should be given 48 hours, over which serum sodium returns to normal.[26]

If serum sodium exceeds 180 mEq/liter, dialysis works far better than IV management.[27] By using a peritoneal dialysate with glucose of 1.5%, the osmolar umbrella induced by moderate hyperglycemia will permit safe reduction of serum sodium. Subsequent metabolism of the glucose leads to a gentle reduction of the hyperosmolar state slowly toward normal. With serum sodium between 155 and 175 mEq/liter, careful IV management should yield a safe outcome, barring preexisting CNS bleeding.

The approach to treatment of hypernatremic dehydration is outlined in Table 35-9. Overall, 48-hour treatment is aimed at replacing the combined fluid deficit and added maintenance but delivered at a steady rate.[28] In acute hypernatremic dehydration, hyperglycemia is common, so glucose load should be monitored to avoid excessive rises. Additionally, with calcium often low, it may be appropriate to monitor ionized calcium and provide calcium if warranted. It is mandatory to review electrolyte and acid-base status every 6 hours in the ICU while carefully following weight. Although the general scheme outlined previously usually works well, individual variation in response may dictate alterations in therapy. Typically, necessary modifications require a slowing of the pace of infusion, due to a fall in serum sodium more rapidly than expected, or more vigorous fluid replacement, because of ongoing losses which prolong the state of dehydration.

Infants and children with diabetes insipidus, especially those with disorders of thirst (the diabetes insipidus/hypodipsia patient), can be challenging to manage. Often, correction of the hypernatremia occurs more quickly than anticipated, and very careful monitoring of these children is necessary when they are given replacement vasopressin—as either parenteral DDAVP or nasal

Table 35-9. Treatment of hypernatremic dehydration

Na⁺ > 175 mEq/liter	Dialysis
Na⁺ 155–175	
Shock	5% albumin 20 ml/kg
1st hr	10–20 ml/kg RL
4 hrs	10 ml/kg RL or 0.5 NS with added NaHCO₃ (35 mEq/liter) per 4 hrs
4–48 hrs	Aim to decrease serum sodium 10 mEq/d using multiple electrolyte solution

RL, Ringer's lactate

spray preparations.[29–31] It is best to avoid use of the vasopressin in oil as delayed release will not be helpful in the acute circumstance.

Hyponatremia

Most children with hyponatremia remain asymptomatic because the drop in serum sodium is relatively small. In the sodium concentration range between 125 and 135 mEq/liter, little trouble occurs. Such a range is commonly encountered in the ICU when treating patients with large volumes of IV fluids, following relief of obstructive uropathy, during the recovery phase of meningitis, and during the course of peritoneal dialysis. Infants undergoing prolonged treatment with IV fluids also can dip into this range. In general, by appropriate upward adjustment of salt intake or mild restriction of water intake, the serum sodium can be restored to a normal range.[32]

When serum sodium falls below 120 mEq/liter, serious clinical symptoms can occur. The more rapid the fall from normal to the hyponatremic value, the more susceptible the brain will be to serious disturbance. Disorientation, seizure, or coma can occur fairly rapidly with a plunging serum sodium. A more chronic lapse into hyponatremia, typically seen in SIADH, allows brain adaptation to occur, and few clinical manifestations will be apparent with the serum even as low as 120 mEq/liter or slightly below. Nonetheless, serum sodium levels between 110 and 120 mEq/liter warrant more urgent intervention, as serious complications may occur at any moment. In addition to the clinical problems caused by the low serum sodium, the underlying disease that causes hyponatremia may contribute further symptoms. For example, in an infant presenting with hyponatremia due to obstructive uropathy, medullary cystic disease, or congenital adrenal cortical hyperplasia, the low sodium typically will be accompanied by a very high serum potassium, which will exert potentially lethal effects on cardiac rhythm. Failure to control the hyperkalemia can lead to a fatal outcome.

A cause of hyponatremia that warrants consideration before proceeding to further investigation is **pseudohyponatremia.** If a flame (lithium) photometric method is used to determine sodium, hyperlipidemia can depress the apparent measurement of serum sodium. The effect could be seen in a case of nephrotic syndrome or when IV lipids are used for parenteral nutrition. In laboratories that utilize an electrode that is selective for sodium ions, this problem is not an issue. When using this method, however, the presence of osmotically active solutes in the plasma can still produce an apparent hyponatremia. For example, urea or glucose in high concentration obligates additional water to enter the intravascular space because of their added oncotic pressure. Similarly, the use of IV mannitol can result in an identical outcome. Diagnosis of this plasma dilutional effect rests on measurement of the osmotically active agent or a determination of serum osmolality, which will be markedly elevated in the absence of any other explanation. As a rule of thumb, serum sodium will be depressed 1.6 mEq/liter for every 100 mg/dl of glucose or mannitol. By reducing glucose or urea to normal levels or discontinuing administration of mannitol, the serum sodium will be returned to a normal value; no other therapy is required.

Diagnosis

In considering hyponatremia, the most important diagnostic consideration is the patient's volume status (i.e., hypovolemic, euvolemic, or hypervolemic). This determination permits the basic distinction between patients who are dehydrated with solute loss exceeding free-water loss, thereby producing hyponatremia, versus those patients who suffer from excess total body water, leading to a relative dilution of ECF solute. In the hypoproteinemic patient (e.g., nephrotic syndrome, protein-losing enteropathy, and kwashiorkor), determination of the patient's volume status will be more difficult because effective circulating volume will be diminished, yet peripheral edema will be evident. Hyponatremia in such a patient requires management of the underlying disorder for its correction.

In those patients with normal plasma proteins and normal colloid oncotic pressure, the overall volume status of the patient can more readily be determined. At the time of admission to the ICU, a review of the patient's weight should aid greatly in distinguishing dehydrated patients from those who are euvolemic or hypervolemic. After a period in the ICU, however, particularly if the patient has been catabolic, determination of volume status can be difficult with changes in the patient's weight often due to several problems, not only gain or loss of fluids. Nonetheless, reviewing history, particularly with respect to changes in weight, and taking into account diseases affecting kidneys, heart, liver, and CNS, one should be able to arrive at a determination of the patient's volume status. Physical examination will help if signs of dehydration or edema are present. Laboratory values may contribute to a volume determination. Useful studies include serum osmolality, urea nitrogen, creatinine, electrolytes, glucose, total protein, and albumin, especially in conjunction with urine urea, creatinine, osmolality, and electrolytes. Table 35-10 indicates some useful diagnostic guidelines for interpretation of serum and urine electrolytes with respect to specific clinical disorders. The broad diagnostic categories of hyponatremic patients are water and sodium losses (hypovolemic), water addition (euvolemic), and water and sodium addition (hypervolemic) (Fig. 35-3).

Hyponatremia: Water and Sodium Losses

When hyponatremia is associated with dehydration, ECF volume contracts as sodium is lost in excess of water. If gastrointestinal losses are causing the dehydration, management is as outlined for dehydration. Hyponatremia that has crept in as a result of ICU treatment typically results from either excessive use of loop diuretics or provision of insufficient solute in IV fluids.[33] Review of urinary electrolytes will reveal inappropriately high sodium from diuretic therapy, or calculating sodium intake in mEq/kg/d will

show that maintenance requirements have not been met. More elusive are the circumstances surrounding renal sodium loss because of an underlying disease. For example, mineralocorticoid deficiency, salt-losing nephropathy (medullary cystic disease), obstructive uropathy, and renal tubular acidosis lead to more subtle sodium wastage. Finally, less apparent sources of sodium and fluid loss occur through excessive sweating in the patient with cystic fibrosis and various drainage arrangements via either fistula or gastrointestinal tubes after surgical procedures. A different and subtle cause of hyponatremic "apparent" dehydration occurs with "third-spacing." In this circumstance, the body deposits fluid and electrolytes in a compartment no longer accessible to the circulation. When the third-space fluid collects, its composition is isotonic. If the loss is replaced with IV or oral hypotonic solution, hyponatremia will develop with signs of dehydration, although weight will not be reduced as one would ordinarily expect.

One typical electrolyte disturbance that presents in the infant warrants special consideration. The case usually involves a 1- to 3-week-old infant presenting with marked dehydration, weight loss, severe hyponatremia, and hyperkalemia. The degree of dehydration and extent of electrolyte disturbance generally falls into the life-threatening range. Major diagnostic considerations include failure to produce sufficient milk in the breast-fed infant, acute tubular necrosis due to severe dehydration, and obstructive uropathy (bilateral, medullary cystic disease, and congenital adrenal cortical hyperplasia). Although time will permit subsequent diagnosis, at the outset this presentation constitutes a dire emergency requiring intensive care management.

The approach to hyponatremic patients with water and salt losses generally involves fluid resuscitation using Ringer's lactate or normal saline until circulatory function stabilizes. Obtaining the first urine for osmolality, sodium, potassium, chloride, and creatinine can be extremely helpful diagnostically once results are available.

Treatment

Before discussing the approach to correction of hyponatremia, a general word of caution is in order regarding rapid correction of hyponatremia. Over the past few years, concern has grown among clinicians caring for adults that the traditional approach to serum sodium concentrations below 120 mEq/liter—rapid elevation of

Table 35-10. Diagnostic guide for serum and urine electrolytes

Condition	Serum values					Urine values			
	Na^+ (mEq/liter)	K^+ (mEq/liter)	Osmolality (mosm/liter)	BUN (mg/dl)	Creatinine	Na^+ (mEq/liter)	K^+ (mEq/liter)	Osmolality (mosm/liter)	Urea (mg/dl)
Primary aldosteronism	140	↓	280	10	N	80	60–80	300–800	Low
Secondary aldosteronism	130	↓	275	15–25	↓	<20	40–60	300–400	
Na^+ depletion	120–130	N or ↑	260	>30	N or ↑	10–20	40	600+	800–1000
Na^+ overload	150+	N	290+	N or ↑	N	100+	60	500+	300
H_2O overload	120–130	↓	260	10–15	↓	50–80	60	50–200	300
Dehydration	150	↓	300	30 or N	N or ↑	40	20–40	800+	800–1000
Inappropriate ADH	<125	↓	<260	<10	↓	90	60–150	$U > P_{Osm}$	300
Acute tubular necrosis									
Oliguric	135	↑	N or ↑	↑↑	↑	40+	20–40	300	300
Polyuric	135	N or ↑	275	↑	↑	20	30	300	100–300

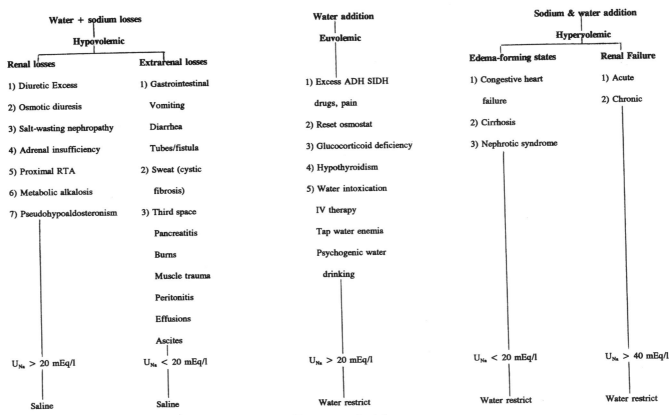

Figure 35-3. Classification, diagnosis, and treatment of hyponatremic states.

serum sodium with hypertonic infusion—may cause serious neurologic sequelae. Particularly when hyponatremia has been chronic, brain adaptation leads to milder cerebral edema than would be expected. Rapid correction then may lead to the "osmotic demyelination syndrome." Although the published literature is almost exclusively based on adult experience, one can extrapolate, with tempered concern, to children.[34–40] In severe cases, central pontine myelinolysis can develop. The typical setting for this potentially fatal complication is the patient who has been hyponatremic for more than 2 days and with serum sodium in the very low range, less than 110 mEq/liter. In the past, standard advice had been to raise the serum sodium in such patients quickly to 125 mEq/liter to avert CNS complications. A more prudent recommendation would be to aim at a correction no greater than 12 mEq/liter/d of the serum sodium, even if the starting value is quite depressed. Obviously, development of new neurologic findings during the early phase of management in hyponatremia warrants very careful review of all changes in order to stop myelinolysis from proceeding, if that is the underlying neurologic disturbance.

In the circumstance of symptomatic hyponatremia, more vigorous restoration of serum sodium becomes necessary. The following is an example for calculating both the sodium deficit and the treatment dose:

1. Sodium deficit in a 10-kg child with a serum sodium of 115 would be

$$10 \text{ kg} \times 0.6 \times (20 \text{ mEq deficit})$$
$$= 120 \text{ mEq sodium (total deficit)}$$

2. To raise serum Na⁺ by 5 mEq/liter acutely requires

$$5 \text{ mEq} \times 0.6 \times 10 \text{ kg} = 30 \text{ mEq};$$

thus, we are correcting no more than one fourth of the deficit over the first several hours.

3. Dose of 3% NaCl solution:

$$30 \text{ mEq Na at } 0.513 \text{ mEq Na}^+/\text{ml} = 60 \text{ ml of 3\% solution}$$

When hyponatremia is due to excess water and excess sodium, patients usually present with pulmonary edema, ascites, or peripheral edema. Usually, they suffer one of three disease states: (1) hypoproteinemia due to nephrotic syndrome or liver cirrhosis, (2) congestive heart failure, and (3) acute and chronic renal failure.[41] In some instances, the underlying predisposition to hyponatremia has been aggravated further by persistent use of high-dose potent diuretics, such as furosemide or zaroxolyn. This treatment depletes sodium further by compelling the tubule to excrete a relatively sodium-rich urine.

Patients with hypoproteinemia or congestive heart failure may have gained fluid weight but have a substantially reduced effective circulating volume due to loss of colloid oncotic pressure. Those with congestive heart failure also have a diminished effective circulating volume because of poor cardiac function. Both circumstances result in generalized edema throughout interstitial spaces. In acute and chronic renal failure, inability to excrete salt and water comes about from the reduction in glomerular filtration rate. For example, in poststreptococcal glomerulonephritis, a particular danger to life is marked fluid retention, marked hypervolemia, and pulmonary edema. Failure to restrict fluid intake in patients with markedly impaired GFR leads rapidly to volume overload. Management of these patients rests on restriction of salt and water. A trial of vigorous diuresis with furosemide, zaroxolyn, or bumetanide is warranted in these patients, despite the hyponatremia. Generally, the excess total body water poses a greater threat than the hyponatremia and may require removal via dialysis or CAVHD.

Intensity of treatment and its tempo must be individualized based on underlying disease, chronicity of problem, and acuteness of symptoms. In general, the patient with reasonably stable clinical and neurologic status and serum sodium above 125 mEq/liter is at greater risk for iatrogenic complications from attempts to raise serum sodium acutely than from the hyponatremia itself. Frequent monitoring of clinical status and laboratory values over the course of the first 48 hours of management will help avert unnecessary complications of treatment.

When hyponatremia is due to water addition, total body sodium is near normal and the hyponatremia is dilutional. Signs of fluid excess are absent, so edema or ascites cannot be demonstrated. Because the circulating volume is normal or expanded, the kidney is not avid for sodium, and urinary concentration exceeds 20 mEq/liter. In fact, in SIADH the urinary sodium may be much higher because the ADH excess leads to inappropriate water reabsorption.

Although water intoxication, glucocorticoid deficiency, and thyroid hormone deficiency may lead to the state of hyponatremia with modest water excess, by far the most common cause—particularly in the ICU—is SIADH secretion. Figure 35-4 illustrates the pathophysiology of SIADH, indicating that both excess ADH **and availability of water** are requisites for the clinical syndrome's development.[42,43]

SIADH secretion presents most commonly in the ICU in children with CNS infections. Although numerous other causes have been identified (Table 35-11), the diagnosis of SIADH rests on excluding a series of other possibilities for hypotonic hyponatremia. The patient should have normal renal function, normal adrenal pituitary and hypothalamic function, normal volume status, no edema, and characteristic urinary findings. The urinary osmolality should be higher than appropriate, given the degree of hyponatremia; the urine osmolality is often greater than the serum osmolality, clearly inappropriate in a hypotonic patient; and urine osmolality should fail to reach maximum dilution, as would be expected. Urinary sodium will be high at the onset of SIADH but can be difficult to interpret if the patient has already received loop diuretics or an infusion of hypertonic saline.

Table 35-11. Causes of SIADH

Central nervous system disorders
  Trauma
  Subdural hematoma
  Abscess
  Meningitis
  Encephalitis
  Subarachnoid hemorrhage
  Guillain-Barré syndrome
  Acute intermittent porphyria
  Systemic lupus erythematosus
  Other CNS disorders
Pulmonary disease
  Tuberculosis
  Pneumonia
  Lung abscess
  Aspergillosis with cavitation
  Chronic chest infections
Tumors
  Bronchogenic carcinoma
  Adenocarcinoma of duodenum
  Adenocarcinoma of pancreas
  Carcinoma of ureter
  Hodgkin's disease
  Thymoma
  Leukemias
Stress

Treatment of SIADH

Treatment of SIADH rests firmly on fluid restriction. Infusion of normal saline or hypertonic 3% saline (513 mEq/liter) is indicated only to correct acute neurologic symptoms.[44] The sodium administered will simply pass through to the urine while causing temporary anatomic fluid shifts. More aggressive therapy for SIADH includes administration of a loop diuretic followed by IV replacement of the fluid loss with 3% saline. The essence of this exchange is to drive out urine with sodium concentration of about half normal (i.e., 60–80 mEq/liter) and to replace it with a solution that is about 3.5 times more concentrated than normal saline. This strategy succeeds only if the restriction of fluid is carried out effectively. Unfortunately, the combination of elevated ADH (because of the syndrome), tight fluid restriction, and infusion of hypertonic saline produces intense thirst in the child who is conscious. Provision of ice chips may be necessary out of humane considerations. **Beware of restricting fluids in hypoproteinemic patients, as this may produce circulatory impairment.**

Drugs associated with SIADH are listed in Table 35-12. While undertaking standard treatment, one should review the absolute necessity of these agents in the hope that they can be eliminated. Finally, before embarking on treatment, consider that other conditions can mimic the clinical and chemical findings in SIADH, as indicated in Table 35-13.

Both absence of glucocorticoid hormone and thyroid insufficiency lead to excess ADH secretion. Consequently, children with Addison's disease or hypothyroidism can present with hyponatremia on a dilutional basis. Treatment of the underlying hormone deficiency will permit excretion of excess water and a return to a normal level of serum sodium.

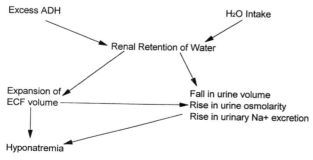

Figure 35-4. SIADH. Pathophysiology of the treatment of the syndrome of inappropriate secretion of ADH.

Table 35-12. Drugs associated with SIADH

Vasopressin

Oxytocin

Chlorpropamide

Vincristine

Cyclophosphamide

Diuretics

Clofibrate

Carbamazepine

Fluphenazine

Amitriptyline

Table 35-13. Conditions mimicking SIADH

Defects in free-water generation
 Chronic renal failure
 Decreased distal delivery, multiple causes, e.g., shock, heptorenal
  syndrome, severe congestive heart failure
 Use of loop diuretics: furosemide, ethacrynic acid
 Chronic severe hypokalemia
 Bartter's syndrome, myxedema
Enhanced distal water reabsorption
 Chlopropamide, tolbutamide therapy
 Phosphodiesterase inhibition
 ? Glucocorticoid deficiency

Potassium

In the ICU, potassium disorders frequently cause major threats to survival. Derangement of hydration, renal function, and endocrine function cause potassium abnormalities. Burns, tissue necrosis, tumor lysis accompanying cancer chemotherapy, and side effects of medication often contribute to disordered potassium balance.[45] Although potassium is the principal intracellular cation, we measure derangements on the basis of plasma or serum determinations reflecting only 5% of total body potassium. Nonetheless, high and low potassium levels in the blood signal abnormal states due to excess, loss, or redistribution of potassium, and demand prompt correction. Failure to restore normal potassium homeostasis can have dire effects on cardiac rhythm, gastrointestinal function, and neuromuscular and CNS activity. Furthermore, when hyperkalemia or hypokalemia combine with other chemical derangements (i.e., calcium disorder in the opposite direction), the danger to life becomes even greater.

Hyperkalemia

Hyperkalemia occurs when serum potassium exceeds 5.5 mEq/liter, and becomes a real threat to life at 7.5 mEq/liter. Note that in the newborn, potassium levels typically run about 0.5 mEq/liter higher. Clinical conditions resulting in hyperkalemia are listed in Table 35-14.

Increased potassium load can result from either excessive intake or endogenous production and release. Common exogenous sources of potassium in the ICU setting include IV solutions, especially those with a potassium concentration exceeding 40 mEq/liter, potassium-containing medicine (e.g., penicillin), or

Table 35-14. Conditions resulting in hyperkalemia

Increased potassium load
 Hemolysis
 Tumor lysis
 Tissue necrosis/burns
 Rhabdomyolysis
 Potassium supplement (oral or intravenous)
 Potassium penicillin
 Blood transfusion (esp. old blood)
 Severe starvation and catabolism
Decreased potassium excretion
 Adrenal failure
  Congenital adrenal cortical hyperplasia (21 and 18 hydroxylase
   deficiencies)
  Addison's disease
  Hypoaldosteronism
 Renal failure, acute or chronic
 Renal tubular disorders
  Obstructive uropathy
  Sickle cell disease
 Interstitial nephritis
 Renal transplant
 Renal tubular acidosis, type 4
Redistribution of potassium
 Acidosis
 Diabetes mellitus
 Familial hyperkalemic periodic paralysis
 Sepsis with ischemia
 Malignant hyperthermia during anesthesia
Medication
 Beta blockers
 Potassium-sparing diuretics
 Potassium penicillin
Pseudohyperkalemia
 Technical difficulties in venipuncture
 Heel-stick samples in nursery
 Hemolysis in vitro (clotted sample)
 Leukocytosis, thrombocytosis

blood transfusions. Ordinarily, such a potassium load would undergo prompt renal filtration and subsequent excretion by the kidney. However, poor circulation coupled with impaired renal plasma flow or acute renal failure rapidly produces a state of potassium intoxication of dangerous proportions.

Any clinical condition producing massive tissue destruction results in the release of large amounts of potassium ion. Crush injuries, multiple trauma, burns, muscle necrosis, rhabdomyolysis, severe ischemia in an extremity, or tumor cell lysis can cause rapidly rising serum potassium levels.

Redistribution of potassium occurs with acidosis because rising levels of blood hydrogen ion are taken up by cells in exchange for the release of potassium ions back into the blood. Thus, severe diabetic ketoacidosis, renal acidosis, and the ischemic acidosis of sepsis lead to hyperkalemia. Rapid catabolism seen in severe starvation and widespread malignancy cause endogenous potassium release as well. Decreased potassium excretion is most commonly seen with renal impairment. Hemolytic-uremic syndrome can produce the worst combination of oliguric renal failure (sometimes anuric) and endogenous potassium release due to widespread hemolysis. In severe instances, the rate of rise of potassium is such that serum levels can reach 8 to 10 mEq/liter over the first 24 to 36 hours of illness. Children admitted to the ICU with this condition must be monitored frequently to initiate early and aggressive therapy for the control of hyperkalemia.

Decreased glomerular filtration rate, whether prerenal in origin or due to acute renal failure, will be accompanied by a rising serum potassium. If this circumstance occurs in the setting of increased exogenous or endogenous potassium load, the problem is compounded. In the case of **non-oliguric renal failure**, ongoing urine production permits sufficient potassium excretion to avoid serious hyperkalemia. Nonetheless, the potassium excretory capacity in non-oliguric renal failure can be readily overcome by injudicious administration of potassium-containing substances, especially blood products.[46]

Renal tubular disorders also can contribute to hyperkalemia. In children with obstructive uropathy and following renal transplantation, tubular dysfunction can give rise to serious hyperkalemia.[47-49] Although the build-up of serum potassium will not occur as dramatically as seen with complete filtration failure, over time the hyperkalemia may require ongoing management.

Adrenal failure leads to hyperkalemia because mineralocorticoids stimulate renin secretin, hence potassium excretion, and any interruption in production can therefore produce serious hyperkalemia. The most common pediatric setting for this circumstance is not Addison's disease but the inherited disorders of mineralocorticoid synthesis. Specifically, congenital adrenal cortical hyperplasia involving a complete 21-hydroxylase deficiency can present early in life with severe hyperkalemia, hyponatremia, and cardiovascular collapse. In addition to controlling potassium, medical management for these infants includes administration of hydrocortisone to shut down the pituitary-adrenal synthetic overdrive resulting from the glucocorticoid blockade and consequent loss of negative feedback to the pituitary.

Obstructive uropathy also can present with a virtually identical chemical picture, with hyperkalemia, hyponatremia, and volume depletion, especially in young infants. Urosepsis may further aggravate the situation.

The toxic effects of hyperkalemia are mainly cardiac. Elevated potassium interferes with normal nodal and bundle conduction. ECG changes include peaked T wave, increased P-R interval and widened QRS complex, depressed S-T segment, and atrioventricular or intraventricular heart block (Fig. 35-5). When serum potassium exceeds 7.5 mEq/liter, danger of heart block, ventricular tachycardia, and ventricular fibrillation becomes grave. ECG monitoring is mandatory. Any evidence of arrythmia requires immediate treatment of the hyperkalemia. Above a serum potassium level of 10 mEq/liter, ventricular fibrillation or asystole become likely, particularly if the rise has been rapid. Also note that hypocalcemia, hyponatremia, and acidosis exacerbate the dangerous effects of hyperkalemia and require separate treatment.

Treatment
The best treatment for hyperkalemia remains prevention. Rapidly rising potassium can be predicted in the setting of acute renal failure, especially anuric situations often found with hemolytic uremic syndrome, rapidly progressive glomerulonephritis, severe acute tubular necrosis, and cortical necrosis. In these instances, avoid administration of any potassium. Measurement of an abnormally high potassium mandates the elimination of artifactual elevation due to heel-stick blood sampling as performed in the newborn or from thrombocytosis, marked leukocytosis, or from hemolysis in the blood-drawing apparatus. If false elevation is not the cause, hyperkalemia must be assessed promptly to determine the urgency

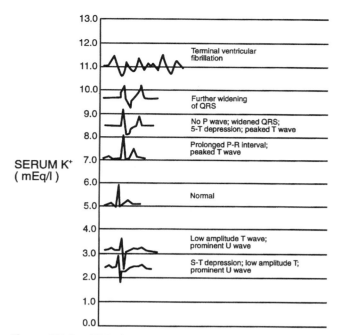

Figure 35-5. ECG changes associated with hyperkalemia.

of treatment. ECG monitoring must continue until serum potassium has been stabilized at a safe level. There are three main approaches available for control: (1) Remove potassium from the body, (2) minimize the harmful effects of hyperkalemia, and (3) sequester the excess ion where it can do no harm.

Figure 35-6 diagrams the approach to hyperkalemia. When serum potassium exceeds 7.5 mEq/liter, the following sequence should be used acutely: Sodium bicarbonate should be administered at 1 to 2 mEq/kg IV. The bicarbonate causes potassium to enter into cells in exchange for hydrogen ion, not buffered by the infusion. For every increase of 0.1 pH units, potassium decreases by about 1 mEq/liter, and the correction occurs within minutes. Calcium infusion (except in digitalized patients) counteracts cardiac toxicity of severe hyperkalemia. At a dose of 10/mg/kg of elemental calcium, the protective effect is prompt. Note that there are different solutions of calcium, each containing a different concentration of calcium. The calcium infusion should run at about 10 mg/kg (elemental Ca^{++}) as a drip, with cardiac monitoring. The use of calcium chloride should be monitored very carefully to be certain that the infusion remains IV; extravasation into local tissues causes severe necrosis because of both the high concentration and the acidity of the preparation.

Cation exchange resins such as Kayexalate (sodium polystyrene sulfonate) sequester potassium ion in the gut by exchange for sodium ions. A dose of 1 g/kg of Kayexalate reduces serum potassium by about 1 mEq/liter. Cation exchange resins are not ion-specific, and excessive use of Kayexalate may cause unwanted hypocalcemia. Another therapeutic approach to moving excess potassium to where it can do no harm involves the combined use of insulin and glucose infusions. This therapy has a limited role in the infant because profound hypoglycemia can result. When used in older children, however, the treatment can be effective, if used cautiously. Over 20 to 30 minutes, potassium will be driven into the intracellular compartment, thereby averting the acute risk of cardiac toxicity.

Ultimate therapy of hyperkalemia may necessitate removal of the

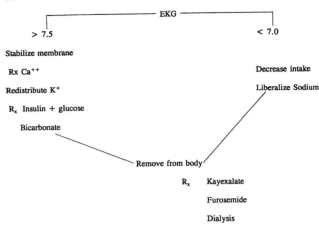

DETERMINE URGENCY

DRUG TREATMENT

(1) Ca⁺⁺ - 10 mg/kg (as elemental Ca⁺⁺)

(2) Insulin - 0.1 u/kg/h

Glucose - 0.5 g/kg/h (adjust prn)

(3) Bicarbonate - 1 mEq/kg

(4) Kayexalate - 1 g/kg in 50-150cc Sorbitol per rectum

(5) Furosemide - 1 mg/kg IV

(6) Dialysis

Figure 35-6. Treatment of hyperkalemia.

Table 35-15. Causes of hypokalemia

Increased potassium excretion

Renal
  Tubulointerstitial disease
  Cystinosis with Fanconi syndrome
  Renal tubular acidosis
  Diuretics
  Diabetic ketoacidosis
  Bartter's syndrome

Gastrointestinal
  Vomiting
  Diarrhea
  Laxative use, abuse

Adrenal
  Hyperaldesteronism
  Congenital adrenal cortical hyperplasia
  Cushing's syndrome
  Excessive steroid therapy

Redistribution of potassium
  Alkalosis
  Insulin
  Hypokalemic periodic paralysis
  Hypochloremia

Medication
  Diuretics
  Insulin
  Amphotericin
  Carbenicillin
  Combinations (e.g., nafcillin, gentamicin, ticarcillin)

potassium if a continuing rise in the serum level can be anticipated. The use of loop diuretics, such as furosemide at 1 mg/kg IV, will hasten urinary excretion of potassium. Obviously, if severe acute renal failure contributes to hyperkalemia, this approach is unlikely to yield results. Peritoneal dialysis can be promptly initiated in the ICU with little delay, because access is simple compared with that of hemodialysis and the patient's other management can proceed without major adjustments. However, if the abdomen is anatomically compromised, or if the patient's respiratory status is marginal, the infusion of large volumes of fluid into the peritoneal cavity may be contraindicated. In the setting of abdominal sepsis or peritonitis, there is no absolute contraindication to peritoneal dialysis. One must consider the anatomic integrity of the abdomen, however, and the likelihood of effective fluid exchange through omentum and peritoneal membranes. Hemodialysis removes potassium more effectively and rapidly. Which approach to take in a given circumstance depends on both the patient's clinical condition and any limits imposed thereby, as well as on general availability of hemodialysis technicians and machinery.

Hypokalemia

The intracellular potassium stores are enormous, and hence, serious dilutional hypokalemia is rare. Most pediatric patients reach a hypokalemic state through depletion of total body stores of potassium. Disease processes such as severe gastroenteritis, persistent vomiting, and renal tubular disorders with electrolyte wastage typically cause clinically important hypokalemia.[50] The use of powerful loop diuretics, such as ethacrynic acid, and furosemide or zaroxolyn can cause urine output of potassium high enough to lead to hypokalemia (Table 35-15).

The multiple medications now commonly prescribed for ICU patients may include multiple renal tubular toxins, which predictably cause K⁺ and Mg⁺⁺ wastage. For example, gentamicin can cause urinary potassium loss, but when combined with nafcillin and ticarcillin, serious kaliuresis will result, with predictable hypokalemia.[52] Always consult patient medication sheets to ascertain the role drug therapy might play in patients with hypokalemia.

Like hyperkalemia, the principal toxic effect of low potassium is the harmful disturbance of cardiac rhythm. Symptoms of hypokalemia are far more common when the cause is acute. Clinically, patients may develop ileus, major muscle weakness, and cardiac rhythm disturbances. Particularly in digitalized patients, arrhythmias can emerge with falling levels of serum potassium. The ECG may show a depressed T wave and U wave.

Oral therapy is best suited for the management for chronic and irreversible causes of hypokalemia, such as renal tubular acidosis. IV therapy becomes necessary, however, if serum potassium acutely falls below 2.5 mEq/liter and is continuing a downward trend. IV therapy may also be necessary if the child cannot take oral medication (if vomiting is severe). When circumstances permit, hypokalemia should be corrected over 2 days by using IV concentrations of potassium no more than 40 mEq/liter. Generally, potassium chloride is the solution of choice, unless there is a specific reason to replace either phosphate, as in diabetic ketoacidosis, or bicarbonate, as in severe acidosis. In those instances, the appropriate anion can be selected or one can use a mixture of both chloride and another anion, as best suits the patient's requirements. In severe potassium depletion, the IV solution may need to exceed a concentration of 40 mEq/liter. In this circumstance, infusion should be through a central vein to avoid irritation of peripheral vessels. ECG monitoring is mandatory throughout the process. It is best never to exceed a potassium infusion rate of 0.5 mEq/kg/hr. Only in dire circumstances (serum potassium level <1.0 mEq/liter) should replacement exceed this limit, and **only** then if authorized by a physician experienced in dealing with this problem. The risk of hyperkalemic arrythmia increases dramatically when a high concentration of potassium is infused into the circulation such that it reaches the heart directly.

Chloride

Chloride rarely proves to be the prime mover in a metabolic disturbance. Usually, chloride is a "fellow traveler" shifting to abnormal values in conjunction with hydration, sodium flux, and acid-base disturbances.

Hyperchloremia

Hyperchloremia usually accompanies hyponatremia and acidosis and will respond to their treatment. In unusual circumstances, such as administration of IV hydrochloric acid or arginine HCl, an excess chloride load may contribute to hyperchloremia.

Hypochloremia

Hypochloremia occurs in all the forms of dilutional hypernatremia, water intoxication, and hyponatremic dehydration.[50] In cases of marked alkalosis, chloride levels will decrease as bicarbonate rises. For example, in the infant with severe pyloric stenosis, the serum chloride can actually fall to the level of the bicarbonate as the latter rises dramatically in response to persistent hydrogen ion loss through vomiting. Thus, one can see the bizarre picture of a chloride in the 70-mEq/liter range and a bicarbonate in the 60-mEq/liter range in the dehydrated infant with severe, untreated pyloric stenosis. Infusion of saline will correct the metabolic disturbance, pending release of the gastric outlet obstruction.

In hypokalemic alkalosis, two interesting states are found. Most patients with this disorder and low urinary chloride respond to a simple infusion of saline. This is the case noted earlier. A subgroup of patients, however, manifests high urinary chloride (typically Cl > 70 mEq/liter and as high as >200 mEq/liter in the urine), and a state of "saline resistance" obtains. This hypochloremia will not correct without administration of large amounts of potassium in conjunction with saline infusion.[53,54] The tip-off for this problem is the setting of severe total body potassium depletion, reported to reach more than 1000 mEq in the adults studied. Correction of the condition often requires very large amounts of potassium, administered over several days, before the hypochloremia is corrected.

Calcium

The key component of plasma calcium with respect to its effectiveness in neuroexcitation and muscle contraction is **ionized calcium**. This component represents 45% to 50% of the plasma ion, the remainder distributed among an equal amount of calcium that is protein-bound to albumin and a small component complexed with anions such as lactate, phosphate, and bicarbonate.

Ionized hypocalcemia has been reported particularly among sick newborn infants and in severely ill pediatric ICU patients.[55,56] An increased mortality rate in critically ill children has been associated with hypocalcemia, and low ionized calcium has been identified both as a marker for sepsis and a contributor to the resulting circulatory impairment.[57] Calcium abnormalities in the ICU setting can be extremely important, as they may suggest

underlying disorders (i.e, genetic, acquired, or iatrogenic), and a high or low serum calcium may seriously disrupt vital functions or even become life-threatening.

The physiology underlying the maintenance of a normal serum calcium level is complicated and includes a number of controlling sites as well as feedback loops. There are two principal factors in the setting of calcium levels: the active bone mass, which serves as the major reservoir for calcium ion, where it is held in place as various salts; and the parathyroid gland, which elaborates PTH, which acts to increase serum calcium and also to cause phosphaturia. Calcitonin is a hormone that acts as a modulator of calcium levels, although routine measurement of calcitonin and clinical use of the hormone tend to be restricted to research centers. Active metabolites of vitamin D arise from a series of synthetic steps initiated by manufacture of the hormone by skin on exposure to ultraviolet light and subsequent modification of this initial structure first by the liver and subsequently by the kidney to produce 1,25 di-OH vitamin D. This active metabolite exerts powerful effects on the gut absorption of calcium and also plays a major role in modulating bone growth and uptake of calcium.

Hypocalcemia

The major causes of hypocalcemia in infants and children are noted in Table 35-16. The clinical manifestations of low calcium include seizures, tetany, depressed cardiac function, and, rarely, laryngospasm.[58] The impairment of cardiac function will be aggravated further if hyperkalemia coexists.[59]

The rhythm disturbance brought about by hypocalcemia produces a prolonged Q-T interval. The standard formula for Q-T interval corrects for heart rate and is especially important in the infant with a normal heart rate—double that of an adult.

Treatment

Investigators have suggested that calcium chloride may confer some advantage over calcium gluconate with respect to bioavailability of the calcium ion. In a prospective randomized double-blind comparison of calcium chloride and calcium gluconate therapies for hypocalcemia in critically ill children, the data presented suggest that calcium chloride produces a greater rise in

Table 35-16. Major causes of hypocalcemia in infants and children

Neonatal
  Hypoparathyroidism
  Idiopathic
  Infant of diabetic mother
Postneonatal
  Hypoparathyroidism
  Idiopathic
  Hypomagnesemia
  Post-exchange transfusion (citrated blood products)
  DiGeorge's syndrome
  Pseudohypoparathyroidism
  Pancreatitis
  Phosphate infusion
  Rickets
    Nutritional
    Renal failure
    Hepatic failure
    Hereditary
  Sepsis

ionized calcium than did calcium gluconate, although other investigators studying the same question have not found any important difference between calcium salts tested for bioavailability.[60] Calcium chloride does carry the advantage of a concentrated solution, making a smaller volume of infusion; on the other hand, the danger of tissue necrosis from extravasation is greatest with this preparation. Usually 10 mg/kg of elemental CaCl is given in a drip over several minutes to treat acute hypocalcemia which may be followed by continuous infusions of calcium as needed. Treatment of the underlying cause is important when appropriate.

Hypercalcemia

The disorders listed in Table 35-17 may present with acute hypercalcemia, requiring aggressive management. In the young infant, familial hypercalcemia can present with a toxic level of calcium, warranting acute intervention with IV medication. In older patients, hyperparathyroidism and malignancy are the conditions with toxic levels of calcium needing intensive care management. Infants with severe hypercalcemia present with neuromuscular symptoms, including lethargy and difficulty feeding as well as hypotonia. Older children may manifest a variety of symptoms, including CNS disturbance, up to and including coma, nausea, and vomiting. Hypertension occasionally presents on the basis of hypercalcemia, especially if present for a prolonged period.

Hypercalcemia constitutes a medical emergency when blood levels exceed 15 mg/dl. Ionized calcium, total protein and albumin, magnesium, phosphorus, and all electrolytes should be determined promptly. With elevated phosphorus complicating hypercalcemia, the risk of metastatic calcification of soft tissue, nephrocalcinosis, and, occasionally, metastatic calcification of the cornea or in the vascular tree may occur.

Treatment

Treatment of hypercalcemia includes the following measures:

1. Direct treatment of any underlying disorder, especially iatrogenic (discontinue any source of vitamin D, thiazide, or excess phosphate).

Table 35-17. Causes of hypercalcemia

Primary hyperparathyroidism

Secondary hyperparathyroidism (rarely, in renal disease)

Hypervitaminosis D

Hypervitaminosis A

Malignancy, especially bone metastases or hormonal tumor products

Familial hypercalcemia with hypocalciuria

Idiopathic infantile hypercalcemia (William's syndrome)

Hypophosphatasia

Hypothyroidism

Hyperthyroidism

Addison's disease

Milk-alkali syndrome

Iatrogenic: Inadequate phosphate during TPN

Excess vitamin D (e.g., calcitriol)

Thiazide diuretic

Excess calcium in dialysate

TPN, total parenteral nutrition

2. Elimination of calcium intake, especially milk and dairy products; infant formula should contain low levels of calcium.

3. IV saline to induce saline diuresis and calciuresis. Infuse at 1500 to 2500 ml/m²/24 hr.

4. Furosemide 1 mg/kg/6–8 hr. Monitor potassium, as both saliuresis and furosemide will produce substantial urinary potassium losses.

5. Glucocorticoid to reduce gut absorption (e.g., prednisone 1–2 mg/kg/d).

6. Phosphate salts. These carry the risk of metastatic soft-tissue calcification; especially with sodium phosphate, give as IV infusion. Reserve this treatment for patients refractory to aforementioned measures. A safer approach is to administer phosphate per rectum as a Fleet enema.

7. Hemodialysis. Utilize a zero calcium dialysate solution while monitoring ionized calcium carefully.

8. In the small infant, an exchange transfusion may prove to be the simplest way to remove calcium promptly.

Phosphorus

Phosphate disorders affecting children in the ICU generally cause the greatest danger when hyperphosphatemia occurs, although hypophosphatemia can reach serious proportions as the phosphate falls towards 1.0 mg/dl. Most of the hypophosphatemic disorders listed in Table 35-18 do not require IV therapy. In the setting of acute diabetic ketoacidosis, hypophosphatemia is commonly seen and can be treated by adding potassium phosphate (rather than potassium chloride) to the saline infusion in a concentration of 20 to 40 mEq/liter. Although this phosphate repletion makes good sense, it is a lower order of priority than the acute metabolic issues in diabetic ketoacidosis. Also, calcium should be monitored carefully when phosphate is infused because an abrupt drop in serum calcium may occur.

Hyperphosphatemia

In the ICU, hyperphosphatemia arises in conjunction with renal failure, dietary excess (especially in the infant), massive tissue destruction such as occurs in the tumor lysis syndrome, rhabdomyolysis, burns, and malignant hyperthermia, and by excess phosphate absorption from a Fleet enema. The major risk of acute hyperphosphatemia is metastatic calcification due to an increased calcium-phosphorus product. When the serum calcium level times the serum phosphorus level exceeds 70, soft-tissue calcification often occurs and may be accompanied by nephrocalcinosis.

Table 35-18. Causes of hypophosphatemia

Nutritional rickets

Hereditary vitamin D–resistant rickets

Cystinosis, Fanconi syndrome

Renal tubular acidosis

Treatment of acute diabetic ketoacidosis

Phosphate-binding antacids

Treatment of severe malnutrition

Total parenteral malnutrition

Hyperparathyroidism

Premature infant fed nonsupplemented breast milk

Treatment

If renal impairment and consequent reduction of urinary phosphate excretion underlies the problem, the use of oral phosphate binders is standard therapy. Dietary phosphate should be reduced to a minimum and should be removed from enteral or parenteral alimentation. A number of oral phosphate binders are available as tablets or liquids. In children, liquid Alternagel contains twice the phosphate binding capacity of Amphojel. Oral preparations containing magnesium, such as Gelusis, present the risk of aggravating preexisting hypermagnesemia, which is often seen in chronic renal failure. Unfortunately, aluminum intoxication continues to be of concern in hemodialysis patients so that constant use of Amphojel or Alternagel also can present problems. Note that in patients receiving oral feeding, the phosphate binder must be given at mealtime to prevent absorption of the dietary phosphate just consumed.

In the circumstance of extreme hyperphosphatemia, as occasionally is seen with tumor lysis syndrome, hemodialysis may be necessary to effect removal of a massive phosphate load arising from intracellular and bone release.

Magnesium

Two groups of patients are especially prone to magnesium disturbances: the newborn infant and the patient with renal failure. As noted with hypokalemia, polyantimicrobial treatment, such as the combination of gentamicin, nafcillin, and ticarcillin, causes renal tubular dysfunction, with K^+ and Mg^{++} leakage sufficient to produce hypokalemia and hypomagnesemia. Hypomagnesemia has symptoms akin to those of hypocalcemia: tetany, muscular weakness, and cardiac rhythm disturbance. Because hypomagnesemia impairs PTH function, hypocalcemia is a common accompaniment. Consequently, calcium, phosphorus, alkaline phosphatase, renal function, and acid-base balance should be surveyed when hypomagnesemia is identified.

In the treatment of hypomagnesemia, magnesium sulfate is given intramuscularly, prepared as a 50% solution of $MgSO_4 \cdot 7H_2O$. The solution contains 48 mg of magnesium/ml and is given at 5 to 10 mg/kg/12–24 hr. Oral repletion can be carried out by giving 10 to 30 mg of magnesium/kg/24 hr as chloride or citrate.

Hypermagnesemia

Hypermagnesemia exerts clinical effects when the concentration exceeds 5 mg/dl. Weakness, neuromuscular abnormalities, including loss of deep tendon reflexes, and paralysis become evident when magnesium rises above 7.5 mg/dl. Abnormal cardiac rhythms become more pronounced, displaying an array of conduction defects on the ECG.

There is no specific drug therapy for hypermagnesemia. One should administer 10 mg/kg of elemental calcium as a slow IV infusion to minimize the effects of hypermagnesemia on the heart. Dialysis may be carried out if neurologic symptoms or cardiac arrhythmias are severe.

Uric Acid

Serum uric acid becomes a problem in the ICU principally in the setting of malignancy, tumor lysis, and renal failure. Normal values for uric acid vary between 3.0 and 5.0 mg/dl and are age-dependent, with higher values in newborns and adults.[61] Although there are many other disorders and drugs that cause elevation or depression of uric acid, severe hyperuricemia is uncommon except in the aforementioned conditions. Hereditary abnormalities, including Lesch-Nyhan syndrome, glucose-6-phosphatase deficiency, familial renal hyperuricemia, and x-linked dominant phosphoribosyl pyrophosphate synthetase overactivity are uncommon causes for hyperuricemia.[62] The greatest danger from excess uric acid is acute uric acid nephropathy, with obstruction of renal tubules due to accumulation of uric acid crystals, and subsequent oliguric acute renal failure. Generally, most children come to this condition after treatment with cytotoxic drugs for childhood lymphoma or leukemia.[63,64]

To prevent the development of acute uric acid nephropathy in children undergoing chemotherapy, the guidelines in Table 35-19 should be followed. In the typical setting for acute urate nephrotoxicity, mild dehydration and consequent oliguria brought on by poor fluid intake during chemotherapy and the tumor cell destruction combine to bring about precipitation of urate sludge in distal renal tubules.[65] Once established, this tubular obstruction is difficult to reverse acutely. The presence of a high level of uric acid in the serum and uric acid crystals in the urine confirms the diagnosis, and a rise in creatinine with reduction in GFR will follow. Once tubular damage is established, treatment with allopurinol, appropriate medical management of the acute renal failure, and hemodialysis are the only effective remedies. Unfortunately, peritoneal dialysis has a low uric acid clearance compared with hemodialysis and so is not the treatment of choice.[66] Note that during hemodialysis, allopurinol is removed and must be replaced. Fortunately, acute uric acid nephropathy in this setting often will resolve with just a few days of hemodialysis treatment as glomerular filtration rate begins to return.

In the setting of renal failure from any cause, uric acid usually rises. Especially in chronic renal failure, allopurinol will be necessary for management, but the hyperuricemia generally responds to oral therapy.

Acid-Base Disturbances

Disturbances of acid-base balance are common in the ICU setting. Maintenance of acid-base homeostasis relies on the proper functioning of many organs—kidney, heart, lung, and liver. Many diseases produce perturbations of acid-base balance, and both surgical manipulations and drug therapy can aggravate imbalances in acid-base status. At times, the disturbance is a feature of a primary disease such as is seen in lactic acidosis or renal tubular acidosis.[67] More commonly, acid-base imbalance is but one of several derangements encountered in the critically ill with systemic disease or multiorgan impairment. At the heart of the matter lies the patient's current measurements of pH (H^+ ion concentration), pCO_2, and bicarbonate (or carbon

Table 35-19. Prevention of acute uric acid nephropathy during cancer chemotherapy

Hydration	3 × maintenance at 4.5–5 l/m²/24 hr with D_5 0.25N saline
Alkalinization	Na HCO_3 1 mEq/kg/dose to maintain urine pH > 6.5
Diuresis	Furosemide 1 mg/kg/dose
	Mannitol 1 g/kg/dose or as steady infusion to maintain high urine flow to keep up with IV fluids
Treatment	Allopurinol 6 mg/kg/loading dose; 3 mg/kg q8h

dioxide content of the blood). For full evaluation of the child's acid-base status, determination of chloride levels, organic anions, electrolytes, and BUN will be helpful. With these measurements in hand and a clinical assessment as to whether the primary organ impairment is renal/metabolic versus respiratory, one can clarify acid-base problems into their underlying etiologies to reach a diagnosis and treatment plan.

General Principles

Hydrogen ion concentration of body fluids is tightly controlled, ranging between pH 7.35 and 7.45. A shift of 0.1 pH units from pH 7.40 represents a change of only 10 nEq/liter in hydrogen ion concentration. This delicate regulation comes about through blood buffering, respiratory activity, and compensatory renal mechanisms, all aimed at maintaining physiologic pH to permit normal mitochondrial enzyme function. In the vital range of pH 6.90 to 7.60, hydrogen ion ranges from 30 nEq/liter up to 126 nEq/liter, or a span of only 100 nEq/liter, encompasses the limits of survival. When one compares hydrogen concentration with other ions (i.e., sodium ion concentration), the difference is startling. Hydrogen ion is monitored at concentrations one millionth that of sodium ion, and corrections occur for concentration changes one millionth the size of the sodium concentration shifts necessary to induce any physiologic correction.

Children ordinarily ingest 1 to 2 mEq/kg/d of "fixed" acid in their diet, as sulfate from amino acids, from nitrate, from phosphate (phosphoprotein), and from incomplete oxidation of fat and carbohydrate, yielding organic acids (e.g., lactic acid). Blood chemical buffers provide an immediate defense against this acid load, but it is ultimately the responsibility of the kidney to maintain long-term pH homeostasis through (1) recovery of filtered plasma bicarbonate, (2) excretion of titratable acid (buffered by phosphate), and (3) NH_4^+ production. To recover plasma bicarbonate, the proximal tubules reabsorb 85% of the filtered load by bulk transfer, and then the distal tubular H^+ gradient permits recovery of the remaining 15% of bicarbonate via H^+ excretion. Ventilation removes thousands of milliequivalents of carbon dioxide per day, thus preventing build-up of the weak acid, H_2CO_3, formed when carbon dioxide remains dissolved in plasma.

Acid-base determination requires measurement of blood pH, pCO_2, and bicarbonate. Bicarbonate, total carbon dioxide content, and carbon dioxide combining power provide the same basic information, with total carbon dioxide (TCO_2) 1 to 2 mEq/liter lower than combining power. Note that bicarbonate can be readily calculated from the pH and pCO_2 measurements available via gas electrode. The following rearrangement of the traditional Henderson-Hasselbalch equation, as originally expressed by Kassirer and Bleich, transforms a logarithmic calculation into a simple algebraic one:[68]

Equation:

$$a. \quad pH = pK + \log \frac{base}{acid} \text{ (where pK = 6.1)}$$

$$b. \quad pH = pK + \log \frac{(HCO_3^-}{\text{dissolved } CO_2}$$

$$c. \quad pH = 6.1 + \log \frac{(HCO_3^-)}{0.03 \times pCO_2}$$

This can be rearranged to

$$d. \quad (H^+) = 24 \times \frac{pCO_2}{HCO_3^-}$$

or

$$e. \quad HCO_3^- = \frac{24 \times pCO_2}{H^+} \text{ or } TCO_2 = \frac{25 \times pCO_2}{H^+}$$

Example of calculation:

Traditional Henderson-Hasselbalch:
$$pH = pK + \log \frac{[HCO_3^-]}{[CO_2 + H_2CO_3}$$

Example
$$HCO_3^- = 24; pCO_2 = 40$$
$$pH = 6.10 + \log \frac{24}{0.03 \times 40}$$
$$= 6.10 + \log \frac{24}{1.2}$$
$$= 6.10 + 1.30 = 7.40 \text{ (i.e., normal)}$$

Useful Kassirer version: $pCO_2 = \frac{[H^+] [HCO_3^-]}{24}$

where pCO_2 is expressed in mm Hg

HCO_3^- is expressed in mEq/liter

H^+ is expressed in nEq/liter

Example: Calculate HCO_3^- when pH = 7.40 and pCO_2 = 40.
$$pH = 7.40$$
$$pCO_2 = 40 \text{ (measured)}$$
$$40 = \frac{40 [HCO_3^-]}{24}$$
$$HCO_3^- = \frac{24 \times 40}{40}$$
$$HCO_3^- = 24$$

where pH is expressed in nEq H^+/liter. Thus, knowing pCO_2 and H^+ (from pH), one can calculate bicarbonate readily. Having the pH and serum bicarbonate values, the extent of a patient's acid-base imbalance can be assessed and the nature of the disturbance determined.

Ideally, arterial samples of blood are run through a blood gas machine to obtain the pCO_2 and pH necessary for calculating bicarbonate. Although venous samples are theoretically acceptable, they may prove inaccurate when patients have impaired circulation, local tissue damage, or blood stasis caused by a tourniquet. The normal values for arterial and venous blood are given in Table 35-20. Note that in infants, pH is lower by approximately 0.05 units.

Definitions

Acid-base disturbances are divided into metabolic versus respiratory, acute versus chronic, simple versus mixed, and pure versus compensated. The clinical state is described as an **acidosis** or an **alkalosis,** depending on the pH, while the isolated change of hydrogen ion concentration in the blood is better described as either **acidemia** or **alkalemia.** Definitions are as follows:

Table 35-20. Normal blood values*

Blood sample	pH	pCO₂	HCO₃⁻	TCO₂
Arterial	7.38–7.45	35–45 torr	23–27 mEq/liter	24–28 mEq/liter
Venous	7.35–7.40	45–50 torr	24–29 mEq/liter	25–30 mEq/liter

*In infants, the normal range for TCO₂ is 20–26, and pH is lower by approximately 0.05.

Table 35-21. Compensation in acid-base disorders

Acid-base disturbances	pH	HCO₃⁻	pCO₂	Compensation
Metabolic acidosis	↓	↓		↓pCO₂; acid urine
Metabolic alkalosis	↑	↑		↑pCO₂; alkaline urine
Respiratory acidosis	↓		↑	Acid urine
Respiratory alkalosis	↑		↓	Alkaline urine

Acidemia	Increased concentration H⁺ in blood
Alkalemia	Decreased concentration H⁺ in blood
Acidosis	Physiologic disturbance due to acid load
Alkalosis	Physiologic disturbance due to alkaline load
Primary	Reflects initial perturbation; uncompensated
Compensated	Results from restorative drive
Simple	One primary disturbance
Mixed	Two primary disturbances
Respiratory	Change in pCO₂; reflects change in ventilation
Metabolic	Change in H⁺ or HCO₃⁻

In "pure" pH imbalances, the disturbance results from a deviation of either pCO₂ (respiratory) or HCO₃⁻ (metabolic) from the normal. Looking at the Henderson equation, one sees that a rise in pCO₂ will increase the denominator, leading to a fall in pH; this defines respiratory acidosis. Conversely, a falling pCO₂ reduces the denominator, and pH rises, producing respiratory alkalosis. Retention of HCO₃⁻ causes alkalosis, while a drop in HCO₃⁻ produces metabolic acidosis. These pure situations will prevail only briefly. The initial change in the internal milieu induces compensatory mechanisms. Ordinarily, the initial disturbance is only partially corrected because compensatory mechanisms are rarely sufficient to offset the primary disturbance completely. Thus, patients typically have a compensated disorder, as is illustrated in Table 35-21.

Respiratory Acidosis

Retention of carbon dioxide gas (↑pCO₂) leads to an increased amount of carbon dioxide dissolved in blood and a consequent increase in H₂CO₃, which produces respiratory acidosis (Table 35-22). Normally, the initial rise in pCO₂ stimulates increased ventilation, thereby eliminating the hypercapnia. In acute respiratory acidosis, buffering mechanisms are minimal, and pH rapidly becomes acidotic as pCO₂ exceeds 50 mm Hg. Acute correction does not occur because the renal compensatory mechanisms require time for induction. In chronic respiratory acidosis, however, renal compensation is very effective through increased ammonium production. By this mechanism of increased hydrogen ion excre-

tion, the kidney is able to raise ECF bicarbonate to a maximum of 40 mEq/liter, thereby compensating for marked hypercapnia.

Respiratory Alkalosis

Respiratory alkalosis is rarely a presenting complaint for the pediatric patient in the ICU. However, mechanical ventilation producing hyperventilation will result in respiratory alkalosis. Respiratory alkalosis may occur in the early phase of salicylate intoxication, Reye's syndrome, and in some hypermetabolic states.[69–71] Other common causes of respiratory alkalosis are noted in Table 35-23.

Rapid correction of metabolic acidosis also can result in respiratory alkalosis, because correction of the pH in cerebral spinal fluid can lag behind correction of acidosis in the ECF, and the continuing CNS acidosis stimulates the medullary ventilatory drive into a state of overcompensation.[72] Diagnosis of respiratory alkalosis rests on the triad of decreased pCO₂, elevated pH, and normal bicarbonate.

Metabolic Acidosis

Increased blood H⁺ produces metabolic acidosis with a concomitant fall in pH. As blood buffers and bicarbonate are consumed, the hydrogen ion concentration increases. In the ICU, metabolic

Table 35-22. Causes of respiratory acidosis

Acute	Chronic
Airway obstruction	Airway obstruction
Respiratory center depression	Depressed respiratory center
Circulatory catastrophe	Neuromuscular defect
Neuromuscular defect	Restrictive defect
Restrictive disease	
Smoke inhalation	
Mechanical ventilation	

Table 35-23. Causes of respiratory alkalosis

Anxiety	Intrathoracic process—congestive heart failure, pneumonitis, emboli
Fever	
Reye's snydrome	Hypoxemia
Salicylate poisoning	Gram (−) sepsis
CNS disease—trauma, cerebrovascular accident, infection, tumor	Pregnancy
	Excessive mechanical ventilation

acidosis may be multifactorial in etiology. There may be (1) an **addition** of hydrogen ion to the patient through medication, (2) **excess production** of hydrogen ion due to disease (i.e., circulatory impairment, diabetes mellitus), (3) **hydrogen ion retention** as in renal failure, and (4) **bicarbonate loss** through diarrhea or renal tubular impairment. The major diagnostic point to consider is the differentiation between accumulation of organic acids contributing to the acidosis versus simple hyperchloremic metabolic acidosis.

Any accumulation of organic acids will be reflected by a rise in the anion "gap"; this (arithmetic) gap reflects unmeasured anions normally present in the plasma. The calculation is as follows: $[Na^+] - [Cl^-] \approx 12$ mEq/liter. In infants, the normal anion gap may reach 16 mEq/liter. When unmeasured organic anions are produced as part of the metabolic disturbance causing acidosis, the anion gap will rise in proportion to the fall in bicarbonate. For example, the large anion gap in lactic acidosis reflects the accumulation of a large amount of "unmeasured anion," which can be quantified by laboratory measurement of lactate and pyruvate. Contrariwise, if the metabolic acidosis is accompanied exclusively by a falling bicarbonate without additional organic anions, the anion gap will change little because chloride rises in proportion to the loss of bicarbonate in serum.

In a patient with an elevated anion gap, the key point is to pursue the diagnosis until the source of the unmeasured organic acid has been identified (Table 35-24). After determining the cause of the metabolic acidosis, treatment should aim first at correcting the underlying disturbance and then at correction of the chemical disturbance, if necessary and possible. Because metabolic acidosis commonly occurs amidst other perturbations, one must also correct problems with circulation, intravascular volume, potassium, chloride, and any organic anion. Over the years, enthusiasm for infusion of sodium bicarbonate versus other substitutes waxes and wanes as concerns about the dangers rise and fall.[73] The use of bicarbonate for correction of diabetic ketoacidosis remains a long-standing controversy.[74] Generally, with metabolic acidosis, if pH falls below 7.15 and serum bicarbonate is below 15 mEq/liter, acute therapy will be indicated.[75] A dose of 0.5 to 2.0 mEq/kg of sodium bicarbonate should be given via rapid IV infusion into a large vein.

One of the major risks of treatment with $NaHCO_3$ is excess sodium administration. Particularly in infants, hypernatremia can result from therapy and may necessitate a change to THAM (Trishydroxymethyl-aminomethane).[76] In a severely hypernatremic patient, dialysis provides an effective treatment for both the sodium excess and the acidosis. One can use bicarbonate in the dialysate, and the dialysis process will remove sodium and acid while replenishing bicarbonate through careful tailoring of dialysate composition.

Table 35-24. Causes of metabolic acidosis

Anion Gap*	
Unchanged	*Increased*
Diarrhea	Lactic acidosis
Renal disease	Salicylate poisoning
Renal tubular acidosis	Ethylene glycol
Carbonic anhydrase inhibition	Diabetic ketoacidosis
Exogenous H+ load	Renal failure
$\quad NH_4Cl$	Paraldehyde
$\quad$ Arginine HCl	Amino acid disorder
Mineralocorticoid deficiency	
Illeal conduit for urinary diversion	

*Anion gap $= Na^+ - [Cl^- + HCO_3^-] \leq 12$.

Metabolic Alkalosis

When bicarbonate rises, metabolic alkalosis results and is reflected in an increased pH. Table 35-25 lists the causes of metabolic alkalosis. Hydrogen ion and chloride depletion result mainly from either gastrointestinal loss through vomiting or excess diuretics. When nasogastric suction is maintained over many days, children can experience substantial losses of HCl, leading to metabolic alkalosis. IV fluid replacement with a higher concentration of saline will help offset the loss of acid. Use of H_2-receptor antagonists such as cimetidine can also help reduce the ongoing loss of HCl.

In addition to gastrointestinal loss, hydrogen ion and chloride can be depleted through diuretic use, mineralocorticoid excess, and Bartter's syndrome. Diuretics such as thiazides and the loop diuretics—furosemide, bumetadine, ethacrynic acid—block reabsorption of chloride either at the distal tubule (thiazides) or in the thin ascending limb of Henle's loop, leading to marked urinary excretion of sodium, chloride, and potassium. This loss of sodium and chloride promotes alkalosis directly because the available anion for reabsorption of cations tends to be bicarbonate in the absence of available chloride. Furthermore, urinary renal kaliuresis (induced by the diuretic) reduces the availability of potassium for

Table 35-25. Metabolic alkalosis

Causes	Comments
H+ depletion	
Chloride depletion	Vomiting, diuretics, nasogastric suction
Mineralocorticoid excess	Congenital adrenal cortical hyperplasia, primary aldosteronism, mineralocorticoid therapy
Bartter's syndrome	
Saline-resistant alkalosis	
Alkaline load	Potassium depletion
ECF contraction	Exogenous HCO_3^- or endogenous metabolism of lactate, acetate, citrate
Diuretics	

sodium exchange in the reabsorption mechanism and leads to further urinary excretion of hydrogen ion in exchange for reabsorbed sodium. This continuing loss of sodium and chloride leads to contraction of the ECF, making the renal tubule more avid for sodium and aggravating hydrogen ion loss through the urine; this physiologic complication contributes to the maintenance of metabolic alkalosis. Together, these mechanisms produce the typical picture of hypokalemic metabolic alkalosis.[77]

The opposite pathophysiology induced by mineralocorticoid excess leads to a similar picture. Excess mineralocorticoid—Cushing's syndrome, congenital adrenal cortical hyperplasia with either the 11-hydroxylase or 17-hydroxylase deficiency—leads to reabsorption of sodium in the distal tubule in exchange for hydrogen ion and potassium, which are excreted in the urine. The excess sodium retention leads to volume expansion rather than the contraction previously noted, but the same hypokalemic metabolic alkalosis results.

In Bartter's syndrome, patients present with a chemical picture of hypokalemic metabolic alkalosis. This disorder is caused by hyperplasia of the juxtaglomerular apparatus in the kidney, with consequent overproduction of renin.[78] This hyperreninemia leads to excess aldosterone and a chemical picture with physiologic mechanisms that are still unclear but an outcome that is hypokalemic metabolic alkalosis. Excess alkaline load will lead to metabolic alkalosis from either direct infusion of bicarbonate intravenously or oral ingestion of medication that contains bicarbonate, such as calcium carbonate in antacid tablets, or from the endogenous metabolism of lactate, acetate, or citrate, usually arising from the IV administration of blood products.

In cases of ECF contraction, mild metabolic alkalosis may result from the mechanism already outlined. In young patients with cystic fibrosis, however, both hyponatremia and metabolic alkalosis have been reported when excess sweating occurs without provision of sodium chloride to replete losses.[79] The mechanism is that of ECF contraction and mineralocorticoid stimulation, leading to metabolic alkalosis by the mechanism previously discussed.

A peculiar form of metabolic alkalosis occasionally develops in patients who are severely potassium-depleted. In this "saline-resistant alkalosis," repletion of sodium and chloride does not correct the alkalosis; rather, the infused saline reappears in the urine. Management of these patients requires provision of large amounts of potassium intravenously as potassium chloride; this will turn off the saline resistance.

Treatment of metabolic alkalosis would seem to be simple, in that provision of an acidifying agent should correct the chemical disturbance. However, the available agents all have problems. Even when dilute, hydrochloric acid (as a 0.1 molar solution) is still difficult to infuse because of the pain it elicits and the risk of hemolysis. Arginine HCl is infrequently used, has produced hyperkalemia, and is contraindicated in renal failure. Ammonium chloride (NH_4Cl) cannot be used in patients who suffer liver failure with elevated ammonia and is also contraindicated in renal failure patients. Rather than employing acidifying agents, one should provide sodium chloride, which both corrects any ECF deficit and reverses the contractional alkalosis, thereby again permitting excretion of excess bicarbonate in the urine. Correction of any underlying defect, provision of saline intravenously, and repletion of potassium are the mainstays of therapy for metabolic alkalosis. When severe alkalosis occurs and pH begins to approach 7.60, one should consider the use of acidifying agents. Alternatively, peritoneal dialysis can be employed with high-chloride and low-

bicarbonate dialysate to correct the alkalosis. Although this approach seems very attractive and makes good sense in the patient who has concomitant renal failure, it has little application. Unfortunately, renal failure far more commonly results in metabolic acidosis than alkalosis. When using peritoneal dialysis in a patient with metabolic alkalosis, it is important to avoid ECF contraction. This would further aggravate the alkalosis and can occur fairly rapidly if the dialysis works efficiently.

Mixed Acid-Base Disorders

Mixed acid-base disturbances are among the most challenging diagnostic and therapeutic cases. Remember that the presence of one (primary) acid-base disturbance does not protect against a second disturbance.[80] There is no simple way to unmask the presence of a mixed disturbance, but the use of a nomogram (Fig. 35-7) may help clarify the problem.[81] The nomogram provides 95% confidence bands for each of the primary acid-base disturbances. The data from which these are derived are based on pediatric cases. As an example of a mixed disturbance, consider a child who presents with pH 7.50, $PaCO_2$ 60 mm Hg, and a bicarbonate of 44 mEq/liter. When plotted on the nomogram, the disturbance falls between metabolic alkalosis and respiratory acidosis and is, in fact, a mixture of both. This common mixed disturbance may occur in infants who have bronchopulmonary dysplasia leading to chronic respiratory acidosis and are treated with furosemide, which induces metabolic alkalosis.

The Pharmacology and Use of Diuretics

While diuretics produce an increase in urine flow, as the term *diuresis* suggests, they also can serve to manipulate changes in body chemistry through changes in sodium, potassium, chloride, acid-base balance, uric acid, and calcium balance by judicious enhancement or depression of urinary solute and water excretion.[82] This requires knowledge of renal tubular physiology and also familiarity with the different major classes of diuretics and their sites of action.[83,84] Drugs that may work with predictable effects in adults may behave quite differently in an infant or young child. Fewer studies are available on the pharmacokinetics of diuretics in infants and small children, as compared with adults.[85,86] Nonetheless, clinical pharmacologic practice has evolved that permits the safe and effective use of diuretic agents in children.

Anatomy and Physiology of the Renal Tubule

The renal tubule can best be considered as comprising several major zones, both structurally and functionally; each of the zones in turn includes subsegments (Fig. 35-8). In the proximal tubule, after filtration by the glomerulus, the ultrafiltrate passes into the proximal tubule, which consists of an initial convoluted segment followed by a straight segment. This portion of the nephron serves to effect bulk transfer of water, glucose, amino acids, bicarbonate, and electrolytes out of the tubule lumen into the interstitium and ultimately back into the circulation to complete the reabsorption process. About 70% of filtered sodium is reabsorbed in this location by using isosmotic mechanisms, leaving a vastly reduced solute and water volume exiting from the proximal tubule into the thin descending limb of the loop of Henle.

The loop of Henle permits concentration of the solute and further reduction of intratubular water volume, particularly in

Figure 35-7. In vivo acid-base nomogram.

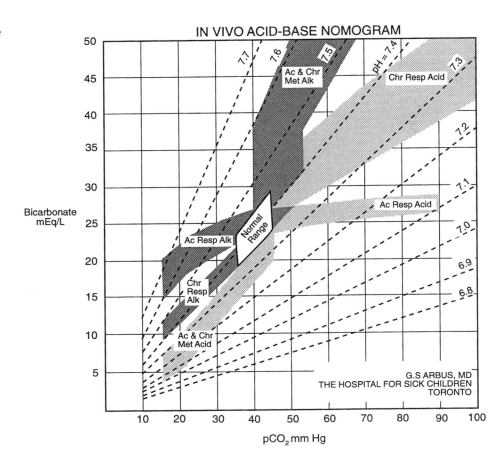

the deep juxtamedullary nephrons. The thin descending limb is permeable to water, sodium, potassium, and chloride. Water reabsorption occurs, leading to a steadily increasing concentration of the tubular contents as Henle's loop descends toward the medulla. After rounding the hairpin turn, the intratubular fluid enters a region relatively impermeable to water but virtually freely permeable to chloride. Along this segment, sodium and chloride are passively absorbed and the ionic concentration of the fluid drops until it is nearly isosthenuric as the fluid reaches the distal tubule.

The ascending limb of the distal tubule acts to absorb about 20% of sodium via active transport mechanisms. Potassium and chloride are also reabsorbed out of the lumen through these mechanisms. The key importance of the transport system is that it operates in a zone of relative water impermeability in the ascending limb. By the time the ultrafiltrate reaches termination of the distal tubule, it is hyposthenuric and enters the collecting duct quite dilute.

A short segment of nephron joins the distal tubule to the collecting duct. This conduit conveys proto-urine all the way from the superficial cortex down through the medulla, terminating at the ducts of Bellini, which open onto the renal papilla. The effluent from the ducts collects in the renal calyces and from there are conveyed through the renal pelvis and thence out of the body. The key feature of the collecting duct is its responsiveness to ADH. Under the influence of ADH, collecting duct cells generate pores permeable to water and permit reabsorption of water out of the collecting duct and back into the interstitium. This produces a concentrated urine. Lack of ADH, or insensitivity to it, permits dilute urine to flow through the impermeable collecting duct on to the renal calyces, resulting in a high-volume, dilute diuresis.

Pharmacology of Specific Diuretics: Indications for Use, Complications, and Dosages

There are four general sites of action in the nephron for the major classes of diuretics: (1) proximal tubule, (2) loop of Henle, (3) distal tubule, and (4) collecting duct. Table 35-26 lists the commonly used diuretic agents, with their sites and modes of action and relative strengths with respect to sodium diuresis.[87]

Loop Diuretics

This group of drugs effects diuresis by altering the normal function of the loop of Henle.

Furosemide (Lasix)

Furosemide affects the thick ascending limb of the loop of Henle by blocking chloride transport. By confining this anion to the tubule lumen, it obligates the cations sodium, potassium, and calcium to remain in the tubule fluid and pass out with the urine. IV administration results in effective diuresis and natriuresis within 30 to 60 minutes; the action usually disappears over 4 hours. Sodium excretion rises 15 to 30 times, and urine flow rises tenfold or more. Furosemide remains the best studied diuretic. Its safety and efficacy are well characterized and predictable.[87-89] To work, furosemide must reach the lumenal border of the tubule; hence,

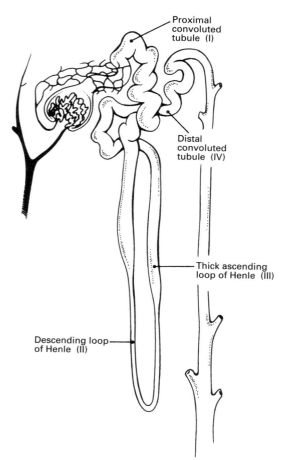

Figure 35-8. The renal tubule. See Table 35-26 for relative sites of action of the diuretics.

in patients with markedly depressed glomerular filtration rate, the drug loses much of its effectiveness.

Furosemide is widely used in bronchopulmonary dysplasia, and this remains one of the common chronic uses for the drug.[90,91] Furosemide proves very effective in the management of congestive heart failure, nephrotic edema, and volume overload in the setting of acute renal failure.[92,93] In the circumstance of acute glomerulonephritis with severe fluid retention, furosemide is invaluable for volume management, control of pulmonary edema, and reduction of hypervolemic hypertension. Furosemide also plays a role in the control of fluid retention in liver failure and for inducing high-volume diuresis in patients treated with nephrotoxic agents for chemotherapy. Despite evidence from animal studies that furosemide can "open up" oliguric renal failure, its use in children has remained disappointing in this clinical setting.[94]

The major side effects of furosemide are the results of its potent diuretic effect on many ions. Hypokalemic metabolic alkalosis follows chronic use. Vigorous diuresis with high doses of furosemide regularly produces hyponatremia and hypokalemia. Persistent use can also produce depletion of calcium and magnesium and has caused nephrocalcinosis, particularly in infants.[95,96] Concern has been raised over the possible aggravated ototoxicity of combined furosemide and aminoglycoside treatment. This circumstance can arise in the ICU when patients with acute renal failure receive aminoglycoside antibiotics for sepsis and furosemide to augment urine production.[97] The aminoglycoside level must be carefully monitored to avoid toxicity.

In patients with severe edema due to the nephrotic syndrome, combined use of albumin and furosemide causes mobilization and removal of fluid. During a 4- to 6-hour infusion of salt-poor albumin, furosemide is infused at 2 and 4 hours to enhance salt and water excretion. In patients requiring minoxidil for severe hypertension, concurrent administration of furosemide can help to avoid the severe salt and water retention that is a side effect of

Table 35-26. Action and potency of diuretics

Diuretic agent	Site of action	Mechanism of action	Natriuretic potency (%)*
Osmotic agent 　Mannitol 　Urea	I	Osmotic diuresis	5
Acetazolamide	I	Carbonic anhydrase inhibitor	5
Loop diuretics 　Ethacrynic acid 　Furosemide 　Bumetanide	II	Block Na, K, and 2 Cl co-transport	15–25
Thiazides 　Chlorothiazide 　Hydrochlorothiazide 　Chlorthalidone 　Metalazone	III	Block isosmotic reabsorption NaCl	5–10
Potassium-sparing agents 　Spironolactone 　Triameterene 　Amiloride	IV	Aldersterone inhibitor Blocks apical sodium reabsorption Blocks apical sodium reabsorption	2–3

*Natriuretic potency refers to maximal ability to increase the functional excretion of sodium.
Adapted from TG Wells. The pharmacology and therapeutics of diuretics in the pediatric patient. *Pediatr Clin North Am* 37:472, 1990. With permission.

minoxidil treatment. Furosemide is also useful in patients with dangerous hypercalcemia because the calciuresis is prompt and large.[98] Furosemide is an excellent treatment for acute hyperkalemia, either to avoid dialysis or as a temporizing measure while awaiting dialysis. Furosemide also is a handy wash-out treatment when using methotrexate or cyclophosphamide as cancer chemotherapy. In severe refractory edema, especially with impaired renal function, the combination of metalazone and furosemide (or another loop diuretic) is especially effective. This combination should be used carefully because large salt and water losses may occur rapidly. In volume overload due to water intoxication, hyponatremia may be treated with furosemide diuresis followed by the infusion of normal saline to begin correction of the hyponatremia.

Ethacrynic Acid (Edecrin)

Ethacrynic acid's action and pharmacokinetics are similar to those of furosemide. It, too, acts on the ascending limb of Henle's loop and also inhibits chloride transport at that site.

Ethacrynic acid is used in the pediatric population for clinical problems similar to those for which furosemide is indicated. When infants and children prove resistant to furosemide, ethacrynic acid is often used as a clinical trial. Like furosemide, ethacrynic acid is unlikely to work if glomerular filtration rate is extremely depressed. For children who are sulfonamide allergic, ethacrynic acid can substitute for furosemide. Ototoxicity has been reported in patients receiving ethacrynic acid, and it is not clear that the toxicity of this agent is significantly different from that of furosemide.[99]

Bumetanide (Bumex)

Experience with bumetanide in the PICU is not extensive. In clinical practice, 1 mg of bumetanide is approximately equal to 40 mg of furosemide orally. Intravenously, bumetanide doses are relatively larger, in the range of 0.05 to 0.1 mg/kg/dose, because of differences in oral versus IV bioavailability.[100]

The use of bumetanide parallels the uses of the other loop diuretics. Like ethacrynic acid, it may achieve successful diuresis in patients resistant to furosemide. The adverse consequences of bumetanide are similar to those of the other loop diuretics. It is thought to be less ototoxic than ethacrynic acid and furosemide.[101]

Osmotic Agents

Small molecules filtered by the glomerulus but not reabsorbed further along in the nephron will obligate water to proceed into the collecting system and thus promote enhanced water excretion. Several agents will cause this effect: mannitol, urea, radiographic contrast agents, and excess filtered glucose. Mannitol is the most common agent used for inducing an osmotic water diuresis. Given intravenously at 0.25 to 1.0 g/kg/dose, mannitol first increases intravascular volume by its plasma oncotic effect. Then after glomerular filtration, it induces a brisk water diuresis. Mannitol works rapidly and is quickly cleared from the body over 2 to 4 hours.

The two major uses for mannitol are (1) increased intracranial pressure, and (2) prerenal acute renal failure; both of these uses of mannitol occur in precariously ill patients. Unfortunately, there may be a rebound in intracranial pressure after treatment. In renal failure, excessive use of mannitol may lead to its accumulation in the blood with consequent disturbance in serum sodium.[102] Hyponatremia may ensue if mannitol remains in the circulation consequent to severe oliguria; or hypernatremia may result from excess free-water loss due to protracted use of mannitol. During cardiac surgery, mannitol is sometimes used prophylactically to maintain a high urine volume in an attempt to avert ischemic renal damage and subsequent acute tubular necrosis.

Use of mannitol may cause electrolyte disturbances either because it obligates water to enter the intravascular space and thereby dilutes electrolytes or because of excess urinary water losses leading to hemoconcentration. Careful monitoring of fluid balance, weight, and BP are essential; electrolyte monitoring may be necessary in cases of repeated mannitol treatments.[103]

Thiazide Diuretics (Diuril, Hydrodiuril, Hygroton)

The thiazide drugs work by blocking chloride transport out of the thick ascending limb of Henle's loop in the distal tubule. Because sodium transport is coupled to chloride transport, the thiazide agents enhance excretion of sodium, chloride, and water, as well as potassium. Unlike the loop diuretics, thiazide agents exert an anticalciuric effect. Generally, thiazides are administered orally and act more slowly than the loop diuretics. Chlorothiazide and hydrochlorothiazide are commonly used in infants and children on a 12-hour schedule. The dose for chlorothiazide is 10 to 20 mg/kg/d, and for hydrochlorothiazide is 1 to 2 mg/kg/d.

Thiazides are an excellent choice of diuretic for chronic use in children. Thus, patients with congestive heart failure, infants with bronchopulmonary dysplasia, and patients with fluid retention due to moderate renal failure are candidates for thiazide treatment.[103] In advanced renal failure, the thiazide diuretics are not effective.

Although thiazides do not induce as vigorous a diuresis as that induced by loop agents, they have a number of side effects that can become serious with chronic treatment. Serious volume depletion, hypokalemia, hyponatremia, and hypercalcemia can result at ordinary therapeutic doses. Hypomagnesemia and marked hypokalemic metabolic alkalosis also can occur with aggressive thiazide treatment. In patients at risk for hyperuricemia, thiazides may exaggerate the problem.

Because thiazides are available in oral suspension, they are particularly attractive in the treatment of infants with either hypertension or fluid retention. In infants or children susceptible to calcium kidney stones, the hypocalciuric effect of thiazides can be exploited as protection against calculi and yet not produce serious levels of hypercalcemia.

Acetazolamide (Diamox)

Acetazolamide works as a carbonic anhydrase inhibitor in the proximal tubule. It is not used very widely for diuresis because its natriuretic effect is mild and newer diuretic agents are more powerful. Because it results in bicarbonate excretion in the urine, however, it is valuable where urinary alkalinization is desired (e.g., in the correction of severe metabolic alkalosis). Urinary alkalinization may increase excretion of salicylate in salicylate poisoning and will also enhance the excretion of cystine or uric acid. Another indication for acetazolamide in children is control of hydrocephalus.[104]

Acetazolamide causes metabolic acidosis if used chronically and in pharmacologic doses. Potassium losses also occur as a result of increased sodium-potassium exchange.

Metolazone (Zaroxolyn)

Metolazone is a moderately long-acting diuretic that works in both proximal and distal tubules to block sodium reabsorption. Unlike thiazides, this agent does not cause kaliuresis.

Metolazone is not commonly used as a single agent in children. Rather, it is combined with furosemide for treatment of refractory edema.[105,106] This potent combination often will be effective in the face of markedly diminished glomerular filtration rate, unlike thiazide or loop diuretics alone. Tablets of 2.5 and 5 mg are available. Dosages are not well established for infants and children. A dose of 1.25 mg can be used in infants, and up to 5 mg is appropriate for older children.

Metolazone has side effects similar to those of other thiazide diuretics, including hypokalemic metabolic alkalosis and hyperuricemia. These complications were noted when metolazone was added to furosemide for resistant edema in children with the nephrotic syndrome.[106] Because metolazone is typically used in combination with a loop diuretic to produce a more potent result, these side effects deserve serious consideration.

Potassium-Sparing Diuretics
Spironolactone (Aldactone)
By competing for aldosterone binding sites in the collecting tubule, spironolactone blocks the action of aldosterone. Consequently, the aldosterone-induced exchange of sodium for potassium, which results in sodium reabsorption and potassium excretion, is reduced, and sodium is excreted while potassium remains in the body. The diuretic efficacy of spironolactone is less than the thiazides or loop diuretics for both water and sodium excretion. Onset of action is slower, and the duration of action persists longer than either thiazides or loop diuretics.

Spironolactone often is used in conjunction with either a thiazide or loop diuretic to reduce potassium losses. Although it can be used for conventional diuresis, it is especially effective in situations of elevated mineralocorticoid. Thus, this drug is effective in children with hyperaldosteronism, edema secondary to liver disease, or congestive heart failure due to congenital heart disease. Hyperkalemia may result from chronic use. Potassium supplementation given with spironolactone poses special dangers.

In children with tubular potassium wasting and impaired renal function, spironolactone can be particularly useful. For example, in children with nephropathic cystinosis with the Fanconi syndrome, refractory hypokalemia commonly occurs. Use of spironolactone or triamterine, coupled with potassium supplements, can help greatly in raising the serum potassium.

Triamterene (Dyrenium) and Amiloride (Midamor)
Triamterene and amiloride are used for their potassium-sparing effects in patients treated with thiazide or loop diuretics. Clinical experience with these two agents in infants and children is limited. Like spironolactone, triamterene has a special use in children treated with digoxin for congenital heart disease and concurrent loop diuretic for diuresis. The addition of triamterene can prevent potential hypokalemia. Also, in children with tubulointerstitial disorders such as cystinosis or the Fanconi syndrome, triamterene markedly improves the refractory hypokalemia from which these children suffer. Neither agent is a powerful diuretic, and they are commonly used in conjunction with thiazides or loop diuretics.

Both of these agents can cause severe hyperkalemia, especially when used in conjunction with potassium supplements. For this reason, great care should be exercised if either agent is used in a child with renal impairment. The combination of hydrochlorizide and amiloride is used to treat congenital nephrogenic diabetes insipidus.[107]

References

1. Smith HW. *The Kidney: Structure and Function in Health and Disease.* New York: Oxford University Press, 1955.

2. Maxwell MH, Kleeman CR, Narins RG. *Clinical Disorders of Fluid and Electrolyte Metabolism* (4th ed). New York: McGraw-Hill, 1987.

3. Kokko JP, Tannen RL. *Fluids and Electrolytes* (2nd ed). Philadelphia: Saunders, 1990.

4. Schrier RW. *Renal and Electrolyte Disorders* (3rd ed). Boston: Little, Brown, 1986.

5. Rose BD. *Clinical Physiology of Acid Base and Electrolyte Disorders.* New York: McGraw-Hill, 1989.

6. Ichikawa I. *Pediatric Textbook of Fluids and Electrolytes.* Baltimore: Williams & Wilkins, 1990.

7. Winters R. *The Body Fluids in Pediatrics.* Boston: Little, Brown, 1973.

8. Shantosham M et al. Oral rehydration therapy of infantile diarrhea: A controlled study of well nourished children hospitalized in the United States and Panama. *N Engl J Med* 306:1070, 1982.

9. American Academy of Pediatrics. Use of oral fluid therapy in post-treatment feeding following enteritis in children in a developed country. *Pediatrics* 75:358, 1985.

10. Klish W. Use of oral fluids in treatment of diarrhea. *Pediatr Rev* 7:27, 1985.

11. Finberg L. The role of electrolyte glucose solutions in hydration for children—International and domestic aspects. *J Pediatr* 96:51, 1980.

12. Link DA. Fluid and electrolytes. In Grafe JW, Cone TW (eds): *Manual of Pediatric Therapeutics* (2nd ed). Boston: Little, Brown, 1980.

13. Friis-Hansen B. Changes in body water compartments during growth. *Acta Paediatr Scand* 110:1–68, 1957.

14. Friis-Hansen B. Body water compartments in children: Changes during growth and related changes in body composition. *Pediatrics* 28:107, 1963.

15. Link DA. Accurate assessment in therapy of pediatric dehydration. In Link DA (ed): *Updates in Acute Pediatrics II.* Atlanta: American Health Consultants, 1987.

16. Kallen RJ, Lonergan JM. Fluid resuscitation of acute hypovolemic hypoperfusion states in pediatrics. *Pediatr Clin North Am* 37:287, 1990.

17. Berl T et al. Clinical disorders of water metabolism. *Kidney Int* 110:117, 1976.

18. Saunders N, Balfe J, Laski B. Severe salt poisoning in an infant. *J Pediatr* 88:258, 1976.

19. Bravo EL, Tarazi RE, Duston HP. Changing clinical spectrum of primary aldosteronism. *Am J Med* 74:641, 1883.

20. Guyton AC et al. Salt balance and longer term blood pressure control. *Annu Rev Med* 31:15, 1980.

21. Arieff AI, Guisado R, Lazarowitz VC. The pathophysiology of hyperosmolar states. In Andreoli TE, Granthan JJ, Rector FC (eds): *Disturbances in Body Fluid Osmolality.* Bethesda, MD: American Physiological Society, 1977.

22. Brucke E, Abal G, Aceto T. Pathogenesis and pathophysiology of hypertonic dehydration with diarrhea. *Am J Dis Child* 115:122, 1968.

23. Arieff AI, Guisado R. Effects on the central nervous system of hypernatremic and hyponatremic states. *Kidney Int* 10:104, 1976.

24. Brenner BM, Stein J. *Sodium and Water Homeostasis.* New York: Churchill Livingston, 1978.

25. Kleeman CR. CNS manifestations of disordered salt and water balance. *Hosp Pract* 14:59, 1979.

26. Brucke E. Fluid and electrolyte therapy. *Pediatr Clin North Am* 12:193, 1972.

27. Miller NL, Finberg L. Peritoneal dialysis for salt poisoning. *N Engl J Med* 263:1347, 1960.

28. Rosenfeld W et al. Improving the management of hypernatremic dehydration. *Clin Pediatr* 5:411, 1977.

29. Robertson GL. Abnormalities of thirst regulation. *Kidney Int* 25:460, 1984.

30. Hayek A, Peake GT. Hypothalamic adipsia without demonstrable structural lesion. *Pediatrics* 70:275, 1982.

31. Schaff-Blass E, Robertson GL, Rosenfield RL. Chronic hypernatremia from a congenital defect in osmoregulation of thirst and vasopressin. *J Pediatr* 102:703, 1983.

32. Berry PL, Belsha CW. Hyponatremia. *Pediatr Clin North Am* 37:354, 1990.

33. Fichman MP et al. Diuretic-induced hyponatremia. *Ann Intern Med* 75:853, 1971.

34. Sterns RH. "Slow" correction of hyponatremia: A break with tradition? *Kidney* 23:1, 1991.

35. Sterns RH, Thomas DJ, Herndon RM. Brain dehydration and neurologic deterioration after rapid correction of hyponatremia. *Kidney Int* 35:69, 1989.

36. Cluitmans FH, Meinders AE. Management of severe hyponatremia: Rapid or slow correction? *Am J Med* 88:161, 1990.

37. Sterns RH. Severe symptomatic hyponatremia: Treatment and outcome: A study of 64 cases. *Ann Intern Med* 107:656, 1987.

38. Sterns RH. The treatment of hyponatremia: First, do no harm. *Am J Med* 88:557, 1990.

39. Ayus JC, Krothapalli RK, Afieff AI. Treatment of symptomatic hyponatremia and its relation to brain damage. *N Engl J Med* 317:1190, 1987.

40. Berl T. Treating hyponatremia: "Damned if we do and damned if we don't." *Kidney Int* 37:1006, 1990.

41. Schrier RW. Pathogenesis of sodium and water retention in high output and low output cardiac failure, nephrotic syndrome, cirrhosis, and pregnancy. *N Engl J Med* 319:1065, 1988.

42. Bartter FC, Schwartz WB. The syndrome of inappropriate secretion of antidiuretic hormone. *Am J Med* 42:790, 1967.

43. Kaplan SL, Feigin RD. Syndrome of inappropriate antidiuretic hormone in children. *Adv Pediatr* 27:247, 1980.

44. Hantman D. Rapid correction of hyponatremia in the syndrome of inappropriate secretion of antidiuretic hormone: An alternative treatment of hypertonic saline. *Ann Intern Med* 78:870, 1973.

45. James JA. *Renal Disease in Childhood* (2nd ed). St. Louis: Mosby.

46. Field MJ, Giebisch GH. Hormonal control of renal potassium excretion. *Kidney Int* 27:379, 1985.

47. Battle DC, Arruda JA, Kurtzman NA. Hyperkalemic distal renal tubular acidosis associated with obstructive uropathy. *N Engl J Med* 304:373, 1981.

48. McSherry E. Renal tubular acidosis in childhood. *Kidney Int* 20:799, 1981.

49. Arnold JE, Healy JK. Hyperkalemia, hypertension and systemic acidosis without renal failure associated with a tubular defect in potassium excretion. *Am J Med* 47:461, 1969.

50. Link DA. Fluid and electrolytes. In Grafe JW, Cone TE (eds): *Manual of Pediatric Therapeutics* (2nd ed). Boston: Little, Brown, 1980.

51. Kassirer JP, Harrington JT. Diuretics and potassium metabolism: A reassessment of the need, effectiveness and safety of potassium therapy. *Kidney Int* 11:505, 1977.

52. Appel GB, Nau HC. Nephrotoxicity of anti-microbial agents. *N Engl J Med* 296:663, 1977.

53. Cirra JP, Schwartz WB. Correction of metabolic alkalosis in man without repair of potassium deficiency. A reevaluation of the role of potassium. *Am J Med* 40:19, 1966.

54. Garella S, Chazan JA, Cohen JJ. Saline-resistant metabolic alkalosis or "chloride-wasting nephropathy". *Ann Intern Med* 73:31, 1970.

55. Venkataraman PS et al. Effect of hypocalcemia on cardiac function in very-low-birth-weight preterm neonates: Studies of blood ionized calcium, echocardiography and cardiac effect of intravenous calcium therapy. *Pediatrics* 76:543, 1985.

56. Broner CW et al. Hypermagnesemia and hypocalcemia as predictors of high mortality in critically ill pediatric patients. *Crit Care Med* 18:921, 1990.

57. Cardenas-Riveri N et al. Hypocalcemia in critically ill children. *J Pediatr* 114:946, 1989.

58. Marx SJ, Bordeau JE. Divalent ion metabolism. In Maxwell MH, Kleeman CR, Narins RG (eds): *Clinical Disorders of Fluid and Electrolyte Metabolism* (4th ed) New York: McGraw-Hill, 1987.

59. Drop LJ. Ionized calcium, the heart and hemodynamic function. *Anesth Analg* 64:532, 1985.

60. Broner CW et al. A prospective, randomized, double-blind comparison of calcium chloride and calcium gluconate therapies for hypocalcemia in critically ill children. *J Pediatr* 117:986, 1990.

61. Baldree LA, Stapleton FB. Uric acid metabolism in children. *Pediatr Clin North Am* 37:391, 1990.

62. Baldree LA, Stapleton FB. Uric acid metabolism in children. *Pediatr Clin North Am* 37:391, 1990.

63. Cohen LF et al. Acute tumor lysis syndrome: A review of 37 patients with Burkitt's lymphoma. *Am J Med* 68:486, 1980.

64. Leradaelli L et al. Acute renal failure in 11 children with non-Hodgkins lymphoma. *Proc Eur Dial Transplant Assoc* 18:531, 1981.

65. Andreoli SP, Clark JH, McGuire WA. Purine excretion during tumor lysis in children with acute lymphocytic leukemia receiving allopurinol: Relationship to acute renal failure. *J Pediatr* 109:292, 1986.

66. Nolph KD, Sorkin M. Peritoneal dialysis in acute renal failure. In Brenner BM, Lazarus JM (eds): *Acute Renal Failure.* Philadelphia: Saunders, 1983.

67. Hood VL, Tannen RL. Lactic acidosis. *Kidney* 22:1, 1989.

68. Kassirer JP, Bleich H. Rapid estimation of plasma carbon dioxide from pH and total carbon dioxide content. *N Engl J Med* 272:1067, 1965.

69. Winters RW. Salicylate intoxication. In Winters RW (ed): *The Body Fluids in Pediatrics.* Boston: Little, Brown, 1973.

70. Corey L, Rubin RJ, Hattwick MAW. Reye's syndrome: Clinical progression and evaluation of therapy. *Pediatrics* 60:708, 1977.

71. Lovejoy RH et al. Clinical staging in Reye syndrome. *Am J Dis Child* 128:36, 1974.

72. Plum F, Price RW. Acid-base balance of cisternal and lumbar cerebrospinal fluid in hospital patients. *N Engl J Med* 289:1346, 1973.

73. Narins RG, Cohen JJ. Bicarbonate therapy for organic acidosis: The case for its continued use. *Ann Intern Med* 106:615, 1987.

74. Morris LR, Murphy MB, Kitabchi AE. Bicarbonate therapy in severe diabetic ketoacidosis. *Ann Intern Med* 105:836, 1986.

75. Garella S, Dana CL, Chasen J. Severity of metabolic acidosis as a determinant of bicarbonate requirements. *N Engl J Med* 289:121, 1973.

76. Simmons MA et al. Hypernatremia, intracranial hemorrhage, and NaHCO3 administration in neonates. *N Engl J Med* 291:6, 1974.

77. Emmett J, Seldin DW. Clinical syndromes of metabolic acidosis and metabolic alkalosis. In Seldin DW, Giebisch G (eds): *The Kidney.* New York: Raven, 1985.

78. Bartter FC et al. Hyperplasia of the juxtaglomerular complex with hyperaldosteronism and hypokalemic alkalosis. *Am J Med* 33:811, 1962.

79. Laughlin JJ, Brady MS, Eigen H. Changing feeding trends as a cause of electrolyte depletion in infants with cystic fibrosis. *Pediatrics* 68:203, 1981.

80. Narins RG, Emmett M. Simple and mixed acid-based disorders: A practice approach. *Medicine* 59:161, 1980.

81. Arbus GS. *In vivo* acid base nomogram for clinical use. *Can Med Assoc J* 109:291, 1973.

82. Weiner IM, Mudge GH. Diuretics and other agents employed in the mobilization of edema fluid. In Gilman AG et al (eds): *The Pharmacological Basis of Therapeutics* (7th ed). New York: MacMillan, 1985.

83. Dirks JH. Mechanisms of action and clinical uses of diuretics. *Hosp Pract* 9:99, 1979.

84. Eknoyan G. Understanding diuretic therapy. *Drug Ther* 3:47, 1981.

85. Wells TG. The pharmacology and therapeutics of diuretics in the pediatric patient. *Pediatr Clin North Am* 37:463, 1990.

86. Chemtob S et al. Pharmacology of diuretics in the newborn. *Pediatr Clin North Am* 36:1231, 1989.

87. Wells TG. The pharmacology and therapeutics of diuretics in the pediatric patient. *Pediatr Clin North Am* 37:463, 1972.

88. Greene TP et al. Prophylactic furosemide in severe respiratory distress syndrome: A blinded prospective study. *J Pediatr* 112:605, 1988.

89. Engelhardt B, Elliot TS, Hazinski TA. Short and long-term effects

of furosemide on lung function in infants with bronchopulmonary dysplasia. *J Pediatr* 109:1034, 1986.

90. Kaol C et al. Effect of oral diuretics on pulmonary mechanics in infants with chronic bronchopulmonary dysplasia. Results of a double-blind cross-over sequential trial. *Pediatrics* 74:37, 1984.

91. Moylan FMB et al. Edema of the pulmonary interstitium in infants and children. *Pediatrics* 55:783, 1975.

92. Pruitt AW, Boles A. Diuretic effect of furosemide in acute glomerulonephritis. *J Pediatr* 89:306, 1976.

93. Repetto HA et al. Renal functional response to furosemide in children with acute glomerulonephritis. *J Pediatr* 80:660, 1972.

94. Brown CB, Ogg CS, Cameron JS. High dose furosemide in acute renal failure: A controlled trial. *Clin Nephrol* 15:90, 1981.

95. Ezezedeen F, Adelman RD, Ahfors CE. Renal calcification in preterm infants: Pathophysiology and long-term sequelae. *J Pediatr* 113:532, 1988.

96. Whitington PF, Black DD. Cholelithiasis in premature infants treated with parenteral nutrition and furosemide. *J Pediatr* 97:647, 1980.

97. Lynn AM et al. Isolated deafness following recovery from neurologic injury and adult respiratory distress. A sequela of intercurrent aminoglycoside and diuretic use. *Am J Dis Child* 139:464, 1985.

98. Najjar SS, Aftimos SF, Kurani RF. Furosemide therapy for hypercalcemia of infants. *J Pediatr* 81:1171, 1972.

99. Pillay BK et al. Transient and permanent deafness following treatment with ethacrynic acid in renal failure. *Lancet* 1:77, 1969.

100. Jacobson HR. Diuretics: Mechanics of action and uses. *Hosp Pract* 22:107, 1987.

101. Brummett RE, Bendrick T, Himes D. Comparative ototoxicity of bumetanide and furosemide when used in combination with kanamycin. *J Clin Pharmacol* 21:628, 1981.

102. Badr K, Ichikawa I. Prerenal failure: A deleterious shift from renal compensation to decompensation. *N Engl J Med* 319:623, 1988.

103. Weiner IM, Mudge GH. Diuretics and other agents employed in the mobilization of edema fluid. In Gilman AG et al. (eds): *The Pharmacological Basis of Therapeutics* (7th ed). New York: MacMillan, 1985.

104. Shinnar S et al. Management of hydrocephalus in infancy: Use of acetazolamide and furosemide to avoid cerebrospinal fluid shunts. *J Pediatr* 107:31, 1985.

105. Arnold WC. Efficacy of metolazone and furosemide therapy in children with furosemide resistant edema. *Pediatrics* 74:872, 1984.

106. Garin EH, Richard GA. Edema resistant to furosemide therapy in nephrotic syndrome: Treatment with furosemide and metolazone. *Int J Pediatr Nephrol* 2:181, 1981.

107. Alon U, Chan JCM. Hydrochlorothiazide-amiloride in the treatment of congenital nephrogenic diabetes insipidus. *Am J Nephrol* 5:9, 1985.

Appendix Medical conditions requiring special intravenous therapy

System and/or disorder	Correction
Central nervous system	
Meningitis (SIADH)	1/2–2/3 maintenance
Trauma	1/2–2/3 maintenance
Tumor	1/2–2/3 maintenance
Renal	
Acute renal failure (except polyuric acute tubular necrosis)	No K+; 350 ml/m²/24 hr + urine output
Chronic renal failure	No IV K+
	Fluid limit
	Na+ limit
Postobstructive diuresis (e.g., valves)	3500 + ml/m²/24 hr for at least first day. Use 1/2 NS + appropriate K+
Tubular dysfunction	Supplemental
Renal tubular acidosis	NaHCO₃, 2–3 mEq/kg/24 hr
Fanconi syndrome/cystinosis	Na+, 2–5 mEq/kg/24 hr
Bartter's syndrome	K+, 2–5 mEq/kg/24 hr
Osmotic diuresis (postangiography)	Replace urine output with 1/2 N saline, 3000–3500 ml/m²/24 h
Endocrine	
Diabetes insipidus	4000 ml/m²/24 hr
Diabetes mellitus in ketoacidosis	supplement K+ after urine produced
Congenital adrenocortical (adrenogenital) with Na+	No K+
	Supplement Na+
Addisonian crisis	No K+
	Supplement Na+
Cardiac	
Congestive heart failure	Reduce Na+
Gastrointestinal	
Liver compromise	Reduce Na+
	May need K+ supplement
Respiratory	
Pneumonitis (SIADH)	2/3 maintenance
Iatrogenic	
Postanesthesia	Reduce fluids
Posthypothermia	Supplement fluids
Postextracorporeal circulation	Close attention to central venous pressure and fluids
Postangiography or IVP	Replace obligatory diuresis with 1/2 NS
Diuretics	May need K+ supplement
	Watch for alkalosis
Accidents	
Poisoning	See Poisonings by Anderson and Shannon, this volume
Burns	Add to maintenance: 2 ml lactated Ringer's × % burn surface area for up to 50% body surface area burn
	Maintenance for AgNO₃ surface therapy: 3000 ml/m²/24 hr NS + 40 mEq/liter; KCl + protein 25 gm/m²/24 hr
Drowning	1/2 maintenance

John T. Herrin
Timothy P. Trompeter

36 ▸ Acute Renal Failure

Renal failure is the loss of ability to maintain fluid and sodium balance and/or to excrete nitrogenous waste products.[1] Clinically, acute renal failure (ARF) is characterized by rapid decrease in glomerular filtration rate (GFR), usually manifested symptomatically as oliguria or azotemia.[2]

ARF is a clinical syndrome commonly encountered in the intensive care unit (ICU), where renal damage may follow resuscitation from circulatory collapse or where patients are medically sustained through extensive injuries or aggressive and complicated surgery. The term *acute renal failure* refers to an abrupt, often temporary loss of renal function following an insult that may or may not be evident at the time of patient presentation.[3]

Although oliguria is the most common situation, attenuated (non-oliguric) renal failure has been recognized more often in recent years.[4] Total anuria, although rare, is usually secondary to bilateral obstruction to vasculature or ureters or to urethral obstruction. Urine volume and composition are both significantly altered in ARF, and patients may succumb to a variety of fluid, electrolyte, or acid-base disorders in the absence of proper monitoring and management.[5] Prognosis for ARF depends on the patient age, underlying condition, and the degree (extent of the precipitating insult) and presence of superinfection.[6]

In general, children have a statistically better outcome than adults for the same insult,[7] and primary nephrologic disorders such as hemolytic uremic syndrome (HUS), poststreptococcal glomerulonephritis (PSGN), or acute interstitial nephritis (AIN) have a better outcome than renal ischemia due to trauma, dehydration, or major surgery.[8]

Cases with multisystem organ failure pose a major problem where renal failure and/or sepsis supervene to produce a markedly diminished prognosis. Therapy is directed at maintaining homeostasis,[9] minimizing the potential for underlying insult to the kidney,[10] optimizing nutrition,[11] and providing prophylaxis or elimination of the presence of infection.[12] Adequate psychological and emotional support to both parent and child is necessary throughout this time of significant decrease in renal function.[13,14]

Pathogenesis

The pathogenesis of ARF is complex and controversial because the initial insult leads to variable change and outcome. No one mechanism is applicable to all experimental models or human clinical ARF.[15]

Four basic pathogenic mechanisms are described[16]: (1) Decrease in renal blood flow, (2) change in filtration constant, (3) intratubular obstruction, and (4) back-leak produce the differing ischemic and toxic insults to the kidney that result in the clinical syndrome. The importance of each factor is controversial.[16] These pathogenic mechanisms result in various injuries and alterations to the nephron including tubular injury, tubular obstruction, vascular alterations, and oxygen starvation. Experimental work suggests that decreased oxygen delivery to the cells of the medullary thick ascending limb may be a common factor in all mechanisms.[17]

Tubular Injury

Damage to the tubular cells results in altered ionic and protein transport and increased cellular permeability. Back-diffusion of tubular fluid into peritubular capillaries and interstitium is ultimately returned to the blood stream. The swollen interstitium with increased pressure causes collapse of intrarenal structures, ultimately reducing GFR. Because of back-leak, creatinine or inulin cannot be used as direct markers of GFR in ARF.

Tubular Obstruction

Obstructive casts form from sloughed microvilli, toxic crystals, necrotic tubular cellular material, and protein pigments. This results in an increased obstruction with back-pressure, further damaging tubular cells and decreasing GFR. Tubular obstruction has been demonstrated in both ischemic and toxic models of ARF.

Vascular Alterations

Intense vasoconstriction in the renal cortex is present in ARF, produced by norepinephrine, renal arterial clamping, and some forms of toxic damage in experimental models. Afferent arteriolar constriction related to changes in renin-angiotensin system, kidney swelling, reduction in prostaglandins, increase in antidiuretic hormone (ADH), or changes in other vasoactive substances (e.g., adenosine or kallikrein-kinins) may result in a depressed GFR.

Oxygen Starvation

Normal renal medullary cells function in a low oxygen environment. Cells of the thick ascending loop of Henle expend a large amount of energy and consequently utilize large quantities of oxygen under normal circumstances. Low oxygen tension in the medulla is the price for increased concentrating ability. Trauma, shock, hypotension, or hypervolemia further decrease oxygen supply, increasing susceptibility to damage. Any increase in work of the thick ascending limb will lead to greater damage.[18] It is possible that protection of this area may be possible by temporarily decreasing the work load, by decreasing sodium transport using mannitol[19] and furosemide[20] or by increasing perfusion[21] (e.g., dopamine).

Pathophysiology

For convenience in diagnosis and therapy, alterations in renal function may be categorized as (1) prerenal azotemia, (2) parenchymal damage, and (3) obstructive disorders. A common mechanism for the biochemical disorders of renal failure may be considered. Prerenal conditions lead to decrease in clearance of substances by decreased renal perfusion and subsequent loss of glomerulotubular balance. Parenchymal damage and obstructive conditions result in renal vessel injury, circulatory insufficiency, and toxic damage, which in turn produce decreased filtration and alterations in glomerulotubular balance. Redistribution of blood flow from cortex to medulla resulting from either poor perfusion or anatomic alteration produces a tendency toward sodium and water retention.[22]

Prerenal Azotemia

This is the most common cause of change in urine volume, character, and chemical composition in the critically ill patient during periods when variations in volume control and fluid replacement occur. The diagnostic manifestation is the production of a low volume of concentrated urine with an increased BUN-creatinine ratio.

Serum protein, hematocrit, and serum osmolality are less helpful than BUN and urine flow in monitoring adequacy of volume replacement. Blood and plasma losses or sequestration and replacement often occur concomitantly, making later indices more difficult to interpret. Adequate circulation may be inferred when BP is stable, peripheral capillary return is normal, and urine output is rising or sustained. It may be necessary to monitor volume status using central venous pressure (CVP) or pulmonary wedge pressure measurement while there is continuing fluid loss, disruption of capillary integrity, or in the presence of cardiac failure. With the restoration of normal circulation, renal function will also return to normal, provided that poor perfusion or anoxia have not produced parenchymal damage. If prerenal factors are not corrected, tubular damage may ensue, changing an easily reversible situation to one requiring more prolonged supportive therapy.[23]

Parenchymal Damage

A number of conditions that cause parenchymal damage leading to acute renal failure require consideration:

1. Glomerulonephritis[6,24]
2. Tubular necrosis (following ischemia, toxins, antibiotics, myoglobin, or hemoglobin)[2,6]
3. Cortical necrosis[25]
4. Interstitial nephritis[26] (from pyelonephritis or drugs, e.g., synthetic penicillin)
5. Hemolytic uremic syndrome[27]
6. Crescentic glomerulonephritis[28,29]

In this group of disorders, urine flow is diminished as the result of glomerular involvement and swelling of capillary endothelium and tubular cells or interstitium. A concomitant fall in renal plasma flow and GFR follows such swelling or necrosis of cortical tissue. A history of recent streptococcal infection (acute glomerulonephritis), diarrhea (HUS), rash or purpura (Henoch-Schoenlein purpura), hypotension, toxins, hemoglobinuria, myoglobinuria, crush damage, and drug or antibiotic administration suggest possible etiology.

Urine flow is usually decreased, and osmolality will vary, being increased in PSGN and isotonic in tubular necrosis or interstitial nephritis. Patient responses to similar stimuli may vary widely. Radiographic definition of kidney size and function, complemented by renal scan, renogram, and biopsy may be required to fully define parenchymal damage and to exclude obstruction.[30]

Urinary Tract Obstruction

In the ICU, obstructive conditions are most common in the postoperative period. Obstruction of a drain tube, ureteric or bladder catheter with blood clot, sediment or other debris (crystalline material, e.g., uric acid), and mechanical kinking or crushing of a drainage tube or catheter will lead to an acute fall in urine output and discomfort, often with voiding or dribbling around the catheter. Other less obvious causes of obstruction include urinary calculi, anatomical lesions, or edema of ureter or urethra often following instrumentation or operative repair.[6] Pain, fever, and often hypertension may be present with acute obstruction. Chemical derangements include elevation of BUN, serum creatinine, and potassium levels, with a fall in serum bicarbonate content secondary to and proportional to the degree of obstruction.

Partial anatomic obstruction is more difficult to diagnose because urine output may be sustained. The rise in BUN and creatinine is slower, and elevation of serum potassium may be minimal in partial obstruction.

Clinical Approach to Diagnosis of Acute Renal Failure

1. Suspect ARF with acute onset of azotemia and/or oliguria.
2. Check serum creatinine or creatinine clearance: These provide the best guides to renal function in the absence of rhabdomyolysis in children apart from the neonatal period. It should be remembered that in situations where back-leak may be expected (tubular injury or obstruction), these indices cannot be used as direct markers of glomerular filtration.[31]
3. Table 36-1 depicts causes of elevated BUN.
4. Carefully review history and physical examination for etiologic factors.
5. Obtain a careful urinalysis, including analysis of sediment and chemical analysis for sodium, creatinine, and osmolality. A flowsheet protocol approach is outlined in Fig. 36-1.[32] Note that the initial phase is the recognition of azotemia and/or oliguria, and the initial separation is to define oliguria less than 0.8 ml/kg/hr of an isotonic urine. Also note lower urine flow, 0.2–0.3 ml/kg/hr, with significantly hypertonic urine does not represent renal failure unless coincident azotemia is present. Hypertonic urine suggests ADH secretion, either appropriate (hypovolemic or hyperosmolar stress) or inappropriate, is present. **Once oliguria has been defined, exclude obstruction before fluid loading or diuretic therapy is initiated.**
6. Collect and examine urine and serum for sodium, BUN, creatinine, and osmolality to allow calculation of fractional excretion of sodium (FENa), urine/plasma osmolar ratio, osmolar excretion, and waste product levels—to check the adequacy of glomerular and tubular function.
7. By reviewing the collected data, a diagnosis as to prerenal azotemia, ARF secondary to parenchymal damage, or obstruction may be obtained. Radiological data from ultrasound, renal scans, or renogram may be helpful. Figure 36-1 and Tables 36-1 and 36-2 will also help in determining the diagnosis.

General Principles of Therapy

General principles of therapy[32] include (1) emergency resuscitation, (2) treatment of correctable conditions, (3) reduction in excretory load or utilization of extrarenal routes of metabolism, (4) compensation for regulatory inadequacy, or (5) artificial replacement of renal function by dialysis.

Emergency Measures

In considering therapy for the child with renal failure, initial life-threatening situations are often the reason for presentation: (1) circulatory collapse from rapid salt and water depletion; (2) sepsis; (3) severe metabolic acidosis from obstruction, infection, and immaturity of tubular functions; (4) hyperkalemia; (5) neurologic

Table 36-1. Causes of elevated BUN

Decreased GFR
Decreased urine volume or flow rate
Increased protein catabolism
Trauma
Inadequate calorie supply
Infection
Drugs (steroid, tetracycline, pressors)

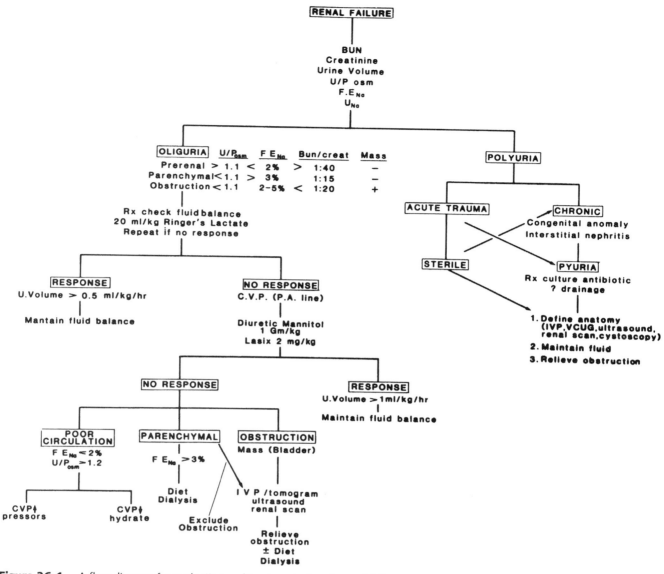

Figure 36-1. A flow diagram for evaluation and treatment of acute renal failure. (From JT Herrin. The kidney. In JF Burke (ed): *Surgical Physiology*. Philadelphia: Saunders, 1983. Pp 187–207. With permission.)

complications of electrolyte disturbances (e.g., hypernatremia, hyponatremia, hypercalcemia, hypocalcemia); (6) pulmonary overload with congestive heart failure and/or pulmonary edema; and (7) hypertensive crisis.

Circulatory Collapse

Intravenous (IV) fluid and electrolyte replacement is the basis of therapy. The circulation should be restored using isotonic solution, such as lactated Ringer's, 0.45% saline with 50 mEq/liter sodium bicarbonate, or 5% albumin in isotonic solution. Commence with rapid infusion of 10–20 ml/kg over 20 to 30 minutes, and repeat if necessary. Replace the measured deficit (weight difference when available) with isotonic fluid and then change to a maintenance solution. Replace measured urine losses of fluid and sodium and correct bicarbonate deficit after circulation has been established and stabilized.

Sepsis

Antibiotics should be given after appropriate cultures have been collected. Broad-spectrum antibiotics like oxacillin, vancomycin, and gentamycin or third-generation cephalosporins will treat most potential pathogens and may be given in standard loading dosage. Subsequent doses are adjusted for degree of excretory impairment.[33]

Severe Metabolic Acidosis

Correction is necessary to stabilize the circulation and to allow cellular metabolism to return to normal. If severe acidosis is associated with dehydration or circulatory collapse, infusion of isotonic (1/6 molar) sodium bicarbonate solution (150 mEq/liter Na) at 10 ml/kg over 15 to 30 minutes, or until the serum carbon dioxide level can be returned to 12 to 15 mEq/liter. Should acidosis persist after isotonic fluid replacement and if

Table 36-2.   Differential features in diagnosis of acute renal failure

Parameter	Physiologic oliguria	Prerenal azotemia	Acute tubular necrosis		Obstructive renal failure	
			Infant	Adult	Acute (48 hr)	Chronic (48 hr)
U_{sg}	1024	1016	1010	1008–1012	1015–1025	1010–1015
U_{osm} (mOsm/liter)	750	500	250–320	300–350	450–700	300–450
U_{osm}/P_{osm}	2.0	1.5	1.0	1.2	1.5	1.2
Urine flow (ml/kg/hr)	0.25	0.25–0.5	Variable	Variable	0.5	1.2
BUN/creat	20:1	20:1	5:1	10:1	20:1	10:1
U_{creat}/P_{creat}	40:1	40:1	10:1	10:1	20–40:1	10:1
U_{Na}	10	20	30–50	40	20	10–50
FE_{Na}	1%	1%	3%	2%	1%	3%
Urine sediment	Pro. trace, hyaline casts	Pro. trace, hyaline/fine gran. casts	Coarse gran. casts, hematuria	Renal tubular cells, coarse gran. pigmented casts	Pro. trace, occasional fine gran. casts	Blood trace
Radiology						
Size	Normal	Normal	Variable	Variable	Variable	Small
Nephrogram	Early	Early	Early, dense	Persistent	Delay	Delay
Calyces	Normal	Normal	Normal	Normal	Dilated	Dilated
Excretion	No delay	Delay	Delay	Delay	Delay	Marked delay
Clinical features	Thirst, mild weight loss	Circulatory failure, weight loss 2–3%			Pain, fever	Dehydration

From JT Herrin. The kidney. In JF Burke (ed): *Surgical Physiology.* Philadelphia: Saunders, 1985. Pp 187–207. With permission.

significant hyponatremia is present, continue to use 1/6 molar sodium bicarbonate solution, giving bicarbonate to correct half of the calculated deficit or to return plasma bicarbonate to 18 to 20 mEq/liter over 12 to 24 hours. If serum calcium levels (particularly ionized calcium) are low, rapid correction of acidosis may precipitate tetany or seizures and is not necessary once circulation has been stabilized.

For the patient with fluid overload and acidosis, hypertonic sodium bicarbonate 5% or 8% may be used in an amount calculated to return serum bicarbonate levels to 15 mEq/liter (bicarbonate deficit × 0.5 × body weight in kilograms). If acidosis persists or fluid overload is marked, dialysis is the therapy of choice.

Hyperkalemia
In hyperkalemia, the urgency of the situation is assessed by review of the electrocardiographic changes. There are three methods of therapy: (1) Stabilize membrane potential, (2) produce a temporary shift in potassium intracellularly, and (3) remove potassium from the body.

1. Calcium will stabilize the membrane potential.
2. (i) Sodium bicarbonate and (ii) glucose and insulin produce potassium shift intracellularly.
3. Potassium removal by (i) resin (e.g., Kayexalate binding, (ii) diuretic to produce potassium loss, e.g., furosemide, or (iii) dialysis may be required if poor renal function is present.

If ECG changes are present (wide QRS–high peak T), calcium chloride or gluconate in a dose of 10 mg/kg elemental calcium is administered over 10 to 30 minutes. Once acute control is obtained, stabilizing measures are instituted. Infusion of hypertonic glucose solution $D_{10}W$ to which sodium bicarbonate 50 mEq/liter is added, administered at a rate to provide 1 to 2 mEq/kg sodium bicarbonate over 2 to 4 hours. Sodium bicarbonate administration is continued to correct any metabolic acidosis and will produce a fall in serum potassium levels of approximately 1 mEq/liter for each 0.1 pH unit elevation. An approximate 2-mEq/liter fall will follow administration of 2.5 mM/kg sodium bicarbonate.

Insulin and glucose regimes (1 U insulin/4 g glucose) may be useful in older children and adolescents, but it has been our experience that insulin is not necessary in younger patients; in fact, in the under 10-kg child, insulin administration may lead to hypotension and hypoglycemia.

Control of serum potassium levels associated with intracellular redistribution of potassium may last 2 to 4 hours. After that time, potassium removal must be undertaken, unless urine output can be reestablished.

Potassium removal can be accomplished with use of (1) sodium polystyrene sulfonate resin as an enema (2 g/kg in 50–100 ml of sorbitol) and concurrent oral administration at 1 g/kg, (2) kaliuresis produced by diuretic therapy (loop diuretic), or (3) dialysis, either hemodialysis or peritoneal dialysis.

Neurologic Complications
Neurologic complications may follow electrolyte disturbances such as hypernatremia, hyponatremia, and hypocalcemia, with altered consciousness, seizures, or impairment of respiratory function. These conditions can be prevented by correction of fluid and electrolyte balance. In the acutely ill and symptomatic child, dialysis may be the therapy of choice.

Pulmonary Overload

Judicious fluid and electrolyte administration will prevent this complication. If pulmonary edema is present, endotracheal intubation and positive-pressure ventilation may be necessary while response to high-dose furosemide (2–4 mg/kg IV) with supplemental metalazone 1.25 to 5.0 mg orally can be assessed. If there is no response in 30 to 40 minutes, peritoneal dialysis, rotating tourniquets, venisection, ultrafiltration, or hemodialysis should be undertaken.

Hypertensive Crisis

Indications for emergency therapy include

1. Hypertensive encephalopathy present or incipient
2. Left ventricular failure
3. Pulmonary edema or incipient pulmonary edema
4. Dry cough with positive chest x-ray (pulmonary congestion or edema)
5. Deteriorating renal function with microangiopathic anemia and hypertension
6. Diastolic pressure over 120 mm Hg without fluctuation

Agents and doses for control of a hypertensive crisis are outlined in Table 36-3.

Treatment of Correctable Conditions

Dehydration, hyponatremia, hypokalemia, hypercalcemia, urinary tract obstruction, and infection predispose to acute decompensation in otherwise compensated renal failure or prerenal azotemia in the presence of previously normal renal function. Table 36-4, section A, gives examples of common medical conditions that are easily correctable and obstructive lesions that usually require surgery.

Reduction of the Excretory Load or Utilization of Extrarenal Methods of Excretion

These methods are most helpful in ARF or for use on a short-term basis (Table 36-41, section B).

Phosphate Load

Phosphate load may be removed from the diet by restricting food rich in phosphate. This makes the diet unpalatable and unacceptable for longer than short periods. Calcium carbonate has largely replaced aluminum gels as a phosphate binder since the recognition of aluminum toxicity syndromes. Chronic administration of aluminum salts can lead to aluminum toxicity, with neurologic symptoms and bony changes. Phosphate binding in the gut pre-

vents phosphate absorption. (In fact, it is possible to effectively deplete the body of phosphate.) Calcium carbonate 100 to 150 mg/kg/d is used in liquid or tablet form. Aluminum hydroxide or aluminum carbonate gel are both successful when used at 150 to 300 mg/kg/d of aluminum and may be used on a short-term basis

Table 36-3. Agents for control of hypertensive crisis

Nifedipine 2–10 mg sublingual

Labetalol 0.1 mg/kg IV intermittent injection each 10–15 min

Hydralazine 0.2 mg/kg IM or IV

Furosemide 1–2 mg/kg IV

Nitroprusside as a drip infusion may be administered in an ICU titrated to control. There are marked dangers in the absence of renal function, low renal flow, or decreased hepatic function requiring strict monitoring of metabolites in addition to the minute-to-minute monitoring of BP and pulse rate.

Diazoxide 2–5 mg/kg IV given as rapid push

Table 36-4. General principles of therapy

A. Treatment of Correctable Conditions

Prerenal	Hypovolemia	Salt depletion
		Dehydration
	Poor perfusion	Congestive cardiac failure
		Sepsis
		Infection
		Increase water loss
		Hypokalemia
		Hypercalcemia
Obstruction	Outlet	Urethral valves
		Neurogenic bladder
		Trauma to urethra
	Bladder	Megacystis
		Neurogenic
	Ureter	Ureteropelvic junction
		Stricture
		Calculus

B. Reduce Excretory Load or Utilize Extrarenal Route of Excretion

Protein restriction	Giovanetti diet
Fluid and sodium	Maintain as high as tolerated; fluid 350 ml/m² + urine output
Phosphate binding	Amphojel 150–300 mg/kg (aluminum, used only short-term) or calcium carbonate 100–150 mg/kg/d
Potassium	List specific exact volumes of juice and food
	List K⁺ free fluids
	Avoid salt substitutes
Modify drug dosage	Antibiotic
	Aminoglycosides
	Avoid tetracycline
	Sedatives
	Antihistamines
	Hypotensive agents
	Nonsteroidal analgesics, aspirin, indomethacin

C. Compensate for Regulatory Inadequacy

Correct acidosis—sodium bicarbonate, Shohl's solution
Calcium
Vitamin D (1,25 OHD3, DHT)
Anemia—washed frozen packed RBC
Calories

D. Artificially Replace Function

Dialysis	Peritoneal	Acute/chronic
	Hemodialysis	Acute/chronic
	Hemofiltration	Acute
Transplantation		Living related donor
		Identical
		Parent
		Sibling
		Cadaver donor

if calcium carbonate is not effective. Patient acceptance of calcium carbonate and aluminum is poor, and a trial of available tablets, liquid, and capsule forms will be necessary. Tablets are less effective in lowering serum phosphorous level unless chewed or dissolved in the mouth. Constipation may occur in the critically ill patient, making careful observation of bowel function during treatment necessary.

In the critically ill patient with minimal or no oral intake, nasogastric suction, antacid therapy, and low phosphate IV solutions can lead to profound hypophosphatemia and respiratory depression. Close monitoring of serum phosphorous is necessary.

Potassium (previously outlined)
Restriction of potassium in diet, IV, fluids, and medications is necessary in ARF. If this is not sufficient to maintain a normal serum potassium level, sodium polystyrene sulfonate resin is the most effective method of control. This can be given either orally or rectally. The oral route is slower in onset of action but more efficient. The dose of 1 g/kg orally or 2 g/kg rectally is usually suspended in 15% to 20% sorbitol to facilitate dispersion of the resin and produce fluid and electrolyte flux into bowel lumen so adequate exchange may occur. Sorbitol also prevents a tendency toward marked constipation. If adequate renal function remains, furosemide can be used as a kaliuretic. Uncontrolled hyperkalemia is an indication for dialysis.

Protein Restriction
Restriction of dietary protein will decrease the rate of rise in nitrogenous waste products and slow the rate of change in the biochemical profile if an adequate caloric intake can be maintained. The diet must provide essential amino acids while restricting nonessential amino acids. Nitrogen from urea and other breakdown products will be used to synthesize nonessential amino acids, leading to a fall in BUN.[34,35] In the child, it is helpful to maintain a higher caloric, mildly restricted protein diet of 0.6 to 1.5 g/kg/d and maintain biochemical control with dialysis if necessary.

To provide adequate nutrition while maintaining appropriate fluid restrictions, either the oral use of a modified high-quality protein diet, the enteral administration of synthetic amino acid mixtures, or the parenteral administration of "renal failure fluid"—a mixture of amino acids in hypertonic glucose—through a centrally placed IV catheter may be used, as clinically feasible.

Salt and Water Restriction
In oliguric renal failure secondary to acute parenchymal disease—glomerulonephritis or acute tubular necrosis (ATN)—both salt and water restriction (2 g sodium; 500 ml/m²/d of fluid plus a volume of water to replace the previous day's urine volume) should be undertaken as a prophylaxis against hypertension and acute pulmonary overload. Restriction may also be necessary in chronic renal failure. BP should be monitored closely. With a decreased number of nephrons in chronic renal failure, salt wasting is expected to occur, and the range for modification of sodium concentration in urine is limited.[26]

Under conditions of net fluid loss or in the presence of hypovolemia (e.g., in nephrotic syndrome), salt restriction may aggravate existing prerenal azotemia or even precipitate circulatory collapse. Under these conditions, sodium replacement rather than restriction is required. Monitoring of sodium losses and daily weights is necessary to guide fluid and electrolyte therapy/replacement.

In acute glomerulonephritis the early high-output congestive heart failure usually responds to diuresis and fluid restriction.

Digitalization is not necessary, except in the presence of severe fluid and/or salt overload. Under these circumstances, failure of response to diuretic therapy is an indication for dialysis or ultrafiltration.

Modification of Dosage of Drugs[33]
This is required for concurrent therapy, particularly antibiotics, digitalis preparations, anticonvulsants, and antihistamines (see Table 36-4, section B).

Compensation for Regulatory Inadequacy
Supplement for inadequacy of present renal mechanisms is important during both acute and chronic care.

Sodium Bicarbonate Supplementation
To control metabolic acidosis, sodium bicarbonate supplementation is often necessary acutely to maintain normal circulation and chronically to allow for growth. If volume replacement in the acutely ill patient does not fully restore circulation and correct acidosis, sodium bicarbonate should be given as an initial bolus to achieve a plasma concentration of 12 to 15 mEq/liter, followed by slower replacement to complete correction of sodium bicarbonate to 18 to 22 mEq/liter over 12 to 24 hours.

In the patient with chronic renal failure, bicarbonate is needed to neutralize the daily intake of acid or potential acid (approximately 2–4 mEq/kg/d). The exact dose is adjusted as necessary to maintain normal serum bicarbonate or carbon dioxide levels.

Calcium Administration
If tetany is symptomatic, calcium may be given intravenously as calcium gluconate, calcium chloride, or calcium glucoheptonate in a dose of 10 mg/kg of elemental calcium over 10 minutes IV and followed by a calcium infusion of 40 to 50 mg/kg of elemental calcium per day. Monitoring of total and ionized calcium levels will guide therapy. If needed after the period of acute care, 100 mg/kg/d of elemental calcium should provide oral supplementation.

Vitamin D Supplements
These may be necessary to assist in maintenance of normal serum calcium levels by enhancing calcium absorption. Vitamin D_3, as 1, 25 dihydroxycholecalciferol or dihydrotachysterol, should be used in the acute setting because of its more rapid onset of action and shorter half-life.

Diet
The methods of providing essential amino acid nitrogen and calories with restriction of nonessential amino acids has been briefly discussed previously. Fuller details are available in many excellent reviews.[34,35]

Artificially Replace Function
Dialysis
Either peritoneal dialysis, hemodialysis, or hemofiltration may be used as a method of either acute or chronic care. In ARF with a reversible cause and in the very small patient, peritoneal dialysis is the method of choice. Technical aspects are described in Peritoneal Dialysis by Link and Fugate, this volume. When longer-term dialysis is anticipated or recent or extensive abdominal surgery has been performed, hemofiltration or hemodialysis is the choice.

Indications for dialysis will vary among units (Table 36-5). Prophylactic dialysis should be considered in any patient with multisystem organ failure to allow adequate nutrition, provision of adequate

Table 36-5. Indications for dialysis

Volume overload with congestive heart failure or pulmonary edema
Hyperkalemia in the presence of acidosis
Markedly disordered metabolic status
    Hypernatremia
    Hypokalemia
    Hyperkalemia
    Hypocalcemia
Severe hyperosmolality with serum sodium >180 mEq/liter or hypo-osmolality serum sodium <115 mEq/liter
Overt clinical uremic symptoms
    CNS disturbance, e.g., twitching, seizures, hyperreflexia, clouding of consciousness
    Bleeding with azotemia
    Pericarditis
Prophylactic dialysis is planned to prevent the symptomatic uremia
BUN level of >100 mg/dl or BUN rising at a rate >20 mg/d in catabolic renal failure

amino acids, and better fluid balance. Prophylaxis against infection should be early and vigorous. Early dialysis should be considered in those conditions where excess fluid compromises the overall outcome; water removal can be of therapeutic value in adult respiratory distress syndrome (ARDS), head trauma, cerebral edema following hypoxia or trauma.

Special Examples of Childhood Renal Failure

Hemolytic Uremic Syndrome

Renal failure in HUS is among the most common causes of renal failure in childhood.[27] HUS is defined clinically as the triad of (1) oligoanuric renal failure, (2) microangiopathic hemolytic anemia, and (3) thrombocytopenia. This triad usually follows a prodromal viral or bacterial illness, most often gastroenteritis, particularly in the younger age group. Preceding upper respiratory tract infection is less common.

Pathophysiology

Although the etiology remains unknown, similarity to the Schwartzman phenomenon exists, particularly in those cases associated with pathogenic strains of *E. coli*. Cortical necrosis is common in this group of patients. An endotoxic phenomenon is likely in some recent outbreaks in which a verotoxin-producing *E. coli* O157:H7[36,37] or shigella[38] had an etiologic role.

Endothelial damage from the endotoxic damage produces secondary damage to platelets and deposition of intravascular fibrin. Hemolysis follows mechanical trauma to the RBCs during flow through the area of damaged endothelium; thrombocytopenia results from consumption and damage during adhesion to the capillary endothelium. Damaged platelets are destroyed rapidly in the liver and spleen. Local thrombosis with distal patchy necrosis and infarction may occur in any body organ. The degree of overall organ involvement approximates that of renal involvement, so that clinical symptoms of renal dysfunction provide an overall guideline of severity.

Pathologic changes are system-related. Renal changes include thrombotic microangiopathy with glomerular lesions, showing hyaline thrombi occluding isolated capillary loops or occasionally glomerular congestion or even total occlusion. Acute ischemic glomerulonephritis with arteriolar necrosis may follow fibrinoid and vessel wall necrosis, similar to changes of severe hypertension. Patchy or total cortical necrosis may also be present. Glomerular vessels, particularly afferent arterioles, and occasionally vessels of interlobular vessel size are involved. Light and electron microscopy show a clear zone beneath the endothelial cell, between the cell and basement membrane. Cellular debris may be present in this space.

Gastrointestinal lesions include thrombosis of submucosal vessels and may be associated with small areas of infarction, ulceration, pseudopolyp formation, or perforation, with late intestinal stricture or stenosis.

Cerebral manifestations may be those of hemorrhagic encephalitis, a "vasculitic" picture with small areas of cerebral infarction, edema, or thrombosis. Signs and symptoms similar to those found in patients with hypertonic dehydration or electrolyte abnormalities may also occur and be associated with functional or structural change.

Clinical Presentation

The patient presents approximately 3 to 7 days after an episode of diarrhea, with pallor, oliguria, and laboratory findings of anemia, thrombocytopenia, and ARF. Males and females are affected equally, and although the mean age is 12 months, patients of any age may be affected.

There is a prodromal illness (usually gastroenteritis) with blood-stained diarrhea. After an apparent mild improvement, the child demonstrates a sudden onset of pallor, increasing lethargy, and anemia. The child is markedly irritable. Purpura occurs in the gastrointestinal tract, skin, and puncture sites.

Oliguria with hematuria and a urinary sediment with occasional cellular casts, pigmented granular casts similar to those found in ATN, numerous hyaline casts, and coarse granular casts are present. The urinary sediment findings are proportional to the degree of renal glomerular involvement.

The intensity of neurologic symptoms varies within epidemics and may result from variations in the disease process,[39,40] with cerebral damage occurring secondary to vascular change, or following chemical imbalances that result from renal failure. Symptoms include neuromuscular irritability, seizure activity, and/or coma.

The child may be mildly jaundiced (total bilirubin <2 dl). Hepatomegaly is common, but splenomegaly is rare. Rectal ulceration, bleeding, and colitis may occur as a result of submucosal infarction, which may also produce prolapse, intussusception, or perforation.

Hypertension (45%–75%) is common and sometimes associated with congestive cardiac failure. Edema follows fluid overload, and pulmonary edema may occur, particularly at the onset of renal failure.

Laboratory findings include a Coomb's negative microangiopathic hemolytic anemia, and mild hyperbilirubinemia. RBC fragments, schistocytes and burr cells are discernible on the characteristic peripheral blood smear. Tests of hemolysis are positive, with markedly decreased plasma haptoglobin and free hemoglobin present.

Thrombocytopenia is usually present, with less than 50,000 platelets/μL, and may show wide variations in platelet counts from hour to hour throughout the day, consistent with the consumptive origin for the thrombocytopenia.

Leukocytosis with a left shift is common (20,000–40,000/μL). Very elevated levels, even 100,000/μL, have occasionally been described. Bone marrow aspirate, when performed, has shown euthyroid hyperplasia with normal thrombocytopenia. Oligoanuria is present with elevation of BUN (usually above 50 mg/dl), with concurrent elevation of serum creatinine, phosphate, and potassium. Metabolic acidosis with decreased serum albumin and serum calcium values may develop.

Coagulation studies have shown factors V and VIII normal or elevated. A consumption coagulopathy is uncommon. Cerebral spinal fluid may show increased protein, xanthochromia, and red cells in the presence of vascular involvement of the CNS. Abdominal radiologic findings reflect the involved organ, so there may be blurring of fat lines, bowel shadows, or the presence of ascites. Barium studies of the gastrointestinal tract may show thumb printing, pseudotumor, and submucosal hemorrhage. Late findings include strictures and stenoses.

Differential Diagnosis

Differential diagnosis of HUS is wide and best segregated by the pattern of clinical syndrome: (1) oliguria, (2) hemolytic anemia with renal shutdown, (3) gastrointestinal syndromes, and (4) purpura and abdominal pain.

Oliguria may be present in other renal diseases, for example, (1) glomerulonephritis; (2) ATN (either toxic or ischemic); (3) mechanical obstruction; and (4) systemic disorders with renal involvement, such as lupus erythematosus or Henoch-Schonlein purpura. It may also be present due to toxic methicillin, aminoglycosides, sulfonamides, cephalosporin, or amphotericin.

Hemolytic anemia with renal shutdown and thrombocytopenia may occur as a result of exogenous toxins including drugs and pesticides, or red cell enzyme defects, as in the case of favism, and occasionally in congenital oxalosis.

Gastrointestinal involvement may mimic ulcerative colitis, intussusception, or pseudomembranous colitis. Purpura and abdominal pain may be seen in Henoch-Shonlein purpura and thrombotic thrombocytopenic purpura, as well as in HUS.

Management

Management principles are similar to those of ATN, with modification occasioned by pathologic differences. The cornerstone of therapy is strict intensive supportive care and early institution of monitoring and support for renal failure. Early dialysis is often necessary, because vigorous hemolysis with relative or absolute oliguria will be associated with increased risk of significant cardiac arrhythmia, even before a significant rise in BUN or creatinine. (Hyperkalemia follows hemolysis with release of high intracellular concentration of potassium and phosphate.) We make a practice of instituting dialysis with severe oliguria of 4 to 6 hours' duration, particularly in the early hemolytic phase of the disease.

Transfusion for anemia is reserved for patients with a rapid fall in hematocrit levels below 15% to 20% or for cardiac failure secondary to edema. Potential complications from transfusion include volume overload, hyperkalemia, HLA sensitization, and the small risk of transmitted infection (hepatitis, cytomegalovirus, AIDS).

Therapy is symptomatic and includes maintenance of circulation, control of BP, correction of electrolyte abnormalities, maintenance of nutrition, and dialysis, if necessary, for fluid or electrolyte control.

No specific treatment has been proven to be very effective for the microangiopathic hemolytic anemia. Anticoagulation,[43,44] plasma infusion,[45,46] and plasmapheresis[47,48] have their advocates, and these therapies may have a place in a small number of patients. The results of conservative therapy are so good that the evaluation of other therapies is difficult to assess.[49] Perhaps early plasmapheresis in HUS associated with cyclosporin toxicity is effective and necessary.[50,51] For those patients with bacterial enteritis (*Salmonella*, *Shigella*, or toxigenic *E. coli*), antibiotic therapy may decrease verotoxin production.

A special case of renal failure in HUS is the patient with familial HUS, which may occur sporadically (epidemic form) or follow a true inherited pattern. In the epidemic form, affected members in the same family develop disease at the same time and in association with a defined epidemic. This form is nonrecurring. A true familial form of HUS may show autosomal dominant or autosomal recessive expression.[27,52,53] In patients with the true familial HUS, episodes may recur, with eventual loss of kidney function.

Recurrences within a transplant occur in both sporadic and familial forms of HUS,[54] although repeat transplantation may be successful.[55]

Prognosis

Patients greater than 2 years of age show a more severe disease pattern.[41] Patients with toxigenic *E. coli* may show cortical necrosis or complete renal infarction. Patients with an upper respiratory tract or other viral prodrome (apart from diarrheal illness) appear to have a worse prognosis.[42]

Posttraumatic Acute Renal Failure

Early recognition and prompt correction of the abnormalities that precede ARF provide the basis of prophylactic therapy in the patient with trauma. Any patient who has suffered significant trauma and who returns from an operating room with significant oliguria should initially be regarded as having ARF.

The patient is reviewed to exclude acute urinary tract obstruction and prerenal causes. The patency of a urinary catheter (if present) is checked, or a catheter is passed to be sure that drainage is possible. Renal and retroperitoneal ultrasound is useful to exclude obstruction to the ureter or vena cava.

Complete anuria is uncommon, but may occur with obstruction to a single ureter, bladder outlet, or urethra secondary to trauma, or with acute bilateral damage to the renal artery or vein.

Sediment analysis, review of renal indices (see Table 36-2), fractional excretion of sodium, concentrating ability, urine/plasma osmolar ratio, and creatinine clearance may be necessary to define the lesion and differentiate these conditions from ATN. BUN and creatinine may be used as surrogates for glomerular filtration, remembering that back-flow or muscle damage will alter the plasma values, making them less useful.[15,56,57]

Prerenal causes, including hypovolemia, or decreased circulation are considered next (after obstruction has been excluded). Volume expansion with 20 ml/kg of isotonic fluid (0.9% saline or lactated Ringer's solution) is given. If urine output is not restored despite a return to normal circulation (normal BP and pulse), circulatory monitoring using a CVP or PA line is undertaken (see Fig. 36-1).

BP should be maintained within the normal range with volume expansion and/or pressors. GFR is a function of mean arterial pressure. Although autoregulation keeps glomerular filtration remarkably constant over a wide pressure range, when a systolic pressure falls below 90 mm Hg, the GFR falls rapidly, so that at a mean pressure of 60 mm Hg, GFR has fallen to 50%, and at 30 mm Hg pressure, glomerular filtration is essentially 0.[57] This also occurs in infants and children but at lower pressures. Return to normal BP reestablishes urine flow, unless prolonged hypotension has produced tubular damage.

Oliguria in the posttraumatic or postsurgical state, with appropriate increases in urine specific gravity/osmolality, suggests a physiologic decrease in urine flow secondary to decreased extracellular fluid (ECF) volume rather than tubular damage.

Administration of diuretics, although producing a transient rise in urine volume, may further deplete ECF volume so that the patient is at greater risk of developing true acute parenchymal renal failure. Diuretics should not be used until volume has been replaced and circulation restored (e.g., by administration of 20 mg/kg of isotonic saline or lactated Ringer's solution over 1–2 hours). Should there be a response, further fluid expansion is continued until circulation and urine output stabilize. If there is no rise in urine volume, but circulation is improved (rise in BP and decreased pulse rate), a second fluid challenge is justified before instituting intravascular monitoring. When the circulation is stable, a trial of diuretic (e.g., mannitol 1 g/kg and/or furosemide 1–2 mg/kg) is justified (see Fig. 36-1). Mannitol is the diuretic of choice if the vascular bed remains underexpanded but is best avoided when there is circulatory overexpansion, as monitored by CVP or pulmonary wedge pressure. Furosemide administration is preferred in the presence of oliguria with an elevated or rising CVP. If an initial response occurs, followed by a fall-off in urine volume, IV mannitol 20% and furosemide 1 to 2 mg/kg may be administered as an infusion and titrated to sustain urine flow, converting the patient from oliguric to non-oliguric renal failure.

If oliguria persists or the urinary osmolality/plasma osmolality ratio is less than 1:1, intravascular volume status should be monitored with CVP or capillary wedge pressure measurements.

Postoperative Acute Renal Failure

ARF is more often the result of a surgical complication rather than the surgery itself.[1,26,58] In the postoperative period of cardiac surgery, in which cardiac output is decreased, toxic drugs or antibiotics (e.g., aminoglycosides) are more likely to lead to tubular damage.

Postsurgical ATN should be expected in those patients with infectious or surgical complications following the operation. It is rare to find an isolated cause of postsurgical ARF. Simple reversible shock of short duration is rarely a cause of postoperative ARF but may increase the risk of damage from nephrotoxic antibiotics and anesthetic agents. Dehydration and electrolyte abnormalities are frequently encountered in the early stages of ARF and should be anticipated.

Although most patients develop oliguric renal failure, a subgroup will show polyuric or non-oliguric renal failure. In the non-oliguric group, the prognosis is excellent. The greatest risk in non-oliguric renal failure is late diagnosis or missed diagnosis, because urine output is sustained. If there is a rise in BUN and creatinine, examination of urinary indices (see Table 36-2) should be made. The patient with non-oliguric renal failure continues to show limited salt and water tolerance, so fluid overload and pulmonary edema may occur if attention to balance, intake, and output is not maintained.[4]

Prophylaxis in severely ill patients in need of surgery includes sustaining circulation and consideration of loop diuretic and/or mannitol administration for prophylaxis,[59] if variations in glomerular filtration with surgery, e.g., cardiac bypass surgery, are expected.

Diagnosis follows review for causes of prerenal, renal parenchymal, or obstructive factors. Early recognition and resolution of correctable causes will protect renal function in the early postoperative period. Improvements in survival have been demonstrated to follow early and vigorous dialysis, increased attention to nutrition, and aggressive treatment of infection. Treatment of established renal failure (see Table 36-4) is described earlier in this chapter.

Modification to a standard treatment regime is coordinated with a phase of postsurgical renal failure. In the early postoperative phase, fluid and electrolyte balance problems are major factors, with mortality risk from fluid overload or hyperkalemia. Later, with established renal failure and continuing oliguria, the major risk is the catabolic state secondary to malnutrition and infection. During the diuretic phase, with returning renal function, fluid and electrolyte balance once again becomes the major problem. Continuing danger of infectious complications, particularly catheter-induced infections (bladder or intravascular catheters), make constant reassessment necessary.

Intense early dialysis combined with adequate caloric and protein intake is helpful in protection of renal function (Tables 36-6 and 36-7). Either hemodialysis or peritoneal dialysis may be used to control the chemical state. Recent use of CAVH and CAVHD has widened the potential spectrum for dialysis and ultrafiltration.[60,61]

Acute Renal Failure in the Burned Patient

In the patient with burns, vigorous early resuscitation and patient stabilization have produced better overall survival and increased the preservation of renal output.[62,63] Oliguric renal failure is uncommon in the acute phase of the burn injury, unless a delay in resuscitative effort is followed by hemodynamically mediated renal failure. Early changes in renal function indices are similar to those seen in other forms of shock and circulatory insufficiency.

Acute tubular injury with oliguric or non-oliguric renal failure and pigment nephropathy may occur. Established oliguric failure in the burn patient carries an increased morbidity and mortality resulting from the severe catabolic state, increased risk of infection, hyperpyrexia, and caloric deficit.

In the second or third week after the injury, a different functional pattern of polyuric renal failure may occur. Differences from other forms of non-oliguric renal failure include a fractional excretion

Table 36-6. Factors improving survival in renal failure

Aggressive dialysis

Peritoneal dialysis

Hyperalimentation

Aggressive surgery

Control of infections

Table 36-7. Indications for dialysis in the postsurgical patient

Chemical indications
   Rapid rise in BUN
   Rapid rise in potassium
   Development of severe acidosis
Fluid status
   Overhydration
   Ultrafiltration (to allow administration of adequate calories and protein)
Clinical signs
   Changing level of consciousness

of sodium in urine which remains low, while the urine to plasma osmolar ratio (Uosm:Posm) remains greater than unity.[64–66] The pattern of urinary indices resembles that seen in radiologic contrast-induced renal failure.[67]

The type of pigments characterize burn injuries sustained within an enclosed area (hemoglobinuria), or myoglobinemia in deep burns with pressure necrosis or interference with blood supply to muscle. Myoglobin and hemoglobin have direct effects on the kidney and produce nontraumatic ATN. In the burn patient, hypotension and hemoconcentration may exacerbate the renal effects of myoglobin released from damaged muscle.[68]

The clinical course of pigment-induced ARF is similar to that of other forms of ARF. Release of creatinine from muscle produces a more rapid rise in serum creatinine and persistently higher average serum values.[69] The BUN-creatinine ratio in rhabdomyolysis is usually lower than in other forms of renal failure because elevated creatinine reflects increased creatinine load from muscle damage in the presence of lowered renal function, while urea levels reflect only renal function.

Prophylaxis for both hemoglobin and myoglobin requires increased administration of fluid to sustain urine output (mannitol, loop diuretics such as furosemide, plus alkalinization). The major risks of therapy are congestive heart failure from overdosage of mannitol or toxicity from loop diuretics, which are not excreted.

The hypercatabolic state linked to muscle injury complicates management and requires careful caloric, fluid, and electrolyte balance, with early dialysis[69,70] if prophylactic therapy is not effective.

Non-Oliguric Renal Failure

Better recognition of non-oliguric renal failure in recent years (20%–50% of all ARF patients) has allowed protection from salt and water overload. Non-oliguric renal failure commonly follows a nephrotoxic insult that is less damaging than complete tubular injury, producing an attenuated renal failure with tubular dysfunction rather than structural damage of oliguric renal failure. Morbidity, mortality, and duration of renal failure are less protracted than seen with oliguric ARF.[2]

Hepatorenal Syndrome

Loss of urinary output in the patient with hepatic failure is often a premorbid event associated with severe liver damage or with declining liver function. Diagnosis of hepatorenal syndrome requires that prerenal factors be excluded. Urinary sediment is within a normal range and urinary indices are "markedly prerenal" in character (i.e., urinary sodium and fractional excretion of sodium are very low while Uoms/Posm remains greater than 1.5:2).

A wide variety of therapeutic agents have been tried, with no consistent effect. Maintenance of adequate circulation, dopamine to increase renal perfusion, diuretic blockage (partial or total), or prostaglandin therapy may be effective in selected cases.[71,72]

Acute Renal Failure Following Transplantation

Failure of adequate function of a transplanted kidney may be due to a variety of possible causes, which are best classified by the time of onset posttransplantation (Table 36-8). Renal failure may follow acute tubular damage (ATN, cyclosporin toxicity), manifestations of rejection or technical failure (ureteric obstruction, leakage or infection on obstruction, or leak to vascular anastomosis), or may be a manifestation of cyclosporin toxicity. It is normal for a profuse diuresis to follow in the first days after transplantation. This derives from excess total body water and osmotic loads and

Table 36-8.   Acute renal failure following transplantation

Early (<48 hours)
 Hyperacute rejection
 Acute tubular necrosis
 Cyclosporine toxicity
 Ureteral obstruction
 Ureteral or bladder leak
 Vascular complication

4–10 days
 Acute obstruction
 Cyclosporine toxicity
 Ureteral obstruction or leak
 Lymphocele

Late renal failure
 Acute rejection
 Cyclosporine toxicity
 Lymphocele
 Ureteral obstruction
 Chronic or subacute rejection
 Recurrence of original renal disease
 De novo glomerulonephritis in the transplant
 Renal artery stenosis

from a decreased tubular reabsorptive capacity in a denervated kidney. Careful monitoring of fluid and electrolyte status to avoid hypovolemia is necessary to avoid hypoperfusion. In the infant and younger child, large-volume diuresis is accompanied with the disparate filtration of an adult kidney and the infant's lower ECF volume. The new transplant has a blunted autoregulation and is more susceptible to hypoperfusion injury. The recipient of an adult kidney must maintain systemic pressures in the adult normal range, at least temporarily, to allow for adequate perfusion of the transplanted organ.

Acute tubular injury manifested by ATN is influenced by warm and cold ischemia time such that 40% to 50% of cadaver kidneys and 10% of living donor kidneys will show evidence of tubular dysfunction in this early phase, occasionally severe enough to require dialysis and more often severe enough to require modification of cyclosporin dosage or avoidance of cyclosporin therapy. Technical complications are infrequent but require radiologic imaging techniques to demonstrate their presence (radionuclide scan for perfusion to exclude significant vascular obstruction or leakage and ultrasound to demonstrate obstructive phenomena). A rapidly rising BUN and creatinine associated with graft tenderness and fever suggests rejection. Fever and graft tenderness are encountered much less frequently since the advent of cyclosporine therapy, and renal biopsy may be required if technical complications can be excluded and there is abnormal or slow response to antirejection therapy.

Management is aimed at identifying and correcting the underlying functional cause. Technical problems need early correction, and immunosuppression is adjusted to renal function. In the presence of potential cyclosporin toxicity or in the presence of early renal tubular damage, cyclosporin dose is decreased or discontinued, with the substitution of monoclonal antibody therapy (OKT 3) or anti-lymphocyte globulin treatment. Steroid and azathioprine dosage is adjusted to compensate for the decrease in cyclosporin dosage to maintain adequate immunosuppression.

In renal allograft dysfunction later than 3 to 4 days, the treatment is to exclude obstruction, check cyclosporin blood trough levels, and if it is not possible to exclude cyclosporin toxicity, administer a pulse dose of steroids and decrease the cyclosporin dosage. If a decrease in serum creatinine and BUN does not follow, differentiation of cyclosporin toxicity from rejection will require early biopsy definition.

Acute Renal Failure Superimposed on Chronic Renal Failure

An initial presentation in ARF may occur when acute renal disease or acute metabolic decompensation occurs in the course of an underlying chronic renal disease. Standard measures for therapy of ARF are instituted. As metabolic stabilization occurs, a lag in return to normal BUN and creatinine should prompt investigation of renal size and renal anatomy to exclude underlying disease. Should a chronic cause be defined, emotional and educational preparation is carried out in preparation for future chronic or end-stage renal failure therapy, as appropriate.

Acute Renal Failure Associated with Sepsis

In the setting of the septic patient, ARF may follow hypoperfusion (prerenal azotemia), acute tubular damage, or necrosis from hypoperfusion or antibiotic therapy. Hypoperfusion will accentuate the potential for renal damage to antibiotic therapy. In the aftermath of sepsis, bleeding phenomena, or superinfection of the urinary tract, the onset of candidiasis may lead to obstructive renal failure.

Prophylactic therapy is aimed at the maintenance of a normal state of hydration and circulation. Administration of potentially nephrotoxic antibiotics (e.g., aminoglycosides) is carried out with great care, particularly in those patients who have shown difficulty in circulatory maintenance. It would appear that sepsis as a cause of renal failure alone is uncommon but can be incriminated in combination with other insults, such as aminoglycoside exposure, hypoperfusion, dehydration, and hypovolemia.[72] Multiple insults tend to produce a picture of oliguric rather than non-oliguric renal failure. Treatment of established ARF follows the generally outlined principles given earlier in this chapter.

Acute Renal Failure Associated with Therapy

A large number of medications used in the critically ill patient act as exogenous nephrotoxins (Table 36-9). Nephrotoxic ARF in these situations is usually preventable, reversible, or correctable if the potential for toxic injury is remembered and adjustments are made to therapy to minimize the nephrotoxic insult by decreasing the concentration of the toxin or the duration of exposure. At times it may be necessary to continue using potentially nephrotoxic agents, even in the presence of dehydration, vascular insufficiency, or circulatory failure. Attention to maintenance of circulation, preservation of urine flow with mannitol or diuretics, and maintenance of appropriate urinary pH may allow the effects of such potential nephrotoxins to be minimized or maintained in an acceptable range so they can be used as therapeutic agents (e.g., aminoglycosides, amphotericin, radiology contrast agents, newer antimetabolites, and antineoplastic agents). An extensive listing of such compounds may be found in the literature.[73–75] An abbreviated listing of potential toxins in common use in the ICU is outlined in Table 36-9.

Acute Renal Failure Associated with Childhood Malignancy

ARF in childhood malignancies may follow such divergent causes as obstruction to the urinary tract from the tumor itself (e.g., rhabdomyosarcoma of bladder or genital tract); invasion of either ureter or bladder, producing obstruction; spontaneous or induced

Table 36-9. Therapeutic agents producing renal failure

Antibiotics
  Aminoglycosides
  Amphotericin β
  Pentamidine
  Sulfonamide/trimethaprim
  Cefalosporins
  Synthetic penicillins
Anesthetic agents
Radiologic contrast media
Diuretics
Chemotherapeutic agents
  Cisplatin
  Methotrexate
Immunosuppressive agents
  Cyclosporine
Analgesics
  Acetaminophen
  Nonsteroidal antiinflammatory agents
  Phenacetin
Vasodilators (in renovascular disease)
  ACE inhibitors
Prostaglandin synthesis inhibitors
  Indomethacin ibuprofen
Converting enzyme inhibitors
  Captopril
Miscellaneous
  Dextrans
  Epsilon-amino caproic acid
  EDTA
  Penicillinamine

Table 36-10. Acute renal failure with childhood malignancy

Obstruction to bladder/ureter
Infiltration of bladder/ureter/kidney
Tumor turnover
  Hyperuricemia
Tumor lysis syndrome
  Hyperuricemia
  Hyperphosphatemia
  Hyperkalemia
Chemotherapy
  Cisplatin
  Methotrexate
Radiation effects
Antibiotics
  Aminoglycerides
  Amphotericin β

toxicity from tumor lysis (e.g., hyperphosphatemia, tumor lysis syndrome); hypercalcemia or renal failure associated with chemotherapy (e.g., cisplatin, methotrexate); late effects of radiation; and secondary effects of sepsis or antibiotic therapy (Table 36-10).

Tumor lysis syndrome[76,77] may occur spontaneously or more commonly in the setting of therapy in the patient with high-turnover tumors with high tumor load. This is often associated with hyperuricemic ARF but may also occur alone.

Management is most effective if prophylactic care is instituted with increased hydration, production, and maintenance of a high urine flow, and phosphate binding gels to reduce the urinary excreted load of phosphate. Aluminum hydroxide gel may be used on a short-term basis in the presence of high urine flow. If the serum phosphate level is markedly elevated (above 10 mg/dl), administration of acetazolamide is helpful in producing a phosphate loss with diuresis by preventing proximal tubular reabsorption. Although there is a potential danger to intratubular phosphate precipitation in the presence of urinary alkalinization, the concurrent hyperuricemia produced in most of these children makes alkalinization necessary to prevent precipitation of uric acid, and hence management is aimed at sustaining a vigorous diuresis.

Concurrent risk of hyperkalemia from rapid lysis of tumor cells is accentuated if renal failure or decreased excretion follows from hyperphosphatemia or uric acid nephropathy. Prophylactic Kayexalate therapy will increase potassium binding and is helpful if commenced 6 to 12 hours prior to the initial chemotherapeutic regime.

Hemodialysis, hemofiltration, or continuous peritoneal dialysis may be used to remove both phosphate and potassium while control is otherwise gained and may be necessary, particularly in those patients with hyperuricemic renal failure.

Hyperuricemic renal failure occurs as a complication of high-turnover tumors (e.g., leukemia, Burkitt's lymphoma, or in the early phase of tumor lysis secondary to therapy). Peak levels of uric acid in untreated patients may be extremely high, and the ratio of uric acid-creatinine in the urine may also be significantly elevated. Because the mechanism for oliguria is most often tubular precipitation of uric acid crystals or ureteral obstruction from uric acid sludge or stones, prophylactic therapy with initiation of a high-flow diuresis prior to the institution of definitive tumor therapy and alkalinization of the urine is most helpful. Allopurinol should be started as soon as practical and maintained together with an alkaline diuresis through the early days of induction chemotherapy. If the serum uric acid rises to levels greater than 10 to 12 mg/d, acetazolamide therapy should be instituted to assist with the alkaline diuresis and maintenance of high flow.

Once the syndrome of hyperuricemic ARF or tumor lysis syndrome is established, prophylactic measures and attempts at attaining a diuresis may be ineffective. Under these circumstances, early and vigorous dialysis should be instituted and maintained until return of renal function. CAVHD or peritoneal dialysis may be used as background therapy, with intermittent hemodialysis aimed at producing normalization of fluid and electrolyte balance in the early catabolic phase of tumor lysis.

Neonatal Renal Failure

In neonatal renal failure, the anabolic state of the neonate provided with adequate calories allows for a blunting of the otherwise active rise in BUN, creatinine, potassium, and phosphate that are seen in the older child and adult population.[78] For this reason the definition of renal failure by standard indices is not valid. A further reason for difficulty is the relative inability of the neonate to conserve sodium so that fractional excretion and urinary sodium figures are expected to be higher than in the older child. Changes in plasma creatinine, creatinine clearance, and sodium handling are proportional to conceptual age and to correlation with hydration status.[79]

A functional definition of renal failure in the nursery is a condition characterized by persisting oliguria of 48-hr duration, BUN > 25 mg/d persisting for 24 hrs, and a serum creatinine of >1.5 mg/dl in the presence of oliguria which fails to respond to a fluid challenge of 20 ml/kg isotonic fluid or 1 to 2 mg/kg furosemide administration. Since the major excretory function is performed by the placenta during intrauterine life, levels of BUN and creatinine from birth to 24 hrs of life reflect the renal function of the mother rather the infant. Thus infants with even renal agenesis will have a normal serum creatinine at birth so that sequential change over the first 24 to 72 hrs will be important in diagnosis. Fluid challenge and furosemide administration are not without their risks because fluid challenge may increase the symptomatology in those patients with respiratory distress and cardiac failure, and may lead to persistence or reestablishment of flow through a patent ductus arteriosus. Furosemide may cause hypotension, and hyperviscosity by raising the hematocrit with hypovolemia. It may also cause hyponatremia with increased sodium losses.

Clinical conditions associated with the development of acute renal failure in the neonatal period are outlined in Table 36-11 and include perinatal anoxia, asphyxia, hypotension, shock, renal ischemia, or sepsis. Renal agenesis and obstructive uropathy may be encountered as causes of renal failure in the nursery, but are more common in association with multiple congenital anomalies or with a relatively asymptomatic early course, and produce an incidental finding. Certainly the combination of renal anomalies and perinatal asphyxia will produce significant renal failure with a poor long-term outlook. Stapleton reports that acute renal failure occurs in approximately 8% of neonates admitted to neonatal intensive care units. Most of the acute renal failure in this period is secondary to major perinatal insults with over 60% reported secondary to perinatal asphyxia, hypoxia, or sepsis.[80] Preexisting renal disease is not present in most infants with acute renal failure although bilateral renal agenesis, bilateral renal dysplasia, or infantile polycystic kidney disease may present in a similar fashion to acquired renal disorders. Patients with congenital heart disease are at a high risk of developing acute renal failure. Uric acid nephropathy has been postulated as a significant cause of renal failure in the newborn and may occur with increased urinary uric

Table 36-11. Causes of neonatal renal failure

Prerenal causes	asphyxia
	anoxic birth damage
	shock
	sepsis
	respiratory distress syndrome
	cardiac failure
Renal parenchymal damage	cortico-medullary necrosis
	asphyxia
	sepsis
	renal arterial damage
	renal venous thrombosis
	aminoglycosides
	cardiac surgery
Congenital abnormalities	multiple systems
	renal agenesis (bilateral)
	renal dysplasia (bilateral)
	infantile polycystic disease
	megacystis/megaureter
	megaureters (obstructive)
Hyperuricemia	hyperuricosuria

acid excretion following hypoxia, asphyxia, hemolysis, rhabdomyolysis (anoxic), cyanotic congenital heart disease, cardiopulmonary bypass surgery, and the administration of hyperosmolar radiographic contrast media.

Mortality rates in neonatal acute renal failure range from 14 to 73%,[81,82,83] survival statistics being related to the various causes of renal failure in the newborn intensive care unit, with survival depending more closely on the etiology of renal failure. Newborns with congenital heart disease or congenital renal anomalies have a higher mortality than patients with hypoxia, shock, or sepsis, where the underlying condition is self-limited or reversible.[83,84] A positive correlation has been shown between renal perfusion and reversibility of acute renal failure; hence the early screening with a radionuclide scan can be helpful.[80] Survivors of acute renal failure have a higher incidence of residual renal dysfunction. Over 40% showed decreased glomerular filtration or tubular dysfunction which will persist. The incidence of residual renal dysfunction is even more marked in those patients who show genitourinary anomalies.

Treatment modalities in the neonate (Table 36-12) include periodic supportive care, close attention to fluids, and electrolyte balance until evidence of renal recovery is present. Careful administration of calories, amino acids, and electrolytes are usually sufficient to sustain the neonate through this period of increased stress. Acute hemodialysis, peritoneal dialysis, or CAVH have been used but are less commonly necessary than in older infants or adults. The decision to utilize early dialysis or to treat conservatively with parenteral nutrition and prophylactic care of electrolyte and fluid balance depends more on the ability to deliver calories, electrolytes, and fluid rather than an arbitrary BUN or creatinine level.

Table 36-12. Therapeutic scheme for neonatal renal failure

Diagnosis: Exclude obstruction	ultrasound
Confirm renal perfusion	nuclide renal scan
Therapy: Monitor	weight
	electrolyte losses
	serum electrolytes
	acid-base status
Provide calories 80–100 cal/kg	
Amino acids 0.6 gm/kg	
Replace measured electrolyte losses	
Control hypertension	
Modify drug dosage	avoid fluid overload
Dialysis/CAVH	excess fluid gain

Table 36-13. Factors influencing neonatal fluid balance

Increased fluid requirements	phototherapy
	warming table
Decreased fluid requirement	respirator therapy
Drugs	furosemide
	phenobarbital
	dopamine
	tolazoline
	antibiotics
	indomethacin

Insensible losses are calculated and fluid balance adjusted frequently to therapeutic need. Electrolyte losses are monitored and replaced. Factors influencing change in fluid and electrolyte need in the neonate are outlined in Table 36-13. Total body weight is carefully monitored and serum electrolyte levels are expected to remain stable within normal range.

Oliguria is usually of shorter duration than in the older infant so that dialysis is less likely to be required as supportive therapy until renal function is restored.

Many therapeutic and physiologic mechanisms influence neonatal renal function and an understanding of these factors is helpful in planning for appropriate prophylaxis and therapy in the neonate.

Summary and Conclusions

ARF is a syndrome with multiple causes. Vigorous therapy in multiple clinical situations and the presence of potent pharmacologic agents, which can be helpful sustaining circulation or treating sepsis, produce a multifactorial risk to the patient who can be sustained or saved by such measures. Presently, supportive therapy is both possible and effective. Reversible causes and prophylaxis against continuing or sequential insults to renal parenchyma require attention to diminish the time taken for restoration of normal renal function.

Meticulous attention to fluid and electrolyte balance is the keystone of therapy. Replacement of renal function by dialysis allows a much easier balance of fluid and electrolytes and can provide a safe margin to fluid, caloric, and drug therapy while awaiting the return of underlying renal function.

The prognosis for survival and for return of normal renal function depends on the underlying cause for renal failure. An etiologic diagnosis and review of potential multifactorial insults are therefore important. A basic supportive regime is outlined and appropriate modifications are suggested for specific etiologies to allow safe, efficient, and comfortable therapy.

References

1. Barratt TM. Acute renal failure. In Halliday MA, Barratt TM, Vernier RL (eds): *Pediatric Nephrology* (2nd ed). Baltimore: Williams & Wilkins, 1987.
2. Anderson RJ, Schrier RW. Acute tubular necrosis. In Schrier RW, Gottschalk CW (eds): *Diseases of the Kidney* (4th ed). Boston: Little, Brown, 1988.
3. Frankel MC, Weinstein AM, Stenzl KH. Prognostic patterns in acute renal failure. The New York Hospital 1981–1982. *Clin Exp Dial Apher* 7:145, 1983.
4. Anderson RJ, Schrier RW. Clinical spectrum of oliguric and non-oliguric acute renal failure. In *Acute Renal Failure* (Contemporary Issues in Nephrology). New York: Churchill Livingstone, 1980.
5. Kennedy AC et al. Factors affecting the prognosis in acute renal failure. *Q J Med* 42:73, 1973.
6. Siegel NJ. Acute renal failure. In Brenner BM, Stein JH (eds): *Pediatric Nephrology*. New York: Churchill Livingstone, 1984.
7. Meadow SR et al. Children referred for acute dialysis. *Arch Dis Child* 46:221, 1971.
8. Offner G et al. Acute renal failure in children. Prognostic features after treatment with acute dialysis. *Eur J Pediatr* 144:482, 1986.
9. Barry KG, Malloy JP. Oliguric renal failure. Evaluation and therapy by the intravenous infusion of mannitol. *JAMA* 179:510, 1963.
10. Kashgarian M et al. Hemodynamic aspects in the development and recovery phases of experimental post ischemic acute renal failure. *Kidney Int* 10:S160, 1976.
11. Abel RM et al. Improved survival from acute renal failure after treat-

ment with intravenous essential amino acid and glucose. *N Engl J Med* 288:695, 1973.

12. McMurray SD et al. Prevailing patterns and predictor variables in patients with acute tubular necrosis. *Arch Intern Med* 138:950, 1978.

13. Sorrels AJ et al. Getting back to reality. Psychosocial adjustments in CAPD. *Nephrol Nurse* 4:22–23, 1982.

14. Trompeter TP, Herrin JT, Slovik L. Chronic renal disease. In Jellinek M, Hersog DB (eds): *MGH Psychiatric Aspects of General Hospital Pediatrics.* Chicago: Year Book, 1990. Pp 119–123.

15. Brezis M, Rosen S, Epstein FH. Acute renal failure. In Brenner BM, Rector FC (eds): *The Kidney.* Philadelphia: Saunders, 1981. P 748.

16. Hostetter TM, Wilkes BM, Brenner BM. Mechanisms of impaired glomerular filtration in acute renal failure. In Brenner BM, Stein JH (eds): *Acute Renal Failure* (Contemporary Issues in Nephrology, Vol. 6). New York: Churchill Livingstone, 1980.

17. Mason J, Thier G. Workshop on the role of medullary circulation in the pathogenesis of acute renal failure. *Nephron* 31:289, 1982.

18. Brezis M et al. Selective vulnerability of the medullary thick ascending limb to anoxia in the isolated perfused rat kidney. *J Clin Invest* 73:182, 1984.

19. Burke TJ, Arnold PE, Schrier RW. Prevention of ischemic acute renal failure with impermeant solutes. *Am J Physiol* 244:F646, 1983.

20. Brezis M et al. Transport-dependent anoxic cell injury in the isolated perfused rat kidney. *Am J Pathol* 116:327–341, 1984.

21. Davis RF, Lappas DG, Kirklin JK. Acute oliguria after cardio-pulmonary bypass; renal improvement with low dose dopamine infusion. *Crit Care Med* 10:852–856, 1982.

22. Stein JH, Boonjarern S, Mauk RC. Mechanism of redistribution of renal cortical blood flow during hemorrhagic hypotension in the dog. *J Clin Invest* 52–39, 1973.

23. Hou S, Bushinsky DA, Wish JB. Hospital-acquired renal insufficiency; a prospective study. *Am J Med* 74:243–248, 1983.

24. Rodriquez-Iturbe B. Epidemic post-streptococcal glomerulonephritis. *Kidney Int* 25:129–136, 1984.

25. Doncherwolcke RA, Chantler C, Broyer M. Paediatric dialysis. In Drukker N, Parsons FM, Maher JF (eds): *Replacement of Renal Function by Dialysis* (2nd ed). Boston: Martinus Nijhoff, 1983.

26. Ellis D et al. Acute interstitial nephritis in children. *Pediatrics* 67:862, 1981.

27. Kaplan BS, Thompson PD, De Chadarevian JP. The hemolytic uremic syndrome. *Pediatr Clin North Am* 23:761–777, 1976.

28. Brown CB et al. Combined immunosuppression and anticoagulation in rapidly progressive glomerulonephritis. *Lancet* ii:1166, 1974.

29. Cole BR et al. Pulse methyl prednisolone therapy in the treatment of severe glomerulonephritis. *J Pediatr* 88:307, 1976.

30. Bastl CP, Rudnick MR, Nairns RG. Diagnostic approaches to acute renal failure. In Brenner BM, Stein JH (eds): *Acute Renal Failure* (Contemporary Issues in Nephrology, Vol. 6) New York: Churchill Livingstone, 1980.

31. Donohoe JF et al. Tubular leakage and obstruction after renal ischemia. Structural-functional correlations. *Kidney Int* 13:208–222, 1978.

32. Herrin JT. The kidney. In Burke JF (ed): *Surgical Physiology.* Philadelphia: Saunders, 1983. Pp 187–207.

33. Bennett WM, Blythe WB. Use of drugs in patients with renal failure. In Schrier RW, Gottschalk CW (eds): *Diseases of the Kidney* (4th ed). Boston: Little, Brown, 1988.

34. Siegel NJ. *Amino-acids and Adenine Nucleotides in Acute Renal Failure.* Philadelphia: Saunders, 1983.

35. Toback FG. Amino acid treatment of acute renal failure. In Brenner BM, Stein JH (eds): *Acute Renal Failure* (Contemporary Issues in Nephrology, Vol. 6). New York: Churchill Livingstone, 1980.

36. Bricker NS. On the meaning of the intact nephron hypothesis. *Am J Med* 46:1, 1969.

37. Karmali MA et al. The association between idiopathic hemolytic-uremic syndrome and infection by verotoxin-producing *Escherichia coli. J Infect Dis* 151:775–782, 1985.

38. Koster F et al. Hemolytic-uremic syndrome after shigellosis. Relation to endotoxemia and circulating immune complexes. *N Engl J Med* 281:1023–1027, 1969.

39. Upadhaya K et al. The importance of non-renal involvement in hemolytic uremic syndrome. *Pediatrics* 65:115–120, 1980.

40. Steele BT et al. Recovery from prolonged coma in hemolytic uremic syndrome. *J Pediatr* 103:402, 1983.

41. Habib R et al. Prognosis of the hemolytic uremic syndrome in children. In Hamburger J et al. (eds): *Advances in Nephrology.* Vol. 11. Chicago: Year Book, 1982. Pp 99–128.

42. Dolislager D, Tune B. The hemolytic-uremic syndrome. *Am J Dis Child* 122:55, 1978.

43. Aronson EB, August CS. Preliminary report: Treatment of the hemolytic uremic syndrome with aspirin and dipyridamole. *J Pediatr* 86:957–961, 1975.

44. O'Reagan S et al. Aspirin and dipyridamole therapy in the hemolytic-uremic syndrome. *J Pediatr* 97:473–476, 1980.

45. Remuzzi G et al. Haemolytic-uraemic syndrome: Deficiency of plasma factor(s) regulating prostacyclin activity. *Lancet* ii:871–872, 1978.

46. Bergstein JM, Kuederli U, Bang NU. Plasma inhibitor of glomerular fibrinolysis in the hemolytic-uremic syndrome. *Am J Med* 73:322–327, 1982.

47. Remuzzi G et al. Treatment of the hemolytic-uremic syndrome with plasma. *Clin Nephrol* 12:279–284, 1979.

48. Mitchell JRA. Prostacyclin—powerful, yes but is it useful? *Br Med J* 287:1824, 1983.

49. Morel-Maroger L et al. Prognostic importance of vascular lesions in acute renal failure with microangiopathic hemolytic anemia (hemolytic-uremic syndrome); clinicopathologic study in 20 adults. *Kidney Int* 15:548–558, 1979.

50. Vanrenterghem Y et al. Thromboembolic complications and haemostatic changes in cyclosporin treated cadaveric kidney allograft recipients. *Lancet* i:999–1002, 1985.

51. Bonser RS et al. Cyclosporin-induced haemolytic uraemic syndrome in liver allograft recipient (letter). *Lancet* 2:1337, 1984.

52. Remuzzi G et al. Familial deficiency of a plasma factor stimulating prostacyclin activity. *Thromb Res* 16:517–525, 1979.

53. Bergstein JM, Michael AF, Kjellstrand CM. Hemolytic-uremic syndrome in adult sisters. *Transplantation* 17:487–490, 1974.

54. Herbert D, Sibley RK, Mauer SM. Recurrence of hemolytic uremic syndrome in renal transplant recipients. *Kidney Int* 30:S51–S58, 1986.

55. Buturovic J et al. Cyclosporine-associated hemolytic uremic syndrome in four renal allograft recipients: Resolution without specific therapy. *Transplant Proc* 22(4):1726–1727, 1990.

56. Lucas CE. The renal responses to acute injury and sepsis. *Surg Clin North Am* 56:953, 1976.

57. Hollenberg NK, Epstein M, Rosen SM. Acute oliguric renal failure in man and evidence for preferential cortical ischemia. *Medicine* 47:455, 1968.

58. Niaudet P, Maher H, Gagnadoux. Outcome of children with acute renal failure. *Kidney Int* 28:S148–S151, 1985.

59. Levinsky NG, Bernard DB, Johnston PA. Enhancement of recovery of acute renal failure: Effects of mannitol and diuretics. In Brenner BM, Stein JH (eds): *Acute Renal Failure* (Contemporary Issues in Nephrology, Vol. 6). New York: Churchill Livingstone, 1980.

60. Lieberman KV, Nardi L, Bosch JP. Treatment of renal failure in an infant using continuous arteriovenous hemofiltration. *J Pediatr* 106:646–649, 1985.

61. Ronco C. Continuous arteriovenous hemofiltration in infants. In Paganini EP (ed): *Acute Continuous Renal Replacement Therapy.* Boston: Martinus Nijhoff, 1986.

62. Sevitt S. Renal function after burning. *J Clin Pathol* 18:572–578, 1965.

63. Demling RH. Burns. *N Engl J Med* 313:1389–1398, 1985.

64. Eklund J. Studies on renal function in burns. II. Early signs of impaired renal function in lethal burns. *Acta Clin Scand* 16:735–740, 1970.

65. Planas W, Wachtel T, Frank H. Characterization of acute renal failure in the burned patient. *Arch Intern Med* 142:2087–2091, 1982.

66. Diamond JR, Yonurn DC. Non-oliguric acute renal failure associated

with a low fractional excretion of sodium. *Ann Intern Med* 96:5970–6000, 1982.

67. Fang LST et al. Low fractional excretion of sodium with contrast media-induced acute renal failure. *Arch Intern Med* 140:531–533, 1980.

68. Walsh MB, Miller SL, Kagen LJ. Myoglobinemia in severely burned patients: Correlations with severity and survival. *J Trauma* 22:6–10, 1982.

69. Bosch JP. Continuous arteriovenous hemofiltration (CAVH). Operational characteristics and clinical use. *Nephrol Lett* 3:15–26, 1986.

70. Lazarus JM. The kidney in health and disease, XXVIII. Dialytic therapy: Principles and clinical guidelines. *Hosp Pract* 17:111, 1982.

71. Fischer JE, Baldessarini RJ. False neurotransmitters and hepatic failure. *Lancet* ii:75, 1971.

72. Zipser RD, Radvan GH, Kronberg IJ. Urinary thromboxane B_2 and prostaglandin E_2 in the hepatorenal syndrome: Evidence for increased vasoconstrictor and decreased vasodilator factors. *Gastroenterology* 84:697–703, 1983.

73. Rasmussen HH, Ibels LS. Acute renal failure: Multivariate analysis of causes and risk factors. *Am J Med* 73:211–218, 1982.

74. Brezis M, Rosen S, Epstein FH. Acute renal failure. In Brenner BM, Rector FC (eds): *The Kidney*. Philadelphia: Saunders, 1981. P 748.

75. Rieselbach RE, Garnick MB (eds). *Cancer and the Kidney*. Philadelphia: Lea & Febiger, 1982.

76. Rieselback RE, Garnick MB. Renal disease induced by antineoplastic agents. In Schrier RW, Gottschalk CW (eds): *Diseases of the Kidney*. Boston: Little, Brown, 1988.

77. Heney D et al. Continuous arteriovenous hemofiltration in the treatment of tumour lysis syndrome. *Pediatr Nephrol* 4:245, 1990.

78. William GS, Klenk EL, Winters RW. Acute renal failure in pediatrics. In Winters RW (ed): *The Body Fluids in Pediatrics*. Boston: Little Brown, 1973.

79. Arant BS. Renal disorders of the newborn infant. In Brenner BM, Stein JH (eds); Tune BM, Mendoza SA (guest eds): *Pediatric Nephrology* (Contemporary Issues in Nephrology, Vol. 12). New York: Churchill Livingstone, 1984. Pp 111–135.

80. Stapleton FB, Jones DP, Green RS. Acute renal failure in neonates: Incidence, etiology and outcome. *Pediatr Nephrol* 1:314–320, 1987.

81. Anand SK, Northway JD, Crussi, FG. Acute renal failure in newborn infants. *J Pediatr* 92:985, 1978.

82. Norman ME, Asadi FK. A prospective study of acute renal failure in the newborn infant. *Pediatrics* 63:475, 1979.

83. Chevalier RL et al. Prognostic factors in neonatal acute renal failure. *Pediatrics* 74:265–272, 1984.

84. Torrado A, Guignard JP. Renal failure in respiratory distress syndrome. *J Pediatr* 85:443–444, 1974.

VI Metabolic Disorders

37 ◆ Metabolic Disorders

William E. Russell　**37.1**　Diabetic Ketoacidosis

Pathophysiology

Diabetic ketoacidosis (DKA) is a state of hyperglycemia and metabolic acidosis that results from insulin deficiency. It is characterized by a depletion of water, electrolytes, and intracellular substrates for normal metabolism. In many instances, infection or other metabolic stresses precipitate decompensation into DKA by antagonizing the marginal levels of insulin present in the child with undiagnosed or inappropriately treated diabetes; severe emotional stress may also produce insulin resistance and precipitate DKA, although noncompliance is probably a more common cause of decompensation.[1]

Although initiated by insulin insufficiency, DKA is propagated by an excess of glucagon and other counterregulatory hormones, which catabolize proteins and lipids in the peripheral tissues to provide substrates for the unrestrained production of glucose (gluconeogenesis) and ketoacids (ketogenesis), primarily in the liver. Decreased renal perfusion, decreased utilization of glucose and fatty acids, and decreased clearance of lactic acid from peripheral tissues are all secondary effects that perpetuate and steadily worsen the hyperglycemia, acidosis, dehydration, and insulin resistance.

Roughly 30% of newly diagnosed diabetics initially present in DKA, while the incidence among known diabetics is between 3 and 8 episodes per 1000 patients per year.[2] DKA is the major cause of diabetic mortality in children, and accounts for 41% of deaths in diabetics under 21 years of age and 70% of deaths of diabetic children under 10 years.[2,3]

The treatment of ketoacidosis consists of insulin administration to reverse lipolysis and protein degradation in the peripheral tissues, and to inhibit glucose and ketoacid production in the liver. At the same time, water, electrolytes, and glucose are replaced to restore tissue perfusion, ionic balance, and substrate supply for normal metabolism.

Gluconeogenesis

A fall in the ratio of insulin to glucagon in blood entering the liver from the splanchnic bed is probably the critical initiator of gluconeogenesis.[4] Other glucose counterregulatory hormones, such as cortisol, growth hormone, and catecholamines, contribute to the physiologic aberrations observed in insulin deficiency. Glucocorticoid therapy, or overproduction of these hormones, in disorders such as Cushing's syndrome, acromegaly, or pheochromocytoma can result in hyperglycemia. In contrast, the underproduction of cortisol and growth hormone in children with pituitary insufficiency contributes to their propensity to hypoglycemia as infants. Some conditions of "brittle" or unstable diabetes are characterized by enhanced sensitivity to the glucose counterregulatory hormones. As acidosis develops and worsens in DKA, insulin action is further antagonized by a negative effect of low pH on insulin binding to its receptor and postreceptor signaling.[5]

The major physiologic aberrations that result from insulin deficiency are illustrated in Fig. 37.1-1. Unopposed by insulin, gluca-

Figure 37.1-1. Pathophysiology of diabetic ketoacidosis.

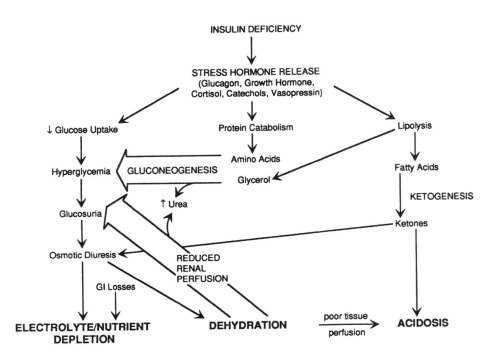

454

gon diverts liver metabolism away from the storage of glucose as glycogen and from its conversion to pyruvate for oxidation in the Krebs cycle (glycolysis). Instead, glycogen is converted to glucose, and gluconeogenic substrates coming to the liver from the periphery are diverted to new glucose production (gluconeogensis). At the periphery, a catabolic state develops: Proteins and fats are degraded in muscle and adipose tissue, leading to a release of gluconeogenic amino acids, glycerol, and fatty acids into the blood. At the liver, and to a small extent, the kidney, these gluconeogenic precursors fuel the synthesis of new glucose. Under experimental conditions, acute insulin deprivation in human diabetic subjects doubles hepatic glucose production within 2 hours.[6]

As gluconeogenic amino acids are presented to the liver for utilization of their carbon skeletons, the amino groups are converted to urea, resulting in elevated levels of BUN. The rise in BUN is further exacerbated by volume contraction and decreased glomerular filtration.

Ketogenesis and Acidosis

Insulin deficiency, coupled with cortisol excess, results in lipolysis in peripheral tissues and a copious supply of free fatty acids (FFAs) for the liver. In the insulin-replete or -fed state, FFAs presenting to the liver are reesterified to triglycerides. In the insulin-deficient state, however, a relative excess of glucagon stimulates FFA oxidation to ketones, largely acetoacetate and beta-hydroxybutyrate. In addition, acetoacetate can be converted to acetone, which gives the characteristic "fruity" odor to the breath in DKA, and is an additional substrate for gluconeogenesis.[7]

Ketoacids are not, however, the sole source of excess acidity in DKA. The catabolism of amino acids and lipids produces increased quantities of phosphoric and sulfuric acids, while diminished tissue perfusion leads to the accumulation of lactic acid as well. All of these substances contribute to the significant anion gap that is measured in DKA. Ketones and other acids contribute to vasomotor instability and the peripheral vasodilation that is prominent in DKA.

As will be discussed later, renal hypoperfusion contributes greatly to the hyperglycemia and acidosis of DKA. In a small percentage of patients in DKA, a significant ion gap is not detected. Instead, they show a hyperchloremic acidosis, which is presumed to result from sufficient fluid intake to permit ketone excretion as sodium-ketone salts, and a consequent chloride retention.[8] In very rare instances of DKA associated with copious vomiting, a metabolic alkalosis can predominate.[9]

Dehydration and Electrolyte Depletion

The hyperglycemic effects of unrestrained gluconeogenesis are magnified by a diminished utilization of glucose in the periphery, and by the progressive volume depletion and renal hypoperfusion that result from osmotic diuresis. Under ordinary hemodynamic circumstances, the renal tubular capacity to reabsorb glucose (Tm) is exceeded when plasma glucose is greater than 180 to 200 mg/dl. Therefore, all of the filtered glucose that is in excess of the Tm should be excreted with the urine, and blood glucose maintained under 200 mg/dl. However, the actual "glucose threshold" of the kidney is determined by the glomerular filtration rate (GFR) as well as the Tm,[10] and the GFR is significantly reduced as fluid losses worsen.

Diminished GFR results from the progressive dehydration that

Table 37.1-1. Approximate fluid and electrolyte losses in diabetic ketoacidosis

Compartment	Deficit (per kg body weight)
Water	100 ml
Sodium	7 mEq
Potassium	5 mEq
Chloride	5 mEq
Magnesium	0.5 mEq
Phosphate	1 mEq

Adapted from D Porter Jr, JB Halter. The endocrine pancreas and diabetes mellitus. In RH Williams (ed): *Textbook of Endocrinology.* Philadelphia: Saunders, 1981. P 811. With permission.

develops in DKA. High concentrations of glucose in the glomerular filtrate produce an osmotic diuresis that facilitates a loss of water and electrolytes, especially sodium and potassium, which form salts with the overabundant ketoacids. Anorexia exacerbates the progressive extracellular fluid volume contraction that results from the osmotic diuresis, vomiting, and other GI losses. The result is dehydration and diminished GFR and, consequently, the loss of a potentially useful "escape valve" for excess glucose. The magnitude of water and electrolyte losses typically observed in DKA are presented in Table 37.1-1. Because of the high glucose content of urinary fluid losses, water is lost in excess of electrolytes (the composition of the excreted fluid approximates 70 mEq/liter of sodium and 50 mEq/liter of potassium), suggesting replacement with hypotonic fluids after the initial correction of hypovolemia.

In addition to the loss of water, sodium, potassium, and energy sources in the form of glucose and fatty acids, an important contributor to the pathophysiology of DKA may be phosphate loss. The Tm for the reabsorption of phosphate is reduced in the presence of high glucose and by glucocorticoids. Phosphorus depletion results in significant muscle weakness, including diaphragmatic dysfunction and possibly cardiomyopathy.[11] The reestablishment of normal renal perfusion to facilitate excretion of the excess glucose can also increase urinary losses of phosphate and other ions. However, prospective studies of phosphate replacement in children with DKA, at doses that do not cause hypocalcemia, have not proven to benefit recovery, and may prolong the hypophosphatemia.[12]

Hyperosmolar, Nonketotic Coma

Hyperosmolar, nonketotic coma (HNKC) is a variant of DKA that is much less common in children than in adults, especially the elderly. In this condition, patients who are typically mild diabetics, or unknown to have diabetes, present with severe dehydration, serum osmolality exceeding 350 mosm/kg, and plasma glucose concentrations frequently in excess of 1000 mg/dl, with absent or minimal elevation of serum ketones. This puzzling entity has been observed in infants and children in a variety of clinical settings, including dialysis, hyperalimentation, acute infection, and burns, and associated with a number of pharmacologic agents, including propranolol, cimetidine, thiazide diuretics, phenytoin, and diazoxide.[13,14]

The reasons for the depressed ketogenesis and tendency to profound dehydration are not clear, but factors that distinguish HNKC from DKA and have been implicated in its pathogenesis include a higher rate of endogenous insulin secretion (plasma FFA concentrations are generally not elevated), a diminished secretion of glucose counterregulatory hormones, an inhibitory effect of osmolality on lipolysis, and drugs, impaired thirst, or preexisting renal disease that worsen the dehydration. Typically, both BUN and creatinine are elevated to a greater extent than is seen in DKA. The profound hyperosmolar state produces a degree of cellular dehydration that may not be reflected in estimates of dehydration based on body weight. The treatment strategy for HNKC in children is not significantly different from DKA, although the water and electrolyte deficits are likely to be greater and the insulin requirement less in HNKC.

Clinical Examination

Initial Evaluation

As in any medical emergency, the evaluation of the patient with suspected DKA must begin with attention to immediate life-sustaining measures, the ABCs of cardiopulmonary resuscitation.

Airway

It is important to recognize that significant drowsiness or obtundation can develop with metabolic decompensation or cerebral edema in DKA, whatever the baseline neurologic status. There remains a strong potential for inability to defend the airway and risk of aspiration. The etiologies of neuromuscular dysfunction in DKA include brain edema, electrolyte imbalances, poor cerebral perfusion, and tissue hypoxia.

Breathing

The classic Kussmaul respirations of DKA, periods of air hunger alternating with brief apnea, become evident as the serum pH falls below 7.2. As the pH continues to fall, however, respiration is depressed and periods of apnea are prolonged. When present, the fragrance of acetone on the breath, which resembles fruit-flavored chewing gum, can be helpful in suggesting the diagnosis, although the breath odor of ethanol can be indistinguishable.

Circulation

Tissue perfusion can be difficult to assess clinically in DKA. The presence of ketones and other acids typically results in peripheral vasodilation and a flushed appearance that often belies profound hypovolemia. The ketoacidotic state is **always** associated with volume depletion and decreased glomerular filtration. In addition to the usual vital signs of BP and pulse, direct measurements of central venous pressure can prove helpful in DKA and should be considered in all children with preexisting cardiopulmonary disease or oliguria, and in those instances in which adequate BP is not rapidly restored with initial fluid resuscitation.

Endocrinopathy

Augmenting the classic ABCs is the reminder that diabetes in children is an autoimmune disease and can coexist with other autoimmune endocrine diseases. When dealing with DKA, one should always consider the possibility of other coexisting undiagnosed, but life-threatening, endocrinopathies, especially of the thyroid, adrenals, and parathyroid glands.

Hypoglycemia

Hypoglycemia should always be ruled out immediately in the known diabetic with altered mental status. Because the time course for the development of DKA is generally several days, the history of a very brief or unheralded clinical decompensation is strongly suggestive of hypoglycemia. The physician should be acquainted with the use of any one of several rapid blood-glucose–determining strips that can be interpreted visually, and have them available in the emergency treatment facility. In the absence of means for a blood glucose measurement, hypoglycemia should be presumed and treated with an intravenous (IV) bolus of glucose, 0.5 ml/kg of a 50% solution. If venous access cannot be rapidly obtained, glucagon may be given: 0.5 mg for children, 1.0 mg for adolescents and adults. These maneuvers will not significantly exacerbate the condition of a ketoacidotic patient, but can be life-saving in a hypoglycemic emergency.

The onset of recurrent hypoglycemia in a known diabetic should suggest the possible advent of autoimmune adrenal insufficiency, which might also be suggested by hyperpigmentation. Confirmatory blood studies include a subnormal cortisol and elevated ACTH at time of hypoglycemic stress.

At the initial evaluation of the nonambulatory patient with DKA, venous access through a suitably large bore catheter should be secured and initial blood studies obtained promptly. Although the insulin and fluid components of the therapy are adjusted independently, they may share a common IV line (discussion follows). However, the frequent blood sampling required in the initial hours of treatment is facilitated by the insertion of a separate sampling catheter through which no glucose is infused.

Physical Signs

With initial stabilization, a flow sheet is established to monitor the response to therapy. Physical signs to be documented, hourly until the patient has stabilized and then every 4 hours, include BP, pulse, and temperature; the state of hydration (central venous pressure, where indicated); the quality of respirations; and neurologic status, especially state of consciousness, pupil size, funduscopic examination, and deep tendon reflexes. The importance of documenting and following neurologic status cannot be overemphasized, and is further discussed in the section, Cerebral Edema.

Differential Diagnosis

The coexistence of hyperglycemia, ketosis, and acidosis is diagnostic of DKA, and very few conditions should confuse the diagnosis. When glucosuria is found, hyperglycemia must be documented by blood studies to be diagnostic, as benign glucosuria of renal origin, resulting from a subnormal Tm for glucose, can be accompanied by ketosis in the fasted or stressed state.

It should be borne in mind that individuals with certain chromosomal disorders are prone to develop autoimmune endocrinopathies, including impaired glucose tolerance and frank diabetes. These include the Turner, Down, and Klinefelter syndromes. More complete listings of diabetes-associated syndromes are available.[15] Hyperglycemia, generally with minimal ketosis, is seen in the context of a number of metabolic disorders, including glucocorticoid therapy or Cushing's syndrome, pheochromocytoma, thyrotoxicosis, hemochromatosis, shock, burns, and hypoxia. In general, these should present no confusion in the diagnosis of DKA. A listing of disorders with greater clinical overlap with DKA is presented in Table 37.1-2.

Table 37.1-2. Differential diagnosis of diabetic ketoacidosis

Condition	Features
Salicylate intoxication	Acidosis with anion gap, hyperventilation, ketosis, polyuria and hyperglycemia
	Distinguishing features: Briefer clinical history than DKA: 5–6 hrs vs. >3 days Blood salicylate level
Hypernatremic dehydration	Significant hypernatremia with variable hyperglycemia
	Distinguishing features: Generally no overlap in sodium concentration with DKA
Postconvulsion in the very young	Infants and children <3 years old
	Distinguishing features: Hyperglycemia is transient, rarely associated with ketosis. Probably catecholamine-mediated
Acute pancreatitis	Prominent abdominal pain with hyperglycemia, elevated amylase
	Distinguishing features: Hyperglycemia, probably of catecholamine origin. In some cases of acute viral pancreatitis, islet cell destruction with insulinopenia can develop. Lipase elevated in pancreatitis, not DKA.
Organophosphate poisoning	Hyperglycemia, ketosis, and acidosis
	Distinguishing features: Sialorrhea, rhinorrhea, watery diarrhea, pupillary constriction, depressed blood cholinesterase activity Response to atropine

Laboratory Studies

After attention to the cardiopulmonary status and documentation of baseline vital signs, venous access is established and laboratory studies rapidly initiated, as they may significantly influence the immediate therapy.

Table 37.1-3 outlines the recommended baseline blood and urine studies. Once again, a preliminary glucose determination should be made at the bedside using a whole-blood glucose strip. It is unnecessary to document the presence of ketones in the blood, as urinary ketone tests are easier to perform and are reflective of blood ketone status.

Of most critical nature in these initial studies are the serum electrolytes, especially potassium. Based on the previous discussion of the pathophysiology of DKA, it should be evident that there will be significant electrolyte depletion, although serum concentrations for sodium and potassium may be normal or even elevated initially. Especially if there is oliguria, the replacement of potassium must be delayed until serum concentrations fall into the normal range and urinary output is established. In the absence of serum measurements, the ECG can be helpful in determining serum potassium status.

During insulin therapy, the most critical blood indices of response to follow are the serum glucose and potassium, which should be measured hourly for the first several hours. As insulin facilitates the transfer of one molecule of glucose to the intracellular space, one potassium ion follows. **Hypokalemia is as likely to cause clinical mischief during the treatment of DKA as is hypoglycemia.** In addition to its effects on cardiovascular function, hypokalemia can result in profound resistance to insulin and other hormones, especially vasopressin. The supervention of a water-losing, diabetes insipidus–like state

secondary to hypokalemia can significantly complicate the recovery from DKA.

Hypomagnesemia is not rare in DKA. In one well-documented instance, depressed magnesium concentrations were associated

Table 37.1-3. Initial laboratory studies in diabetic ketoacidosis

Blood

Glucose. **Always** perform a bedside glucose measurement using a visually interpreted rapid measurement strip.

Na, K, Cl, Ca, PO₄, BUN

Serum bicarbonate of pH: Can use either direct bicarbonate measurement on a fully filled blood tube (to prevent CO_2 diffusion) **or** calculate the bicarbonate from the pH and pCO_2 on heparinized venous or arterial blood obtained without exposure to air.

Serum osmolality: May be measured directly or calculated using the formula: osmolality $= 2 \times [\text{Na}^+ + \text{K}^+] + [\text{glucose}]/18 + \text{BUN}/2.8$ where osmolality is expressed as mosm/kg; [Na$^+$] and [K$^+$] as mEq/liter; and [glucose] and [BUN] as mg/dl.

CBC

Culture, if indicated

Urine

Glucose and acetone

Examine sediment

Culture, if indicated

Cerebrospinal fluid: Unless there is very strong evidence of meningitis, and CSF is required for diagnosis and therapy, lumbar punctures are contraindicated in patients with DKA. See discussion of Cerebral Edema.

ECG: Especially useful if laboratory results are unavailable. Scrutinize for indications of potassium status.

Table 37.1-4. Laboratory artifacts in diabetic ketoacidosis

Observation	Causes
Hyponatremia	Dilutional, from osmotic swelling of extracellular space Hyperlipidemia, producing a large plasma compartment to which ions do not distribute, but influencing the calculated ion **concentration**
Elevated MCV, hematocrit	Swelling of cells taken from their hypertonic environment and diluted in isotonic buffers for automated counting Not seen on manual hematocrit
Elevated creatinine	Cross-reactivity of ketones in creatinine assays that employ picrate
Elevated ketones	Captopril
Depressed ketones	A strong predominance of betahyroxybutyrate over acetoacetate, the form of ketoacid that is measured by the nitroprusside reaction
Elevated amylase	Salivary, pancreatic, and possibly hepatic origin; lipase may be more specific for acute pancreatitis.

with an insulin resistance that could not be corrected until normal serum magnesium was restored.[16] A number of laboratory artifacts are commonly encountered in the serum of patients with DKA. Some of these are outlined in Table 37.1-4.

History and Physical Examination

Once initial assessment and stabilization of the patient have occurred and laboratory studies initiated, a more complete history and physical examination are in order. As indicated in the discussion of pathophysiology, the ketoacidotic state commonly develops in an undiagnosed or marginally treated diabetic patient who develops an infection or other metabolic stress that requires increased insulin secretion. It is, therefore, important to direct the history and physical examination toward the diagnosis of the precipitating event, including head trauma and poisoning in the comatose patient.

Fever is **not** a nonspecific feature of the ketoacidotic state. Because body temperature is often slightly subnormal in DKA, fever is suggestive of infection or disordered CNS temperature regulation, as seen in cerebral edema. Bacterial infections, especially streptococcal pharyngitis and urinary tract infections in girls, are common precipitants of DKA. Major sunburn or contact dermatitis, such as poison ivy, can also cause decompensation of diabetic control.

The classic history of polydipsia, polyphagia, and polyuria is almost always present but can be so overshadowed by other complaints, such as abdominal pain, nausea, and fever, as to be forgotten by patients and family. These features must be specifically probed in the history. An attempt should be made to determine the most recent reliable body weight. With increasing public awareness of the symptoms of diabetes, many pediatricians find themselves in the position of having the diagnosis of glucosuria made for them by astute parents with access to urine dipsticks.

Except in those patients with the hyperosmolar, nonketotic form of diabetic decompensation, dehydration should be evident in loss of skin turgor and sunken eyes. As discussed previously, the presence of ketones results in peripheral vasodilation and a distinct malar flush, which can persist well into the second or third day of treatment. This reflects the relatively slow clearance of ketones, even after ketogenesis has been halted with insulin therapy.

Abdominal pain and distention with ileus, often mimicking a surgical condition, are very common secondary events in DKA, but

they must never be passed over as a normal part of the syndrome. Abdominal emergencies, such as appendicitis, or pelvic emergencies, such as ruptured ectopic pregnancy in the female adolescent, must be considered because they can precipitate DKA.

Therapy

The Therapeutic Approach in Four Stages

Based on the pathophysiology of the ketoacidotic state, the treatment of DKA can be divided into four (arbitrary) stages, which are outlined in Table 37.1-5.

Stage 1

The initial resuscitation aims to restore the intravascular volume with isotonic, glucose-free fluid to reestablish adequate tissue perfusion and to present the excess glucose load of the blood to the kidneys for filtration and excretion. During this stage, insulin therapy is initiated to begin to stop the production of new glucose and ketones. Even in the absence of insulin therapy, however, rehydration alone will reduce the blood glucose to the range of the renal Tm, and must be initiated even if insulin is not available. The beneficial influence of fluid therapy on serum glucose has been particularly well documented in hyperosmolar coma.[17]

If BP is not stabilized after a total of 30 ml/kg of isotonic fluids over 1 to 2 hours, consideration should be given to the use of colloids to prevent tissue swelling. Exogenous catecholamines may, in extreme circumstances, prove essential in restoring BP, but their effectiveness is much diminished in acidosis. Transition to stage 2 occurs when urine output has been established and BP stabilized, generally within 1 to 2 hours.

Stage 2

Once BP has been stabilized and tissue perfusion restored, the process of cellular rehydration begins. As indicated in the discussion of pathophysiology, the osmotic pull of glucose results in the loss of water in DKA in **excess** of electrolytes. However, there is disagreement as to the appropriate fluid tonicity for this stage of rehydration. Out of concern for the possible consequences of rapid drops in serum osmolality, some centers continue to employ isotonic fluids at this stage to prevent rapid changes in plasma osmolality.[18]

It is our recommendation, and it has been the practice at the

Table 37.1-5. The therapeutic approach in four stages

Stage	Goals	Insulin[a]	Fluids	Endpoint
1	Expansion of intravascular volume Renal perfusion Inhibit catabolism Inhibit gluconeogenesis and ketogenesis	0.1 U/kg hr IV or IM	N saline, Ringer's lactate 10–30 ml/kg over 1 hr Colloid, if required	Urine flow Adequate BP
2	Rehydration of intracellular space Restoration of depleted ions Continued insulinization	0.1 U/kg/hr IV or IM	1/2 N saline with KCl/PO$_4$: 10–40 mEq/liter[b] 3000 ml/m^2/d	BS < 200 mg/dl
3	Continued rehydration Provision of energy substrates	1 U/100 mlD$_5$W titrated to BS IV, IM, SC	D$_5$ 1/2 N saline with electrolytes 3000 ml/m^2/d	Bowel sounds
4	Transition to oral rehydration and alimentation	SC	Oral liquids Soft solids	Normal food intake

[a]Only crystalline insulin may be dissolved in electrolyte solutions for IV infusion. See text for details.
[b]Potassium concentration determined by serum potassium.
BS, blood sugar; SC, subcutaneously, IV, intravenously, IM, intramuscularly.

Pediatric Endocrine Unit of the Massachusetts General Hospital for the past 15 years, to continue rehydration at this stage with hypotonic fluids, at a rate of 3,000 ml/m^2/d (roughly, twice maintenance). Because glucose levels in the blood at this stage of treatment are generally still in excess of the renal threshold, glucose-free, 0.5 N saline is administered, with potassium salts as required to maintain normokalemia. With respect for the possible contribution of vigorous rehydration in worsening cerebral edema (discussion follows), fluid administration should be limited to a rate not faster than twice the maintenance rate. Transition to stage 3 occurs when the combined effects of renal perfusion and insulin therapy have reduced the blood glucose to the range of the renal threshold, approximately 200 mg/dl.

Stage 3

Once blood glucose has fallen into a range that can be reabsorbed after glomerular filtration, insulin therapy will be more effective in restoring intracellular transport. During this phase, 5% dextrose in 0.5 N NaCl with added potassium remains a suitable fluid for continued rehydration at a continued rate of 3,000 ml/m^2/d.

Insulin requirements in this stage of therapy can be quite variable and are aimed at maintaining the blood glucose below the renal threshold. A rough estimate of insulin needs can be calculated by estimating that 1 unit will be required for each 4 to 5 gm of glucose infused, or roughly 1 U/100 ml of a 5% dextrose solution. The infusion rate will approximate 0.05 U/kg/hr, but will be governed by the blood sugar response. However, in those instances (generally younger children) in which acidosis (pH < 7.2) persists after the blood sugar has fallen below 200 mg/dl, the insulin infusion rate is maintained at 0.1 U/kg/hr and the concentration of dextrose in the infusate increased to maintain the blood sugar in the normal range.

The transition to stage 4 is largely determined by a number of clinical variables, including the presence of bowel sounds and the patient's state of consciousness and appetite. Generally, the latter two factors are in favor of oral alimentation before the former.

Stage 4

Once blood glucose has stabilized at a concentration below the renal Tm, and the patient has recovered sufficient GI and neurologic function, oral alimentation and a transition to subcutaneous

insulin can begin. Stage 4 is characterized by a gradual decrease in IV fluids as oral intake of initially **glucose-free** liquids is increased. Once it is clear that oral fluids will be tolerated, soft solids may be introduced in multiple small meals. At this point, IV insulin may be discontinued and injections of subcutaneous regular insulin begun. Practical points of this transition are discussed next.

Practical Considerations in Fluid and Insulin Therapy

It is possible, and often preferable, to administer fluids and insulin through a common IV line; however, this should be accomplished with two converging, but separately controlled infusion systems. The dilution of insulin **in** the resuscitation fluid, as recommended by some authors, necessitates changes in fluid infusion rates with each change in the insulin rate and greatly limits therapeutic flexibility.

Fluids

Although the fluid administration rates during stages 1 to 3 are relatively stable, the most critical variable is generally the potassium concentration of the infusate. Serum potassium is very sensitive to insulin administration and is monitored on a 1- to 2-hour basis initially. Therefore, it is best to add potassium to a small quantity of fluid, generally a 1- to 2-hour aliquot, so that rapid changes can be made based on serum potassium concentrations. Potassium is generally administered 50% as the chloride salt and 50% as buffered phosphate salt to prevent chloride overload and to restore depleted phosphate.

Insulin

The doses of insulin used to treat the acutely ill child with DKA are generally referred to as "low-dose" therapy to contrast them with practices of more than a decade ago, which employed insulin administration rates 10 times greater. Although insulin is ideally administered intravenously and in an intensive care setting, comparable success can be attained using intramuscular crystalline insulin on an hourly schedule when the requisite infusion equipment and nursing care are not available.

The advantage of IV insulin is the extreme flexibility in altering the administration rate: The actions of IV insulin abate within 20 minutes of discontinuation, as opposed to about 2 hours when deposited intramuscularly, or 3 to 4 hours subcutaneously. IV insulin administration, however, requires appropriately accurate, low-volume infusion pumps and constant nursing supervision. Comparable results, with minimal sacrifice in control, can be attained with the intramuscular administration of insulin at a dose of 0.1 U/kg each hour. Intramuscular insulin will require use of a tuberculin syringe with a 1.5-inch needle and, in the absence of an insulin-specific scale, careful attention to the dose administered: 10 U/0.1 ml.

Only crystalline (CZI, regular, actrapid) insulin is soluble in electrolyte solutions; cloudy suspensions of insulin (NPH, lente, semilente, ultralente) are for subcutaneous use only and must never be infused intravenously. Crystalline insulin is a clear liquid in the stock solution and is universally available at a concentration of 100 U/ml (U-100). Given the recommended starting dose of 0.1 U/kg/hr, the size of the patient and the pumping rate of the available infusion pumps will determine the most practical concentrations to employ at the bedside.

1 U/ml:	1 ml U-100 regular insulin in 100-ml normal saline
10 U/ml:	10 ml U-100 regular insulin plus 90-ml normal saline

The insulin molecule has a weak affinity for glass and plastic; therefore, a certain amount of insulin in any diluted solution will bind to tubing and lower the insulin concentration in the initial infusate. It is not necessary to add albumin or other blood products to the insulin solution to prevent insulin binding. It is advisable, however, to discard the first 20 ml of infusate that comes through the line in order to saturate the capacity of the tubing to bind further insulin.

Many of the in-line particle and air-trapping filters that have come into increasing use have a very high affinity for insulin in solutions passing through them, and also the capacity to absorb large amounts of insulin. Merely running through a quantity of insulin solution, therefore, may not result in their complete saturation and the delivery of appropriate insulin doses to the patient. Although this issue must be addressed on a product-by-product basis, it is advisable to **omit** these filters from the insulin-infusing line.

An insulin dose of 0.1 U/kg/hr is recommended when initiating therapy. In patients with extreme insulin resistance, however, it may be necessary to increase the dose in the absence of a response to the initial dose. If in stage 2 of therapy, the rate of fall in blood glucose exceeds 100 mg/dl/hr, it is advisable to reduce the insulin infusion rate by 25% or more to prevent rapid changes in serum osmolality. **When it has been established that other factors, especially the presence of in-line filters or pump malfunction, are not responsible for diminishing the delivered insulin dose,** it is permissible to double the insulin infusion rate if the blood sugar has not begun to fall after 2 hours of therapy.

Similarly, a halving of the insulin infusion rate will generally produce a noticeable slowing in the rate of glucose fall. There is a tendency among inexperienced physicians to overreact when the blood glucose falls into the normal range and discontinue the insulin infusion while administering boluses of dextrose. Unless a massive overdose of insulin has been given, this is almost never necessary and usually results in a rebound hyperglycemia that will require several hours to bring back into control.

Table 37.1-6. Hazards associated with bicarbonate therapy

Hypernatremia and hyperosmolality

Hypokalemia leading to tissue refractoriness to insulin and other hormones

CNS acidosis: When H^+ ions are rapidly neutralized by bicarbonate, CO_2 enters the CNS, leading to acidosis and acute respiratory depression. Similar depressive effect on myocardium.

Diminished O_2 dissociation from hemoglobin (anti-Bohr effect), leading to tissue hypoxia

Decreased ionized calcium concentration

Deactivation of catecholamines

Precipitation of Ca salts in IV solutions.

Monitoring and Supportive Care

Until glucose-containing solutions are introduced into the regimen, it is essential to monitor the blood glucose and potassium every 1 to 2 hours. Other electrolytes and serum pH should be checked every 4 to 6 hours. Urine output must be followed hourly until the patient has made the transition to stage 4 of therapy.

Decreased GI motility is very common in DKA. Nasogastric suction should be considered in all patients with depressed sensorium, especially in the early stages of treatment. Later in the course of treatment, it is commonly observed that patients will begin to complain of thirst and hunger before there is evidence of sufficient GI motility to allow feeding.

Another frequently overlooked problem during the transition to oral alimentation is the presence of fecal impaction caused by dehydration. Glycerin suppositories or enemas are frequently useful in comforting the patient and facilitating feeding.

Bicarbonate

Probably no aspect of DKA therapy has engendered more controversy than the role of bicarbonate administration. Without being dogmatic, it has been our policy that there is no clear benefit to bicarbonate therapy, and we have discouraged its use.

Considerations that have been invoked in limiting bicarbonate administration, some theoretical and some quite real, are outlined in Table 37.1-6. Our policy has evolved from the lack of documented efficacy of bicarbonate[19] in treating DKA, coupled with the significant hypernatremia that is encountered as a consequence of its use. In acute cardiopulmonary resuscitation situations, bicarbonate administration has been associated with lethal increases in serum osmolality.[20] Largely, for those reasons, recommendations for bicarbonate administration have been greatly curtailed in the standards for cardiopulmonary resuscitation published by the American Medical Association.[21]

In situations of extreme acidosis **and** cardiovascular compromise, the infusion of 1 mEq/kg sodium bicarbonate (1 ml/kg of the 8.4% solution) over 10 to 30 minutes may be considered, but with close attention paid to response to pH, sodium, and potassium concentrations.

Complications

Acute Complications

Cerebral Edema

Cerebral edema is a complication of DKA that is seen in the very young, and predominantly in children experiencing their first episode of DKA. All but two of 69 patients were less than 20 years old, with 30% less than 5 years old.[22] Furthermore, 62% of occurrences were associated with new-onset diabetes. Initial reports of this complication stressed its rapid occurrence, unheralded by clinical indicators, generally in the first 12 hours of treatment.[23–26] Subsequently, reports began to surface of successful intervention to reverse cerebral edema in DKA.[27] Rosenbloom's comprehensive review of the published clinical experience (up to 1990) indicates that one third of cases showed clinical evidence of neurologic decompensation at least 1 hour before collapse.[22] The onset of deterioration ranged from 2.5 to 48.0 hours after the start of treatment, and roughly one half of the children who received early intervention were saved from severe or fatal brain damage. Warning signs of impending cerebral edema documented in that retrospective study are listed in Table 37.1-7.

Although all previously reported cases of cerebral edema have occurred during the course of treatment with fluids and insulin, and assumed by many to be "complications" of therapy, a 1991 report documented a case of fatal cerebral edema that developed precipitously in a 33-month-old child who was unknown to be diabetic, and in whom no therapy had been initiated.[28]

All children with DKA should be considered to be at risk for this complication. Previous studies had documented increased cerebrospinal fluid pressure in adults with DKA.[29] A prospective study in children found CT evidence of brain swelling in each of six patients studied in the first 12 hours after presentation to the hospital; follow-up scans showed resolution in all six. However, in no case were abnormal neurologic signs detected.

Earlier reviews of this subject implicated bicarbonate therapy, rapid rates of glucose decrease, the use of isotonic saline, high rates of fluid replacement, and hyponatremia as precipitating causes of cerebral edema. However, the large review of Rosenbloom failed to implicate any of these factors as predictive.[22]

The clinical lessons for physicians treating DKA are several: (1) All children with DKA are at risk for developing cerebral edema, with the very young and the newly diagnosed at greatest risk; (2) the period of risk precedes the institution of therapy and extends for 2 days after diagnosis; (3) neurologic signs and symptoms must be routinely monitored and recorded, because a substantial number of children exhibit warning signs of impending decompensation; and (4) mannitol and the means for intubation and hyperventilation must be available at the bedside. Although not rigorously substantiated by the aggregate published clinical experi-ence, it is our strong recommendation to avoid rates of fluid administration in excess of 3000 ml/m²/d, unless there is a clear clinical indication.

Vascular Thrombosis

The extreme dehydration seen in DKA can lead to a hypercoagula-ble state that results in thrombosis. Blood levels of clotting factors are elevated and there is evidence that platelets become activated in DKA. The consequences of this process are generally more severe in the elderly, in whom myocardial infarction and stroke are seen with much higher frequency than in children, and for whom prophylactic heparin therapy is sometimes advocated.

Infection

Infection should be considered less a complication of DKA than a precipitating event. Unless promptly identified in the initial evaluation, evidence of infection should be sought throughout the course of recovery. In newly diagnosed patients with altered sensorium or meningeal irritability, CNS infections should be entertained. In light of the probability that some degree of cerebral swelling is present in all patients in DKA, however, extraordinary precautions must be taken if a diagnostic lumbar puncture is contemplated.

Long-standing diabetes is known to predispose to certain infec-tions, especially of the skin, external auditory canal, and the urinary tract in females. Because of altered chemotaxic and phagocytic function in diabetes, opportunistic infections must always be con-sidered in known diabetic children who decompensate into DKA. Mucormycosis, which can cause devastating disease of the nasal passages and meninges, must be considered in those patients who persist in a comatose or obtunded state or who have eye findings after metabolic correction, and in those with facial pain or cell-ulitis.

Leukemoid Reaction

A leukemoid reaction is not unusual in DKA and should not be a cause for concern. However, glucose intolerance or frank DKA has been observed in children with leukemia, even before the institution of chemotherapy.

Rhabdomyolysis

Rhabdomyolysis with acute renal failure is a rare complication of DKA, although laboratory evidence of myoglobinemia with elevations of muscle creatine kinase may be found more commonly than expected.[30]

Adult Respiratory Distress Syndrome

This is another rare complication of DKA that is seen with greater frequency in younger adults, although it has been reported in children. Developments that are suggestive of this condition during the recovery from DKA include sudden dyspnea, profound hypo-xemia, decreased lung compliance, and diffuse pulmonary infil-trates.[31] Spontaneous pneumomediastinum has also been reported in DKA.

Later Sequelae

Blurred Vision

Blurred vision is a common complaint during the first several days of recovery from DKA and results from osmotic deformation of the lens. Patients respond well to reassurance that this condition is anticipated and transient. Persistence of blurred vision, however,

Table 37.1-7. Signs and symptoms of decompensating cerebral edema

Severe headache

Incontinence

Dramatic change in arousal or behavior

Pupillary changes

BP changes

Seizures

Bradycardia

Disturbed temperature regulation

Diabetes insipidus

Adapted from AL Rosenbloom. Intracerebral crises during treatment of diabetic ketoacidosis. *Diabetes Care* 13:22, 1990. With permission.

should prompt ophthalmologic examination for cataract formation.

Transient Ascites, Peripheral Edema, and Hepatomegaly

These will occur in rare instances up to several weeks after treatment for DKA and should be of little clinical consequence. Liver enlargement generally reflects insulin-induced accumulation of lipids and glycogen. The fluid retention that follows treatment of DKA is similar to the "refeeding edema" that develops during recovery from malnutrition and is associated with sodium retention. The mechanism remains unclear, but renal effects of insulin coupled with altered secretion or sensitivity to aldosterone have been implicated.

Hyperphagia

Hyperphagia is commonly observed in the first several weeks of new-onset diabetes, regardless of whether the initial presentation included DKA. While this response is transient and appears related to insulin therapy, the mechanism remains unclear.

The Transition to Ambulatory Status

Within 24 to 36 hours, the vast majority of children with DKA will be normalized with regard to blood sugar, electrolytes, and pH, although ketonemia may persist for an additional 24 to 48 hours. In addition, most will begin to complain of thirst and hunger relatively early in the course of treatment. As indicated earlier, the craving for food generally precedes adequate GI motility to handle food. Once adequate bowel sounds have been detected, however, the time has come for transition to oral food and subcutaneous insulin.

This transition is made most smoothly if, coincident with the first meal, the glucose-containing IV fluid infusion is discontinued (or locked), while the insulin is allowed to infuse at its previous rate for about 30 minutes after a subcutaneous dose of short-acting insulin. Subcutaneous insulin should be given 30 minutes before the first meal. This overlap should provide adequate insulin coverage between cessation of IV insulin and attainment of adequate blood levels from subcutaneous insulin. Management of blood sugar at this stage is very much frustrated by continued IV infusion of glucose. If IV fluids are required for medications, they should be free of glucose.

The insulin needs of children with new-onset diabetes will generally range between 0.5 and 1.0 U/kg day, although this will be determined by the competing and rapidly changing forces of caloric intake, activity, and state of insulin resistance. For the first 12 to 24 hours, we have found it most useful to administer only short-acting (regular) insulin every 4 to 6 hours in response to blood sugar. A summation of the total number of units of insulin required over the previous 24 hours will serve as a useful guide to the insulin requirements of the second day on subcutaneous insulin, in which short and intermediated insulins are introduced. In most children, day-to-day therapy of diabetes consists of two injections, one before breakfast and one before supper. The morning dose contains about two thirds of the total daily insulin units, and the evening dose contains one third. For each dose, the short- and intermediate-acting insulins are generally in a ratio of 1:2. For small children and those in whom a single daily injection is planned, 30% of the insulin is given as a short-acting preparation and 70% as intermediate-acting. For children with previously diagnosed diabetes who have had a relatively rapid recovery, it may be practical to simply resume their usual insulin regimen.

Home Management of Hyperglycemia with Ketosis

While the emergency room or intensive care physician typically sees the most sick of children with DKA, many patients with decompensating diabetes can be managed safely at home. Early diagnosis is critical, and it is our practice to instruct parents and children to test for urinary ketones at any time a blood sugar is detected over 240 mg/dl, especially when there are signs of infection. The presence of ketones is indicative of significant insulin resistance and suggests the need for increased insulin doses.

With the guidance of the experienced primary care pediatrician or pediatric endocrinologist, a therapeutic plan is established using subcutaneous insulin, oral hydration, and frequent blood glucose monitoring. For each successive 4-hour period, a fluid intake goal of approximately 500 ml/m^2 is established. Clear broths are preferable to flattened glucose-free sodas, because they contain significantly higher concentrations of sodium and other electrolytes. Only short-acting insulin is administered, and each succeeding 4-hour dose is adjusted by the blood sugar response to the previous one. *At any time that vomiting supervenes, fever develops, or there is a change in mental status, emergency room evaluation and care must be sought promptly.*

References

1. White K, Kolman ML, Wexler P. Unstable diabetes and unstable families: A psychosocial evaluation of diabetic children with recurrent ketoacidosis. *Pediatrics* 73:749, 1984.
2. Fishbein HA. Diabetic ketoacidosis, hyperosmolar nonketotic coma, lactic acidosis and hypoglycemia. In Harris MI, Hamman RF (eds): *Diabetes in America: Diabetes Data Compiled 1984.* US DHHS XII, 1985, Pp 1–22.
3. Goto Y, Sato S-I, Masuda M. Causes of death in 3151 diabetic autopsy cases. *Tohoku J Exp Med* 112:339, 1974.
4. Foster DW, McGarry JD. The metabolic derangements and treatment of diabetic ketoacidosis. *N Engl J Med* 309:159, 1983.
5. Van Putten JPM, Wieringa TJ, Krans HMJ. Low pH and ketoacids induce insulin receptor binding and postbinding alterations in cultured 3T3 adipocytes. *Diabetes* 34:744, 1985.
6. Miles JM et al. Effects of acute insulin deficiency on glucose and ketone body turnover in man: Evidence for the primacy of overproduction of glucose and ketone bodies in the genesis of diabetic ketoacidosis. *Diabetes* 29:926, 1980.
7. Reichard GA Jr. Acetone metabolism in humans during diabetic ketoacidosis. *Diabetes* 35:668, 1986.
8. Adrogue HJ et al. Plasma acid-base patterns in diabetic ketoacidosis. *N Engl J Med* 307:1603, 1982.
9. Prando R, Odetti P, Defarrari G. Metabolic alkalosis in diabetic ketosis: A case report. *Diabete Metab* 10:218, 1984.
10. Pitts RF. Tubular reabsorption. In (ed): *Physiology of the Kidney and Body Fluids* (2nd ed). Chicago: Year Book, 1971. Pp 71–93.
11. Knochel JP. The clinical status of hypophosphatemia. *N Engl J Med* 313:447, 1985.
12. Becker DJ et al. Phosphate replacement during treatment of diabetic ketosis: Effects on calcium and phosphorus homeostasis. *Am J Dis Child* 137:241, 1983.
13. Gordon EE, Kabadi UM. The hyperglycemic hyperosmolar syndrome. *Am J Med Sci* 271:252, 1976.
14. Khardori R, Soler NG. Hyperosmolar hyperglycemic nonketotic syndrome: Report of 22 cases and brief review. *Am J Med* 77:899, 1984.
15. Rimoin DL, Rotter JI. Genetic syndromes associated with diabetes mellitus and glucose intolerance. In Kobberling J, Tattersall R (eds): *Genetics of Diabetes Mellitus.* London: Academic, 1982. Pp 149–181.
16. Moles KW, McMullen JK. Insulin resistance and hypomagnesaemia: Case report. *Br Med J* 285:262, 1982.
17. West ML et al. Quantitative analysis of glucose loss during acute

therapy for hyperglycaemic, hyperosmolar syndrome. *Diabetes Care* 9:465, 1986.

18. Marshall SM, Alberti KGMM. Diabetic ketoacidosis. In Alberti KGMM, Krall LP (eds): *The Diabetic Annual.* New York: Elsevier, 1987. Pp 498–526.
19. Lever E, Jaspan JB. Sodium bicarbonate therapy in severe diabetic ketoacidosis. *Am J Med* 75:263, 1983.
20. Mattar JA et al. Cardiac arrest in the critically ill. *Am J Med* 56:162, 1974.
21. Standards for cardiopulmonary resuscitation and extracorporeal circulation. Part IV: Pediatric basic life support. *JAMA* 255:2954, 1986.
22. Rosenbloom AL. Intracerebral crises during treatment of diabetic ketoacidosis. *Diabetes Care* 13:22, 1990.
23. Winegrad AI, Kern EFO, Simmons DA. Cerebral edema in diabetic ketoacidosis. *N Engl J Med* 312:1184, 1985.
24. Young E, Bradley RF. Cerebral edema with irreversible coma in severe diabetic ketoacidosis. *N Engl J Med* 276:665, 1967.
25. Duck SC et al. Cerebral edema complicating therapy for diabetic ketoacidosis. *Diabetes* 25:111, 1976.
26. Rosenbloom AL et al. Cerebral edema complicating diabetic ketoacidosis in childhood. *J Pediatr* 96:357, 1980.
27. Franklin B, Liu J, Ginsberg-Fellner F. Cerebral edema and ophthalmoplegia reversed by mannitol in a new case of insulin-dependent diabetes mellitus. *Pediatrics* 69:87, 1982.
28. Glasgow AM. Devastating cerebral edema in diabetic ketoacidosis before therapy. *Diabetes Care* 14:77, 1991.
29. Clements RS et al. Increased cerebrospinal-fluid pressure during treatment of diabetic ketoacidosis. *Lancet* Sep 25:671, 1971.
30. Buckingham BA, Roe TF, Yoon JW. Rhabdomyolysis in diabetic ketoacidosis. *Am J Dis Child* 135:352, 1981.
31. Carroll P, Matz R. Adult respiratory distress syndrome complicating severe uncontrolled diabetes mellitus: Report of 9 cases and a review of the literature. *Diabetes Care* 5:574, 1982.
32. Porte D Jr, Halter JB. The endocrine pancreas and diabetes mellitus. In Williams RH (ed): *Textbook of Endocrinology.* Philadelphia: Saunders, 1981. P 811.

Marco Danon **37.2**   # Adrenocortical Insufficiency

Acute adrenal insufficiency or adrenal crises are rare in the pediatric intensive care unit (PICU) but may produce a confusing and stormy course. The clinical manifestations include those of both mineralocorticoid and glucocorticoid insufficiency.

Mineralocorticoid Deficiency

Mineralocorticoid deficiency causes hyponatremia, hypovolemia, and hyperkalemia by leading to inadequate resorption of sodium and water and decreased excretion of potassium.[1] This mineralocorticoid lack leads to a loss of extracellular fluid (ECF) volume, presenting clinically as weight loss, dehydration, hypotension, or shock. Abnormal neurologic manifestations, including quadriplegia, have been described in such cases. The shock (or preshock) state has some unusual features, in that it may be poorly responsive to volume and catecholamine infusions.

Glucocorticoid Deficiency

Glucocorticoid deficiency is responsible for a wide range of signs and symptoms. Children and adolescents have heightened sensory acuity or may be apathetic, confused, or psychotic. Young patients suffer from anorexia, nausea, vomiting, diarrhea (or constipation), and abdominal pain. A febrile state may be present. Disturbance of normal gluconeogenesis and impaired fat utilization may lead to hypoglycemia and, potentially, seizures. Eosinophilia or lymphocytosis may occur. Cardiac output is depressed, and there is a blunted or diminished response to catecholamines. Any additional stress further aggravates the adrenal crisis. Sudden death has been described in adrenal hypofunction.

Etiology of Adrenal Failure

The etiology of adrenal failure varies at different ages. The newborn infant may have adrenal hypoplasia or intrapartum adrenal hemorrhage, associated with a traumatic birth, as a cause for sudden cardiovascular collapse. A more subacute onset of signs is charac-

teristic of the congenital adrenal hyperplasia (CAH) syndrome, a varied group of disorders inherited as autosomal recessive traits. The salt-losing, severe, 21-hydroxylase deficiency variety usually manifests as an adrenal crisis.[2] These infants may present in the first weeks of life with progressive irritability or lethargy, poor feeding, and vomiting and progress to frank circulatory collapse. The dehydrated infant suspected of having pyloric stenosis may indeed be a patient with congenital adrenal hyperplasia. The infant with pyloric stenosis is not hyponatremic and usually demonstrates a metabolic alkalosis due to chloride loss in vomiting. In contrast, the infant with CAH will be hyponatremic and hyperkalemic as well as in metabolic acidosis. Pyloric stenosis is not a surgical emergency; rather, it is more a medical illness requiring rehydration and electrolyte supplementation. Therefore, an infant in shock or with severe dehydration should be appropriately rehydrated, with particular attention paid to correcting potentially life-threatening hyponatremia or hyperkalemia. Infants who present with extreme hyperkalemia but with no ECG change may do well with conservative fluid therapy. The "shocky" or "floppy" infant invokes a wide differential diagnosis, including infection, congenital heart disease, inborn errors of metabolism, and trauma. Although CAH may be rare, it must not be forgotten. Urgent volume expansion and Na+ and glucose support should be provided; this therapy alone can correct the hyperkalemia. No mineralocorticoid therapy is needed as long as the sodium supply is adequate. Emergency administration of "stress glucocorticoids" is unlikely to be detrimental to infants not suffering from CAH, but it may be useful to one who does have CAH.

Appearing at any age, the Waterhouse-Friderichsen syndrome represents acute hemorrhage into the adrenal glands as the result of a coagulopathy associated with sepsis (classically, meningococcemia).[3] It has been suggested that the association of petechiae with meningococcemia is a sign that the adrenals are at risk. The adrenal hemorrhage can thus result in cardiovascular collapse from acute adrenal failure. Reduced adrenocorticosteroid output may also be due to poor adrenal perfusion in shock, although more recent data demonstrate that the adrenal medulla is protected during shock and the adrenal cortex and medulla are protected during hypoxia.

Addison's disease is a clinical syndrome of chronic hypoadrenalism in the majority of cases.[4] However, 20% present in adrenal crises. Addison's disease is usually secondary to autoimmune adrenal atrophy in up to 80% of cases. Ten percent is secondary to tuberculosis and the remaining percentage to a large variety of causes[5–7] (Table 37.2-1). Certain drugs are also known to inhibit adrenal steroidogenesis, including trimethoprin-sulfamethoxazole, ketoconazole, and etomidate (Table 37.2-2). However, the most common cause of adrenal insufficiency in older children and young adults is the autoimmune adrenal failure either isolated or associated with the autoimmune polyglandular deficiency syndromes. These comprise two forms, one with chronic mucocutaneous candidiasis and a second with chronic autoimmune thyroiditis and insulin-dependent diabetes mellitus.

An important group of causes for adrenal hypofunction comprises those due to deficient ACTH production. The lack of ACTH secretion is usually due to either primary pituitary disease (tumor, infarction, surgery, irradiation) or hypothalamic-pituitary-adrenal (HPA) axis suppression by exogenously administered corticosteroids. In either case, the failure of ACTH production causes cortisol deficiency with all of its attendant features. It does not affect the aldosterone production, and volume depletion is therefore not as much of a problem for these patients as for those with primary

Table 37.2-1.   Etiology of adrenal insufficiency

Primary hypoadrenocorticism
  Congenital hypoplasia of adrenals
  Bilateral adrenal hemorrhage of the newborn
  Congenital deficiency of aldosterone biosynthesis
  Congenital adrenocortical unresponsiveness to ACTH
  Adrenal crisis of acute infection
  Chronic hypoadrenalism: Addison's disease
    Idiopathic
    Autoimmune destruction, types I and II polyglandular failure
    Peroxisomal disorders

Secondary hypoadrenocorticism due to insufficient CRH/ACTH secretion
  Hypopituitarism
  Cessation of glucocorticoid therapy
  Hypothalamic-pituitary tumors
  Anencephaly
  Infants born of steroid-treated mothers (10)

CRH, corticotropin-releasing hormone.

Table 37.2-2.   Drugs causing hypoadrenalism

Inhibition of steroidogenesis
  Ketoconazole
  Etomidate
  Metyrapone
  Mitotane (o,p = DDD)
  Aminoglutethimide

Enhancement of steroid metabolism
  Rifampin
  Phenytoin
  Phenobarbital
  Mitotane (o,p = DDD)
  l-thyroxine

adrenal insufficiency. The cortisol deficiency reduces the kidney's ability to excrete a water load, and so the patient with free fluid excess may become hyponatremic. However, hypovolemia may occur secondary to significant fluid losses or poor intake, because cortisol normally supplies about half of the mineralocorticoid effect responsible for fluid homeostasis. Besides the clinical manifestations of ECF volume problems, pituitary insufficiency can be distinguished from primary adrenal failure in that ACTH is not produced in the former, so the hyperpigmented skin of the Addisonian patient is not seen in the hypopituitary patient. Despite appropriate aldosterone secretion, the child with hypopituitarism may be in danger because of multiple hormone deficiencies (growth hormone [GH], thyroid-stimulating hormone [TSH], ACTH from the adenohypophysis, and vasopressin from the neurohypophysis).

Diagnostic Tests

The Cortrosyn stimulation test, in which cortisol is measured at baseline and 60 minutes after the intravenous (IV) administration of 250 μg of synthetic ACTH, is an excellent diagnostic test for patients suspected of having adrenal insufficiency.[8] Although this test directly measures only the functional integrity of the adrenal glands, it also provides an indirect assessment of hypothalamic and pituitary function, because the adrenal glands depend on endogenous ACTH for its trophic effect. When ACTH production is impaired by pituitary or hypothalamic disease, the adrenal gland loses the capacity to respond to exogenous stimulation. The normally responsive adrenal glands produce a peak cortisol level ranging from 15 to 25 μg/dl and double the baseline value. Differentiation between pituitary and hypothalamic hypofunction may be obtained by administering a bolus of corticotropin-releasing hormone (CRH) of 1 μg/kg intravenously, which produces a brisk (30-minute) rise in plasma ACTH levels in patients with an intact pituitary gland. This effect may be blunted by previous long-term, high-dose, glucocorticoid therapy, indicating a direct feedback mechanism of glucocorticoids on pituitary ACTH secretion. For the PICU patient, the ACTH and CRH stimulation tests provide safer testing of adrenal and pituitary ACTH reserve than do stimulation tests such as insulin-induced hypoglycemia or adrenal crisis secondary to metyrapone blockade of cortisone secretion.

Interpretation of a plasma cortisol level, however, is complicated by a number of factors. Hydrocortisone, methylprednisolone, and prednisone, but not dexamethasone, cross-react in the cortisol assay.[9] The 250-μg dose of ACTH is supraphysiologic, and children could probably be tested with 1 μg/kg, because a dose as low as 3 μg has produced a normal adrenal response in the adult.

Stress and Corticosteroid Needs

Any stress sufficient to bring the child with known adrenal hypofunction to the PICU requires additional corticosteroid coverage. Fever and nontrivial infections deserve a doubling of the maintenance cortisol dosage (to 24 mg/m²/d IV). Sepsis, major trauma, or surgery should be covered with cortisol at a minimum of 3 to 4 times the maintenance dose (36–50 mg/m²/d IV). It is always more dangerous, acutely, to administer inadequate corticosteroids than to administer an excess. When in doubt, the clinician could reasonably give 100 mg of cortisol (hydrocortisone) per square meter per day IV as a continuous infusion or in divided dosages. This coverage should begin the day before scheduled surgery, and the patient should be weaned from the medication over 3 days, beginning when the child's condition is stable.

Children admitted to the PICU with a history of steroid requirement for nonadrenal disease (e.g., asthma, systemic lupus) should have their pharmacologic doses of steroids continued. There is no evidence to suggest the need to increase their steroid doses if the dosage is already pharmacologic or supraphysiologic. Acute exacerbation of their systemic disease may occur as a result of the acute insult (trauma or surgery). To the contrary, patients on long-term steroids may be functionally immunosuppressed and require tapering of dosage of steroids to the "minimum stress dosage" of 3 to 4 times physiologic maintenance.

References

1. White PC. Disorders of aldosterone biosynthesis and action. *N Engl J Med* 331:250, 1994.

2. New MI. Steroid 21-hydroxylase deficiency (congenital adrenal hyperplasia). *Am J Med* 98:2S, 1995.

3. Rao RH. Bilateral massive adrenal hemorrhage. *Med Clin North Am* 79:107, 1995.

4. Werbel SS, Ober KP. Acute adrenal insufficiency. *Endocrinol Metab Clin North Am* 22:303, 1993.

5. Schwartz LJ et al. Endocrine function in children with human immunodeficiency virus infection. *Am J Dis Child* 145:330, 1991.

6. Oberfield SE et al. Steroid response to adrenocorticotropin stimulation in children with human immunodeficiency virus infection. *J Clin Endocrinol Metab* 70:578, 1990.

7. Sadeghy-Nejad A, Senior B. Adrenolmyeloneuropathy presenting as Addison's disease in childhood. *N Engl J Med* 322:13, 1990.

8. Danon M et al. Adrenal response to intravenous ACTH in premature infants. *Pediatr Res* 25:741, 1990.

9. Grinspoon SK, Biller BMK. Laboratory assessment of adrenal insufficiency. *J Clin Endocrinol Metab* 79:923, 1994.

10. Hadden DR. Adrenal disorders of pregnancy. *Endocrinol Metab Clin North Am* 24:139, 1995.

John T. Herrin   **37.3**   # Treatment of Life-Threatening Metabolic Derangements Secondary to Inherited Metabolic Disorders

Metabolic derangement secondary to inherited metabolic disorders may present to the intensive care unit (ICU) as (1) multiorgan dysfunction or failure, (2) acute neurologic dysfunctional syndromes (seizure, irritability, or coma), or (3) cardiac dysfunction in the setting of significant metabolic acidosis or electrolyte abnormalities. If uncontrolled, the impairment to cellular function and energy supply in these patients may lead to cardiac or respiratory failure, permanent neurologic damage, or death.[1,2]

A diagnosis of inherited metabolic disease should be excluded in any infant who becomes acutely ill after a period of normal behavior or feeding, with seizures and/or hypotonia or a peculiar odor, particularly if progression of these symptoms occurs in the absence of apparent sepsis, intracranial hemorrhage, or other congenital anomaly. Metabolic acidosis, hyperammonemia, and reducing substances in the urine are common accompaniments of these disorders. Other clinical situations that should raise a suspicion of inherited metabolic disease include a history of unexplained neonatal death in the family, neonatal signs and symptoms of jaundice, hepatomegaly, poor weight gain or weight loss, anorexia, "Kussmaul" respirations, dehydration, coarse facial features, or unusual odor to sweat or urine.

Admission criteria to an ICU include criteria similar to standard admission (i.e., circulatory insufficiency, hypoventilation, inability to maintain ventilation, intractable seizures, or coma), thus making differentiation difficult unless consideration is given to inherited metabolic disorders in all patients (Fig. 37.3-1)

Sepsis and cardiac failure remain the major causes for metabolic abnormalities seen in the ICU and dictate initial investigation and therapy. Severe electrolyte or acid-base abnormalities are usually obvious from routine standard chemical monitoring, and standard electrolyte patterns may suggest diagnosis in patients with hypernatremia, adrenal insufficiency, hypocalcemia, hypercalcemia, or hypomagnesemia. Drug intoxication is usually suggested in the history and should be considered in the patient with coma or rapid unexplained deterioration.

Differential Diagnosis

An inborn error of metabolism should be suspected if (1) rapid metabolic control is not attained with standard therapy to optimize respiratory and cardiac support, and (2) there are obvious mixed patterns of acid-base disturbance or markedly elevated anion gap acidosis.

Combinations of features may be approached, as outlined in Fig. 37.3-1 and Table 37.3-1. If the electrolyte profile is normal, but there are obvious discrepancies in osmolality and/or acid-base

Table 37.3-1. Common diagnostic patterns of metabolic disorders

Disorder	Urinary reducing substance	Hypoglycemia	Ketosis	Metabolic acidosis	Respiratory alkalosis	Hyperammonemia
Carbohydrate	+	+	+	+	−	−
Organic acidemia	−	−	−	+	−	−
Respiratory chain defect	−	+	+	+	−	−
Aminoacidopathy	−	+	+	+	+	+
Urea cycle abnormality	−	+	+	+	+	+

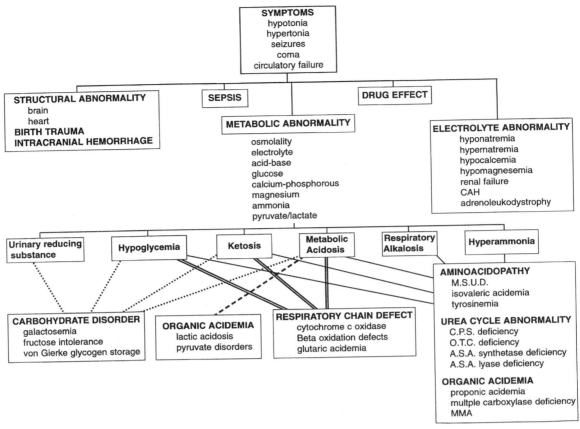

Figure 37.3-1. An approach to the differential diagnosis of metabolic disorders in the ICU. CAH, congenital adrenal hyperplasia; MSUD, maple syrup urine disease; MMA, methylmalonic acidemia.

metabolism, the initial chemical profile should be extended to include serum glucose, serum ketones, blood ammonia, toxic screens of "blood and urine," blood and urine levels of amino-acids, and/or organic acids.[2,3] An aliquot of urine should be sent for reducing substances (glucose, galactose, fructose), ketones, urinary amino-acid pattern, urinary pH, urinary sediment analysis, urinary protein excretion, and urinary organic acid profile. Rapid urine testing with ferric chloride or Phenistix should be made. A further aliquot of the urine should be frozen for later examination if necessary. It is important to use an aliquot of urine from the time of acute illness for gas chromatography and mass spectroscopy in patients with defects in fatty-acid metabolism.[4]

If hyperammonemia or severe acidosis is present, a liver function profile and serum pyruvate and lactate level should be performed early.[5] Specific testing is instituted on the basis of screening results guided by consultation with a metabolic specialist. Certain associated symptoms and features from a careful physical examination may assist in determining further testing (See Fig. 37.3-1 and Table 37.3-2).

Physical examination for jaundice, hepatosplenomegaly, body or skin odor, hair structure, formal ophthalmologic examination, and careful review of body or urinary odor is needed and a room-temperature urine sample is required because very cold urine may mask potential emission of characteristic odor. Further physical examination and chemical review of the child are necessary after feedings have commenced. Protein feeding will produce decompensation in urea cycle and hyperammonemic syndromes,[6,7] while

milk feeding may produce decompensation in galactosemia.[2] *E. coli* sepsis is a common presentation in galactosemia, may be an associated feature in other metabolic disorders,[2] and should be sought at baseline testing or for deterioration in infants suspected of inherited metabolic disease. Leukopenia may occur in organic acidemia, particularly propionic acidemia, which needs consideration in the differential diagnosis of "sepsis" if the urine is clear of reducing substances.

Acid-base data and anion gap measurement are important in the differentiation of (1) endogenous (organic) acidemia (e.g., propionic acidemia, methylmalonic acidemia, congenital lactic acidosis), (2) acidosis following bicarbonate losses in renal tubular acidosis or with diarrhea, and (3) exogenous acid ingestion (e.g., salicylate poisoning, methanol, or ethylene glycol ingestion).

Combinations of symptoms can assist in focusing further workup (see Table 37.3-1). A combination of hyperammonemia with metabolic acidosis occurs in organic acidemia, while hyperammonemia with respiratory alkalosis is the pattern seen in urea cycle abnormalities.[2,6] Vomiting, hypotonia, hypoglycemia, and acidosis may also be seen in mixed carboxylase deficiency and congenital lactic acidosis.[2,5,8]

Lactic acidosis may be a primary (inherited) condition or secondary to sepsis, critical cardiac failure, or "shock"-adrenal insufficiency from congenital adrenal hyperplasia or hemorrhage. The clinical pattern, culture, and electrolyte profile help in differentiation. Organic acid screening is indicated in patients who do not respond to restoration of circulation, glucose, and oxygenation.

Table 37.3-2. Clinical clues to presence of inherited metabolic disorders

Sympton	Disorder	Associated features	Testing
Seizures/coma	Galactosemia	HG, K, milk ingestion, *E. coli* spesis, U. Red, jaundice	Urine galactose (if milk feeding), Assay RBC galactose 1-phosphate, uridyl transferase
	Fructose intolerance	HG, K	Fructose tolerance test, hepatic fructose-1-phosphate aldolase
	MSUD	HG, K, MA, odor (urine)	DNP, paper chromatography, ion exchange chromatography
	Congenital lactic acidosis		
	Abnormalities of pyruvate;		Fibroblast enzymes
	pyruvate dehydrogenase;	HG, MA	
	pyruvate carboxylase deficiency	HG, MA	
	Gluconcogenesis;		Blood, fibroblast enzymes
	biotinidase;	HG, K, MA	
	fructose 1-6 diphosphate deficiency	HG, MA	
	glucose 6 phosphate deficiency;	HG	
	Mitochondrial myopathy		Muscle enzymes
	Leigh's syndrome	HG, MA	
	Electron transport deficiency	HG, MA	
	Organic acidemia	HG, HA, MA, K, leukopenia (propionic acid)	Gas chromatography–mass spectrometry
	Urea cycle disorder	HG, HA, R AIK	High-voltage electrophoresis, amino acid chromatography, citrulline, orotic acid
	Glycogen storage	HG, hepatomegaly	Serum enzymes, liver biopsy
	Biotinidase	HG, lactic acidosis, MA, K	Blood, fibroblast enzymes
	Pyridoxine-dependent seizures		EEG response to IV pyridoxine
Choreoathetosis	Glutaric acidemia	HG, MA, K	Fibroblast enzymes, gas chromatography
Pyramidal signs	Sulfite oxidase	Fanconi syndrome; lens dislocation	Urinary sulfate/thiosulfate
"Reye's syndrome–like" presentation	β oxidation defects	HG, MA, HA	Gas chromatography–mass spectroscopy on urine and blood
	MCACDD	HG, MA, HA	
	LCACDD	HG, MA, HA	Fibroblast and/or muscle emzymes
	Glutaric acidemia type 2	HG, MA, HA	Mitochondrial enzyme
	β ketothiolase deficiency	HG, MA, HA	
Jaundice/liver disease	Galactosemia	See above	
	Hereditary fructose intolerance	See above	
	Alpha-1 antitrypsin deficiency	Pulmonary fibrosis	Serum levels
	Glycogen storage	See above	
Unusual odor	MSUD	Maple syrup odor (urine)	See above
	Isvaleric acidemia	Sweaty feet odor (skin)	
	β-methyl-crotonyl glycinuria	Cat urine odor	
	Tyrosinemia	Rancid butter odor (skin/urine); Fanconi syndrome HG, MA, R AIK	
Cardiomyopathy	Mitochondrial myopathies		Gas chromatography–mass spectroscopy
	Carnitine deficiency		

HG, hypoglycemia; K, ketosis; MSUD, maple syrup urine disease; MA, metabolic acidosis; U. Red, reducing substance in urine; DNP, dinitrophenyl testing urine; R AIK, respiratory alkalosis; HA, hyperammonemia; MCACDD, medium-chain acyl CoA dehydrogenase deficiency; LCACDD, long-chain acyl CoA dehydrogenase deficiency.

Primary lactic acidosis[4,5,7] may result from abnormalities of pyruvate dehydrogenase, abnormalities of gluconeogenesis, or unknown (undefined) defects in Leigh's syndrome (subacute necrotizing encephalomyelopathy) and mitochondrial myopathies. A markedly elevated serum lactate with a lactate-pryuvate ratio of less than 50:1 is suggestive of primary lactic acidosis or disorders of pyruvate metabolism, while lower serum lactate levels and a ratio greater than 50:1 is seen in oxidative phosphorylation disorders, biotinidase deficiency, or as a secondary phenomen in

other metabolic disorders. In patients with abnormalities of pyruvate dehydrogenase, coarse dysmorphic features may be present.

Hypoglycemia, metabolic acidosis, and ketosis are common features of carbohydrate disorders and respiratory chain defects. Mixed acid-base disturbances with hyperammonemia are common in aminoacidopathies.

Disorders of mitochondrial fatty-acid oxidation[9,10] should be considered in patients who present with (1) muscle pain, myoglobinuria, muscle weakness, or cardiomyopathy; (2) coma, hypoglycemia, and acidosis, particularly with fasting; (3) developmental delay; or (4) a Reye's syndrome–like illness.[4,9,11] A urine specimen taken at the time of acute illness should be examined by gas chromatography–mass spectroscopy.[2,11,12] Plasma and tissue carnitine levels and studies of fatty-acid oxidation in cultured skin fibroblasts or muscle biopsy complete a profile in this group of disorders.[4,8,11,13] Carnitine is a required cofactor in the rate-controlling step in fatty-acid oxidation, and discussion as to its exact role in primary versus secondary deficiency awaits further definition.[4,9,10,13] Secondary carnitine deficit may occur in acyl CoA block,[14,15] other genetic defects such as cystinosis,[16] cytochrome-C oxidase deficiency[9,17] or homocystinuria, and may be acquired during valproate therapy, liver disease (cirrhosis), and hemodialysis.[4] Adaptation to fasting is limited in patients with carnitine deficiency and fatty-acid oxidation defects and may produce life-threatening illness[4] if fasting is prolonged.

Most patients with aminoacidopathy (e.g., maple syrup urine disease) have screening data available (identified during phenylketonuric screening), and this is a common reason for referral, often before significant symptoms develop. In patients with no obvious screening abnormality, such as hyperammonemia, hypoglycemia, unusual odor, or metabolic acidosis, diagnosis is more difficult and relies on clinical findings to suggest appropriate testing, for example, (1) peroxisomal diseases such as Zellweger's syndrome or neonatal adrenoleukodystrophy, (2) galactosemia, and (3) sulfite oxidase deficiency.[2]

Therapy

Therapy is based on acute symptoms. Initially standard symptomatic intervention is instituted: control of seizures, protection of the airway, adequate oxygenation, and circulatory support. Correction of acid-base and electrolyte abnormality is necessary, and nonspecific therapy should proceed in parallel with the continuing investigations. Early consultation with a metabolic specialist is appropriate to guide biochemical review.

Prospective diagnostic and therapeutic protocols have been designed[7] and, when instituted at birth, produce a more favorable prognosis for survival and neurologic outcome.[17,18] Protocoled diagnostic studies and therapy commence at birth in patients identified prenatally at high risk for urea cycle abnormalities. Although such a medical regime is complex and requires preparation for transfer of the infant at birth, this option should be offered along with genetic counseling to families with potential life-threatening inherited errors of metabolism, particularly early urea cycle enzyme abnormalities.[17]

The scheme outlined in Fig. 37.3-1 uses simple, readily available screening tests to differentiate between diagnostic groups of inherited abnormalities, so that nonspecific therapeutic interventions can be initiated while more definitive testing proceeds. This scheme uses a database of ammonia levels, glucose level, and acid-base data as the initial screen. Review of symptoms and careful physical examination identifies features (see Table 37.3-2) that can guide further testing. A simplified general scheme for initial therapy is outlined in Table 37.3-3.

Hyperammonemia is often profound, and permanent neurologic damage is possible. Neurologic recovery is proportional to the duration of hyperammonemia, thus a scheme to allow rapid institution of therapy is necessary.[18] Table 37.3-4 outlines common causes of hyperammonemia in childhood.[1,2] Urea cycle abnormalities, organic acidemia, and transient hyperammonemia of the newborn produce elevation of ammonia levels to greater than 500

Table 37.3-3. Therapeutic considerations: A simplified approach to treatment

Acute symptomatic therapy for circulatory failure hypoventilation, intractable seizures, or coma

Consider inherited abnormalities in initial evaluation based on symptoms

Extend laboratory profile (Fig. 37.3-1)

Institute nonspecific supportive therapy
  Calories
  Glucose
  Protein restriction
  Lipid restriction
  Provision of cofactors
  Correction of acidosis
  Treatment of hyperammonemia
  Carnitine supplementation
  Consideration of dialysis (peritoneal or hemodialysis dialysis or peritoneal perfusion)

Collect specimens for diagnosis

Specific therapy
  Prospective
  Based on enzyme/chemical analysis

Consider transplantation liver, leukocytes to provide enzyme replacement

Table 37.3-4. Causes of hyperammonemia in children

Urea cycle abnormalities

Organic acidemia

Transient hyperammonemia of newborn

Acyl-CoA dehydrogenase deficiency

Carnitine deficiency

Liver failure

Portocaval shunt procedures

Table 37.3-5. Treatment of hyperammonemia

Provide glucose for calories—minimum 40 kcal/kg/24 hr (7–10 mg/kg/min)

Protein-free diet (Nil Prote [R])

Activation alternative pathways for waste nitrogen excretion
  Sodium benzoate 250 mg/kg in 30 ml/kg D10W priming over 1–2 hr, 500 mg/kg/24 hr in D10W
  Sodium phenylactate 250 mg/kg in 30 mg/kg D10W priming over 1–2 hr, 500 mg/kg/24 hr in D10W
  Reduce sodium benzoate and sodium phenylactate to 250 mg/kg/24 hr as serum ammonia falls

Arginine 10% 210 mg/kg prime over 1hr; 210 mg/kg/24 hr sustaining (in arginosuccinase deficiency 840 mg/kg rather than 210 mg/kg)

Dialysis if not responsive to initial therapy or marked elevation ammonia level

Carnitine supplementation in patients reveiving sodium benzoate therapy or with low serum carnitine levels

µg/dl. Other causes of hyperammonemia usually produce lower serum levels of ammonia (200–500 µg/dl). Treatment should be initiated using a scheme similar to that outlined by Brusilow et al.[6] (Table 37.3-5). Dialysis should be instituted concurrently if levels of plasma ammonia are greater than 500 μg/dl or response to therapy is not attained within 24 hours of therapy aimed at activating alternative pathways of excretion of waste nitrogen.[6,19] Carnitine levels should be monitored and, if necessary, carnitine supplementation provided in patients treated with sodium benzoate.[20]

Nonspecific Therapy

Calories are provided as glucose (7–10 mg/kg/min) and lipid (0.25–0.5 gm/kg/24 hr), initially with a protein-free intake if there is a suggestion of aminoacidopathy or urea cycle enzyme deficiency.[1,2,3] Protein restriction is also necessary in the organic acidopathies, particularly those in which there is an association of hyperammonemia. Later, when control of ammonia levels is present, protein intake may be slowly titrated to tolerance.[1,2,3]

Lipid restriction may be necessary in patients with beta-oxidation defects or respiratory chain enzyme defects.[2] Mitochondrial fatty-acid oxidation defects and carnitine deficiency (primary or secondary) in patients who present with (1) muscle pain, cardiomyopathy, rhabdomyolysis, or chronic weakness; and (2) coma and hypoglycemia require that lipid intake be limited. If such symptoms occur with introduction of lipid supplements, a trial of lipid restriction, riboflavin, carnitine, or coenzyme Q supplementation is appropriate.[9,10]

Coenzyme supplements may be given empirically after metabolic consultation if rapid clinical deterioration is occurring. Such administration will not affect other disease processes adversely. IV administration of 100 mg thiamine, 100 μg vitamin B12, and 2 mg qid biotin orally is a reasonable initial empiric cover. Riboflavin 100 mg, lipoic acid, carnitine 50 to 100mg/kg orally, or 20 mg/kg IV, increasing to 40 to 60 mg/kg IV until oral administration is possible and coenzyme Q10 (ubiquinone) 25 mg may be considered under special circumstances.[2,3]

In patients with severe metabolic derangements, coma, or seizures, dialysis may be helpful in (1) gaining control of hyperammonemia and markedly increased aminoacid levels (leucine, isoleucine, tyrosine), or (2) reducing lactate levels, and (3) allowing correction of acidosis while maintaining electrolyte (particularly sodium balance) and fluid volume control. Hemodialysis requires specialized care to balance osmolar changes, which occur with removal of these relatively small molecular-weight solutes (ammonia, leucine, propionic acid, lactic acid). Peritoneal dialysis will remove solute at a lower rate and, if rapid generation of ammonia organic acid or amino acid is present, may lack the efficiency to produce control. Efficiency can be increased by using a peritoneal dialysis catheter and a constant flow of dialysate in and out. Peritoneal perfusion, peritoneal dialysis, or continuous veno-venous hemodialysis or hemofiltration (CVVH or CVVHD) may be necessary to stabilize the patient between hemodialysis treatments initially and should be continued until dietary and pharmacologic support produces long-term control.

Dialysis can be used in patients with (1) severe hyperammonemia (urea cycle enzyme deficits [e.g., carbamyl phosphate synthetase deficiency, ornithine transcarbamylase deficiency]); (2) organic acidemia (e.g., propionicacidemia, severe lactic acidosis, methylmalonic acidemia); or (3) amino acid disorders, pratically maple syrup urine disease.

Exchange transfusion, although a relatively inefficient method of control, may be helpful in reducing plasma levels of ammonia or branch-chain amino acids in a single treatment before or during transfer to a definitive treatment center, where more efficient techniques of dialysis can be instituted.

Carnitine supplementation is used in patients with significant decrease of the total carnitine levels below (25 nmol/ml). IV carnitine 20-mg/kg has been used when oral supplementation is not possible. The dose is then increased over 4 to 6 days to 40 to 60 mg/kg IV until oral administration is possible.

An approximation of the definitive enzyme system deficiency can be made by extending biochemical studies in many cases.[1,2,3,5] Full definition, however, may require biopsy and enzyme analysis of skin (fibroblast), liver, and/or muscle to provide evidence of a definitive enzyme defect and allow planning for rational therapy.

Therapy with biotin is necessary in all potential biotin-deficient syndromes, inherited conditions such as isolated apocarboxylase deficiency, holocarboxylase synthetase deficiency, or biotinidase[21] deficiency, or in severe acquired biotin deficiency. Twelve to 20 mg/d biotin (orally) is usually effective in patients with multiple carboxylase deficiency. Within 24 to 48 hours, organic aciduria can be reversed, but neurologic response and clearing of dermatologic manifestations may take 7 to 10 days. In patients with isolated 3-methyl crotonyl-CA carboxylase deficiency, therapy with biotin is not effective, and a leucine-restricted diet is necessary as therapy.[22]

Pharmacologic-dose vitamin therapy, dietary manipulation, and bicarbonate administration to control metabolic acidosis still remain the major foci of therapy. Definitive enzyme replacement therapy may be available by transplantation of leukocyte or liver. Liver transplantation may replace urea cycle enzyme deficiencies and may be considered for other metabolic abnormalities (e.g., tyrosinemia and alpha-1-antitrypsin deficiency) as definitive therapy.

Despite optimal care, a number of children with inherited metabolic disorders will continue to show ongoing metabolic deterioration, leading to death. Autopsy in these cases most often fails to show any specific findings. Because these conditions have a genetic basis, it is important to the family to have an accurate metabolic diagnosis to allow appropriate genetic counseling. The importance of such a diagnosis should be discussed with the family, and appropriate diagnostic tissue samples should be obtained during deterioration or as soon as possible after death.[23] Table 37.3-6 outlines tissue samples of importance. To optimize diagnostic results, proper handling (temperature, volume, culture media or special anticoagulant, packing and delivery arrangements) should be discussed with a metabolic consultant and the potential reference laboratory where the tests will be performed.

Table 37.3-6. Tissue samples for metabolic diagnosis

Plasma frozen
  Initial
  Late

Leukocytes or other tissue for DNA enzyme

Enzyme and molecular diagnosis
  Skin (fibroblast)
  Liver (frozen, liquid nitrogen)
  Muscle (frozen, liquid nitrogen)

Urine
  Aliquot of initial sample frozen (pretreatment)
  Aliquot after feeding introduced

Cerebrospinal fluid for chemistry

Cord blood

Blood and urine at 12, 24, and 48 hrs for electrophoresis, chromatography, and mass spectrometry

References

1. Batshaw M, Thomas H, Brusilow S. New approaches to diagnosis and treatment of inborn errors of urea synthesis. *Pediatrics* 68:290–297, 1981.
2. Goodman SI. Inherited metabolic disease in the newborn, approach to diagnosis and treatment. *Adv Pediatr* 33:197–223, 1986.
3. Rosenberg L. Diagnosis and management of inherited aminacidopathies in the newborn and unborn. *Clin Endocrinol Metab* 3:145, 1974.
4. Stanley CA. New genetic defects in mitochondrial fatty acid oxidation and carnitine deficiency. *Adv Pediatr* 34:59–88, 1987.
5. Robinson B. Inborn errors of metabolism leading to lactic acidemia. *Trends Biochem Sci* 7:151, 1982.
6. Brusilow SW et al. Treatment of episodic hyperammonemia in children with inborn errors of urea synthesis. *N Engl J Med* 310:1630–1634, 1984.
7. Maestri NE et al. Prospective treatment of urea cycle disorders. *J Pediatr* 119:923–928, 1991.
8. Robinson BH, Sherwood WG. Lactic acidemia. *J Inherited Metab Dis* (Suppl 1):69, 1984.
9. DeVivo DC, DiMauro S, Rapin I. Mitochondrial disorders. In Rudolph A (ed): *Pediatrics* (18th ed). Norwalk, CT/Los Altos, CA:Appleton & Lange, 1987. Pp 1736–1737.
10. DiMauro S, Hays AP. Myopathies. In Rudolph A (ed): *Pediatrics* (18th ed). Norwalk, Ct/Los Altos, Ca: Appleton & Lange, 1987. Pp 1674–1675.
11. Stanley CA, Coates PM. Inherited defect of fatty acid oxidation which resembles Reye's syndrome: IV. Reye's syndrome. *J Natl Reye's Syndrome Found* 5:190–200, 1985.
12. Goodman SI. An introduction to gas chromatography-mass spectometry and the inherited organic acidemias. *Am J Hum Genet* 32:781, 1980.
13. Coates PM et al. Systemic carnitine deficiency simulating Reye syndrome (letter). *J Pediatr* 105:679, 1984.
14. Roe CR et al. Diagnostic and therapeutic implications of medium-chain acylcarnitines in the medium-chain acyl-CoA dehydrogenase deficiency. *Pediatr Res* 19:459–466, 1985.
15. Stanley CA et al. Medium-chain acyl-CoA dehydrogenase deficiency in children with non-ketotic hypoglycemia and low carnitine levels. *Pediatr Res* 17:877–884, 1983.
16. Bernardini I et al. Plasma and muscle free carnitine deficiency due to renal Fanconi syndrome. *J Clin Invest* 75:1124–1130, 1985.
17. Muller-Hocker J et al. Fatal lipid storage myopathy with deficiency of cytochrome-C oxidase and carnitine: A contribution to the combined cytochemical-fine structural identification of cytochrome-C oxidase in long term frozen muscle. *Virchows Arch [A]* 399:11–23, 1983.
18. Msall M et al. Neurologic outcome in children with inborn errors of urea sythesis. *N Engl J Med* 310:1500, 1984.
19. Rutledge SL et al. Neonatal hemodialysis: Effective therapy for the encephalopathy of inborn errors of metabolism. *J Pediatr* 116:125–128, 1990.
20. Sakuma T. Alteration of urinary carnitine profile induced by benzoate administration. *Arch Dis Child* 66:873–875, 1991.
21. Wolf B et al. Biotinidase deficiency: Initial clinical features and rapid diagnosis. *Ann Neurol* 18:614–617, 1985.
22. Ring E, Zobel G. Hemofiltration in acute metabolic crisis. *Wien Klin Wochenshr* 104:674, 1992.
23. Kronick JB et al. A perimortem protocol for suspected genetic disease. *Pediatrics* 71:960–963, 1983.

VII ◆ Infectious Diseases

Leticia Castillo

38.1 Septic Shock

Septic shock is a complex syndrome that has become an increasingly important cause of morbidity and mortality in the intensive care unit (ICU).[1] Sepsis is the host's inflammatory response to infection, and it is a continuous progression from a localized infection without systemic manifestations (e.g., otitis media or gastroenteritis) to an infection with systemic manifestations (e.g., fever, tachycardia, leukocytosis, chills, and bacteremia) to an infection with systemic manifestations and hemodynamic instability (e.g., hypotension, poor perfusion, and cardiorespiratory arrest). Septic shock is the final stage of the dynamic process of sepsis.[2] To identify a population of patients at risk for developing sepsis earlier, the term *clinical sepsis syndrome* was first used by Bone in 1987.[3] Sixty-four percent of 191 patients identified with clinical sepsis syndrome subsequently developed shock, while only 45% of the patients had positive blood culture. Clinical sepsis syndrome uses clinical criteria to diagnose sepsis, including a high suspicion of infection (confirmation by blood culture is not required), fever, tachypnea, tachycardia, and impaired organ system function as indicated by oliguria, abnormal mentation, hypoxemia, or increased plasma lactate. When we apply this concept to the pediatric population, a large proportion of our patients, many with uncomplicated viral infections, may meet the sepsis syndrome criteria without necessarily progressing toward septic shock. This definition is significant, however, because it is an effective warning to carefully assess, treat, and follow patients at risk for developing septic shock. The mortality for those patients who will progress to shock is 60% to 90%, despite current antibiotic therapy and sophisticated techniques of life-support.[4,5] Under these circumstances, the early diagnosis and aggressive management of septic patients is of utmost importance in the outcome of septic shock.[5] Table 38.1-1 shows the characteristics of sepsis syndrome in children. The concept of systemic inflammatory response syndrome (SIRS) has been introduced to differentiate those patients that present with a systemic inflammatory response of unknown etiology (e.g., trauma, hypoxemic ischemic events, etc.), but in this case, sepsis may or may not be responsible.[6]

Pathogenesis

Traditionally, it had been considered that septic shock occurs as the result of released lipopolysaccharide (LPS) by gram-negative bacteria; however, exotoxin from gram-positive bacteria and fungal and viral products is able to produce the same clinical picture.[7,8] It is now known that these bacterial, viral, and fungal products possess no profound toxicity of their own; instead, they elicit the production of highly toxic endogenous mediators by the host.[9–11] LPS, for instance, activates leukocytes, macrophages, endothelial cells, and possibly other cells. The activated leukocytes release peptides known as cytokines. These cytokines, particularly tumor necrosis factor (TNF)[2] and interleukin-1 (IL-1), are responsible for the physiologic changes observed in septic shock.[12,13] TNF and IL-1 elicit the release of nitric oxide (NO), an oxygen radical product of arginine metabolism synthesized by macrophages, neutrophils, CNS cells, endothelial cells, and probably others. NO is a signal transducer produced by a low-output constitutive pathway and by a high-output inducible pathway. Both pathways are mediated by the action of the nitric oxide synthase (NOS). NO has cytotoxic activity and is a potent endogenous vasodilator responsible for the hypotension observed in septic shock.[14,15] TNF induces fever, lactic acidosis, and hypotension and suppresses lipoprotein lipase, resulting in hypertriglyceridemia. If TNF is administered at sublethal doses, it induces fever, anorexia, cachexia, anemia, and leukocytosis.[12,16] IL-1 also has widespread systemic effects.[17,18] At the CNS level, it induces lethargy, release of ACTH, and neuropeptides and decreases appetite. IL-1 also has profound metabolic effects as it increases the synthesis of acute-phase reactant proteins such as C-reactive protein and fibrinogen and decreases the synthesis of structural proteins, mainly albumin and transferrin. A fraction of IL-1, known as proteinolysis-inducing factor, is responsible for the protein breakdown observed in septic patients, also known as septic autocannibalism. IL-1 elicits the release of glucagon, catecholamines, and other counterregulating hormones, resulting in hyperglycemia.[18] The vascular effects of IL-1 are of great significance in septic shock because it increases leukocyte adherence, degranulation, and release of proteases and free radicals. These elements will cause lipid peroxidation of the phospholipid layer in the cellular membranes, resulting in widespread tissue and organ injury.[19] During this process, both pathways of arachidonic acid metabolism become activated. The lipooxygenase pathway will result in the production of leukotrienes, which induce enhanced capillary permeability, vasoconstriction, bronchoconstriction, and leukocyte aggregation. Activation of the cyclooxygenase pathway leads to production of prostaglandin (PG) and thromboxane. Some PGs, such as PGE and PGI or prostacyclin, are synthesized primarily by vascular endothelium and induce vasodilation and inhibit platelet aggregation. Thromboxane is mainly produced by platelets and results in vasoconstriction and platelet aggregation.[20] The main pathophysiologic events of septic shock are summarized in Fig. 38.1-1.

There are many other mediators of the inflammatory process of sepsis, such as platelet activating factor, fibronectin, complement, proteases, and endogenous opioids (Table 38.1-2). It is likely that some others have not been discovered. Hence, the pathogenesis

Table 38.1-1. Clinical sepsis syndrome in children*

Fever	Bounding pulses
Irritability	Oliguria
Tachycardia	Capillary refill > 3 sec
Flushed, warm skin	

*The most frequent clinical manifestations of sepsis syndrome in children are listed.

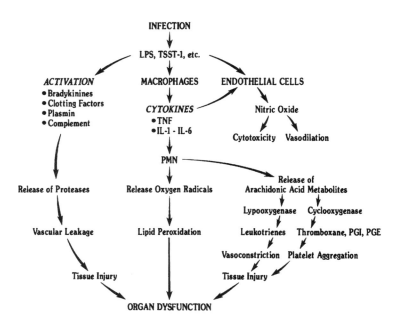

Table 38.1-2. Mediators of septic shock

Cytokines
   Tumor necrosis factor
   Interleukins

Eicosanoids
   Leukotrienes
   Thromboxane A_2
   Prostaglandins

Others
   Platelet-activating factor
   Nitric oxide
   Complement fragments C_{3a}, C_{5a}
   Toxic oxygen radicals
   Proteases
   Fibrin
   Thrombin
   Bradykinin
   Plasminogen activator inhibitors
   Beta-endorphins
   Myocardial depressant factor

of sepsis is multifactorial, and once the inflammatory cascade is activated, no single "magic bullet" will prevent it from progressing; thus, a wide comprehensive approach is necessary if we are to reduce the morbidity and mortality of septic shock.

Clinical Manifestations

The clinical manifestations of sepsis are widespread, involving multiple organs and systems.

Central Nervous System

At the CNS level, sepsis may induce varying mental changes, coma, seizures, and focal neurologic alterations. Septic encephalopathy may be caused by toxic and metabolic changes or diffuse impairment of cerebral perfusion.[21] A severe peripheral neuropathy characterized by axonal degeneration of motor and sensory nerves is found in 50% of septic patients. This peripheral neuropathy may contribute to the failure in successfully weaning a patient from the ventilator.[22]

Cardiovascular

Sepsis may manifest itself with hemodynamic instability. Children, however, have remarkable compensatory mechanisms, and hypotension is often a late sign. Diagnosis of septic shock in children should not be based on hypotension, but on early hemodynamic changes such as persistent tachycardia; flushed, warm skin; and bounding pulses and wide-pulse pressure. This has been known as the "early" hyperdynamic or "warm" phase of septic shock. Poor capillary refill, metabolic acidosis, and evidence of organ hypoperfusion (e.g., oliguria or lethargy) supervene later. Initially, cardiac output may be increased severalfold, and the systemic vascular resistance may be low. If hypovolemia secondary to the peripheral maldistribution of the circulating volume is not aggressively corrected, the patient will progress toward the late, hypodynamic ("cold") phase of septic shock, characterized by hypotension and cold, clammy skin. In this situation, the cardiac output is decreased and the systemic vascular resistance is high.

Hypotension is the result of multifactorial events affecting preload (circulating volume), afterload (systemic resistances), and myocardial contractility.[23] Some mediators (e.g., nitric oxide, leukotrienes, activated complement, prostacyclin, etc.) play a role in the vasodilation of sepsis.[24] Down regulation of alpha-adrenergic receptors, resulting in a decreased capacity for vasoconstriction, also contributes. In addition, despite the initial increase in cardiac output, there is myocardial depression manifested by decreased left ventricular ejection fraction.[25] Myocardial dysfunction is secondary to down-regulation of beta-receptors. Some mediators, such as TNF or NO, may possibly be responsible for the depressed cardiac function.

A controversial hemodynamic event in septic shock is the development of flow-dependent oxygen consumption ($\dot{V}O_2$).[26–29] Oxygen delivery (DO_2) is the result of cardiac output (CO) and the arterial oxygen content (CaO_2) (i.e., $DO_2 = CO \times CaO_2$). Cardiac output is dependent on preload, afterload, and contractility. Arterial oxygen content is the sum of the oxygen chemically bound to hemoglobin and the oxygen physically dissolved in the plasma:

$$CaO_2 = Hb \times 1.34 \times SaO_2 + PaO_2 \times 0.003$$

where 1.34 is the volume of oxygen that binds to 1 g of hemoglobin when it is fully saturated, 0.003 is the solubility coefficient of oxygen in human plasma, Hb is hemoglobin concentration, and SaO_2 is the percentage of arterial oxygen saturation. In healthy individuals, the oxygen uptake is independent of oxygen supply. As shown in Fig. 38.1-2, if DO_2 is acutely reduced, oxygen extraction ratio (VO_2/DO_2) increases, so that VO_2 (oxygen consumption) may be maintained. It is only when DO_2 values fall below a critical point (8 ml/kg/min) that the oxygen extraction capabilities are overwhelmed and VO_2 falls; at this point, lactic acidosis may develop.

During sepsis, the ability of tissues to extract oxygen is impaired by microvascular and cellular abnormalities, and oxygen delivery is decreased due to myocardial depressant factors and/or abnormal CaO_2 (hypoxemia, anemia, etc.).[27] DO_2 may need to be increased to achieve adequate oxygen uptake by the tissues. This is known as an abnormal dependency of oxygen consumption on oxygen delivery. Fig. 38.1-3 shows the relationship between VO_2 and DO_2 under physiologic conditions and during septic shock. Recently, however, the concept of pathologic VO_2/DO_2 dependency has been challenged.[30] Mathematical coupling measured errors in shared variables has been advocated as responsible for dependency of VO_2 or DO_2, which results in a false correlation between VO_2 (as determined by the Fick principle) and DO_2.[31]

Respiratory

Initially, hyperventilation and respiratory alkalosis are present during the early stages of septic shock; later, hypoxemia may develop as

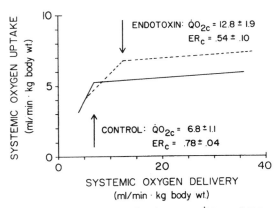

Figure 38.1-3. The relationship between VO_2 and DO_2 under physiologic conditions and during septic shock.

a result of pulmonary shunting. Adult respiratory distress syndrome (ARDS) may be a severe complication of septic shock. Persistent hypoxemia, low-pressure pulmonary edema, and pulmonary hypertension are important features of ARDS.[26,32]

Gastrointestinal

There may be some degree of liver dysfunction induced by sepsis. Abnormal plasma amino acid patterns characterized by an increase in aromatic amino acids, such as phenylalanine and tyrosine, and decreased branched-chain amino acids are seen in later stages of septic shock.[33] Redistribution of blood flow may result in GI ischemia with translocation of bacteria and/or endotoxin that may set the stage for chronic inflammation and multiorgan failure.[34] Stress ulcers occasionally complicate the clinical course of critically ill septic children. Hypoperfusion and oxygen radical injury are major factors in the development of stress ulcers and GI bleeding under these conditions.[35]

Metabolic

Energy expenditure is greatly increased in septic shock. Oxygen consumption may be high, normal, or low, depending on the hemodynamic state. Metabolic acidosis due to excessive production of lactic acid carries a poor prognosis.

Gluconeogenesis is also increased and does not resolve with exogenous administration of glucose. There is some degree of insulin resistance and increased proteolysis that supplies amino acids for gluconeogenesis, with these events leading to glucose intolerance.[36] Hyperglycemia frequently is an early manifestation of sepsis in infants; hypoglycemia may present in later states of septic shock if metabolic support is not provided. Hypertryglyceridemia is often present as a result of increased lipolysis.

Septic patients exhibit massive weight loss due to increased protein breakdown, which supplies amino acid substrate for gluconeogenesis. Nitrogen balance under these circumstances is negative.[36]

Disseminated Intravascular Coagulation

Disseminated intravascular coagulation (DIC) is a common manifestation of sepsis and is characterized by coexistent hemorrhage and microvascular thrombosis. Clinically, it may present with per-

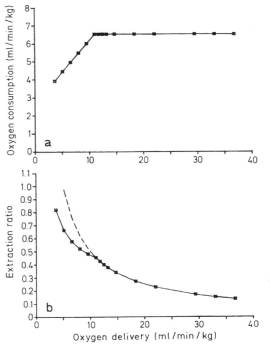

Figure 38.1-2. As seen in this figure, if DO_2 is acutely reduced, oxygen extraction ratio increases so that VO_2 may be maintained.

sistent GI bleeding, hematuria, and bleeding at previous puncture sites and membrane mucosae. If DIC is severe, areas of necrosis may occur. A prolonged prothrombin and partial thromboplastin time (PT, PTT), thrombocytopenia, increased fibrin degradation products, and microangiopathic hemolytic anemia are usually found in DIC.[37]

Renal

Sepsis often manifests with hypoperfusion and oliguria, and if the hypovolemic state is not corrected promptly, morphologic and functional disturbances of the kidneys will occur. Prerenal disease due to hypovolemia and poor perfusion is the most frequent cause of the renal dysfunction. Activation of mediators and local inflammatory response in the kidneys may lead to tubular necrosis. Drug toxicity, such as that caused by aminoglycoside antibiotics, may also contribute to tubulointerstitial disease. Decreased urine output to less than 1 ml/kg/hr in children or 30 ml/hr in adolescents should alert the clinician to potential problems. Rising BUN and creatinine, metabolic acidosis, and hyperkalemia may appear later. Fractional excretion of sodium is less than 1% during prerenal states, due to appropriate sodium retention. In the presence of tubular damage, the kidneys fail to retain sodium, and high urinary sodium excretion results in a fractional excretion greater than 1%.[38]

Treatment

In view of the multiple pathophysiologic events in septic shock, its treatment must be focused at every organ system, and therefore a broad approach is necessary. In any critically ill patient, basic principles of resuscitation (airway, breathing, and circulation) are vital in the initial management of these patients. If the patient is diagnosed early and successfully fluid-resuscitated, endotracheal intubation and mechanical ventilation may not be necessary. In contrast, if the patient appears to have an increased work of breathing, regardless of normal arterial blood gases, and presents with hemodynamic instability (e.g., persistent tachycardia, poor capillary refill, mottled skin or hypotension), endotracheal intubation should be performed. The use of mechanical ventilation, sedation, and muscle relaxation will avoid "wasting" cardiac output and oxygen delivery to respiratory muscles and prevent respiratory arrest.[39]

Endotracheal intubation, if elective, should always be performed under controlled conditions. The patient should receive preoxygenation, sedation, and, if necessary, muscle relaxation. Some sedatives, such as morphine or its derivatives, may aggravate hypotension. Careful consideration to the side effects of any drugs should always be given. Benzodiazepines (e.g., diazepam 0.2 mg/kg, or midazolam 0.1 mg/kg) or synthetic narcotics such as fentanyl 1 to 3 μg/kg IV will provide adequate sedation with less risk of hemodynamic instability.

Once the patient is intubated and muscle-relaxed, optimal ventilation should be achieved by using the necessary tidal volume to appropriately expand the chest. High positive end-expiratory pressure (PEEP) may be necessary, because of pulmonary edema, to achieve adequate arterial oxygenation. Concomitant to the management of airway and ventilation is the support of the circulation. Immediate venous access via peripheral or central lines should be gained for fluid resuscitation. If venous access becomes a problem due to hypotension, intraosseous access should be initiated. In addition to airway, breathing, and circulation, antibiotic treatment is of paramount importance in the treatment of septic shock. Blood cultures should be obtained quickly and antibiotic coverage started according to the clinical situation. After the initial stabilization has been completed, individual organ systems should be evaluated.

Central Nervous System

Critically ill patients should be adequately sedated. Anxiety or pain leads to cathecholamine release and increased metabolic demands under conditions of already precarious oxygen delivery. Continuous IV infusion of sedatives achieves better sedation than sporadic IV boluses. Morphine 0.05 mg/kg/hr, fentanyl 3 to 5 μg/kg/hr, or midazolam 0.1 mg/kg/hr may be used. Sedatives should be titrated to achieve the desired effect. Some patients may require larger amounts or even combinations of two drugs, particularly those patients with protracted clinical courses in whom tolerance has developed.[40] If the patient remains muscle-relaxed, the neurologic examination, with exception of pupillary reflexes, will be negated. At our institution, we use phenobarbital to achieve a prophylactic anticonvulsant effect, particularly on those patients with severe hypoxemic-ischemic events or meningitis that may predispose to seizure activity. In the critically ill muscle-relaxed patient, seizure activity may manifest only as episodes of hypertension, tachycardia, or desaturation. A therapeutic level of phenobarbital of about 20 to 40 mg/dl should be maintained under these circumstances, unless continuous EEG monitoring is available.

Cardiovascular

Cardiovascular support is dependent on the clinical stage of septic shock. Early and aggressive fluid resuscitation is paramount for survival because it increases CO, DO_2 and $\dot{V}O_2$. An initial bolus of crystalloid solution (lactated Ringer's or normal saline) of 20 ml/kg should be administered rapidly if there are signs of shock. Continuous reassessment of the patient's perfusion status (capillary refill time, pulses, heart rate, mentation, BP) is mandatory. If there is no improvement, IV fluid boluses should be repeated, and 60 ml/kg may be given in the first hour. Other patients, especially those with meningococcemia will require larger amounts of fluid resuscitation. Garcillo et al.[5] reported that a more aggressive fluid resuscitation approach in the first hours of management is associated with an improvement in survival and does not increase the risk of cardiogenic pulmonary edema or ARDS. If after adequate fluid resuscitation the patient remains hypotensive, invasive monitoring with a central venous catheter or pulmonary artery catheter is required. Assessment of central venous pressure; CO; pulmonary capillary wedge pressure; systemic and pulmonary vascular resistances; DO_2, $\dot{V}O_2$, and oxygen extraction; and mixed venous saturation is important to guide management. Elevation of systemic oxygen delivery to supranormal values was previously advocated[2] but is not warranted and may have detrimental effects.[41] It may be more advisable to investigate tissue hypoxia by tonometry to guide therapy. Close observation of the patient's clinical response to any therapeutic maneuver is necessary to integrate the hemodynamic assessment and the clinical states. Sophisticated monitoring should be complemented with good clinical judgement and dedication to the patient.

When hemodynamic support is no longer achieved by fluid administration, pharmacologic support of the circulation should be initiated.[42–44] This subject is reviewed in Pharmacologic Support of the Circulation, by Ziegler, Englander, and Fugate, this volume.

Respiratory

The goal of respiratory management is to maximize DO_2. If hypoxemia secondary to ARDS develops, increased levels of PEEP may be required. It is important to keep in mind that high PEEP levels will decrease CO by (1) reducing preload secondary to higher intrathoracic pressure, (2) increasing right ventricular afterload due to increase in pulmonary vasculature resistance, and (3) decreasing left ventricular end-diastolic volume (LVEDV) due to ventricular interdependence. If the right ventricle becomes enlarged, it will displace the ventricular septum and decrease the LVEDV. Therefore, further fluid resuscitation or increasing inotropic support may be necessary when using high levels of PEEP.[39,45]

Supplemental oxygen should be weaned as soon as possible. Tolerance for lower PaO_2 (50–60 torr), hypercapnea (50–60 torr), and mild respiratory acidosis (pH 7.28–7.30), (permissive hypercapnea) will allow for survivors with lesser morbidity with ARDS. Permissive hypercapnea should be gradually achieved.[46] However, these parameters should be used only after hemodynamic stability has been achieved for several hours.

Gastrointestinal

Due to their unique metabolic states, septic patients may require "tailoring" of their nutritional support according to their individual needs.[47] Early enteral feedings are of major importance in preventing multiorgan failure. The enteral route can provide a larger amount of calories, avoids gut atrophy, and may prevent bacterial translocation.[34] Bronchial aspiration may be a risk, even for those patients with cuffed endotracheal tubes. Use of nasojejunal feedings should prevent this complication. Continuous diluted feeding in small volumes should be started as soon as possible, often within 24 to 36 hours of the initial septic episode. Although muscle relaxation is not a contraindication for enteral feedings, narcotic sedatives may decrease intestinal motility; thus a change in sedative drugs may be necessary. Gastric pH should be monitored and if the pH is less than 4.5, antacid medications, H_2 blocker agents, or sucralfate should be administered.

Renal and Metabolic

The preservation of renal function in the management of the shock states is important. This is done by maintaining an adequate intravascular volume with the administration of fluids and the use of dopamine at low doses (3 μg/kg/min) to maintain renal blood flow. A Foley catheter should be placed to obtain an accurate estimation of renal function. In the presence of persistent oliguria, it is important to rule out decreased CO or hypovolemia before diuretics are used. Despite multiple fluid boluses, septic patients may remain hypovolemic due to capillary leak syndrome, in which the infused fluids escape into the interstitial space, with resultant oliguria. If fluid challenge does not resolve oliguria and there is hemodynamic evidence of euvolemia, diuretics such as furosemide and/or mannitol may be indicated.[35]

Fluids and Electrolytes

Once the acute episode is controlled, patients with septic shock usually require management with two-thirds to full maintenance fluids. In view of the requirement for blood products, multiple medications, and fluid boluses, it is likely that during the initial 24 hours, patients will have an excessively positive fluid balance.

The objective of fluid therapy is to achieve an euvolemic state while avoiding fluid overload. Electrolyte abnormalities should be corrected promptly. Hypocalcemia often develops in patients with septic shock and frequently needs to be corrected to improve BP and perfusion. Hypophosphatemia and hypomagnesemia are often found. The latter occurs particularly in patients that have received aminoglycoside therapy. Hyperglycemia and glucose intolerance are often seen early in the course of the disease and are usually resolved by decreasing endogenous glucose supply.[36] The use of insulin in septic hyperglycemic patients is controversial; although it will decrease the blood glucose, insulin does not increase glucose oxidation and utilization in the critically ill patient.[48] Metabolic acidosis is a sign of poor perfusion and impaired DO_2. Under these conditions, fluid challenge and improving CO may prove beneficial. If metabolic acidosis persists despite adequate fluid resuscitation and DO_2, sodium bicarbonate may be used. Parenteral nutrition should be initiated whenever enteral nutrition is not possible.

Disseminated Intravascular Coagulation

Rapid recognition and treatment of the primary underlying disease continues to be the most important aspect of successful management of DIC. Replacement therapy with fresh frozen plasma (factors II, V, VII, VIII, IX, X, XI, XII, antithrombin III, etc.), cryoprecipitate (factors VIII, von Willebrand factor, fibronectin, fibrinogen), RBCs, and platelets is necessary.[37] Heparin is not used to treat DIC unless there is evidence of thrombosis and severe ischemia that may lead to necrosis of the affected area. This is often seen in patients with severe meningococcemia. Inhibitors of fibrinolysis, such as ε-aminocaproic acid, may foster the appearance of thrombosis and are not routinely used.

Experimental Therapy

During past years, there has been an explosion of potential therapies for septic shock. When corticosteroids are given to animals **before** a challenge injection of a lethal endotoxin dose, septic shock does not develop.[49] Nevertheless, in human studies, high-dose corticosteroid therapy failed to improve morbidity or mortality from infection.[3] Corticosteroids are used only in those septic patients with established or suspected adrenal insufficiency.

Nonsteroidal antiinflammatory drugs (NSAIDs) have proved to be useful in different animal models of septic shock and lung injury. Preliminary studies in human sepsis indicate possible benefits. A National Institutes of Health–sponsored multicenter trial is in progress to determine the efficacy of NSAIDs in the treatment of patients with septic shock. Currently, these drugs are still considered experimental.[50] Controlled studies using naloxone, an endorphin inhibitor, have failed to prove a beneficial effect, and there is still controversy regarding its use.[51,52]

Pharmacological inhibition of NO synthesis has restored BP in patients with septic shock. Nevertheless, in view of the complex pharmacodynamic effects of drugs that inhibit NO synthase, this potential therapy will need to be evaluated carefully before it can be widely applied to the clinical setting.[53,54]

Therapeutic use of human (HA-1A) monoclonal antilipid A antibody or murine-derived IgM monoclonal antibody has shown beneficial effects in selected populations of septic patients. The cost of this therapy is very expensive and patient selection is still controversial.[55,56]

Monoclonal antibodies to TNFα have proved to be efficacious

in experimental animals, and preliminary results in human studies are encouraging.[57,58] Receptor antagonists to IL$_1$ (IL$_1$-a), or to PAF, are also potential beneficial therapies.[59,60] Other inhibitors of inflammation, such as complement C$_1$ and C$_5$ inhibitors, neutrophil and protease inhibitors (pentoxifylline, adenosine, etc.), antioxidants, and oxygen-radical scavengers may play a role in the management of complex pathophysiologic events of sepsis.[19] Further studies are necessary to confirm their benefit and to determine proper clinical use.

The treatment of septic shock is no longer limited to supportive care and antibiotic administration. Better understanding of the concepts of oxygen delivery and uptake from the tissues and of the mechanisms of tissue and cellular injury has opened new opportunities to an earlier diagnosis and improved treatment of this disease.

References

1. Jacobs PR et al. Septic shock in children: Bacterial etiologies and temporal relationships. *Pediatr Infect Dis* 9:196–200, 1990.
2. Shoemaker W. Hemodynamic and oxygen transport patterns in septic shock: Physiologic mechanism and therapeutic implications. In Sibbald W, Sprung CH (eds): *Prospective on Sepsis and Septic Shock*. Fullerton, CA: Society of Critical Care Medicine, 1986. Pp 203–234.
3. Bone R, Fisher C, Clemmer T. A controlled clinical trial of high-dose methyl prednisolone in the treatment of severe sepsis and septic shock. *N Engl J Med* 317:653–658, 1987.
4. Parker M, Parrillo J. Septic shock-hemodynamics and pathogenesis. *JAMA* 250:3324–3327, 1983.
5. Garcillo J, Davis A, Zaritsky A. Role of early fluid resuscitation in pediatric septic shock. *JAMA* 266:1242–1245, 1991.
6. Bone R et al. Definitions for sepsis and organ failure and guidelines for the use of innovative therapies in sepsis. *Chest* 101:1644–1645, 1992.
7. Dal Nogare A. Septic shock. *Am J Med Sci* 302:50–65, 1991.
8. Thijs L, Schneider A, Groeneveld A. The haemodynamics of septic shock. *Intensive Care Med* 16:S182–S186, 1990.
9. Michalek S et al. The primary role of lymphoreticular cells in the mediation of host response to bacterial endotoxin. *J Infect Dis* 141:55–63, 1980.
10. Glauser M et al. Septic shock: Pathogenesis. *Lancet* 338:732–736, 1991.
11. Dunn D. Role of endotoxin and host cytokines in septic shock. *Chest* 100:1645–1685, 1991.
12. Beutler B, Cerami A. Cachectin: More than a tumor necrosis factor. *N Engl J Med* 316:379–385, 1987.
13. Fong Y, Lowry S, Cerami A. Cachectin/TNF: A macrophage protein that induces cachexia and shock. *JPEN* 12:725–775, 1988.
14. Moncada S, Palmer RM, Higgs EA. Nitric oxide physiology, pathophysiology and pharmacology. *Pharmacol Rev* 43:109–142, 1991.
15. Joulou-Shaeffer G et al. Loss of vascular responsiveness induced by endotoxin involves the L-arginine pathway. *Am J Physiol* 259:H1038–H1043, 1990.
16. Rock C, Lowry S. Tumor necrosis-α. *J Surg Res* 51:434–445, 1991.
17. Dinarello C, Mier J. Current concepts: Lymphokines. *N Engl J Med* 317:940–945, 1987.
18. Dinarello C. Biology of interleukin. *FASEB J* 2:108–115, 1988.
19. Zimmerman J, Ringer T. Inflammatory host responses in sepsis. *Crit Care Clin* 8:163–189, 1992.
20. Zimmerman J, Dietrich K. Current perspectives on septic shock. *Pediatr Clin North Am* 34:131–163, 1987.
21. Jackson A et al. The encephalopathy of sepsis. *Neurology* 14:141–146, 1983.
22. Bolton C, Broun J, Sibbald W. The electrophysiologic investigation of respiratory paralysis in critically ill patients. *Neurology* 33:2–18, 1983.
23. Crone R. Acute circulatory failure in children. *Pediatr Clin North Am* 27:525–538, 1980.
24. Bone R. Sepsis syndrome: New insights into its pathogenesis and treatment. *Intensive Crit Care Dig* 10:49–56, 1991.
25. Suffredini A et al. The cardiovascular response of normal humans to the administration of endotoxin. *N Engl J Med* 321:280–287, 1989.
26. Schumacker P, Cain S. The concept of a critical oxygen delivery. *Intensive Care Med* 13:223–229, 1987.
27. Tuschschmidt J et al. Elevation of cardiac output and oxygen delivery improves outcome in septic shock. *Chest* 102:216–220, 1992.
28. Wysocki M et al. Modification of oxygen extraction ratio by change in oxygen transport in septic shock. *Chest* 102:221–226, 1992.
29. Nelson DP et al. Pathological supply dependence of systemic and intestinal O$_2$ uptake during endotoxemia. *J Appl Physiol* 64:2410, 1988.
30. Ronco JJ et al. Oxygen consumption is independent of increased in oxygen delivery by dobutamine in septic patients who have normal or increased plasma lactate. *Am Rev Respir Dis* 147:25–31, 1993.
31. Phang PT et al. Mathematical coupling explains dependence of oxygen consumption on oxygen delivery in ARDS. *Am J Respir Crit Care Med* 150:318–323, 1994.
32. Demling R. Current concepts on the adult respiratory distress syndrome. *Circ Shock* 30:297–309, 1990.
33. Sprung C et al. Amino acid alterations and encephalopathy in sepsis syndrome. *Crit Care Med* 19:753–757, 1991.
34. Fiddian-Green R, Baker S. Nosocomial pneumonia in the critically ill: Product of aspiration or translocation. *Crit Care Med* 19:763–769, 1991.
35. Konturek S et al. Role of nitric oxide and prostaglandins in sucralfate-induced gastroprotection. *Eur J Pharmacol* 211:277–279, 1992.
36. Cerra F. Metabolic manifestations of multiple systems organ failure. *Crit Care Clin* 5:119–131, 1989.
37. Watson K, Vercelotte G. Issues in hemostasis: Surgery and critical care. In Cerra F (ed): *Perspectives in Critical Care*. QMP, Inc.: St. Louis, MO, 1989. Pp. 115–139.
38. Neild G. Manifestations of L cellular injury: Tubuloglomerular dysfunction in multiple organ failure. In Bihari D, Cerra T (eds): *Critical Care State of the Art*. Fullerton, CA: Society of Critical Care Medicine, 1989. Pp 263–276.
39. Lee R, Balb R, Bone R. Ventilatory support in the management of septic patients. *Crit Care Clin* 5:157–175, 1989.
40. Brill J. Control of pain. *Crit Care Clin* 8:203–218, 1992.
41. Hayes MA et al. Elevation of systemic oxygen delivery in the treatment of critically ill patients. *N Engl J Med* 330:1717–1727, 1994.
42. Natanson C, Hoffman W. Septic shock and other forms of distributive shock. In Parillo J (ed): *Current Therapy in Critical Care Medicine* (2nd ed). Philadelphia: Decker, 1991. Pp 62–70.
43. Schreuder W et al. Effect of dopamine vs norephinephrine on hemodynamics in septic shock. *Chest* 95:1282–1288, 1989.
44. Chernow B, Kasinski M, Salem M. Catecholamines in critical illness. In Lumb P, Shoemaker W (eds): *Critical Care State of the Art*. Fullerton, CA: Society of Critical Care Medicine. 1990. Pp 75–113.
45. Pinky M. The hemodynamic effects of artificial ventilation. In Snyder D, Pinsky M (eds): *Oxygen Transport in the Critically Ill*. Chicago: Year Book, 1987. Pp 319–332.
46. Hickling K, Henderson S, Jackson R. Low mortality associated with low pressure limited ventilation with permissive hypercapnia in severe adult respiratory distress syndrome. *Intensive Care Med* 16:372–377, 1990.
47. Castillo L et al. Phenylalanine and tyrosine kinetics in critically ill children with sepsis. *Pediatr Res* 35:580–588, 1994.
48. Burke JF et al. Glucose requirements following burn injury. *Ann Surg* 190:274–285, 1979.
49. Hinshaw L, Beller-Todd B, Archer L. Current management of the septic shock patient. Experimental basis for treatment. *Cir Shock* 9:543–553, 1982.
50. Petrak R, Balk R, Bone R. Prostaglandins, cyclooxygenase inhibitors,

and thromboxane synthesis inhibitors in the pathogenesis of multiple organ failure. *Crit Care Clin* 5:303–314, 1989.

51. Rock P et al. Efficacy and safety of naloxone in septic shock. *Crit Care Med* 13:28–33, 1985.

52. Napolitano L, Chernow B. Endorphins in circulatory shock. *Crit Care Med* 16:566–567, 1988.

53. Petros A, Bennett D, Vallance P. Effect of nitric oxide synthase inhibitors on hypotension in patients with septic shock. *Lancet* 338:1557–1559, 1991.

54. Hotchkiss R et al. Inhibition of NO synthesis in septic shock. *Lancet* 339:434–435, 1992.

55. Ziegler E et al. Treatment of gram negative bacteremia and septic shock with HA-IA human monoclonal antibody against endotoxin. A randomized, double blind, placebo control trial. *N Engl J Med* 324:429–436, 1991.

56. Warren H, Danner R, Munford R. Antiendotoxin monoclonal antibodies. *N Engl J Med* 326:1153–1157, 1992.

57. Walsh C et al. Monoclonal antibody to tumor necrosis factor α attenuates cardiopulmonary dysfunction in porcine gram negative sepsis. *Arch Surg* 127:138–145, 1992.

58. Vincent J et al. Administration of anti-TNF antibody improves left ventricular function in septic shock patients. *Chest* 101:810–815, 1992.

59. Ohlsson K et al. Interleukin-1 receptor antagonist reduces mortality from endotoxin shock. *Nature* 348:550–552, 1990.

60. Yue T, Farhat M, Rabinovici R. Protective effect of BN 50739, a new platelet-activating factor antagonist, in endotoxin-treated rabbits. *J Pharmacol Exp Ther* 254:976–981, 1990.

James W. Ziegler   **38.2** # Hemorrhagic Shock and Encephalopathy Syndrome

In 1983, Levin et al. described a series of ten patients with what he called a "new" disease, the hemorrhagic shock and encephalopathy syndrome (HSES).[1] This syndrome, consisting of the acute onset of shock, encephalopathy, and bleeding diasthesis in previously well infants, subsequently began surfacing throughout Europe and the United States. Also, two reports from France[2,3] and one from Great Britain[4] in the late 1970s described series of infants with all of the characteristics of those in Levin's series. To date, well over 100 cases have been reported throughout the western world.[5] Although there are many controversies and unanswered questions surrounding this disease, it does appear to be a new syndrome, one that is increasing in frequency and with a very high incidence of mortality and long-term morbidity.

Clinical Presentation

Table 38.2-1 lists the 11 clinical features described by the British Pediatric Association and Communicable Disease Surveillance Centre seen in patients presenting with HSES. The majority of patients so far reported have been less than 1 year old, with the average age being approximately 3 to 5 months.[1,6,7] The typical history is that of a previously well infant who may or may not have a mild prodromal illness consisting of upper respiratory or GI symptoms. The infant then acutely develops high fever, cardiovascular collapse, seizures, coma, and irregular respirations. Multiple organ systems become involved over the subsequent hours, with the development of hepatic and renal dysfunction and disseminated intravascular coagulation (DIC). The development of watery diarrhea progressing to bloody diarrhea has been a consistent feature in most patients.

The typical laboratory findings are listed in Table 38.2-2. Leukocytosis without a left shift has been a common finding. Normal hemoglobin and hematocrit values on admission rapidly fall by an average of greater than 3 grams percent[6] over the first several hours. Liver enzymes are usually elevated, but bilirubin and am-

Table 38.2-1. The percentage of patients with eleven different diagnostic criteria*

Feature	% of patients with feature
Encephalopathy	100
Liver dysfunction	100
Negative cultures for bacteria	100
Shock	97
Acidosis	97
Falling platelets	94
Diarrhea	92
Falling hemoglobin	91
Disseminated intravascular coagulation	90
Renal impairment	86
Normal ammonia	82

*Includes only percentage out of total tested for each particular feature.
Data from PHLS Communicable Disease Surveillance Centre.[7]

Table 38.2-2. Major laboratory findings

Laboratory feature	Presence in HSES
Metabolic acidosis	Almost always
Elevated SGOT and SGPT	Almost always
Near normal alk. phos. and bilirubin	Almost always
Ammonia 130 μmol/liter	Almost always
Falling hemoglobin	Almost always
Falling platelets	Almost always
Elevated PT and PTT	Almost always
Normal CSF profile	Almost always
Negative blood and CSF cultures	Almost always
Hypernatremia	Usually
Hypokalemia	Occasionally
Hypocalcemia	Occasionally
Hypoglycemia	Rarely

alk. phos., alkaline phosphatase; PT, prothrombin time; PTT, partial thromboplastin time; CSF, cerebrospinal fluid.

monia levels tend to remain normal or just slightly above normal limits. Clotting profiles are consistent with DIC. BUN and creatinine values reflect renal involvement, although they usually normalize with repletion of the intravascular space and correction of shock.[5] Metabolic acidosis with compensatory respiratory alkalosis can be profound and difficult to treat. Cerebrospinal fluid analysis is unremarkable and blood cultures are negative. Hypernatremia occurs in over half of those described[1,6,7]; hypoglycemia and hypocalcemia have been reported less frequently.

The mortality of this syndrome is high, greater than 65% in series so far reported.[1,6,7] In addition, those who survive have a very high incidence of profound neurologic damage; however, there have been case reports of patients with normal outcomes, suggesting that a milder form of this disease does exist.[8,9]

Etiology

The cause of this devastating disease is unknown, although several theories have been put forth. Bacon et al., in their description of five infants with features identical to those seen in HSES, blamed overwrapping and thus a heat stroke–like reaction as the causative factor.[4] All five patients were hyperpyrexic and had a history of being overwrapped. Three of the five also had symptoms of a viral illness prior to their acute deterioration. Bacon et al. hypothesized that the combination of a mild infection plus enforced insulation resulted in a rapid rise in temperature and heat stroke. Other authors[10,11] support this concept for several reasons. First, several patients with HSES present with marked hyperpyrexia, and its absence does not rule out heat stroke, as infants and children, with their relatively large body surface areas, cool rapidly, and thus may be normothermic by the time they arrive at the hospital. Second, the course of heat stroke is very similar to the course of HSES, that is, multisystem involvement resulting in death, or in survivors, resulting in a high incidence of neurologic damage.[12–14]

Last, autopsy findings in HSES are very similar to those seen in heat stroke.

Other authors have speculated that HSES is infectious in etiology. Morris and Mathews suggest that HSES results from a toxin produced by a "common" bacterium, one that might be encountered by the normal host.[15] This would explain the seeming immunity from HSES noted in the newborn and older child because of protective antibody. Others have suggested a new, unrecognized bacterium or virus.[1] In the absence of both temporal and geographic clustering, however, this seems unlikely. Also, exhaustive searches for an infectious agent have proven fruitless, although several common viruses have been isolated, suggesting HSES may be an abnormal response in the genetically susceptible patient to a common triggering agent.[1,6,7,16]

In Levin's series of 25 patients,[6] no evidence of overwrapping was found. Thus, he felt classic heat stroke as the cause of HSES was unlikely. He did, however, find diminished levels of circulating alpha-1 antitrypsin and elevated levels of circulating trypsin, suggesting that the etiology of HSES might be related to an overabundance of proteolytic enzymes. It is known that experimental infusion of proteolytic enzymes into the circulation results in widespread intravascular coagulation,[17] and Levin hypothesized that the diminished levels of circulating alpha-1 antitrypsin in HSES patients could be overwhelmed by massive release of proteolytic enzymes, leading to uncontrolled coagulation and activation of the kinin and complement pathways.[6] More work in this area is needed to further elucidate this potential etiology.

Differential Diagnosis

The differential diagnosis of HSES is listed in Table 38.2-3 and includes overwhelming sepsis and viremia, toxic shock syndrome, hemolytic uremic syndrome, viral hemorrhagic fevers, and Reye's

Table 38.2-3. Differential diagnosis

Disease	Similarities	Differences
Sepsis	Multisystem failure; fulminant course	Positive cultures Autopsy evidence of generalized infection
Viremia	Multisystem involvement; occasionally with acute fulminant course	Positive viral culture or positive serology or evidence of virus on autopsy
Toxic shock syndrome	Multisystem involvement; occasionally with acute fulminant course	Presence of rash Isolation of toxin producing staph More common in older children Outcome in survivors usually good
Hemolytic uremic syndrome	Multisystem involvement Anemia Falling platelets	Microangiopathic hemolytic anemia Kidneys primary site of involvement Outcome usually good
Viral hemorrhagic fever	Multisystem involvement Fulminant course Coagulopathy	Presence of rash Pleural effusions Rare in Western world Positive serology Encephalopathy rare Outcomes in those surviving good
Reye's syndrome	Multisystem involvement Occasionally runs fulminant course	Elevated ammonia Rare in infancy Fatty infiltration of viscera

syndrome. Also included in Table 38.2-3 are features of those diseases that differentiate them from HSES.

When elevated ammonia occurs, differentiation from Reye's syndrome may be difficult. However, age range, absence of hypoglycemia, and pathologic findings help make the distinction.

Pathology

Table 38.2-4 lists the histopathologic findings present on autopsy in 17 patients with HSES. Taken alone, none of these findings is pathognomonic of HSES, but together they form a fairly characteristic picture.

Treatment

Because the etiology of HSES is unknown, treatment is mainly supportive. In the hyperpyrexic patient, rapid lowering of core temperature should be an early priority, especially because cerebral edema is a common finding and the long-term morbidity is dependent on the extent of irreversible neurologic injury. The following approach reviews the therapy for the various organ systems involved.

Cardiovascular

As mentioned, the majority of patients with HSES present with cardiovascular collapse. This is always associated with a low central venous pressure and thus is reflective of a severe hypovolemic state. Massive amounts of colloid and isotonic crystalloid, sometimes as high as 200 cc per kilogram, are required to correct this fluid deficit. Usually, with repletion of the intravascular space, the hemodynamic status stabilizes. Direct myocardial involvement per se is not a feature of this disease, and long-term requirement for pressors in the face of intravascular fluid repletion is distinctly unusual.

The etiology of the large fluid loss in HSES is probably multifactorial. Generalized vasodilation, third spacing of fluid into the gastrointestinal tract with resultant diarrhea, and increased insensible fluid losses secondary to fever and hyperventilation probably all contribute. Capillary leak is not thought to be present in these patients.[6]

Table 38.2-4. Findings on autopsy: 17 cases

Finding	% of time present
Cerebral edema/liquefaction necrosis	88
DIC	88
Centrilobar hepatic necrosis	82
Hemorrhage into skin	76
Hemorrhage into GI mucosa	65
Hemorrhage into other organs	65
Hemorrhage into lungs	59
Evidence of acute tubular necrosis	53
Mild fatty change in liver	41
Pituitary necrosis	35

Data from Levin et al.[6]

Respiratory

The lungs are not directly affected in HSES. However, most patients are found hyperventilating to compensate for the marked metabolic acidosis usually present. Airway management may be a problem, especially in comatose or obtunded patients who are unable to maintain their airways. Intubation and mechanical ventilation is usually necessary in this setting.

Gastrointestinal

Profuse diarrhea, initially watery and later bloody, seems to be a common feature of HSES. Its etiology has not been worked out but may be related to pooling of hypotonic fluid within the GI tract.[8] Treatment is supportive, with measurement and replacement of stool losses being the most important goal. Because ulcerations in the stomach and small intestine are common autopsy findings, the use of antacids and H_2 receptor antagonists would seem reasonable.

Renal

Renal dysfunction in HSES is secondary to cardiovascular collapse and hypoperfusion. It usually improves with correction of shock. Occasionally, severe renal tubular necrosis occurs, and in Levin's series, 6 of 25 patients needed peritoneal dialysis.[6]

Hepatic

The typical laboratory picture of the hepatic involvement in HSES is one of cellular injury with elevated SGOT and SGPT but normal or only slightly elevated levels of bilirubin, alkaline phosphatase, and ammonia. Again, though part of this injury may be a primary insult, maintenance of adequate oxygen delivery with the correction of shock provides the best chance of recovery. Extensive involvement with hepatic failure probably occurs only in fatal cases. Of note is that a firm, enlarged liver is frequently noted in patients with HSES.[5]

Metabolic

Marked metabolic acidosis is an almost universal feature of HSES. Its etiology is most likely secondary to hypoperfusion of tissues, resulting in anaerobic metabolism and the accumulation of lactic acid in tissue beds; most authors have found a satisfactory result with correction of shock and infusion of sodium bicarbonate. We have seen one patient with a persistent hyperchloremic, metabolic acidosis into the fifth day of therapy secondary to excessive losses of alkali into both stool and urine. This resolved with time.

Hypernatremia is commonly seen in HSES and, if present, necessitates slow correction to avoid osmotic shifts into the brain. After initial correction of shock with isotonic fluids, the hypernatremia should be slowly corrected over a 24- to 48-hour period. Careful monitoring of serum sodiums is essential.

Hypocalcemia is seen occasionally and may be a reflection of the frequency with which this metabolic abnormality is noted in critically ill patients in general. Maintenance of a normal ionized calcium is important, especially if hemodynamic instability is present.

Hematologic

As mentioned, hemoglobin and hematocrit values are usually normal on admission but then dramatically fall over the ensuing few hours. This rapid fall in hematocrit is probably secondary to blood loss into the GI tract and elsewhere. In addition, dilution of the RBC mass by fluids used during resuscitation plays a role. Because maintenance of oxygen delivery is the primary goal in treating shock, transfusions of RBCs to maintain a hematocrit greater than 30 are required.

Disseminated intravascular coagulation occurs at some point in most patients with HSES, although some authors question whether it is really an integral part of the syndrome.[18] Treatment consists of infusion of fresh-frozen plasma, cryoprecipitate, and platelets as needed to minimize bleeding and correct the laboratory abnormalities.

Neurologic

The encephalopathy of HSES manifests itself as seizures and alterations in level of consciousness. Because damage to the brain is more severe relative to other organs, some wonder whether the brain is the site of the primary insult of this disease. Also, because severity of the CNS insult determines eventual long-term outcome, close attention to optimizing brain recovery is mandatory. Aggressive control of seizures is crucial and may require the use of multiple anticonvulsants. Refractory seizures are occasionally encountered; these patients usually die.

Because cerebral edema is a consistent finding on autopsy specimens, at least conservative measures to control rising intracranial pressure would seem prudent. Fluid restriction after resuscitation, mild hyperventilation, maintenance of adequate oxygen delivery, keeping the head in the midline and elevated 30 degrees, and avoiding painful procedures unless adequately medicated are rational treatment goals without deleterious side effects. Avoidance of hyperthermia and control of seizures have already been emphasized.

Summary

HSES is a recently described, devastating disease affecting infants and young children. Its etiology remains unclear, and therefore, treatment relies mainly on supportive care. Outcomes to date have been poor, with the vast majority of patients either dying or surviving with profound neurologic deficits.

In England, HSES has been a reportable disease since 1984. It appears to be more common than some of the other "new" devastating diseases of children, including Reye's syndrome and toxic shock syndrome[5]; thus the pediatrician needs to be well acquainted with this disease entity.

References

1. Levin M et al. Haemorrhagic shock and encephalopathy: A new syndrome with a high mortality in young children. *Lancet* ii:64, 1983.
2. Beaufils F et al. Syndrome d'hyperthermie majeure de l'enfant. In *Monographie de la Societe de Reanimation de Langue Francaise*. Paris: Expansion Scientifique Francaise, 1975. Pp 244–427.
3. Aujard Y et al. Hyperthermie majeure de l'enfant. *Arch Fr Pediatr* 35:477–485, 1978.
4. Bacon C, Scott D, Jones P. Heatstroke in well-wrapped infants. *Lancet* i:422–425, 1979.
5. Chesney PJ, Chesney R. Hemorrhagic shock and encephalopathy; Reflections about a new devastating disorder that affects normal children. *J Pediatr* 114:254–256, 1989.
6. Levin M et al. Hemorrhagic shock and encephalopathy: Clinical, pathologic, and biochemical features. *J Pediatr* 114:194–203, 1989.
7. PHLS Communicable Disease Surveillance Centre. Joint Paediatric Association and Communicable Disease Surveillance Centre surveillance scheme for haemorrhagic shock encephalopathy syndrome: Surveillance report for 1982–4. *Br Med J* 290:1578, 1985.
8. Whittington LK, Roscelli JD, Parry WH. Hemorrhagic shock and encephalopathy: Further description of a new syndrome. *J Pediatr* 106:599–602, 1985.
9. McGucken RB. Hemorrhagic shock and encephalopathy syndrome (letter). *Lancet* ii:1087, 1983.
10. Beaufils F, Aujard Y. Hemorrhagic shock and encephalopathy syndrome (letter). *Lancet* ii:1086, 1983.
11. Sofer S et al. Hemorrhagic shock and encephalopathy syndrome, its association with hyperthermia. *Am J Dis Child* 140:1252–1254, 1986.
12. Ziegler JW. Heatstroke in infancy. *Am J Dis Child* 130:1250, 1976.
13. Roberts K, Roberts E. The automobile and heat stress. *Pediatrics* 58:101–104, 1976.
14. Danks DM, Webb DW, Allen J. Heat illness in infants and young children. *Br Med J* ii:287–293, 1962.
15. Morris JA, Mathews TS. Haemorrhagic shock and encephalopathy: A new syndrome in young children. *Lancet* ii:278, 1983.
16. Weibley R, Pimentel B, Ackerman N. Hemorrhagic shock and encephalopathy syndrome of infants and children. *Crit Care Med* 17:335–338, 1989.
17. Kwaan HC, Anderson MC, Gramatica L. A study of pancreatic enzymes as a factor in the pathogenesis of disseminated intravascular coagulation during acute pancreatitis. *Surgery* 69:663–672, 1971.
18. Shrager GO, Shah A. Hemorrhagic shock encephalopathy syndrome in infancy (letter). *Lancet* ii:396, 1983.

Ruth Lynfield
H. Shaw Warren

39 ▸ Antimicrobial Treatment of Sepsis

This chapter is a guide for the pediatric intensive care specialist in choosing appropriate antimicrobial therapy for patients in the pediatric intensive care unit (PICU). We concentrate on the treatment of bacterial infections because they are the most common cause of sepsis in the PICU, and we include brief sections on the use of antifungal and antiviral agents. We start the chapter with the empiric use of antibiotics in several different clinical settings before the diagnosis is confirmed. We next address issues relating to the antibiotics themselves, such as dosing, choice of beta-lactam and aminoglycoside antibiotics, allergies, and treatment of several specific bacteria. We conclude with a section on the use of antibiotics for the chemoprophylaxis of close contacts of patients in the PICU.

Management of patients with sepsis includes recognition of the site(s) and microbial agent(s) causing infection, drainage if appropriate and possible, administration of effective antimicrobial therapy, and maintenance of aggressive supportive care. In patients with severe infections, antimicrobial therapy should be directed against the most likely organisms as determined by history, physical examination, and laboratory results (including rapid diagnostic tests such as examination of Gram stains of infected body fluids). Definitive therapy can then be instituted when culture data and sensitivities become available.

Empiric Antibiotic Therapy When There Is No Focal Source Identified

When there is no identifiable focus of infection in a previously well child (i.e., a "community-acquired" infection), empiric therapy for sepsis of possible bacterial origin is in part guided by the age of the patient. The young infant (1 to 3 months of age) is at risk for late-onset neonatal sepsis as well as infection from the pathogens that commonly afflict older infants. Consequently, it is reasonable to empirically treat for infections caused by group B streptococci, gram-negative enteric bacilli, *Listeria monocytogenes*, *Streptococcus pneumoniae*, *Haemophilus influenzae*, and *Neisseria meningitidis*. Other organisms, including salmonella, nonenteric gram-negative bacteria, and *Enterococcus* are occasionally a cause of sepsis. Infants in this age group with bacteremia are at a relatively high risk for developing secondary tissue infections, including meningitis. Therefore, the antibiotic regimen should include drugs that penetrate into the cerebrospinal fluid (CSF). An empiric regimen often used is ampicillin and a third-generation cephalosporin. Ampicillin is included both to cover *L. monocytogenes* and because clinical experience suggests that ampicillin is preferable to cephalosporins against group B streptococci. In older infants or children, *S. pneumoniae* and *N. meningitidis* are the predominant pathogens. Prior to the widespread use of conjugate vaccines to *H. influenzae*, infections with these bacteria were common and humoral immunity to *H. influenzae* was usually acquired naturally by the age of 5 years. Invasive infections caused by *H. influenzae* are now relatively rare in populations that have been fully vaccinated. Initial therapy with a third-generation cephalosporin such as ceftriaxone is increasingly used for broad-spectrum coverage that includes the CNS. Addition of an aminoglycoside or specific antistaphylococcal therapy may be added if there is a desire to bolster the coverage until culture results are known.

In addition to the common causes of bacterial sepsis, there are several other severe infections that need to be considered for empiric therapy in relevant epidemiologic settings in order to institute prompt and life-saving therapy. Rocky mountain spotted fever, malaria, typhoid fever, toxic shock syndrome, and disseminated tuberculosis would fit into this category. Each of these diseases mandates specific and emergent treatment different from that mentioned previously.

Empiric Antibiotic Therapy When There Is a Focal Source

Meningitis

In any patient suspected of meningitis, a lumbar puncture with Gram stain as well as appropriate cultures, chemistries, and cell count provide important diagnostic information. Gram stain may yield a preliminary diagnosis. If the Gram stain is negative, therapy is logically guided by the organisms most commonly involved in the patient's age group or clinical setting. In general, in the absence of a contiguous focus of infection, the bacterial pathogens involved are those that have seeded the meninges from the blood. Consequently, empiric therapy mirrors that discussed in the previous section. Coverage may be narrowed when the organism and sensitivities are definitively known. For a detailed discussion of infection of the CNS see Infections of the Central Nervous System by Pasternack, this volume.

Infections of the Head and Neck

Infections of the head and neck can be life-threatening because of their location and tendency to spread rapidly to critical tissues. Accordingly, there is less of a margin of error in antibiotic choice, and therapy needs to be started early and at relatively high doses. Of equal importance to the choice of antimicrobial therapy is the need to protect the airway from obstruction and to evaluate possible spread of infection into the deep structures of the neck and mediastinum.

Infections within the Oral Cavity

The organisms most frequently isolated from pharyngeal space infections are group A streptococci, *Staphylococcus aureus*, and anaerobic bacteria. There are many antibiotic combinations used to treat these infections, including but not limited to ampicillin/ sulbactam, chloramphenicol plus nafcillin, clindamycin, and penicillin with consideration of an additional anaerobic and/or antistaphylococcal agent. Most odontogenic infections are polymicrobial, with anaerobes playing a leading role. Infections with spread to orofacial soft tissues are usually caused by a mixture of anaerobic and aerobic bacteria, especially if trauma or surgical manipulation is involved. Although earlier teaching suggested that penicillin G alone was sufficient to cover most bacterial mouth flora, some oral anaerobic bacteria have become resistant to penicillin. Accordingly, in severe infections thought to be caused by anaerobic bacteria, the physician should consider adding another agent. *H. influenzae* is rarely a cause of infections within the oral cavity, with the singular exception of acute supraglottitis in young children. Other organisms, including streptococci or staphylococci, rarely but occasionally cause acute supraglottitis. Protection of the airway is important. Empiric treatment might include ampicillin/sulbactam, a third-generation cephalosporin, cefuroxime, or ampicillin with chloramphenicol.

Sinusitis

Sinusitis is more often a cause of fever than of sepsis with bacteremia. Its complications, however, can be severe and include meningitis; epidural, subdural, brain, and orbital abscesses; and cavernous sinus thrombosis. In children, the most common pathogens of acute sinusitis are *H. influenzae*, *S. pneumoniae*, *Moraxella catarrhalis*, *S. aureus*, and *Streptococcus pyogenes*. In more chronic infections, anaerobic bacteria play a predominant role. In patients who have been in the hospital or who have been on antibiotics, gram-negative organisms or, very rarely, fungi may be involved, especially in patients who are immunocompromised. Sinusitis is more common in children who have had nasogastric or nasotracheal tubes. Therapy in patients who have acquired an acute infection outside of the hospital might initially include antibiotics tailored to these organisms, such as ampicillin/sulbactam, a third-generation cephalosporin, or an antistaphylococcal penicillin with chloramphenicol. In a patient who develops sinusitis in the ICU setting, and who has been on multiple antibiotics, coverage should be broad and should take into consideration the likelihood of gram-negative organisms or the possibility of antimicrobial resistance. Collaboration with an otolaryngologist is useful, as patients with severe infection or with secondary complications often need surgical drainage. In this case, surgical specimens should be sent for stains and bacterial and fungal cultures so that antimicrobial therapy can be adjusted accordingly.

Mastoiditis

Mastoiditis is rarely a problem that requires intensive care unless there is intracranial spread of infection. Group A streptococci, *S. pneumoniae*, *S. aureus*, and less commonly *H. influenzae* are organisms that are frequently isolated from the middle ear and mastoid during acute mastoiditis. In contrast, gram-negative bacteria, especially *Pseudomonas*, anaerobic organisms, and *S. aureus* are important pathogens in chronic mastoiditis. Ideally, surgically obtained cultures will help guide therapy. Frequently, however, empiric therapy is necessary. For acute mastoiditis, this might be an antibiotic regimen similar to that suggested for acute sinusitis. In more chronic infections, empiric coverage should treat gram-negative bacteria, including *Pseudomonas*.

Orbital Cellulitis

Infection of the orbit often occurs because of secondary spread of infection from contiguous structures such as the ethmoid, frontal, or maxillary sinuses. Occasionally, intraorbital infection can result from progression of preseptal cellulitis or secondary hematogenous seeding. Complications include blindness, septic thrombosis of the cavernous sinus, and intracranial suppuration. The bacterial flora reflect the initial source of infection and thus are similar to those causing sinusitis. Infections with streptococci, staphylococci, *H. influenzae*, and anaerobes are common. There are several options for an initial antibiotic regimen to cover these organisms. Examples include ampicillin/sulbactam, a third-generation cephalosporin, alone or together with an antistaphylococcal penicillin or clindamycin, or chloramphenicol with an antistaphylococcal penicillin. An early computed tomography (CT) scan to define the anatomy and collaboration with an otolaryngologist/ophthal-

mologic surgeon are important to diagnose and treat an orbital abscess that requires rapid drainage. Stains and cultures (aerobic, anaerobic, and fungal) of the abscess will help direct therapy. Antimicrobial therapy can then be modified, depending on the culture results and sensitivities.

Infections of the Lower Respiratory Tract

Infections of the lower respiratory tract are common and are a frequent cause of sepsis. A decision regarding appropriate antimicrobial therapy depends on understanding the etiology of the infection so that the likely pathogenic organisms can be treated while a diagnostic workup is underway. Assessment of such infections are complex and require the integration of multiple historical and clinical clues. Some of the many factors that are useful are knowledge of where the infection was acquired, the patient's age, history of infectious exposures, assessment of the patient's immune status, and history of prior respiratory infections. The radiographic picture may be helpful in constructing a differential diagnosis. Bacterial pneumonias generally have radiographic consolidation. As a group, pneumonia caused by viruses, *Chlamydia*, *Mycoplasma*, and *Pneumocystis* tend to have an interstitial pattern. Unfortunately, none of the radiologic patterns are diagnostic. An effort should be made to obtain sputum for smears and culture prior to beginning antimicrobial therapy. In the appropriate settings, respiratory washings can be sent for rapid diagnostic tests (e.g., respiratory syncytial virus, *Chlamydia*, and pertussis) and for culture. Pleural effusions should be tapped and samples sent for smears, culture, pH, cell count, and chemistries. If the diagnosis is still unclear in a worsening, critically ill patient, bronchoscopy or open-lung biopsy may be indicated.

An important clue regarding the etiology of severe pneumonia, which may affect the choice of antimicrobial agents utilized, is whether the infection was acquired in a community setting. Pneumonia acquired in the community is more likely to have a viral etiology than infection acquired in the hospital, and is particularly common during the winter months. Among the more common viral agents in children are respiratory syncytial virus, parainfluenza, influenza, and adenovirus. In part because of denuding of the respiratory tree, patients with viral pneumonia are at risk for becoming superinfected with bacterial pathogens, especially staphylococci and streptococci.

The age of the child is helpful in the differential diagnosis of pneumonia that is acquired as an outpatient. In all age groups, *S. pneumoniae* is a very common cause of bacterial pneumonia that is acquired as an outpatient. A rare but important cause of pneumonia acquired in outpatients is group A streptococci, which can cause a rapid and severe pneumonia often with an accompanying pleural effusion. Infections of infants with *Bordetella pertussis* can be severe and require intensive care monitoring and possibly tracheal intubation. Prior to the recent widespread use of vaccines to *H. influenzae*, this organism was an important pathogen in children younger than 5 years of age. In older children, *Mycoplasma pneumoniae* is a frequent pathogen, as is *Chlamydia pneumoniae*, strain TWAR, which is an underappreciated cause of pneumonia although not typically severe in children.[1,2] *S. aureus* is rarely the cause of a primary respiratory infection, except following an antecedent viral illness, especially influenza. The empiric treatment of severe community-acquired pneumonia is pragmatic and is based on covering the likely pathogens discussed earlier. Because a microbiologic diagnosis may be difficult to make or may lag behind the time of admission, it is reasonable to base antimicrobial therapy on the treatable possibilities, realizing that in many cases, the underlying cause may be viral. Erythromycin with a second- or third-generation cephalosporin or ampicillin/sulbactam provides good empirical coverage. In children with underlying cardiac or pulmonary compromise in whom infection with respiratory syncytial virus has been documented, inhalant therapy with ribavirin may be helpful.[3]

There are many other less common or rare causes of pneumonia acquired in the community that are not previously addressed. Some examples of such atypical pneumonias include pulmonary tularemia, plague, Q fever, and psittacosis. Three other infections that need to be considered in this category are tuberculosis, legionellosis, and *Pneumocystis carinii* pneumonia. A history regarding epidemiologic factors or exposure is helpful. Ordinarily, it is preferable to await diagnostic evidence of tuberculosis before treating, unless there is a history of definite exposure and the patient is critically ill. Skin testing for tuberculosis may be helpful. Infection of children with legionella is rare, and some coverage is provided with the doses of erythromycin ordinarily administered, although high doses of erythromycin are necessary for established infection with legionella. Clarithromycin also has activity against *Mycoplasma*, *Chlamydia*, and legionella and may be better tolerated than erythromycin, although it is not yet licensed for use in community-acquired pneumonia and is only available in oral form. *P. carinii* almost exclusively infects patients with defects in cellular immunity. Often, such defects are previously known, although occasionally children may present to the hospital with pneumonia caused by *P. carinii* as the presenting illness associated with AIDS. Therefore, treatment with trimethoprim/sulfamethoxazole might be considered in patients who present with hypoxemia and pulmonary interstitial infiltrates in an appropriate epidemiologic setting until diagnostic tests for *Pneumocystis* and HIV can be completed.

A different problem is the management of patients who have acquired pneumonia in the hospital, including chronically ill patients who develop chest manifestations. History, clinical course, and evolution of the pulmonary x-rays are helpful in sorting out the diagnostic possibilities and the consequent need and choice of antimicrobial therapy. Empiric therapy in the event of infection should be guided by Gram stain of the sputum and previous sputum cultures and sensitivities. Gram-negative bacilli that are often highly resistant to antibiotics are frequently present, and careful deliberation needs to be made whether a culture result represents colonization or infection. Overtreatment will result in the selection of yet more resistant organisms and superinfection.

Pulmonary aspiration of gastric contents and mouth organisms is a cause of pneumonia in both inpatients and outpatients. Usually there is a predisposing cause or event that has led to aspiration. Infection with anaerobic bacteria is common. Penicillin G or clindamycin is sufficient and appropriate antimicrobial treatment for pneumonia due to aspiration that has occurred in the community. Pneumonia from aspiration occurring in the hospital often involves hospital-acquired gram-negative bacteria as well as anaerobic bacteria. In this situation, antibiotics are used that provide coverage for both anaerobic and gram-negative bacteria.

Gastrointestinal Infections

Perforated Viscus

Many antibiotic regimens designed to treat leakage of intestinal contents into the peritoneum are based on experiments performed by Bartlett et al. in the 1970s.[4] It was clearly demonstrated in animal models that optimal therapy consisted of the treatment of both aerobic gram-negative bacilli and intestinal anaerobic bacteria. Animals that were treated with antimicrobials aimed at only anaerobic bacteria had a higher early mortality from septic shock, whereas animals who received only antimicrobials for aerobic gram-negative bacilli developed late abdominal abscesses. To achieve a high probability of killing aerobic gram-negative bacilli, many regimens for clinical use include two antibiotics of different types with activity against gram-negative bacilli, one of which is an aminoglycoside. The necessity of empirically treating *Enterococcus* (*Enterococcus faecium* or *Enterococcus faecalis*) is unclear, although many infectious disease consultants choose to do so. A commonly used regimen that takes these principles into account is ampicillin with gentamicin plus clindamycin or metronidazole. There are many other broad-spectrum antibiotic combinations that accomplish the same goal. Blood cultures and swabs taken at the time of surgery for Gram stain and culture are helpful in identifying possible untreated or resistant organisms. In this setting, the decision to narrow coverage based on these culture results should be taken with considerable caution.

Spontaneous Bacterial Peritonitis

Children with ascites are at risk for spontaneous bacterial peritonitis, which is often caused by pneumococci, other streptococci, and enteric gram-negative bacilli. In the absence of other complications, anaerobic bacteria are rarely involved. Because the presentation is usually indolent, a high index of suspicion is necessary for paracentesis. Bacteremia is common.[5] Once specimens have been obtained, empiric antimicrobial therapy based on the likely organisms can be started and then tailored to the results of the cultures. Initial treatment with ampicillin or vancomycin together with an aminoglycoside may be preferable to a cephalosporin to provide broader coverage. Peritonitis may occur in patients who have a catheter in place for peritoneal dialysis. In this case, organisms found on the skin play a predominant role.

Gastroenteritis

The causes of gastroenteritis are multiple and include bacteria and their toxins, viruses, and parasites. Disease severe enough to warrant admission to the ICU is rare, and sepsis may be difficult to distinguish from severe dehydration. The decision to treat with empiric antibiotics depends on the clinical situation. In some cases, such as uncomplicated gastroenteritis caused by salmonella, treating with antibiotics may prolong the duration of intestinal carriage. In cases of severe clinical illness, however, it is appropriate to treat with empiric antibiotics until the diagnosis is clear. This is particularly important in young infants. Bacterial etiologies of gastroenteritis include salmonella, shigella, campylobacter, *E. coli* (including enterotoxic, invasive, enteropathic, and enterocytotoxic strains), and yersinia. Evaluation of the patient with enteritis should include an examination of the stool for fecal leukocytes and a stool culture. Empiric therapy pending cultures might include ceftriaxone, trimethoprim/sulfamethoxazole, or ampicillin.

Antibiotic-Induced Colitis

Colitis induced by antibiotic use is thought to result from an alteration of the intestinal flora. Overgrowth of some bacterial strains, such as *Clostridium difficile*, leads to the production of cytotoxins that can cause severe colitis if not recognized and treated. The diagnosis of colitis can be made by assaying the stool for toxin. Current treatment consists of oral vancomycin or metronidazole to eradicate or suppress *C. difficile*.

Genitourinary Infections

Pediatric patients with pyelonephritis rarely develop sepsis unless there is obstruction of urinary drainage. Renal infections are frequently caused by enteric gram-negative organisms or enterococci. Because there is infection of tissue, a systemic level of antibiotics should be attained. The initial antibiotic choice should depend on Gram stain of the urine and prior cultures. If there is not a strong likelihood of infection with resistant organisms, initial broad therapy with ampicillin and gentamicin may be started while awaiting culture information.

A more common occurrence in the ICU is the development of urinary tract infection following instrumentation of the urinary tract or secondary to the presence of a urinary catheter. Infection in this setting is often caused by resistant nosocomial flora. The high concentrations of antibiotic achieved in the bladder make treatment relatively easy once the organism is identified. Cystitis due to *Candida* in the absence of upper tract involvement often responds rapidly to changing the catheter and irrigating the bladder with amphotericin B or nystatin, a procedure that avoids the use of systemic antifungal agents.

Infections in Postoperative Wounds, Burns, and Trauma

Infections in Surgical Wounds

Postoperative wound infections may involve any of the tissue layers within the incision. If the surgery did not involve infected tissue, the infecting organism was presumably introduced at the time of surgery and commonly represents host flora. Accordingly, infections with organisms normally found on the skin, such as *Staphylococcus* and *Streptococcus*, are frequent. Previous cultures of other sites and the patient's history over the prior days and weeks may give some clues regarding the possible presence and sensitivities of less likely organisms, such as gram-negative bacilli, which may need to be empirically treated. Infection with anaerobic bacteria should be considered in deep surgical wounds. Gram stain and culture of any draining fluid is worthwhile, although it is difficult to distinguish between infection and colonization unless there are bacteria within granulocytes. Initial antibiotic regimens vary with the setting. Choices may include a first-generation cephalosporin or an antistaphylococcal penicillin alone or with an aminoglycoside.

Infections in Patients with Burns

The development of infection in patients with burns is a result of the interaction between the organisms present, inoculum size, and host defenses. The decision to use antibiotics and the choice depends on the particular setting. In the absence of documented or suspected infection, there is no reason to start empiric antibiotics, and indeed the overzealous use of antibiotics in patients with burns will lead to the development of superinfection and to the selection of resistant organisms that may be more difficult to treat should infection develop. Decades ago, the incidence of early severe infections with group A streptococci prompted the use of prophylactic penicillin during the first several days following the burn injury. The incidence of streptoccal infections today is low, and it not clear that the allergic risks of empiric treatment of all children on admission to the ICU outweigh the potential benefit of treatment. Burn wounds are prone to infection with *Clostridium tetanus*, and early consideration of the need for a tetanus booster or tetanus immune globulin is important. Modern therapy of burn

injuries consists of aggressive, early wound closure. This practice is widely believed to have reduced mortality, in part through reducing the incidence of severe infections. In many burn centers, prophylactic antibiotics based on the sensitivities of prevalent wound organisms are given for a short course (18–24 hours) beginning with debridement of the burn wound, with the hope of decreasing bacteremia. This approach seems logical, although there are few concrete data addressing the issue. Secondary infections in burn patients are common and involve, but are not limited to, burn wounds, intravenous catheters, the respiratory tree, and the urinary tract. These infections should be treated on an individual basis. Dosing of antimicrobial agents in this patient population needs to be adjusted for their altered drug metabolism.[6,7]

Use of Antimicrobial Agents in Trauma

Injury predisposes patients to infection in multiple ways, and an effort should be made to identify potential locations of infection so that infections can be diagnosed and treated rapidly. As with burns, an early assessment should be made concerning the immune status against tetanus. The initial evaluation may identify sites of bacterial contamination induced by the trauma either through direct inoculation in a penetrating injury, or through disruption of normal body barriers with introduction of microorganisms into tissues. In the case of inoculation of microorganisms from the external environment through penetrating trauma, antimicrobial agents should be administered based on the best estimate of which organisms may be present. A detailed history of the location of the trauma and of the objects involved is therefore very important. Antibiotics should provide coverage against skin flora that might have been carried into the wound at the time of the trauma. In the case of blunt trauma, an educated guess can be made regarding the type of organisms inoculated into tissues based on the known normal flora of body sites, such as the oral cavity, sinuses, and intestine.

Infections of Intravascular Catheters

Any unexplained fever in a patient with an IV catheter may be related to infection of the catheter. There may be no external signs of infection, especially in patients with a central line in place. Blood cultures should be obtained peripherally and through the catheter. If the catheter is removed, the tip should be sent for culture. Infection is often caused by resident skin flora, such as *Staphylococcus* or *Streptococcus*, although in chronically ill patients, almost any bacteria, or yeast may be involved. Perhaps because it is a rich culture medium, infections associated with IV hyperalimentation are common and can be associated with fastidious organisms that are not ordinarily pathogens. Single blood cultures that grow organisms that normally reside on the skin may be difficult to interpret because of the possibility of contamination of the culture at the time the blood was obtained. Multiple positive cultures that grow early after inoculation are suggestive of infection.

Long-term, surgically placed catheters are tunneled beneath the skin before entering a large blood vessel. A thorough examination of the skin is important in a patient who may have a catheter infection. Physical findings of the skin are variable and depend on whether the infection involves the tip of the catheter (no skin findings), the tunnel site (redness along the subcutaneous catheter tunnel), or the exit site (local cellulitis). Complications include septic thrombophlebitis, seeding of other sites, and endocarditis. Empiric therapy, if needed, is started only after numerous blood cultures are obtained. Vancomycin is frequently used alone or in combination with an aminoglycoside pending results of cultures. Previously, it was thought that all infected catheters needed to be removed. In some instances, however, the catheter can be cleared of infection without removing it, particularly with infections caused by *streptococci* or *staphylococci*.[8–10] Attempts to leave the line in place are much less likely to be successful if cellulitis or tunnel site infection[11] is present or gram-negative bacteria or yeast[10,12] are involved. If a decision is made to treat with antibiotics but to attempt to salvage the line, the patient should be closely observed for defervesence of fever and sterilization of the blood. In the absence of rapid clinical improvement, the catheter should be removed. Ideally, a peripheral catheter should be utilized until the fungemia or bacteremia has definitively cleared before replacement of a more permanent catheter.

Empiric Therapy in Patients with Fever and Neutropenia

Patients with immunodeficiencies are at increased risk for infection by pathogens that infect normal hosts in addition to opportunistic organisms. Symptoms may be subtle, and focal signs may be minimal in patients who cannot mount a normal inflammatory response. A particularly sensitive and thorough history and physical examination is thus especially important in the search for occult infection.

Empiric antibiotic therapy decreases mortality in neutropenic patients with less than 500 granulocytes/μL who are febrile, even if there is not an obvious source of infection. Empiric antibiotics should be provided against invasive disease from endogenous flora, especially gram-negative organisms. Antistaphylococcal therapy should also be considered, especially in those patients who have an indwelling catheter. Multiple regimens in this setting have been described.[13] An approach for initial treatment might include a beta-lactam (either a cephalosporin, antipseudomonal penicillin, or carbapenem) paired with an aminoglycoside. It is logical to base therapy on frequently isolated hospital pathogens. If a localized source of infection is found, consideration should be made to treat broadly, in addition to treating the diagnosed infection. If fever persists with negative cultures and no clear source of fever, antifungal therapy is often added, typically after 7 days. If the patient responds to therapy, antibiotics are generally continued until granulocytes return, because recurrent infection is not rare and may be life-threatening.

Antibiotic Issues

Dosing

Rational dosing of the wide variety of antibiotics currently available depends on the potency, pharmacokinetics, and toxicity of each drug). The dose needs to be diminished if excretion or metabolism of the antibiotic is slowed by renal or hepatic failure. Suggested doses of most antibiotics in varying degrees of renal failure can be found in many available handbooks and texts. The dose of some antibiotics should be decreased or the antibiotic avoided in liver failure. Antibiotics included in this group are cefoperazone, chloramphenicol, clindamycin, erythromycin, isoniazid, metronidazole, nafcillin, pyrazinamide, and rifampin. Conversely, dosing of antibiotics should be increased if excretion or metabolism of the drug is increased, such as in patients with burns[6,7] or cystic fibrosis.[14] For several frequently utilized agents in the ICU, it is possible and advisable to monitor serum levels to ensure that

Table 39-1. Antibiotics commonly used to treat serious infections

Drug	Daily Dose
Aminoglycosides	
Gentamicin	Ped: 5–7.5 mg/kg/d ÷ q8h
	Adult: 5 mg/kg/d ÷ q8h
Tobramycin	same as gentamicin
Amikacin	15–22 mg/kg/d ÷ q8–12h
	Adult: 15 mg/kg/d
Penicillins	
Penicillin G	100,000–300,000 u/d ÷ q4–6h
	max dose 24 million u/d ÷ q4h
Ampicillin	Ped: 100–200 mg/kg/d ÷ q6h
	200–300 mg/kg/d (meningitis)
	Adult: 4–12 g/d
Nafcillin	Ped: 100–150 mg/kg/d ÷ q4–6h
	Adult: 9–12 g/d
Oxacillin	Ped: 100–200 mg/kg/d
	Adult: 9–12 g/d
Ticarcillin	Ped: 200–300 mg/kg/d ÷ q4–6h
	Adult: 18g/d
Mezlocillin	200–300 mg/kg/d ÷ q4–6h
	Adult: 18g/d
Piperacillin	200–300 mg/kg/d ÷ q4–6h
	Adult: 18g/d
Cephalosporins	
Cefazolin	Ped: 50–100 mg/kg/d ÷ q6–8h
	Adult: 3–6 g/d
Cephalothin	Ped: 100–150 mg/kg/d ÷ q4–6h
	Adult: 6–12 g/d
Cefoxitin	Ped: 80–160 mg/kg/d ÷ q4–6h
	Adults: 4–12 g/d
Cefuroxime	Ped: 100–150 mg/kg/d ÷ q8h (severe, nonmeningitis)
	Adults 3–6 g/d ÷ q6–8h
Cefotaxime	Ped: 100–200 mg/kg/d ÷ q4–6h
	Adult: 4–12 g/d
Ceftriaxone	Ped: loading dose for meningitis 75 mg/kg, then 100 mg/kg/d ÷ q12h other serious infections: 50–100 mg/kg/d ÷ q12h Adult: 1–2 g q12–24h; max dose 4 g/d
Ceftazidime	Ped: 90–150 mg/kg/d ÷ q8h
	Adult: 3–6 g/d ÷ q8–12h
Others	
Chloramphenicol	50–100 mg/kg/d ÷ q6h
	Adults: 2–4 g/d
Clindamycin	Ped: 25–40 mg/kg/d ÷ q6–8h
	Adult: 1.2–2.7 g/d ÷ q6–8h
Metronidazole	Loading dose 15 mg/kg followed by 30 mg/kg/d q6h
Erythromycin	Ped: 20–50 mg/kg/d ÷ q6h
	Adult: 1–4 g/d ÷ q6h
Trimethoprim/ Sulfamethoxazole	15–20 mg/kg/d ÷ q6h of trimethoprim component
Vancomycin	Ped: 30–40 mg/kg/d ÷ q6–8h 45–60 mg/kg/d for CNS
	Adult: 2 g/d ÷ q6–12h

Note that this is only a partial listing. For a particular patient the dose may differ depending on the clinical situation. To adjust dosing in the presence of renal or hepatic failure and for information on precautions, side effects and interactions, the reader is referred to a pharmacology textbook.

adequate drug is being delivered while minimizing toxicity. Assessment of peak and trough serum levels of the aminoglycosides after several doses is particularly helpful because of their toxicity. A range of acceptable levels is often considered safe. It is reasonable to aim for the low end of the range to minimize toxicity if the infection is not severe and to adjust the dose to the upper end of the range if high levels are needed for an infection whose consequences may outweigh the risk of antibiotic toxicity. Serum levels of vancomycin are helpful if there is abnormal or changing renal function or when it is given together with an aminoglycoside or when there is uncertainty regarding the adequacy of the serum level.[15-17] Other antibiotics for which serum levels can be measured include chloramphenicol, sulfonamides, and flucytosine. Dosing recommendations for antibiotics for which no blood levels are available are often suggested as a range given in milligrams per kilogram (Table 39-1). A decision to use the top or bottom of this range depends, other factors being equal, on the severity of the potential or documented infection, the need to penetrate the CSF, and the toxicity of the drug. Because many of the doses have been estimated for smaller children, some caution needs to be applied in simply multiplying the dose by the child's weight. In particular, in an older or overweight child, a dose should be carefully examined to be sure that it is not greater than the maximum dosage recommended.

Many antibiotics interfere in some way with other drugs and can lead to adverse effects. The large number of different antibiotics make it difficult to generalize regarding the numerous potential toxic effects. Some side effects may be due to synergistic toxicity between drugs. For example, the combination of an aminoglycoside with some cephalosporins has been proposed by some authors to lead to the potentiation of drug-induced nephrotoxicity.[17] A similar effect has been described for the use of aminoglycosides with vancomycin.[18] Other side effects may be due to the effect of the antibiotic altering the effect or metabolism of a second drug. Examples are antibiotics (including chloramphenicol, isoniazid, metronidazole, trimethoprim/sulfamethoxazole, and some cephalosporins) that lead to an increased anticoagulant effect of oral anticoagulants and to the increase in blood levels of theophylline caused by erythromycin.[19]

Choice between Beta-Lactam Antibiotics

Penicillin was described by Flemming in the late 1920's[20] and was put into clinical use in the 1940's. Since then, many other antibiotics of different chemical structures have been discovered. Nonetheless, the penicillins and related antibiotics which share the beta-lactam ring (cephalosporins, carbapenems, and monobactams) remain useful because of their wide spectrum of activity against diverse bacteria and their relatively low toxicity. The choice of which beta-lactam antibiotic to use is based upon spectrum, toxicity concerns, availability, and cost. As with other antibiotics, therapy should be tailored to provide the narrowest spectrum possible in order to diminish the selection of resistant organisms and the incidence of superinfection.

Choice between Penicillins

Despite the availability of newer derivatives, penicillin G remains the drug of choice for many organisms. Penicillin G provides excellent coverage for most streptococci (including group A streptococci and pneumococcus), most of the organisms in the oral cavity, clostridia, and *N. meningitidis*. The resistance of many streptococci to penicillin G has been increasing in recent years. Clinically

important resistance is still somewhat unusual in most clinical settings; however, this problem should be kept in mind when using penicillin as a single agent for streptococci before antibiotic sensitivities are available. Some conditions for which penicillin G may be administered to patients in the PICU include: 1) infections due to meningococcus, Group A streptococcus, or pneumococcus (that is sensitive to penicillin), 2) synergistic therapy (with an aminoglycoside) for enterococcal infections, and 3) aspiration pneumonia (together with an aminoglycoside to cover colonizing gram-negative organisms). Ampicillin provides coverage against some enteric gram-negative bacilli but is destroyed by the beta-lactamases that are produced by many gram-negative organisms. The antistaphylococcal penicillinase-resistant penicillins (methicillin, nafcillin, and oxacillin) are primarily useful in treating infections with *S. aureus*. Each also provides good coverage against streptococci but no coverage for gram-negative organisms or many coagulase-negative staphylococci. In vitro testing for sensitivity is usually measured using methicillin, although the results are applicable to each of the three drugs. Sensitivity testing is important because a low percentage of strains of *S. aureus* have become resistant to all of the antistaphylococcal penicillins. These strains are known as methicillin-resistant *S. aureus* (MRSA). Vancomycin, a drug that is not a beta-lactam, is generally needed to treat these infections. Several penicillins (carbenicillin, ticarcillin, piperacillin, azlocillin, and mezlocillin) have been developed to expand the gram-negative spectrum and to provide coverage against *P. aeruginosa*. In general, these antibiotics are given in high doses, leading to a considerable salt load. They are usually used in combination with another antibiotic, typically an aminoglycoside, to achieve optimal killing and to diminish the emergence of resistant organisms. Each of these penicillins has anaerobic activity. Each of the latter three (ureido penicillins) can be used in combination with an aminoglycoside for the treatment of severe enterococcal infections[21] although other agents are preferred.

Choice between Cephalosporins

The large number of different cephalosporin antibiotics with almost identical-sounding names often cause confusion. Fortunately, the cephalosporins can be classified into several broad categories. The first-generation cephalosporins generally cover *S. aureus*, most streptococci that are sensitive to penicillin G, and some aerobic gram-negative bacilli (including many strains of *E. coli* and *Klebsiella*). They do not provide adequate coverage for enterococci.[22] Examples of this class include cephalothin and cefazolin. Second-generation cephalosporins were developed to increase the spectrum of the first-generation agents. While there are several in this category, the most useful for the pediatric patient population is cefuroxime. Cefuroxime is relatively resistant to beta-lactamase and provides coverage for beta-lactamase-producing *H. influenzae*, *Moraxella catarrhalis*, and many *Enterobacteriaciae*, yet maintains coverage for *S. aureus*. Although it was initially hoped that cefuroxime would treat meningitis, some failures have been described.[23] In general, coverage of methicillin-sensitive *S. aureus* is diminished in many of the second- and higher generation cephalosporins. The third generation of cephalosporins includes agents that have an even larger spectrum of activity. Two properties that were successfully sought were the ability to penetrate the CSF and the ability of some agents (e.g., ceftazidime and cefaperazone) to treat infections with *P. aeruginosa*. Ceftriaxone, one of the third-generation cephalosporins, has a long serum half-life, which allows single or twice daily dosing. Ceftriaxone provides some coverage of *S. aureus*, although an antistaphylococcal penicillin or a first-generation cephalosporin is preferable for this purpose.

Newer Beta-Lactam Antibiotics

Several agents have become available that have an increased spectrum of antibacterial activity, which may be useful in certain settings in the PICU.

Beta-Lactamase Inhibitors

One approach in broadening the spectrum of therapy is to combine a penicillin with a compound that inhibits beta-lactamase activity. Two such compounds are clavulanic acid and sulbactam. Clavulanate is a compound that itself has only a low level of antibacterial activity, but it can inhibit certain beta-lactamases and thereby expand the spectrum of beta-lactam antibiotics. Clavulanate acts as a "suicide inhibitor" by forming an acyl enzyme intermediate with the beta-lactamase, blocking its enzymatic activity in the process. Sulbactam has some antibacterial activity by itself (primarily against *Neisseria*, bacteroides, and some species of acinetobacter), but is used to expand the spectrum of other beta-lactam antibiotics in a manner similar to clavulanate by acting as a beta-lactamase inhibitor. Because there are different types of beta-lactamase, not all bacteria become susceptible to combination therapy. Organisms of particular relevance to pediatric infections that produce beta-lactamases and that can be inhibited include *S. aureus*, *H. influenzae*, *Neisseria gonorrheae*, *M. catarrhalis*, and bacteroides. In addition, most of the plasmid-mediated beta-lactamases present in gram-negative bacilli are inhibited by clavulanate or sulbactam. The inducible chromosomal beta-lactamases of enterobacter, proteus, serratia, *Pseudomonas*, acinetobacter, and citrobacter are not inhibited.

The beta-lactam/clavulanate combination that is currently available for IV use is ticarcillin/clavulanate. It is available in a fixed ratio combination of 3 g of ticarcillin with 100 mg of clavulanate. This combination increases the spectrum of ticarcillin against beta-lactamase-producing strains of *S. aureus* (but not MRSA), *M. catarrhalis*, *H. influenzae*, bacteroides, and some gram-negative bacilli. It does not significantly increase activity against organisms resistant to ticarcillin by mechanisms other than the production of beta-lactamase.[24] It may be helpful in the setting of mixed infections, where *S. aureus*, aerobic, and anaerobic gram-negative bacilli are present. The safety, efficacy, and dosage for children less than 12 years of age has not been definitively established. The adult dose is 3 g q4–6h (if < 60 kg, 50 mg/kg q4–6h) of the ticarcillin component. The dose needs to be modified in the presence of renal impairment.

The beta-lactam/sulbactam combination that is currently available is ampicillin/sulbactam in a fixed combination of 2 g of ampicillin with 1 g of sulbactam. Inclusion of sulbactam expands the spectrum of ampicillin to include beta-lactamase-producing strains of *S. aureus*, *H. influenzae*, *M. catarrhalis*, some Enterobacteriaceae, and many anaerobic bacteria, including bacteroides.[25] It is useful in the setting of mixed bacterial infections, but it is not active against *Pseudomonas*. Efficacy and safety in children less than 12 years of age has not been definitively established. The adult dose is 1 to 2 g of the ampicillin component given q6h and is modified in the setting of renal failure. Dosing in children should be based on the ampicillin component.

Monobactams

Aztreonam is a monocyclic beta-lactam whose spectrum of activity is limited to aerobic gram-negative bacilli. It is not hydrolyzed by most beta-lactamases and has activity against most *Enterobacteriaceae*, *H. influenzae*, *Neisseria*, and *P. aeruginosa*.[26] In vitro synergy of aztreonam with aminoglycosides has been demonstrated.[27] There is minimal allergic cross-reactivity with other beta-lactam antibiotics.[28,29] Aztreonam is particularly useful in settings in which there are resistant gram-negative bacilli or in which the patient is allergic to other beta-lactam antibiotics. In many cases, its narrow spectrum of activity precludes its use as a single agent. Aztreonam has not been approved for use in children. The adult dose is up to 2 g given q6–8h for severe infections. A dose that has been used in children with severe infections is 30 mg/kg given q6h. Doses need to be reduced when renal impairment is present.

Carbapenems

Imipenem is a carbapenem that is used in combination with a dehydropeptidase inhibitor called cilastatin, which blocks the destruction of imipenem by renal depeptidases. Imipenem is resistant to most beta-lactamses, although it is hydrolyzed by the beta-lactamses produced by *Xanthomonas maltophilia*, and some strains of bacteroides.[27] Imipenem has an extremely broad spectrum of activity. It is active against most gram-positive cocci. Exceptions include methicillin-resistant *S. aureus*, *S. epidermidis*, and some tolerant strains of group D streptococci. Imipenem is likewise effective against most gram-negative organisms, including *P. aeruginosa*, and against anaerobic organisms. It is useful for mixed infections or in cases in which there are multiple, resistant gram-negative organisms. It should be used in combination with other agents to treat serious infections, especially those due to *P. aeruginosa*, because the emergence of resistance was observed when it was used alone.[30,31] Seizures have been reported in a little more than 1% of patients receiving the drug, especially in patients receiving high doses or in the presence of renal failure or underlying neurologic disorders.[32] Imipenim has not been approved for use in children. The adult dose is up to a maximum of 1 g given q6h and the pediatric dose is 10 to 15 mg/kg q6h.

Choice between Aminoglycosides

The broad spectrum of activity of the aminoglycoside antibiotics against gram-negative organisms makes them useful in the ICU setting. Toxicity is probably equivalent between gentamicin, tobramycin, and amikacin if serum levels are monitored. For most situations, these three antibiotics are equal in efficacy. There are, however, a few situations in which one may be preferable to the others. Gentamicin provides better synergy with penicillin against *S. faecium* than the other aminoglycosides.[33] Tobramycin is slightly more active in vitro against *P. aeruginosa* and may cover a slightly higher percentage of *P. aeruginosa* than gentamicin.[34] Because constant use of aminoglycosides in the ICU leads to a population of antibiotic-resistant organisms, many institutions choose to hold amikacin in reserve for resistant organisms.

Allergies

Patients admitted to the ICU not infrequently have a history of allergy to one or several antimicrobial agents, limiting the choices for an antibiotic regimen. Every effort needs to be made to obtain as much information as possible concerning the history of allergy to assess the risk that a rechallenge with the antibiotic would entail. The easiest, and safest, solution is simply to avoid all antimicrobial drugs from the class to which the patient has an allergy. Sometimes, however, this is not possible in the setting of a life-threatening infection. In general, a history of an immediate-type hypersensitivity reaction or of a Stevens-Johnson-type reaction precludes rechallenge in all but the most extreme cases. On the other hand, the risk of rechallenging a patient who had a macular-papular eruption while on a number of different drugs needs to be weighed against the need for the antibiotic. Allergies to penicillins are a particular problem. In urgent situations, patients can be skin tested with a penicillin derivative to determine the risk of an immediate-type hypersensitivity reaction. A negative skin test makes the chance of a life-threatening reaction highly unlikely.[35] In general, all beta-lactam antibiotics should probably be avoided in patients with a history of a severe drug reaction to any other beta-lactam antibiotic. A useful exception is aztreonam, which is a monocyclic beta-lactam antibiotic with activity for gram-negative organisms that does not cross-react with most other beta-lactam antibiotics.[28,29]

Use of More Than One Antimicrobial Agent to Treat a Specific Organism

Although there are few carefully controlled studies, in most situations little is gained by using more than a single antibiotic to treat an infection caused by an organism known to be sensitive by routine in vitro testing. There are some exceptions to this rule. In certain settings, some organisms are not easily killed by a single antibiotic alone and require doses of two synergistic antibiotics to achieve adequate or more rapid killing. Examples are the use of penicillin or vancomycin together with an aminoglycoside to treat severe infections with enterococci, and the addition of rifampin or an aminoglycoside to vancomycin to treat persistent or difficult infections with coagulase-negative *Staphylococcus*. A second rationale for the use of more than one antibiotic is to reduce the chance of the selection of resistant organisms in settings in which this is likely. An example is the use of several different antibiotics to treat infections with mycobacteria. Finally, many infectious disease consultants employ two antibiotics with different mechanisms of action for the treatment of severe infections with gram-negative bacteria, especially in patients who have infections caused by *Pseudomonas* or who have a compromised immune system.[13,36–39]

Antimicrobial Therapy of Specific Organisms

Infections with Pseudomonas

Infections with *Pseudomonas* species are common in the ICU setting because of the inherent virulence of *Pseudomonas*, because of its tendency to cause illness in patients who are immunocompromised, and because it can colonize the water traps of sinks in the ICU, thereby providing a constant source for nosocomial spread by personnel. To treat infections with *Pseudomonas*, generally two antibiotics of different classes are used in relatively high doses. In part because of their presence in the ICU, where antibiotics are used constantly, *Pseudomonas* species tend to be relatively resistant to commonly used antibiotics. Of the species of *Pseudomonas* seen in the PICU, *P. aeruginosa* is usually the most frequently isolated. Other species, such as *P. cepacia* or *X. maltophilia*, occasionally cause infections and may be highly resistant. Antibiotics that are useful for the treatment of *P. aeruginosa* include aminoglycosides, antipseudomonas penicillins (carbenicillin, ticarcillin, azlocillin, mezlocillin, and piperacillin), certain third-generation cephalosporins (such as ceftazidime and cefoperazone), imipenem, and aztreonam.

Infections with Coagulase-Negative Staphylococci

Staphylococci are separated in the bacteriology laboratory on the basis of coagulase production. *S. aureus* is an organism of high virulence and is coagulase-positive. There are currently greater than 20 recognized species of coagulase-negative staphylococci.[40] All of these are, in general, of low virulence. One of these, *S. epidermidis*, is part of the normal flora of skin. Because coagulase-negative staphylococci behave similarly, it is not usually necessary to separate each subspecies. Coagulase-negative staphylococci are often contaminants of blood and other cultures. However, they are frequently pathogens in certain circumstances, including very young or immunocompromised patients or as an established infection on foreign bodies such as catheters.[41] Antibiotic sensitivity testing can be complicated by the presence of subpopulations of organisms that are resistant to methicillin, a phenomenon called heteroresistance. Strains that are resistant to methicillin are resistant to all beta-lactam antibiotics. Caution is needed because routine testing may indicate sensitivity when there are in fact some resistant bacteria present. Because of these difficulties, vancomycin is usually utilized for the primary antibiotic therapy for infections with coagulase-negative staphylococci. Vancomycin-resistant organisms have been described, but are rare. Gentamicin and rifampin are active against coagulase-negative staphylococci, but if used alone, there is rapid emergence of resistance. Although controversial, it may be reasonable to add an aminoglycoside and/or rifampin to vancomycin to achieve better killing of the organism in patients who have refractory infections.

Infections with Enterococci

Most enterococcal infections are due to *E. faecalis* or *E. faecium*. *E. faecalis* commonly colonizes the gastrointestinal tract and causes a variety of infections, including urinary tract infections, intraabdominal abscesses, bacteremia, and endocarditis. Soft-tissue infections are rare. The pathogenic role of *Enterococcus*, which is cultured from mixed infections, is not clear. The treatment of *Enterococcus* is difficult because the organism is resistant to most clinically achievable levels of antibiotics in blood. *E. faecium* tends to be more resistant than *E. faecalis*.[33] The combination of an aminoglycoside together with certain penicillins or vancomycin is synergistic for killing *Enterococcus*, perhaps because cell wall damage induced by penicillin or vancomycin permits better penetration of the aminoglycoside.[42] Therefore, in systemic infections in which a bacteriocidal effect is needed, both an aminoglycoside together with a penicillin or vancomycin should be used. In general, for infections with *E. faecium*, gentamicin has better activity than tobramycin or amikacin.[33] Penicillin G, ampicillin, and the ureido penicillins provide better synergy than the antistaphylococcal penicillins. Cephalosporins are not synergistic.[22] High-grade plasmid-mediated aminoglycoside resistance has been reported in some strains of *E. faecium* and *E. faecalis*.[43] Additionally, several aminoglycoside-resistant strains of *E. faecalis* have been found that also produce beta-lactamases.[44] Susceptibility to a particular aminoglycoside should be checked in cases of severe infection. Inducible resistance to vancomycin has also been described in several strains of *E. faecalis* and *E. faecium*.[45,46] These strains are still uncommon, but are increasing in frequency. For uncomplicated urinary tract infections, penicillin or ampicillin alone is sufficient because of the high concentration of drug that is achieved in urine.

Infections with Penicillin-Resistant Streptococci pneumoniae

Although penicillin G has classically been the drug of choice for pneumococcal infections, the number of pneumococcal strains that are resistant to penicillin is increasing,[47] and isolates of pneumococcus from the blood, CSF, or other infected body fluids should be screened for resistance. An oxacillin disk is used for the initial screening, followed by the determination of the MIC of the isolate to penicillin G. Isolates with an MIC 0.1 to 1.0 μg/ml are considered to have intermediate-level resistance to penicillin. Isolates with an MIC greater than 1 μg/ml are considered to have high-level resistance to penicillin. Antibiotics that can be useful in treating infections caused by resistant pneumococci include vancomycin, cefotaxime, and ceftriaxone. Isolates with intermediate resistance to penicillin can sometimes be treated by using very high doses of penicillin G, although this should be done very cautiously, and probably not in cases of meningitis. Careful testing is needed, because some strains may be resistant to multiple antibiotics (including chloramphenicol, trimethoprim-sulfamethoxazole, erythromycin, and clindamycin). Strains that have a very high MIC to penicillin may also have a high MIC to other beta-lactam antibiotics (e.g., cefotaxime or ceftriaxone). These strains are usually sensitive to vancomycin. Vancomycin may be the preferred antibiotic for these strains, although in some cases of infection of the CNS, vancomycin together with a third-generation cephalosporin may be a better choice because of ceftriaxone's superior penetration of the CSF. This complex area is rapidly evolving. For a detailed discussion, see Infections of the Central Nervous System by Pasternack, this volume.

Antimicrobial Therapy of Fungal Infections

Invasive infections with fungi occur primarily in patients whose immunity is altered and/or those who have been on an extended course of antibiotics. The diagnosis of tissue infections is difficult and requires a high index of suspicion, often coupled with an aggressive approach to obtain appropriate material for pathology and culture. It is convenient to separate infections caused by *Candida* from those caused by other fungi. Infections with *Candida* are relatively common, are often diagnosed by positive urine or blood cultures, and frequently can be treated medically. Other fungal pathogens are seen less frequently in the ICU setting and in general are more difficult to culture and treat.

Infections with Candida Species

Candida species grow readily on culture media utilized to isolate bacteria, although the sensitivity and speed of isolation can be enhanced by using special fungal media. Because the skin and mucosal surfaces of patients in the ICU are frequently colonized with *Candida*, cultures of sputum and wounds are often positive in the absence of infection. Ordinarily, these cultures have little diagnostic value, although a report has suggested that the isolation of *Candida* from three or more other sites in patients who are immunocompromised correlates with disseminated infection.[48] Special blood-culturing techniques are available that increase the yield of isolation of fungus from the blood by concentrating microorganisms before planting the cultures so that they can be directly plated on appropriate media. Blood cultures that are positive for *Candida* may indicate infection of an IV catheter or tissue. In this situation, more cultures should be obtained from blood and other relevant sites. False-positive blood cultures due to skin contamination are rare, and in most cases it is prudent to start specific antifungal therapy pending further investigations, even if the patient looks relatively well. Therapy can then be adjusted if subsequent cultures are negative. On the other hand, the diagnosis of disseminated candidasis is difficult; less than half of patients with disseminated candidasis have positive blood cultures.[49] A positive urine culture for *Candida* with pyuria suggests cystitis, although contamination of the culture by the perineum is frequent. *Candida* cystitis is often easily treated with irrigation of the bladder with dilute amphotericin B or nystatin urinary solutions. For refractory infections, another option is fluconazole. Still another possibility is a low dose of flucytosine, which is primarily excreted by the kidneys. Treatment by irrigation of the bladder with an antifungal agent is theoretically preferable because there is little associated toxicity. Ultrasound should be considered to rule out infection that has ascended to involve the ureters and renal pelvis.

In vitro testing of fungi for antimicrobial sensitivity is difficult to perform and interpret and is generally not helpful. There are only a few antifungal agents available that can be given systemically and that are effective.[50-54] Amphotericin B has been the mainstay of therapy for several decades and continues to be the drug of choice for most severe fungal infections. Flucytosine is occasionally included in certain situations to provide synergy. Fluconazole is a newly developed imidazole. Its role in the prophylaxis and therapy of fungal infection is still evolving. A short synopsis of each drug with dosing parameters is given next.

Amphotericin B

Amphotericin B is a broad antifungal agent that binds to ergosterol and leads to leaky fungal cell membranes. It requires IV administration and is toxic, causing dose-dependent nephrotoxicity (decreased glomerular filtration, potassium and magnesium wasting) and anemia. It may be associated with systemic reactions during its administration. Some experts suggest a test dose of 0.1 mg/kg (up to 1 mg), followed by an initial dose of 0.25 mg/kg if the test dose is not accompanied by toxicity. Doses are gradually increased by 0.05 mg/kg/d until a final dose of 0.6–0.8 mg/kg/d is reached. In severely ill patients, the dose may be increased more rapidly. A single daily dose of 0.8 to 1.0 mg/kg may be required, although this dose is accompanied with a higher incidence of toxic side effects. Premedication with acetaminophen and diphenhydramine hydrochloride and coadministration of hydrocortisone may decrease the incidence of systemic reactions that may occur during the infusion. Levels of creatinine, potassium, magnesium, and hemoglobin or hematocrit should be monitored during therapy. Although renal wasting of cations and anemia often occur with long-term treatment, usually therapy can be continued with potassium and magnesium supplementation unless there is a rapidly rising creatinine, in which case the dose should be held until renal function has improved.

Flucytosine

Flucytosine is an orally administered drug that interferes with fungal nucleic acid synthesis. Flucytosine should not be used alone, except in urinary candidasis, because resistant yeast may emerge. Under some circumstances, such as in persistent, severe infections with *Candida*, torulopsis, or *Cryptococcus*, it may be desirable to use flucytosine (50–150 mg/kg/d divided q6h) in combination with amphotericin B. The dose is limited by toxicity to the kidneys and bone marrow, especially when given with amphotericin B. Accordingly, serum levels should be monitored while on therapy.

Fluconazole

Fluconazole is an imidazole that inhibits ergosterol biosynthesis. It has been approved for the treatment of candidasis and cryptococcal meningitis.[55] Three advantages are that it may be given orally or intravenously, that it is well tolerated with little toxicity, and that it has excellent CNS penetration. For these reasons, fluconazole appears to be a very promising alternative to the two older antifungal agents. The recommended dose for children aged 3 to 13 years is 3 to 6 mg/kg/d (the dose for children has not been definitively established and higher doses are being evaluated), given orally or intravenously as a single dose. The dose is 200 to 400 mg/d for adults. Fluconazole interacts with or alters the metabolism of several commonly used drugs, including warfarin, phenytoin, rifampin, and sulfonylureas. Resistance to fluconazole is observed most frequently in species other than candida albicans including candida Krusei, candida tropicalis, and Torulopsis glabrata.

Antiviral Therapy

Antiviral therapy is still evolving. At present, there are few antiviral agents that are useful in the PICU setting. The two agents most frequently used are acyclovir, for the treatment of certain herpes viruses, and ribavirin, for the treatment of severe infections with respiratory syncytial virus.

Acyclovir is an acyclic nucleoside analogue of guanosine that has activity against herpes simplex virus (HSV) and varicella zoster virus (VZV). The decision to treat depends on the clinical setting, because infections with each of these herpes viruses may not require systemic therapy. Two commonly encountered situations in the ICU in which treatment with acyclovir is clearly beneficial are disseminated infection with HSV or VZV in an immunocompromised host and encephalitis caused by HSV in a normal host. Acyclovir is also used for the treatment of progressive cutaneous disease or esophagitis caused by HSV. Slightly higher doses are needed for VZV than for HSV. The dose of acyclovir for disseminated varicella is 10 mg/kg q8h for patients less than 1 year of age, and 500 mg/m² IV q8h for older children. The dose for herpes simplex (disseminated herpes or herpes encephalitis) is 10 mg/kg IV q8h. Doses of acyclovir should be adjusted in the presence of renal impairment. Acyclovir is generally well tolerated. Therefore, a risk-benefit analysis favors treatment in the frequent situation in which the diagnosis is suggestive but not definite. Crystallization in the renal collecting system can occur and is diminished by administering the drug with adequate fluid over an hour. Resistant strains of herpes have been reported, but have not as yet become a widespread problem.

Ribavirin is a guanosine analogue that has been studied primarily for use as a continuous aerosol in children who have severe infections caused by respiratory syncytial virus. Multiple studies suggest that the patient populations that may benefit from therapy are children at high risk for severe disease (particularly patients with underlying cardiac or pulmonary disease[56] or immunodeficiency[57]), premature or very young infants, or patients with progressive respiratory distress.[3] Technological advances now permit its safe use in ventilated patients.[58,59]

Chemoprophylaxis for Contacts of Patients with Infections in the Pediatric Intensive Care Unit

For a limited number of infections that are seen in the PICU, antimicrobial chemoprophylaxis is thought to be of value in reducing the incidence of secondary infection in close contacts. This is a subject of considerable controversy and few data. Guidelines for prophylaxis for many situations can be found in the *Red Book—Report of the Committee on Infectious Diseases* of the American Academy of Pediatrics.[60] It should be kept in mind that some of the agents used in prophylaxis may have unknown or toxic effects in a particular individual. An example is the use of rifampin in pregnancy.

Meningococcal Disease

Surveillance studies of nonepidemic situations have demonstrated that a small percentage of untreated household contacts of patients who have infection with *N. meningitidis* may develop meningococcal infection.[61] Some evidence suggests that treating close contacts with an appropriate antibiotic may decrease the risk of colonization or infection.[62] Medical personnel who have had heavy exposure to respiratory and oral secretions prior to the initiation of antibiotics in the index patient should also be treated. Rifampin is suggested at a 10-mg/kg dose (maximum dose 600 mg) every 12 hours for 2 days. Infants younger than 1 month should receive a 5-mg/kg dose twice a day for 2 days. Alternative agents include a single dose of ceftriaxone or ciprofloxacin (adults only), although there is less experience with these agents, or sulfasoxazole if the isolate is susceptible. The index patient should also receive prophylaxis prior to discharge to eradicate colonizing organisms.

Haemophilus influenzae *Type B*

Treatment of close contacts of patients with invasive infections caused by *H. influenzae* type B may decrease the occurrence of secondary disease in these individuals and their susceptible household contacts. Young children less than 4 years of age who have not acquired antibody are at the highest risk. Prophylaxis is suggested for all household contacts (irrespective of age) when there is one child less than 4 years of age who is unvaccinated (with *Hemophilus* conjugate vaccine) or who is immunosuppressed. All members of a household with a child less than 12 months of age should receive prophylaxis. The theory behind the treatment of contacts older than 4 years is not to protect these individuals but to eradicate the organism so that susceptible children will not be exposed to the organism. Patients with invasive infections caused by *H. influenzae* should receive prophylaxis prior to discharge. Rifampin is recommended at a dose of 20 mg/kg (maximum dose 600 mg) once daily for 4 days. The dose may be adjusted to 10 mg/kg in contacts less than 1 month of age. The need to treat daycare and nursery school groups is controversial and complex. For this situation and in special circumstances not outlined here, detailed guidelines can be found in the *Red Book—Report of the Committee on Infectious Diseases* of the American Academy of Pediatrics.[60]

Bordetella Pertussis

Mortality in patients with pertussis is highest in the first 6 months of life. Furthermore, immunity induced by vaccination is not absolute in its protection against pertussis. It is therefore recommended that all household and close contacts of patients with pertussis receive erythromycin. This is important in older children and adults to diminish the likelihood that they will transmit infection to younger children who may develop severe disease. Erythromycin is thought to eliminate carriage of the organism and may halt the development of disease if given very early in the course of illness. The dose is 40 to 50 mg/kg/d divided q6h (maximum dose 2 g/day) for 14 days. Close contacts under 7 years of age should receive a booster or a scheduled dose of vaccine.

Mycobacterium tuberculosis

Most contacts of patients with tuberculosis can be simply evaluated for the presence of active or incubating infection with a PPD skin test. In infants and young children, however, *M. tuberculosis* may cause disseminated disease and/or meningitis at presentation. Accordingly, close contacts of patients admitted with active tuberculosis should be evaluated for their risk of exposure, either from the patient or through a common source (e.g., a parent or relative). Children less than 4 years of age who have a history of exposure should have a PPD planted and should be treated for presumptive tuberculosis, even in the absence of clinical or laboratory findings of infection. If the PPD is negative, treatment should continue for 12 weeks after the contact has been made, and the PPD should be repeated. Then, if the PPD is still negative, and the patient is not anergic, the treatment can be stopped. Further details can be found in the Red Book—Report of the Committee on Infectious Diseases of the American Academy of Pediatrics.[60]

Acknowledgment

The authors thank Mark Pasternack, M.D., and George Jacoby, M.D., for their thoughtful comments.

References

1. Grayston JT et al. A new respiratory tract pathogen: *Chlamydia pneumoniae* strain TWAR. *J Infect Dis* 161:618–625, 1990.
2. Grayston JT. Chlamydia pneumoniae (TWAR) infections in children. *Pediatr Infect Dis J* 13:675–85, 1994.
3. Smith DW et al. A controlled trial of aerosolized ribavirin in infants receiving mechanical ventilation for severe respiratory syncytial virus infection. *N Engl J Med* 325:24–29, 1991.
4. Bartlett JG et al. Lessons from an animal model of intra-abdominal sepsis. *Arch Surg* 113:853–857, 1978.
5. Wilcox CM, Dismukes WE. Spontaneous bacterial peritonitis: A review of pathogenesis, diagnosis, and treatment. *Medicine* 66:447–456, 1987.
6. Glew RH, Moellering RC Jr, Burke JF. Gentamicin dosage in children with extensive burns. *J Trauma* 16:819–823, 1976.
7. Loirat P et al. Increased glomerular filtration rate in patients with major burns and its effect on the pharmacokinetics of tobramycin. *N Engl J Med* 299:915–919, 1978.
8. Prince A et al. Management of fever in patients with central vein catheters. *Pediatr Infect Dis* 5:20–24, 1986.
9. Flynn PM et al. *In situ* management of confirmed central venous catheter related bacteremia. *Pediatr Infect Dis* 6:729–734, 1987.
10. Decker MD, Edwards KM. Central venous catheter infections. *Pediatr Clin North Am* 35(3):579–612, 1988.
11. Press OW et al. Hickman catheter infections in patients with malignancies. *Medicine* 63:189–200, 1984.
12. Eppes SC, Troutman JL, Gutman LT. Outcome of treatment of candidemia in children whose central catheters were removed or retained. *Pediatr Infect Dis* 8:99–104, 1989.
13. Hughes WT et al. Guidelines for the use of antimicrobial agents in neutropenic patients with unexplained fever. *J Infect Dis* 161:381–396, 1990.
14. de Groot R, Smith AL. Antibiotic pharmacokinetics in cystic fibrosis differences and clinical significance. *Clin Pharmacokinet* 13:228–253, 1987.
15. Cantu TG, Yamanaka-Yuen NA, Lietman PS. Serum vancomycin concentrations: Reappraisal of their clinical value. *Clin Infect Dis* 18:533–543, 1994.
16. Moellering RC. Monitoring serum vancomycin levels: Climbing the mountain because it is there. *Clin Infect Dis* 18:544–546, 1994.
17. Wade JC et al. Cephalothin plus an aminoglycoside is more nephrotoxic than methicillin plus an aminoglycoside. *Lancet* 2:604–606, 1978.
18. Goetz MB, Sayers J. Nephrotoxicity of vancomycin and aminoglycoside therapy separately and in combination. *J Antimic Chemother* 32:324–334, 1993.
19. Paulsen O et al. The interaction of erythromycin with theophylline. *Eur J Clin Pharmacol* 32:493–498, 1987.
20. Fleming A. On the antibacterial action of cultures of a penicillium, with special reference to their use in the isolation of *B. influenzae*. *Br J Exp Pathol* 10:226–236, 1929.
21. Donowitz GR, Mandell GL. Beta-lactam antibiotics (first of two parts). *N Engl J Med* 318:419–426, 1988.
22. Moellering RC, Swartz MN. Drug therapy: The newer cephalosporins. *N Engl J Med* 294:24–28, 1976.
23. Marks WA et al. Cefuroxime versus ampicillin plus chloramphenicol in childhood bacterial meningitis: A multicenter randomized controlled trial. *J Pediatr* 109:123–130, 1986.
24. Sutherland R et al. Antibacterial activity of ticarcillin in the presence of clavulanate potassium. *Am J Med* 79 (Suppl 5B):13–24, 1985.
25. Retsema JA et al. Sulbactam/ampicillin: *In vitro* spectrum, potency, and activity in models of acute infection. *Rev Infect Dis* 8 (Suppl 5):S528–S534, 1986.
26. Lebel MH, McCracken GH Jr. Aztreonam: Review of the clinical experience and potential uses in pediatrics. *Pediatr Infect Dis* 7:331–339, 1988.
27. Donowitz GR, Mandell GL. Beta-lactam antibiotics (second of two parts). *N Engl J Med* 318:490–500, 1988.
28. Adkinson NF Jr, Swabb EA, Sugerman AA. Immunology of the monobactam aztreonam. *Antimicrob Agents Chemother* 25:93–97, 1984.
29. Saxon A, Swabb EA, Adkinson NF Jr. Investigation into the immunologic cross-reactivity of aztreonam with other beta-lactam antibiotics. *Am J Med* 78 (Suppl 2A):19–26, 1985.
30. Krilov LR et al. Imipenem/cilastatin in acute pulmonary exacerbations of cystic fibrosis. *Rev Infect Dis* 7 (Suppl 3):S482–S489, 1985.
31. Acar JF. Therapy for lower respiratory tract infections with imipenem/cilastatin: A review of worldwide experience. *Rev Infect Dis* 7 (Suppl 3):S513–S517, 1985.
32. Wang C et al. Efficacy and safety of imipenem/cilastatin: A review of worldwide clinical experience. *Rev Infect Dis* 7(Suppl 3):S528–S536, 1985.
33. Moellering RC et al. Species-specific resistance to antimicrobial synergism in *Streptococcus faecium* and *Streptococcus faecalis*. *J Infect Dis* 140:203–208, 1979.
34. Brogden RN et al. Tobramycin: A review of its antibacterial and pharmacokinetic properties and therapeutic use. *Drugs* 12:166–200, 1976.
35. Weiss ME, Adkinson NF. Immediate hypersensitivity reactions to penicillin and related antibiotics. *Clin Allergy* 18:515–540, 1988.
36. Andriole VT. Antibiotic synergy in experimental infection with pseudomonas. II. The effect of carbenicillin, cephalothin or cephanone combined with tobramycin or gentamicin. *J Infect Dis* 129:124–133, 1974.
37. Allan JD, Moellering RC. Antimicrobial combination in the therapy of infections due to Gram-negative bacilli. *Am J Med* 78(Suppl 2A):65–76, 1985.
38. Rahal JJ. Antibiotic combinations: The clinical relevance of synergy and antagonism. *Medicine* 57:179–195, 1978.
39. Klastersky J, Meunier-Carpentier F, Prevost JM. Significance of antimicrobial synergism for the outcome of Gram-negative sepsis. *Am J Med Sci* 273:157–167, 1977.
40. Patrick CC. Coagulase-negative staphylococci: Pathogens with increasing clinical significance. *J Pediatr* 116:497–507, 1990.
41. Noel GJ, O'Loughlin JE, Edelson PJ. Neonatal *Staphylococcus epider-*

midis right-sided endocarditis: Description of five catheterized infants. *Pediatrics* 82:234–239, 1988.

42. Moellering RC, Wennersten C, Weinberg AN. Studies on antibiotic synergism against enterococci. *J Lab Clin Med* 77:821–827, 1971.

43. Patterson JE, Zervos MJ. High-level gentamicin resistance in *Enterococcus*: Microbiology, genetic basis, and epidemiology. *Rev Infect Dis* 12:644–652, 1990.

44. Rhinehart E et al. Rapid dissemination of beta-lactamase-producing, aminoglycoside-resistant *Enterococcus faecalis* among patients and staff on an infant-toddler surgical ward. *N Engl J Med* 323:1814–1818, 1990.

45. Shlaes DM et al. Inducible, transferable resistance to vancomycin in *Enterococcus faecalis* A256. *Antimicrob Agents Chemother* 33:198–203, 1989.

46. Williamson R et al. Inducible resistance to vancomycin in *Enterococcus faecium* D366. *J Infect Dis* 159:1095–1104, 1989.

47. Friedland IR, McCracken GH Jr. Management of infections caused by antibiotic-resistant *Streptococcus pneumoniae*. *N Engl J Med* 331:377–382, 1994.

48. Young RC et al. Fungemia with compromised host resistance. *Ann Intern Med* 80:605–612, 1974.

49. Meunier F. Fungal infections in the compromised host. In Rubin RM, Young SL (eds): *Clinical Approach to Infection in the Compromised Host*. New York: Plenum, 1988. Pp 193–220.

50. Medoff G, Kobayashi GS. Strategies in the treatment of systemic fungal infections. *N Engl J Med* 302:145–155, 1980.

51. Gallis HA, Drew RH, Pickard WW. Amphotericin B: 30 years of clinical experience. *Rev Infect Dis* 12:308–329, 1990.

52. Bennett JE. Flucytosine. *Ann Intern Med* 86:319–322, 1977.

53. Como JA, Dismukes WE. Drug therapy: oral azole drugs as systemic antifungal therapy. *New Engl J Med* 330:263–272, 1994.

54. Presterl E, Graninger W, Multicentre study group. Efficacy and safety of fluconazole in treatment of systemic fungal infections in pediatric patients. *Eu J Clin Micro Infect Dis* 13:347–51, 1994.

55. Fluconazole for fungal infections. *FDA Drug Bull* 20:7–8, 1990.

56. Hall CB et al. Ribavirin treatment of respiratory syncytial viral infection in infants with underlying cardiopulmonary disease. *JAMA* 254:3047–3051, 1985.

57. McIntosh K et al. Treatment of respiratory viral infection in an immunodeficient infant with ribavirin aerosol. *Am J Dis Child* 138:305–308, 1984.

58. Outwater KM, Meissner HC, Peterson MB. Ribavirin administration to infants receiving mechanical ventilation. *Am J Dis Child* 142:512–515, 1988.

59. Frankel LR et al. A technique for the administration of ribavirin to mechanically ventilated infants with severe respiratory syncytial virus infection. *Crit Care Med* 15:1051–1054, 1987.

60. 1994 Red Book. *Report of the Committee on Infectious Diseases*. Elk Grove Village IL: American Academy of Pediatrics, 1994.

61. The Meningococcal Disease Surveillance Group. Meningococcal disease: Secondary attack rate and chemoprophylaxis in the United States, 1974. *JAMA* 235:261–265, 1976.

62. Meningococcal Disease Surveillance Group. Analysis of endemic meningococcal disease by sero group and evaluation of chemoprophylaxis. *J Infect Dis* 134:201–204, 1976.

Andrew L. Salzman

40 ▶ Acquired Immune Deficiency Syndrome

With the emergence of HIV infection in the early 1980s, AIDS has become one of the landmark medical events of the twentieth century. In the space of 10 years, the death of 100,000 young adults and children in the United States[1] has exerted a profound impact on medical, religious, and political institutions. Although the extent of childhood mortality in Western countries does not rival the consequences of the influenza outbreak of the 1920s or the polio epidemics of the 1950s, the dire prognosis of the disease and its particular means of transmission have captured international attention and concern.

At the beginning of the 1980s, as AIDS was first reported, it was not recognized as a significant threat to children but was thought to be concentrated in the homosexual and intravenous (IV) drug-abusing adult populations.[2] It soon became evident, however, that heterosexual transmission to women occurred with some regularity and that there was a major but ill-defined risk of subsequent vertical transmission.[2] Today, AIDS is increasing more rapidly among children than adults in the United States,[3] and AIDS-related mortality represents the ninth leading cause of death in the 5- to 14-year-old age group.[4] Since its recognition, AIDS has been diagnosed in 5000 American children and adolescents, and asymptomatic viral infection with HIV is estimated to include an additional 10,000 children.[5] In other continents, such as Africa, where heterosexual transmission of the disease is more prominent, AIDS has become a childhood killer on a pandemic scale.[6,7] The World Health Organization, for example, estimates that during the 1990s there will be several hundred thousand new pediatric cases worldwide and that more than a million uninfected children will be orphaned by the death of their HIV-infected parents.[6] Even in the unlikely event that an effective vaccine were to become available in the near future and further new HIV infections were prevented, existing children with HIV infection will increasingly place a demand on the medical system for the next several decades. As AIDS prophylaxis and supportive therapy improves, moreover, survival into late childhood and adolescence may be expected,[8] thereby further increasing the need for pediatric critical care.[4] Thus, the pediatric intensivist must become proficient in the recognition, diagnosis, and treatment of the myriad clinical features of HIV-related disease.

Epidemiology

HIV infection is thought to be transmitted by human immune cells in which the virus resides, whether in the form of an intact virion or in a latent form in which viral DNA is incorporated into the cellular genetic material.[9] Transmission of the virus is rather inefficient,[2] not occurring by means of fomites, aerosols, arthropods, bathing, casual contact, or limited mucosal contact such as kissing or sharing of toothbrushes. Successful transmission occurs only when infected cells of semen or blood enter the circulation directly via a needle stick or transfusion or indirectly via contact with a broken area of the skin or mucosa.[10] In the adult population, these modes of disease transmission occur in several well-defined groups.

1. Blood-borne transmission between IV drug abusers occurs when hypodermic needles contaminated with infected blood are shared.[10] Perhaps no other means of transmission is as effective, because the inocula of infecting cells is placed directly into the recipient's bloodstream. The great majority (85%) of such disease transmission occurs in the inner city African-American and Hispanic populations.[1,4]

2. Sexual transmission may occur during vaginal or anal intercourse.[10] HIV-infected male bisexuals and IV drug abusers are the major groups in the United States and Europe that transmit the disease to women by the sexual route.[2] In Africa and increasingly in developed countries, however, AIDS has entered the mainstream heterosexual population, so that the disease is less confined to certain geographic and subgroup enclaves. This widespread dissemination of HIV has contributed to the rapid rate of new infection in the general African population.

3. Blood-borne transmission by infected commercial blood products may occur, leading to a massive inoculation of virus and frequent disease transmission.[4] This route of infection led to an epidemic in the hemophiliac population in the early 1980s, prior to the period when blood products were screened routinely for the presence of HIV.[2] Recipients of cryoprecipitate were exposed to blood products pooled from thousands of donors, and the majority developed HIV infection. Since 1985, transfusions have been screened serologically for HIV, but there remains a finite probability, estimated as 1:38,000,[4] that infected blood may escape detection if the donor recently infected with HIV has yet to generate a serologic response. These facts should serve as a caution that the transfusion of blood products, while extremely safe, carries a a small but real risk of HIV transmission.[4] Transfusion of blood products must thus be reserved only for strong clinical indications and should involve, whenever possible, a discussion of this risk with the parents and their formal consent. In other countries, such as Romania, which lag in transfusion standards, transfusion-associated HIV infection is still of great concern.

The infant and childhood epidemiology of HIV infection differs most from that of the adult due to the route of transmission. Ninety percent of HIV infection in childhood is via a congenital route.[4,11] Adolescents may also have a similar route of transmission as adults if they are involved in drug abuse, promiscuity, and homosexual behavior,[5] or if they have received tainted blood products. Although rare, pediatric HIV infection may be acquired as a result of sexual abuse inflicted by infected adults.[2,4] Infection may be transmitted from the mother to her offspring in utero, at the time of delivery, or in the postpartum period.[2,4,11] The placenta is rich in CD4 T-cell receptors that bind the HIV virion and can allow the virus to reach the developing fetus as early as 12 weeks of gestation in a manner reminiscent of rubella.[4,12] Infection during early embryogenesis may result in fetal demise or survival with a recognizable microcephalic morphology, although the issue of dysmorphism has been questioned.[12,13] Infants may also acquire infection during parturition as they come into contact with the birth canal, as is typical in congenital hepatitis B infection.[4,11] Postpartum acquisition of HIV may occur via the ingestion of infected breast milk.[2,4,11] This has led to the recommendation in developed nations, where alternative milk sources are readily available,[11] that infected mothers refrain from breast feeding.

The relative contribution of these three different modes of vertical transmission to the current epidemic is unclear.[11] It is known that the rate of vertical transmission is variable, with the highest risk of congenital infection occurring when mothers have T4 cell counts of less than 200 (i.e., in mothers with the most advanced stage of immunosuppression in whom viral titers are the greatest).[4,14] In aggregate, vertical transmission has been found to range from 15% to 45%.[11] It is important to note than many mothers with HIV infection have not yet developed AIDS and may be unaware of their own infection until such time as their offspring become ill. It is not uncommon, therefore, for a family to be informed that their child has AIDS and to face the prospect that they and their siblings may be undiagnosed carriers of HIV infection. As a corollary to this, parents may refuse to consent to HIV testing of their children out of fear that such information might unmask undiagnosed parental disease.

The particular time of onset of vertical transmission has implications for viral burden, organ injury, and probably the time of onset and course of clinical disease.[7] In general, a bimodal incidence of AIDS is recognized in the pediatric population.[4,11] Some children present in the first years of life, with evidence of failure to thrive, loss of developmental milestones, recurrent infection, persistent thrush, and generalized lymphadenopathy and hepatosplenomegaly.[12,15] Often the initial presentation of this group of children is a fulminant opportunistic infection.[16] Even with aggressive support and a successful outcome, the prognosis for long-term survival is poor and rarely exceeds 1 year.[4] A second group of children appears to do well at first, but then develops insidious complaints of poor growth, chronic diarrhea, progressive dementia, developmental failure, and frequent respiratory infections superimposed on a picture of lymphocytic interstitial pneumonitis.[12] Such children may survive into late toddlerhood or early childhood before presenting with a major opportunistic infection. For unclear reasons, some children with congenital HIV infection present as late as 7 to 10 years of age.

The prognostic factors governing the onset and severity of childhood AIDS are not fully known. In adults, the CD4 count has been shown to define the relative risk in terms of acquiring *Pneumocystis carinii* pneumonia (PCP), and P24 antigen levels are predictive of the risk of progression to AIDS.[17] The situation is less clear in the pedatric age group due to the normal developmental changes in CD4 values. The ability to predict accurately the clinical course of HIV infection will become even more difficult in the future with the advent of effective prophylactic and treatment regimens.[17] Patients will be living longer, surviving previously fatal complications, and developing more of the multisystem dysfunction of HIV disease.

Immunology

Blood-borne HIV-infected cells are thought to transmit infection rapidly to immune cells of the host via the uptake by the T-cell CD4 receptor on the helper T-cell subset. The accumulation of virus in this manner leads to the progressive depletion of this cell population, resulting in a reversal of the normal helper (T4) to suppressor (T8) T-cell ratio.[12] The absolute number of remaining T4 cells is important prognostically in that those with more severe and long-standing disease will have fewer cells and are at greater risk of acquiring opportunistic infections.[12] The natural history of T-cell subpopulations has been only recently well characterized, and it appears that HIV-infected infants, particularly those less than 1 year of age, may develop opportunistic disease despite the presence of significantly higher T4 cells than their adult counter-

parts.[18] The function of the remaining T4 cells is also disturbed,[2] with a decline in the production of T-cell lymphokines, which regulate and support the immune response of other cells.[19] Lack of IL-2 production from T4 cells, for example, means that T cells that recognize specific pathogens may not proliferate appropriately and trigger corresponding B cells to mature into plasma cells and secrete antigen-specific immunoglobulins.[19] The high levels of IgG and IgM, often detected early in the course of childhood HIV infection,[2,12] represent a nonspecific surfeit of antibodies with no immune benefit.[19,20] The deficiency of IL-2 is also detrimental to the function of natural killer cells and cytotoxic T lymphocytes in the eradication of viral disease.[19] Common viral pathogens, such as cytomegalovirus (CMV), herpes simplex, varicella, and Ebstein-Barr virus (EBV), may thereby produce life-threatening infection in children with AIDS.[21]

The mononuclear phagocyte system, essential for the removal of opsonized pathogens and the formation of granulomas, is also impaired in HIV-infected children and may serve as a reservoir of HIV.[9,19] Infected macrophages are unable to adequately express Fc and complement receptors on their surface and cannot, therefore, clear opsonized pathogens.[19] The paucity of specific immunoglobulin and the down-regulation of immunoglobulin Fc receptors render the patient functionally asplenic, not unlike the child with advanced sickle cell disease.[19] Effective phagocytosis is also compromised by the marked deficiency in B-cell function and humoral immunity early in the course of the disease.[2] Children with AIDS are susceptible, therefore, to the development of cellulitis, impetigo, skin abscesses, otitis media, sinusitis, pneumonia, and fulminant sepsis produced by encapsulated organisms such as *Streptococcus pneumoniae*, *Hemophilus influenzae*, *Salmonella* sp, and *Staphylococcus aureus*.[2,19]

Although most HIV-infected children are not neutropenic, there is reason to believe, on the basis of adult data, that neutrophil chemotaxis and phagocytosis may not be optimal.[19] It is common for patients with AIDS to present with fulminant bacterial sepsis and mucocutaneous candidal infection,[12] suggesting a defect in neutrophil function.[19]

It is not known to what extent HIV infection affects the developing immune system in utero, but it is clear, by several months of age, that there is a broad derangement of multiple arms of the immune response, affecting the recognition of pathogens, the amplification of appropriate immune cell subpopulations in response to infection, and ultimately the delivery of an adequate effector cell response. The infant with HIV infection is, therefore, susceptible to serious disease from a wide range of viral, bacterial, fungal, and protozoal agents.[19]

Diagnosis

The differential diagnosis of a suspected immune dysfunction should include malignancy and congenital diseases, such as adenosine deaminase deficiency, DiGeorge syndrome, Wiskott-Aldrich syndrome, agammaglobulinemia, hypogammaglobulinemia, combined immunodeficiency, and TORCH infections.[2] In the patient greater than 15 months of age, a diagnosis of HIV infection is established by detecting the presence of antibodies directed at the HIV virion. An ELISA analysis is used as a rapid screen, followed by a Western blot study for confirmation.

In infants less than 15 months of age, these serologic-based methods may be confounded by residual maternal antibody acquired via a transplacental route.[11] Confirmation of HIV infection in this age group is made by viral culture of body fluids or by identifying the presence of genetic material from the HIV virion, using the highly sensitive technique of polymerase chain reaction (PCR).[22–24] These diagnostic methods are not universally available, so some patients are left with only a clinical suspicion of infection until the age of 9 to 12 months, by which time maternally transmitted antibody is no longer present.[22] Screening of immunoglobulins, T-cell subpopulations, and monitoring of clinical signs has been shown to identify HIV infection in half of infected children of this age group, with a specificity of 99%.[17]

Clinical Manifestations

Sepsis

The HIV-infected child is subject to a broad range of clinical infections[19,26] leading to sepsis and hemodynamic instability.[2,12] A focal source of infection may be identified in the lungs or gastrointestinal (GI) tract or a child may present with clinical evidence of sepsis without a localizing source. Given the broad spectrum of immunologic deficits in the child with AIDS, it is not surprising that such patients frequently become infected and develop fulminant sepsis. Thus, the response to the febrile child with AIDS should be aggressive, with a low threshold for diagnostic evaluation and rapid introduction of broad-spectrum antibiotic therapy and hemodynamic support.

For the child with a mild febrile illness acquired in the community, in the absence of a focal source of infection, it is reasonable to initiate therapy with a second-generation cephalosporin, such as cefuroxime, or with the combination agent ampicillin/sulbactam, after obtaining a complete blood count, blood culture, and chest roentgenogram. In the child under the age of 2, a urine culture should also be obtained. Hospital-acquired infections require broader antibiotic coverage, particularly if the patient has been admitted to the intensive care unit (ICU), where there is an increased incidence of infection with resistant gram-negative bacilli. In such instances, it is reasonable to initiate empiric therapy with ampicillin, to cover *Listeria* and *Enterococcus*, and a third-generation cephalosporin, such as cefotaxime (or ceftazadime, depending on the institutional prevalence of *Pseudomonas*). Children with more severe illness, as evidenced by toxicity or cardiovascular instability, should also receive vancomycin and antipseudomonal therapy. In the presence of pulmonary infiltrates, trimethoprim/sulfamethoxazole (TMP/SMX) should be added to this regimen to ensure coverage of *P. carinii*. A thorough examination for a febrile source is mandatory, and any localized infection should be treated aggressively. Due to the frequent finding of multiple pathogens and infectious processes in childhood AIDS, it is unwise to narrow therapy initially, even when a clear-cut source of infection is discovered. At all times, consideration must be given to the possibility of an opportunistic viral, fungal, parasitic, or mycobacterial infection that would escape treatment by the aforementioned empiric antibiotic regimen. The decision to expand therapy to cover such pathogens should be guided by clinical signs, laboratory data, and epidemiology. The risk of PCP, for example, may be estimated by comparing the T4 count to age-adjusted norms (Table 40-1).

Pulmonary Disease

Acute respiratory failure is one of the major causes of death in the pediatric HIV patient, with a reported mortality rate of greater than 90%.[25,26] Although the incidence of fulminating respiratory

Table 40-1. Increased risk of *Pneumocystis carnii* pneumonia by comparing T4 count to age-adjusted norms

Age (yrs)	CD4 count
0–1	<1500
1–2	<750
2–6	<500
>6	<200

Data from The Working Group on PCP Prophylaxis in Children. Guidelines for prophylaxis against *Pneumocystis carinii* pneumonia in children infected with the human immunodeficiency virus. *Morbidity and Mortality Weekly Report* 40:1–13, 1991.

disease may diminish in the future with the routine use of prophylaxis for PCP, it is likely that it will continue to represent the most common admitting diagnosis requiring intensive care.[14,26] Most acute respiratory failure in childhood AIDS results from infection with the protozoan *P. carinii* (13 of 31 cases in one series).[26] Pneumonia is also frequently associated with infection by CMV, *Aspergillus* sp, *Candida albicans*, and pyogenic, mycobacterial, and gram-negative nonenteric bacteria.[26] In one study, 48% of children with HIV who required mechanical ventilation had histologic evidence of PCP, 15% had lymphocytic interstitial pneumonitis (LIP), 7% had respiratory syncytial virus (RSV), and the remainder had evidence of infection with CMV, *Mycobacterium avium-intracellulare* (MAI), and *Pseudomonas aeruginosa*.[25] In a second series, the incidence of bacterial infections was much greater, second only to PCP.[26] It is, therefore, essential that children with HIV infection presenting with pulmonary disease receive broad spectrum empiric therapy pending a diagnostic study to define the responsible pathogen. Empiric therapy for the leading cause of acute respiratory failure, PCP, suggested by typical chest roentgen findings, an elevated serum lactate dehydrogenase, or a previous history of PCP,[18] should be followed by definitive pathologic diagnosis, for the following reasons:

1. Therapy with TMP/SMX is often toxic, although less in children than in adults.[18] Salvage therapy with pentamadine, eflorithane, or trimetrexate also involves the risk of significant toxicity and should not be considered unless the diagnosis is certain.[27]

2. Adjunctive use of steroids for PCP, which is now recommended in adults, may exacerbate fungal, viral, bacterial, and particularly mycobacterial disease.

3. Many pathogens are potentially treatable but would not be addressed routinely by the typical agents selected for empiric broad-spectrum coverage. Examples of such therapy would include the use of amphotericin for aspergillus infection, the combination of 5FC and amphotericin for severe candidiasis, ganciclovir for invasive CMV, isoniazid for tuberculosis, and ribavirin for RSV.[12]

Pulmonary disease severe enough to produce significant hypoxemia, or suggestive of a process other than an uncomplicated bacterial pneumonia, should lead to a diagnostic evaluation. This should include examination of sputum or tracheal secretions by Gram and acid-fast stains for the presence of polymorphonuclear leukocytes, bacteria, and fungi. Unless the child is neutropenic, the absence of moderate to abundant polymorphs suggests either an inadequate sampling of bronchial secretions, if a bacterial pneumonitis is present, or the absence of such infection. Deep endotracheal aspirates should also be stained for *P. carinii*, although the sensitivity in detecting cysts from this source was only 55% to 78% in an adult series, compared with a 90% recovery from fluid obtained by bronchoalveolar lavage.[26] Chest x-rays may reveal a lobar infiltrate characteristic of a bacterial pneumonia, a coarse granular pattern suggestive of LIP, or a bilateral diffuse alveolitis without hilar adenopathy typical of PCP.[23] The variability in roentgenographic findings of pneumonia in the immunocompromised patient is great enough, however, that the chest film should serve only as a screening process for pulmonary pathology.

If a deep tracheal aspirate is unrevealing, the workup should proceed to a bronchoalveolar lavage (BAL).[18,28] Fiberoptic bronchoscopy with lavage has been shown to be invaluable in identifying PCP, and the procedure is generally well tolerated by the child when performed by an experienced pediatric bronchoscopist.[26] Staining of BAL samples with Gomori's methenamine silver or toluidine blue[12] offers a diagnostic sensitivity approaching 90%.[28] Reference laboratories and tertiary research centers may employ monoclonal and other stains, but the routine methods previously described usually suffice. A diagnosis of PCP made by BAL should not discourage further evaluation for additional pathogens because coinfection may occur. PCP may present, for example, in conjunction with RSV,[12] parainfluenzae, influenza, CMV, and a wide range of typical childhood bacterial pathogens, as well as enteric and nonenteric gram-negative bacilli. BAL is equally important as a means of excluding PCP and defining the presence of bacterial and viral pathogens that are amenable to therapy.[28] Certain fungal infections, such as candidiasis and aspergillosis, are not readily diagnosed by BAL and require tissue diagnosis to distinguish colonization from infection.

In some series of immunocompromised children, therapy has been altered on the basis of the results of BAL in up to 80% of patients studied.[28] If a BAL is unrevealing, a repeat study should be performed after several days. In the event that the BAL remains nondiagnostic and the patient has severe and worsening respiratory disease, an open-lung biopsy may be considered.[26] Biopsies in this setting are nearly always diagnostic and may, therefore, permit aggressive and possibly toxic therapy when there is no doubt as to the etiology of the pulmonary failure.[26] The decision to proceed with such a procedure should take into account the adverse effects of a thoracotomy and general anesthesia, as well as the potential for creating air leaks and prolonging mechanical ventilation. If the child has not yet developed acute respiratory failure, the postoperative course is generally uneventful, requiring mechanical ventilation for only several days. In the setting of acute respiratory failure, however, the procedure is not without considerable risk. It should also be noted that there are no studies that have shown a clinical benefit from the procedure in terms of increased survival.[28] In centers without an experienced bronchoscopist, openlung biopsy may need to play an earlier role in the diagnostic evaluation of acute respiratory failure.[26] Alternative procedures that appear to be less aggressive, such as transbronchial or transthoracic biopsy, pose a significant risk of air leak in children and should not be attempted.[12]

Treatment of PCP is initiated with high-dose IV trimethoprim (15–20 mg/kg/d) and sulfamethoxazole (100 mg/kg/d) administered in four divided doses.[18] The preference by most clinicians for TMP/SMX is based on the relatively lower incidence and severity of drug toxicity.[18] TMP/SMX is, however, associated with dose-dependent bone marrow suppression, which may become significant in patients on zidovudine, an antiviral agent that inhibits HIV replication.[29] Exanthems, hepatic transaminase elevations,

and GI toxicity are common, but rarely severe and typically resolve following the discontinuation of the drug.[2] Overall, the incidence of significant adverse reactions of TMP/SMX is approximately 15%.[18] Parenteral pentamadine, an alternative therapy for PCP, is associated with the development of hypotension, neutropenia and azotemia.[12] Loss of glucose homeostasis, although uncommon, may be significant. There is no evidence to suggest that the failure to respond to TMP/SMX constitutes an indication to change therapy to IV pentamadine,[12] because almost 90% of patients with a poor response to TMP/SMX will show no better response with pentamadine.[27] The proper duration of therapy for PCP is still unclear, but there is a general consensus that a 2- to 3-week course is optimal.[19] There are no clinical trials, however, comparing 14 versus 21 days of therapy, nor are there studies in pediatric AIDS patients directed at resolving this question.

Respiratory support of the child with PCP should be guided by the degree of hypoxemia and ventilatory failure. Evidence of mild arterial desaturation and minimal respiratory distress is an indication for oxygen delivered by nasal cannula or face mask, advancing to a nonrebreather apparatus as required. With increasing severity of disease, there is a loss of functional residual capacity and vital capacity, resulting in a mismatch of ventilation and perfusion and the development of profound hypoxemia and increased work of breathing.[30] In the majority of pediatric patients with PCP, who are infants between 3 and 6 months of age, mechanical ventilation will be required. In many older children and adolescents, the degree of respiratory failure will clearly demand prompt intubation and mechanical ventilation, whereas in others the judicious use of face mask or nasal CPAP may suffice.[30] CPAP may need to be increased slowly in a stepwise fashion, allowing time for equilibration with each change and titrating pressure to the clinical response. Avoidance of high pressures is desirable in order to decrease the risk of barotrauma.[30] A requirement for CPAP in excess of 15 cm H_2O or the development of hypercarbia is an indication for endotracheal intubation and mechanical ventilation.[30]

Face-mask CPAP is usually tolerated in adult AIDS patients with PCP, but complications of barotrauma and aspiration may occur.[30] In a series of 18 adults with PCP, face-mask CPAP was associated with the development of a pneumothorax in only one patient.[30] The presence of an air leak and a tension pneumothorax should be considered in any patient on face-mask CPAP when a sudden deterioration in respiratory and hemodynamic variables occurs in association with decreased air entry and increased difficulty in obtaining good chest wall movement by bag-and-mask ventilation. Emergent evacuation of pleural air by the placement of a 14-gauge catheter through the second intercostal space in the midclavicular line may be life-saving in this setting. Gastric insufflation is an additional complication of face-mask CPAP therapy, because the increased air pressure in the pharynx may result in esophageal passage of gas.[30] On occasion, this may lead to gastric distension, which interferes with the provision of nutrition by nasogastric tube feedings and may precipitate emesis and pulmonary aspiration. Avoidance of excessive CPAP and venting of gastric air by a nasogastric catheter will reduce the risk of these complications. Placement of a fine-bore nasojejunal feeding catheter will often permit successful continuous enteral nutrition during CPAP therapy, despite some unavoidable gastric insufflation.[30]

PCP that progresses to respiratory failure requiring mechanical ventilation carries a poor prognosis, with an estimated mortality of 50% to 95%.[25] Respiratory failure from other pathogens, such as CMV, RSV, LIP, MAI, or *Pseudomonas* sp, is also associated with a bleak outcome, with an overall mortality of 81% in one series.[25] Pediatric AIDS patients who are intubated for indications other than acute respiratory failure, however, have a low incidence of mortality, reported as 9% in one series,[25] consistent with the prognosis in the general PICU patient population.

The management of mechanical ventilation in the AIDS patient with PCP or other causes of acute respiratory failure is not fundamentally different from that in children with adult respiratory distress syndrome (ARDS) or severe pneumonitis. Elevated levels of positive end-expiratory pressure (PEEP) are often required to maintain oxygenation without employing excessive levels of inspired oxygen. The deleterious effect of PEEP on systemic venous return may result in decreased preload and cardiac output. To some extent, this may be mitigated by volume loading and inotropic support. Both measures usually require the placement of a Swan-Ganz catheter to optimize left ventricular filling pressure and contractility. There is an impression that respiratory failure due to PCP is associated with the development of barotrauma more frequently than with other types of pulmonary infection; thus, the level of PEEP should be raised cautiously, and adequate sedation should be provided.[33] Muscle relaxants should be administered to prevent the development of air leak in children exposed to PEEP greater than 12 or a peak inspiratory pressure greater than 30 in the young infant or greater than 40 in the adolescent. Barotrauma is best avoided by using relatively low tidal volumes and accepting moderate levels of hypercarbia.

Despite their poor long-term prognosis, most HIV-infected patients with PCP will demonstrate a favorable response to IV TMP/SMX or pentamadine by the fifth day of therapy, with defervescence and a reduction in hypoxemia.[27] Prior to this time, the clinical status may actually worsen, probably due to the inflammatory effect elicited by antibiotic-mediated destruction of organisms. The adjunctive use of early corticosteroid therapy may alter this typical scenario by exerting an antiinflammatory effect on the alveolitis. Two randomized, prospective, double-blind studies in adults with PCP have demonstrated that the early use of steroids can improve survival and decrease the occurrence of respiratory failure.[31,32] In a nonrandomized prospective study, which included only adults with PCP requiring CPAP or mechanical ventilation, there was a decreased mortality with the addition of corticosteroids.[33] A consensus statement by an expert National Institutes of Health (NIH) panel now recommends the early adjunctive treatment with methylprednisolone in AIDS patients greater than 13 years of age with documented or suspected PCP, if there is moderate to severe pulmonary dysfunction (i.e., an AaDO$_2$ gradient >35 mm Hg or a PaO$_2$ of <70 mm Hg in room air). Adjunctive use of steroids should be started within 72 hours of the initial antipneumocystis therapy.[34] To date, there have been no prospective randomized trials of steroid use in pediatric or infant AIDS patients with PCP. It would seem reasonable, however, to extrapolate the results of the adult studies, given the magnitude of the observed effect and the lack of any serious toxicity noted.[18,21] Some studies have found that patients demonstrated a favorable initial response to adjunctive corticosteroid therapy, only to have limited survival owing to a high relapse rate once steroids were discontinued.[35] This may have resulted from steroid-mediated immunosuppression of macrophage function, which may be necessary to eradicate alveolar pneumocystic infection.[36] Steroids are well known to impede the clearance of fungal and mycobacterial infection, so their use should be restricted to settings in which the presence of additional pathogens has been excluded. The potential for the relapse of PCP after the conclusion of steroid therapy has led some centers to recommend a steroid taper.[31]

Treatment of other opportunistic pathogens presenting with acute respiratory failure has a particularly poor prognosis. CMV pneumonitis, which may present with hypoxia and nonspecific diffuse pulmonary infiltrates, has a mortality of 86%, and even higher if present in combination with PCP.[37] The antiviral agent ganciclovir has had some success in this setting, but its use is associated with a high rate of relapse.[37] Treatment, therefore, with this potentially toxic drug should proceed only after tissue biopsy confirmation, because the mere presence of CMV in BAL fluid may reflect colonization rather than parenchymal infection.

MAI pneumonia presents late in the course of AIDS, with fever, drenching sweats, weight loss, cough, dyspnea, and hemoptysis, and with chest roentgen findings of diffuse infiltrates.[21,38] Adult patients typically demonstrate profound immune dysfunction by the time they present with MAI, with the mean number of T4 cells less than 60/μL.[39] Focal pneumonia may occur in isolation, but dissemination usually ensues, involving blood, bone marrow, liver, spleen, and variety of other organs. Diagnosis is best established by the culture of bone marrow, lymph node, or liver.[39] Blood is cultured by special techniques, involving the lysis of the cellular fraction, with a sensitivity of 98% in one study.[39] Antibiotic therapy can provide significant symptomatic relief and may clear the bacteremia. Combination regimens with ethambutol, clofazamine, ciprofloxacillin, and rifampin are well tolerated and effective if given for greater than 3 months' duration. Death rarely results directly from infection with MAI, but instead is the consequence of immunosuppression and sepsis from emaciation induced by the infection.[39]

LIP is a chronic pulmonary process seen in older HIV-infected children.[4] The etiology of LIP is unclear but may be related to EBV infection, leading to the hyperplasia of bronchial-associated lymphoid tissue.[40] The onset of symptoms tends to be insidious, unlike the typically fulminant presentation of PCP.[15] Lung biopsy remains the only definitive means to establish the diagnosis, but clinical and laboratory data may show suggestive symptoms and signs: parotid gland enlargement, lymphadenopathy, clubbing, reticulonodular interstitial infiltrates on chest x-ray, hyperglobulinemia, lymphocytosis, and increased gallium uptake on radionuclide lung scan.[12,41] Clinical symptoms of hypoxemia are typically mild, with rare instances of respiratory failure reported in the presence of a coexistent pulmonary infection.[42] Bronchodilator therapy and supplemental oxygen are sufficient in the majority of cases.[12] Steroids may also be effective in hypoxemic patients and are given as a 2-mg/kg daily bolus of methylprednisolone[42] for 2 to 4 weeks, followed by a taper.[21,43]

Cardiac Disease

Cardiac disease develops in the HIV-infected child as a primary response to viral infection of cardiovascular tissue or as a secondary response to pulmonary failure.[12] As a primary entity, clinically significant cardiac impairment is estimated to occur in 27% of HIV-infected children, with the majority of patients presenting after the age of 1 year but with reports of heart failure in infants as young as 2 months.[43] The initial symptoms reflect a disturbance in vascular tone, manifested as a hyperdynamic circulation with diminished peripheral vascular resistance and increased contractility. Later in the course of the infection, a dilated, poorly contractile ventricle may be recognized by echocardiography, with pathologic diagnosis revealing the presence of hypertrophy, necrosis of myocardial fibers, and an inflammatory infiltrate.[12] Cardiac disease often remains clinically silent until precipitated by sepsis, anemia, or hypoxemia.[37] Given the high incidence of cardiac and vascular pathology, it is advisable to obtain an ECG and to initiate central venous pressure monitoring early in the course of shock or acute respiratory failure to diagnose compromised ventricular function and guide cardiovascular management.

Autonomic dysfunction may also contribute to abnormal vascular tone and chronotropy secondary to a sympathetic neuritis or direct HIV infection of the atrial wall. Arrhythmias are common, ranging from sinus arrhythmia with a wandering atrial pacemaker to high-grade ventricular ectopy. It appears that patients with significant ectopy have increased left ventricular contractile function with decreased afterload.[43] It is unclear whether arrhythmias in HIV-infected children result from a primary myocardial pathology or an underlying autonomic and vascular dysfunction. Ventricular tachycardia and fibrillation have also been reported in association with the use of pentamadine in the treatment of PCP.[43]

Patients with PCP and severe hypoxemia may have electrocardiographic evidence of myocardial ischemia.[27] When this occurs, left ventricular failure may be precipitated by PEEP and excessive fluid administration. Careful use of diuretics may lessen the risk of cardiac decompensation in the critically ill patient with PCP and underlying myocardial disease.[27]

Gastrointestinal Disease

Pathology may occur along any aspect of the GI tract, contributing to diarrhea, dehydration, failure to thrive, abdominal pain, and, rarely, an acute abdomen with obstruction, perforation, or hemorrhage.[44] The oral cavity is often involved, but rarely in a critical way, with viral or fungal disease, which may result in odontophagia and exacerbate an underlying malnourished state. *C. albicans* infection of the oral mucosa may cause thrush,[2] characterized by the presence of white adherent plaques that leave bleeding points when forcibly scraped off of the underlying mucosa.[2,4] KOH preparations of the scrapings will confirm the presence of budding yeasts. Treatment with ketaconazole or clotrimazole may temporarily reduce or clear the infection.[45] On occasion, thrush may be confused with herpes simplex virus (HSV), which presents with oral vesicular lesions of gingivostomatitis.[2,12] Diagnosis of HSV may be established by viral culture, immunofluorescent staining, or Tzanck smear. Treatment with acyclovir, if needed, should continue until all lesions have crusted and there is no evidence of disseminated HSV disease.

Esophagitis, causing dysphagia and substernal chest pain, may result from infection by *C. albicans*, HSV, and CMV, although the latter agent more commonly infects the colon rather than the esophagus and small intestine.[46] Confirmation of esophagitis may reliably be made by barium swallow, but identity of the responsible pathogen requires endoscopy with biopsy.[46] Candidal infection that fails to respond to oral antifungal agents may be treated with low-dose IV amphotericin B at 0.1 mg/kg/d, which is usually effective and well tolerated, free of the nephrotoxic complications often seen with dosing regimens employed for deep tissue infection.[21] HSV esophagitis requires treatment with IV acyclovir until lesions have resolved, at least for a minimum of 2 weeks. CMV infection of the esophagus is less common and, at present, has no approved therapy available, although trials with the nucleoside ganciclovir have shown it to be especially effective in the treatment of GI infections.[46]

Clinical hepatic disease is uncommon in HIV-infected children, although many will have evidence of hepatic enlargement and transaminase elevations.[12] Initial evaluation should include (1)

serologic studies to rule out common viral pathogens; (2) bacterial, fungal, and mycobacterial cultures of blood; and, on occasion, (3) cultures of biopsied liver. Pathologic examination may reveal infiltrates of lymphocytes and plasma cells, granulomas, and cholestasis, reflecting the wide range of pathogens that may contribute to hepatic disease in the HIV-infected child. The differential diagnosis includes viral agents, such as EBV; CMV; HSV; varicella; hepatitis A, B, and C; mycobacterial pathogens, such as *Mycobacterium tuberculosis* and MAI; and fungi or yeasts.[12] In septic states, liver failure may occur in the context of multiple-organ failure so that biopsies may be less revealing and associated with a substantial risk of hemorrhage from any underlying coagulopathy.

Gastroenteritis may result from the full range of opportunistic pathogens as well as more typical bacterial agents. Children with AIDS often present with long-standing malabsorption and diarrheal syndromes, with failure to thrive.[37] On occasion, intestinal disease may present acutely with a surgical abdomen or a gastroenteritis characterized by abdominal pain, vomiting, and watery diarrhea. Typical pathogens include *Entamoeba histolytica*, *Giardia lamblia*, *Salmonella* sp, *Shigella* sp, CMV, HSV, *Campylobacter* sp, *Cryptosporidium*, *Isospora belli*, and, rarely, MAI.[15] *Clostridium difficile*–related pseudomembranous colitis may follow the extensive use of antibiotic therapy. Direct HIV invasion of the base of intestinal crypts has also been described.[37] Examination of the stool often yields the appropriate diagnosis and should precede any invasive investigation. In addition to cultures for standard bacterial stool pathogens, the evaluation should include viral cultures for CMV and HSV, microscopy for ova and parasites, and a modified acid-fast stain to screen for *Cryptosporidium* and *I. belli*. Terminal patients with very low CD4 counts should also have stool cultures for MAI.

Treatment of gastroenteritis requires supportive fluid and electrolyte therapy, in addition to antibiotic therapy when appropriate. Given the high incidence of invasive bacteremia in HIV patients during *Salmonella* gastroenteritis, it is reasonable to treat aggressively for positive stool cultures. Infection with *Cryptosporidium* is without a specific therapy but is usually self-resolving. Infections with *I. belli* are sensitive to treatment with TMP/SMX. GI infection with MAI is usually a component of disseminated disease, involving the liver, lung, and bone marrow.[21] Eradication of systemic MAI is difficult, requiring long-term therapy with clofazamine, rifampin, ciprofloxacillin, ethambutol, and amikacin.[21]

GI hemorrhage may occur in the setting of severe small- or large-bowel ulceration. Several reports of infants presenting with GI disease as their first manifestation of HIV infection describe massive hemorrhage and perforation of the bowel secondary to CMV.[44,47] As with any patient experiencing severe GI bleeding, evaluation should include endoscopy, gastric lavage, supine and upright abdominal x-rays, and possibly a Meckel's scan and arteriography, depending on the presumptive location and the extent of hemorrhage, respectively. Therapy is initially supportive, with infusion of crystalloid and blood products and correction of coagulopathy and thrombocytopenia, followed by exploratory laparotomy if bleeding is significant or if evidence exists of obstruction, perforation, or the loss of intestinal viability. Although ganciclovir has been found in trials to be effective in reducing the pain and diarrhea of chronic CMV colitis, it has no place yet in the acute management of disease.[46] Where a specific pathogen has been identified that may be contributing to GI hemorrhage, such as *Yersinia*, *Salmonella*, or *Shigella*, antibiotic therapy is indicated.

The chronic malnutrition in HIV-infected children places them at risk during an acute intervening illness.[37] Inadequate nutritional stores can be expected to have a debilitating effect on the immune system in the setting of sepsis, in which caloric requirements may double and immune cells may be starved of essential nutrients such as arginine. Emaciation of respiratory muscles during a pulmonary infection may compromise vital capacity and cough, leading to the pooling of secretions, atelectasis, respiratory failure, and the inability to clear infection. Aggressive nutritional support should be administered early in the course of critical illness.[37] The enteral route is preferred for its simplicity, lack of catheter-associated infections, ability to deliver sufficient calories in low volume, and better maintenance of immune function.[48] This ideal is not always achievable in the HIV-infected child, given the possible presence of malabsorption, nausea, vomiting, and diarrhea, as well as ileus from sepsis, low cardiac output, or narcotics. After the placement of a nasogastric or a nasojejunal feeding tube, one should monitor abdominal girth, the volume of gastric contents, and stool output in order to assess the adequacy of enteral therapy. As a last resort, parenteral nutrition may be necessary.

Renal Disease

Primary renal disease has been reported in 7.7% of HIV-infected children,[12] presenting with proteinuria, edema, and frank nephrotic syndrome. Two types of disease are equally prevalent:

1. An HIV-associated nephropathy has been described, with global involvement of glomeruli and tubules, progressing ultimately to end-stage renal disease within 2 years.[12] Hemodialysis has not been shown to be effective in prolonging survival.[37]

2. A mesangial proliferative glomerulonephritis with a similar clinical presentation occurs in older children and carries a better prognosis.[12]

Neither form of renal disease appears responsive to therapy.[12] Renal involvement may also take place in the setting of sepsis and multiple-organ failure, or as a consequence of drug toxicity.

Neurologic Disease

Children with HIV infection may present with a spectrum of neurologic impairment, ranging from a chronic progressive encephalopathy to an acute fulminant infection. It is estimated that 70% to 90% of adult AIDS patients have evidence of subacute encephalitis, with impairment of behavioral and motor function, which progresses to frank dementia, ataxia, abnormal tone, and seizures.[37] Associated clinical findings include a cerebral spinal fluid (CSF) pleocytosis, brain atrophy on CT scan, and attenuation in white matter on MRI. The most common pathologic finding, seen in 84% of autopsied infants and children with AIDS, is a dystrophic calcification of blood vessels in the basal ganglia and deep cerebral white matter. Subacute encephalitis was detected in 60% of patients, with microglial nodules and multinucleated giant cells. Corticospinal tract degeneration was noted in 80% of spinal cords examined, some with delayed myelination and others with evidence of axonal injury.[49] Focal neurologic disease may also occur from encephalitis or meningitis due to non-HIV viral pathogens, bacteria, fungi, or protozoa, but the incidence of opportunistic CNS infections in the pediatric AIDS patients is less than 10%.[49]

Patients with CNS infection may present clinically with a mild headache and fever, a focal neurologic deficit, or seizure activity and coma. Diagnostic evaluation of the CSF should include KOH preparation, Gram and acid-fast stains, and viral, bacterial, and fungal cultures. In the adolescent, one should also test for cryptococcal antigen and toxoplasmosis IgM. CT and MRI may be helpful in defining lesions from toxoplasmosis and brain abscess.

Empiric therapy of meningitis should include a third-generation cephalosporin, as well as ampicillin, to cover *Enterococcus* and *Listeria*. Additional agents are added when the clinical assessment and aforementioned studies suggest a nonbacterial etiology. Suspicion of cryptococcal meningitis, which develops at some time in approximately 10% of adult AIDS patients,[50] should lead to the prompt inclusion of amphotericin B and flucytosine, still the agents of choice despite the promising results with fluconazole.[36,50] Treatment for toxoplasmosis is typically based on serologic evidence, without resort to tissue diagnosis. Long-term therapy with pyrimethamine and sulfadiazine may be of limited benefit. Detection of tuberculous meningitis requires prolonged therapy with isoniazid, rifampin, and ethambutol. When the evidence points to a diagnosis of viral encephalitis, an empiric course of acyclovir should be administered for 3 weeks. Fluids should be administered cautiously in a setting of CNS disease, so as not to exacerbate cerebral swelling and to avoid hyponatremia if SIADH is present. Insufficient fluid administration carries a risk, however, when treating with acyclovir, due to the precipitation of the drug in the renal tubules during hypovolemia.

Hematologic Disease

All three hematologic cell lines may be impacted by HIV infection and associated therapy.[12] Anemia is common, although usually mild, and results from a combination of chronic disease due to HIV infection, iron deficiency, malnutrition, and myelosuppressive medications.[51] Severe anemia requiring transfusion may be seen with chronic parvovirus infection, which directly inhibits erythropoiesis, and as a consequence of drug toxicity in 20% of children receiving zidovudine.[51] Neutropenia occurs in 10% to 25% of pediatric HIV patients,[12,52] although surprisingly, such children do not have an increased risk of sepsis during febrile episodes, as is the case for children immunocompromised by malignancy or chemotherapy.[12] Lymphopenia, particularly of the helper T-cell subset, is frequent and progressive. Thrombocytopenia occurs in 10% of patients and has been associated with clinical bleeding and even fatal hemorrhage.[12] The etiology remains unclear but antiplatelet antibodies have been identified in some patients.[52] Treatment includes platelet transfusions to maintain levels of greater than 20,000 to 40,000/μL and specific immunosuppressive or immunomodulating therapy. IV gammaglobulin has been shown to be effective in 40% of patients on a transient basis, and some nonresponders may benefit from a course of steroid therapy.[12] Zidovudine leads to a rise in the platelet count, which is maintained for the duration of drug therapy, but the onset of the effect occurs 2 weeks after the introduction of the drug.[12] Clinical hemorrhage requires immediate therapy, however, so the treatment of choice in the critical care setting is typically a platelet transfusion.

Intensive Care Unit Utilization

The decision to admit AIDS patients to ICUs has generated controversy since the beginning of the epidemic in the early 1980s.[53–55] This issue has not been confined to the medical sphere and has involved the political, social, and legal concerns of the larger community.[55] Little has been written regarding the merits of intensive care for the infant or child with AIDS.[25]

A major area of debate revolves around the value of critical care for patients with acute lung failure, in whom the life expectancy is very low.[25] Intubation and mechanical ventilation have been regarded by some physicians as "futile" and wasteful of limited ICU resources. Until recently, this view has been supported by mortality data, with short-term survival limited to 10% to 20% of patients with severe PCP.[25] Several new advances in the care of AIDS patients have altered this outlook favorably[53]: (1) HIV suppression with zidovudine, (2) PCP prophylaxis with TMP/SMX or aerosolized pentamadine, and (3) adjunctive use of steroids in PCP. With aggressive ICU care, the prognosis of PCP survivors has been lengthened to years rather than months. The data supporting this conclusion are sparse[53] but have provided some encouragement for aggressive intensive care management. Compared with other diseases requiring extensive medical support, such as malignancy or hypoplastic left heart, the utilization of ICU resources for the treatment of PCP does not seem unreasonable.[53] For indications other than acute respiratory failure, such as infection, hemodynamic instability, or encephalopathy, the mortality of adult AIDS patients is 20% to 43%,[55] even less than for PCP. Given the overall trend toward greater survival and the introduction of more effective prophylaxis and treatment, it is no longer justifiable to exclude children with AIDS from ICU care, even when a life-threatening infection with PCP is present.

The frequent exposure of ICU personnel to blood, secretions, and excretions poses potential risks for staff.[10,57] To date, fortunately, this has been extremely rare. In one series examining ICU personnel exposed to 129 needle sticks and 213 mucosal splashing incidents, there were no HIV seroconversions after 10 months.[10] On a global scale, seroconversion of health care workers is reported to have occurred only 14 times after a needle stick and 3 times after mucosal or cutaneous exposure.[10] To avoid any potential contact with HIV, health care workers are required by OSHA to wear gloves, masks, gowns, and protective eye goggles with all patients, regardless of HIV status, when engaged in activities in which contact with secretions or blood is possible.[57] The incidence of occult HIV infection varies with geographic location but has been reported to be as high as 3% in one study of emergency room admissions who were not suspected of being seropositive.[37] In practice, the level of precaution taken in most ICUs does not meet OSHA standards, and proper leadership is necessary to implement these sensible recommendations.

The issue of privacy regarding HIV status is undergoing debate and change. Initially, the homosexual community prevailed over the public health establishment in an effort to exclude HIV infection from consideration as a sexually transmitted disease in the traditional framework of syphilis and gonorrhea.[58] As a result, partners were not required to be informed of contact with infected individuals, nor were they required to undergo testing. ICU patients suspected of HIV infection could not have serologic status determined routinely, despite the potential risk of transmission of disease to health care workers. The pendulum is now shifting toward a more balanced view, incorporating the concerns of privacy with the reasonable protection of the community.[53]

References

1. Gayle JA, Selik RM, Chu LY. Surveillance for AIDS and HIV infection among black and hispanic children and women of childbearing age. *MMWR CDC Surveill Summ* 39(3):23–30, 1990.

2. Straka BF et al. Cutaneous manifestations of the acquired immunodeficiency syndrome in children. *J Am Acad Dermatol* 18(5):1089–1102, 1988.

3. Conviser R, Grant C, Coye MJ. Pediatric acquired immunodeficiency syndrome hospitalization in New Jersey. *Pediatrics* 87(5):642–653, 1991.

4. Caldwell MB, Rogers MF. Epidemiology of pediatric HIV infection. *Pediatr Clin North Am* 38(1):1–16, 1991.

5. Van Dyke RB. Pediatric human immunodeficiency virus infection and the acquired immunodeficiency syndrome. *Am J Dis Child* 147: 524–525, 1993.

6. Chin J. Current and future dimensions of the HIV/AIDS pandemic in women and children. *Lancet* 336(8709):221–224, 1990.

7. Rubinstein A. Introductory remarks. *Ann NY Acad Sci* 693:1–3, 1993.

8. Moore R et al. Zidovudine and the natural history of the acquired immunodeficiency syndrome. *N Engl J Med* 324(20):1412–1416, 1991.

9. Laurence J. Reservoirs of HIV infection or carriage: Monocytic, dendritic, follicular dendritic, and B cells. *Ann NY Acad Sci* 693:52–64, 1993.

10. Gerberding JL et al. Risk of transmitting the human immunodeficiency virus, hepatitis B virus, and cytomegalovirus to health care workers exposed to patients with AIDS and AIDS-related conditions. *J Infect Dis* 156(1):1–8, 1987.

11. Wara DW et al. Maternal transmission and diagnosis of human immunodeficiency virus during infancy. *Ann NY Acad Sci* 693:14–19, 1993.

12. Burroughs M, Edelson P. Medical care of the HIV infected child. *Pediatr Clin North Am* 38(1):45–67, 1991.

13. Joshi VV. Pathology of pediatric AIDS: Overview, update, and future direction. *Ann NY Acad Sci* 693:71–92, 1993.

14. European Collaborative Study. Children born to women with HIV-1 infection: Natural history of risk and infection. *Lancet* 337 (8736):253–260, 1991.

15. Scott G et al. Survival in children with perinatally acquired HIV type 1 infection. *N Engl J Med* 321:1791–1796, 1989.

16. Greenwald BM. Update: AIDS in the pediatric ICU. In Gioia F, Yeh T (eds): *Pediatric Critical Care Clinical Review Series*. Part 3. Boston: Little Brown, 1991. Pp 113–131.

17. Phillips AN, Lee CA, Elford J. Serial CD4 lymphocyte counts and development of AIDS. *Lancet* 337(8738):389–398, 1991.

18. Hughes W. *Pneumocystis carinii* pneumonia: New approaches to diagnosis, treatment, and prevention. *Pediatr Infect Dis* 10(5):391–399, 1991.

19. Noel G. Host defence abnormalities associated with HIV infection. *Pediatr Clin North Am* 38(1):37–43, 1991.

20. Pahwa S, Fikrig S, Pahwa R. Pediatric acquired immunodeficiency syndrome: Demonstration of B lymphocyte defects in vitro. *Diagn Immunol* 4:24, 1986.

21. Van Dyke RB. Opportunistic infections in pediatric HIV disease. *Ann NY Acad Sci* 693:158–16, 1993.

22. Manak MM et al. Use of PCR for detection of HIV-1 sequences in babies born to seropositive mothers. *Ann NY Acad Sci* 693:255–257, 1993.

23. George JR, Parekh BS, Shaffer N. Detection of HIV-1 IgA by an IgA capture enzyme immunoassay for early diagnosis in infants. *Ann NY Acad Sci* 693:272–274, 1993.

24. Brandt CD et al. Detection of human immunodeficiency virus type 1 infection in young pediatric patients by using polymerase chain reaction and biotinylated probes. *J Clin Microbiol* 30:36–40, 1992.

25. Notterman DA, Greenwald BM, Di Maio-Hunter A. Outcome after assisted ventilation in children with acquired immunodeficiency syndrome. *Crit Care Med* 18(1):18–20, 1990.

26. Vernon DD et al. Respiratory failure in children with acquired immunodeficiency syndrome and acquired immunodeficiency syndrome-related complex. *Pediatrics* 82(2):223–228, 1988.

27. Miller RF, Mitchell DM. Management of respiratory failure in patients with the acquired immune deficiency syndrome and *Pneumocystis carinii* pneumonia. *Thorax* 45:140–146, 1990.

28. Winthrop AL, Waddell T, Superina RA. The diagnosis of pneumonia in the immunocompromised child: Use of bronchoalveolar lavage. *J Pediatr Surg* 25(8):878–880, 1990.

29. Gershon AA. Antiviral therapy for HIV infection in infants and children. *Ann NY Acad Sci* 693:166–177, 1993.

30. Gregg RW, Friedman BC, Williams JF. Continuous positive airway pressure by face mask in *Pneumocystis carinii* pneumonia. *Crit Care Med* 18(1):21–24, 1990.

31. Gagnon S et al. Corticosteriods as adjunctive therapy for severe pneumocystitis carinii pneumonia in the acquired immunodeficiency syndrome. *N Engl J Med* 323(21):1444–1450, 1991.

32. Bozzette SA et al. A controlled trial of early adjunctive treatment with corticosteroids for *Pneumocystis carinii* pneumonia in the acquired immunodeficiency syndrome. *N Engl J Med* 323(21):1451–1457, 1990.

33. Friedman Y, Franklin C, Weil M. Use of systemic corticosteroids in patients with AIDS, *Pneumocystis carinii* pneumonia, and acute respiratory failure. Abstract at 29th Educational and Scientific Symposium, Society of Critical Care Medicine, Washington, D.C., 1991.

34. National Institutes of Health. University of California expert panel for corticosteroids as adjunctive therapy for pneumocystis pneumonia: Consensus statement. *N Engl J Med* 323(21):1500–1504, 1991.

35. Schiff MJ, Farber BF, Kaplan MH. Steroids for *Pneumocystis carinii* pneumonia and respiratory failure in the acquired immunodeficiency syndrome. *Arch Intern Med* 150:1819–1821, 1990.

36. Sugar AM, Stern JJ, Dupont B. Overview: Treatment of cryptococcal meningitis. *Rev Infect Dis* 12(3):338–348, 1990.

37. Singer P et al. Reassessing intensive care for patients with the acquired immunodeficiency syndrome. *Heart Lung* 19(4):387–394, 1990.

38. Gleason-Morgan D, Church JA, Ross LA. *Mycobacterium avium* complex in HIV-infected children. *Ann NY Acad Sci* 693:288–290, 1993.

39. Horsburgy CR Jr. *Mycobacterium avium* complex infection in the acquired immunodeficiency syndrome. *N Engl J Med* 324(19):1332–1338, 1991.

40. Zuckier L, Ongsend F, Goldfarb CR. Lymphocytic interstitial pneumonitis: A cause of pulmonary gallium-67 uptake in a child with acquired immunodeficiency syndrome. *J Nucl Med* 29:707–711, 1988.

41. Schiff RG, Kabat L, Kamani N. Gallium scanning in lymphoid interstitial pneumonitis of children with AIDS. *J Nucl Med* 28:1915–1919, 1987.

42. Pitt J. Lymphocytic interstitial pneumonitis. *Pediatr Clin North Am* 38(1):89–95, 1991.

43. Lipshultz SE et al. Cardiovascular manifestations of HIV infection in infants and children. *Am J Cardiol* 63:1489, 1989.

44. Schwartz DL et al. A case of life-threatening gastrointestinal hemorrhage in an infant with AIDS. *J Pediatr Surg* 24(3):313–315, 1989.

45. Larsen RA. Azoles in AIDS. *J Infect Dis* 162:727–730, 1990.

46. Pau AK, Pitrak DL. Management of cytomegalovirus infection in patients with acquired immunodeficiency syndrome. *Clin Pharma* 9:613–630, 1990.

47. Dolgin SE et al. CMV enteritis causing hemorrhage and obstruction in an infant with AIDS. *J Pediatr Surg* 25(6):696–698, 1990.

48. Zaloga GP. Nutrition and prevention of systemic infection. In Taylor R, Shoemaker W,(eds): *Critical Care: State of the Art*. Anaheim: SCCM Fullerton, 1987. Pp 31–79.

49. Dickson DW et al. Central nervous system pathology in pediatric AIDS: An autopsy study. *APMID* 8(Suppl):40–57, 1989.

50. Larsen RA, Leal ME, Chan LS. Fluconazole compared with amphotericin B plus flucytosine for cryptococcal meningitis in AIDS. *Ann Intern Med* 13:183–187, 1990.

51. McKinney RE Jr, Pizzo PA, Scott GB. Safety and tolerance of intermittent intravenous and oral zidovudine therapy in human immunodeficiency virus-infected pediatric patients. Pediatric Zidovudine Phase 1 Study Group. *J Pediatr* 116(4):640–647, 1990.

52. Sandhaus LM, Scudder R. Hematologic and bone marrow abnormalities in pediatric patients with human immunodeficiency virus infection. *Pediatr Pathol* 9(3):277–288, 1989.

53. Friedman Y, Franklin C. Admission of AIDS patients to a medical intensive care unit: Causes and outcomes (letter to the editor). *Crit Care Med* 18(3):346–347, 1990.

54. Layon AJ, D'Amico R. Intensive care for patients with acquired immunodeficiency syndrome: Medicine versus ideology. *Crit Care Med* 18(11):1297–1299, 1990.

55. Sprung CL. Acquired immunodeficiency syndrome and critical care. *Crit Care Med* 18(11):1300–1302, 1990.

56. Friedman Y et al. Improved survival in patients with AIDS, *Pneumocystis carinii* pneumonia, and severe respiratory failure. *Chest* 96:862, 1989.

57. Rogers PL et al. Admission of AIDS patients to a medical intensive care unit: Causes and outcomes. *Crit Care Med* 17(2):113–117, 1989.

58. Angel M. A dual approach to AIDS epidemic. *N Engl J Med* 324(21):1498–1500, 1991.

VIII Hematopoietic System

John T. Truman

41 Hemostasis

Bleeding in the critically ill patient must be arrested as quickly as possible. This requires diagnostic tests that are initially rapid and ultimately specific. It then requires therapeutic measures that are initially broad-based and then ultimately precise.

Hemostasis involves two entirely different sets of physiologic reactions. The first and most important is the formation of a stable blood clot. The second is the cessation of small blood vessel bleeding by means of thrombus formation. The initial battery of screening tests addresses both of these phenomena.

1. Prothrombin time (PT) measures the integrity of the extrinsic coagulation system, which consists of factors VII, X, V, prothrombin, and fibrinogen (Fig. 41-1). Normal is approximately 12 seconds, with a prolongation of up to 2 seconds beyond control as acceptable.

2. Partial thromboplastin time (PTT) is a measure of the intrinsic coagulation system, which consists of factors XII, XI, IX, VIII, X, V, prothrombin, and fibrinogen. Normal is approximately 35 seconds, with any prolongation beyond the upper limit of normal requiring further investigation.

3. Platelet count measures only the number of platelets rather than functional ability, with normal in the 200 to 400,000/μL range.

4. Bleeding time measures the function of platelets and/or the integrity of small blood vessels. Normal by the forearm or template method is up to 10 minutes. The bleeding time should not be measured if the platelet count is less than 100,000, as it will always be prolonged.

5. Fibrin split product assay is a measure of fibrin degradation. Several different assays are available, and the presence of any but a minimal concentration of split products is indicative of either disseminated intravascular coagulation or fibrinolysis. The thrombin time is an indirect way of assessing the presence of fibrin by-products.

Depending on the abnormalities in screening tests, more specific coagulation tests can be ordered. These can focus on specific factor assays, such as factors V and VIII, which may be consumed in disseminated intravascular coagulation or which may be absent because of congenital deficiencies. Fibrinogen may also be consumed in disseminated intravascular coagulation (DIC) or be absent congenitally. Factors IX, XI, and XII may be measured if the PTT is prolonged and the PT is normal. Factor VII should be measured if the PT is prolonged and the PTT normal. Specific inhibitors to factors VIII, IX, and XI may be assayed if a patient otherwise known to be deficient in these factors fails to respond to proper replacement. Factor VIII antigen can be assayed to differentiate hemophilia from von Willebrand's disease. Von Willebrand factor can also be quantified. Platelet function tests can be done if the bleeding time is prolonged but the platelet count is normal.

Broad-spectrum treatment can be administered as soon as the results of the initial screening tests are available. Fresh-frozen plasma is a rich source of all clotting factors and should be given in a loading dose to any patient who is actively bleeding, with a prolonged PT or PTT. More specific replacement can be done as the results of more precise testing become available. Platelet infusions can be given to the thrombocytopenic patient until it is clear whether the problem is due to decreased production or increased destruction.

Screening tests should provide a reasonable point of therapeutic departure within 20 minutes of a critical care event. Plasma and platelets can be made available in the same period so that broad-based treatment can begin in short order. More accurate diagnosis will take a longer time, but specific replacements or interventions now make intractable bleeding almost unreported. No patient should bleed to death, given current knowledge and technology. The demands on laboratories and blood banks may be very severe, but with resourcefulness and cooperation, virtually all challenges can be met.

Clot Formation: Factor Abnormalities

When damaged subendothelial tissue activates platelets, nonspecific activating factors are released that initiate the process of converting soluble clotting factors to an insoluble protein clot. This takes somewhat longer than platelet plug formation but is more durable and acts as the infrastructure on which tissue repair can occur. Limiting reactions are also initiated that prevent the clot from extending too far, and thus lead to its ultimate dissolution. This delicate balance can be upset by the absence of any of the necessary factors, by abnormalities in their structure, by inhibitors of their activity, or by excesses in their functional capacities.

Clotting factors act as either enzymes or cofactors. In their resting state, the enzymes are present as inactive enzyme precursors, or zymogens. When activated, they undergo conformational alteration or peptide cleavage to become proteases that act on the zymogen substrate of the next clotting factor in the clotting sequence. As enzymes, they are not consumed in the process but can move on to other zymogen substrates in a process of amplification or cascading. Factors VIII and V act as cofactors and are consumed in the process (see Fig. 41-1). There are two

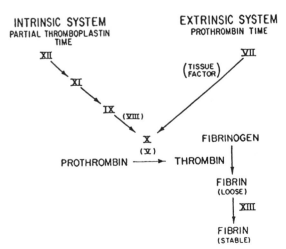

Figure 41-1. Clotting factors. Parentheses indicate cofactors that are consumed in the process of coagulation. Fibrinogen is also consumed in the formation of the clot.

independently activated systems that link together with the activation of factor X. Events beyond that point are common to both systems and are known as the common pathway. The faster of the two systems is initiated by the release of subendothelial tissue factor, often secondary to profound external trauma. This is the extrinsic system. Factor VII becomes activated and in turn binds to factor X. The events in the extrinsic system and common pathway are measured by the PT. The slower system is activated by the exposure of collagen or a variety of intracellular factors that activate circulating factor XII. This is the intrinsic system. Activated factor XII initiates three reactions: (1) activation of factor XI; (2) activation of kallikrein, which is chemotactic for the cellular repair system; and (3) activation of plasminogen to prevent the clot from overextension. Factor XI then activates factor IX, which interacts with factor VIII to bind factor X. The events in the intrinsic system and common pathway are measured by the PTT. Activated factor X, with factor V as a cofactor, then cleaves prothrombin at several sites to form a distinct protein, thrombin. This in turn cleaves fibrinogen into a slightly smaller molecule, fibrin, which interacts with neighboring fibrin molecules to form a loose fibrin clot. A transpeptidation reaction mediated by factor XIII converts this to a stable fibrin clot.

A parallel system of clot limitation is mediated by plasmin, which diffuses into the fibrin network and breaks it down into smaller nonclottable proteins, the fibrin split products. A further limiting reaction is that of antithrombin III, which slowly neutralizes thrombin by forming a complex with it. This effect is markedly enhanced by heparin, which also binds to factor IX. Its effect is detected most sensitively by the PTT.

Structural similarity exists among prothrombin, VII, and X at one point on each molecule. This is mediated by vitamin K and is inhibited by coumarin anticoagulants.

Hemophilia: Factor VIII Deficiency (Hemophilia A)

Though not a common disorder, hemophilia A occurs frequently enough that a physician involved with critically ill children should be adept in both diagnosis and treatment.[1] Factor VIII is present in an antigenically normal amount but is functionally deficient in its measurable activity as a clot-promoting cofactor. The carrier female may have a normal amount of clot-promoting VIII activity but will have roughly twice as much antigenically measurable VIII protein. This is the basis of carrier testing. Neonatal diagnosis can easily be made on cord blood if there is a positive family history. However, it is more often made because of easy bruising when the child is learning to walk. Hemarthroses, mucous membrane bleeding, deep hematomas, and abdominal pain mimicking appendicitis are the other major problems of childhood.

The PTT will be prolonged, the PT normal, and the VIII level constant throughout life. Clinical severity is related to the factor VIII concentration.

Severe (less than 1% factor VIII): Spontaneous bleeding may occur; bleeding always follows trauma; average 20 to 100 infusions annually.

Moderate (1% to 5% factor VIII): No spontaneous bleeding; usually bleeding after trauma; average few to 40 infusions annually.

Mild (5% to 20% factor VIII): Unpredictable bleeding after trauma; none or few infusions per year.

Subclinical (20% to 50% factor VIII): PTT may be normal; bleeding only after major trauma, if ever.

Treatment should be directed to early and vigorous factor replacement whenever bleeding is suspected rather than proved. Factor VIII is available in two forms:

1. Factor VIII concentrate. This is commercially available and is produced by many different methods, all of which are now free of HIV. It is easily stored, transported, and administered; each bottle contains 200 to 1000 units and is accurately labeled.

2. Cryoprecipitate. This must be kept frozen and is more difficult to administer. Each bag contains 60 to 100 units, but the precise amount is usually not known. For any form of factor VIII, the infusion of 1 unit per kilogram of body weight will increase the circulating VIII level by 2%. For hemarthrosis and soft-tissue bleeding, the infusion of 25 U/kg will result in a 50% level, with a half-life of 6 to 8 hours; this may be repeated in 24 hours. For CNS bleeding, 100 U/kg will yield a 200% level; this should be repeated at 8-hour intervals.

Mucous membrane bleeding may be treated by blocking salivary plasmin activity with epsilon-aminocaproic acid (EACA; Amicar). The initial dose is 200 mg/kg by mouth, followed by 100 mg/kg every 4 to 6 hours, around the clock. This should be continued for 8 to 10 days, as rebleeding is common. It should not be given for genitourinary bleeding, because insoluble clots may form.

The major problem in hemophilia is the formation of factor VIII inhibitors.[2] This appears to be inevitable in 10% to 20% of patients, regardless of how many infusions they receive. Thus, the fear of inducing an inhibitor should never be a reason for delaying a necessary factor VIII infusion. An inhibitor can be suspected when an infusion fails to arrest bleeding or correct the PTT. Specific assays are available. Low-titer inhibitors can be treated by high-factor VIII infusions. High-titer infusions require factor IX concentrates or factor VIII inhibitor–bypassing activity (FEIBA), which appear to contain small quantities of thrombin. This bypasses the inhibitor.

Home infusion has been a great advance in the management of hemophilia. Parents readily learn how to give intravenous (IV) concentrates to children as young as 3 years old, and 12-year-old children may learn self-administration. Careful records must be kept, and there must be close supervision of possible joint, dental, and psychosocial problems.

For patients with moderate or mild hemophilia, IV DDAVP will increase the baseline factor VIII level two- to fourfold. The dosage is 0.3 μg/kg IV q12–24h given over 20 minutes. Peak response occurs within 1 hour. Aspirin and other platelet-inhibiting drugs must be avoided.

Mucous membrane bleeding, such as a cut lip or tongue, can be very frustrating because of its intermittent nature over many days. It is wise to give EACA (Amicar) as soon as bleeding starts and continue for 10 days. It acts as a substrate for fibrinolysis and thus prevents a clot from being dissolved. The dose is 200 mg/kg by mouth initially, then 100 mg/kg q6h.

Von Willebrand's Disease

This is a deficiency of the von Willebrand factor (VWF) multimer that binds platelets to subendothelial tissue and acts as a carrier of factor VIII. Patients thus have both a prolonged bleeding time and a prolonged PTT, although there is considerable variability of expression within families and within the same person from time to time. Inheritance is usually autosomal dominant, but can be recessive. It is the most common hereditary hemostatic disorder.[3]

Clinically, there is a greater tendency for bruising and postoperative or postpartum bleeding, consistent with the platelet function defect. However, there is a lesser tendency for hemarthroses or intraabdominal bleeding, because the factor VIII coagulant activity is usually greater than 1%.

Confirmation of diagnosis requires the demonstration of absence of VWF or the failure of platelet aggregation in response to ristocetin. Differentiation from the hemophilia carrier can be made by demonstrating an equimolar concentration of VIII coagulant and VIII antigen in von Willebrand's disease.

Treatment consists of factor replacement with cryoprecipitate, which is a much richer source of VWF than is factor VIII concentrate. The only exception to this is Humate-P (Boeringer), which contains VWF. IV DDAVP may also be used in non-life-threatening situations at a dose of 0.3 μg/kg IV over 20 minutes. These correct both the platelet adhesive defect and the deficiency of VIII coagulant.

Factor IX Deficiency (Christmas Disease, Hemophilia B)

Factor IX deficiency is much less common than factor VIII deficiency but is clinically identical. Inheritance is sex-linked. Factor IX replacement in mild cases is most safely given as fresh-frozen plasma 10 ml/kg every 6 to 8 hours. In moderate or severe cases, commercially available concentrates provide a reliable source of high-potency factor IX. An infusion of 1 U/kg gives an increment of only 1%, but the half-life is 30 hours. Thus, more must be given initially in severe bleeding, but the dose is repeated less frequently.

Factor XI Deficiency (Hemophilia C)

A rare, autosomal recessive disorder with carriers having a prolonged PTT, factor XI deficiency is seen in females as well as males. Bleeding is rarely a problem, but should it occur, fresh-frozen plasma, 10 ml/kg, is required every 6 to 8 hours.

Factor XII Deficiency

PTT is prolonged, but there is no clinical bleeding whatever, hence no treatment is necessary. Variants such as Fletcher factor deficiency and high-molecular-weight kininogen deficiency likewise have no clinical significance, in spite of the markedly prolonged PTT.

Factor XIII Deficiency

Poor wound healing, easy bruising, and late umbilical stump bleeding characterize this disorder. PT, PTT, and bleeding time are normal. Diagnosis is by specific assay of clot solubility in 5M urea. Treatment is administration of fresh-frozen plasma.

Miscellaneous Deficiencies

Fibrinogen, prothrombin, factor V, and factor X deficiencies have a prolonged PT and PTT. Factor VII deficiency has a prolonged PT but normal PTT. All are exceedingly rare.

Vitamin K Deficiency

This is usually a dietary deficiency seen in infants who fail to receive a prophylactic vitamin K injection. It is also seen with biliary atresia, cystic fibrosis, chronic diarrhea, and long-term antibiotic administration. Often, there is concomitant dietary deficiency. Prothrombin, factors VII, IX, and X fail to develop their homologous Ca^{2+} binding sites, and hence the PT is selectively prolonged. Intramuscular administration of 5 mg vitamin K corrects the PT within hours.

Circulating Anticoagulants

Circulating anticoagulants occasionally develop with lupus erythematosus or in the postpartum state. Bleeding is uncommon in spite of marked derangements of PTT or PT.

Nephrotic Syndrome

Factors IX and XII may be lost in the general proteinuria of the nephrotic syndrome. Factor IX must be replaced prior to renal biopsy.

Cessation of Bleeding: Platelet Abnormalities

There is a dynamic interplay between circulating platelets and blood vessel endothelial cells. The presence of platelets enhances the continuity of the endothelial lining, and a decrease in platelets predisposes to loss of vascular integrity and thus petechiae.

Under normal circumstances, platelets are produced by megakaryocytes in the bone marrow to survive for 8 days in the peripheral blood and to be present in a concentration of 200,000 to 400,000/ μL. When trauma exposes subendothelial tissue, platelets adhere to the site of damage. In actual fact, this adhesion is mediated by von Willebrand's factor (VWF), which itself is closely related to, but distinct from, the antihemophilic factor (factor VIII). Following adhesion, the platelets undergo a phase of primary aggregation in which there is a physical transformation from a discoid to spheroid shape, plus an extension of pseudopods. This occurs in response to collagen and adenosine diphosphate (ADP) released from damaged subendothelial cells. These same stimuli cause endogenous ADP, which is stored in cytoplasmic platelet granules, to be released via canaliculi that connect with the platelet surface. This, in turn, enlarges the platelet plug by causing nearby platelets to aggregate and undergo a release reaction.

The platelet plug takes only minutes to form and is stable for several hours. At that time, however, it undergoes dissolution, and the continuance of hemostasis thereafter depends on the interim formation of the fibrin clot.

Quantitative Platelet Disorders: The Thrombocytopenias

Decreased platelet counts will be seen when there is increased destruction of platelets, decreased production, abnormal distribution, or dilutional loss. Although the platelet count may be very low for any of these reasons, there is much less morbidity or mortality when the underlying problem is increased platelet destruction. This is due to the fact that the bone marrow is able to produce normal platelets that, though diminished in number, are young and metabolically active. Thus, a platelet count of 5,000/ μL in a child with idiopathic thrombocytopenic purpura (ITP) does not have the worrisome significance it would have in a marrow failure syndrome such as leukemia or aplastic anemia. The exception to this rule is disseminated intravascular coagulation in which platelet function is abnormal and the soluble clotting factors are partially depleted as well.

Increased Destruction of Platelets

Idiopathic Thrombocytopenic Purpura

This is the most common acquired disorder of hemostasis in pediatric practice. It is most often seen in children ages 2 to 8, but it may be seen at any age. The onset is usually sudden, often 1 to 3 weeks following a viral infection. Presumably, this triggers an immune response in which the platelet is coated with antibody, and the platelet-antibody complex is removed from the circulation within minutes or hours by the reticuloendothelial system. Transfused platelets suffer the same fate, so are of no therapeutic value. A variety of tests for antiplatelet antibodies have been developed but are still of little practical value in directing therapy.

Petechiae are extensive, especially on the legs and ankles and frequently about the face and eyes if the child has been crying. There is no splenomegaly. The platelet count is usually below 40,000/μL, often below 10,000/μL. The white cell count is normal, as is the hemoglobin, unless there has been significant blood loss. In the peripheral smear, the only abnormality is the number of platelets, 0 to 1 per oil immersion field instead of the usual 15 to 30. The few platelets present are larger than normal because they are newly formed.

Bone marrow aspiration is advisable to exclude acute leukemia if there is any deviation from normal in physical examination, Hgb, WBC, or WBC morphology. Serious bleeding is anecdotally rare in prepubertal children, and this author has never encountered it in three decades of pediatric hematology practice. Spontaneous recovery occurs within 3 weeks in about three of four patients and within 6 months in nine out of ten patients. Whether to use IV gammaglobulin or corticosteroids is largely a matter of judgment. With children under 18 months and those over 12 years, it is usual to give IV gamma globulin, as the risk of bleeding is somewhat greater. The usual dose is 1.0 g/kg for 2 days or 400 mg/kg for 5 days. The response is very prompt, often within 24 hours. However, for most children with ITP who are between ages 2 and 12 and have only moderate petechiae and bruising, it is doubtful that treatment has any long-term value. This is a short-term disorder with virtually no morbidity or mortality, and though treatment clearly works, it may be unnecessary. This author advises nothing more than prudence in daily activities, the avoidance of aspirin, and weekly platelet counts to ascertain when the disease has run its course. Others suggest IV gamma globulin when the platelet count is below 20,000/μL.[4] The use of IV anti-D in patients who are Rh-positive may simplify future decision making of this sort because of the ease of administration and relative lack of expense.[5]

If the platelet count remains below 40,000/μL 2 years after diagnosis, and a trial of IV gamma globulin or corticosteroids is ineffective, splenectomy should be considered. The success rate is 80% to 90%, although preoperative pneumococcal, *Hemophilus influenzae*, and *Neisseria meningitides* vaccinations should be given. Postoperative penicillin prophylaxis 250 mg bid will also minimize the risk of overwhelming sepsis.

Neonatal Alloimmune Thrombocytopenia

This is seen in one in 3000 births, so it is a predictable occurrence in a newborn nursery. Correct management is of great importance. These newborns have extensive petechiae at birth or shortly thereafter, and a platelet count below 20,000/μL. The etiology is analogous to that in erythroblastosis fetalis: The fetus and mother are of differing platelet types, the mother is PL^A1-negative and the fetus is PL^A1-positive. The mother develops an antibody that crosses the placenta to destroy the fetus's platelets. Fetal mortality may be 15% and morbidity a further 15%. Washed maternal platelets must be given to the neonate as soon as possible. Random blood bank platelets and IV gamma globulin are appropriate temporizing measures, pending the preparation of maternal platelets. Once it has occurred in a family, however, every effort must be made to predict accurately any future occurrences and treat appropriately antepartum.[6]

Drug-Induced Thrombocytopenia

Even though rare in pediatrics, thrombocytopenia may be associated with almost any drug, especially those used in critical care pediatrics. It is most commonly seen with the following:

1. Antibiotics, sulfonamides, and sulfonamide derivatives: penicillin, ampicillin, nafcillin, cephalothin, rifampicin, INH, PAS, sulfisoxazole, trimethoprim-sulfamethoxazole, thiazides, acetazolamide, diazoxide, chlorpropamide, furosemide

2. Analgesics: acetylsalicylic acid, acetaminophen, phenylbutazone

3. Anticonvulsants: phenytoin, barbiturates, sodium valproate, benzodiazepines

4. Miscellaneous: quinidine, alpha-methyldopa, chlorpheniramine, digoxin, gold salts, heparin, propylthiouracil, penicillamine, spironolactone

Various diagnostic tests are available but are not wholly reliable. Removal of likely drug offenders will result in a rise in platelet count within a few days. Corticosteroids are of little or no value, but IV gamma globulin sometimes hastens recovery. Valproate is a special situation in which the extent of thrombocytopenia is often dose-specific. Thus, a modest decrease in dosage (i.e., by one third) may result in a prompt rise in platelet count to a safe range.

Bacterial Sepsis

The presence of circulating bacteria, especially in neonates, often causes thrombocytopenia. This is probably a combination of shortened platelet survival plus marrow suppression. Platelet transfusions should be given if there is active bleeding or if the platelet count falls below 20,000/μL.

Hemolytic-Uremic Syndrome

The renal vasculature is the target organ in a process of accelerated coagulation with entrapment and deposition of platelets. A platelet count less than 80,000/μL is present in nearly all patients, though bleeding is rarely a problem. This is a process of localized intravascular coagulation that is largely uninfluenced by anticoagulants or antiplatelet drugs. Treatment should be directed at sustaining kidney function until the process expends itself. Platelet transfusion is rarely, if ever, necessary.

Thrombotic Thrombocytopenia Purpura

This is a much rarer, though much more devastating, disease of localized intravascular coagulation in which the target organ is the CNS. The etiology is unknown; the onset is fulminant in teenagers and young adults. Thrombocytopenia and hemolytic anemia occur together with bizarre and variable neurologic signs. Plasma exchange transfusion or massive plasma infusion should be performed promptly.

Cyanotic Congenital Heart Disease

Platelet counts of 60,000/μL to 100,000/μL, with mild prolongations of PT and PTT, are common in secondary polycythemia. The etiology is multifactorial—some shortening of platelet survival and clotting factor half-life and some suppression of synthesis. Bleeding is rarely, if ever, a problem. It is important to decrease the volume of anticoagulant in blood collection tubes in proportion to the increased hemoglobin concentration (and hence decreased plasma volume).

Indwelling Prosthesis

Arterial catheters, arteriovenous fistulas, and prosthetic heart valves may absorb platelets or cause activation with shortened survival. This rarely causes any clinical problems.

Giant Hemangioma (Kasabach-Merritt Syndrome)

Thrombocytopenia occurs as a result of localized intravascular coagulation, but rarely results in bleeding. It should be treated expectantly, pending decrease in size of the hemangioma.

Phototherapy

Phototherapy may cause mild thrombocytopenia in the jaundiced neonate. It is clinically unimportant, but other causes of thrombocytopenia must be given proper consideration.

Decreased Production of Platelets

Marrow Replacement

Thrombocytopenia is the most common abnormal laboratory finding in children with leukemia. The risk of bleeding is much greater than in ITP, so the decision to use prophylactic platelet transfusions must be individualized. In the presence of sepsis, it is advisable to transfuse platelets to keep the platelet count above 20,000/μL.

Metastatic cancer (e.g., neuroblastoma or rhabdomyosarcoma) myelofibrosis, or miliary tuberculosis may also result in bone marrow failure due to marrow replacement. In the neonate, the TORCH infections may cause decreased platelet production.

Radiation Therapy

Moderate thrombocytopenia is quite common, but the platelet count rarely falls below 20,000/μL.

Marrow Aplasia

Bone marrow aplasia that is secondary to intensive cancer chemotherapy is much commoner than primary bone marrow failure. With bone marrow aplasia, the likelihood of bleeding with a platelet count below 20,000/μL is very much higher than bleeding due to ITP. Therefore, it is usual to transfuse platelets regardless of bleeding status for a platelet count below 20,000/μL. In aplastic anemia due to primary bone marrow failure, however, it is wise to avoid platelet or blood transfusions as much as possible if bone marrow transplantation is contemplated. Exposure to blood products compromises the success rate of bone marrow transplantation. On the other hand, platelet transfusion is necessary for uncontrollable bleeding.

Thrombocytopenia-Absent Radius Syndrome

Apparent at birth, this syndrome is uncommon. There is a lifelong decrease in platelet count that is due to a decrease in megakaryocytes.

Wiscott-Aldrich Syndrome

Only males are affected by this syndrome. It is part of a complex immune deficiency state involving helper T cells and is associated with eczema and decreased IgM production. Bone marrow transplantation is the definitive treatment.

Megaloblastic Anemias

Characterized by vitamin B_{12} or folic acid deficiency, these anemias are associated with marrow underproduction that can involve megakaryocytes as well as the red cell and white cell lines.

Abnormal Platelet Distribution

Any condition causing giant splenomegaly (e.g., Gaucher's disease, portal hypertension, or thalassemia major) can result in sequestration of large numbers of platelets. These are unavailable for hemostasis and may be removed prematurely by the reticuloendothelial system.

Dilution of Circulating Platelets

Extensive blood loss followed by replacement with non-platelet-containing blood products results in dilution of a normal platelet pool. It is frequently seen postoperatively and is correctable by platelet transfusion.

Qualitative Platelet Disorders: The Thrombocytopathias

Abnormal platelet function may be acquired or congenital. There may be increased bruisability and postoperative or mucous membrane bleeding, but rarely petechiae. The platelet count is normal, but the bleeding time is invariably prolonged. There are specific disorders for each of the three phases of the process that leads to the formation of the platelet plug: adhesion, primary aggregation, and secondary aggregation.

Disorders of Adhesion

Von Willebrands' disease: Strictly speaking, the platelets are normal but are unable to adhere to the subendothelium because the bridging protein, VWF, is decreased. (See previous section, Von Willebrand's Disease, this chapter).

Disorders of Primary Aggregation

Glanzmann's thrombasthenia: In this rare disorder, the membrane receptor sites for ADP, collagen, and epinephrine are absent. Platelets will adhere to subendothelium but will not aggregate to form a plug. Clinical bleeding is a serious problem, and treatment is platelet transfusion. Inheritance is autosomal recessive. Milder variants with only partial dysfunction of the receptor sites may be more common than realized and the reason for some children's easy bruisability or postoperative bleeding.

Disorders of Secondary Aggregation

Aspirin effect: Aspirin inhibits the enzyme cyclooxygenase that mediates the release of endogenous ADP. This in turn retards the formation of the definitive platelet plug. Aspirin affects some patients more than others, but the effect is universal. All platelets are affected by a single ingestion of as little as 60 mg, and the inhibition is irreversible for the lifetime of the platelet. Thus, some prolongation of the bleeding time can be expected for 8 to 10 days following ingestion. All families should be advised to avoid aspirin for 10 full days prior to elective surgery, especially tonsillectomy and adenoidectomy.

Storage Pool Diseases

There are a variety of inherited diseases in which secondary aggregation cannot occur because of a lack of intracellular ADP. There may be an isolated platelet defect, or there may be additional clinical findings, as in oculocutaneous albinism, Wiscott-Aldrich syndrome, or Chediak-Higashi syndrome.

Miscellaneous Disorders of Platelet Function

There are a wide variety of conditions in which abnormal platelet function may be encountered. Bleeding may or may not be a problem, but when it is, the bleeding time is always prolonged. The precise effect on the platelets may not be clear, or the effect may be at several sites. Platelet transfusion will be of temporary benefit. These conditions include

1. The neonate
2. Uremia
3. Liver disease
4. Cyanotic congenital heart disease, with or without thrombocytopenia
5. Myeloproliferative syndrome: acute and chronic myelocytic leukemia, myelofibrosis, polycythemia vera
6. Intake of various drugs:
    indomethacin
    sulfinpyrazone
    depyridamole (Persantine)
    naproxen
    penicillin, ampicillin, carbenicillin, ticarcillin
    tricyclic antidepressants
    phenothiazines
    antihistamines
    guaifenesin (Robitussin)
    nitrofurantoin
    sodium valproate
    ethyl alcohol

Henoch-Schönlein Purpura (Allergic Vasculitis)

Henoch-Schönlein purpura may be trivial or severe. It is a multisystem disorder in which petechiae are the most prominent manifestation. These tend to cluster in the buttocks, along the lower limbs, or on the arms below the elbows. In children under 2 years, they may be generalized. Often the petechiae are raised and thus palpable. Later they become brownish. Polyarthralgia and arthritis are seen in two of three patients, and abdominal pain in one of two. Renal involvement with gross or microscopic hematuria is seen in one of three children. This may persist for months or years, with or without functional impairment.

This disorder often follows a minor infection, viral or streptococcal, and appears to result from the deposition of antigen-antibody complexes. It usually runs its course spontaneously in 1 to 3 weeks but has a frustrating tendency to wax and wane. There is no specific treatment, although prednisone is effective for severe abdominal pain to avoid intussusception. Prednisone should be given for as short a period as possible and should not be given for rash or joint involvement alone.

Miscellaneous Causes of Vascular Purpura

1. Gram-negative sepsis; Rocky Mountain spotted fever
2. Ehlers-Danlos syndrome
3. Scurvy
4. Heredity hemorrhagic telangiectasia

Combined Factor and Platelet Abnormalities

Disseminated Intravascular Coagulation

DIC is a common acute problem in critical care pediatrics. Almost any pathologic process can trigger the activation of factor XII and thus the entire coagulation cascade. In its most malignant form, purpura fulminans, the resultant fibrin clots can occlude peripheral arterioles, resulting in gangrene of fingers, toes, nose, and skin. More commonly, the clinical manifestation is bleeding because of consumption of fibrinogen, prothrombin, factors V and VIII, and platelets in an uncontrolled clotting sequence. Conditions that may trigger DIC are

1. Infections
    a. Any gram-negative or gram-positive sepsis
    b. Any viremic process
    c. Malaria, kala-azar
    d. Histoplasmosis, aspergillosis
    e. Rocky Mountain spotted fever
2. Liberation of tissue factor
    a. Intravascular hemolysis
    b. Malignant disease, especially acute promyelocytic leukemia
    c. Abruptio placentae, amniotic fluid embolus, toxemia
    d. Respiratory distress syndrome
    e. Fat embolism
3. Endothelial damage
    a. Shock
    b. Heat stroke
    c. Acute glomerulonephritis
    d. Giant hemangioma (Kasabach-Merritt syndrome)

In DIC's full-blown form, the PT and PTT are prolonged; the platelet count, factor VIII, and fibrinogen concentration are decreased; and fibrin split products are increased. Often the laboratory findings are more erratic. The platelet count is most frequently involved, and if two additional tests are abnormal, the diagnosis is almost certain.

Treatment requires replacement of consumed clotting factors with fresh-frozen plasma, 10 ml/kg every 6 to 8 hours, and platelets, 4 to 8 units every 6 to 8 hours. If active bleeding continues, cryoprecipitate should be added as an additional source of fibrinogen and factor VIII. However, cryoprecipitate cannot replace fresh-frozen plasma because cryoprecipitate lacks factor V, which is consumed in DIC.

Purpura fulminans presents a special problem because of direct tissue necrosis. As soon as the diagnosis is made, heparinization should be started to arrest fibrin deposition. The dosage is 50 U/kg as a loading dose, followed by 10 to 20 U/kg/hr by continuous infusion. Fresh-frozen plasma and platelets can be given as described previously.

Table 41-1.   Conditions associated with hypercoagulability

Familial antithrombin III deficiency

Protein C and protein S deficiency

Estrogen-containing oral contraceptives

Pregnancy

Cigarette smoking

Diabetes mellitus

Thrombocytosis in adolescents (platelet count >10⁶ per cubic mm)

Kawasaki syndrome

Malignancy

Hyperbetalipoproteinemia type II

Hypercholesterolemia

Homocystinuria

Prosthetic devices in circulation

Early stages of DIC

Nephrotic syndrome

Primary antiphospholipid syndrome

Hypercoagulability

A much greater problem in adult than in pediatric medicine, hypercoagulability remains poorly understood. Spontaneous arterial or venous thromboses may occur. The criteria used in adults must be used in the treatment of children. The patient with deep venous thromboses should receive heparin for 1 week, followed by coumarin for 8 to 12 weeks. Underlying associations should be sought and corrected when possible and consideration given to antiplatelet drugs where indicated. Conditions associated with hypercoagulability are noted in Table 41-1.

References

1. Furie B, Limentani SA, Rosenfield CG. A practical guide to the evaluation and treatment of hemophilia. *Blood* 84:3–9, 1994.
2. Lusher JM et al. Recombinant factor VIII for the treatment of previously untreated patients with hemophilia A: Safety, efficacy and development of inhibitors. *N Engl J Med* 328:453–459, 1993.
3. Werner EJ et al. Prevalence of Von Willebrand's disease in children: A multiethnic study. *J Pediatr* 123:893–898, 1994.
4. Blanchette VS et al. A prospective, randomized trial of high-dose intravenous immune globulin G therapy, oral prednisone therapy, and no therapy in childhood acute immune thrombocytopenic purpura. *J Pediatr* 123:989–995, 1994.
5. Andrew M, Blanchette VS. A multicenter study of the treatment of childhood chronic thrombocytopenic purpura with anti-D. *J Pediatr* 120:522–527, 1992.
6. McFarland JG et al. Prenatal diagnosis of neonatal alloimune thrombocytopenia using allele-specific oligonucleotide probes. *Blood* 78:2276–2282, 1991.

William S. Ferguson

42 Hematologic Disorders

Although hematologic abnormalities are common in children, they rarely are responsible for severe acute illness. Thus, in the intensive care unit (ICU) setting, it is likely that any hematologic problem is **not** the primary cause for the patients condition, although it may have a great impact on the patient's care and prognosis. Those caring for a patient with a hematologic disorder must continuously weigh the often conflicting demands of diagnosis and treatment in the context of the patient's overall condition. While hasty treatment may interfere with efforts to establish a diagnosis, there are times when intervention must take precedence to prevent severe injury or death. A proper balance requires an appreciation for the severity and tempo of the patient's illness and the ability to quickly and accurately establish an appropriate differential diagnosis.

General Approach to the Patient

It is easy to focus too narrowly on the patient's major symptom. A systematic review of the patient's history and physical examination, together with a few initial laboratory determinations, should provide a good idea of the general underlying process. Armed with this information, one can then gather any further diagnostic specimens and proceed with any needed therapeutic intervention, even if the results of such tests are not immediately forthcoming.

Personal History

The personal medical history should document the presence, duration, and frequency of

- fatigue (suggestive of anemia or systemic illness)
- pallor (suggestive of anemia)
- jaundice (suggestive of hemolysis)
- bruising or bleeding (suggestive of thrombocytopenia or a coagulopathy)
- cyanosis (which occasionally is due to methemoglobinemia)
- pain (sickle crisis, bone pain from marrow infiltration, splenic engorgement or infarct, etc.)
- hematuria/hemoglobinuria (suggestive of hemolysis or genitourinary bleeding)
- melena or hematochezia (acute or chronic GI blood loss)
- known or possible exposure to drugs, chemicals, or toxins
- symptoms suggestive of acute, chronic, or recurrent infection (either bacterial, viral, or protozoal)
- diet (nutritional deficiency, toxin exposure)
- growth (retarded growth might suggest a dietary deficiency or a constitutional abnormality)
- for infants, the prenatal and perinatal history

Family History

Many hematologic diseases are hereditary; others can be due to environmental causes that may be common to members of the same household. Be sure to ask

- if there are other members who have (or have had) similar problems
- whether other family members have a history of some other hematologic disease or a history of a nonhematologic disease that might have hematologic manifestations (e.g., collagen vascular disorders, malabsorption)
- about ethnic background (many disorders are concentrated in certain ethnic groups)

Physical Examination

Particular note should be made of

- pallor (suggestive of anemia)
- jaundice/icterus (suggestive of hemolysis)
- bruising (suggestive of a bleeding disorder)
- glossitis, changes in skin or nails (suggestive of nutritional deficiencies)
- neurologic defects (constitutional disorder, metabolic disorder, vitamin B_{12} deficiency)
- skeletal abnormalities (constitutional disorders, dietary deficiencies)
- genitourinary abnormalities (constitutional disorders, e.g., Fanconi's syndrome)
- lymphadenopathy (suggestive of infection or malignancy)
- hepatomegaly and/or splenomegaly (suggestive of malignancy or storage disease)
- signs suggestive of an abnormal mass effect (e.g., swelling, obstruction, peripheral nerve dysfunction)

Initial Laboratory Tests

- Complete blood count, including indices and platelet count
- WBC with differential and platelet count
- Reticulocyte count
- Examination of the peripheral smear, noting:
  - RBC morphology
  - WBC morphology
  - platelet size and appearance
  - presence and appearance of any abnormal cells
  - the WBC differential (particularly important when the differential is performed by machine, because certain morphologic changes can "fool" the instrument)
- If a bleeding disorder is suspected, then one should also obtain
  - prothrombin time/partial thromboplastin time (PT/PTT)
  - bleeding time
  - If any aspect of the history or physical exam suggests the presence of hemolysis (sudden onset of pallor, jaundice, hemoglobinuria), then it is wise to include
  - direct and indirect Coombs' (Coombs'-positive hemolytic anemia is a medical emergency)
  - direct and indirect bilirubin (metabolites of released hemoglobin; to confirm presence of hemolysis)
  - lactic dehydrogenase (LDH), SGOT (released from lysed RBC; to confirm presence of hemolysis)

- other liver function tests (to exclude liver disease as cause for jaundice)
- haptoglobin (decreased with intravascular hemolysis; to confirm presence of hemolysis)

Conceptual Approach to Hematologic Disorders

The history, physical examination, and initial laboratory tests should provide the answers to the following questions:

1. Which elements of the blood (erythrocytes, leukocytes, platelets, soluble clotting factors) are affected?
2. Is the process predominately **quantitative** or **qualitative?**
3. If quantitative, is the affected cell line **increased** or **decreased?**
4. Is a decreased number of cells due to **decreased production** or **increased destruction?**

5. Is the process **constitutional** or **acquired?** This is not always obvious. Many constitutional disorders can first manifest symptoms later in life or be manifested only in response to an exogenous stimulus; conversely, acquired defects may be present early in life if due to prenatal or perinatal influences.

Figure 42-1 provides a diagnostic flow-chart.

Quantitative Hematologic Disorders

Table 42-1 provides indices for age-adjusted normal values for hemoglobin, hematocrit, and red cells.

Pancytopenia

By the strictest definition, *pancytopenia* means a combination of anemia, leukopenia, and thrombocytopenia, and in practice is almost always due to decreased production. Pancytopenia can be

Figure 42.1. Algorithm for the initial evaluation of a patient suspected of having a hematologic disorder. Hb, hemoglobin; Hct, hematocrit; wbc, white blood cell count; anc, absolute neutrophil count = (total wbc) × (%polys + % bands)/100); PT, prothrombin time; PTT partial thromboplastin time; DIC, disseminated intravascular coagulation.

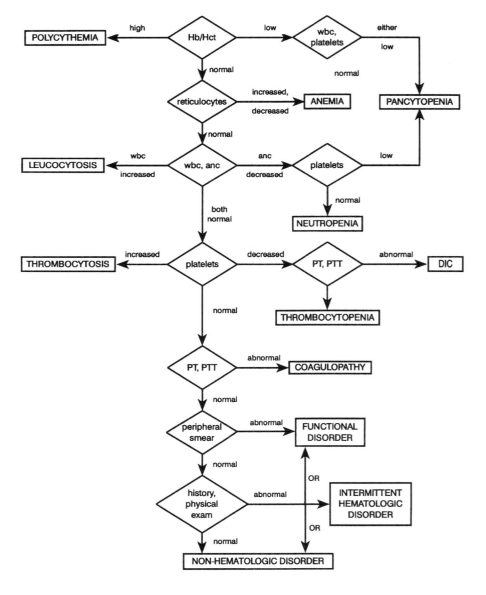

Table 42-1. Red blood cell values at various ages: Mean and lower limit of normal (-2SD)

Age	Hemoglobin (g/dl) Mean	-2 SD	Hematocrit (%) Mean	-2 SD	Red cell count (10^{12}/l) Mean	-2 SD	MCV (fl) Mean	-2 SD	MCH (pg) Mean	-2 SD	MCHC (g/dl) Mean	-2 SD
Birth (cord blood)	16.5	13.5	51	42	4.7	3.9	108	98	34	31	33	30
1–3 days (capillary)	18.5	14.5	56	45	5.3	4.0	108	95	34	31	33	29
1 week	17.5	13.5	54	42	5.1	3.9	107	88	34	28	33	28
2 weeks	16.5	12.5	51	39	4.9	3.6	105	86	34	28	33	28
1 month	14.0	10.0	43	31	4.2	3.0	104	85	34	28	33	29
2 months	11.5	9.0	35	28	3.8	2.7	96	77	30	26	33	29
3–6 months	11.5	9.5	35	29	3.8	3.1	91	74	30	25	33	30
0.5–2.0 years	12.0	10.5	36	33	4.5	3.7	78	70	27	23	33	30
2–6 years	12.5	11.5	37	34	4.6	3.9	81	75	27	24	34	31
6–12 years	13.5	11.5	40	35	4.6	4.0	86	77	29	25	34	31
12–18 years: Female	14.0	12.0	41	36	4.6	4.1	90	78	30	25	34	31
Male	14.5	13.0	43	37	4.9	4.5	88	78	30	25	34	31
18–49 years: Female	14.0	12.0	41	36	4.6	4.0	90	80	30	26	34	31
Male	14.5	13.5	47	41	5.2	4.5	90	80	30	26	34	31

MCV, mean corpuscular volume; MCH, mean corpuscular hemoglobin; MCHC mean corpuscular hemoglobin concentration.
From PR Dallman. In A Rudolph (ed): *Pediatrics* (16th ed. New York: Appleton-Century-Croft, 1977. P 1111. With permission.

due to either **marrow replacement** or **marrow failure** (i.e., aplastic anemia), and be either **congenital** or **acquired.** The processes that can cause pancytopenia need not affect all cell lines to the same extent or at an equal rate; thus, when faced with a decrease in a cell line that is not clearly due to increased destruction, one should include the causes of pancytopenia in the differential diagnosis (Fig. 42-2).

Congenital aplastic anemia (Fanconi's anemia) usually manifests hematologic abnormalities during the first decade in life; many patients exhibit skeletal or genitourinary abnormalities.[1] The chromosomes of these patients are exceptionally prone to breakage either spontaneously or by chemical damage, which is used as a diagnostic test.[2] **Acquired aplastic anemia** can be caused by chemicals, drugs, radiation, and infections, although the majority of cases in children have no discernible cause.[3] Many such cases of idiopathic aplastic anemia may actually represent an autoimmune phenomenon, because various forms of immunosuppression have been successfully employed in reversing the disease.

The most common acquired form of marrow replacement in children is **acute leukemia,** but both lymphomas and sarcomas can also involve the marrow. In contrast to leukemia—in which the marrow is literally packed with neoplastic cells—the marrow of patients with metastatic tumor can occasionally be relatively hypocellular, implicating some form of local myelosuppressive effect. Nonneoplastic causes of marrow replacement include **Langerhans histiocytosis** and infections, such as **tuberculosis.** Congenital disease leading to marrow replacement includes **osteopetrosis** and the storage diseases, such as **Gaucher's disease** and **Niemann-Pick.**

Evaluation

Examination of the bone marrow should be performed in all cases of pancytopenia, unless there is unequivocal evidence for a process that involves destruction of all cell lines (e.g., overwhelming sepsis or hypersplenism). An aplastic marrow should prompt further search for an infectious or toxic cause. The most common cause of marrow replacement is acute leukemia, and samples of aspirated marrow should be obtained for evaluation of surface and cytoplasmic markers and karyotype analysis. On occasion, the hematologic abnormalities resulting from marrow involvement will be the presenting symptoms of metastatic tumors. Because it is unlikely that the bone marrow alone would provide sufficient tissue with which to secure a diagnosis, an aggressive search for the primary tumor should be undertaken.

Treatment

Any necessary supportive care for the various cellular deficiencies should be given, as outlined later in this chapter. Any possible agent that might cause aplastic anemia—in particular, any drug that has been reported to cause marrow suppression—should be removed immediately. For severe aplastic anemia and Fanconi's anemia, bone marrow transplantation is the current treatment of choice[4–6]; unfortunately, many children will not have a fully compatible sibling donor, and transplantation from unrelated donors or related, partially matched donors poses an increased risk of life-threatening graft-versus-host disease.[7] Immunosuppressive therapy, using either antithymocyte globulin,[8–12] high-dose corticosteroids,[5,8,9–14] or cyclosporine,[10,11,15–17] can be effective in many cases; unfortunately, the time to marrow recovery can be quite prolonged (months to years). Acyclovir has been reported to reverse a few cases of aplastic anemia, although these were cases probably caused by a sensitive viral agent.[18] For many years, androgenic steroids were the only treatment available for aplastic anemia; although they may have some beneficial effect in mild or moderate cases,[1] they appear to be no better than supportive care alone for severe cases.[3,4,8] Although the currently available recombinant growth factors (G-CSF and GM-CSF) can temporarily raise the

Figure 42.2. Evaluation of a patient with suspected pancytopenia. DIC, disseminated intravascular coagulation; PT, prothrombin time; PTT, partial thromboplastin time; FSP, fibrin split products.

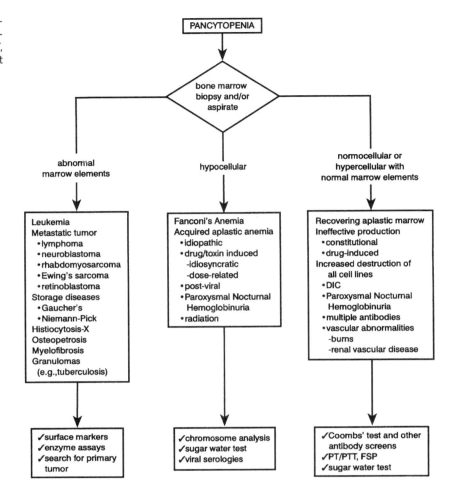

neutrophil count in some patients with aplastic anemia, they have little effect on other cell lines; however, they should be considered in a patient with serious infections in the context of neutropenia.[19,20] *In vitro* data suggest that the recently described stem cell growth factor may provide more generalized marrow recovery.[21,22]

The treatment of marrow replacement is determined by the underlying disorder. Acute leukemia in children generally has a quite good prognosis and usually responds promptly to chemotherapy.[23–26] Although marrow involvement with metastatic lymphomas or sarcomas denotes quite advanced disease, it does **not** preclude long-term survival or even cure and should not be used to justify withholding appropriate antineoplastic therapy.[27–33]

Anemia

The normal ranges for hemoglobin and hematocrit vary widely with age (see Table 42-1). Mild, transient decreases in erythrocyte production are common following even minor infections or other illnesses; thus, mild anemia in this context need not lead automatically to an extensive evaluation, but rather can be followed. In contrast, anemias that are persistent, severe (e.g., Hb more than 10% below the age-adjusted lower limit of normal), or that occur without concurrent illness should prompt a more thorough investigation. The evaluation should be guided by the **mean corpuscular volume** (MCV) and the **reticulocyte count** (see Table 42-1 for the normal range for the MCV, Table 42-2 for the method of

determining the corrected reticulocyte count, and Figs. 42-3 and 42-4 for a diagnostic flowchart).

General Care of the Patient with Anemia

The major function of the RBC is the transport of oxygen by intracellular hemoglobin. A decrease in the concentration of hemoglobin normally is compensated by increased cardiac output and an increase in the percentage of oxygen that is removed from the blood (AV O_2 gradient). An otherwise healthy child or young adult should be minimally symptomatic with a hematocrit greater than 20; a slow drop, particularly in young children, can be reasonably tolerated down to a hematocrit of 10 to 13.

Transfusion of erythrocytes (either whole blood or packed RBC) is the most direct way to augment oxygen-carrying capacity of the blood. The increased concerns about the infectious risks of blood transfusions make it especially important to decide whether a transfusion is actually needed. Remember to treat the patient, not the numbers: Many anemias either will respond rapidly to specific therapy (e.g., iron deficiency) or are self-limited (e.g., hemolysis due to G-6-PD deficiency), whereas concurrent disease may justify maintaining a patient's hematocrit higher than would otherwise be necessary. Because RBC transfusion has the potential of affecting the characteristics of the circulating RBC, any necessary diagnostic tests should be drawn prior to transfusion, if at all possible. In the absence of ongoing blood loss or hemolysis, a transfusion of 10 ml/kg of packed

Table 42-2. Calculation of the corrected reticulocyte count and the reticulocyte production index

$$\text{Corrected reticulocyte count} = \text{observed reticulocyte count} \times \frac{\text{observed hematocrit}}{\text{normal hematocrit for age}}$$

$$\text{Reticulocyte production index} = \frac{\text{corrected reticulocyte count}}{\text{blood reticulocyte maturation time}}$$

Blood reticulocyte maturation time:

Hematocrit	Maturation time (d)
>40	1.0
35	1.5
25	2.0
15	2.5

The normal value for both the corrected reticulocyte count and the reticulocyte production index is 1; the latter number corrects for the tendency toward earlier release of reticulocytes from the marrow to the peripheral blood during periods of anemia, and thus is a more accurate assessment of erythrocyte production during such episodes. Values less than 1 indicate relative underproduction of RBC, and values greater than 1 indicate overproduction of RBCs.[145]

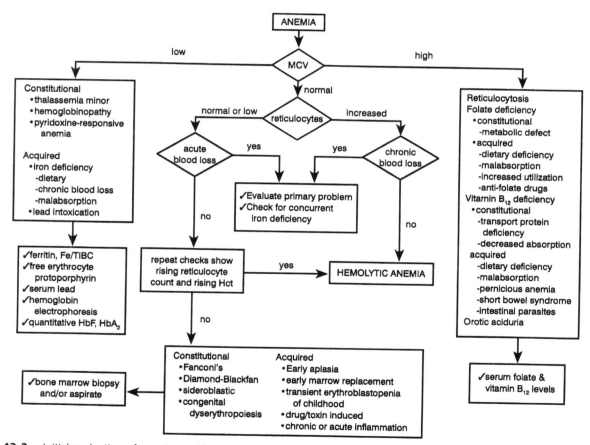

Figure 42.3. Initial evaluation of a patient with anemia. MCV, mean corpuscular volume.

RBCs should raise hematocrit by 7 to 10. Transfusion therapy is discussed more fully in Transfusion Therapy and Apheresis, by Perry and Ilstrup, this volume.

Supplemental oxygen will provide little help to an anemic child with normal pulmonary and cardiac function, because under normal circumstances the hemoglobin in erythrocytes leaving the pulmonary circulation is almost fully saturated with oxygen, and the amount of extra oxygen that can be dissolved in plasma is

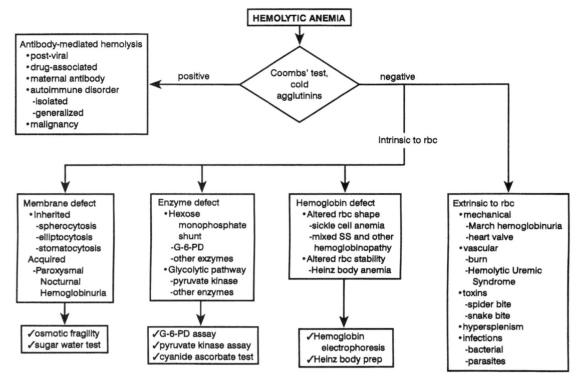

Figure 42.4. Evaluation of a patient with hemolytic anemia.

minimal. However, oxygen may be useful in the context of pulmonary or cardiac disease, or in the presence of hemoglobin with an abnormal oxygen-dissociation curve.

Microcytic Anemias

The vast majority of microcytic anemias involves iron deficiency, lead intoxication, or thalassemia minor. Because these are all common, they will frequently coexist; thus, establishing one diagnosis does not preclude the presence of another. Although the erythrocyte morphology can vary among these disorders (e.g., prominent basophilic stippling in lead intoxication and target cells in thalassemia minor), these differences are not pathognomonic. Microcytosis can also be caused by the sideroblastic anemias, which are rare in children; some hemoglobinopathies are characterized by microcytosis but without anemia.

Iron deficiency is the only cause of microcytosis likely to cause severe anemia. Although lead intoxication can cause significant anemia, other symptoms will probably be more prominent; the thalassemia minor syndromes should cause only mild anemia — indeed, many children with thalassemia minor will have normal hemoglobin levels.

Evaluation

Evaluation should include a measurement of iron status and a hemoglobin electrophoresis (including quantitation of HbA_2 and HbF, which will be increased in beta-thalassemia minor). The serum ferritin provides a better estimate of total body iron stores than the ratio of serum iron to iron-binding capacity, but can be falsely normal in the presence of acute infection or hepatitis.[34,35] Patients with beta-thalassemia minor can have a normal level of HbA_2 and HbF in the context of concurrent iron deficiency, and so these may need to be repeated if microcytosis persists despite iron repletion. If lead intoxication is a possibility, determination of serum lead and the free erythrocyte protoporphyrin level is necessary.

Treatment

Iron deficiency anemia should respond quickly to iron replacement therapy, with a reticulocytosis appearing within 2 to 3 days. Oral iron therapy is preferable to parenteral iron therapy unless there is a condition that precludes enteral feeding or that severely interferes with absorption. The usual dose of oral iron is 6 mg/kg/d in three divided doses, based on the elemental iron content of the particular iron salt. Although ferrous sulfate is felt to be the most bioavailable form of iron, some patients tolerate it poorly; an alternative iron preparation (ferrous gluconate or ferrous fumarate) may be more palatable. An occasional patient will absorb oral iron poorly; switching to an alternative salt, or adding vitamin C, may enhance iron absorption. Iron dextran is a parenteral form of iron that may be given either intramuscularly or intravenously. Intramuscular (IM) injections are painful and can lead to staining of the skin. Intravenous (IV) therapy may thus be better tolerated, although there have been reports of severe adverse reactions to IV iron dextran. Transfusions should be used only for profound iron deficiency anemia or if there is a complicating medical problem that mandates immediate correction of the anemia.

The anemia of lead intoxication should respond rapidly to chelation therapy; it is likely that the other symptoms of lead intoxication will be more severe than the anemia.

Thalassemia minor and other hemoglobinopathies leading to microcytosis should cause, at worst, only a mild anemia that under normal circumstances should require no treatment. More severe anemia in patients known or suspected of having these disorders should prompt a search for an additional etiology.

Macrocytic Anemias

Because reticulocytes have a higher MCV than mature erythrocytes, mild macrocytosis can be seen in the presence of reticulocytosis. True megaloblastic anemias may also have a modestly elevated reticulocyte count, but in addition will demonstrate hypersegmented neutrophils and have characteristic changes in the morphology of erythrocyte precursors in the bone marrow. Neurologic symptoms resulting from dysfunction of the posterior columns of the spinal cord can be seen with vitamin B$_{12}$ deficiency.

Essentially all cases of megaloblastic anemia are due to deficiencies of either folic acid or vitamin B$_{12}$. Primary dietary deficiencies of these vitamins are unusual in developed countries, and so **malabsorption** should be strongly suspected in all cases of megaloblastic anemia. In rare instances, disordered vitamin transport or metabolism is responsible for congenital megaloblastic anemia.[36–40] Equally rare as a cause of congenital megaloblastic anemia is **orotic aciduria,** which combines megaloblastic anemia, crystals of orotic acid in the urine, and typically growth and/or developmental delays and other congenital defects.[41] Antifolate drugs (methotrexate, pentamidine, sulfamethoxazole/trimethoprim) can also cause megaloblastosis, although significant anemia would be unusual when these are given in conventional doses.

Evaluation
Direct measurement should be made of the serum levels of both folic acid and vitamin B$_{12}$. A dietary history may reveal the origin of a deficiency, but evaluation for a generalized malabsorption syndrome should be considered. Although pernicious anemia is rare in children, a Schilling test should be performed in cases of vitamin B$_{12}$ deficiency.

Treatment
Deficiencies of folic acid and vitamin B$_{12}$ should respond quite rapidly to vitamin replacement. If therapy must be instituted prior to making a definitive diagnosis, it is important to replace both folic acid and vitamin B$_{12}$; administration of folic acid alone can exacerbate the neurologic deficits of vitamin B$_{12}$ deficiency.

Normocytic Anemias of Underproduction
The various causes of pancytopenia should be considered when there is a normocytic anemia and an inappropriately low reticulocyte count; although erythrocyte turnover is much slower than that of either platelets or granulocytes, occasionally anemia will be the most prominent presenting symptom of leukemia or aplastic anemia.

The most common cause of acquired red cell aplasia in children is **transient erythroblastopenia of childhood** (TEC), a temporary suppression of red cell production that typically follows a viral infection; some children with TEC will also have moderate neutropenia.[42] Many drugs can also selectively suppress erythrocyte production. Congenital red cell aplasia (Diamond-Blackfan anemia) usually becomes symptomatic during the first year of life; if untreated, it is persistent.[43]

Evaluation
Examination of the bone marrow is the essential first step in the evaluation of these anemias, both to rule out the presence of malignancy or aplasia and to determine the presence or absence of red cell precursors. There will be a complete absence of red cell precursors in Diamond-Blackfan anemia; this can also be seen in TEC, although many patients will already be starting to recover at the time they come for medical attention and will have early red cell precursors in their marrow. Although the distinction between Diamond-Blackfan anemia and TEC can usually be made on the basis of age and marrow morphology, it can sometimes be difficult to make in infants. There are biochemical differences between

Diamond-Blackfan anemia and TEC; although erythrocyte adenine deaminase activity appears to discriminate well between the two disorders,[44] it is not widely available, and those tests that can be routinely measured can be equivocal. Often, the final diagnosis is only determined with time.

Treatment
Any drugs that may contribute to marrow suppression should be discontinued. By definition, TEC spontaneously resolves; some patients, however, will become so anemic that a red cell transfusion is necessary. The course of TEC is usually such that only a single transfusion is necessary, and so a more prolonged anemia should bring the diagnosis into question.

Diamond-Blackfan anemia will usually respond to treatment with corticosteroids.[45] Typically, high doses (1–2 mg/kg/d of prednisone) are required to induce a reticulocytosis, but then more modest doses will suffice to maintain an adequate hematocrit. A few patients seem to eventually outgrow their dependence on glucocorticoids, or are able to periodically discontinue therapy. In those patients who do not respond to steroids, or in whom unacceptably high doses are required to maintain erythropoiesis, chronic transfusions are necessary. Early studies with stem cell growth factor suggest that this particular colony-stimulating factor may eventually be useful in the treatment of Diamond-Blackfan anemia.[22]

Hemolytic Anemias
A significant reticulocytosis is the hallmark of anemias resulting from increased erythrocyte destruction; although usually normocytic, they may be mildly macrocytic due to the relatively high MCV of reticulocytes. Depending on the severity, there may be other signs and symptoms resulting from the accelerated release of erythrocyte contents. Conceptually, a hemolytic process can be either **extrinsic** or **intrinsic** to the erythrocyte. Extrinsic causes of hemolysis include mechanical destruction, toxins, infections (e.g., parasites), and immunologic processes. Intrinsic causes of hemolysis involve defects of the erythrocyte membrane, intracellular enzymes, hemoglobin, or disordered erythrocyte maturation (see Fig. 42-4).

Mechanical destruction can result from diverse causes, such as artificial heart valves and abnormal capillaries or blood vessels.[46] **March hemoglobinuria** is the term used for mechanical hemolysis caused by prolonged walking or running and is not uncommon among long-distance runners.[47] Anemias caused by mechanical destruction are generally limited in severity.

Although many chemicals have been implicated as direct causative agents of hemolysis, few are likely to be readily accessible in the home. **Spider bites** can cause significant hemolysis[48,49]; although some snake venoms can cause hemolysis *in vitro*, the venoms from snakes endemic to North America do not seem to cause significant clinical hemolysis.[50] Inhalation of fresh water can alter the osmolality of blood enough to cause hemolysis, as can the IV or intraperitoneal instillation of distilled water.[51]

Thermal injury has been implicated as a cause of hemolysis in patients with burns, although some degree of microangiopathic anemia is also common.[52] There have been a few reported cases of hemolysis following excessive warming of blood during transfusions.[53,54]

Both bacterial and parasitic infections can directly cause hemolysis; **malaria** is probably the most widespread such infection and should certainly be suspected among anyone with hemolysis who has visited an endemic area of the world.

Immunologic red cell destruction is often instigated by an external stimulus, such as drug exposure, viral infections, or bacterial infections; it can also be seen as part of a more generalized autoimmune disorder. The presence of antierythrocyte antibodies is demonstrated by the **Coombs' test;** the direct Coombs' test detects the presence of antibodies on the red cell, whereas the indirect Coombs' test detects red cell antibodies in the serum. Refinements of the basic test allow determination of the type of reacting antibody. Among adults, Coombs'-positive hemolytic anemias are usually secondary to medications (e.g., penicillins, alpha-methyl dopa); the degree of hemolysis tends to be mild or moderate, and the process quickly reverses once the offending drug is removed. In contrast, Coombs'-positive hemolytic anemias among children are most commonly triggered by a viral infection; they tend to be exceptionally severe and have a significant degree of mortality, even with optimum management.[55] **Coombs'-positive hemolytic anemias in children constitute a true medical emergency and require immediate treatment** (discussion follows).

The most common intrinsic membrane defect is **hereditary spherocytosis;** it is the most common cause of hemolytic anemia among Caucasians. The reticuloendothelial system—primarily in the spleen—treats the spherocytes as it would damaged red cells and removes them prematurely from the circulation. The same process is present in the less common disorders of **hereditary elliptocytosis** and **hereditary stomatocytosis,** although usually less severe than for spherocytosis.[56] All of these disorders typically cause only moderate hemolysis, and there is usually sufficient marrow reserve that the resulting anemia is mild; however, any concurrent depression of red cell production—such as that which can follow parvovirus infections—will rapidly lead to severe anemia.

Paroxysmal nocturnal hemoglobinuria (PNH) is a rare disorder characterized by increased sensitivity of the red cell membrane to the effects of complement. As the name implies, hemolysis tends to be episodic and self-limited; because the membrane defect is not limited to red cells, other cytopenias can be present. In children, PNH can initially present as anemia or pancytopenia without significant signs of hemolysis.[57]

Unstable hemoglobins can also lead to chronic hemolysis.[58,59] Although conceptually the thalassemia major syndromes are anemias of underproduction, in reality they manifest as hemolytic anemias. In part, this is due to actual hemolysis of the misshapen erythrocytes. In addition, there is ineffectual erythropoiesis, which results in erythroid hyperplasia and extramedullary hematopoiesis in an attempt to maintain sufficient red cell mass. The rare **dyserythropoietic** anemias, in which red cell maturation is disordered, can range in severity; the more severe forms mimic thalassemia major.

The most common enzyme defect leading to hemolysis is deficiency of **glucose-6-phosphate dehydrogenase** (G-6-PD).[60–62] This deficiency is widespread, but especially common among Mediterraneans and Africans; the Mediterranean form is more severe. The gene for G-6-PD is on the X chromosome, and so the deficiency is much more common among males. G-6-PD deficiency impairs the production of NADPH and renders erythrocytes more susceptible to oxidant stress. Hemolysis can occur in the context of infections, but is most common following the ingestion of certain drugs or foods (Table 42-3). Because levels of G-6-PD decline as the red cell ages, hemolysis episodes tend to be self-limited as older cells are lysed and only young (relatively enzyme-replete) cells remain. Other defects of the hexose monophosphate shunt, although much rarer, have the same manifestations. Defects of the enzymes of the glycolytic pathway can also lead to hemolysis; the most common such defect, that of pyruvate kinase, is much less common than deficiencies of G-6-PD.

Table 42-3. Drugs and chemicals associated with lysis of G-6-PD-deficient erythrocytes

Drugs with a high risk of hemolysis in conventional clinical doses:

Acetanilid	Niridazole	Sulfacetamide
Diaminodiaphenylsulfone	Nitrofurantoin	Sulfamethoxazole
(Dapsone)	Pamaquine	Sulfanilamide
Fava beans	Pentaquine	Sulfapyridine
Furazolidone	Phenazopyridine	Thiazolesulfone
Methylene blue	Phenylhydrazine	Toluidine blue
Nalidixic acid	Primaquine	Trinitrotoluene
Naphthalene		

Drugs that might cause hemolysis when given to neonates or to individuals with severe variants of G-6-PD deficiency, or when given in doses greater than the usual therapeutic range:

Chloramphenicol	Doxorubicin	Sulfadimidine
Chloroquine	Sulfamethoxypyridazine	Vitamin K analogues

Drugs that are unlikely to cause hemolysis in conventional doses:

Acetaminophen	Phenacetin	Quinine
Aminopyrine	Phenylbutazone	Streptomycin
Aspirin	Phenytoin	Sulfadiazine
Colchicine	Probenicid	Sulfamerizine
Diphenhydramine	Procainamide	Sulfaxone
Dimercaprol	Pyrimethamine	Sulfisoxazole
L-dopa	Quinacrine	Trimethoprim
Isoniazid	Quinidine	Tripelannamine
PAS		Vitamin C

Data from Sullivan and Glader,[61] Beutler,[62] and Luzzatto and Mehta.[63]

Evaluation

The most important test in the evaluation of hemolytic anemia is the Coombs' test; as mentioned earlier, Coombs'-positive hemolytic anemias in children are frequently severe and require immediate therapy.[63]

If the Coombs' test is negative, the history should be reviewed for clues to any extrinsic cause of hemolysis (e.g., March hemoglobinuria, spider bites). In any patient who has been in an area where a parasitic disease such as malaria is endemic, examination of a thick blood smear should be performed. Lacking an extrinsic cause of hemolysis, a reasonable battery of tests would include the osmotic fragility test, G-6-PD assay, and Heinz body test.

The **osmotic fragility test** will detect hereditary spherocytosis. Although the diagnosis of hereditary spherocytosis was originally made on the basis of erythrocyte morphology, the presence of spherocytes in the peripheral smear is neither sensitive nor specific. Red cell morphology will be essentially normal in Wright-stained peripheral smears of about half of patients with hereditary spherocytosis; conversely, spherocytes can be seen in other disorders, particularly Coombs'-positive hemolytic anemia. In contrast, the osmotic fragility test is usually normal in hereditary elliptocytosis and stomatocytosis, and these entities are diagnosed on the basis of the peripheral smear.

Direct measurement of a low erythrocyte enzyme level can confirm a deficiency of G-6-PD. A normal level, however, should be interpreted with caution; because a hemolytic event can remove all but the youngest erythrocytes (those with the highest enzyme levels), a spuriously normal level can be seen during or immediately after a hemolytic episode. If no other cause of hemolysis is found and an individual is felt to be at risk of G-6-PD deficiency on the basis of family history or ethnic background, a repeat determination is probably warranted in 2 to 3 months. Pyruvate kinase deficiency can also be detected by direct enzyme assay; other enzyme deficiencies can be detected by the cyanide-ascorbate test. Although some unstable hemoglobins might be detected by hemoglobin electrophoresis, the Heinz body test is more reliable.

Treatment

Patients with Coombs'-positive hemolytic anemias should be started immediately on high-dose corticosteroids (e.g., 10 mg/kg/d). If the anemia is severe—which is typical—transfusions of packed RBC should be given. Although it may be impossible to find completely compatible units of blood, the best available units should be given; the risks of profound anemia outweigh those of increased hemolysis.[55] Plasmapheresis can be useful in patients with IgM-mediated hemolysis,[64] but it is useless in the more common IgG-mediated episodes. IV gammaglobulin may provide some benefit in patients who do not respond to corticosteroids, but it appears to be less effective in the treatment of immune-mediated hemolysis than it is in the treatment of immune-mediated thrombocytopenia.[65–67]

Drug-mediated hemolysis, whether resulting from a direct toxic effect of the drug or an immune-mediated mechanism, should respond promptly to cessation of the offending substance. Likewise, removal of the instigating food or drug in patients with G-6-PD deficiency will halt the hemolysis; these episodes tend to be self-limited anyway, however, as the older (enzyme-depleted) cells are selectively destroyed. Red cell transfusion may be necessary in patients with the more severe forms of G-6-PD deficiency who develop profound anemia.

Membrane defects and unstable hemoglobins tend to result in mild, chronic anemia. Concurrent suppression of erythropoiesis, however, can rapidly lead to severe anemia, for which red cell transfusions may be necessary.[68–70] Splenectomy will ameliorate the hemolysis caused by hereditary spherocytosis and is usually performed around 8 years of age, unless the degree of hemolysis is quite mild. Hereditary elliptocytosis and stomatocytosis typically cause only very mild hemolysis; in the minority of patients with significant hemolysis, splenectomy will also be helpful.

Neutropenia

Neutropenia can be due to **underproduction** or **increased destruction/utilization** of neutrophils; decreased production can be either acquired or inherited. Because the normal lifespan of a neutrophil in the circulation is only about 12 hours, neutropenia is a frequent early sign of a more generalized marrow suppression.

Congenital neutropenias can range in severity from severe (Kostmann's neutropenia[71]) to relatively benign; the latter can be either familial—benign familial neutropenia—or sporadic.[72–74] Neutropenia can also exist as part of a more generalized disease (e.g., Schwachmann's syndrome,[75] cartilage-hair syndrome[76]). In all of these there is an inborn defect in the maturation of neutrophils. An interesting variation is presented by **cyclic neutropenia,** in which episodes of neutropenia alternate with periods of normal white cell counts.[77]

Many bacterial and viral infections can cause transient cessation of neutrophil production; significant infections also cause consumption of neutrophils. Many drugs can interfere with neutrophil production, either as an idiosyncratic reaction or as a dose-related phenomenon. Antineoplastic chemotherapy is probably the most common cause for severe neutropenia seen in tertiary pediatric centers. These patients will also frequently suffer from a decreased number of monocytes, disordered cell-mediated immunity, and some compromise of antibody production, all of which further decrease their ability to fight infection.

Increased neutrophil utilization can outpace production in the course of severe infections; other mechanisms of increased neutrophil loss include **hypersplenism** and **immune-mediated destruction.**[78] Antineutrophil antibodies can be transferred placentally and cause neonatal neutropenia; although this is a transient neutropenia, significant infections can arise because other segments of the body's defenses against infection are immature.[79] Later in life, antineutrophil antibodies can arise after viral infections, secondary to drug exposure, or as part of a more generalized autoimmune disorder. The so-called *benign neutropenia of childhood* is probably antibody-mediated; the instigating stimulus is unclear in most cases, and the neutropenia usually resolves by the age of 5 years.[80] Postviral antibody-mediated neutropenia can be quite severe and persist for years, but monocytes are usually spared and can carry on some of the phagocytic function usually provided by neutrophils. Although these patients are still at some risk of developing severe, rapidly progressive infection, the risk appears to be less than for patients with impaired neutrophil production.

Evaluation

Significant sepsis or hypersplenism may provide sufficient reason for the observed neutropenia and obviate the need for further specific evaluation (Fig. 42-5) unless correction of the underlying disorder does not result in a concomitant rise in the neutrophil count. A careful drug history should be taken and any medications evaluated for their potential to cause either underproduction or antibody formation.

If there is no obvious cause for the neutropenia, examination of the bone marrow should be performed. This will serve to rule

Figure 42.5. Evaluation of a patient with neutropenia. ANA, anti-nuclear antibody; anc, absolute neutrophil count; ESR, erythrocyte sedimentation rate.

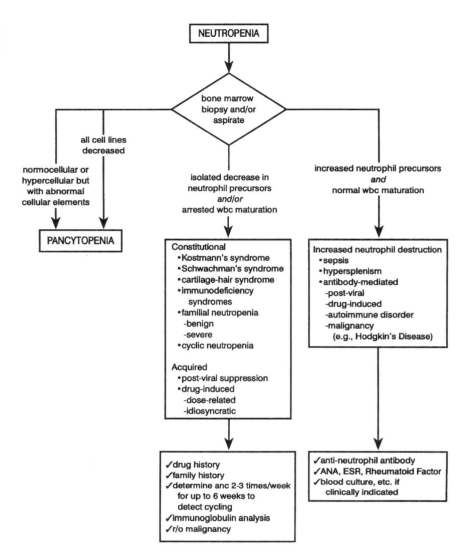

out more generalized marrow failure or replacement and also determine the presence, number, and maturation of any granulocyte precursors. Primary neutrophil underproduction should be manifested by either a decreased total number of myeloid precursors or a failure of complete maturation (although a similar appearance might be seen early in the course of marrow recovery). Cyclic neutropenia can be diagnosed only by observing the periodic rise and fall of the peripheral WBCs; twice-weekly blood counts over a period of 6 to 8 weeks may be necessary to establish this diagnosis.

An increased number of granulocyte precursors implies the presence of increased peripheral destruction. **Anti-neutrophil antibodies** can be detected either in serum or on the surface of neutrophils, but the assays are relatively insensitive, and so a negative test does not rule out the possibility of immune-mediated destruction. Although isolated neutropenia in the absence of any other symptoms would be an unusual presentation for a collagen vascular disorder, such disorders should be considered carefully if there are any other suggestive signs or symptoms.

General Treatment of Neutropenia

As the neutrophil count drops, the risk of developing a bacterial infection rises, the body's ability to limit infection diminishes, and the common inflammatory manifestations of infection are

decreased or absent.[81] The combination of neutropenia and infection is a potentially life-threatening event. Fortunately, fever remains a sensitive (although not specific) indicator of bacterial infection, even in the setting of profound neutropenia. **Regardless of etiology, the combination of fever (>102°F) and neutropenia (absolute neutrophil count <500) represents a potential medical emergency and requires prompt evaluation and therapy.**

The vast majority of bacterial infections in immunocompromised patients results from endogenous flora. Prophylactic hospitalization or antibiotics are useless for the majority of patients, and by altering the endogenous flora to more drug-resistant forms may actually be harmful. One exception is patients with chronic isolated neutropenia or neutrophil dysfunction, for whom prophylactic antibiotics appear to decrease the incidence of serious *Staphylococcus* infections.

Evaluation of the febrile and (potentially) neutropenic patient should include a history exploring the possible symptoms of infection and a complete physical examination.[82,83] Due to their decreased inflammatory response, these patients may have minimal symptoms other than fever. Although the physical examination may be remarkably unrevealing, particular attention should be paid to the skin, mouth, and perirectal area, all common potential sites for bacterial invasion. Many patients undergoing chemotherapy will have permanent indwelling venous catheters, and the site of entry should be examined carefully for signs of infection.

Laboratory studies should include

- CBC, differential and platelet count
- PT/PTT (to check for disseminated intravascular coagulation [DIC] secondary to sepsis)
- CXR (although pneumonia may not manifest an infiltrate when granulocytopenia is severe)
- blood culture (both peripheral and central, if an indwelling catheter is present)
- throat culture
- urinalysis and urine culture
- culture of any other potential sites of infection (e.g., skin abscess)
- electrolytes, BUN, and serum creatinine, if the use of an aminoglycoside antibiotic (or other nephrotoxic agent) is considered

Because the risk of meningitis does not appear to be significantly increased in these patients, lumbar puncture is **not** routinely indicated and should be performed only if there are signs or symptoms suggestive of meningeal infection. If a lumbar puncture is performed, make sure the platelet count is adequate (e.g., >70,000).

The survival of patients with fever and neutropenia is markedly enhanced by the prompt initiation of empiric broad-spectrum antibiotic therapy, which should be started immediately after all appropriate cultures are obtained.[82,83] In the 1970s and early 1980s, most infections in which a causative organism could be identified (which actually comprise a minority of cases—in most, a causative organism is never isolated) were due to enteric gram-negative rods (particularly *Pseudomonas*), *Streptococcus*, or *Staphylococcus*. To provide adequate coverage of these organisms, antibiotics combinations such as carbenicillin-cephalothin-gentamicin or ticarcillin-nafcillin-gentamicin were commonly used.[82] In the late 1980s, the incidence of *Pseudomonas* infection decreased, while the number of infections due to gram-positive cocci increased; concurrently, newer cephalosporins demonstrating broader spectrum and good anti-staphylococcal coverage have been developed.[83] Recent trials at the NCI have shown that single-agent therapy with a broad-spectrum cephalosporin (in their trials, ceftazidime) provided results comparable to combination therapy, and monotherapy with one of the newer broad-spectrum antibiotics would appear to be an acceptable choice in institutions where the incidence of *Pseudomonas* infection is low.[83–87] However, a combination of drugs is usually warranted for any documented infection. For patients with an indwelling venous catheter, who are at particular risk of staphylococcal infection (including *S. epidermatis*, which is commonly nafcillin-resistant), the combination of vancomycin and an aminoglycoside may be preferable. The actual choice of drugs must depend on both the relative incidence of various organisms at any given institution and their pattern of drug sensitivity. Furthermore, frequent reassessment of the adequacy of antibiotic coverage must be made in light of the patient's clinical status and bacteriologic culture data; bacteriologic cultures should be repeated regularly for continuing fever.

Patients experiencing prolonged neutropenia, particularly those who receive extended antibiotic therapy, are also at risk of developing fungal infections. Obviously, a positive fungal culture should prompt initiation of antifungal therapy. In addition, empiric antifungal therapy with amphotericin has been shown to increase survival in neutropenic patients with persistent fever (>7 days) or in whom fever recurs after an afebrile period.[83,88,89]

Documented infections should be treated as appropriate for the particular site and organism.[83,90] The duration of empiric antibiotic coverage in the patient with persistently negative cultures is less clear cut. The most conservative approach would be to continue empiric therapy until the anc is greater than 500; however, this may not be either practical or necessary in patients who have prolonged or chronic neutropenia.[91] In such patients, it has become acceptable practice to stop antibiotic therapy if the patient has been afebrile (<101°F) for at least 24 hours, if all cultures are negative (after a duration of at least 72 hours for the initial set of cultures), and there are neither symptoms nor physical signs of infection. If the patient remains afebrile for 24 hours and there is adequate home care, the patient is discharged; if fever recurs, new cultures are drawn and antibiotics are reinstituted.

Although granulocyte transfusions have theoretical appeal in the treatment of infected neutropenic patients, in practice, the short lifespan of transfused granulocytes limits their utility, and modern antibiotic and antifungal therapy provides adequate treatment in the majority of cases. However, granulocyte transfusions might be worth considering as a temporizing measure in the context of life-threatening infection and severe, but imminently reversible, neutropenia.

Specific Treatment of Neutropenia

If at all possible, any medications that might contribute to neutropenia should be stopped; drug-induced neutropenia should resolve fairly quickly, regardless of the mechanism responsible for the neutropenia. Treatment of hypersplenism should be guided by the clinical situation.

The treatment of familial neutropenia should be guided by the severity of the disorder and the patient's clinical course. Milder neutropenias may require no specific treatment, because infections can be rare and the marrow might still respond to infections with increased granulocyte production.[72,73] More severe familial neutropenias lead to greater risks; prophylactic anti-staphylococcal antibiotics and aggressive treatment of overt infection have increased the lifespan for these patients. Granulocyte colony-stimulating factor (but not granulocyte-macrophage colony-stimulating factor) has been shown to markedly increase neutrophil production in at least some of these patients[92–94] and in some patients with acquired chronic neutropenia.[95,96] Therefore, a therapeutic trial of G-CSF should be used in any patient with a severe defect in neutrophil production and recurrent infections.

The treatment of antibody-mediated neutropenia can be frustrating. Many (but not all) cases will respond to glucocorticoid treatment, although often at a dose that precludes chronic treatment.[78] IV gammaglobulin has been effective in some cases,[67,97–99] but with less consistent success than for immune-mediated thrombocytopenia. The risks of more severe immunosuppressive therapy would seem to outweigh the potential benefits, because these patients often do well with specific treatment of infections.

Thrombocytopenia and Clotting Disorders

These are covered in Hemostasis in Pediatric Critical Care, by Truman, this volume. Figure 42-6 provides a guideline for evaluating thrombocytopenia.

Polycythemia

In evaluating a patient with apparent polycythemia, a true increase in total red cell mass must be distinguished from a rise in hemoglobin concentration resulting from dehydration. Primary polycythe-

Figure 42.6. Evaluation of a patient with thrombocytopenia. DIC, disseminated intravascular coagulation; ANA, antinuclear antibody; ESR, erythrocyte sedimentation rate; PT, prothrombin time; PTT, partial thromboplastin time; FSP, fibrin split products; TAR, thrombocytopenia with absent radii syndrome.

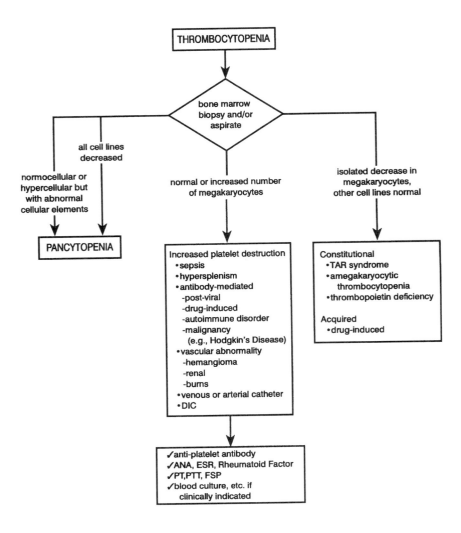

mia is rare in children; secondary polycythemia is usually the compensatory response to decreased oxygen delivery. Causes of secondary polycythemia include

1. Impaired pulmonary oxygenation
   a. decreased ventilation
   b. increased alveolar-arterial oxygen gradient
2. Mixture of oxygenated blood with deoxygenated blood
   a. intrapulmonary shunting
   b. intracardiac-intravascular shunting
3. Decreased blood delivery
   a. generalized, due to cardiac or aortic disease
   b. renal vascular disease
4. Decreased peripheral off-loading of oxygen
   a. abnormal hemoglobin with increased oxygen affinity
   b. severe methemoglobinemia
   c. decreased levels of erythrocyte 2,3-DPG
5. Inappropriate secretion of erythropoietin
   a. renal tumors or cysts
   b. endocrine disorders/tumors
   c. cerebellar hemangiomas

Evaluation

A careful evaluation of the patient's pulmonary and cardiovascular status is most likely to uncover the cause for polycythemia. Hemo-globin electrophoresis will reveal some but not all of the hemoglobins with increased oxygen affinity; direct measurement of oxygen affinity is a less widely available test but would confirm the presence of an electrophoretically normal hemoglobinopathy.[58,59]

Treatment

Moderate secondary polycythemia represents an appropriate compensatory response and should require no specific treatment (although the underlying cause may be amenable to correction). Blood viscosity rises along with the hematocrit, however, and at some point this increased viscosity will cause decreased blood flow through small vessels and an overall drop in oxygen delivery. A significant increase in viscosity usually occurs at a hematocrit between 65 and 70 and may be accompanied by symptoms of tissue hypoxia. Although treatment of any causative factors should be undertaken, acute symptoms may require more rapid correction of the polycythemia. In cases of spurious polycythemia due to decreased plasma volume, fluid replacement is the most appropriate measure. Fluid therapy alone is unlikely to cause a significant or durable response for actual polycythemia; in such patients, removal of blood or partial exchange transfusion may lead to improved tissue oxygenation. Repetitive phlebotomy may be required for secondary polycythemia resulting from disorders for which there is no effective treatment, and for the rare patient with primary polycythemia.

Leukocytosis

The clinical significance of leucocytosis is related not only to the degree of increase but also to the type of cell that is increased. **Lymphocytosis** is common following viral illnesses; during infectious mononucleosis or other viral infections, **atypical lymphocytes** may predominate. To an experienced observer, there should be no confusion between atypical lymphocytes and **lymphoblasts.** Under normal circumstances, lymphoblasts are almost never seen in the peripheral smear and never in significant numbers; their presence should suggest acute leukemia (although only a minority of patients with acute leukemia have lymphoblasts present in their peripheral blood at the time of diagnosis). Patients whose leukemia presents with a high white count are more likely to relapse than patients with a low or normal white count. Very high white counts (e.g., >100,000) can cause tumor lysis syndrome (discussion follows); the risk of venous stasis is also increased, although some patients with spectacularly high peripheral WBC counts are asymptomatic.

An increase in peripheral granulocytes is a common response to infection and to many noninfectious inflammatory disorders. Such **leukemoid reactions** can lead to WBC counts in excess of 50,000 and include some immature neutrophil precursors (metamyelocytes, myelocytes, and even promyelocytes), although mature neutrophils and bands will predominate. Acute myeloid leukemia, in contrast, will usually manifest anemia and/or thrombocytopenia, and the population of myeloid cells will be more monotonous and immature. The degree of peripheral leukocytosis is less of a prognostic indicator in myeloid leukemia than for lymphoid leukemia, but the risk of leukostasis is higher, particularly as the WBC exceeds 100,000.

The only neoplastic-disease that might mimic a leukemoid reaction is **chronic myelogenous leukemia** (CML); in the adult form of CML, there are a variety of mature and immature leukocytes, anemia is absent or mild, and the platelet count is frequently increased. However, CML accounts for only about 1% of childhood leukemias.

Evaluation

Any suspicion of acute leukemia is sufficient cause for bone marrow aspiration and biopsy. The diagnosis of acute leukemia can usually be made from the morphologic appearance of the marrow, although subclassification may depend on characterization of surface or biochemical markers. CML may not present a distinctive morphologic appearance to the marrow; however, karyotypic analysis will reveal the presence of the Philadelphia chromosome, and the level of alkaline phosphatase in peripheral leucocytes will be decreased (as compared with an increased level in nonneoplastic leukemoid reactions).

Lymphocytosis is usually a self-limited manifestation of viral illness; a serologic test for infectious mononucleosis may be warranted if atypical lymphocytes are present.

The cause of a significant leukemoid reaction will often be obvious, particularly among critically ill patients. However, the lack of obvious cause or failure to resolve as the presumptive cause abates should prompt a search for an occult inflammatory process.

Treatment

Acute leukemias will usually respond quickly to the initiation of appropriate antineoplastic chemotherapy. A slower response will be seen in patients with CML. In patients with symptomatic leukostasis, especially for whom specific therapy must be delayed (e.g., pending final identification of the leukemia), **leukopheresis** can effect a prompt and dramatic decrease in peripheral WBC and ameliorate symptoms. The high white count of leukemoid reactions should not primarily cause symptoms; therapy should be directed to the underlying disorder.

Thrombocytosis

An increase in platelet count can be seen in a wide variety of inflammatory states. It is also common as a rebound phenomenon following thrombocytopenia (e.g., following acute idiopathic thrombocytopenic purpura [ITP]), in patients who have undergone splenectomy, and with iron deficiency anemia (and occasionally hemolytic anemias). Thrombocytosis is a late symptom of Kawasaki's syndrome. Chronic myelogenous leukemia can also present with thrombocytosis, but it is usually less impressive than the concomitant leukocytosis, and because the platelets are often dysfunctional there can be increased bruising or bleeding. Primary thrombocythemia, like primary polycythemia, is rare in children.

The major theoretical concern for patients with thrombocytosis is an increased risk of thrombosis. In practice, there appears to be little risk in any patient unless the platelet count exceeds one million, and among otherwise healthy children, there appears to be little risk even at platelet count over one million.[100]

Evaluation

Given the wide variety of benign conditions that can cause thrombocytosis, mild transient elevations of the platelet count can usually be ignored. Persistent unexplained thrombocytosis should prompt some consideration of an occult inflammatory process. Occult malignancies, which can cause thrombocytosis in adults, are uncommon among children.

Treatment

Specific therapy is rarely necessary, because the risk of thrombosis appears to be minimal in children, even with platelet counts over one million. Antiplatelet therapy should be necessary only if a concomitant condition increases the risk of venous thrombosis. Such conditions would include

1. Disordered vascular endothelium (secondary to injury or malformation)
2. Extensive tissue injury
3. Prolonged immobilization or other cause for venous stasis
4. Central venous catheter

If antiplatelet therapy is necessary, aspirin is usually the drug of choice; the addition or substitution of dipyridimole offers no benefit.[101] A single dose of 10 to 15 mg/kg/d should suffice. Aspirin therapy also has been used in Kawasaki's syndrome to prevent coronary artery aneurysms, although the combination of aspirin and IV gamma globulin is more effective.[67]

Qualitative Hematologic Disorders

Erythrocyte Disorders

Many of the qualitative disorders of erythrocytes lead to increased susceptibility to hemolysis, and thus present as hemolytic anemias. Although there is a component of hemolysis in the sickle syndromes, the other clinical manifestations are usually more obvious and severe. Other qualitative red cell disorders that can be symptomatic include methemoglobinemia, sulfhemoglobinemia, and hemoglobins with abnormal oxygen affinity.

Sickle Cell Anemia

Sickle cell anemia is the most common hemoglobinopathy and the most common genetic disease among African-Americans.[102] It is most common in those whose ancestors came from sub-Saharan Africa, but is also found through the Middle East and the Indian subcontinent, and occasionally will be seen in persons of other ethnic backgrounds. Sickle cell anemia results from a single base pair substitution in the hemoglobin beta-chain (HbS). The deoxygenated HbS can form long polymers, which in turn cause a change in the shape of the erythrocyte; this shape change is initially reversible but becomes irreversible with prolonged or repeated sickling. Sickled erythrocytes are less deformable than normal erythrocytes, and so the presence of a significant number of sickled erythrocytes leads to "sludging" in capillaries and small vessels and subsequent obstruction of blood flow. The major manifestations of sickle cell anemia are direct or indirect results of the resulting tissue infarction.

The propensity to sickle and the rate at which hemoglobin polymers form depend on both the absolute concentration of HbS and the relative concentration and type of other hemoglobins. Temperature, pH, and ionic strength also have an effect on the initial stages of polymer formation. Erythrocytes from a normal heterozygote (i.e., HbAS) can be made to sickle only under extreme conditions of deoxygenation; thus, such heterozygotes are almost always asymptomatic. HbC has less inhibitory effect on sickling than HbA; although such double heterozygotes have relatively mild disease, they are considerably more symptomatic than patients with HbAS. HbF, in contrast, exhibits more inhibitory effect than HbA; patients who combine homozygous HbS disease with persistence of fetal hemoglobin (a combination common in the Middle East) can show quite mild disease, even when the concentration of HbF is only 15% to 20% of the total hemoglobin.[103–106]

Patients with homozygous sickle cell disease exhibit a moderate chronic hemolytic anemia; a typical patient will have a hematocrit of 25 to 30 and a moderate reticulocytosis. The anemia itself is largely asymptomatic, although as for any patient experiencing chronic hemolysis, gallstones can form relatively early in life. More important, these patients have a greatly increased risk of infection, and most will also experience the periodic "crises" that are the hallmark of the disease. These episodes can be characterized as vaso-occlusive, sequestration, and aplastic crises.

Vaso-Occlusive Crises

Vaso-occlusive or painful crises are the major clinical manifestation of sickle cell anemia, and are the direct result of small blood vessel occlusion and subsequent tissue infarction.[107] The bones are most commonly involved, but other common locations of vaso-occlusive events include the lungs, spleen, liver, brain, and penis.

A typical vaso-occlusive crisis may involve diffuse pain involving many areas of the body.[102,108] In young children, the pain in small bones of the hands and feet (hand-foot syndrome) is common and may be the initial presentation. In some cases, pain may be localized with point tenderness, swelling, effusion in adjacent joints, fever, and leucocytosis; distinguishing vaso-occlusive crisis from osteomyelitis or septic arthritis, both of which have increased incidence among patients with sickle cell disease, can be difficult.

The **acute chest syndrome** can mimic pneumonia, with fever, cough, pleuritic pain, and infiltrate on chest x-ray.[109] Pneumonia is also common among patients with sickle cell disease, particularly younger patients. Either vaso-occlusive crisis or pneumonia can result in hypoxia, which in turn can exacerbate the tendency to sickle.

Sickling in the **CNS** can occur either spontaneously or in the context of other vaso-occlusive symptoms; the symptoms depend on the site of occlusion and can include paresis, seizures, comas, and disturbances of vision or speech. Mortality from CNS events is approximately 20%, and as many as 70% of survivors will have persistent neurologic abnormalities.[102]

The relatively deoxygenated conditions in the spleen invariably lead to splenic infarction of infancy, although the infarctions may be asymptomatic. Such infarction leads to functional **asplenia** at an early age and contributes to the increased risk of infection that these patients experience.

Priapism affects as many as 40% of males with sickle cell disease, although many of these will have only brief, repetitive episodes that resolve without specific treatment. Painful episodes that persist longer than 3 hours are likely to last for days or even weeks without medical intervention and are likely to cause impotence.

Sequestration Crises

These result from the rapid, progressive pooling of blood in the spleen or liver. Because autosplenectomy occurs at a young age among patients with HbS disease, sequestration crises are common only in young children. Patients with HbSC disease or a combination of HbS and beta-thalassemia are likely to retain splenic function to a later age, and thus are at risk until later in life. Splenic sequestration can rapidly lead to life-threatening hypovolemia and anemia.[102]

Aplastic Crises

Like any patient with chronic hemolysis, even a temporary decrease in red cell production can rapidly lead to profound anemia. Such episodes of aplasia can follow viral infections, although the antecedent infection may be trivial and barely noticed; parvovirus B19 is a particular agent that has been implicated in aplastic crises.[68] In theory, folate deficiency can develop in patients with chronic hemolysis and contribute to erythrocyte underproduction; for this reason, prophylactic folate supplementation should be prescribed for patients with sickle cell anemia.

Infection

From an early age, patients with sickle cell disease are at a significantly increased risk of infection.[110–113] This is due in part to the functional asplenia, which most affected individuals develop during infancy, and for this reason infections with encapsulated organism—particularly *Pneumococcus* and *H. influenzae*—are especially dangerous. The incidence of bacteremia is particularly increased, as is the risk of osteomyelitis. The accurate evaluation of infection is complicated because many of the hallmarks of infection—fever, leukocytosis, increased erythrocyte sedimentation rate (ESR), local inflammation—can also be seen with vaso-occlusive crises; a high index of suspicion should be maintained for patients with sickle cell disease.

Other Manifestations

Many patients will exhibit bony changes of the vertebrae (cod fish deformity), although this rarely has a significant effect on stature. More significant is the development of aseptic necrosis, particularly of the femoral head. All patients will develop some degree of hyposthenuria within the first decade of life, and the obligatory renal fluid loss can increase any tendency to dehydration, which in turn can exacerbate a crisis. Renal tubular dysfunction, hematuria, and papillary necrosis can also be seen in children. The heart is frequently increased in size, usually because of left ventricular hypertrophy. The chronic hemolysis can lead to gallstones, which may become symptomatic as early as the first decade of life. Neovascularization of the retina can be seen in patients with sickle cell anemia but is much more common in patients with HbSC disease. In addition, patients with sickle hemoglobinopathies who develop hyphema secondary to trauma have an increased risk of developing increased intraocular pressure and resultant visual loss.

Evaluation

In many patients, sickle cell anemia is discovered during routine screening performed either prenatally or in the neonatal period; although routine hemoglobin electrophoresis in the newborn will show a predominance of HbF, the presence or absence of HbS and HbA is possible if the test is performed carefully. Sickle cell disease should be considered in any person of African ancestry in whom the diagnosis has not been definitely excluded. In addition, some index of suspicion should exist for those from a non-African ancestry who exhibit suggestive clinical symptoms or chronic hemolytic anemia. The so-called sickle prep, which exposes cells to a solution of sodium metabisulfite, will cause sickling of erythrocytes from both homozygous and heterozygous individuals. Thus, although a negative sickle prep will exclude the diagnosis of sickle cell disease, a positive prep will not distinguish between sickle cell disease and sickle trait. Hemoglobin electrophoresis will confirm the presence of a sickle hemoglobin and distinguish sickle disease from sickle trait; it will also identify double heterozygotes (e.g., HbSC and HbSD).

The evaluation of a patient in crisis must be guided by the presenting signs and symptoms. A complete blood count and reticulocyte count should be performed on all patients. Vaso-occlusive crises can be relatively free of objective findings, and further evaluation may be unnecessary. Although fever, leukocytosis, and a high ESR can be seen during an uncomplicated vaso-occlusive crisis, any of these signs suggest the presence of infection. Fever that is high (e.g., >102°F), rapidly rising, or that occurs in the absence of significant pain is particularly suggestive of bacterial sepsis.[110] In young children, the acute chest syndrome is more often pneumonia than pulmonary infarction.[109] Focal pain, tenderness, and erythema can be seen with bone infarctions but are suggestive of osteomyelitis. Although osteomyelitis is not the usual cause of hand-foot syndrome, a prolonged course should increase the suspicion of infection.

If infection is suspected, blood and throat cultures should be obtained, and, if possible, a urine culture. If osteomyelitis is considered, direct culture of the affected bone should performed. Adequate sputum cultures may help in the subsequent management of suspected pneumonia but are difficult to obtain in young children. A lumbar puncture should be performed if there are any signs of meningitis. Significant right upper quadrant pain should suggest gallstones or biliary tract disease,[107] which can be confirmed by ultrasound.

CNS events can present with dramatic and unmistakable signs and symptoms; however, it may be more difficult to assess patients who are receiving narcotics for pain medication. Significant headache or any specific neurologic sign should arouse suspicion of a CNS event. A CT scan should be obtained in these cases, although in younger children, cerebral infarctions are more common than hemorrhage, and the CT scan may not reveal any abnormality early in the course of the event. A lumbar puncture may be useful for patients in whom a subarachnoid hemorrhage or meningitis is being considered.

Treatment

Preventive Care

An effective and safe means of preventing vaso-occlusive crises remains elusive. Several different compounds that inhibit sickling in vitro have undergone clinical trials but either have demonstrated little success or been accompanied by unacceptable toxicity.[114,115] It is obviously prudent for patients to avoid conditions that would predispose to sickling—cold, dehydration, hypoxia. Because fetal hemoglobin retards sickling,[103-106] there has been research into agents that increase the relative production of fetal hemoglobin in vivo. **5-Azacytidine** is effective but requires parenteral administration and has the potential for severe myelosuppression.[116,117] **Hydroxyurea**—either alone[118-121] or in combination with erythropoietin[122]—has been shown to cause a significant elevation in fetal hemoglobin levels in patients with sickle cell disease with modest myelosuppression; clinical trials in adult patients have shown that hydroxyurea can decrease the frequency and severity of painful crises.[123] Trials of the efficacy and safety of hydroxyurea in children are underway. Preliminary studies have also shown that derivatives of butyrate can also increase HbF levels.[124,125]

Functional asplenia occurs early in life, and patients with sickle cell disease should be on prophylactic antibiotics (e.g., penicillin).[126] They should also be immunized with pneumococcal vaccine as well as a vaccine against *H. influenzae* type B.[127] As in any patient with chronic hemolysis, a relative folic acid deficiency can develop and contribute to erythrocyte underproduction; accordingly, supplemental folic acid (1 mg/d) is also recommended. Iron supplements are **not** indicated unless there is proven iron deficiency.

Painful Crises

Pain control and hydration are the mainstays of the treatment of vaso-occlusive crises.[102,128] Crises can have few objective findings but still be extremely painful. Because painful crises tend to be repetitive, the potential for narcotics abuse or addiction does exist; unfortunately, this concern is often used as an excuse for providing inadequate pain control. Moderate pain can often be controlled at home with nonnarcotic analgesics or Percocet (or its equivalent). If these are not providing adequate pain relief, admission for parenteral narcotics is necessary. At least modest comfort should be attainable with either morphine or Demerol; in teenagers or adults, patient-controlled anesthesia can provide some degree of patient control while allowing careful monitoring of the amount of analgesia required. Total fluid intake should approximate one and one-fourth maintenance; because of the hypothesnuria that is common in sickle cell disease, urine output or osmolality may be a poor guide to hydration status. For similar reasons, diuretics such as furosemide are generally contraindicated because the hyposthenuria can lead to excessive urine losses and rapid dehydration.

For most patients, supplemental oxygen will be of little utility in decreasing the duration or intensity of painful crises, because in the absence of pulmonary or cardiac disease, the hemoglobin will be fully saturated while the patient is breathing room air.[128] Supplemental oxygen may be helpful for patients with acute or preexisting pulmonary disease, who can have significant arterial desaturation, which in turn can exacerbate intravascular sickling.[102,109,128] Monitoring of oxygen saturation can be extremely helpful in the management of these patients.

Infections

A low threshold should exist for suspecting infection, and empiric antibiotic therapy should be started immediately after the appropriate cultures have been obtained.[102,110–112,129] There should be adequate coverage of pneumococcal infections, which are especially common among asplenic patients. Coverage for *H. influenzae* should continue until the second decade of life and be considered in all patients with pulmonary symptoms. Thus, appropriate choices for initial antibiotic coverage include ampicillin or a third-generation cephalosporin. *Mycoplasma* infections can occur in older patients, and positive cold agglutinins should prompt the **addition** of erythromycin to the antibiotic regimen. Bone infections require treatment for both *Staphylococcus* and *Salmonella*.

Transfusions

Aplastic crises can occur alone or be superimposed on vaso-occlusive crises or infection. Simple transfusion of packed RBCs should be performed once the hematocrit falls below 20, or in any patient exhibiting significant symptoms related to the anemia (e.g., heart failure, dyspnea, mental status changes). Patients undergoing sequestration crises may exhibit catastrophic declines in hematocrit, with subsequent shock and death; immediate and massive blood transfusions and fluid support can literally be life-saving.[102,128] Subsequent splenectomy should be strongly considered in any patient who experiences a significant sequestration crisis, because there is a tendency for them to recur.

Partial exchange transfusions can speed resolution of vaso-occlusive crises by lowering the concentration of erythrocytes susceptible to sickling. Because of the associated risks, transfusions are not indicated for the treatment of uncomplicated painful crises or minor infections. The goal of partial exchange transfusions is to reduce the percentage of susceptible erythrocytes to less than 30%; however, the total hematocrit should be kept at less than 45%, because above that level, viscosity increases and may itself contribute to prolonged capillary transit time and increased sickling.

Indications for **immediate** partial transfusion include[102]

- any CNS event
- severe infection
- progressive pulmonary disease
- acute priapism that fails to respond to medical management within 6 hours
- fat embolization

Less urgent indications for partial exchange include

- general anesthesia
- surgery not requiring general anesthesia but requiring placement of a tourniquet
- painful crises lasting more than 7 days
- acute chest syndrome lasting more than 4 days
- administration of contrast material

Often, these subacute transfusions can be effected by repeated simple transfusions of packed RBCs over 2 to 3 days, without the necessity of removing blood; this is particularly true if significant hemolysis is occurring.

Chronic transfusion therapy should be performed on all patients following a CNS event for a minimum of 3 years, and perhaps for life.[130,131] Chronic transfusions have also been advocated during pregnancy because of the high risk of complications to both mother and infant; although the incidence of painful crises during pregnancy can be reduced, it is not clear that the probability of other complications is similarly decreased.[132] Although the risks of chronic transfusion preclude their general use in the prevention of painful crises, for some patients who suffer from especially frequent and severe crises—particularly if complicated by dependency on narcotics—the benefits of chronic transfusion will outweigh the risks.

Methemoglobinemia

The reversible association of oxygen with hemoglobin requires that the heme iron atom be maintained in the ferrous state. There is a continual tendency for oxidation to ferric iron, which can be exacerbated by many substances with oxidative potential (Table 42-4). Ferric iron is reduced by a NADH-dependent **methemoglobin reductase**, which normally keeps the level of methemoglobin under 1%. An inherited deficiency of this enzyme is responsible for most cases of congenital methemoglobinemia.[133,134] Because there is normally a considerable excess of reducing capacity in the erythrocyte, heterozygotes do not spontaneously demonstrate increased levels of methemoglobin, although, as might be expected, they will be more susceptible to the effects of oxidant stress. Structural changes of the globin molecule, which increase the tendency for the heme iron atom to be oxidized, are a much less common cause for methemoglobinemia.

Congenital methemoglobinemia is a rare disorder. Aside from cyanosis, most patients will be asymptomatic. Symptoms, if they occur, are related to the loss of oxygen-carrying capacity and are most likely to exist following exposure to oxidizing substances. Concentrations of methemoglobin up to 30% should be asymptomatic unless there is concurrent anemia. As the level increases to 50%, symptoms of hypoxemia will appear; levels above 50% will cause significant symptoms, and levels above 70% can lead rapidly to death.

Ingestion of drugs that oxidize hemoglobin can also cause methemoglobinemia in the absence of a biochemical disorder. See Table 42-4 for a listing of drugs implicated as possible causes of methemoglobinemia.

Evaluation

Methemoglobin causes observable cyanosis at a lower level than deoxy-hemoglobin (2 g/dl vs. 3 to 5 g/dl). Cyanosis in the absence of pulmonary or cardiac disease should suggest the presence of methemoglobinemia. Although quantitative measurement of the amount of methemoglobin can be performed, a rapid bedside test consists of exposing a sample of blood (either in a test tube or applied to a piece of paper) to air. Deoxy-hemoglobin should reoxygenate promptly; a persistent dark color supports the presence of either methemoglobin or sulfhemoglobin. In any patient suspected of having methemoglobinemia, a careful review of any possible chemical exposure should be done.

Treatment

Mild methemoglobinemia (<30% methemoglobin) requires no treatment, although the cyanosis may prompt therapy for cosmetic reasons. Patients with mild symptoms can be treated with oral methylene blue at an initial dose of 2 to 4 mg/kg/d; the dose can then be titrated empirically. More severe symptoms should be treated with 1 to 2 mg/kg of IV methylene blue, which should cause resolution or diminution of the methemoglobinemia within an hour.[133,134] Methylene blue causes reduction of methemoglobin via the hexose monophosphate shunt, and so will not be effective for individuals with G-6-PD deficiency.[135] Symptomatic patients

Table 42-4. Drugs that have been implicated as causes of methemoglobinemia

Acetanilid	Hydroquinone	Phenols
Acetophenetidin	Hydroxyamine	Phenylazopyridine
Acilinoethanol	Hydroxylacetanilid	Phenylenediamine
Alloxans	Inks, marking	Phenylhrazine
Alpha naphthylamine	Kiszka	Phenyhydroxylamine
Aminophenols	Lidocaine	Phenytoin
Ammonium nitrate	Menthil	Piperzine
Amyl nitrite	Meta-chloraniline	Plasmoquine
Antipyrine	Methylacetanilid	Prilocaine
Arsine	Methylene blue	Primaquine
Benzocaine	Monochloroaniline	Propitocaine
Bismuth subnitrate	Moth balls	Pyridine
Chloranilines	Naphthylamines	Pyridium
Chlorates	Nitrates	Pyrogallol
Chlorobenzene	Nitrites	Quinones
Chloronitrobenzene	Nitrobenzene	Resorcinol
Cobalt preparations	Nitrofurans	Shoe dye or polish
Corning extract	Nitrogen oxide	Spinach
Crayons, wax (red or	Nitroglycerine	Sulfonal
orange; no longer	Nitrosobenzene	Sulfonamides
manufactured)	Pamaquine	Sulfones
Dapsone	Para-aminopropiophenone	Tetrain
Diaminodiphenylsulfone	Para-bromoaniline	Tetranitromethane tetronal
Diesel fuel additives	Para-chloroaniline	Toluenediamine
Dimethylamine	Para-nitroaniline	Toluidine
Dimethyl aniline	Para-toluidine	Toluyhydroxylamine
Dinitrobenzenes	Pentaerythritol tetranitrate	Trichlorocarbanilide
Dinitrophenol	Phenacetin	Trinitrotoluene
Dinitrotoluene	Phenetidin	Trional

From S. Curry. Methemoglobinemia. *Ann Emerg Med* 11:214–220, 1982. With permission.

who do not respond to methylene blue should be treated with exchange transfusion.

Sulfhemoglobinemia

Ingestion of sulfur-containing drugs can lead to formation of sulfhemoglobin.[136] Like methemoglobin, low concentrations of sulfhemoglobin can cause clinical cyanosis. Sulfhemoglobinemia should be suspected when blood cyanosis is not affected by oxygenation or the administration of methylene blue; its presence can be confirmed by spectroscopic analysis. The level of sulfhemoglobin is rarely so high that the oxygen-carrying capacity of the blood is compromised; therefore treatment is rarely necessary. Because there is no known mechanism by which sulfhemoglobinemia can be reversed, the only effective treatment for symptomatic sulfhemoglobinemia would be blood transfusion.

Altered Oxygen Affinity

Hemoglobin mutations resulting in both increased and decreased oxygen affinity have been described.[58,59] Increased hemoglobin affinity for oxygen results in decreased tissue off-loading, and the compensatory response is polycythemia (the evaluation and treatment of polycythemia was discussed earlier). Moderately decreased oxygen affinity leads to increased tissue off-loading of oxygen; such patients tend to be mildly anemic. With a larger decrease of oxygen affinity there can be cyanosis resulting from the incomplete saturation of arterial hemoglobin. The diagnosis of these abnormal hemoglobins depends on either the demonstration of a characteristic change in the electrophoretic mobility or direct measurement of the oxygen affinity. Except for patients with severe secondary polycythemia, treatment is rarely necessary.

White Cell Disorders

The defensive function of neutrophils is dependent on the proper functioning of a complex set of cellular activities, including chemotaxis, neutrophil adhesion, phagocytosis, fusion of granules with phagocytic vacuoles, and subsequent destruction of ingested bacteria. Multiple mechanisms contribute to the neutrophil's bactericidal activity, including the generation of reactive superoxide and hydrogen peroxide. Defects in any of these cellular functions can lead to an increased susceptibility to bacterial infection.[137] In some disorders (e.g., Chediak-Higashi syndrome) the cellular defect also affects other cells. Disorders affecting granule formation or function may demonstrate distinctive morphologic changes.

The most consistent feature of qualitative granulocyte disorders is recurrent bacterial infections, which may respond slowly to antibiotic therapy. Staphylococcal infections, in particular, are common in these patients. The signs of acute inflammation may be minimal; granuloma formation is seen in several of these disorders and can contribute to their morbidity.

Evaluation

A qualitative granulocyte disorder should be considered in the differential diagnosis of any patient with recurrent or chronic bacterial infections. All the disorders of granulocyte function are all quite rare, however, and abnormalities in the production of immunoglobulins or complement proteins are more likely causes of recurrent infections. HIV infection must also be considered in a child with recurrent infections.

The defect in superoxide production that exists in chronic granulomatous disease can be detected by the nitroblue tetrazolium test[138]; specific evaluation of other potential defects in granulocyte function requires specialized laboratory facilities and expertise.

Treatment

Few specific therapeutic options exist for patients with neutrophil dysfunction, although gamma-interferon has recently been shown to decrease the incidence and severity of infections in patients with chronic granulomatous disease.[139] Prophylactic antibiotics, either with trimethoprim-sulfamethoxazole or an anti-staphylococcal penicillin, can help reduce the incidence of infections.[140] When infections do occur, prolonged courses of IV antibiotics may be required; obviously, a reasonable attempt at isolating a causative organism should be made prior to initiating antibiotic therapy. Patients with chronic granulomatous disease may require surgical drainage of granulomas; glucocorticoids have been useful in rapidly shrinking granulomas that are causing acute obstruction.[141]

Platelet Disorders

Qualitative platelet disorders are covered in Hemeostasis in Pediatric Critical Care by Truman, this volume.

Oncologic Emergencies

Tumors can cause morbidity either through a direct mass effect or by metabolic disturbances. The entities considered here are the **superior mediastinum syndrome** and the **tumor lysis syndrome.**

Superior Mediastinum Syndrome

Masses in the superior mediastinum can cause symptoms by compressing the trachea, leading to stridor and respiratory distress, and by impeding venous return from the head (SVC syndrome).[142,143] Lymphoid malignancies—in particular, lymphoblastic lymphoma and T-cell leukemia—are the most common primary cause of the superior mediastinum syndrome in children. Other malignancies that present with a superior mediastinal mass include teratomas, thymomas, and thyroid carcinomas; other possibilities include primary tumors of the chest wall, including Ewing's sarcoma, primitive neuroectodermal tumor, and rhabdomyosarcoma. Granulomas are the most common nonneoplastic cause of superior mediastinal syndrome; isolated SVC syndrome can result from intravascular thrombosis, which is usually secondary to surgery or the presence of a central venous catheter. Because lymphoid malignancies grow rapidly and the thorax is a relatively confined space, the airway or vascular compromise can rapidly progress to a life-threatening state.

Evaluation

Chest x-ray will usually confirm the presence of a mediastinal mass; sometimes a relatively asymptomatic mass is detected on chest x-ray obtained for unrelated reasons or during the evaluation of cervical adenopathy. The precise size and location of tumor is usually best evaluated by a CT scan; additional images of the neck and abdomen may be useful in delineating the spread of disease. A complete blood count may suggest the presence of leukemia, in which case a bone marrow aspiration and biopsy would be the next diagnostic step. Ideally, a tissue diagnosis is preferred prior to giving any antineoplastic therapy. Unfortunately, the degree of tracheal compromise often makes it impossible to perform a biopsy safely, and empiric therapy might be necessary.

Treatment

Significant airway compromise requires immediate therapy aimed at shrinking the tumor mass. Corticosteroids (e.g., 1–2 mg/kg of methylprednisolone, followed by 2 mg/kg/d) will cause rapid shrinkage of either a non-Hodgkin's lymphoma (NHL) or a thymus enlarged by lymphoblastic leukemia; unfortunately, the histologic and biochemical features of these neoplasms will be obscured equally rapidly. If a tissue diagnosis cannot be made prior to starting therapy, a rapid response to steroids can be taken as strong evidence favoring NHL, and a full course of appropriate chemotherapy should be given. Radiation therapy is equally effective against lymphoid malignancies and will usually have an effect on other tumors. Under some circumstances, the radiation port can be tailored to spare peripheral tissue for later diagnostic sampling, a theoretical advantage that must be weighed against the long-term risks of radiation exposure. In severely compromised patients, both steroids and emergency radiation therapy should be given.

Tumor Lysis Syndrome

Tumor lysis syndrome refers to the combination of metabolic derangements resulting from the rapid cytolysis of malignant cells.[142,144] These changes include elevations in serum levels of uric acid, potassium, and phosphorus; symptomatic hypocalcemia can result from the hyperphosphatemia. Hyperuricemia can cause renal failure, with a subsequent inability to correct the metabolic abnormalities. Tumor lysis syndrome is most commonly seen in rapidly growing malignancies, which also tend to exhibit the most rapid cell kill in response to chemotherapy. It is particularly likely in large NHL (especially Burkitt's lymphoma) and in acute leukemias when the peripheral WBC exceeds 100,000; indeed, some degree of tumor lysis syndrome can be seen in patients with these diseases even before the initiation of treatment.

Evaluation

The following initial laboratory tests should be obtained:

Na, K, Cl, CO_2

BUN/creatinine

Ca, P, Mg

uric acid

urinalysis

Repeat testing should be performed as warranted by individual circumstances.

Treatment

The primary goal of treatment is to maintain adequate renal function. All patients with lymphoid malignancy or bulky nonlymphoid tumor should receive adequate alkaline hydration (e.g., 2 to 3 times maintenance, including 50–100 mEq/liter of $NaHCO_3$) and allopurinol. At this time, IV allopurinol is available only on an experimental basis; in patients unable to take oral medication, the pills can be crushed and given rectally. Placement of a Foley catheter may be necessary to follow urine output and prevent urethral obstruction by uric acid crystals. Hyperkalemia should be treated with cation exchange resins, and aluminum hydroxide antacids should be given for hyperphosphatemia. An algorithm for the management of tumor lysis syndrome is given in Fig. 42-7.

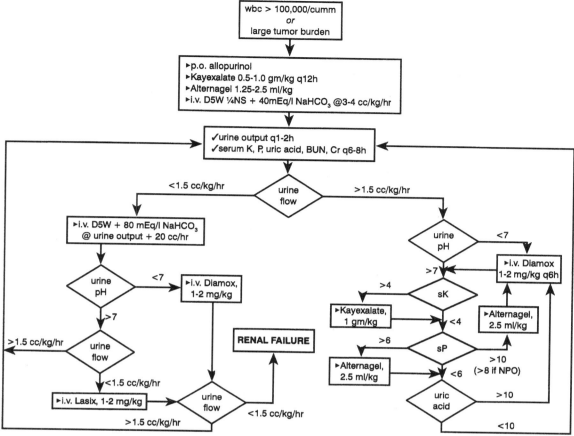

Figure 42.7. Algorithm for the treatment of tumor lysis syndrome.

References

1. Fanconi G. Familial constitutional panmyelocytopathy, Fanconi's anemia (F.A.). I. Clinical aspects. *Semin Hematol* 4:233–240, 1967.
2. Schmid W. Familial constitutional panmyelocytopathy, Fanconi's anemia (F.A.). II. A discussion of the cytogenetic findings in Fanconi's anemia. *Semin Hematol* 4:241–249, 1967.
3. Camitta BM, Storb R, Thomas ED. Aplastic anemia: Pathogenesis, diagnosis, treatment, and prognosis. *N Engl J Med* 306:645–652, 712–718, 1982.
4. Camitta BM et al. A prospective study of androgens and bone marrow transplantation for treatment of severe aplastic anemia. *Blood* 53:504–514, 1979.
5. Wemer EJ et al. Immunosuppressive therapy versus bone marrow transplantation for children with aplastic anemia. *Pediatrics* 83:61–65, 1989.
6. Gluckman E et al. Bone marrow transplantation in 107 patients with severe aplastic anemia using cyclophosphamide and thoraco-abdominal irradiation for conditioning: Long-term follow-up. *Blood* 78:2451–2455, 1991.
7. Camitta B et al. Bone marrow transplantation for children with severe aplastic anemia: Use of donors other than HLA-matched siblings. *Blood* 74:1852–1857, 1989.
8. Gluckman E et al. Results of immunosuppression in 170 cases of severe aplastic anaemia. *Br J Haematol* 51:541–550, 1982.
9. Champlin R, Ho W, Gale RP. Antithymocyte globin treatment in patients with aplastic anemia. *N Engl J Med* 308:113–118, 1983.
10. Frickhofen N et al. Treatment of aplastic anemia with antilymphocyte globulin and methylprednisolone with or without cyclosporine. *N Engl J Med* 324:1291–1304, 1991.
11. Gluckman E et al. Multicenter randomized study comparing cyclosporine-A alone and antithymocyte globulin with prednisone for treatment of severe aplastic anemia. *Blood* 79:2540–2546, 1992.
12. Doney K et al. Immunosuppressive therapy of aplastic anemia: Results of a prospective, randomized trial of antithymocyte globulin (ATG), methylprednisolone, and oxymethalone to ATG, very high-dose methylprednisolone, and oxymethalone. *Blood* 79:2566–2571, 1992.
13. Bacigalupo A et al. Bolus methylprednisolone in severe aplastic anemia. *N Engl J Med* 300:501, 1979.
14. Bacigalupo A et al. Treatment of severe aplastic anemia with bolus 6-methylprednisolone and anti-lymphocyte globulin. *Blut* 41:168–171, 1980.
15. Stryckmans PA et al. Cyclosporine in refractory severe aplastic anemia. *N Engl J Med* 310:655–666, 1984.
16. Wisloff F, Godal HC. Cyclosporine in refractory severe aplastic anemia. *N Engl J Med* 312:1193, 1985.
17. Kojima S et al. Cyclosporine and recombinant granulocyte colony-stimulating factor in severe aplastic anemia. *N Engl J Med* 323:920–921, 1990.
18. Bacigalupo A, Frassoni F, Van Lint MT. Acyclovir for the treatment of severe aplastic anemia. *N Engl J Med* 310:1606–1607, 1984.
19. Vadham-Raj S et al. Stimulation of myelopoiesis in patients with aplastic anemia by recombinant human granulocyte-macrophage colony-stimulating factor. *N Engl J Med* 319:1628–1634, 1988.
20. Guinan EC et al. A phase I/II trial of recombinant granulocyte-macrophage colony-stimulating factor for children with aplastic anemia. *Blood* 76:1077–1082, 1990.
21. Wodnar-Filipowicz A et al. Stem cell factor stimulates the in vitro growth of bone marrow cells from aplastic anemia patients. *Blood* 79:3196–3202, 1992.

22. Alter BP et al. Effect of stem cell factor on in vitro erythropoiesis in patients with bone marrow failure syndromes. *Blood* 80:3000–3008, 1992.

23. Clavell LA et al. Four-agent induction and intensive asparaginase therapy for treatment of childhood acute lymphoblastic leukemia. *N Engl J Med* 315:657–663, 1986.

24. Steinherz PG et al. Improved disease-free survival of children with acute lymphoblastic leukemia at high risk for early relapse with the New York regimen—A new intensive therapy protocol: A report from the Children's Cancer Study Group. *J Clin Oncol* 4:744–752, 1986.

25. Krance RA et al. A pilot study of intermediate-dose methotrexate and cytosine arabinoside, "spread-out" or "up-front," in continuation therapy for childhood non-T, non-B acute lymphoblastic leukemia: A Pediatric Oncology Group study. *Cancer* 67:550–556, 1991.

26. Steuber CP et al. A comparison of induction and maintenance therapy for acute nonlymphocytic leukemia in childhood: Results on a Pediatric Oncology Group study. *J Clin Oncol* 9:247–258, 1991.

27. Ziegler JL. Treatment results of 54 American patients with Burkitt's lymphoma are similar to the African experience. *N Engl J Med* 297:75–80, 1977.

28. Patte C et al. Improved survival rate in children with stage III and IV B cell non-Hodgkin's lymphoma and leukemia using multi-agent chemotherapy: Results of a study of 114 children from the French Pediatric Oncology Society. *J Clin Oncol* 4:1219–1226, 1986.

29. Maurer HM et al. The intergroup rhabdomyosarcoma study–I: A final report. *Cancer* 61:209–220, 1988.

30. Miser JS et al. Preliminary results of treatment of Ewing's sarcoma of bone in children and young adults: Six months of intensive combined modality therapy without maintenance. *J Clin Oncol* 6:484–490, 1988.

31. Cangir A et al. Ewing's sarcoma metastatic at diagnosis: Results and comparisons of two intergroup Ewing's sarcoma studies. *Cancer* 66:887–893, 1990.

32. Shafford EA, Rogers DW, Pritchard J. Advanced neuroblastoma: Improved response rate using a multiagent regimen (OPEC) including sequential cisplatin and VM-26. *J Clin Oncol* 2:742–747, 1984.

33. Philip R et al. High-dose chemoradiotherapy with bone marrow transplantation as consolidation therapy in neuroblastoma: An unselected group of stage IV patients over 1 year of age. *J Clin Oncol* 5:266–271, 1987.

34. Lipschitz DA, Cook JD, Finch CA. A clinical evaluation of serum ferritin as an index of iron stores. *N Engl J Med* 290:1213–1216, 1974.

35. Elin RJ, Wolff SM, Finch CA. Effect of induced fever on serum iron and ferritin concentrations in man. *Blood* 49:147–153, 1977.

36. Hakami N et al. Neonatal megaloblastic anemia due to inherited transcobalamin II deficiency in two siblings. *N Engl J Med* 285:1163–1171, 1971.

37. MacKenzie IL et al. Ileal mucosa in familial selective vitamin B₁₂ malabsorption. *N Engl J Med* 286:1021–1025, 1972.

38. Fenton WA, Roxenberg LE. Inherited disorders of cobalamin transport and metabolism. In Scriver CR et al (eds): *The Metabolic Basis of Inherited Disease.* New York: McGraw-Hill, 1989. Pp 2065–2081.

39. Erbe RW. Inborn errors of folate metabolism. *N Engl J Med* 293:753–757, 807–812, 1975.

40. Rosenblatt DS. Inherited disorders of folate transport and metabolism. In Scriver CR et al (eds): *The Metabolic Basis of Inherited Disease.* New York: McGraw-Hill, 1989. Pp 2049–2064.

41. Suttle DP, Becroft DMO, Webster DR. Hereditary orotic aciduria and other disorders of pyrimidine metabolism. In Scriver CR et al (eds): *The Metabolic Basis of Inherited Disease.* New York: McGraw-Hill, 1989. Pp 1095–1126.

42. Freedman MH, Sanders EF. Transient erythroblastopenia of childhood: Varied pathogenesis. *Am J Hematol* 14:247–254, 1983.

43. Diamond LK, Allen DM, Magill FB. Congenital (erythroid) hypoplastic anemia: A 25-year study. *Am J Dis Child* 102:403–415, 1961.

44. Glader BE, Backer K, Diamond LK. Elevated erythrocyte deaminase

45. Allen DM, Diamond LK. "Congenital (erythroid) hypoplastic anemia: Cortisone treated. *Am J Dis Child* 102:416–423, 1961.

46. Marsh GW, Lewis SM. Cardiac haemolytic anaemia. *Semin Hematol* 6:133–149, 1969.

47. Davidson RJL. Exertional haemoglobinuria: A report on three cases with studies on the hemolytic mechanism. *J Clin Pathol* 17:536–540, 1964.

48. Nance WE. Hemolytic anemia of necrotic arachnidism. *Am J Med* 31:801–807, 1961.

49. Madrigal GC, Ercolani RL, Wenzl JR. Toxicity from a bite of the brown spider (*Loxosceles reclusus*), skin necrosis, hemolytic anemia, and hemoglobinuria in a nine-year old child. *Clin Pediatr* 11:641–644, 1972.

50. Reid HA. Cobra bites. *Br Med J* 2:540–545, 1964.

51. Landsteiner EK, Finch CA. Hemoglobinemia accompanying transurethral resection of the prostate. *N Engl J Med* 237:310–312, 1947.

52. Ham TH et al. Studies on the destruction of red blood cell, IV. *Blood* 3:373–403, 1948.

53. Phillips WA, Pottinger LA, DeWald RL. Extracorporeal hemolysis in orthopedic patients. *Clin Orthop* 238:241–244, 1989.

54. Opitz JC et al. Hemolysis of blood in intravenous tubing caused by heat. *J Pediatr* 112:111–113, 1988.

55. Screiber AD. Autoimmune hemolytic anemia. *Pediatr Clin North Am* 27(2):253–267, 1980.

56. Lux SE, Wolfe LC. Inherited disorders of the red cell membrane skeleton. *Pediatr Clin N Am* 27:463–486, 1980.

57. Ware RE, Hall SE, Rosse WF. Paroxysmal nocturnal hemoglobinuria with onset in childhood and adolescence. *N Engl J Med* 325:991–996, 1991.

58. Miller DR. The unstable hemoglobins, hemoglobins M, and hemoglobins with altered oxygen affinity. In Schwartz E (ed): *Hemoglobinopathies in Children.* Littleton, MA: PSG, 1980. Pp 149–185.

59. Vichinski EP, Lubin BH. Unstable hemoglobins, hemoglobins with altered oxygen affinity, and M-hemoglobins. *Pediatr Clin North Am* 27:421–428, 1980.

60. Sullivan DW, Glader BE. Erythrocyte enzyme disorders in children. *Pediatr Clin North Am* 27:449–462, 1980.

61. Beutler E. Glucose-6-phosphate dehydrogenase deficiency. *N Engl J Med* 324:169–174, 1991.

62. Luzzatto L, Mehta A. Glucose-6-phosphate dehydrogenase deficiency. In Scriver CR et al (eds): *The Metabolic Basis of Inherited Disease.* New York: McGraw-Hill, 1989. Pp 2237–2265.

63. Alter BP, Young NS. The bone marrow failure syndromes. In Nathan DG, Oski FA (eds): *Hematology of Infancy and Childhood* (4th ed). Philadelphia: Saunders, 1992. Pp 216–316.

64. Shumak KH, Rock GA. Therapeutic plasma exchange. *N Engl J Med* 310:762–771, 1984.

65. Oda H et al. High-dose intravenous intact IgG infusion in refractory autoimmune hemolytic anemia (Evan's syndrome). *J Pediatr* 107:744–746, 1985.

66. Pocecco M et al. High-dose IVIgG in autoimmune hemolytic anemia. *J Pediatr* 109:726, 1986.

67. Dwyer JM. Manipulating the immune system with immune globulin. *N Engl J Med* 326:107–116, 1992.

68. Pattison JR et al. Parvovirus infections and hypoplastic crisis in sickle cell anemia. *Lancet* 1:664, 1981.

69. Kelleher JF et al. Human serum "parvovirus": A specific cause of aplastic crisis in children with hereditary spherocytosis. *J Pediatr* 102:720–722, 1983.

70. Kurtman GJ et al. Chronic bone marrow failure due to persistent B19 parvovirus infection. *N Engl J Med* 317:287–294, 1987.

71. Kostmann R. Infantile genetic agranulocytosis: A review with presentation of ten new cases. *Acta Paediatr Scand* 64:362–368, 1975.

72. Cutting HO, Lang JE. Familial benign chronic neutropenia. *Ann Intern Med* 61:876–887, 1964.

73. Pincus SH, Boxer LA, Stossel TP. Chronic neutropenia in childhood. *Am J Med* 61:849–861, 1976.

74. Dale DC et al. Chronic neutropenia. *Medicine* 58:128–144, 1979.

75. Schwachman H et al. The syndrome of pancreatic insufficiency and bone marrow dysfunction. *J Pediatr* 65:645–663, 1964.

76. Lux SE et al. Chronic neutropenia and abnormal cellular immunity in cartilage-hair hypoplasia. *N Engl J Med* 282:231–236, 1970.

77. Page AR, Good RA. Studies on cyclic neutropenia: A clinical and experimental investigation. *Am J Dis Child* 94:623–661, 1957.

78. Boxer LA et al. Autoimmune neutropenia. *N Engl J Med* 293:748–753, 1975.

79. Boxer LA, Yokoyama M, Lalezari P. Isoimmune neonatal neutropenia. *J Pediatr* 80:783–787, 1972.

80. Lalezari P, Khorshidi M, Petrosova M. Autoimmune neutropenia of infancy. *J Pediatr* 109:764–769, 1986.

81. Howard MW, Strauss RG, Johnston RB. Infections in patients with neutropenia. *Am J Dis Child* 131:788–790, 1977.

82. Pizzo PA. Infectious complications in the child with cancer. I. Pathophysiology of the compromised host and the initial evaluation and management of the febrile cancer patient. *J Pediatr* 98:341–354, 1981.

83. Pizzo PA et al. The child with cancer and infection. I. Empiric therapy for fever and neutropenia, and preventive strategies. *J Pediatr* 119:679–694, 1991.

84. Pizzo PA et al. A randomized trial comparing ceftazidime alone with combination antibiotic therapy in cancer patients with fever and neutropenia. *N Engl J Med* 315:552–558, 1986.

85. Granowetter L, Wells H, Lange BJ. Ceftazidime with or without vancomycin vs. cephalothin, carbenicilln and gentamicin as the initial therapy of the febrile neutropenic pediatric cancer patient. *Pediatr Infect Dis* 7:165–170, 1988.

86. Morgan G, Duerden BI, Lilleyman JS. Ceftazidime as a single agent in the management of children with fever and neutropenia. *J Antimicrob Chemother* 12 (Suppl A):347–351, 1983.

87. Rikonen P. Imipenem compared with ceftazidime plus vancomycin as initial therapy for fever in neutropenic children with cancer. *Pediatr Infect Dis* 10:918–923, 1991.

88. Pizzo PA et al. Empiric antibiotic and antifungal therapy for cancer patients with prolonged fever and granulocytopenia. *Am J Med* 72:101–111, 1982.

89. Commers JR, Pizzo PA. Empiric antifungal therapy in the management of the febrile-granulocytopenic cancer patient. *Pediatr Infect Dis* 2:56–60, 1983.

90. Pizzo PA et al. The child with cancer and infection. II. Nonbacterial infections. *J Pediatr* 119:845–857, 1991.

91. Griffin TC, Buchanan GR. Hematologic predictors of bone marrow recovery in neutropenic patients hospitalized for fever: Implications for discontinuation of antibiotics and early discharge from the hospital. *J Pediatr* 121:28–33, 1992.

92. Bonilla MA et al. Effects of recombinant human granulocyte colony-stimulating factor on neutropenia in patients with congenital agranulocytosis. *N Engl J Med* 320:1574–1580, 1989.

93. Welte K et al. Differential effects of granulocyte-macrophage colony-stimulating factor and granulocyte colony-stimulating factor in children with severe congenital neutropenia. *Blood* 75:1056–1063, 1990.

94. Hammond WP et al. Treatment of cyclic neutropenia with granulocyte colony-stimulating factor. *N Engl J Med* 320:1306–1311, 1989.

95. Jakabowski AA et al. Effects of human granulocyte colony-stimulating factor in a patient with idiopathic neutropenia. *N Engl J Med* 320:38–42, 1989.

96. Gauser A et al. The effect of recombinant human granulocyte-macrophage colony-stimulating factor on neutropenia and related morbidity in chronic severe neutropenia. *Ann Intern Med* 111:887–892, 1989.

97. Pollack S et al. High-dose intravenous gamma globulin for autoimmune neutropenia. *N Engl J Med* 307:253, 1982.

98. Bussel J et al. Reversal of neutropenia with intravenous gammaglobulin in autoimmune neutropenia of infancy. *Blood* 62:398–400, 1983.

99. Bussel J, Lalezari P, Fikrig S. Intravenous treatment with gamma-globulin of autoimmune neutropenia in infancy. *J Pediatr* 112:298–301, 1988.

100. Chan KW, Kaikov Y, Wadsworth LP. Thrombocytosis in children: A survey of 94 patients. *Pediatrics* 84:1064–1067, 1989.

101. Fitzgerald GA. Dipyridimole. *N Engl J Med* 316:1247–1257, 1987.

102. Charache S, Lubin B, Reid CD (eds). Management and therapy of sickle cell disease. NIH publication No. 85-2117, 1985.

103. Jackson JF, Odom JL, Bell WN. Amelioration of sickle cell disease by persistent fetal hemoglobin. *JAMA* 177:867–869, 1961.

104. Conley CL et al. Hereditary persistence of fetal hemoglobin: A study of 79 affected persons in 15 negro families in Baltimore. *Blood* 21:261–281, 1963.

105. Ali SA. Milder variant of sickle-cell disease in Arabs in Kuwait associated with unusually high level of foetal haemoglobin. *Br J Haematol* 19:613–619, 1970.

106. Perrine RP et al. Natural history of sickle cell anemia in Saudi Arabs: A study of 270 subjects. *Ann Intern Med* 88:1–6, 1978.

107. Rennels MG et al. Cholelithiasis in patients with major sickle hemoglobinopathies. *Am J Dis Child* 138:66–67, 1984.

108. Platt OS et al. Pain in sickle cell disease: Rates and risk factors. *N Engl J Med* 325:11–16, 1991.

109. Sprinkle R et al. Acute chest syndrome in children with sickle cell disease: A retrospective analysis of 100 hospitalized cases. *Am J Pediatr Hematol Oncol* 82:105–110, 1986.

110. McIntosh S et al. Fever in young children with sickle cell disease. *J Pediatr* 96:199–204, 1980.

111. Powars D, Overturf G, Turner E. Is there an increased risk of *Haemophilus influenzae* septicemia in children with sickle cell anemia? *Pediatrics* 71:927–931, 1983.

112. Zarkowsky HS et al. Bacteremia in sickle hemoglobinopathies. *J Pediatr* 109:579–585, 1986.

113. Leikin SL et al. Mortality in children and adolescents with sickle cell disease. *Pediatrics* 84:500–508, 1989.

114. Dean J, Schechter AN. Sickle cell anemia: Molecular and cellular bases of therapeutic approaches. *N Engl J Med* 299:752–763, 804–811, 863–870, 1978.

115. Abraham DJ et al. Vanillin, a potential agent for the treatment of sickle cell anemia. *Blood* 77:1334–1341, 1991.

116. Ley TJ et al. 5-azacytidine selectively increases γ-globin synthesis in a patient with β+-thalassemia. *N Engl J Med* 307:1469–1475, 1982.

117. Ley TS et al. 5-azacytidine increases γ-globulin synthesis and reduces the proportion of dense cells in patients with sickle cell anemia. *Blood* 62:370–380, 1983.

118. Letvin NL et al. Augmentation of fetal-hemoglobin production in anemic monkeys by hydroxyurea. *N Engl J Med* 310:869–873, 1984.

119. Veith R et al. Stimulation of F-cell production in patients with sickle-cell anemia treated with cytarabine or hydroxyurea. *N Engl J Med* 313:1571–1575, 1985.

120. Rodgers GP et al. Hematologic responses of patients with sickle cell disease to treatment with hydroxyurea. *N Engl J Med* 322:1037–1045, 1990.

121. Charache S et al. Hydroxyurea: Effects on hemoglobin F production in patients with sickle cell anemia. *Blood* 79:2555–2565, 1992.

122. Rodgers GP et al. Augmentation by erythropoietin of the fetal-hemoglobin response to hydroxyurea in sickle-cell disease. *N Engl J Med* 328:73–80, 1993.

123. Charache S et al. Effect of hydroxyurea on the frequency of painful crises in sickle cell anemia. *N Engl J Med* 332:1317–1322, 1995.

124. Dover GJ, Brunsilow S, Samid D. Increased fetal hemoglobin in patients receiving sodium 4-phenylbutyrate. *N Engl J Med* 327:596–570, 1992.

125. Perrine SP et al. A short-term trial of butyrate to stimulate fetal-globin gene expression in the β globin disorders. *N Engl J Med* 328:86–81, 1993.

126. Gaston MH et al. Prophylaxis with oral penicillin in children with

sickle cell anemia: A randomized trial. *N Engl J Med* 314:1593–1599, 1986.

127. Frank AL et al. *Haemophilus influenzae* type b immunization of children with sickle cell disease. *Pediatrics* 82:571–575, 1988.

128. Charache S. Treatment of sickle cell anemia. *Annu Rev Med* 32:195–206, 1981.

129. Rogers ZR et al. Outpatient management of febrile illness in infants and young children with sickle cell anemia. *J Pediatr* 117:736–739, 1990.

130. Wiliams J et al. Efficacy of transfusion therapy for one to two years in patients with sickle cell disease and cerebrovascular accidents. *J Pediatr* 96:205–208, 1980.

131. Cohen AR et al. A modified transfusion program for prevention of stroke in sickle cell disease. *Blood* 79:1657–1661, 1992.

132. Koshy M et al. Prophylactic red cell transfusions in pregnant patients with sickle cell disease: A randomized cooperative study. *N Engl J Med* 319:1447–1452, 1988.

133. Jaffe ER. Hereditary methemoglobinemias associated with abnormalities in the metabolism of erythrocytes. *Am J Med* 41:786–798, 1966.

134. Curry S. Methemoglobinemia. *Ann Emerg Med* 11:214–220, 1982.

135. Dolan MA, Luban NLL. Methemoglobinemia in two children: Disparate etiology and treatment. *Pediatr Emerg Care* 3:171–174, 1987.

136. Park CM, Nagel RL. Sulfhemoglobinemia: Clinical and molecular aspects. *N Engl J Med* 310:1579–1584, 1984.

137. Baehner RL. Neutrophil dysfunction associated with states of chronic and recurrent infection. *Pediatr Clin North Am* 27:377–401, 1980.

138. Gallin JI et al. Recent advances in chronic granulomatous disease. *Ann Intern Med* 99:657–674, 1983.

139. The International Chronic Granulomatous Disease Cooperative Study Group. A controlled trial of interferon gamma to prevent infection in chronic granulomatous disease. *N Engl J Med* 324:509–516, 1991.

140. Margolis DM et al. Trimethoprim-sulfamethoxazole prophylaxis in the management of chronic granulomatous disease. *J Infect Dis* 162:723, 1990.

141. Chin TW et al. Corticosteroids in the treatment of lesions of chronic granulomatous disease. *J Pediatr* 111:349–352, 1987.

142. Lange B et al. Oncologic emergencies. In Pizzo PA, Poplack DG (eds): *Principles and Practice of Pediatric Oncology.* Philadelphia: Lippincott, 1989. Pp 799–822.

143. Issa PY et al. Superior vena cava syndrome in childhood. *Pediatrics* 71:337–341, 1983.

144. Cohen LF et al. Acute tumor lysis syndrome. *Am J Med* 68:486–491, 1980.

Elizabeth H. Perry

Sarah J. Ilstrup

43 ▶ Transfusion Therapy and Apheresis

Whole blood drawn from healthy volunteer donors is collected in an anticoagulant-preservative solution and separated into blood components at blood collection facilities or hospital blood banks. The most commonly transfused blood components are listed in Table 43-1. In critically ill pediatric patients, components derived from whole blood are transfused for two primary reasons: (1) to increase oxygen delivery to the tissues and (2) to obtain and maintain hemostasis in patients with coagulopathies. It is rare that physicians order granulocyte transfusions for infected patients with severe neutropenia or white cell dysfunction. Manufactured plasma derivatives, such as albumin and plasma protein fraction, are transfused to increase intravascular volume. Transfusion guidelines and the recommended amount of each blood component to transfuse have been well established for routine transfusion episodes.[1-3] Although transfusion is relatively safe, the associated risks include allergic, febrile, and hemolytic reactions, alloimmunization, and disease transmission.[4]

Selection of Compatible Blood

After blood has been collected from volunteer donors, samples undergo testing at the processing facility.[5] These tests include typing the donor blood for ABO and Rh blood groups, screening the donor serum for unexpected antibodies, and performing multiple infectious disease tests. In the United States, infectious disease testing includes screening tests for antibodies to hepatitis B core antigen, hepatitis C, human immunodeficiency virus (HIV1/2), and human T-cell lymphocytotrophic virus (HTLVI/II). Additional tests include hepatitis B surface antigen and a serologic test for syphilis. The whole blood is usually separated into three components: red blood cells (RBCs), platelets (PCs), and plasma.

ABO and Rh blood groups also are determined on blood samples from all patients who have a transfusion ordered. Units of RBCs for transfusion are matched to the patient's ABO and Rh blood groups. The ABO blood group is the most important blood group

in transfusion medicine because naturally occurring antibodies bind complement and may result in intravascular hemolysis if ABO incompatible blood is transfused.[6] There are two antigens in the ABO blood groups system, A and B attached to precursor substance H, and four major ABO blood groups: A, B, AB, and O. Group O people lack both A and B antigens but have precursor substance H. Antibodies to the ABO blood group are formed after exposure to antigens in the gut flora and environment, rather than by direct stimulation from incompatible red cell antigens, and are therefore called "naturally occurring antibodies." Table 43-2 lists ABO red cell antigens, antibodies, and the compatible RBC types for transfusion. In an emergency situation, if there is not time to determine an ABO blood group on an exsanguinating patient, group O RBCs can be transfused because they do not carry the A or B antigen. There are potential serious side effects if group O whole blood is transfused to a non-O patient because whole blood contains plasma, which in a group O blood donor contains naturally occurring anti-A and anti-B. If these antibodies are present in low titer, there may be no complications. If, however, the antibodies are present in high titer, and the patient is type A, B, or AB, there may be a significant hemolytic transfusion reaction.

After ABO, the most important red cell antigen is the Rh or D antigen. The terms *Rh-positive* and *Rh-negative* refer to the presence or absence of the D antigen. Unlike the ABO blood group, antibody to Rh (D) occurs in Rh-negative individuals only after exposure to Rh-positive red cells through transfusion or pregnancy. The Rh blood group is important because it is highly immunogenic. An Rh-negative person who is inadvertently or emergently transfused with Rh (D) positive red cells or whole blood has a 50% to 100% chance of mounting an immune response and producing anti-D.[7-9] This antibody may be responsible for delayed hemolytic transfusion reactions and is a cause of hemolytic disease of the newborn. The antepartum and peripartum use of Rh immune globulin in Rh-negative women has markedly decreased the incidence of Rh hemolytic disease of the newborn. When

Table 43-1. Blood components

Component	Indication	Dose	Volume	Preparation time
RBCs	Increase oxygen-carrying capacity	3 ml/kg increases Hct 3%		1.0–1.5 hrs for ABO, Rh, antibody screen, cross-match (if negative antibody screen)
CPDA-1			250 ml	
Additive solution			350 ml	
Platelets	Improve hemostasis			If ABO group known: 10 min for pooling
Concentrate (PC)		1 U/10 kg	50 ml	
Apheresis		Same as 6–8 PC	200 ml	Immediate
Fresh frozen plasma	Improve hemostasis	15 ml/kg	75–100 ml (peds)	45 minutes to thaw
			200 ml (adult)	
Cryoprecipitate	Improve hemostasis:		10 ml	45 minutes to that and pool
80–120 U factor VIII	Factor VIII deficiency	1 unit factor VIII/kg		
		Increases factor VIII 2%		
80 U VWF	von Willebrand's	1 bag/10 kg		
250 mg fibrinogen	Hypofibrinogenemia or dysfibrinogenemia	2–4 bags/10 kg		

Hct, hematocrit; VWF, von Willebrand's factor.

Table 43-2. ABO blood group system

Blood group	Red cell antigens	Naturally occurring antibodies in plasma	Compatible RBCs
A	A	Anti-B	A, O
B	B	Anti-A	B, O
AB	A,B	None	A, B, AB, O
O	None	Anti-A and anti-B	O

uncrossmatched blood is released for transfusion, Rh-negative is provided, if available, until Rh typing can be done on the patient. Once the patient's ABO and Rh groups are determined, group-specific blood is given.

A third laboratory test done before a routine transfusion is a screen of the plasma for clinically significant "unexpected" antibodies, which might cause hemolysis of transfused red cells. Antibodies to ABO are "expected" antibodies and not detected in this test because the red cells used for screening are group O and do not have A or B antigen on them. This test is performed by incubating the patient's serum with two different screening-group O red cells that are positive for clinically significant red cell antigens. After checking for agglutination or hemolysis after immediate spin and 37°C incubation, the cells are washed with normal saline to remove unbound globulins. Anti-human globulin serum (Coombs' serum) is added to the washed screening cells to detect the presence of nonagglutinating antibody or complement on the cells. The indirect Coombs' test is negative if there is no agglutination. If the antibody screen on the patient is negative, a unit of red cells can be crossmatched for transfusion. If the antibody screen is positive, the "unexpected" antibody must be identified before crossmatching RBCs.[10]

The final step in pretransfusion compatibility testing is the major crossmatch. The goal of pretransfusion compatibility testing is to crossmatch donors and recipients so that transfused RBCs have an acceptable survival time in the recipient.[11,12] The blood donor's red cells are mixed with patient serum, and the mixture is examined for agglutination or hemolysis of the red cells. If the patient does not have unexpected antibodies, the crossmatch is done primarily as a final check that the unit is ABO-compatible. If the patient has an unexpected antibody detected in the antibody screen, which has been identified using a panel of red cells with known antigens, red cells selected for crossmatching must be negative for the antigen corresponding to the patient's antibody, and a complete crossmatch through the indirect Coombs' phase must be done. A complete crossmatch may take up to 1 hour to perform, so extra time must be allowed if a patient is known to have an unexpected antibody.

When a transfusion is necessary, the written order includes the name of the blood component, number of units requested, and indication for transfusion. The Joint Commission for Accreditation of Healthcare Organizations (JCAHO) requires documentation of informed consent for transfusion. The time of anticipated transfusion is indicated in the order. Routine ABO and Rh red cell grouping, screen for unexpected antibodies and cross-match takes 60 to 90 minutes if there are no unexpected antibodies to identify. In an emergency situation, ABO group-specific red cells (e.g., A negative) can be available 5 to 20 minutes after a blood specimen is received in the laboratory. In life-threatening hemorrhage, if the blood groups are unknown, and there is no time to wait for

ABO and Rh typing, group O Rh-negative red cells may be transfused without cross-match.[13–15] However, a properly labeled tube of blood is sent to the laboratory as soon as possible so that ABO and Rh-specific red cells can be provided.

The plasma components of fresh-frozen plasma (FFP), cryoprecipitate (CRYO), and platelet components do not require cross-matching; however, the ABO group of the patient must be known so that ABO compatible units can be selected for transfusion in order to prevent ABO antibody–mediated immune hemolysis. FFP and CRYO are frozen for storage, so 45 minutes should be allowed for thawing or pooling of units. Platelet concentrates require pooling, which takes 10 minutes to perform. Apheresis platelets need no preparation.

Blood Components and Indications for Transfusion

Components for Increasing Oxygen Carrying Capacity

RBCs are indicated for increasing oxygen carrying capacity in anemic patients. One unit of red cells has the same red cell mass as a unit of whole blood. The hematocrit of packed red cells collected in standard anticoagulant-preservative solutions ranges from 70% to 80% while the hematocrit of red cells stored in additive solutions to extend the shelf life is 50% to 60%. As with any transfusion, the decision to transfuse RBC must be made on clinical grounds rather than any preset numerical transfusion trigger. The transfusion of 1 unit of red cells increases the hematocrit in a stable 70-kg patient by 3%. Transfusion of 3 ml/kg of RBCs increases the hematocrit 3% and hemoglobin 1 g/dl in a nonbleeding pediatric patient.

With the advances in blood component therapy, whole blood is often not available. Whole blood transfusion simultaneously replaces oxygen carrying capacity and volume. Some hospitals specializing in trauma stock an inventory of whole blood for use following crystalloid resuscitation. Refrigerated whole blood that has been stored more than 24 hours has few viable granulocytes and platelets; however, viable lymphocytes may persist throughout storage. The levels of labile coagulation factors V and VIII decrease to 30% and 20%, respectively, in whole blood stored for 21 days, and these levels are not considered adequate to correct deficiencies in bleeding patients with either factor V or factor VIII deficiency.[16,17] In nonbleeding pediatric patients, 8 to 10 ml/kg of whole blood increases the hematocrit by 3%. In addition to the possible adverse effects associated with RBC transfusion, whole blood transfusion can cause volume overload.

Components for Hemostasis

Blood components used to obtain and maintain hemostasis include platelets, FFP, and CRYO[3] (Table 43-1). Coagulation factor concentrates are produced from pools of human plasma that have been treated to reduce viral transmission and, more recently, by recombinant technology.

Platelet transfusions are given to control or prevent bleeding episodes associated with thrombocytopenia or platelet dysfunction. Detailed guidelines for appropriate platelet transfusion practice have been published[1,18,19] (Table 43-3). Patients with appropriate indications may receive one platelet transfusion a day.

Platelet concentrates (PCs) made from whole blood and apheresis platelets collected from random single donors are stored at room temperature on a rotator for up to 5 days. The standard dose for PCs is 1 unit (5.5×10^{10} platelets) per 10 kg of body weight. Some transfusion services supply platelets in standard pools for patients weighing more than 60 kg (e.g., "6-pack" of pooled PCs) and 1 unit of PCs per 10 kg for patients weighing less than 60 kg. Other blood banks provide 1 U/10 kg for all patients. In general, one PCs is expected to increase the platelet count by 10,000/m² in an otherwise stable patient.

Blood centers also collect platelets from single donors, using apheresis technology. A unit of apheresis platelets is equivalent to 6 to 8 pooled PCs. The advantages of transfusing apheresis platelets include saving technical time in the blood bank, because pooling is not necessary, and limiting the number of blood donor exposures. Additionally, apheresis platelets collected by specified validated technology may meet the current standard for leukocyte reduction to prevent febrile transfusion reactions. At this time, transfusion of a unit of apheresis platelets costs significantly more than a transfusion of pooled PCs.

A corrected count increment (CCI) using pretransfusion and 10- to 60-minute posttransfusion platelet counts is a useful tool to determine if a patient has an adequate response to platelet transfusion (Table 43-4). Patients can become refractory to transfusions of platelets from random donors and may respond with better increments to platelets collected by apheresis from an HLA-matched donor or platelets that are compatible by cross-matching techniques.[20] If the expected CCI is not obtained with appropriate platelet transfusions on two separate occasions, the patient is considered refractory to platelet transfusion.[21,22] Causes of refractoriness include alloimmunization to HLA or platelet-specific antigens, splenomegaly, bleeding, sepsis, disseminated intravascular coagulation (DIC), and certain medications. When causes other than alloimmunization have been excluded, the patient's serum should be tested in the laboratory for the presence of HLA or platelet-specific antibodies at the same time the first HLA-matched or cross-match-compatible platelets are being ordered. The patient's HLA type must be known before the blood bank can order HLA-matched platelets from a blood collection center. It is a serious problem, beyond the scope of this chapter, when the patient who is refractory on the basis of alloimmunization does not respond to HLA-matched or cross-match-compatible platelets. Consultation with a specialist in transfusion medicine or hematology is recommended.[20,23] Because alloimmunization has dire consequences for the patient, the National Institutes of Health is conducting a multisite study (Trial to Reduce Alloimmunization to Platelets [TRAP]) to determine if leukocyte-reduction or UVB irradiation of platelets and leukocyte-reduction of red cells will prevent alloimmunization in patients with acute myelogenous leukemia.

FFP is a plasma component separated from whole blood, frozen within 8 hours of collection, and stored for up to 1 year. FFP contains 100% of all normal plasma constituents, including coagulation factors, complement components, and other plasma proteins. FFP is indicated to correct bleeding due to multiple coagulation factor abnormalities or single deficiencies when specific therapy (concentrate) is unavailable. Each unit of FFP contains 200 to 250 ml of plasma with 1 unit of coagulation factor per milliliter of plasma. The usual initial dose of FFP for treatment of coagulopathy is 10 to 20 ml/kg.[24] A prothrombin time (PT) or international normalized ratio (INR) and activated partial thromboplastin time (aPTT) should be performed before and after the transfusion. Clinical bleeding due to coagulation factor deficiency is not expected unless the PT and/or aPTT are greater than 1.5 times the mean normal value, or the INR is 1.6 or greater. FFP is also indicated for treatment of thrombotic thrombocytopenic purpura (TTP) and hemolytic-uremic syndrome (HUS) and replacement of plasma anticoagulant factors, such as protein C, protein S, and antithrombin III, when specific concentrates are not available or advisable.[1] FFP is contraindicated for volume expansion or replacement of colloidal losses in postoperative patients, such as chest tube drainage, because the risk of possible transfusion reactions and viral transmission outweighs the benefit. Alternatives to FFP for volume expansion include albumin and plasma protein fraction derived from human plasma and synthetic colloids such as hetastarch (HES) and dextran.

CRYO, another blood component used for hemostasis, is the cold-insoluble portion of FFP.[25] CRYO is stored frozen at $-18°C$ or lower as single units or pools of 4 units. Each unit of CRYO contains factor VIII (80–120 U/bag), von Willebrand's factor (80 U/bag), factor XIII (40–60 U/bag), fibrinogen (250 mg/bag), and fibronectin.[3] CRYO contains insignificant amounts of other coagulation factors and must not be used to treat factor IX deficiency (hemophilia B). CRYO is used to treat bleeding episodes due to hemophilia A (factor VIII deficiency) and von Willebrand's disease, when noninfectious concentrates are not available; decreased or dysfunctional fibrinogen; and factor XIII deficiency. CRYO is used as a source of fibrinogen for hypofibrinogenemic patients with DIC and for topical fibrin glue. CRYO has been reported to shorten the prolonged bleeding time in uremia; however, use of synthetic vasopressin (desmopressin, DDAVP) shows similar clinical improvement in bleeding and a decrease in the bleeding time without the risks associated with transfusion of blood compo-

Table 43-3. Criteria for platelet transfusion

Platelet count < 5,000–20,000/μL in a nonbleeding patient

Platelet count < 50,000/μL with active bleeding, coagulopathy, fever, sepsis, or neonate

Platelet count < 50,000/μL with surgery or invasive procedure pending

Platelet count < 100,000/μL in patient with diffuse bleeding after cardiopulmonary bypass

Bleeding time > 20 min, regardless of platelet count

Table 43-4. Corrected count increment to determine response to platelet transfusions

$$\text{CCI at 10–60 min} = \frac{\text{(Posttransfusion platelet count} - \text{pretransfusion platelet count)} \times \text{BSA(m}^2)}{\text{Number of PCs transfused}}$$

CCI > 4,000–5,000 is adequate.

CCI, corrected count increment; BSA, body surface area; PCs, platelet concentrates.

nents.[26] Desmopressin may also be used in mild or moderate hemophilia A and type I von Willibrand's disease to achieve hemostasis.

Coagulation and anticoagulant factor concentrates produced from human plasma include factor VIII and IX concentrates for treatment of hemophilia A and B, respectively, and antithrombin III concentrate, used for prevention of thrombosis in patients with inherited or acquired antithrombin III deficiency. Consultation with a hematologist or specialist in the use of these products is necessary before use.

Granulocytes

Granulocyte transfusions may be indicated for the following groups of patients: patients with infections and documented functional defects of granulocytes, such as chronic granulomatous disease, and severely neutropenic patients ($<0.5 \times 10^9$ granulocytes/liter) with fever and suspected or documented sepsis who have not responded to 48 hours of appropriate antibiotic therapy.[27,28] Granulocytes must be transfused as soon as possible after collection to maximize effectiveness. The component can be ordered as "buffy coats" collected from whole blood donations or granulocytapheresis collected from a single donor. The standard dose is 1 buffy coat per 10 kg of body weight or one granulocytapheresis transfused once a day. Some experts believe that granulocyte colony stimulating factors given to donors prior to granulocytapheresis will increase the number of neutrophils collected and thus the efficacy of granulocyte transfusions.

Plasma Derivatives

Five percent albumin is frequently used for restoration of intravascular volume and colloid replacement in hypovolemic patients. Albumin is prepared by cold ethanol fractionation and heat inactivation and does not carry the same risks of disease transmission as blood components. Albumin may, however, cause allergic and febrile nonhemolytic transfusion reactions.[29] Plasma protein fraction (PPF) is a plasma derivative made by fractionation and heat treatment and contains 83% albumin and 17% globulins. New manufacturing processes have decreased the incidence of hypotensive episodes due to activation of the kinin system, which had been reported to occur with rapid infusion of PPF.[30] Synthetic colloids such as HES and dextran are also used to restore intravascular volume. Both of these agents can cause abnormalities in the coagulation screening tests, with slight prolongation of the PT and PTT, and marked shortening of the thrombin time and dextrans have been associated with abnormal bleeding. Anaphylactic reactions and bleeding have been reported with dextrans and HES.[31]

Several gamma globulin preparations, including intravenous immunoglobulin (IVIgG), immune serum globulin (ISG), and hyperimmune globulins such as Rh immune globulin, are available for clinical use. Gamma globulins are prepared by modified cold ethanol fractionation of pooled human blood donor plasma. The intramuscular preparations have not been reported to transmit infectious diseases. One manufacturer's IVIgG prepared without a viral inactivation step has been implicated in hepatitis C transmission.[32] All IVIgG products currently available in the United States have a viral inactivation step in the manufacturing process. The use of IVIgG has expanded over the past several years.[33,34] Potential indications for IVIgG include congenital immune deficiencies, prophylaxis or treatment of infectious diseases, acquired antibody deficiency (e.g., in bone marrow transplant patients), immune

thrombocytopenic purpura, Guillain-Barré syndrome, Kawasaki syndrome, and posttransfusion purpura. A frequently used dose is 0.4 g/kg for 5 days. Transfusion of IVIgG has been associated with generally mild reactions that include headache, fever, chills, nausea, vomiting, and urticaria. Anaphylaxis may occur in the rare IgA-deficient patient with antibody to IgA.

ISG is used primarily for viral prophylaxis, primarily against hepatitis A. Hyperimmune globulins are prepared from the plasma of donors with high titers of the desired antibody. Rh immune globulin (RhIG) is a concentrated solution of anti-D gamma globulin. RhIG used antepartum and postpartum has markedly decreased the incidence of hemolytic disease of the newborn due to Rh incompatibility between the Rh-negative mother and Rh-positive fetus. RhIG has also been used to prevent immunization of Rh-negative patients after they receive blood components containing Rh-positive RBCs, such as PC. Other hyperimmune globulins are hepatitis B immunoglobulin (HBIG) and varicella zoster immune globulin (VZIG). Side effects of intramuscular preparations include fever, allergic reactions, and pain at the injection site. Intramuscular preparations cannot be given intravenously because of anaphylactic reactions. An intravenous (IV) preparation of RhIG has recently been introduced into clinical trials. The IV preparation of RhIg is now available commercially (trials over) for use in patients with ITP. This product is less expensive than IVIgG and works equally well. There have not been recommendations to prevention of immunization to Rh D during pregnancy, but some will probably use it for this purpose.

Special Components

Certain patients have requirements for leukocyte-reduced or cytomegalovirus (CMV)-safe or irradiated components, and these must be specifically ordered.

Leukocyte-Reduced Components

Leukocyte-reduced components are used to prevent fegrile, nonhemolytic transfusion reactions; transmission of CMV; and possibly allo-immunization.

CMV-Safe Components

CMV disease is a serious problem in immunosuppressed patients (i.e., bone marrow and solid organ transplant patients). CMV-antibody seronegative cellular components (red cells, platelets, and granulocytes) have been shown to decrease the incidence of transfusion-transmitted CMV disease in patients with negative CMV antibody tests.[35,35a] FFP and CRYO are acellular components and do not transmit CMV. Recent studies show that infection with CMV can be prevented by using leukocyte-reduction filters that remove 99.0%–99.9% of white cells. In areas where CMV-antibody seronegative donors are rare, the use of leukocyte-reduction filters to provide CMV-safe RBC and platelets has become a practical alternative.

Irradiated Components

Transfusion-associated graft-versus-host disease (TA-GVHD) occurs when viable lymphocytes in blood components are transfused into susceptible patients and these lymphocytes engraft and attack recipient tissues.[36,37] Gamma irradiation at 2500 cGy interferes with the lymphocytes' ability to proliferate and prevents TA-

GVHD.[38] The clinical syndrome of TA-GVHD includes fever, skin rash, hepatitis, diarrhea, and bone marrow suppression with infection usually leading to a fatal outcome. It is necessary to order irradiated cellular blood components (red cells, platelets, and granulocytes) for patients at high risk for TA-GVHD. High-risk situations include congenital immunodeficiency syndromes, intrauterine transfusions, intrauterine transfusion followed by exchange transfusion, bone marrow transplant recipients, and Hodgkin's disease. TA-GVHD may be seen in immunocompetent recipients when blood from an HLA-homozygous donor is given to a recipient who is haploidentical.[39] This is most likely to occur in donations from blood relatives and with HLA-matched apheresis platelets, and both of these require irradiation. Other indications for use of gamma-irradiated blood components continue to evolve.

Washed Red Cells and Platelets

Washing red cells and platelets to remove most of the plasma may be requested for patients with severe allergic reactions due to unspecified plasma proteins or for IgA-deficient patients with antibodies to IgA and anaphylactic reactions to transfusion. In the case of IgA deficiency with anaphylaxis, plasma for FFP and CRYO transfusions must be collected from IgA-deficient donors.[40,41]

Volume Reduction

Reduction in the volume of platelets is occasionally requested. Volume reduction might be indicated when volume overload is a critical clinical problem. For neonatal transfusion, the volume of red cells and single units of platelets cannot be reduced further by the laboratory. For older children, the volume of pooled units of PCs or apheresis platelets can be reduced to approximately 50 ml.[42] This has been associated with 15% to 55% platelet loss.[43,44] The volume of FFP and CRYO cannot be reduced.

Frozen-Deglycerolized Red Cells

Transfusion of frozen-thawed-deglycerolized red cells once was a popular way to provide leukocyte-reduced cells primarily for the prevention of alloimmunization to HLA antigens. With the leukocyte-reduction filters now available, red cell cryopreservation is limited to storage of rare or selected red cell units. Once red cell units are thawed and deglycerolized, they are stored at 1°C to 6°C and must be used within 24 hours.

Adverse Effects of Transfusion

Transfusion Reactions

Classifications of transfusion reactions include acute and delayed, acute and chronic, hemolytic and nonhemolytic, immunologic

Table 43-5. Current estimated transfusion risks

Complication	Risk per unit transfused
Hepatitis C	1:6,000–1:70,000
Hepatitis B	1:200,000
HIV	1:400,000
Fever, chills, urticaria	1:1,000
Fatal hemolytic reaction	1:600,000

and nonimmunologic, and a combination of these.[45,46] Estimated risks for some serious adverse effects are listed in Table 43-5. Immediate reactions generally occur within minutes up to 4 hours after transfusion, while delayed reactions occur days to years later. Patients who are being transfused must be monitored closely so that transfusion reactions can be recognized and prompt appropriate management initiated. Symptoms such as fever and chills may signal the onset of a hemolytic transfusion reaction, bacterial contamination of the unit, or a less serious, febrile, nonhemolytic transfusion reaction.[47] When there is an alteration in the patient's vital signs or if symptoms develop during a transfusion, the transfusion must be stopped immediately. The IV line is kept in place until the situation has been fully assessed. Shock, anaphylaxis, pulmonary edema, and circulatory overload must be aggressively treated. After the patient has been stabilized, the labels on the blood bag are rechecked with the patient's identification to make certain there has not been a clerical error. The discontinued bag of blood, the entire transfusion set, and all forms and labels are sent to the blood bank with a report of suspected transfusion reaction.

Immediate hemolytic transfusion reactions occur by immune and nonimmune mechanisms. Fifty-one percent of transfusion-associated deaths reported to the Food and Drug Administration (FDA) from 1976 to 1985 were due to acute hemolysis resulting from ABO incompatibility.[48] The major cause of ABO incompatibility is clerical error in either patient identification or labeling of crossmatch tubes or RBCs for transfusion.[49] The risk of death from a hemolytic transfusion reaction is estimated to be 1:600,000 per unit transfused.[50] Immediate hemolysis of RBC following an ABO-incompatible transfusion results from naturally occurring antibodies binding to red cell antigens, with subsequent activation of the complement, coagulation, and kinin systems, and can result in shock, acute renal failure, and DIC. Hemolysis must always be considered when fever, an increase in temperature of 1°C or 2°F or more, is associated with transfusion, because fever is the most common initial manifestation of a hemolytic transfusion reaction. Fever occurs in about 75% of hemolytic transfusion reactions.[47] Other signs and symptoms of immediate hemolytic transfusion reactions include hemoglobinuria, chills, flank pain, nausea, vomiting, tachycardia, tachypnea, and hypotension. Hemoglobinuria is often the first indication of a hemolytic transfusion reaction in unconscious patients. Nonimmune hemolysis of red cells is rare and may result from simultaneous infusion of hypotonic or hypertonic solutions, mechanical damage from pumps or needles, or overwarming of blood.[51,52]

The most common immediate transfusion reactions, febrile nonhemolytic and allergic transfusion reactions (FNHTRs), occur in 0.1% of units transfused.[50] FNHTRs are usually caused by antibodies in the patient's plasma to HLA or granulocyte antigens in the transfused component and occur most often in multiply transfused or previously pregnant patients. The role of cytokines is under intensive study as a potential cause of FNHTR to stored platelets.[53] FNHTRs recur in 10% to 12% of patients, and leukocyte-reduced red cells are recommended when a patient has had two or more reactions despite premedication. The concern when fever is associated with transfusion is that a life-threatening reaction has occurred. The transfusion must be stopped and specimens sent to the laboratory so that a hemolytic reaction or bacterial contamination of the unit can be excluded. Whether the transfusion can be restarted once hemolysis has been excluded is currently being debated by transfusion medicine specialists.[54,55]

Most allergic reactions are due to patient antibodies to unidentified donor plasma proteins. If the only manifestation of the allergic reaction is urticaria, which completely resolves after treatment with an antihistamine, the transfusion may be restarted. Even if the transfusion reaction is mild, and the transfusion is completed without further incident, a report of suspected transfusion reaction should be sent to the blood bank so that the episode can be evaluated and the reaction documented. Thorough evaluation of anaphylactic reactions to transfusion includes an IgA level and possibly antibodies to IgA.

Transfusion-related acute lung injury (TRALI) or noncardiogenic pulmonary edema is a rare adverse effect of transfusion due to passive transfer of donor antibody directed against the patient's white cells, resulting in leukoagglutination and stasis in the pulmonary microvasculature.[56] Aggressive management includes intubation, positive pressure ventilation, fluid resuscitation, and high-dose corticosteroids.

Delayed hemolytic transfusion reactions are frequently detected by the blood bank when an unexpected antibody is identified in a blood sample sent to the laboratory for routine type, screen, and cross-match 10 days after transfusion. With delayed hemolytic transfusion reactions, the patients have formed a red cell antibody some time in the past, as a response to transfusion or pregnancy, which had fallen to undetectable levels at the time of the initial antibody screening test prior to transfusion. Because the antibody was undetectable, and there was no history in the blood bank of its ever being present, red cells carrying the antigen were transfused and an anamnestic response of antibody production occurred. Delayed reactions may also occur following primary exposure to a foreign red cell antigen. With delayed hemolytic transfusion reactions, the patient generally presents with fever, anemia, and indirect hyperbilirubinemia.[57] In general, the transfused red cells are destroyed extravascularly in the spleen.

Infectious Complications

Viruses, bacteria, and protozoans can be transmitted by blood transfusion. The most commonly transmitted disease causing serious clinical problems is viral hepatitis. Up to 10% of cases of posttransfusion hepatitis are caused by hepatitis B, despite sensitive screening tests for hepatitis B surface antigen and antibody to hepatitis B core antigen.[58] The other 90% of cases are caused by non-A, non-B hepatitis, with 85% to 90% of these caused by the hepatitis C virus (HCV).[59,60] Infection with HCV may not be apparent clinically in the months following transfusion because as many as 75% of cases are anicteric. Up to half of patients with HCV develop chronic hepatitis, and of these, 10% to 15% develop cirrhosis, which is a major health problem. Blood collection centers started screening donor blood for antibody to HCV in 1990. With the introduction of this screening test, the risk of transfusion-transmitted hepatitis has markedly decreased, with a current risk of 1 in 6,000 to 1 in 70,000 per unit transfused. Clinicians are responsible for notifying the blood bank or transfusion service if a patient who has been transfused develops hepatitis, so that the donors of all the transfused blood components can be investigated.

AIDS is known to be transmitted by transfusion, and all blood donors are asked specific health history questions to determine if they are in high-risk groups. Each unit of donated blood is tested for antibody to HIV-1 and HIV-2. The risk of acquiring AIDS from a blood transfusion is less than 1 in 400,000 per blood component transfused.[50] This risk occurs because there is a window period between the time the donor is exposed to the virus and the time of seroconversion. There is no test currently available to consistently detect infectious donors in the window period, so blood collection centers rely on screened volunteer donors who do not have known risk factors associated with HIV infection.

Transmission of malaria and Chagas disease by transfusion is rare in the United States but is a major issue in endemic areas. Bacterial contamination of red cells and platelets continues to be a rare occurrence, but fatal complications have been reported.[61,62] Bacterial growth in platelets is most often due to contaminating skin flora that multiply during room temperature storage, while contamination of red cells is most often caused by gram-negative bacteria that proliferate at refrigerator temperature. Bacterial contamination should be suspected in patients who have a transfusion reaction that consists of fever, chills, and hypotension. If bacterial contamination is suspected, a culture is performed on the patient's blood, and a Gram stain and culture are done on the donor blood remaining in the bag. Broad-spectrum antibiotic coverage and supportive therapy are provided until transfusion-associated sepsis can be excluded.

Therapeutic Apheresis

Apheresis is derived from a Greek word meaning "to take away from." Therapeutic apheresis or hemapheresis has its roots in the ancient practice of bloodletting to "relieve the pressure" or "remove bad humors." In 1950, exchange transfusion for hemolytic disease of the newborn was first reported. Subsequently, exchange transfusion was performed for sickle cell disease and rheumatoid arthritis. Modern hemapheresis started in the 1940s when the Cohn fractionator, based on the cream separator used in the dairy industry, was used by the military to separate plasma from whole blood. Subsequently, in the late 1950s, an IBM engineer who had a relative undergoing cancer therapy with extended periods of neutropenia, helped design the NCI-IBM Blood Cell Separator to more effectively collect granulocytes for transfusion. Today, apheresis is a tool useful in collection of normal plasma or cellular elements, reduction of abnormal or clinically significant cells, and therapeutic plasma exchange (TPE) for removal of nondialyzable plasma factors. Indications for newer applications, such as immunoadsorption and photopheresis, continue to evolve.

Automated hemapheresis is performed using one of several commercially available blood cell separators, the majority of which use centrifugal force for the separation of whole blood into plasma and cellular elements. Either cells or plasma can be collected for transfusion from a healthy blood donor or removed and discarded from a patient. Advantages of automated blood separators include preprogramming, efficiency, versatility in collection of cells or plasma, and smaller fluid shifts in adult patients. However, the process is expensive and requires skilled, well-trained staff and venous access that will withstand the drawing forces of the separator. Therapeutic hemapheresis instrument technology has improved over the past few years. Very small pediatric patients (<10 kg) can now have therapeutic apheresis procedures performed safely. The ability to perform automated apheresis procedures will decrease the number of time-consuming, inefficient, push-pull whole blood exchanges historically performed on small pediatric patients.

In healthy blood donors, automated apheresis technology permits collection of plasma for production of plasma derivatives, such as factor VIII concentrate and albumin, and collection of platelets and granulocytes for patients requiring these cellular elements. Primary applications of therapeutic apheresis for pediatric patients are cytapheresis and TPE. Table 43-6 lists diseases and

Table 43-6. Acceptable indications for therapeutic apheresis

Cytapheresis	Therapeutic plasma exchange

Leukemia with hyperleukocytosis syndrome
Thrombocytosis, symptomatic
Sickle cell disease syndromes
Hyperparasitemia
Peripheral blood progenitor cell collections
	Major indications
	    Coagulation factor inhibitor
	    Goodpasture's disease
	    Guillain-Barré syndrome
	    Hemolytic-uremic sydrome
	    Hyperviscosity syndrome
	    Myasthenia gravis
	    Posttransfusion purpura
	    Rapidly progressive glomerulonephritis
	    Thrombotic thrombocytopenic purpura
	Other indications
	    Cold agglutinin disease
	    Cryoglobulinemia
	    Drug overdose and poisoning (protein bound)
	    Homozygous familial hypercholesterolemia
	    Pemphigus vulgaris
	    Systemic vasculitis

conditions in which use of therapeutic apheresis is considered acceptable and often standard medical practice.[63,64] Therapeutic apheresis can be used as a primary therapy or in conjunction with other medical treatment.

Cytapheresis is used for reduction of malignant WBC, to decrease the number of circulating platelets, to exchange hemoglobin A for hemoglobin S, to collect circulating mononuclear cells for stem cell transplant or gene therapy, and in rare instances, for removing parasitized red cells. Cytapheresis generally does not require replacement fluid. If greater than 20% of the blood volume is removed as plasma with the collected cells, however, colloid replacement is indicated. Cytapheresis procedures have target goals that include less than 100,000 blasts/uL in acute myelogenous leukemia, less than 1,000,000 platelets/uL, less than 50% hemoglobin S in sickle cell disease, and a transplantable dose of peripheral blood progenitor cells. The procedure may be repeated several times to achieve or maintain adequate cytareduction or cell collection. Although a cytareduction procedure may prove beneficial until definitive therapy can be instituted, it does not supplant treatment of the underlying disease or disorder.

In TPE, a nondialyzable plasma factor, which may be antibody, immune complex, metabolite, toxin, or unknown mediator of disease, is removed or replaced. The majority of plasma exchanges currently are done for immunologic disorders.[65] Most commonly, TPE involves exchange of 1.0 to 1.5 plasma volumes. A one-volume TPE should reduce the substance being removed to approximately 30% of its initial value. The second plasma volume exchanged during the same procedure is less efficient, reducing the concentration of the unwanted factor from 30% to 10%.[66] The amount of plasma factor removed depends on the rate of synthesis of the factor, fractional catabolic rate, tissue exchange rate, and reequilibration rate. The frequency of exchange depends on the disorder being treated. For example, patients with TTP or HUS should undergo TPE daily until there is evidence of a clinical response, while a patient with myasthenia gravis may undergo TPE every other day.

Practical Considerations

When therapeutic apheresis is being considered, there are several important things that the clinician and apheresis service need to

Table 43-7. Practical considerations of therapeutic apheresis

Who provides apheresis service

Indication for procedure, type of procedure, and coverage by payer

Clinical condition of patient; emergent or routine scheduling

Venous access: always assess peripheral access

Replacement fluid, type and volume

Adverse effects

Informed consent

consider together before embarking on a course of apheresis, and some of these considerations are listed in Table 43-7 and discussed here. Many facilities contract apheresis services through their blood bank or transfusion service, dialysis unit, or off-site consultant. The type of procedure to be performed is determined by the condition being treated. Most payers provide reimbursement lists of indications for therapeutic apheresis procedures. It is advisable to check with the payer prior to initiating therapy. The clinical condition of the patient and the disorder being treated determine where the procedure is performed (patient care unit, intensive care unit, or outpatient clinic), how often the procedure is performed, and how soon apheresis is begun.

Venous access is always a concern when automated therapeutic apheresis instruments are used. Large, good-condition peripheral veins can be used and should always be assessed by the apheresis team prior to central access placement. Central venous access can be obtained using short, rigid, large-bore double lumen catheters, such as those used for dialysis. Some apheresis instruments can be adapted to use a single venous access. Replacement fluid type and volume is dependent on the disorder being treated. The amount of plasma to be exchanged is calculated using the following formula: (blood volume) $\times$ (1 − Hct) = 1 plasma volume. For quick calculations, the plasma volume is equal to about 40 ml/kg in patients with normal hematocrit. Potential adverse effects of therapeutic apheresis include reactions to the replacement fluid, especially if blood components (FFP or RBCs) are used, citrate toxicity, bleeding, chills, and hypotension. Specific informed consent for the apheresis procedure should be obtained and documented in the patient chart.

References

1. Stehling L et al. Guidelines for blood utilization review. *Transfusion* 34:438–448, 1994.
2. Voak D et al. Guidelines for administration of blood products: Transfusion of infants and neonates. *Transfusion Med* 4:63–69, 1994.
3. Fresh-Frozen Plasma, Cryoprecipitate, and Platelets Administration Practice Guidelines Development Task Force of the College of American Pathologists. Practice parameter for the use of fresh-frozen plasma, cryoprecipitate and platelets. *JAMA* 271:777–781, 1994.
4. Adverse effects of blood transfusion. In Branch DR et al (eds): *Technical Manual* (11th ed). Bethesda, MD: American Association of Blood Banks, 1993.
5. Klein HG (ed). *Standards for Blood Banks and Transfusion Services* (16th ed) Bethesda, MD: American Association of Blood Banks, 1994. P 14.
6. ABO, Lewis, Ii, and P groups. In Mollison PL, Engelfriet CP, Contreras M (eds). *Blood Transfusion in Clinical Medicine* (9th ed). Oxford: Blackwell, 1993. Pp 149–175.
7. The Rh Blood Group System (and LW). In Mollison PL, Engelfriet CP, Contreras M (eds): *Blood Transfusion in Clinical Medicine* (9th ed). Oxford: Blackwell, 1993. Pp 204–245.
8. Pollack W et al. Studies on Rh prophylaxis. II. Rh immune prophylaxis after transfusion with Rh-positive blood. *Transfusion* 11:340–344, 1971.
9. Woodrow JC, Donohue WTA. Rh-immunization by pregnancy: Results of a survey and their relevance to prophylactic therapy. *Br Med J* 4:139–144, 1968.
10. Giblett ER. Blood group antibodies: An assessment of some laboratory practices. *Transfusion* 17:299–308, 1977.
11. Holland PV (ed). *Standards for Blood Banks and Transfusion Services* (13th ed). Arlington, VA: American Association of Blood Banks, 1989.
12. Mintz PD et al. Expected hemotherapy in elective surgery. *NY State J Med* 76:532–573, 1976.
13. Barnes A. The blood bank in hemotherapy for trauma and surgery. In Barnes A, Umlas J (eds). *Hemotherapy in Trauma and Surgery*. Washington, DC: American Association of Blood Banks, 1979. Pp 77–87.
14. Blumberg N, Bove J. Un-cross-matched blood for emergency transfusion. *JAMA* 240:2057–2059, 1978.
15. Hebert PC et al. Transfusion requirements in critical care: A pilot study. *JAMA* 273:1439–1444, 1995.
16. Bowie EJW, Thompson JH, Owen CA. The stability of antihemophiliac globulin and labile factor in human blood. *Mayo Clin Proc* 39:144, 1964.
17. Counts RB et al. Hemostasis in massively transfused patients. *Ann Surg* 190:91, 1979.
18. Beutler E. Platelet transfusions: The 20,000/uL trigger. *Blood* 81:1411–1413, 1993.
19. McCullough J et al. Platelet utilization in a university hospital. *JAMA* 259:2414–2418, 1988.
20. Friedberg RC, Donnelly SF, Mintz PD. Independent roles for platelet crossmatching and HLA in the selection of platelets for alloimmunized patients. *Transfusion* 34:215–220, 1994.
21. Bishop JF et al. The definition of refractoriness to platelet transfusion. *Transfusion Med* 2:35–41, 1992.
22. Lee EJ, Schiffer CA. ABO compatibility can influence the results of platelet transfusion. Results of a randomized trial. *Transfusion* 29:384–389, 1989.
23. Meryman HT. Transfusion-induced alloimmunization and immunosuppression and the effects of leukocyte depletion. *Tran Med Rev* 3:180–93, 1989.
24. Contreras M, Ala FA, Greaves M et al. Guidelines for the use of fresh frozen plasma. *Transfusion Med* 2:57–63, 1992.
25. Poon MC. Cryoprecipitate: Uses and alternatives. *Trans Med Rev* 180–192, 1993.
26. Mannucci PM et al. Deamino-8-D-arginine vasopressin shortens the bleeding time in uremia. *N Engl J Med* 308:8, 1983.
27. Strauss RG. Therapeutic granulocyte transfusions in 1993. *Blood* 81:1675–1678, 1993.
28. Bhatia S et al. Granulocyte transfusions: Efficacy in treating fungal infections in neutropenic patients following bone marrow transplantation. *Transfusion* 34:226–232, 1994.
29. Alexander MR et al. Albumin utilization in a university hospital. *Drug Intell Clin Pharm* 23:214–217, 1989.
30. Alving BM et al. Hypotension associated with prekallikrein activator (Hageman-factor fragments) in plasma protein fraction. *N Engl J Med* 299:66–70, 1978.
31. Ring J, Messmer K. Incidence and severity of anaphylactoid reactions to colloid volume substitutes. *Lancet* 1:466, 1977.
32. Yu MW et al. Hepatitis C transmission associated with intravenous immune globulins. *Lancet* 345:1173–1174, 1995.
33. Dwyer JM. Manipulating the immune system with immune globulin. *N Engl J Med* 326:107–116, 1992.
34. NIH Consensus Conference. Intravenous immunoglobulin: Prevention and treatment of disease. *JAMA* 264:3189–3193, 1990.
35. Andrew O. Role of leukocyte depletion in the prevention of transfusion induced cytomegalovirus. *Semin Hemotol* 28:26–31, 1991.
35a. Hillyer CM, Emmers RK, Zago-Novaretti M, Berkman EM. Methods for the reduction of transfusion-transmitted cytomegalovirus infection: filtration versus the use of seronegative donor units. *Transfusion*, 34:929–934, 1994.
36. Anderson KC, Weinstein HJ. Transfusion-associated graft-versus-host disease. *N Engl J Med* 323:315–321, 1990.
37. Sanders MR, Graeber JE. Posttransfusion graft-versus-host disease in infancy. *J Pediatr* 117:159–163, 1990.
38. Holland PV. Prevention of transfusion-associated graft-vs-host disease. *Arch Pathol Lab Med* 113:285–291, 1989.
39. Thaler M et al. The role of blood from HLA-homozygous donors in fatal transfusion-associated graft-vs-host disease after open-heart surgery. *N Engl J Med* 321:25–28, 1989.
40. Sandler SG et al. IgA anaphylactic transfusion reactions. *Trans Med Rev* 9:1–8, 1995.
41. Fox SM, Stavely-Haiber LM. Immunoglobulin A (IgA) levels in blood products and plasma derivatives. *Immunohematology* 4:5–9, 1988.
42. Walker RH (ed). *Technical Manual* (10th ed). Arlington, VA: American Association of Blood Banks, 1990. Pp 640–641.
43. Moroff G et al. Reduction of the volume of stored platelet concentrates for use in neonatal patients: *Transfusion* 24:144–146, 1984.
44. Simon TL, Sierra ER. Concentration of platelet units into small volumes. *Transfusion* 24:173–175, 1984.
45. Walker RH (ed). *Technical Manual* (10th ed). Arlington, VA: American Association of Blood Banks, 1990. Pp 411–432.
46. Beauregard P, Blajchman MA. Hemolytic and pseudo-hemolytic transfusion reactions: An overview of the hemolytic transfusion reactions and the clinical conditions that mimic them. *Trans Med Rev* 8:184–199, 1994.
47. Pineda AA, Brzica SM, Taswell JG. Hemolytic transfusion reaction: Recent experience in a large blood bank. *Mayo Clinic Proc* 53:378, 1978.
48. Sazama K. Reports of 355 transfusion-associated deaths: 1976 through 1985. *Transfusion* 30:583–590, 1990.
49. NIH Consensus Conference. Perioperative red blood cell transfusion. *JAMA* 260:2700–2703, 1988.
50. Dodd RY. Transfusion risk figures updated. Presentation at AABB Annual Seminar, 1994.
51. Davey R, Lee B, Coles S. Acute intraoperative hemolysis following rapid infusion of hypotonic solution. *Lab Med* 17:282, 1986.
52. Wilcox GJ, Barnes A, Modanlou H. Does transfusion using a syringe infusion pump and small-gauge needle cause hemolysis? *Transfusion* 21:750–751, 1981.
53. Heddle NM et al. The role of the plasma from platelet concentrates in transfusion reactions. *N Engl J Med* 331:625–628, 1994.
54. Oberman HA. Controversies in transfusion medicine: Should a febrile

transfusion reaction occasion the return of the blood component to the blood bank? *Con Transfusion* 34:353–355, 1994.

55. Widmann FK. Controversies in transfusion medicine: Should a febrile transfusion reaction occasion the return of the blood component to the blood bank? *Pro Transfusion* 34:3556–3558, 1994.

56. Eastlund T et al. Fatal pulmonary transfusion reaction to plasma containing donor HLA antibody. *Vox Sang* 57:63–66, 1989.

57. Pineda AA, Taswell HF, Brzica SM. Delayed hemolytic transfusion reaction: An immunologic hazard of blood transfusion. *Transfusion* 18:1–7, 1978.

58. Holland PV (ed). *Standards for Blood Banks and Transfusion Services. Screening Tests.* (13th ed). Arlington, VA: American Association of Blood Banks, 1989. P 15.

59. Polesky HF, Hanson MR. Transfusion-associated hepatitis C virus (non-A, non-B) infection. *Arch Pathol Lab Med* 113:232–235, 1989.

60. Alter HJ et al. Detection of antibody to hepatitis C virus in prospectively followed transfusion recipients with acute and chronic non-A, non-B hepatitis. *N Engl J Med* 321:1494–1500, 1989.

61. Goldman M, Blajchman MA. Blood product-associated bacterial sepsis. *Trans Med Rev* 5:73–83, 1991.

62. Tipple MA et al. Sepsis associated with transfusion of red cells contaminated with *Yersinia enterocolitica*. *Transfusion* 300:207–213, 1990.

63. MacPherson JL, Kasprisin DO (ed). *Therapeutic Hemapheresis* Vols. 1 and 2. Boca Raton, FL: CRC Press, 1985.

64. *Guidelines for Therapeutic Hemapheresis.* Bethesda, MD: American Association of Blood Banks, 1992.

65. Chopek M, McCullough J. Protein and biochemical changes during plasma exchange. In Berkman EM, Umlas J (eds): *Therapeutic Hemapheresis.* Washington, DC: American Association of Blood Banks, 1980.

66. McCullough J, Chopek M. Therapeutic plasma exchange. *Lab Med* 12:745–753, 1981.

IX ◆ Gastrointestinal System

Tracie L. Miller
Ronald E. Kleinman

44 ▸ Gastrointestinal Hemorrhage

Gastrointestinal (GI) hemorrhage in infants and children is common and can be life-threatening. In the past, the etiology of GI hemorrhage went undiagnosed in up to 50% of pediatric patients.[1] Recent advances in both the diagnosis and management of GI hemorrhage have allowed the practitioner to make definitive diagnoses and effect appropriate therapy. Ten percent of children with GI hemorrhage bleed from a site proximal to the ligament of Treitz, 33% from the small intestine, and 50% from the colorectal area.[1] An organized, systematic approach, with a complete history and physical examination, is essential to best localize the site of bleeding and initiate appropriate therapy.

Approach to Gastrointestinal Hemorrhage

A complete history often reveals the cause of hemorrhage. Usually the history is obtained as the physical examination is performed and preliminary stabilization is initiated. Key questions involve the patient's age; history of fevers; bleeding diatheses (e.g., hemophilia); medications, including aspirin or nonsteroidal antiinflammatory drugs; and preexisting acute or chronic diseases that predispose the child to intestinal hemorrhage, such as chronic liver disease. It is also important to determine if the patient has been vomiting, the appearance and consistency of the patient's stool, as well as any abdominal complaints. One must also confirm the reports of blood. The presence of blood in the vomitus or stool is often quite frightening to both the patient and the family, and what is red may not be blood. Red food coloring, fruit juices, or beets may resemble blood. Iron-containing medications as well as bismuth may make the stool black[2] and may even turn stool hemoglobin test cards positive if the stool pH is acidic.[3] Thus, the presence of hemoglobin should be confirmed chemically. In addition, blood may not be the patient's own. Swallowed maternal blood from a fissured nipple may appear in the gastric fluid or stool of a nursing infant. Finally, one must also determine that the blood has originated from the GI tract. Blood from the lung, as well as from oropharyngeal lesions, may result in heme-positive stools or emesis.

The character of blood in either the vomitus or stool will often suggest the site of bleeding. *Hematemesis* refers to the vomiting of recognizable blood, either bright red or coffee ground-like material. *Melena* describes stool that is black and tar-like. In both of these conditions, the site of hemorrhage is usually proximal to the ligament of Treitz, although conditions such as enterogastric fistula, gastrocolic fistula, and high jejunal obstruction can occasionally cause hematemesis.[4] Additionally, with slow intestinal transit time, melanotic stool may result from small intestinal lesions. The passage of maroon-colored stool is more suggestive of bleeding in the distal small bowel or colon. *Hematochezia* is a term used to describe stool containing bright red blood. The source of bleeding is usually colonic, although more rarely, because blood is a potent cathartic and if the bleeding is brisk, the location may be as proximal as the esophagus. Bright red blood streaked around the stool suggests an anorectal source.

When presented with an infant or child who is bleeding from the GI tract, one must quickly determine the rate of blood loss and the child's hemodynamic stability. The child's color is a crucial sign; pallor is more suggestive of a large blood loss, which may be either acute or chronic. Vital signs, including postural changes, should be recorded immediately, although previously healthy children, with excellent vascular tone, are in general able to maintain their BPs until cardiovascular collapse is near. Thus, the pulse rate as well as orthostatic changes are often more reliable than BP in detecting hypovolemia. The presence of a large amount of blood passed rectally or aspirated through a nasogastric tube also indicates brisk bleeding. The evaluation should include a complete physical examination, with special evaluation of the oropharyngeal area for any signs of blood, the skin for any abnormal pigmentation, jaundice, petechiae, ecchymoses, purpura, or rashes. The abdomen should be examined for masses, ascites, and hepatosplenomegaly; the stool should be tested for overt or occult blood, and the rectum examined for hemorrhoids, fissures, or polyps. In patients with significant hypovolemia, hepatosplenomegaly, which may otherwise suggest bleeding varices, may be absent. The vagina should also be examined for the presence of blood.

Pertinent laboratory studies include a complete blood count, platelet count, reticulocyte count, peripheral smear, electrolytes, type and cross-match, coagulation studies, liver function tests, BUN, arterial blood gas, and urinalysis. A hematocrit during a significant acute bleed often will not accurately reflect the extent of blood loss because equilibration may not have occurred.

Stabilization

Postural hypotension, tachycardia, or shock in a previously healthy patient indicates a loss of 20% or more of the blood volume. A patient in this state requires rapid attention. The patient should be positioned with the legs elevated. Preferably, more than one large-bore intravenous (IV) catheter should be inserted. If IV access is difficult, a person adept in performing cutdown catherizations or subclavian punctures should be called. Central venous access is helpful in monitoring blood volume and the need for further fluid replacement therapy. If the patient is actively vomiting blood and is hypotensive, early elective endotracheal intubation is advised because aspiration of blood may lead to further pulmonary complications. Regardless, supplemental oxygen should be used to optimize the oxygen-carrying capacity in the remaining RBCs.

Blood volume expansion should be accomplished with packed RBCs; colloid and crystalloid solutions, however, are routinely administered initially. Normal saline, 5% albumin, or lactated Ringer's solution should be infused at the rate of 20 ml/kg/hr, just until BP is stabilized. Excessive hydration in this setting may lead to pulmonary edema and, in a patient with esophageal varices due to portal hypertension, may exacerbate the bleeding. Complications of massive red cell transfusions include hypocalcemia, hyperkalemia, lactic acidemia, thrombocytopenia, and loss of clotting factors. Thus, serum calcium, potassium, serum pH, and blood coagulation should be monitored carefully. Five to 10 mg of vitamin K should be injected intramuscularly or intravenously. A urinary catheter should be placed to accurately assess urine output (Table 44-1).

Table 44-1. Stabilization

Assessment of acuity
  Vital signs
    Tachycardia
    Orthostatic changes
  Mental status changes
  Visible bleeding
    Hematemesis
    Hemoptysis
    Rectal bleeding

Laboratory assessment
  Complete blood count
  Reticulocyte count
  Platelet count
  Coagulation profile
  Type and cross-match
  Electrolytes, renal function
  Liver function
  Arterial blood gas
  Urinalysis

Intervention
  Elevation of legs
  Two large-bore IV lines
  Airway protection
  Fluid replacement
  Vitamin K, 5–10 mg IV/IM
  Urinary catheter
  Diagnose etiology of hemorrhage

Upper Gastrointestinal Hemorrhage

Diagnosis

Bleeding from the upper GI tract in pediatric patients is usually due to one of a limited number of causes that are typically readily diagnosable. These include Mallory Weiss tears, esophagitis, varices, and variants of peptic ulcer disease. Examples of more unusual causes, such as gastric teratomas, polypoid lesions, or arteriovenous malformations, have been reported,[5] but these are rare (Fig. 44-1)

Nasogastric Lavage

Any child with significant GI blood loss should have a nasogastric (NG) tube placed to assess the degree and location of bleeding. Even if a lower source seems most likely, the gastric aspirate may be helpful. Blood in the NG aspirate usually indicates hemorrhage proximal to the ligament of Treitz.[6] On occasion, blood may be absent from the stomach with upper tract hemorrhage, because the pylorus is in spasm, thus preventing blood from refluxing into the stomach.[7] The use of NG lavage to control bleeding and to facilitate endoscopy is controversial.[8] Normal saline is most often used, although studies suggest that tap water can be used in adults without any untoward effects.[9] The use of iced as opposed to room-temperature lavage fluid is also controversial.[10] Studies in canines have found no difference between the two. Hypothermia is thought to decrease gastric blood flow, but has also been shown to decrease platelet function.[11] In small infants, one needs to consider the effect of iced lavage on core body temperature. The addition of norepinephrine to the lavage may be helpful in controlling the hemorrhage, although there have been no controlled studies to date.[12] Finally, esophageal varices are not a contraindication to placing an NG tube. Thus, NG lavage may aid in localizing but probably not controlling hemorrhage from the upper GI tract. Persistent brisk bleeding after 15 to 20 minutes of lavage is an indication to pursue other alternatives.

Endoscopy

Esophagogastroduodenoscopy (EGD) is the diagnostic procedure of choice in patients with upper GI hemorrhage who fail to stabilize. The small, flexible pediatric endoscopes have revolutionized the ability to make accurate diagnoses and effect interventions. A source may be found in up to 100% of patients[13]; barium contrast studies yield a diagnosis in 50% to 60% of patients.[14] Thus, in an acute setting, barium contrast x-rays should not be the first diagnostic study because they are less accurate and may obscure visualization during endoscopy. Disorders such as Mallory Weiss tears, esophagitis, gastritis, peptic and duodenal ulcers, and varices are readily diagnosable by EGD. Endoscopy should be performed within 12 to 24 hours in those patients who fail to achieve hemostasis.[13] However, routine early endoscopy in patients who are bleeding from the upper intestinal tract for the first time and who stop bleeding spontaneously has not been useful in altering the

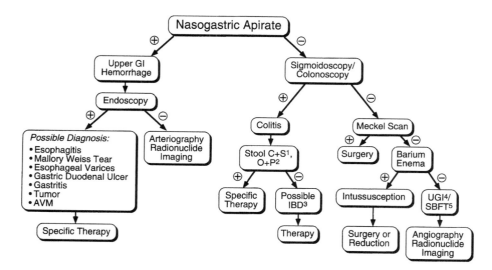

Figure 44-1. Diagnostic algorithm for gastrointestinal bleeding: (1) culture and sensitivity, (2) ova and parasite, (3) inflammatory bowel disease, (4) upper gastrointestinal barium study, (5) small bowel follow through.

management, reducing transfusions, shortening hospitalizations, or prolonging survival.[15] Endoscopy is considered a safe procedure in pediatric patients, with relatively few complications.[16]

Upper Gastrointestinal Fluoroscopic Contrast Studies

Upper GI fluoroscopic contrast studies should not be the initial diagnostic test at the time of acute and life-threatening bleeding. They can be inaccurate in up to 50%[13] of patients and may obscure endoscopic visualization of a bleeding site. Contrast studies may delineate pathology but cannot accurately diagnose the source of the bleed. In one study, up to 50% of patients who had documented varices were not bleeding from them at the time of an acute upper GI bleed, but instead were bleeding from a mucosal lesion.[17]

Radionuclide Studies

Radionuclide studies have been helpful in localizing the source of intestinal hemorrhage or in directing angiographic injections. The ^{99m}technetium-sulfur colloid (^{99m}Tc-SC) and the ^{99m}technetium-pertechnetate-labeled RBC scan are both commonly used. These techniques are applicable to both upper and lower GI hemorrhage, but are more often used in patients with lower intestinal tract hemorrhage. This is due to the fact that the causes of upper tract hemorrhage are more readily diagnosed by endoscopy. In general, for the radionuclide study to demonstrate optimum sensitivity, the patient must be bleeding briskly. Blood loss must be at least 0.1 ml/min for the ^{99m}Tc-SC scan to be useful.[18]

^{99m}Tc-SC is injected intravenously and is cleared by the liver and spleen, making it useful for scanning the liver and spleen. With rapid blood loss, the colloid extravasates at the bleeding site and is imaged as a "hot" spot. Images are taken frequently because the circulating half-life is less than 2.5 minutes. Thus, this examination is only sensitive if the patient is bleeding at the time of injection and is not valuable for intermittent bleeding. Repeated injections may be necessary. Additionally, because the colloid is concentrated in the liver and spleen, it is difficult to localize bleeding sites in the vicinity of these organs, such as colonic lesions. Normal liver function and clearance are necessary, and if these functions are diminished, there may be a high level of background activity, which may make the study less sensitive.[19]

The ^{99m}Tc-labeled RBC scan was first described by Winzelberg et al.[20] as a useful way to detect GI bleeding over a longer period. RBCs from the patient's own blood are labeled in vitro. After injecting the labeled cells, images are taken at 5-minute intervals for the first 30 minutes and can be repeated for up to 24 hours after injection. A scan may not become positive for up to 4 to 6 hours after injection.[21] The scan is 91% accurate for true-positives and has a 5% false-positive and 9% false-negative rate.[21] This technique is advantageous for intermittent hemorrhage, but localizing the exact site of bleeding is not as sensitive as angiography. Thus it should be used optimally as a screening procedure or in conjunction with angiography.

Angiography

Angiography is a useful technique to delineate areas of active bleeding in both the upper and lower GI tract. Due to improved endoscopic and radionuclide technology, however, its use has diminished. This technique may also detect vascular anomalies such as arteriovenous malformations and their variants. Angiography is used commonly to diagnose the etiology of massive GI hemorrhage that is not apparent by other less invasive methods. Accurate angiography requires at least 0.5 to 2.0 ml/min of blood loss.[22] The yield is highest in patients who require greater than 3 units of

blood to maintain cardiovascular stability and is further enhanced when pharmacologic agents such as heparin, tolazoline, or streptokinase are being used or when indwelling catheters are in place during the acute bleed.[23] For suspected upper GI hemorrhage, the celiac axis and superior mesenteric artery are injected. For lower GI hemorrhage, the superior mesenteric artery as well as the inferior mesenteric artery are injected. Transumbilical aortography in a newborn may lead to the diagnosis of an acute hemorrhage.[24] Angiography may also be used for therapeutic maneuvers such as selective embolization of an active bleeding vessel or direct infusion of a vasoconstrictive agent.

Although angiography is very sensitive, younger patients suffer greater morbidity.[25] There is an increased risk of arterial spasm in children, which may compromise blood flow in a catheterized vessel, such as the femoral artery. The child is also at risk for a thrombotic event of the catheterized limb; thus perfusion in the catheterized extremity should be observed closely after angiography.

Management

Hemodynamic stabilization should be the first priority in the initial management of upper intestinal hemorrhage. The sources of upper GI hemorrhage (i.e., those proximal to the ligament of Treitz) may be subdivided into either mucosal or vascular lesions. Mucosal lesions include disorders such as esophagitis, gastritis, Mallory Weiss tears, or ulcer disease. These disorders rarely produce massive hemorrhage, although on occasion they may erode into a major artery and cause significant blood loss. Most mucosal lesions are amenable to management that aims at neutralizing the gastric pH. Topical and acid-blocking agents are the two mainstays of therapy.

Antacids contain either aluminum or magnesium hydroxide, or a combination of the two. A dose of 0.5 ml/kg per dose hourly will maintain the gastric pH at greater than 5 in a setting of an acute hemorrhage.[26] Gastric pH should be monitored hourly in aspirates from the NG tube and antacids titrated accordingly. After the bleeding is well under control, the frequency may be decreased to doses at 1 and 3 hours after meals and at bedtime. Antacids have also been shown to be effective in the prevention of acute GI hemorrhage in critically ill patients and appear to be more effective than H_2 receptor antagonists, such as cimetidine, in this setting.[27] The main disadvantages of antacids are diarrhea (with magnesium) and constipation (from aluminum-based antacids). Both the magnesium and aluminum components of the antacid are absorbed into the systemic circulation, but there are usually no adverse effects.

There are several histamine receptor antagonists available to treat peptic disease. The most commonly used agents are cimetidine, ranitidine, and famotidine. These medications have no role in the setting of an acute upper GI hemorrhage.[28] Cimetidine is useful in the chronic treatment or prophylaxis of many upper GI tract mucosal disorders and is given at a dose of 20 to 40 mg/kg/d in four divided doses. Oral cimetidine and topical antacids should not be given **simultaneously** because topical antacids may block the absorption of cimetidine.[29] However, cimetidine is generally administered intravenously in the intensive care unit (ICU). Sucralfate is a medication that binds to exposed glycosidic residues on injured gastric and duodenal epithelium and forms a barrier to acid at the injured site. This medication also has no role during acute upper GI hemorrhage. It has minimal side effects, the major one being constipation. The recommended dose for adults is 1 g four times daily. The optimal dose for children remains to be established. Ranitidine is also used for the treatment of peptic disorders and is given at a dose of 2 to 4 mg/kg/24 hr twice daily orally and 1 to 2 mg/kg/24 hr intravenously every 6 to 8 hours. Omeprazole, a proton pump inhibitor, is a potent acid-blocking agent that may be used in children, although the experience with this agent is more established in adults. There are currently no recommended dosages for children.

Endoscopy may be useful in the management of upper GI hemorrhage. For mucosal lesions such as gastric and duodenal ulcers with a visible vessel, electrocauterization with the bipolar electrode or heater probe may achieve rapid hemostasis in a patient who might otherwise need surgical intervention. The bipolar electrode has multiple hot and ground points on the end of the probe, which lessen the extent of devitalized tissue.[30] Electrocauterization may achieve hemostasis in up to 92% of patients.[31] Selective transcatheter embolic angiography can also be employed to control massive hemorrhage from mucosal lesions. Additionally, intraarterial infusions of vasopressin have been shown to decrease bleeding in hemorrhagic gastritis.[32] Surgery should be considered in patients who require over 85 ml/kg of blood to keep up with blood loss.[33] A decision regarding surgical intervention in this setting should be made swiftly because the mortality associated with emergency surgery ranges between 15% and 25%.[34]

Bleeding from esophageal varices is another major cause of morbidity and mortality in pediatric patients. Esophageal varices in children are usually due to extrahepatic portal venous obstruction resulting from umbilical venous catheters, necrotizing enterocolitis, and peritonitis,[35] or from serious fibrotic liver disease. Often the cause of portal obstruction is unknown. Major symptoms of portal obstruction include ascites, hypersplenism, and hemorrhage. Bleeding is rare during the first year of life, but 66% of patients bleed by 5 years and 85% by 10 years. Fifty percent of the bleeding is associated with viral syndromes or aspirin therapy. The mortality following a variceal hemorrhage ranges between 2% and 10%.[36]

The administration of IV pitressin or vasopressin can be the first approach in controlling variceal hemorrhage. Pitressin decreases portal pressures by decreasing portal blood flow in the splanchnic circulation. When used alone, IV pitressin may control variceal hemorrhage as often as 50% of the time.[37] In contrast to bleeding gastric mucosal lesions, esophageal varices appear to be as well controlled by IV infusions of pitressin as by arterial infusions, thereby reducing the complications from intraarterial infusions.[38,39] Pitressin is administered as a bolus infusion of 20 to 40 U/1.73 m² diluted in 5% dextrose water over 20 minutes, followed by a constant infusion of 0.1 U/1.73 m²/min. The dose may be increased to 0.4 U/1.73 m²/min in gradual fashion, carefully monitoring for side effects. Increasing the dose over 0.7U/1.73 m²/min significantly increases the incidence of side effects.[37] Toxicity may be severe and includes hypertension, myocardial ischemia, arrhythmias, anuria or oliguria, and tissue necrosis. Once bleeding stops, the pitressin infusion is maintained for approximately 24 hours and then is gradually tapered over the next 12 to 24 hours.

Endoscopic sclerotherapy is an important technique in controlling acute variceal hemorrhage and subsequently preventing recurrent variceal bleeding. In the past, sclerotherapy was not thought to be useful in stopping acute hemorrhage, but more recent experience with this procedure points to its efficacy. During sclerotherapy, a sclerosing agent such as 5% sodium morrhuate, ethanolamine oleate, or 3% tetradecyl sulfate is injected either directly into the varix or in the paravariceal area. Each injection should not exceed 2 to 4 ml. Initially, the most distal esophageal varices are sclerosed. In another 3 to 4 days, the sclerotherapy is repeated on the remaining distal varices, and this procedure is repeated every 2 to 4 weeks until the varices are obliterated. In many pediatric patients, general anesthesia is used because adequate sedation is imperative. The patient is usually observed in the hospital overnight following the procedure.

Children often complain of retrosternal chest pain following sclerotherapy. This usually reflects esophageal spasm, although the patient must be carefully monitored for other complications. Bleeding esophageal ulcerations and ulceration with stricture are the most common complications, occurring in fewer than 5% of patients.[40] Esophageal perforation has also been a reported complication. Hemorrhage during sclerotherapy may result from injected varices or those that remain to be injected. In adult patients, postmortem studies reveal venous thrombosis and necrosis within 24 hours of therapy. Ulceration may occur after 7 days and fibrosis within 1 month.[41] The degree of ulceration correlates with the depth of injection and the volume of sclerosant used at a single site.[42] Other known but rare complications of sclerotherapy include pleural effusions, pulmonary infiltrates, pneumomediastinum, and pericardial effusions. In general, a child who undergoes sclerotherapy needs to monitored very closely for the complications of the procedure.

Recently endoscopic ligation has been employed to control bleeding esophageal varices in both adults and children. Using this technique, esophageal varices are ligated with small elastic O rings. In a study of adults with cirrhosis and bleeding esophageal varices, patients who were randomized to receive endoscopic ligation for treatment had fewer treatment-related complications and better survival rates than those patients treated with sclerotherapy.[42a]

The use of propranolol in the prevention of variceal hemorrhage is controversial. Unfortunately, no controlled studies have been performed in children. In adults with severe liver disease, propranolol alone may reduce the risk of recurrent GI bleeding and mortality in those patients with cirrhosis but without evidence of ascites, jaundice, or encephalopathy.[43]

Balloon tamponade with either the Sengstaken-Blakemore tube or Linton tube is an alternative method that may be used in controlling active variceal hemorrhage. Significant complications can occur with the use of this tube. These include esophageal rupture, mediastinitis, aspiration pneumonia, and esophageal tears. Routine use of balloon tamponade as a first-line approach to control bleeding varices is not advised, because pharmacologic and endoscopic intervention usually accomplish hemostasis with less morbidity.

Surgical portosystemic shunts have been useful in decreasing the bleeding complications of portal hypertension that cannot be controlled by nonsurgical methods.[44] Their use has not been advocated as a prophylactic procedure. Patients who are older than 6 years or greater than 25 kg are considered more suitable surgical candidates because the shunt should be greater than 1 cm in diameter for the best function and fewest complications. Younger or smaller children should be managed by alternative therapies, because they are at greater risk for thrombosis and subsequent nonfunction of the shunt. Recurrent episodes of bleeding despite maximal medical therapy is an indication for a shunting procedure. The complications of portosystemic shunts include hepatic encephalopathy due to decreased blood flow through the liver and decompensation of hepatic synthetic function due to shunting of blood away from the liver. Placement of transjugular intrahepatic portosystemic shunts (TIPS) using expandable metallic stents has been used to control variceal bleeding by creating a shunt between the hepatic and portal veins within the liver. This procedure decompresses the portal system and has been used effectively in patients prior to liver transplantation.[44a]

Lower Gastrointestinal Hemorrhage

Lower GI hemorrhage is defined as intestinal bleeding distal to the ligament of Treitz. Unlike upper GI hemorrhage, the diverse causes of lower hemorrhage make the diagnostic workup more challenging. Limitations in techniques to visualize most of the small bowel may contribute to the difficulty in diagnosis. As with any major hemorrhage, hemodynamic stability is the first goal. The age of the patient is a primary concern in lower GI tract hemorrhage, as the differential diagnosis of bleeding is different in various age groups (Table 44-2).

Etiology and Pathogenesis

The most common cause of rectal bleeding in an infant is an anal fissure. The patient may be entirely well but pass a normal or hard stool that is streaked with bright red blood. Often, the fissure can be easily diagnosed by careful manual inspection. Other causes of lower tract bleeding in the infant include hemorrhagic disease of the newborn, necrotizing enterocolitis, infectious diarrhea, or congenital anomalies such as midgut volvulus. These processes may lead to significant blood loss. Milk or soy allergy may present with marked anemia, but the anemia is usually due to chronic blood loss. This is best diagnosed on rectal biopsy, which demonstrates increased eosinophils in the lamina propria. Occasionally, the infant will also have peripheral eosinophilia.

Intussusception and Meckel diverticulum are the most common causes of rectal bleeding in the infant and preschooler. Intussusception usually occurs between 6 and 18 months of age, but patients may be much younger or older. The infant presents with episodes

Table 44-2. Cause of lower gastrointestinal hemorrhage by age

Infancy
    Vitamin K deficiency
    Anal fissure
    Necrotizing enterocolitis
    Volvulus
    Allergic colitis
    Infectious diarrhea
    Stress ulcer
    Vascular malformation

Toddler/preschool
    Infectious diarrhea
    Meckel diverticulum
    Intussusception
    Polyp
    Vascular malformations
    Henoch-Schönlein purpura
    Hemolytic-uremic syndrome
    Varices

School age
    Inflammatory bowel disease
    Infectious diarrhea
    Varices
    Polyps

of colicky abdominal pain and vomiting and may have a mass in the right lower quadrant. The child will often pass currant jelly-like stools several hours after abdominal symptoms begin. The intussusception is most often ileocecal. Repeated episodes of intussusception in the same patient or an episode in a patient over 5 years of age suggests that there may be a lead point, such as a Meckel diverticulum or polyp. Further diagnostic studies are warranted in this circumstance. Intussusception results in impaired venous drainage in the GI tract, with edema, hemorrhage, incarceration, and necrosis that may lead to perforation and peritonitis if allowed to progress. Intussusception is best diagnosed and often treated with a barium enema, although this is contraindicated in patients with a perforation. Intussusception can be reduced by hydrostatic pressure in up to 80% of patients.[45]

Meckel diverticulum is seen in a slighter older age group. The mean age at presentation is approximately 2 years; it occurs in approximately 2% of the population and is found usually within 2 feet of the ileocecal junction. The majority of patients with a Meckel diverticulum do not bleed. The diverticulum contains heterotopic gastric mucosa that causes ulceration in surrounding tissue. These patients present with painless rectal bleeding that may be significant. The bleeding Meckel diverticulum is fairly easily diagnosable by radionuclide imaging using ^{99m}Tc pertechnetate. This tracer is selectively concentrated by thyroid, salivary, and gastric mucosa, including that which is contained in up to 50% of Meckel diverticula.[19] A positive scan usually shows activity in the right lower quadrant that parallels activity of the gastric mucosa. This technique has a sensitivity of 85%, a specificity of 95%, and an accuracy of 90%.[46] Lesions that give false-positive results include duodenal ulcers, hemangiomas, ureteral obstruction, small bowel obstruction, or any lesions, such as enteric duplications, that may contain ectopic gastric mucosa.[47] Because barium is dense and may interfere with the detection of gamma rays, barium contrast studies should not be performed for suspected Meckel diverticulum. The administration of pentagastrin may enhance the sensitivity of the study.[48] Cimetidine may also have the same effect, although this is controversial.[49]

Polyps in pediatric patients are usually of the hamartomatous juvenile type. Most are located in the rectosigmoid region and are accompanied by painless rectal bleeding. These polyps rarely cause massive hemorrhage, and there is only a small chance for malignant degeneration.

Other disorders that present with rectal bleeding include vasculitic lesions such as Henoch-Schönlein purpura (HSP) and hemolytic-uremic syndrome (HUS). HSP is a hypersensitivity vasculitis that presents with a characteristic purpuric rash that is often localized to the buttocks and posterior aspect of the legs. Patients complain of significant crampy abdominal pain, joint swelling, and GI hemorrhage. The GI symptoms are attributed to a small vessel vasculitis that results in hemorrhage into the bowel wall. This leads to pain and bleeding. The patient is also at high risk for intussusception. Occasionally, HSP presents with upper intestinal hemorrhage,[50] but more often, bloody diarrhea that may occasionally be life-threatening.

HUS comprises a constellation of symptoms. These include a microangiopathic anemia, thrombocytopenia, renal compromise, acute bloody diarrhea, and colitis. The etiology of this disorder is unclear but has been associated with several bacterial agents, including *E. Coli* 0157:H7 and toxins such as verocytotoxins 1 and 2 (shigatoxins), which are produced by bacteria.[51] The colitis, which occurs in up to 50% of patients,[52] may be due to thrombosis of small vessels in the submucosa that results in ischemic bowel disease. In both HSP and HUS, bloody diarrhea may precede the development of other symptoms and may often be misleading.

The most common disorder presenting with rectal bleeding in the school-age years is inflammatory colitis. Infectious agents such as *Salmonella, Shigella, Campylobacter,* and *Yersinia* may be responsible. Pseudomembranous colitis should be considered in patients with rectal bleeding who are receiving antibiotics. Chronic inflammatory bowel disease, ulcerative colitis or Crohn's disease, is now being seen with increasing frequency and may be life-threatening. Acute dilation of the colon with significant protein and blood loss is known as toxic megacolon and may be the initial presentation in both forms of idiopathic inflammatory bowel disease.

Diagnosis

Many of the diagnostic procedures used in delineating the etiology of upper GI hemorrhage may be used to diagnose bleeding from the lower GI tract. A flat-plate x-ray examination of the abdomen will often yield information about the presence of a toxic megacolon, perforation, obstruction, or pneumatosis. If the patient has bloody diarrhea, the stool should be examined for neutrophils and organisms by Wright stain. It should also be cultured for pathogenic bacteria and assayed for *Clostridium difficile* toxin. An examination for ova and parasites should be performed, although the more common parasitic infections in the United States do not present with rectal bleeding. Contrast x-ray studies are important in the diagnosis and therapy of an intussusception. Air contrast is more sensitive than column barium examinations in the diagnosis of polyps. Contrast x-rays should be performed initially if there is a very strong suspicion that an intussusception is present. A contrast examination will preclude other studies because barium often obscures direct visualization and radionuclide imaging.

Sigmoidoscopy can reveal the presence of polyps, determine mucosal integrity, detect a pseudomembrane, and be used to obtain accurate cultures. Colonoscopy may be of added benefit, even if sigmoidoscopy is negative, because the bleeding lesion may be located proximal to the reach of the sigmoidoscope.[53,54] Visualization may be limited if bleeding is brisk, and one should not persist if the rate of bleeding is such that visualization is obscured. This is an indication for pursuing an alternate means of diagnosis and stabilization, such as angiography or nuclear imaging.

The value of radionuclide scanning and angiography have already been discussed in the section on upper GI hemorrhage. Angiography, as well, has already been discussed and should be pursued in the patient whose diagnosis is unclear after the aforementioned procedures. If the source of the bleeding has not been diagnosed and is persistent, surgical intervention may be necessary. The surgeon, together with the gastroenterologist, may localize bleeding at the time of a laparotomy with the use of an enteroscope. This is a longer upper endoscope that passes into the small bowel and can be guided by the surgeon and gastroenterologist jointly during a laparotomy to identify the bleeding site and expedite surgery.

Therapy

The therapy for lower intestinal hemorrhage depends on which lesion is causing the bleeding. More often than not, with significant lower hemorrhage, the therapy of choice is surgical intervention. Disorders that require surgery include a Meckel diverticulum, midgut volvulus, malrotation, nonreducible intussusception, non-

viable bowel resulting from necrotizing enterocolitis, arteriovenous malformations, and occasionally, an uncontrollably bleeding polyp.

Corticosteroids are the mainstay in the treatment of inflammatory bowel disease. Often, steroid therapy (prednisone or methylprednisolone 1–4 mg/kg/d) can control even major GI hemorrhage. In patients with severe colitis, which is described as bloody diarrhea greater than 5 times a day, fever, tachycardia, anemia, and albumin less than 3 g/dl, the majority of patients require surgery within 2 years of initial presentation; only 30% respond initially to medical management.[55]

Conclusion

GI hemorrhage in childhood occurs in all age groups and can be life-threatening. Regardless of the etiology, the primary concern in an intensive care setting is establishing hemodynamic stability. Once established, localizing the source of bleeding is important to effect the best therapy. This can often be done with an accurate history and physical examination. Endoscopic assessment and intervention often play a major role. Other methods, such as angiography and nuclear medicine scans, can give important information regarding localization of bleeding that is beyond the reach of the endoscope.

References

1. Spencer R. Gastrointestinal hemorrhage in infancy and childhood: 476 cases. *Surgery* 55:718, 1964.
2. Stillman AE. Black heme-positive stools without gastrointestinal hemorrhage. *J Pediatr* 100:414, 1982.
3. McDonald WM et al. The effect of iron on the guaiac reaction. *Gastroenterology* 96:74, 1989.
4. Bynum TE. Axioms on gastrointestinal bleeding. *Hosp Pract* 12:52, 1977.
5. Cairo MS, Grosfeld JL, Weetman RM. Gastric teratoma: Unusual cause for bleeding of the upper gastrointestinal tract in the newborn. *Pediatrics* 67:721, 1981.
6. Dent TL. Evaluation of bleeding patients. *Surg Gynecol Obstet* 151:817, 1980.
7. Luk GD, Bynum TE, Hendrix TR. Gastric aspiration in the localization of gastrointestinal hemorrhage. *JAMA* 241:576, 1979.
8. Gilbert DA, Saunders DR, Peoples J. Failure of iced saline lavage to suppress hemorrhage from experimental bleeding ulcers. *Gastroenterology* 76:1138A, 1979.
9. Ruldoph JP. Automated gastric lavage and a comparison of 0.9% normal saline solution and tap water irrigant. *Ann Emerg Med* 14:1156, 1985.
10. Ponsky JL, Hoffman M, Swayngin DS. Saline irrigation in gastric hemorrhage: The effect of temperature. *J Surg Res* 28:204, 1980.
11. Waterman NG, Walker JL. The effect of gastric cooling on hemostasis. *Surg Gynecol Obstet* 137:80, 1973.
12. LeVeen HH et al. Control of gastrointestinal bleeding. *Am J Surg* 123:154, 1972.
13. Cox K, Ament ME. Upper gastrointestinal bleeding in children and adolescents. *Pediatrics* 63:408, 1979.
14. Cichowicz E, Alvarez-Ruiz JR. Acute upper gastrointestinal bleeding in children. *Bol Asoc Med PR* 75:214, 1983.
15. Peterson WL et al. Routine early endoscopy in upper-gastrointestinal tract bleeding. A randomized, controlled trial. *N Engl J Med* 304:925, 1981.
16. Prolla JC et al. Upper gastrointestinal fiberoptic endoscopy in pediatric patients. *Gastrointest Endosc* 29:279, 1983.
17. Buset M et al. Bleeding esophagogastric varices: An endoscopic study. *Am J Gastroenterol* 82:241, 1987.

18. Alvi A. Scintigraphic demonstration of acute gastrointestinal bleeding. *Gastrointest Radiol* 5:205, 1980.

19. Winzelberg GG et al. Scintigraphic detection of gastrointestinal bleeding: A review of current methods. *Am J Gastroenterol* 78:324, 1983.

20. Winzelberg GG et al. Evaluation of gastrointestinal bleeding by red blood cells labeled in vivo with technetium-99m. *J Nucl Med* 20:1080, 1979.

21. Winzelberg GG et al. Radionuclide localization of lower gastrointestinal hemorrhage. *Radiology* 139:465, 1981.

22. Baum S et al. The preoperative radiographic demonstration of intraabdominal bleeding from undetermined sites by percutaneous selective celiac and superior mesenteric arteriography. *Surgery* 58:797, 1965.

23. Koval G et al. Aggressive angiographic diagnosis in acute lower gastrointestinal hemorrhage. *Dig Dis Sci* 32:248, 1987.

24. Fliegel CP et al. Bleeding gastric ulcer in a newborn infant diagnosed by transumbilical aortography. *J Pediatr Surg* 12:589, 1977.

25. Jacobson B et al. Complications of angiography in children and means of prevention. *Acta Radiol* 21:257, 1980.

26. Simoman SJ et al. Non-surgical control of massive acute gastric mucosal hemorrhage with antacid neutralization of gastric contents. *Surg Clin North Am* 56:21, 1976.

27. Priebe HJ et al. Antacid versus cimetidine in preventing acute gastrointestinal bleeding. A randomized trial in 75 critically ill patients. *N Engl J Med* 302:426, 1980.

28. Welch R et al. Effect of cimetidine on upper gastrointestinal hemorrhage. *Gastroenterology* 80:1313, 1981.

29. Steinberg WM, Lewis JH, Katz DM. Antacids inhibit absorption of cimetidine. *N Engl J Med* 307:400, 1982.

30. Donahue PE et al. Endoscopic control of upper gastrointestinal hemorrhage with a bipolar coagulation device. *Surg Gynecol Obstet* 159:113, 1984.

31. Gaisford WD. Endoscopic electrohemostasis of active upper gastrointestinal bleeding. *Am J Surg* 137:47, 1979.

32. Filston HL, Jackson DC, Johnsrude IS. Arteriographic embolization for control of recurrent severe gastric hemorrhage in a 10-year-old boy. *J Pediatr Surg* 14:276, 1981.

33. Morden R et al. Operative management of stress ulcers in children. *Ann Surg* 196:8, 1982.

34. Protell RL et al. Severe upper gastrointestinal bleeding; I. Causes, pathogenesis and methods of diagnosis. *Clin Gastroenterol* 10:17, 1981.

35. Mitra SK et al. Extrahepatic portal hypertension: A review of 70 cases. *J Pediatr Surg* 13:51, 1978.

36. Stevenson RJ. Gastrointestinal bleeding in children. *Surg Clin North Am* 65:1455, 1985.

37. Tuggle DW et al. Intravenous vasopressin and gastrointestinal hemorrhage in children. *J Pediatr Surg* 23:627, 1988.

38. Chojkier M et al. A controlled comparison of continuous intraarterial and intravenous infusions of vasopressin in hemorrhage from esophageal varices. *Gastroenterology* 77:540, 1979.

39. Johnson WC et al. Control of bleeding varices by vasopressin: A prospective randomized study. *Ann Surg* 186:369, 1977.

40. Howard ER, Stamatakis JD, Mowat AP. Management of esophageal varices in children by injection sclerotherapy. *J Pediatr Surg* 19:2, 1984.

41. Evans DMD et al. Oesophageal varices treated by sclerotherapy: A histopathological study. *Gut* 23:615, 1982.

42. Sugawa C et al. Endoscopic sclerosis of experimental oesophageal varices in dogs. *Gastrointest Endosc* 24:114, 1978.

42a. Stiegmann GV et al. Endoscopic sclerotherapy as compared with endoscopic ligation for bleeding esophageal varices. *N Engl J Med* 326:1527–1532, 1992.

43. Lebrec D et al. A randomized controlled study of propranolol for prevention of recurrent gastrointestinal bleeding in patients with cirrhosis: A final report. *Hepatology* 4:355, 1984.

44. Fonkalsrud EW. Surgical management of portal hypertension in childhood. *Arch Surg* 115:1042, 1980.

44a. Ring ER et al. Using transjugular intrahepatic portosystemic shunts to control variceal bleeding before liver transplantation. *Ann Intern Med* 116:304–309, 1992.

45. Liu KW et al. Intussusception—Current trends in management. *Arch Dis Child* 61:75, 1986.

46. Sfakianakis GN, Conway JJ. Detection of ectopic gastric mucosa in Meckel's diverticulum and in other aberrations by scintigraphy: A pathophysiology and 10-year experience. *J Nucl Med* 22:647, 1981.

47. Munroff LR, Casarella WJ, Johnson PM. Preoperative diagnosis of Meckel diverticulum: Angiographic and radionuclide studies in an adult. *JAMA* 229:1900, 1974.

48. Treves S, Grand RJ, Eraklis AJ. Pentagastrin stimulation of technetium-99m uptake by ectopic gastric mucosa in a Meckel's diverticulum. *Radiology* 128:711, 1978.

49. Petrokubi RJ, Baum S, Rohrer GV. Cimetidine administration resulting in improved pertechnetate imaging of Meckel's diverticulum. *Clin Nucl Med* 3:385, 1978.

50. Weber TR et al. Massive gastric hemorrhage: An unusual complication of Henoch-Schonlein purpura. *J Pediatr Surg* 18:576, 1983.

51. Gransden WR et al. Further evidence associating hemolytic uremic syndrome with infection by verotoxin-producing *Escherichia coli* 0157:H7. *J Infect Dis* 154:522, 1986.

52. Brasher C, Seigler RL. The hemolytic-uremic syndrome. *West J Med* 134:193, 1981.

53. Cucchiara S et al. Sigmoidoscopy, colonoscopy, and radiology in the evaluation of children with rectal bleeding. *J Pediatr Gastroenterol Nutr* 2:667, 1983.

54. Holgersen LO, Mossberg SM, Miller RE. Colonoscopy for rectal bleeding in childhood. *J Pediatr Surg* 13:83, 1978.

55. Werlin SL, Grand RJ. Severe colitis in children and adolescents: Diagnosis, course and treatment. *Gastroenterology* 73:828, 1977.

Gary J. Russell
Ronald E. Kleinman

45 Fulminant Hepatic Failure

Fulminant hepatic failure is often defined as the development of encephalopathy and severe coagulopathy within 8 weeks of the onset of hepatic symptoms and is the result of massive hepatocellular injury and necrosis. This may occur in the absence of preexisting hepatic disease or in the setting of chronic liver disease that progresses or is exacerbated by an acute illness. The prognosis is grave in both situations; however, patients without preexisting liver disease may have complete recovery of hepatocyte function. Both viral infections of the liver and hepatotoxic drugs are frequently implicated in liver failure. Worldwide, viral hepatitis B is the most common infectious cause of hepatic failure,[1] and in Western countries, non-A, non-B hepatitis is frequently associated.[2-4] Although hepatitis A viral infection is common, it seldom leads to fulminant hepatic failure, especially among children.[2,5,6] It is doubtful that the hepatitis C virus is a cause of liver failure.[7,8] Among common pharmaceutical agents frequently used, acetaminophen,[9] isoniazid, methyldopa, halothane, sodium valproate,[10] and nicotinic acid have been associated with hepatic failure.[4] Tetracycline can cause a unique form of liver failure with extensive fatty infiltration of the liver, similar to that seen in fatty liver of pregnancy.

Table 45-1. Causes of fulminant hepatic failure

Newborn and infant
  Herpesvirus
  Hepatitis B virus
  Echoviruses
  Adenoviruses
  Epstein-Barr virus
  Tyrosinemia
  Galactosemia
  Fructose intolerance
  Zellweger syndrome
Childhood and adolescents
  Viral infections
  Hepatitis A
  Hepatitis B
  Hepatitis non-A, non-B
Drugs
  Acetaminophen
  Carbamazepine
  Valproic acid
  Isoniazid
  Tetracycline
  Methyldopa
  Halothane
  Chemical toxins
  Carbon tetrachloride
  Phosphorus
  Amanita phalloides
Miscellaneous
  Ischemia/hypotension
  Wilson disease
  Leukemia/lymphoma
  Alpha-1-antitrypsin deficiency

Adapted from GJ Russell, JF Fitzgerald, JH Clark. Fulminant hepatic failure. *J Pediatr* 111:313–319, 1987. With permission.

The age of the patient may be important when considering possible causes of hepatic failure[11] (Table 45-1). Congenitally transmitted infections, including herpesvirus, adenovirus, echovirus, as well as hepatitis B virus, may lead to hepatic failure in the neonate. Congenital fructose intolerance, galactosemia, and tyrosinemia, rare inborn errors of metabolism, should be considered when hepatic failure presents in the perinatal period.

Although patients with fulminant hepatic failure may not initially appear acutely ill, progression of multiorgan dysfunction occurs rapidly, and the associated complications must be anticipated. The potential benefit of an orthotopic liver transplant should be considered early due to the risks of transporting a critically ill patient with cerebral edema to a transplant center and the unpredictable availability of donor organs.

Clinical and Laboratory Findings

Anorexia and icterus are the most common presenting symptoms[12] (Table 45-2). The icterus progresses rapidly and usually precedes the onset of encephalopathy, except when the hepatic necrosis is massive, as in acetaminophen toxicity or *Amanita phalloides* poisoning. Hepatic encephalopathy, if not present initially, usually ensues within 6 to 8 weeks of the onset of symptoms.[13,14] The neuropsychiatric changes observed may be objectively monitored by serial EEGs. Seizures may occur at any stage of encephalopathy.[15]

The laboratory findings indicative of hepatocellular injury include hyperbilirubinemia, increased serum transaminases, hyperammonemia, and hypoglycemia. Impairment of hepatic synthetic function is indicated by vitamin K–resistant prolongation of the prothrombin time. Serum albumin levels are usually normal initially. Hypoalbuminemia presents early in the course of hepatic failure, in association with a low BUN, is suggestive of an underlying chronic hepatopathy.

Coagulopathy

Bleeding is a common complication of hepatic failure and is due in part to impaired hepatic synthesis of fibrinogen and coagulation

Table 45-2. Clinical and laboratory findings

Clinical
  Anorexia
  Progressive icterus
  Ascites
  Encephalopathy
Laboratory
  Elevated serum transaminase levels
  Vitamin K–resistant prolongation of prothrombin time
  Hypoglycemia
  Hypophosphatemia
  Hyponatremia
  Hyperammonemia
  Thrombocytopenia
  Leukocytosis

Adapted from GJ Russell, JF Fitzgerald, JH Clark. Fulminant hepatic failure. *J Pediatr* 111:313–319, 1987. With permission.

factors II, V, VII, IX, and X. Prolongation of the prothrombin time is a sensitive index of hepatocyte dysfunction.[15] Factor VII, with the shortest half-life of the coagulation factors, is the first factor to be depleted and the first to return to normal with improved hepatic function. A low factor V level suggests impaired vitamin K–independent hepatic synthesis and a poor prognosis for survival.[16] In contrast, increased serum levels of fibrin and fibrinogen degradation products, decreased plasminogen activator and plasminogen, and thrombocytopenia without bone marrow suppression are indicative of intravascular coagulation.[17]

Renal Function and Electrolytes

Renal dysfunction, marked by oliguria and an elevated serum creatinine, is a frequent complication of hepatic failure and may be due to prerenal azotemia, acute tubular necrosis, or functional renal failure. Prerenal azotemia can result from dehydration or from increased intestinal absorption of nitrogen when GI hemorrhage occurs. Prerenal azotemia often responds to intravascular volume expansion. Acute tubular necrosis does not respond to a fluid challenge. Additionally, granular and cellular casts are present in the urinary sediment. The etiology of functional renal failure associated with hepatic failure is unknown. Functional renal failure, in contrast to acute tubular necrosis, is characterized by a normal urinary sediment, a urine sodium concentration less than 20 mEq/liter, and a glomerular filtration rate greater than 3 ml/min.[18] Hyponatremia from hemodilution and an impairment of the sodium potassium pump[19] is common, as is hypokalemia from increased renal potassium excretion, which may be exacerbated by diuretic therapy.

Infection

Hepatic failure is complicated by infection in as many as 80% of cases and is frequently a cause of death.[20,21] Nosocomial bacterial infections, such as pneumonia, peritonitis, and meningitis, are most common, but opportunistic fungal infections also occur.[22,23] Patients with hepatic failure have impaired host defenses resulting from serum complement deficiencies and multiple defects in neutrophil function (phagocytosis, opsonization, adherence, and chemotaxis).[20,24–26] It is unclear whether these defects in host defense are the result of hepatic failure and the loss of hepatic synthetic and phagocytic function, or possibly the consequence of preexisting liver disease.

Hypoglycemia

Hypoglycemia often complicates fulminant hepatic failure, especially in children. Hepatic glycogen stores are severely depleted and gluconeogenesis is significantly impaired when hepatic necrosis is massive. Impaired degradation of insulin by the liver leads to elevated serum insulin levels. Increased circulating levels of insulin, glucagon, and growth hormone increase the catabolic drive for gluconeogenesis. When the hypoglycemia persists, pancreatic glucagon synthesis increases, resulting in a decrease in the insulin-glucagon ratio.[27,28] This produces muscle protein catabolism and the release of large amounts of amino acids, which the failing liver is unable to utilize. Impaired hepatic gluconeogenesis results in increased anaerobic metabolism and a subsequent lactic acidosis.

Encephalopathy

Encephalopathy is a prominent clinical feature of hepatic failure and is a manifestation of physiologic rather than morphologic changes in the CNS. The encephalopathy may progress through four stages, which are classified according to neurologic symptoms and signs (Table 45-3). Patients progressing to stage IV hepatic encephalopathy have a mortality rate of 80%.[29] The pathophysiology of the encephalopathy remains elusive.

Ammonia, a putative toxin, is generated in the GI tract by the action of colonic bacteria and mucosal enzymes on enteric proteins. A dramatic increase in the blood ammonia level accompanies GI hemorrhage, which occurs commonly in these patients.[30] Ammonia, alone or in conjunction with other potential toxins such as mercaptans and short-chain fatty acids, causes a disturbance in cerebrocyte energy metabolism, which leads to brain swelling. Blood ammonia levels rise when the liver is unable to incorporate ammonia into urea. Ammonia reduces postsynaptic inhibitory neurotransmission by inhibiting chloride conductance across the cell membranes of postsynaptic neurons.[31] This promotes neural excitation, convulsions, and postictal coma. Ammonia is detoxified by astrocytes that utilize adenosine triphosphate in the conversion of ammonia to glutamine.[30,32] In experimental animals, however, acute ammonia intoxication does not produce the clinical and neuropathologic changes of hepatic encephalopathy. Further, arterial ammonia levels do not correlate with the level of encephalopathy, and in fact, the encephalopathy of fulminant hepatic failure often precedes a demonstrable increase in the blood ammonia level.

Table 45-3. Stages of hepatic encephalopathy

	Stage 1	*Stage 2*	*Stage 3*	*Stage 4*
Clinical symptoms	Normal level of consciousness with periods of euphoria or depression; some lethargy and disorder in sleep pattern	Increased drowsiness, inappropriate behavior, disorientation, agitation, and wide changes in affect	Stuporous, sleeping most of the time; arousable, marked confusion; incoherent speech	Comatose; may not respond to painful stimuli
Signs	Asterixis may be present; patient may have difficulty with line drawings	Asterixis easily elicited	Asterixis; hyperflexia and extensor reflexes elicited; rigidity	Reflexes disappear; asterixis cannot be elicited; flaccid limbs
Electroencephalogram	Normal	Abnormal with generalized slowing	Abnormal	Abnormal

Adapted from GJ Russell, JF Fitzgerald, JH Clark. Fulminant hepatic failure. *J Pediatr* 111:313–319, 1987. With permission.

Patients with hepatic failure demonstrate an alteration in their concentration of plasma amino acids that is characterized by an increase in the aromatic amino acids (phenylalanine, tyrosine, and free tryptophan) and methionine and a decrease in the branched-chain amino acids (leucine, isoleucine, and valine). All of the plasma amino acids, with the exception of the branched-chain amino acids, are increased in hepatic failure.[33–35] Although this disturbance in the plasma amino acid profile has been well documented, a pathogenic relationship between this observation and the development of hepatic encephalopathy has not been established. It is also not clear whether the administration of branched-chain amino acid–enriched solutions alters hepatic encephalopathy.[36,37]

For many years, research efforts focused on the possibility that some of the neurologic manifestations of liver disease could be explained by the accumulation of inhibitory neurotransmitters (e.g., serotonin) or false neurotransmitters (e.g., octopamine).[38] These aromatic amino acids are normally catabolized by monoamine oxidases, primarily in the liver. When hepatic function is impaired, they may be hydroxylated to false or relatively inactive neurotransmitters. For example, excessive tyrosine is converted to tyramine, which competes with dopamine for dopamine beta-hydroxylase. This enzyme converts tyramine to octopamine, a weak neurotransmitter capable of replacing norepinephrine in presynaptic vesicles. Likewise, tryptophan is also increased in hepatic failure and is a precursor of the inhibitory neurotransmitter serotonin. Thus, cerebral dysfunction results when inhibitory neurotransmitters exceed excitatory neurotransmitters in the CNS.

The γ-aminobutyric acid$_A$ (GABA$_A$)-benzodiazepine receptor complex is considered to be the principal inhibitory neurotransmitter system in the brain.[39] It has been speculated that increased activation of this receptor system contributes to the pathogenesis of hepatic encephalopathy. The GABA$_A$ and benzodiazepine receptors are distinct proteins that have a physical as well as a functional association.[40,41] An increase in serum levels of GABA-like activity has been demonstrated in a rabbit model of hepatic encephalopathy.[42] This may be the result of enteric bacterial production, intestinal absorption, and impaired hepatic catabolism of GABA,[42] in addition to an increased transfer of GABA across the blood-brain barrier.[43] In contrast, others have found no changes in GABA levels in the plasma or cerebral spinal fluid of patients with chronic liver disease, with or without accompanying encephalopathy.[44] Even without an increase in GABA levels, however, enhanced neuroinhibitory signals could be effected by agonists of the benzodiazepine receptor, which potentiate the action of GABA.[45] Some evidence has been reported supporting the existence of an endogenous compound that binds to central benzodiazepine receptors present in the cerebrospinal fluid of patients with hepatic encephalopathy.[46] Pharmacologic antagonism of the GABA$_A$-benzodiazepine receptor complex has been shown to improve hepatic encephalopathy in the rabbit model of hepatic failure[47] as well as in humans with stage II–IV hepatic encephalopathy caused by decompensated cirrhosis.[48] Although GABA$_A$-benzodiazepine receptor antagonists may at least temporarily lessen the severity of encephalopathy, there is no effect on the underlying disease process, thus limiting a potential benefit in fulminant hepatic encephalopathy.

Cerebral Edema

Cerebral edema is evident in 80% of patients with fulminant hepatic failure and is a significant cause of death.[49–51] Although experimental animal models suggested a potential effect of steroid therapy in preventing an increase in intracranial pressure, controlled studies in humans with fulminant hepatic failure have demonstrated no benefit.[52,53] IV administration of mannitol, however, does decrease intracranial pressure, reverse clinical signs of cerebral edema, and improve survival.[53] Intracranial pressure monitoring has been recommended once stage III encephalopathy develops in order to optimize medical therapy and guide consideration of liver transplantation.[4,14] The use of epidural pressure transducers appears to have the lowest risk of complications from hemorrhage.[54]

Management

There is no specific therapy for fulminant hepatic failure. These patients require intensive supportive care and diligent anticipation of the associated complications. A central venous catheter and an arterial line allow monitoring of central venous pressure and frequent monitoring of blood chemistries, coagulation, and hematocrit. Initial IV fluids should contain 10% dextrose and be administered at 60 to 80 ml/m^2/hr. Blood glucose levels must be initially monitored every 4 hours to maintain euglycemia. Serum and urinary sodium concentrations are monitored at 8-hour intervals so that sodium retention can be identified early and managed appropriately.[55] Treatment of impaired free-water excretion, which may depress the serum sodium level, is fluid restriction rather than the addition of free sodium, which may promote the development of ascites in the face of renal sodium retention. Unfortunately, hypotension frequently requires administration of colloid volume expanders and blood products with a high sodium content. Potassium must be provided as needed to maintain a serum potassium level greater than 3 mEq/liter. Up to 3 mEq potassium/kg/d can be provided as the phosphate salt if the patient has hypophosphatemia. Provision of calcium and magnesium may be necessary if blood levels indicate deficiencies.

Hypotension, associated with a decrease in central venous pressure, must be treated promptly with fluid volume expanders. Blood products are also necessary when hemorrhage is a contributing factor. Hypotension without evidence of hemorrhage may also occur as a result of inappropriate systemic vasodilatation.[56] Persistent decreased arterial pressure may precipitate renal failure, with or without acute tubular necrosis. Hypotension, especially when associated with increased intracranial pressure, results in decreased oxygen delivery to the brain.[57] Vasopressors are therapeutically indicated to control hypotension.

Vitamin K should be provided parenterally at 1 mg per year of age, up to 10 mg daily for 3 days, and then every other day. Impaired hepatic synthetic capacity is the major cause of the coagulopathy, thus it is unlikely that providing vitamin K will initially have a significant effect on the prothrombin time. Continuing coagulation defects, especially with demonstrated bleeding, must be corrected with fresh-frozen plasma, fresh blood, and platelets. Intravascular coagulation is diagnosed when fibrin split products are identified in the blood in association with a decline in the platelet count. Plasmapheresis has also been suggested for the short-term management of patients with severe coagulopathy and may be particularly helpful in patients with renal failure or oliguria.[58] Exchange plasmapheresis results in rapid improvement in coagulation without increasing the intravascular volume.

A nasogastric tube should be allowed to drain by gravity or by low intermittent suction. Histamine II receptor blockers should be utilized to maintain gastric pH at less than 4 and reduce blood loss from acute gastric erosions common in fulminant hepatic failure. An antacid with a high neutralizing capacity may provide additional gastric mucosal protection. Prophylactic antibiotic therapy has not been shown to be beneficial,[59] but antibiotics should be administered when infection is suspected. Respiratory tract infections are frequent, especially in patients requiring tracheal intubation.

Clinical detection of cerebral edema causing increased intracranial pressure is difficult because papilledema is rarely detected. The neurologic status of the patient must be monitored carefully. Computed tomography may be helpful in early detection of cerebral edema. Sudden changes in consciousness, loss of the oculovestibular reflex, or sluggishness of the pupillary light reflex dictate the immediate administration of mannitol, 0.25 to 0.5 g/kg. Surgical placement of an epidural intracranial pressure monitor, when cerebral edema is suspected or demonstrated, may be necessary to accurately assess intracranial pressure and to provide osmotherapy judiciously.[4,14,54] Maintaining the PCO_2 between 25 and 30 mm Hg while cerebral edema is present is also helpful in reducing the intracranial pressure. The use of corticosteroids has no benefit in the management of cerebral edema associated with fulminant hepatic failure and cannot be recommended.[60]

The administration of poorly absorbed antibiotics and purgatives has long been used in the management of hepatic encephalopathy.[61] The primary intent is to reduce the production and the absorption of potentially toxic enteric substances. Neomycin decreases the urealytic and proteolytic microflora in the colon and consequently the generation of ammonia and other potential toxins. Lactulose is a nondigestible disaccharide that produces an osmotic diarrhea. It can be administered orally, intragastrically, or as an enema (20% solution). The initial oral or intragastric dose of lactulose is 15 to 30 ml every 4 to 6 hours and is titrated to produce two to four loose stools daily. The effectiveness of lactulose is not fully explained by its cathartic action.[62] Metabolism of lactulose by the colonic microflora may retard the production of ammonia[63] or short-chain fatty acids.[64] Another nonabsorbable disaccharide, lactitol, has also been shown to be as beneficial as lactulose in the treatment of hepatic encephalopathy.[65,66]

The use of prostaglandin E for the treatment of fulminant hepatic failure was suggested after an encouraging report of the survival among patients with viral hepatic failure following therapy with prostaglandin E_1.[67] A subsequent controlled trial, however, failed to demonstrate a benefit from prostaglandin E_2 therapy in fulminant hepatic failure.[68] Insufficient data exist at this time to recommend the use of prostaglandin E in fulminant hepatic failure prior to transplantation.

Transplantation

Artificial support for the failing liver may maintain the patient until hepatic regeneration occurs. Various forms of artificial support, including exchange transfusion, cross circulation, charcoal hemoperfusion, and hemofiltration have been evaluated.[69,70] None has been shown to improve the survival rate. An extracorporeal liver assist device has been described that uses cultured hepatoblastoma cells within the filter device.[71] While not yet able to improve the chance of survival, these forms of artificial liver support may be a useful treatment modality to stabilize the patient with hepatic failure before orthotopic liver transplantation.

Orthotopic liver transplantation is being performed more frequently with improved success in patients with fulminant hepatic failure who have not responded to intensive medical therapy. The prognosis of patients with fulminant hepatic failure undergoing liver transplantation remains poor. Although survival rates of greater than 50% have been reported,[16,72,73] many patients die while waiting for transplantation, reducing the overall survival of these patients.[72] Fulminant hepatic failure resulting from viral hepatitis is not a contraindication for liver transplantation. Survival of these patients is also greater than 50%.[72,73] Although evidence of recurrent infection in the donor liver is common, fulminant hepatopathy is rare.[74]

Prognosis

No predictive criteria currently exist to aid in the initial assessment of patients with fulminant hepatic failure. The prognosis remains poor whether patients are treated medically or surgically. The survival of children is no better than that of adults with fulminant hepatic failure. Collapse of the hepatic ultrastructure is manifested by a rapidly shrinking liver, rapid elevation of the serum bilirubin value, and progressive decline of serum transaminase levels. These findings strongly suggest a fatal outcome in the absence of an orthotopic liver transplant. Measurement of serum fetoprotein levels to monitor hepatocyte regeneration is not helpful and does not correlate with outcome.[74] Quantitative liver function tests, such as galactose elimination capacity and colic acid conjugation, have been assessed in patients with hepatic failure,[75,76] but survival criteria have not been determined. A rapid deterioration of the neurologic status in addition to a factor V level less than 20% has been reported to indicate imminent death and the need for immediate liver transplantation.[16,77] Serial factor VII levels may best indicate a return of hepatic synthetic function. Rapid elevation of this factor virtually always accompanies survival.[78]

Summary

Fulminant hepatic failure remains one of the most difficult conditions managed by intensive care personnel. Unfortunately, the mortality rate remains very high despite advances in supportive care. The most serious complications are persistent coagulopathy, hemorrhage, encephalopathy, and cerebral edema. Plasmapheresis can correct the coagulation defects and possibly improve the encephalopathy. Thus, plasmapheresis may stabilize the patient until hepatic regeneration occurs or orthotopic liver transplantation can be accomplished. Liver transplantation has emerged as an important therapeutic intervention for patients who have not responded to medical support. Reliable prognostic indicators are still needed to determine when liver transplantation offers the best chance of survival for patients with hepatic failure.

References

1. Mathieson LR et al. Hepatitis type A, B, and non-A non-B in fulminant hepatitis. *Gut* 21:72–77, 1980.
2. Bernuau J, Rueff B, Benhamou J-P. Fulminant and subfulminant liver failure: Definitions and causes. *Semin Liver Dis* 6:97–106, 1986.
3. Rakela J et al. Fulminant hepatitis: Mayo Clinic experience with 34 cases. *Mayo Clin Proc* 60:289–292, 1985.
4. Riegler JL, Lake JR. Fulminant hepatic failure. *Med Clin North Am* 77(5):1057–1083, 1993.
5. Hepatitis surveillance report no. 53: Atlanta: Centers for Disease Control, 1990.
6. Romero R, Lavine JE. Viral hepatitis in children. *Semin Liver Dis* 14:289–302, 1994.

7. Williams R, Gimson AES. Intensive liver care and management of acute hepatic failure. *Dig Dis Sci* 36:820–826, 1991.

8. Liang TJ et al. Fulminant or subfulminant non-A, non-B viral hepatitis: The role of hepatitis C and E viruses. *Gastroenterology* 104:556–562, 1993.

9. Black M. Acetaminophen toxicity. *Gastroenterology* 78:382–392, 1980.

10. Suchy FJ et al. Acute hepatic failure associated with use of sodium valproate. *N Engl J Med* 300:962–966, 1979.

11. Russell GJ, Fitzgerald JF, Clark JH. Fulminant hepatic failure. *J Pediatr* 111:313–319, 1987.

12. Psacharopoulos HT et al. Fulminant hepatic failure in childhood. *Arch Dis Child* 55:252–258, 1980.

13. Pappas SC. Fulminant hepatic failure. *Mayo Clin Proc* 63:198–200, 1988.

14. Lee WM. Acute liver failure. *Am J Med* 96 (Suppl 1A):3S–9S, 1994.

15. Jones EA, Schafer DF. Fulminant hepatic failure. In Zakim D, Boyer TD (eds): *Hepatology*. Philadelphia: Saunders, 1990.

16. Bismuth H et al. Emergency liver transplantation for fulminant hepatitis. *Ann Intern Med* 107:337–341, 1987.

17. Hillenbrand P et al. Significance of intravascular coagulation and fibrinolysis in acute hepatic failure. *Gut* 15:83–88, 1974.

18. Wilkinson SP et al. Abnormalities of sodium excretion and other disorders of renal function in fulminant hepatic failure. *Gut* 17:501–505, 1976.

19. Alam AN et al. A study *in vitro* of the sodium pump in fulminant hepatic failure. *Clin Sci Mol Med* 55:355–363, 1978.

20. Bailey RJ et al. Metabolic inhibition of polymorphonuclear leukocytes in fulminant hepatic failure. *Lancet* 1:1162–1163, 1976.

21. Rolando N et al. Prospective study of bacterial infection in acute liver failure: An analysis of fifty patients. *Hepatology* 11:49–53, 1990.

22. Triger DR et al. Systemic candidiasis complicating acute hepatic failure in patients treated with cimetidine. *Lancet* 2:837–838, 1981.

23. Walsh TJ, Hamilton SR. Disseminated aspergillosis complicating hepatic failure. *Arch Intern Med* 143:1189–1191, 1983.

24. Wyke RJ et al. Defective opsinisation and complement deficiency in serum from patients with fulminant hepatic failure. *Gut* 21:643–649, 1980.

25. Larcher VF et al. Bacterial and fungal infection in children with fulminant hepatic failure: Possible role of opsinisation and complement deficiency. *Gut* 23:1037–1043, 1982.

26. Altin M et al. Neutrophil adherence in chronic liver disease and fulminant hepatic failure. *Gut* 24:746–750, 1983.

27. Fisher JE et al. The effect of normalization of plasma amino acids on hepatic encephalopathy in man. *Surgery* 80:77–91, 1976.

28. Rossi-Fanelli F et al. Effect of glucose and/or branched chain amino acid infusion on plasma amino acid imbalance in chronic liver failure. *J Parenter Nutr* 5:414–419, 1981.

29. Saunders SJ et al. Acute liver failure. In Wright R et al (eds): *Liver and Biliary Disease*. Philadelphia: Saunders, 1977.

30. Schenker S, Hoyumpa AM Jr. Pathophysiology of hepatic encephalopathy. *Hosp Pract* 19:99–121, 1984.

31. Kvamme E. Ammonia metabolism in the CNS. *Prog Neurobiol* 20:109–132, 1983.

32. Fraser CL, Arieff AI. Hepatic encephalopathy. *N Engl J Med* 313:865–873, 1985.

33. Zieve L. Amino acids in liver failure. *Gastroenterology* 76:219–221, 1979.

34. Fischer JE. Amino acids in hepatic coma. *Dig Dis Sci* 27:97–102, 1982.

35. Cascino A et al. Plasma and cerebrospinal fluid amino acid patterns in hepatic encephalopathy. *Dig Dis Sci* 27:828–832, 1982.

36. Wahren J et al. Is intravenous administration of branched-chain amino acids effective in the treatments of hepatic encephalopathy? A multicenter study. *Hepatology* 3:475–480, 1983.

37. Cerra FB et al. Disease-specific amino acid infusion (FO80) in hepatic encephalopathy: A prospective, randomized, double-blind, controlled trial. *J Parenter Nutr* 9:288–295, 1985.

38. Fischer JE, Baldessarini RJ. False neurotransmitters and hepatic failure. *Lancet* 2:75–80, 1971.

39. Jones EA et al. The neurobiology of hepatic encephalopathy. *Hepatology* 4:1235–1242, 1984.

40. Deng L, Ransom RW, Olsen R: [³H] muscinol photolabels the γ-aminobutyric acid receptor binding site peptide subunit distinct from that labeled with benzodiazepines. *Biochem Biophys Res Commun* 128:1308–1314, 1986.

41. Skolnick P. The γ-aminobutyric acid A (GABA$_A$)-benzodiazepine receptor complex. *Ann Intern Med* 110:534–536, 1989.

42. Ferenci P et al. Metabolism of the inhibitory neurotransmitter γ-aminobutyric acid in a rabbit model of fulminant hepatic failure. *Hepatology* 3:507–512, 1983.

43. Bassett ML et al. Increased brain uptake of γ-aminobutyric acid in a rabbit model of hepatic encephalopathy. *Gastroenterology* 98:747–757, 1990.

44. Moroni R et al. Hepatic encephalopathy: Lack of changes of γ-aminobutyric acid content in plasma and cerebrospinal fluid. *Hepatology* 7:816–820, 1987.

45. Paul SM, Marangos PJ, Skolnick P. The benzadiazepine-GABA-chloride ionophore receptor complex: Common site of minor tranquilizer action. *Biol Psychiatry* 16:213–229, 1981.

46. Mullen KD. Evidence for an endogenous benzodiazepine ligand in cerebrospinal fluid. *Ann Intern Med* 110:541–542, 1989.

47. Bassett ML et al. Amelioration of hepatic encephalopathy by pharmacologic antagonism of the GABA$_A$-benzodiazepine receptor complex in a rabbit model of fulminant hepatic failure. *Gastroenterology* 93:1069–1077, 1987.

48. Bansky G et al. Effects of the benzodiazepine receptor antagonist flumazenil in hepatic encephalopathy in humans. *Gastroenterology* 97:744–750, 1989.

49. Ware AJ, D'Agostino A, Combes B. Cerebral edema: A major complication of massive hepatic necrosis. *Gastroenterology* 61:877–884, 1971.

50. Canalese J et al. Controlled trial of dexamethasone and mannitol for the cerebral edema of fulminant hepatic failure. *Gut* 23:625–629, 1982.

51. Ede RJ et al. Controlled hyperventilation in the prevention of cerebral oedema in fulminant hepatic failure. *J Hepatol* 2:43–51, 1986.

52. Hanid MA et al. Intracranial pressure in pigs with surgically induced acute liver failure. *Gastroenterology* 76:123–131, 1979.

53. Canalese J et al. Controlled trial of dexamethasone and mannitol for the cerebral oedema of fulminant hepatic failure. *Gut* 23:625–629, 1982.

54. Blei AT et al. Complications of intracranial pressure monitoring in fulminant hepatic failure. *Lancet* 341:157–158, 1993.

55. Wyllie R, Arasu TS, Fitzgerald JF. Ascites: Pathophysiology and management. *J Pediatr* 97:167–176, 1980.

56. Trewby PN et al. The role of the false neurotransmitter octopamine in the hypotension of fulminant hepatic failure. *Clin Sci Mol Med* 52:305–310, 1977.

57. Trewby PN et al. Effects of cerebral edema and arterial hypotension on cerebral blood flow in an animal model of hepatic failure. *Gut* 19:999–1005, 1978.

58. Munoz SJ et al. Treatment of coagulopathy of severe liver disease with plasmapheresis. *Gastroenterology* 94:A574, 1988.

59. Rolando N et al. Prospective controlled trial of selective parenteral and enteral antimicrobial regimen in fulminant liver failure. *Hepatology* 17:196–201, 1993.

60. Rakela J et al. A double-blind, randomized trial of hydrocortisone in acute hepatic failure. *Dig Dis Sci* 36:1223–1228, 1991.

61. Weber FL Jr. Therapy of portal-systemic encephalopathy: The practical and the promising. *Gastroenterology* 81:174–181, 1981.

62. Crossley IR, Williams R. Progress in the treatment of chronic portasystemic encephalopathy. *Gut* 25:85–98, 1984.

63. Vince AJ, Burridge SM. Ammonia production by intestinal bacteria: The effects of lactose, lactulose and glucose. *J Med Microbiol* 13:177–191, 1980.

64. Mortensen PB, Rasmussen HS, Holtug K. Lactulose detoxifies *in vitro*

short chain fatty acid production in colonic contents induced by blood: Implications for hepatic coma. *Gastroenterology* 94:750–754, 1988.

65. Morgan MY, Hawley KE. Lactitol vs lactulose in the treatment of acute hepatic encephalopathy in cirrhotic patients: A double-blind, randomized trial. *Hepatology* 7:1278–1284, 1987.

66. Uribe M et al. Lactitol, a second generation disaccharide for treatment of chronic portal-systemic encephalopathy. A double-blind, crossover, randomized clinical trial. *Dig Dis Sci* 32:1345–1353, 1987.

67. Sinclair SB, Levy GA. Treatment of fulminant viral hepatic failure with prostaglandin E. A preliminary report. *Dig Dis Sci* 36:791–800, 1991.

68. Sheiner P et al. A randomized control trial of prostaglandin E₂ (PGE₂) in the treatment of fulminant hepatic failure (FHF). *Hepatology* 16:88A, 1992.

69. O'Grady JG et al. Controlled trials of charcoal hemoperfusion and prognostic factors in fulminant hepatic failure. *Gastroenterology* 94:1186–1192, 1988.

70. Matsubara S et al. Continuous removal of middle molecules by hemofiltration in patients with acute liver failure. *Crit Care Med* 18:1331–1338, 1990.

71. Development of reliable artificial liver support (ALS)–plasma exchange in combination with hemodiafiltration using high-performance membranes. *Dig Dis Sci* 38:469–476, 1993.

72. Peleman RR et al. Orthotopic liver transplantation for acute and subacute hepatic failure in adults. *Hepatology* 7:484–489, 1987.

73. Emond JC et al. Liver transplantation in the management of fulminant hepatic failure. *Gastroenterology* 96:1583–1588, 1989.

74. VanTheil DH. Liver transplantation. *Pediatr Ann* 14:474–480, 1985.

75. Ranek L, Andreasen PB, Tygstrup N. Galactose elimination capacity as a prognostic index in patients with fulminant liver failure. *Gut* 17:959–964, 1976.

76. Bremmelgaard A et al. Colic acid conjugation test and quantitative liver function in acute liver failure. *Scand J Gastroenterol* 18:797–802, 1983.

77. Bernuau J et al. Multivariate analysis of prognostic factors in fulminant hepatitis B. *Hepatology* 6:648–651, 1986.

78. Gazzard BG, Henderson JM, Williams R. Factor VII levels as a guide to prognosis in fulminant hepatic failure. *Gut* 17:489–491, 1976.

Ronald E. Kleinman

46 Postoperative Management of Pediatric Recipients of Hepatic Allografts

Between 1963 and 1979, survival for as long as 1 year could be expected for only 4 of 10 patients undergoing liver transplantation. Since that time, long-term actuarial survival rates of 65% to 80% have been reported.[1] Although there are several liver diseases that affect both children and adults, most liver transplants during infancy and childhood involve disorders unique to the pediatric age group, such as extrahepatic biliary atresia,[2] inborn errors of metabolism, and intrahepatic biliary hypoplasia. In addition to performing the operation, a successful liver transplant program must incorporate careful procedures for evaluation of transplant candidates, ongoing assessment, support of patients prior to transplantation, and provide the extremely complex and intensive postoperative support, including immunosuppression and its attendant complications. This chapter focuses on the postoperative management of pediatric recipients of hepatic allografts. Although such patients may require the intensive care unit (ICU) setting preoperatively, the management of hepatic failure per se is discussed in Fulminant Hepatic Failure by Russell and Kleinman, this volume.

Monitoring

Following engraftment, the intubated patient is taken to the ICU with arterial and central venous catheters in place (Fig. 46-1). Hemodynamic stability is monitored by pulmonary artery and central venous pressure and cardiac output determinations to ensure optimal perfusion of the liver and kidneys. On rare occasions, vasopressors are required; more often, fluid replacement using a combination of colloid, crystalloid, fresh-frozen plasma, and packed red cells suffices to maintain adequate perfusion. Because patients are usually in positive fluid balance, fluid administration and fluid output from nasogastric suction, abdominal drains, and urine must be carefully balanced. Fluids from the biliary stent and drains are quantitated and examined for the presence of blood

and bile and cultured daily to twice weekly for microorganisms, including fungi. Large amounts of bile in any of the three abdominal Jackson-Pratt drains implies damage to the bile duct, which must be promptly investigated by radionuclide or other imaging techniques or surgical exploration. Urine output is often diminished postoperatively, due in part to cyclosporine toxicity but possibly also to preoperative and intraoperative renal dysfunction and the use of nephrotoxic antibiotics. The patient is ventilated to maintain optimal blood oxygenation and monitored by arterial sampling. Sputum is cultured daily.

A parenteral broad-spectrum antibiotic is given (e.g., cefazolin) for 5 days, and then antibiotics are given only for specific indications. Once the patient is extubated and oral intake resumes, nystatin is administered along with trimethoprim/sulfamethoxazole as a prophylaxis for *Candida* and *Pneumocystis carinii*. Blood is sampled every 6 hours for blood gases, electrolytes, CBC, platelets, prothrombin and partial thromboplastin times, glucose, and ionized calcium. Hyperkalemia and alkalosis are common findings that result from large-volume packed-cell transfusions during the procedure. BUN, creatinine, alanine and aspartate amino transferase, alkaline phosphatase, bilirubin, calcium, phosphorous, and albumin are monitored daily.

Complications and Their Management

Hypertension

The most common medical complication in our patients following liver transplantation has been hypertension. This has occurred in 90% of our recipients within the first 2 months following the operation. The pathogenesis of posttransplant hypertension is probably multifactorial. It has been observed in patients not treated with cyclosporine and in patients undergoing cardiac or renal transplantation. Occasionally, hypertension is severe enough to

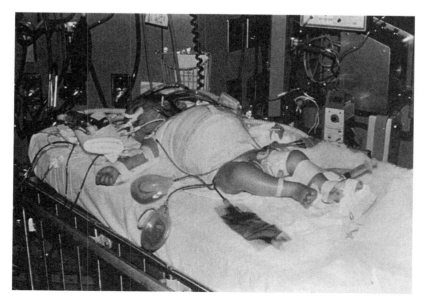

Figure 46-1. Thirteen-month-old infant 6 hours following completion of hepatic allograft.

precipitate hypertensive encephalopathy. Multiple antihypertensive medications may be necessary, including diuretic therapy, angiotensin-converting enzyme inhibitors (e.g., captopril), or vasodilators (e.g., hydralazine). The prevalence of hypertension often declines with increasing time from the operative procedure, and often at 2 years following transplantation antihypertensive medications are no longer needed.

Infections

Infections are the second most common complication that we have seen in our series of patients. The risk of developing infection following transplantation is related to the presence of infection and the repeated use of antibiotics before transplantation, to contamination of the donor liver, to the immunization status of the graft recipient, and finally, and perhaps most important, to the immunocompetence of the graft recipient. In some cases, the underlying liver disease may have been caused by an infectious agent, such as hepatitis B, cytomegalovirus (CMV), Epstein-Barr (EB) virus, or HIV. Some of these same viral infections may be present in the recipient as subclinical infections identified only by serologic evidence of humoral immunity to one or another of the viral antigens. Immunosuppression may lead to reactivation of the infection following transplant with devastating effects, both on the graft and on other organ systems of the recipient. Primary infections with these viral agents occur when the recipient acquires the infection as a result of the transplantation procedure itself, often as a result of transplantation of an organ or transfusion of blood that contains a virus such as CMV.

Chronic liver disease is often complicated by recurrent gram-negative infections. This is particularly true for chronic biliary tract disease. Patients with biliary atresia, who have undergone a portoenterostomy, often have episodes of recurrent cholangitis. The use of multiple antibiotics for prolonged periods directly correlates with the emergence of resistant organisms, which may be exceptionally difficult to treat following transplantation when the patient is immunosuppressed. In particular, it is these patients who often develop life-threatening septicemia due to resistant gram-negative bacteria or opportunistic organisms, such as fungi.

The donor liver should be cultured during the transplant procedure for bacterial contamination and for subclinical viral infections. As mentioned, perioperative cultures of bile, tracheal aspirate, intraperitoneal drainage, the nasal mucosa, and stool are part of routine surveillance for potentially life-threatening infections. The signs of infection following transplantation may be very difficult to discern and even more difficult to differentiate from other complications, such as rejection. Fever, increasing white blood count, and worsening liver functions may be signs of infection or of other complications noted, such as rejection. The sources of infection following transplantation may be in virtually any organ system. Liver transplant recipients appear to be especially predisposed to oral, pharyngeal, and systemic candidiasis.[3] Dehiscence of the biliary anastomosis or operative trauma to the intestine has been identified in many of the patients developing disseminated candidal infections. Patients with biliary tract obstruction or obstruction of the hepatic artery or portal vein may also develop bacteremia, seeding from ischemic abscesses within the liver. This complication is almost universal in those patients with vascular obstruction to the liver and must be recognized promptly. Although retransplantation may be necessary, percutaneous drainage of the abscess with ultrasound guidance has been performed (Fig. 46-2), allowing the successful treatment of these lesions with systemic antibiotics.[4]

After initial perioperative coverage with broad-spectrum antibiotics, antibiotic coverage is directed at specific infectious complications that develop. Once oral intake is not restricted and GI function resumes, oral nystatin may reduce the incidence of oral pharyngeal candidiasis. Although protective isolation may be possible in some transplant centers, it is not known if isolation alone without filtered laminar flow systems and rigorous disinfection of foods, skin, and mucosa reduce the incidence of infection in the immunocompromised host.[5]

CMV and EB virus infections may be treated by reducing immunosuppression and with the use of specific viral chemotherapeutic agents, such as acyclovir, or the investigational agent DHPG. The use of high-titer anti-CMV immune globulin is under investigation in the pretransplant period to reduce reactivation of CMV infection following transplantation. Hyperimmune globulin has been given during or immediately after surgery to hepatitis B surface antigen–positive patients undergoing transplantation, but viral markers inevitably return.

Vascular Complications

Vascular occlusion by thrombi is a major complication, particularly in patients who weigh less than 12 kg. With deteriorating liver functions in the first week following transplantation, compromise of blood flow to the liver should be suspected. This can be evaluated with Doppler ultrasound, CT scan, or angiography. The absence of flow through both the portal vein and hepatic arteries indicates the urgent need for retransplantation. With the presence of blood flow through one or the other vessel, the patient may be treated expectantly, observed for ischemic abscesses and bile duct integrity, and retransplanted only if liver functions progressively deteriorate. Anticoagulants are not routinely used in the absence of vascular obstruction. If obstruction does occur, an antiplatelet agent (e.g., salicylic acid) may be of benefit.

Pulmonary Complications

Pulmonary complications following liver transplant are common.[6] Infection, hemodynamic instability, surgical technique, and chemotherapeutic agents used in immunosuppression may all result in respiratory compromise. Dysmotility of the right hemidiaphragm due to injury of the diaphragm itself or due to denervation of the

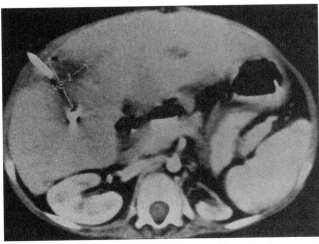

Figure 46-2. Transcutaneous drainage of hepatic abscess following portal venous occlusion in a hepatic allograft recipient.

diaphragm may result in pulmonary insufficiency and atelectasis. We have successfully treated one patient with prolonged diaphragmatic dysfunction with the negative pressure respirator. Pulmonary infections, particularly with opportunistic organisms, contribute to morbidity following surgery. Both azathioprine and cyclosporine may produce interstitial pneumonitis and noncardiogenic pulmonary edema.

Gastrointestinal Complications

GI bleeding is another major complication affecting patients following transplantation.[7] Ulcers, gastritis, bleeding from the enterostomy site, and bleeding from varices in patients who develop portal vein thrombosis are the most frequent GI complications. H2 blockers are routinely administered prophylactically. Perforation or fistula formation, usually at the site of a biliary anastomotic leak, is a less frequent but serious GI complication. Because of immunosuppression, the presentation of these complications may be subtle. Pancreatitis may arise as a result of pancreatotoxic immunosuppressive agents or severe malnutrition. In the early period after liver transplantation, patients are in a state of hypercatabolism with increased tissue breakdown.[8] Careful attention to nutritional requirements is extremely important for healing and rehabilitation following the operation. Patients are initially supported with parenteral nutrition and then with enteral nutrition as intestinal function returns following the surgery.

Neurologic Complications

Seizures are the most common neurologic complication following transplantation. In a series of adult patients, 25% developed seizures, half of them within the first week after surgery.[9] Cyclosporine has been implicated in the development of seizures, particularly in conjunction with hypomagnesemia and hypocholesterolemia. In addition CNS infection, embolus, and vascular accidents must be considered, particularly in the immediate posttransplant period. Cerebral abscess is an almost inevitably fatal disorder.

Primary Graft Nonfunction

Primary graft nonfunction is a generic term indicating that a transplanted liver, once reperfused, is unable to function satisfactorily. If retransplantation is not performed urgently, death results. Damage can occur from instability in the donor, inadequate preservation, or reperfusion injury. The role of vascular thrombosis in primary graft nonfunction is controversial. However, damage to the microcirculation or hepatic swelling from rejection or fluid overload may cause high vascular resistance and lead to retrograde occlusion of arterial inflow in some cases of arterial thrombosis. Whatever the initiating event, the use of current donor organ preservation solutions has dramatically decreased the incidence of primary graft nonfunction.

Rejection

In spite of the introduction of cyclosporine and more recently FK 506, which dramatically diminish the incidence of both early and late rejection, rejection remains a major obstacle in liver transplantation. The clinical manifestations of rejection are nonspecific and variable in both severity and timing. Although hyperacute rejection in the first 24 hours after liver transplantation has been described, it appears to be a rare phenomenon. Furthermore,

graft acceptance and patient survival in the short term between an ABO incompatible donor and a recipient do not appear to differ from matched donors and recipients. Alloantibodies are commonly found in the serum of recipients of ABO mismatched organs. These antibodies may be produced by B lymphocytes, transplanted with the graft, or by the recipient's B cells. The significance of these antibodies remains to be determined. The hemolysis and anemia that may be seen in some of these patients is generally self-limited but occasionally may be prolonged. This phenomena is usually controlled by the immunosuppressive agents used to control rejection. The incidence of late rejection and graft loss is higher among ABO mismatched liver transplant recipients.[10,11]

Fever, enlargement of the liver, and elevation of serum transaminases, bilirubin, and alkaline phosphatase with deterioration of hepatic synthetic function may all herald rejection. Edema of the liver and poor uptake of radioisotope are observed when CT scans and radionuclide studies performed during these episodes. As mentioned, it is important to determine that ischemia from vascular obstruction, infection, and/or drug toxicity are not responsible for the deterioration in liver function.

Liver biopsy may be useful for histologic examination and for culture. The characteristic histologic features of rejection include portal and lobular infiltration by lymphocytes, degeneration of biliary epithelium with progression to paucity of bile ducts, and endothelialitis of both venules and arterioles. Polymorphonuclear leukocytes may be seen within the bile duct epithelia along with epithelial ballooning degeneration and cholestasis. With severe rejection or chronic rejection, obliterative endarteritis; hepatocellular necrosis with fibrosis or cirrhosis and infiltration of portal triads with polymorphonuclear leukocytes, eosinophils, and lymphocytes is seen. Absence of bile ducts is also a common feature.[12]

Immunosuppression

Both helper and cytotoxic T-lymphocytes, recognizing class I and class II alloantigens, play an important role in graft rejection.[13] Although the rapidity of rejection and the relevance of preexisting immunity to donor histocompatibility antigens may be different for liver grafts than for the transplantation of the kidney or heart, a combination of immunosuppressive agents has been standard therapy for all liver graft recipients.

Modern immunosuppressive therapy for liver grafts usually involves the use of several different agents, each of which interrupts the elaboration of the rejection reaction at a different point. Since the introduction of cyclosporine for liver transplants was reported in 1979, it, in combination with other agents, including corticosteroids, azathioprine, and now monoclonal antilymphocyte globulin, has been the mainstay of immunosuppressive therapy.

Glucocorticoids

The mechanism of glucocorticoid-induced immunosuppression is controversial. Although ineffective in preventing liver rejection when used alone, corticosteroids may act synergistically with the other previously mentioned agents to diminish rejection. Proliferating antigen-activated lymphocytes are decreased in number after exposure to corticosteroids, which are known to activate suppressor cells. Both of these actions may be important in ameliorating the active immune response to the heterologous liver graft. In addition to lymphopenia, corticosteroid administration in humans produces redistribution of circulating peripheral lymphocytes preferentially removing the helper-inducer (CD-4) lymphocyte subset from the circulating intravascular lymphocyte pool. Other effects of corticosteroids, especially on the production of interleukins, may explain the synergy between corticosteroids and other agents, such as cyclosporine.

The adverse effects of prolonged, high-dose corticosteroid use in children are well known and will not be reviewed here. Because of the synergism between corticosteroids and cyclosporine, the dose of corticosteroid can be decreased in a relatively short period and the drug administered at low dose in an alternate-day regimen to markedly reduce the toxicity. During the first posttransplant week, doses of 60 to 200 mg of intravenous (IV) methylprednisolone or its equivalent are administered in four divided doses per day, and then tapered over 4 days to 10 to 80 mg/d. Oral prednisone is administered once the intestinal tract is functional at 10 to 40 mg/d. Episodes of rejection are treated with IV boluses of high-dose corticosteroid.

Antilymphocyte Globulin

Polyclonal antilymphocyte globulin (ALG), produced in animals, has been used with conflicting results as an adjunct immunosuppressive agent in hepatic, renal, and cardiac transplants in humans. An important development is the use of monoclonal anticytotoxic/inducer T cell antibodies, produced by murine plasmacytomas. These antibodies selectively destroy host cells active in rejection and theoretically eliminate the adverse effects of irrelevant antibodies found in polyclonal ALG. The pan-T monoclonal antibody, OKT-3, has proved to be the most effective of these monoclonal antibodies investigated to date. In a multicenter controlled trial, OKT-3 reversed rejection episodes more effectively than did corticosteroids.[14] Current trials are in progress to evaluate the use of monoclonal antibodies as initial immunosuppressive therapy in place of cyclosporine. The repeated use of these antibodies is limited by the development of host antibodies against the OKT-3 antibody. A number of other monoclonal antibodies that react only with activated lymphoblasts are currently being evaluated. Antibodies aimed at specific T cell subsets that can be used in sequence or combination and that will avoid the development of antimonoclonal antibodies by the host are goals for the future.[15]

Azathioprine

Until the late 1970s, the combination of azathioprine and prednisone was the principal regimen used to suppress rejection following liver transplantation. The high failure rate in the first year after transplantation of livers and cadaveric kidneys dampened enthusiasm for liver transplantation. Since the advent of cyclosporine, azathioprine has become an adjunct immunosuppressant in most centers and is used as initial therapy when cyclosporine-toxicity precludes the further use of cyclosporine. Azathioprine is similar to its parent compound 6-mercaptopurine, which affects purine nucleotide synthesis and metabolism. Oral doses of the drug vary from 1 to 4 mg/kg/d. Doses must be lowered when the drug is used together with allopurinol. The most common toxic effect of azathioprine is myelosuppression, and it has also caused severe hepatitis and cholestasis.

Cyclosporine/FK 506

Cyclosporine is metabolized in the liver via the cytochrome P450 microsomal enzyme system. It is not clear whether these metabolites are able to enhance immunosuppression or produce toxic complications. A variety of techniques are available to measure cyclosporine in biologic fluids. Fifty percent to 60% of cyclosporine in the systemic circulation is bound to erythrocytes. Another 1% to 9% is bound to lymphocytes, and the remainder is found in the plasma fraction, virtually all of which is bound to plasma proteins. Trough levels of cyclosporine are usually measured for therapeutic decisions, with measurements on whole blood samples running 4 to 6 times the levels detected in serum. The therapeutic range for trough cyclosporine A levels by radioimmunoassay is from 50 to 250 ng/ml for serum.[16] Cyclosporine acts by complexing with a cellular receptor called an immunophilin. This complex then interferes with activation of a protein active in the transcription of the interleukin-2 and other cytokine genes.[17]

Cyclosporine is eliminated principally by excretion through bile. Less than 10% of cyclosporine is excreted through the kidney.[18] The absorption of cyclosporine through the GI tract is quite variable, as reflected by systemic drug levels measured after oral administration. Graft recipients receive cyclosporine by the IV route intraoperatively and in the immediate postoperative period, then by a combination of oral and IV administration, and finally by oral administration. Our experience, and that of others, has been that oral requirements for cyclosporine are significantly higher in pediatric patients than in adult patients.[19] IV doses are usually 4 to 6 mg/kg/d, administered continuously or as two to three bolus infusions, and oral doses vary from 15 mg/kg/d to as high as 45 mg/kg/d for some of our pediatric patients. Dosing must be individualized to minimize side effects such as nephrotoxicity and hypertension.[20]

Once bile flow is completely internalized, drug absorption frequently improves. A number of other drugs are known to affect cyclosporine concentrations in the systemic circulation. Decreased serum concentrations are seen with the concurrent use of phenytoin, phenobarbital, rifampicin, isoniazid, and trimethoprim. In contrast, ketoconazole, erythromycin, and methylprednisolone increase serum concentrations of cyclosporine. Finally, the nephrotoxicity of cyclosporine may be potentiated by other known nephrotoxic medications, such as aminoglycosides. A list of the most common side effects of cyclosporine are found in Table 46-1. Cyclosporine may produce hepatotoxicity with histopathology similar to rejection. In patients receiving cyclosporine, hepatotoxicity and most of the acute metabolic derangements often rapidly reverse when the cyclosporine dose is lowered.[21] Discontinuing or lowering the dose of cyclosporine after significant nephrotoxicity has occurred does little to reverse the renal damage, however, and carries a significant risk of graft rejection.

FK 506 produces immunosuppression in a manner similar to that produced by cyclosporine. Initially, it was principally used as "rescue" therapy for patients experiencing rejection unresponsive

Table 46-1. Adverse effects of cyclosporine

Nephrotoxicity

Hepatotoxicity

Hirsutism

Tremors/seizures

Gingival hyperplasia

Hypertension

Hemolytic anemia

Thrombocytopenia

Lymphoma

to cyclosporine, prednisone, and monoclonal antibody therapy.[22] Some centers currently use FK 506 as primary immunosuppressive therapy without adjuvant steroid therapy. Encephalopathy and nephrotoxicity are among the more serious complications of this drug.[23]

Summary

Intensive care management of liver transplant recipients may be complicated by preexisting disease in vital organs, by the consequences of complex surgery involving massive fluid shifts and multiple vascular anastomoses, and by immunosuppression. With the combined experience at this time, from several thousand liver transplants worldwide, the attendant postoperative complications may be managed expertly. This has in turn contributed importantly to decreased morbidity and mortality following liver transplantation in pediatric patients.

References

1. Starzl TE, Demetris AJ, VanThiel D. Liver transplantation. *N Engl J Med* 321:1014, 1989.
2. Beath S, Pearmain G, Kelly D. Liver transplantation in babies and children with extrahepatic biliary atresia. *J Pediatr Surg* 28:1044, 1993.
3. George DL et al. Patterns of infection after pediatric liver transplantation. *Am J Dis Child* 146:924, 1992.
4. Hoffer SA et al. Infected bilomas and hepatic artery thrombosis in infant recipients of liver transplants. Interventional radiology and medical therapy as an alternative to retransplantation. *Radiology* 169:435, 1988.
5. Nauseef WM, Maki DG. A study of the value of simple protective isolation in patients with granulocytopenia. *N Engl J Med* 304:448, 1981.
6. Kroka MJ, Cortese DA. Pulmonary aspects of chronic liver disease and liver transplantation. *Mayo Clin Proc* 60:407, 1985.
7. Koep LJ, Starzl TE, Weil R. Gastrointestinal complications of hepatic transplantation. *Transplant Proc* XI:257, 1979.
8. Shanbhogue RLK et al. Increased protein catabolism without hypermetabolism after human orthotopic liver transplantation. *Surgery* 101:146, 1987.
9. Stein DP et al. Neurological complications following liver transplantation. *Ann Neurol* 31:644, 1992.
10. Gugenheim J et al. Liver transplantation across ABO blood group barriers. *Lancet* 336:519, 1990.
11. Renard TH et al. ABO incompatible liver transplantation in children: A prospective approach. *Transplant Proc* 25:1953, 1993.
12. Snovar DC et al. Liver allograph rejection. *Am J Surg Pathol* 1:1, 1987.
13. Bach FH, Sachs DH. Current concepts: Immunology. Transplantation immunology. *N Engl J Med* 317:489, 1987.
14. Ortho Multicenter Transplant Study Group. A randomized clinical trial of OKT-3 monoclonal antibody for acute rejection of cadaveric renal transplants. *N Engl J Med* 313:337, 1985.
15. Delmonico FL, Cosimi AB. Monoclonal antibody treatment of human allograft recipients. *Surg Gynecol Obstet* 166:89, 1988.
16. Kahan BD. The pivotal role of the liver in immunosuppression by cyclosporine. *Viewpoints Dig Dis* 19:2, 1987.
17. McCaffrey PG et al. Isolation of the cyclosporin-sensitive T cell transcription factor NFATp. *Science* 262:750–754, 1993.
18. Maurer G et al. Disposition of cyclosporine in several animal species and man. I. Structural elucidation of its metabolites. *Drug Metab Dispos* 12:120, 1984.
19. Whitington PF et al. Small-bowel length and the dose of cyclosporine in children after liver transplantation. *N Engl J Med* 322:733, 1990.
20. Porter GA et al. Cyclosporin-associated hypertension. *Arch Intern Med* 150:280, 1990.
21. Klintmalm GB, Iwatsuki S, Starzl TE. Cyclosporine A. Hepatotoxicity in 66 renal allographed recipients. *Transplantation* 32:488, 1981.
22. Jain AB et al. Comparative study of cyclosporine and FK 506 dosage requirements in adult and pediatric orthotopic liver transplant patients. *Transplant Proc* 3:2763, 1991.
23. Reding R et al. Compassionate use of FK 506 in pediatric liver transplantation: A pilot study. *Transplant Proc* 23:3002, 1991.

Kristy M. Hendricks
Ronald E. Kleinman

47 ▶ Enteral and Parenteral Nutrition

Providing optimal nutrition to infants and children requiring intensive care is a major challenge. Surveys of hospitalized pediatric patients document the prevalence of protein energy malnutrition to range from 20% to 40%, and the prevalence could potentially be much higher in acutely and chronically ill patients.[1-3] Primary protein-energy malnutrition is associated with a high mortality rate, and if accompanied by infection, this risk is increased.[4] Malnutrition is also associated with increased morbidity and prolonged hospitalization.[5] Thus, provision of optimal nutrition is essential to infants and children requiring intensive care. Techniques are currently available to provide adequate parenteral or enteral nutritional support for the majority of these patients, although more research is needed to determine optimal nutrition therapy for specific disease states.

Determination of Need: Nutritional Assessment

The goal of nutritional assessment is to identify those patients with nutritional or metabolic deficiencies or excesses, plan nutrition therapy, and evaluate the effectiveness of such therapy. Although increasingly sophisticated methods are available for performing nutritional assessment, objective clinical judgement remains an important component. Nutritional assessment generally encompasses the four major areas of (1) anthropometry, (2) biochemical evaluation, (3) clinical assessment, and (4) dietary evaluation.[6]

Anthropometric measures repeated over time provide excellent objective data on overall health and well-being of an individual and, dependent on the parameter chosen, may evaluate acute or chronic nutritional status. Biochemical studies may confirm nutrient deficiencies suggested by clinical or dietary evaluation or define deficiencies that are clinically inapparent. Clinical signs of severe malnutrition are easily detected in most cases, occur in later stages of deficiency, and include abnormalities of skin, skeleton, hair, mucous membranes, and eye changes. More subtle early signs of nutrient deficiency may be found on thorough physical examination and are important to look for in patients known to be at risk because of disease or social situation. Dietary evaluation of nutrient intake and estimated needs play an important role in comprehensive nutritional assessment. The recommended dietary allowances (RDAs) are the most appropriate general standards used to evaluate nutrient intake.[7] They are designed for maintenance of good nutrition in a healthy population and are meant to be applied to population groups. More precise methods for estimating energy and nutrient requirements are often needed in acute and chronically ill patients. However, the RDAs provide a basis for evaluation, compared with healthy individuals. In all cases, evaluation of a patient's progress toward established goals (i.e., weight gain or loss, increased albumin, intact immunity) can aid the clinician in modifying the prescribed nutrition therapy. A detailed description of each methodology, indications of use, and standards for assessment is beyond the scope of this chapter but may be found in pediatric nutrition texts.[6] Major components of each are outlined in Table 47-1.

A number of disorders that occur in pediatric patients have been documented to increase nutritional risk and require careful nutrition assessment and intervention.[3] Examples of conditions frequently requiring nutrition support are listed in Table 47-2.

Table 47-1. Nutritional assessment guidelines

Anthropometry
 Weight, weight change
 Weight for height
 Height, height velocity
 Head circumference
 Triceps skinfold thickness
 Arm circumference

Biochemical
 Serum albumin
 Total protein
 Hematocrit
 Hemoglobin
 Total lymphocyte count
 Serum vitamin, mineral, and trace element levels
 Skin tests (to determine delayed-type hypersensitivity immune
  competence)

Clinical
 Complete medical history and physical examination for evaluation of
  changes consistent with nutrient deficiencies (e.g., skin, hair, eyes,
  mucous membranes, sexual maturity in adolescents)

Dietary
 Estimated intake of energy, protein, carbohydrate, fat, vitamins, minerals,
  and trace elements
 Evaluation of appetite, feeding skills
 Estimation of nutrient needs
 Drug-nutrient interactions

Table 47-2. Conditions frequently requiring nutrition support

Increased nutrient losses
 AIDS
 Cystic fibrosis
 Protracted diarrhea
 Inflammatory bowel disease
 Liver disease
 Malabsorption
 Renal disease

Increased nutrient requirement
 Bronchopulmonary dysplasia
 Burns
 Infection
 Congenital heart disease
 Fever
 Surgery

Decreased nutrient intake
 Chronic neurologic disorders
 Nonorganic failure to thrive
 Malignancy
 Altered level of consciousness
 Anorexia
 Nausea/vomiting

Table 47-3. Indicators of increased nutritional risk

Weight	<80% of 50th percentile for height
Height	<85% of 50th percentile for age
Weight loss	>5%
Albumin	<2.5 g/dl
NPO	>3 days

Infants or children at highest risk for malnutrition, and therefore potentially in need of parenteral (PN) or enteral nutrition (EN) support, will frequently have one of the findings listed in Table 47-3.

Complete nutritional assessment, recommended therapy, and establishment of short- and long-term goals are essential to the care of these patients. Both enteral and parenteral nutritional support is available for patients who cannot meet their needs orally. General guidelines for development of such a treatment plan are outlined in Fig. 47-1.

Enteral Nutrition

Enteral nutrition (EN) or alimentation, which is the provision of nutrition via the GI tract, has advantages over intravenous (IV) nutrition that include lower cost and less risk of infection and metabolic abnormalities. In addition, the presence of nutrients within the intestinal lumen appear to be important for maintenance of GI integrity and the stimulation of factors that contribute to intestinal adaptation and recovery, such as enteric secretions, hormones, and intestinal blood flow.[8] Also, EN may contain specific factors that are currently unable to be provided parenterally, and these may facilitate nutritional recovery.[9]

Candidates for EN are those patients who have a functioning GI tract but are unable to meet their nutrient requirements spontaneously through oral intake. The spectrum of clinical indications is broad and includes entities that increase nutrient losses (malabsorption), increase nutrient needs (hypermetabolism), limit oral intake, or require EN for primary management of the candidates' disease.[10]

Feeding Composition

In addition to human milk, a large number of manufactured formulas are available to support the nutrient needs of infants requiring intensive care. They vary in caloric density, nutrient composition, and cost. The Infant Formula Act of 1983 provides specific standards for infant formulas based on what is known about human milk.[11] The composition of currently available formulas is outlined in Table 47-4.[6] General guidelines for use based on composition are the following: (1) Modified cow milk formulas contain lactose and cow milk protein and are recommended for feeding of infants without maldigestion or malabsorption; (2) soy-based formulas, which are lactose free, are recommended for infants with lactose intolerance; and (3) special formulas with modified composition are available for patients with malabsorption and/or maldigestion, renal disease, and specific inborn errors of metabolism. Currently, only two formulas are expressly formulated to meet all of the nutritional needs of children 1 to 6 years of age; these feedings also are included in Table 47-4. Other available formulas are intended for adults and differ significantly in nutrient source, composition, and vitamin, mineral, and trace element content.

Formula choice and method of delivery to the patient are dependent on the patient's past and present nutritional status and the presence of acute or chronic disease. General guidelines regarding the approach to EN are depicted in Fig. 47-2. The initiation and

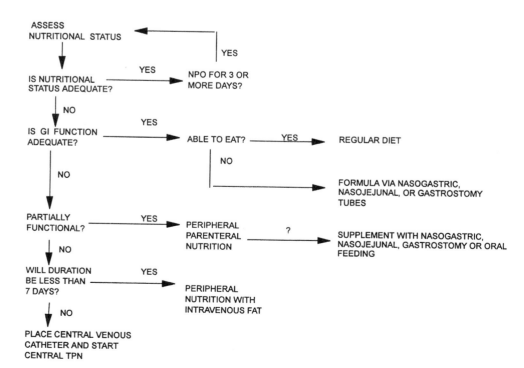

Figure 47-1. Development of a treatment plan. (From A Carlin et al. [eds]. *Handbook of Parenteral Nutrition* (5th ed). Boston: Children's Hospital, 1993. With permission.)

Table 47-4. The composition of currently available standard infant formulas

	kcal/ml	Protein	g/dl	%cal	cho	g/dl	%cal	FAT	g/dl	%cal	Osmolality	Na (mEq/liter)	K (mg/liter)	Ca (mg/liter)	P (mg/liter)	Indications
Milk-based formulas*																
Human milk	0.67	Human	1.05	6	Lactose	7.2	42	Human	4.0	52	290	7.8	13.4	250	140	Normal feeding
Enfamil (Mead Johnson)	0.67	Whey, skim milk	1.5	9	Lactose	7.0	41	Coconut oils, soy	3.8	50	300	8	19	470	320	Normal feeding
Similac (Ross)	0.67	Skim milk	1.5	9	Lactose	7.2	43	Soy, coconut oils	3.6	48	300	8	18	493	380	Normal feeding
SMA (Wyeth)	0.67	Skim milk	1.5	9	Lactose	7.2	43	Coconut oils, soy, oleo	3.6	48	300	6.5	14	420	280	Normal feeding Cardiac conditions
PM 60/40 (Ross)	0.67	Whey, cassein	1.6	9	Lactose	6.9	41	Coconut oils, soy	3.8	48	300	7	15	380	190	Normal feeding Renal conditions
Soy-based formulas																
Prosobee (Mead Johnson)	0.68	Soy protein isolate, L methionine	2.0	12	Corn syrup solids, sucrose	6.8	40	Coconut oil, soy	3.6	48	200	10	21	640	500	Lactose or sucrose intolerance, galactosemia
Isomil (Ross)	0.67	Soy protein isolate, L methionine	1.8	11	Corn syrup solids, sucrose	6.8	40	Coconut oil, soy	3.7	49	240	13	19	710	510	Lactose intolerance, galactosemia
Nursoy (Wyeth)	0.67	Soy protein isolate	2.1	12	Sucrose	6.9	40	Coconut oil, soy, oleo	3.6	47	296	9	18	600	420	Lactose intolerance, galactosemia
RCF (Ross)	0.40	Soy protein isolate, L methionine	2.0	20	Add carbohydrate of choice	0	0	Coconut oil, soy	3.6	80	74	13	19	700	500	Carbohydrate intolerance

Semi-elemental feedings

Nutramigen (Mead Johnson)	0.67	1.9	11	Casein hydrolysate, added amino acids	9.1	54	Corn syrup solids, modified corn starch	Corn oil	2.9	35	320	14	19	640	430	Hypoallergenic
Pregestimil (Mead Johnson)	0.67	1.9	11	Casein hydrolysate, added amino acids	6.9	41	Corn syrup solids, modified corn starch, dextrose	MCT (60%), corn (20%), safflower (20%) oils	3.8	48	320	12	19	640	430	Malabsorption Maldigestion
Alimentum (Ross)	0.67	1.9	11	Casein hydrolysate	6.9	41	Sucrose, modified tapioca starch	MCT (50%), safflower (40%), soy (10%) oils	3.8	48	370	13	20.5	710	510	Malabsorption Maldigestion
Portagen (Mead Johnson)	0.67	2.4	14	Sodium caseinate	7.8	46	Corn syrup solids, sucrose, carbohydrate of choice	MCT (85%), corn oil (12.5%)	3.2	40	230	16	22	635	473	Fat malabsorption

Enteral feeding for older children

Pediasure (Ross)	1	3	12	Whey, protein and sodium caseinate	11	44	Corn syrup solids, sucrose	Safflower oil, MCT oil	5	44	310	17	34	48	800	Children 1–6 years
Kindercal (Mead Johnson)	1	3.4	13	Casein	13.5	50	Maltodextrin, sucrose	Canola, sunflower, corn, and MCT oil	4.4	37	310	16	34	43	850	Children 1–10 years

[a]All formulas are available with or without iron, except SMA "premie" only without iron.
Data from "Composition of feedings for infants and young children in the hospital" (Ross Laboratories, 1991).

advancement of enteral feedings should be individualized and proceed according to a clearly established plan. Initially, monitoring should focus on patient tolerance and fluid and electrolyte balance. Once the recommended intake has been established, the patient should be evaluated for appropriate growth and weight gain. The transition from enteral to oral feeding should be part of the established plan.

Parenteral Nutrition

For those pediatric patients requiring intensive care, enteral alimentation is often not possible or is inadequate to completely support their nutritional needs. In such cases, parenteral nutrition (PN) can be given to provide total or supplemental support. General indications for the use of PN are (1) recent weight loss of 10% or greater of usual body weight, (2) severe GI tract dysfunction, (3) absence of oral intake for greater than 3 to 5 days in a patient with suboptimal nutritional status, (4) markedly increased nutrient requirements, or (5) anticipated need for PN for greater than 3 to 5 days.[12] Patients with intestinal disorders requiring surgical intervention, hypermetabolic states (e.g., burns, sepsis, ischemic bowel injury, multiorgan system failures), and inflammatory bowel disease are examples of conditions often requiring parenteral nutritional support.[12–14]

Total Parenteral Nutrition: General Guidelines

Total parenteral nutrition has the advantage of being able to deliver a higher calorie and protein intake than peripheral PN (PPN) but carries a greater risk of infection and metabolic complications. It is recommended for patients (1) who will be without EN for more than 2 weeks, (2) whose nutrient requirements are greater than can be provided by peripheral PN, or (3) with marked fluid restriction requiring hypertonic solution to provide optimal nutritional support.

Dextrose is the most common source of carbohydrates used in PN solutions. The total quantity of carbohydrate tolerated is variable, particularly in the acutely ill patient.[15] Concentrations of dextrose should be provided in incremental amounts each day to allow appropriate insulin response and tolerance. This can be achieved by initiating the glucose infusion with 5 mg carbohydrate/kg/min and gradually increasing to approximately 15 mg/kg/min.[13] However, 7 to 10 mg/kg/min of dextrose maximally suppresses gluconeogenesis in some pediatric patients, and excessive amounts may contribute to hepatic steatosis.[16] The dextrose concentration that can be delivered by peripheral vein is limited to 10% due to osmolarity with more concentrated solutions. Central vein access allows greater glucose concentrations to be delivered because the dilutional factor is greatly increased in a central vein. Fluid restriction may necessitate provision of a 30% dextrose concentration to provide optimal energy intake.

Crystalline amino acids are the source of nitrogen in PN solutions. The recommended intake of protein for normal growth in infancy is 2 to 3 g/kg/d. Greater amounts of protein may result in azotemia and hyperammonemia, particularly in those infants and children with renal and/or hepatic dysfunction. Some amino acid solutions are formulated to maintain plasma amino acid patterns similar to those of normal, breast-fed infants.[17] The maximum amino acid concentration for peripheral access is 2%; with central venous access, this can rise to 4%. An attempt is usually made to maintain the calorie-nitrogen ratio at approximately 200:1.

Parenteral lipid solutions are a concentrated source of energy and provide essential fatty acids (EFA). Currently available products contain lipid at a concentration of 10% or 20%. The daily requirement of EFA can be provided by infusing 0.5 to 1.0 g/kg/d of IV lipids. In general, the maximum tolerated dose of fat is 3 to 4 g/kg/d or 40% to 50% of total calories from fat. The infusion should occur over a 24-hour period for optimal tolerance and should not exceed 0.15 g fat/kg/min. IV lipids contribute minimally to the osmolarity of the solutions, and although complications have been reported, particularly when excessive amounts are infused, in general lipids are well tolerated and promote positive nitrogen balance as well as glucose. It may be necessary to provide only

Figure 47-2. Approach to enteral nutrition. (Data from JL Rombeau, LR Barot. Enteral nutrition therapy. *Surg Clin North Am* 61:605, 1981. With permission.)

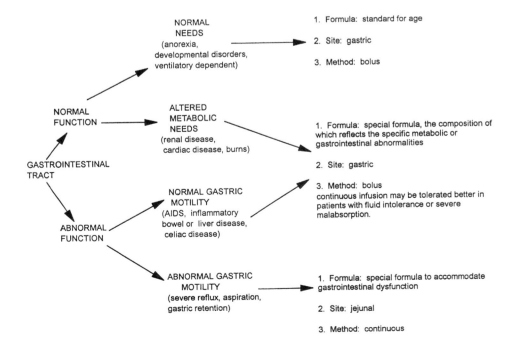

the amount of lipid necessary to meet EFA requirements in such conditions as hyperbilirubinemia and sepsis.[18]

In patients with compromised pulmonary function, the proportion of energy provided by fat or dextrose is particularly important, as metabolic end products of nutrient metabolism (most notably carbon dioxide) affect respiratory function. The respiratory quotient (RQ) is the ratio of the amount of carbon dioxide expired to the amount of oxygen inspired.[19] When only glucose is being metabolized to meet basal requirements, the RQ equals 1.0 because the amount of carbon dioxide produced equals the amount of oxygen consumed. When fat is metabolized, extra oxygen is necessary for the formation of water; this lowers the RQ to an average of 0.7. The average RQ for proteins is 0.82.

In starvation, there is a decrease in basal metabolic rate and a resultant decrease in both oxygen consumption and carbon dioxide production.[20] When glucose is provided in excess of 15 mg/kg/min (as is often the case with total PN), a shift from fat to glucose oxidation occurs and carbon dioxide production may increase twofold or more.[21] Excessive glucose is converted to fat. Under these circumstances, the amount of carbon dioxide produced is greater than the oxygen consumed, the RQ is increased, and because the excess carbon dioxide generated must be removed by the lungs, energy expenditure is increased due to an increased tidal volume and respiratory rate.[22] Thus, at these high levels, a relatively small increase in the IV glucose delivery rate creates a marked increase both in RQ and in carbon dioxide production in relation to oxygen consumption. For the ventilator-dependent patient, and in particular the patient being weaned from the ventilator, these metabolic changes may be significant.

The metabolic response to IV carbohydrate and fat varies with each clinical situation. Septic and injured patients preferentially utilize endogenous fat as an energy source, and this results in an RQ that is significantly lower because there is a large increase in both carbon dioxide production and oxygen consumption; the RQ in these hypermetabolic patients is generally less than 1.0, but the ratio may not reflect these increases in total carbon dioxide production.[22,23] In addition, although carbohydrate and fat significantly influence metabolism, the metabolism of protein may also affect respiratory function.

In summary, the optimal proportions of glucose, fat, and protein needed for acutely ill patients remain controversial. Starvation, hypermetabolic states, and excessive calories may adversely affect the respiratory function of these patients; thus, accurate estimation of nutrient requirements is needed. Steinhorn et al. have documented the feasibility and cost effectiveness of utilizing modular indirect calorimetry for sequential monitoring of multiple pediatric intensive care unit (ICU) patients.[24] Used in combination with other assessment parameters (e.g., urinary nitrogen excretion), such methods will allow nutrition support regimes to be tailored more specifically to the needs of the patient.[25] Each admission to a pediatric ICU will vary significantly for severity and type of illness, degree of preexisting or acquired nutritional deficit, clinical course, and requirements for growth. The ability of standard nutrition assessment tools to accurately predict requirements is therefore limited and, as the astute clinician knows, requirements must be determined specifically for each patient. Ultimately, the goals should include restoration of lean body mass and, in children, promotion of growth.

Protein requirements for critically ill patients, like those for healthy infants, are based on the RDA for age or 10% to 15% total calorie intake, with the remaining calories equally divided between fat and carbohydrate. Protein intake must often be decreased in patients with chronic renal insufficiency and decompensated liver function. Vitamins, minerals, and trace elements must be supplied in parenteral solutions to meet the RDAs and are generally added to the glucose–amino acid infusate. Current recommendations are based on what is known about enteral requirements for these nutrients.[26–28]

PPN is best utilized for patients who had normal nutritional status prior to hospital admission, who can tolerate 1.5 to 2.0 times maintenance fluid, who do not have greater than normal nutrient requirements, and who will be NPO for less than 7 to 10 days. PPN may also be used to supplement enteral nutrient intake. The 10% dextrose and 2% amino acid concentrations keep the osmolality acceptable for peripheral veins, yet limit energy intake. Therefore, PPN cannot support a very malnourished patient or one who has increased requirements. The length of time for PPN administration is limited by difficulty in maintaining peripheral access and the frequent need to provide greater than basal requirements as illness progresses.

The advantages of higher caloric and protein intake must be balanced against the increased risk of infection and metabolic complications (Table 47-5) associated with central access. Risk factors can be minimized if an assessment plan is outlined and implemented, following predetermined protocols for administration and monitoring, whether it is PPN or central PN. Patients on PN must be routinely monitored (Table 47-6) to prevent potential metabolic or catheter-related complications. It may be necessary to obtain certain tests more frequently, depending on the condition and stability of the patient.

Transition from Parenteral to Enteral Nutrition

The transition from parenteral to enteral feedings requires selection of an appropriate enteral formula and method of delivery that is based on individual requirements. The transition may be gradual or rapid, with the goal being maintenance of adequate energy and protein intake and tolerance to enteral feedings. Patients who

Table 47-5. Complications of parenteral nutrition

Metabolic	Technical
Glucose imbalance	Catheter dislodgement
Electrolyte imbalance	Central vein thrombosis
Sodium	Catheter obstruction
Potassium	Catheter leakage
Chloride	Uncoupling of infusion system
Mineral imbalance	Air embolus
Calcium	Local inflammation
Phosphorus	Phlebitis
Magnesium	
Acid-base disorders	
Protein intolerance	
Hyperammonemia	
Abnormal amino acid profile	
Disordered lipid metabolism	
Hypertriglyceridemia	
Essential fatty-acid deficiency	
Trace element deficiency	
Hepatic dysfunction	
Bone demineralization	
Sepsis	

Table 47-6. Monitoring parenteral nutrition

	Daily	Weekly*	Periodically*
Parameter			
Weight	X		
Fluid balance	X		
Vital signs	X		
Urine sugar/acetone	X		
Catheter site/function	X		
Laboratory tests			
Sodium		X	
Potassium		X	
Chloride		X	
TCO₂		X	
Glucose		X	
BUN		X	
Creatinine		X	
Triglycerides		X	
Calcium		X	
Magnesium		X	
Phosphorous		X	
Albumin		X	
Total protein		X	
SGPT		X	
Alkaline phosphatase		X	
Bilirubin (direct/total)		X	
Selenium			X
Copper			X
Zinc			X
Iron			X

*More often as necessitated by clinical course.
From A Carlin et al. (eds). *Handbook of Parenteral Nutrition* (5th ed). Boston: Children's Hospital, 1993.

experience no complications can usually complete the transition to full enteral feedings over several hours or days. Often, because of intestinal dysfunction, the patient may experience intolerance to enteral formulas, and the transition to full enteral feeds may take several weeks. The usual practice is to begin half-strength or full-strength formula in a small volume (continuous infusion or bolus) and increase to full strength, then to advance the volume gradually while decreasing the PN infusion.

Summary

Due to the high incidence of malnutrition in hospitalized patients and the associated increased morbidity and mortality accompanying it, determination of need for nutrition intervention is essential in the acutely ill pediatric patient. Nutritional assessment by a combination of anthropometric, biochemical, clinical, and dietary parameters helps determine need, monitor tolerance, and assess outcome. Depending on the individual patient's degree of malnutrition, medical status, GI function, and nutrient requirements, either EN or PN may be used to support the patient nutritionally. Advances in the technical administration, composition of solutions, and increased understanding of nutrient needs for patients receiving both EN and PN have made it possible to provide adequate nutritional support to many of these patients.

References

1. Merritt RJ, Suskind RM. Nutritional survey of hospitalized pediatric patients. *Am J Clin Nutr* 32:1320, 1979.

2. Parsons HG et al. The nutritional status of hospitalized children. *Am J Clin Nutr* 33:1140, 1980.

3. Hendricks KM et al. Prevalence of malnutrition in hospitalized pediatric patients. *Arch Ped Adol Med* (in press).

4. MacLean WC Jr et al. Nutritional management of chronic diarrhea and malnutrition: Primary reliance on oral feeding. *J Pediatr* 97:315, 1980.

5. Weinsier RL et al. Hospital malnutrition: A prospective evaluation of general medical patients during the course of hospitalization. *Am J Clin Nutr* 32:418, 1979.

6. Hendricks KM, Walker WA. *Manual of Pediatric Nutrition*. Toronto: Decker, 1990.

7. *Recommended Dietary Allowances* (10th ed). Washington, DC: National Academy Press, 1989.

8. Levine GM, Helineli G. Role of nutrition in intestinal adaptation. In Walker WA, Watkins J (eds): *Nutrition in Pediatrics*. Boston: Little, Brown, 1985.

9. Daly JM et al. Enteral nutrition with supplemental arginine, RNA, and omega-3 fatty acids in patient after operation; immunologic, metabolic and clinical outcome. *Surgery* 112:56, 1992.

10. Guideline for the use of enteral nutrition in the adult patient. *JPEN* 11:435, 1987.

11. American Academy of Pediatrics Committee on Nutrition. *Pediatric Nutrition Handbook* (2nd ed). Elk Grove Village, IL: American Academy of Pediatrics, 1985.

12. Carlin A et al. (eds). *Handbook of Parenteral Nutrition* (5th ed). Boston: Nutrition Support Service, The Children's Hospital, 1993.

13. American Academy of Pediatrics Committee on Nutrition. Commentary on parenteral nutrition. *Pediatrics* 71:547, 1983.

14. Kerner JA (ed). *Manual of Pediatric Parenteral Nutrition*. New York: Wiley, 1983.

15. Kalhan SC et al. Role of glucose in regulation of endogenous glucose reduction in the human newborn. *Pediatr Res* 20:49, 1986.

16. Merritt RJ. Cholestasis associated with total parenteral nutrition. *J Pediatr Gastroenterol Nutr* 5:9, 1986.

17. Heird WC et al. Amino acid mixture designed to maintain normal plasma amino acid patterns in infants and children requiring parenteral nutrition. *Pediatrics* 80:401, 1987.

18. American Academy of Pediatrics Committee on Nutrition. Use of intravenous fat emulsions in pediatric patients. *Pediatrics* 68:738, 1981.

19. Harper HA, Rodwell VW, Mayes PA (eds). *Review of Physiological Chemistry* (17th ed). Los Altos, CA: Lange, 1979.

20. Doekel RC Jr et al. Clinical semi-starvation: Depression of hypoxic ventilatory response. *N Engl J Med* 295:358, 1976.

21. Wolfe RR, Allsop JR, Burke. Glucose metabolism in man: Responses to intravenous glucose infusion. *Metabolism* 28:10, 1979.

22. Askanazi J et al. Nutrition for the patient with respiratory failure: Glucose vs. fat. *Anesthesiology* 54:373, 1981.

23. Askanazi J et al. Influence of total parenteral nutrition in fuel utilization in injury and sepsis. *Ann Surg* 191:40, 1980.

24. Steinhorn DM et al. Modular indirect calorimeter suitable for long term measurements in multipatient intensive care unit. *Crit Care Med* 19:963, 1991.

25. Steinhorm DM, Green TP. Severity of illness correlates with alterations in energy metabolism in the pediatric intensive care unit. *Crit Care Med* 19:1503, 1991.

26. Greene AL et al. Guidelines for the use of vitamins, trace elements, calcium, magnesium, and phosphorus in infants and children receiving total parenteral nutrition: Report of the Subcommittee on Pediatric Parenteral Nutrient Requirements for the Committee on Clinical Practice Issues of the American Society for Clinical Nutrition. *Am J Clin Nutr* 48:1324, 1988.

27. American Medical Association Department of Foods and Nutrition. Multivitamin preparations for parenteral use: A statement by the Nutrition Advisory Group. *JPEN* 3:258, 1979.

28. American Medical Association Nutrition Advisory Group. Guidelines for essential trace-element preparations for parenteral use. *JPEN* 3:263, 1979.

X Pharmacology and Poisoning

M. Claire McManus

Myron B. Peterson

48 ▶ Developmental Pharmacology

When one chooses a drug therapy, major emphasis is placed on the selection of the drug of choice, and there is a tendency to ignore other pharmacologic aspects that may profoundly influence the outcome. To select the dosage regimen of choice, one must know something of the drug's pharmacokinetics and pharmacodynamics. Operationally, pharmacokinetics is the discipline that describes what the body does to the drug. It encompasses absorption, distribution, metabolism, and excretion. Pharmacodynamics is the science that defines what the drug does to the body in terms of its effects and mechanism of action. Pharmacokinetics and pharmacodynamics have been well described for many agents in the adult, and various dosage guidelines are defined. This has not been done for children. The sick pediatric patient is unique because of ongoing development, and dosage needs can change as growth continues. It is important that the intensivist be aware not only of the pharmacologic aspects of drug therapy, but also of the consequences of the child's developmental stage and of disease on the final response. We will review certain aspects of development from birth to early childhood that affect the child's handling of and, where different from the adult, response to drugs. Equipped with this information, the intensive care physician should feel more at ease in the effort to design the safest and most efficacious regimen for the young patient.

Pharmacokinetics

The Effect of Development on Drug Absorption

Absorption is the transfer of a drug from its site of administration into the bloodstream and depends on the physicochemical properties of the xenobiotic (foreign, anutrient substance) and certain patient variables.[1] There are two facets to absorption: the rate and the extent. Drug bioavailability involves the **extent** of absorption and is important in determining the dose. It is influenced by many factors, including first-pass effect (FPE). An FPE exists if a majority of the oral dose is metabolized by the liver en route to the systemic circulation. This reduces the bioavailability by the oral route. The **rate** of absorption, on the other hand, refers to how quickly a drug is absorbed from its site of administration and is a major factor in determining the peak effect. Both the rate and extent of absorption must be considered when a drug is given, for example, by the oral, intranasal (IN), intramuscular (IM), subcutaneous (SC), rectal, and percutaneous routes.

Oral Absorption

When a drug is administered orally, the rate and extent of absorption will be affected by some or all of the following: gastric pH, gastric emptying time, GI motility, absorptive surface area, bile acid pool, bacterial colonization of the gut, and the presence of disease.[2,3] There is great variability in gastric acid secretory rates in infants.[4] At birth, the gastric pH is close to neutrality. Within the next few hours, it falls to pH 1.5 to 3.0 but returns to neutrality in the following 24 hours. This early decrease is not evidenced in the premature newborn less than 32 weeks' gestational age.[1,2] For the first 10 to 15 days of life, the pH remains stable at 7, and from then on gradually declines to reach adult levels by 2 to 3 years.[2,5] With such a relatively high pH present in the newborn

(day 0 to 15), the absorption of acidic drugs will be reduced and that of basic drugs will be enhanced. Increased bioavailabilities of drugs such as the penicillins have been noted in neonates,[6–8] whereas delayed absorption and/or reduced bioavailability of phenobarbital, phenytoin, acetaminophen, and riboflavin [9–12] have been noted in this same age group. The high gastric pH probably contributes.

The rate of gastric emptying also affects drug absorption. Gastric emptying is affected by the type of feeding, composition of the meal, gestational maturity, and postnatal age.[13–15] Gastric emptying times are longer in the neonate and infant, and some authors have reported that they reach adult values by age 6 to 8 months.[3,5]

Generally, the overall extent and rate of absorption is quite variable between patients. In one study,[5] the rates of absorption of digoxin, phenobarbital, and certain sulfonamides were slow in the infant and increased with age. The bioavailabilities, however, were similar in both adults and infants. Interestingly, in infants over 3 months of age, the oral absorption rate of various drugs is higher than that seen in grown children and adults.[2]

Intranasal, Sublingual, Transmucosal, and Buccal Absorption

Absorption across mucosal surfaces in the mouth and nose can provide effective drug concentrations rapidly and bypass obstacles associated with low bioavailability via the oral route, such as FPE and enzymatic destruction in the gut. The onset for sedation after sublingual (SL) and IN midazolam is 10 to 15 minutes, compared with 20 to 30 minutes when given orally. Smaller doses can be given as the FPE is minimized. Transmucosal (TM) fentanyl, 15 to 20 μg/kg, reliably induces preoperative sedation in children.[16] However, buccal absorption of morphine was found to be slower in adults than the slow-release oral form,[17] implying less reliable absorption by this route than previously suggested.[18] Overdosage may occur with topical mucosal application of drugs also. This is evident from a reported case of seizures in a child treated with TAC (tetracaine:adrenaline:cocaine), applied to mucosa for tongue laceration. Absorption occurred despite the presence of a vasoconstrictor in the preparation.[19]

Intramuscular and Subcutaneous Absorption

The degree of absorption from the injection site will be governed by both **physicochemical** and **physiologic** factors. The drug should be fairly lipophilic so that it passes easily through membranes; it should also be hydrophilic in nature to avoid precipitation at the injection site. Phenytoin has low water solubility and may precipitate at the site, ascribing to it poor IM absorption characteristics.[20] The surface area and blood flow to the site will also determine the degree of absorption. The neonate displays vasomotor instability and insufficient muscular contractions, and this, in concert with reduced muscle mass and SC fat, may reduce absorption rates substantially.[2] Drugs that can be given IM in the neonate and infant are listed in Table 48-1. Diazepam is readily and efficiently absorbed in the neonate[3] and infant,[2] but IM is slower than the oral route in the former. In contrast to diazepam, bioavailabilities for phenobarbital in children and adults showed no significant difference between IV, IM, oral, or rectal routes.[21] Although similar studies have not been carried out in neonates, some feel that for

Table 48-1. Drugs demonstrating effective systemic absorption following intramuscular administration in neonates

Antimicrobials	Sedative/tranquilizers
Amikacin	Chlorpromazine
Ampicillin	Midazolam
Benzathine penicillin G	Cardiovascular drugs
Benzylpenicillin	Hydralazine
(penicillin G)	Procainamide
Carbenicillin	Pyridostigmine
Cefazolin	Diuretics
Cefotaxime	Acetazolamide
Ceftazidime	Furosemide
Ceftriaxone	Bumetanide
Clindamycin	Endocrine
Gentamicin	Corticotrophin (ACTH)
Kanamycin	Cortisone
Methicillin	Glucagon
Oxacillin	Pituitary
Nafcillin	Vasopressin (tennate oil)
Piperacillin	Narcotics
Ticarcillin	Meperidine
Tobramycin	Morphine
Antituberculous agents	Vitamins
Isoniazid	K
Streptomycin	D
Anticonvulsants	
Diazepam	
Phenobarbitone	

maintenance therapy, parenteral phenobarbital offers little therapeutic advantage over oral dosing.[22] IM midazolam[23] has good bioavailability also, but absorption may be delayed. It is water-soluble and, unlike diazepam, the injection is not painful. The absorption of IM digoxin is variable in pediatric patients, with reports of similar rates in infants and adults[24] and reduced and delayed absorption in neonates.[3] This latter effect may be due to associated tissue necrosis. Generally, the absorption of IM and SC aminoglycosides are equal to that of the intravenous (IV) route. Scarring may occur with repeated IM injections in **small premature babies,** causing erratic absorption.[25] The parenteral nonsteroidal antiinflammatory agent, ketorolac, has equal bioavailabilities for all routes.[23]

Epidural Absorption

Epidural administration of narcotics and local anesthetics can be used in infants and children as a technique to provide analgesia and anesthesia. Caudal anesthesia is frequently used in young infants. The drug is infused into the epidural space where it crosses the dura to act on nerve roots and the spinal cord in the subarachnoid space.[26] Lipophilic narcotics such as fentanyl and sufentanil cross the dura rapidly and have a quick analgesic onset. They also have a short duration, as they are reabsorbed and eliminated systemically. Morphine is more hydrophilic in nature and thus penetrates the CNS more slowly, resulting in a slower onset, and stays there longer, resulting in prolonged duration of action.[27] Morphine has the potential for rostral spread and delayed respiratory depression. The rostral spread also has efficacy implications, as caudal/lumbar block with morphine will alleviate pain from thoracic dermatomes. The volume of the epidural space, on a milliliter-per-kilogram basis, decreases with age, implying that the initial bolus in older children should be one third to one half that in younger patients.[28]

Percutaneous Absorption

The extent of absorption for compounds applied to the skin is increased in the newborn and young infant. Percutaneous absorption is inversely related to the thickness of the stratum corneum and directly related to skin hydration.[2] The barrier function of neonatal and infant skin appears to be intact and probably does not allow substantially more absorption per square centimeter than adult rates. However, because the ratio of body surface area to weight is increased, the infant receives **2.7 times** the adult dose in milligrams per kilogram. This may be doubled with an occlusive dressing.[29,30] In premature neonates, on the other hand, the barrier function of the skin appears not to be intact until 21 days.[31] Cutaneous diseases may increase skin permeability and further interfere with barrier function. An awareness of possible systemic absorption with topical agents is prudent in the neonate. In one study, topical lidocaine cream, 30% for neonatal circumcision in full-term babies, did not result in significant absorption.[32] Percutaneous application is indeed a useful drug delivery route, especially for lipophilic agents such as fentanyl, which is available in the form of skin patches.[33]

Rectal Absorption

The rectal route is a viable alternative for drug administration and, in some cases, can be efficient and complete. This route may be important in regard to bioavailability for drugs with a high FPE, such as lidocaine, morphine, and propranolol,[34] because the blood supply from the lower rectum bypasses the liver on its way to the systemic circulation. Rectal diazepam solution yielded good concentrations in 1–2-year-olds and was found to be beneficial in the prophylaxis of recurrent febrile seizures.[35–37] Valproate solution administered rectally has been used successfully in intractable status epilepticus.[38] Ketamine and thiopental produce satisfactory sedation when given rectally, as does midazolam (bioavailability is 0.5 rectally vs. 0.3 for oral) and methohexital, the latter's absorption being rapid but somewhat irregular.[23]

The Effect of Development on Drug Distribution

The Effect of Body Composition on Drug Distribution

The process whereby a drug reversibly diffuses from one location in the body to another is known as drug distribution. This is described pharmacokinetically as the volume of distribution (Vd) and can vary substantially between adults and children, depending on the drug. Many age-related factors govern distribution and include compartmental size and composition, protein binding, membrane permeability, and hemodynamic factors such as cardiac output, regional blood flow, and, in the newborn, persistence of fetal circulation.[1,39,40]

In the premature neonate, total body water (TBW) comprises 85% of body weight and in the full-term infant, around 75%. Then, it decreases rapidly in the first year of life, and adult values of 60% are attained at 12 years of age.[41,42] Aminoglycosides are confined to the extracellular fluid (ECF), and thus larger doses need to be given in the neonate than in older children, on a milligram-per-kilogram basis. The Vd of the central compartment for propofol (ECF and brain) appears to be larger in children than in adults, as children require larger induction doses.[43] In contrast to conventional pharmacodynamics, wherein drug distribution must occur for a response to be elicited, propofol's action is of interest because it occurs before the drug distributes widely to other tissues (i.e., the targeted brain receptors are reached first). Termination of its CNS effect is a result of rapid redistribution from the brain to other less well perfused tissues, such as fat, rather than due to drug elimination per se.[43] This is true for diazepam also. Unlike diazepam, however, cumulative sedative effects have not been shown to occur with propofol, despite a relatively large final Vd (sequestration in fat) and, consequently, a long terminal half-life. This is due to the fact that concentrations of propofol will have declined to levels below the threshold for sedation before mobilization from fat depots occurs. This, plus its rapid clearance, which appears to be even faster in children, ensures that, on mobilization, serum drug concentrations (SDC) do not rise appreciably and reenter the CNS.[44] Children over 2 years of age tolerate it well. Other factors in the newborn and infant, such as a relative increase in brain, GI tract, and liver and a relative decrease in skeletal muscle mass and fat tissue, also affect distribution. As mentioned previously, diazepam is lipophilic and distributes readily in adipose tissue.[4] In the neonate, diazepam has a decreased volume of distribution, and maintenance dosage requirements are less with respect to the adult. On average, because the developing infant is "composed" differently than the mature adult, dosages are different depending on the physicochemical nature of the drug and the type of tissue it favors.

Developmental Aspects of Protein Binding

The degree to which a drug is protein bound will profoundly affect its distribution. Albumin is by far the most important binding protein and binds many different drugs and other molecules (ligands), such as fatty acids and bilirubin. Some globulins (lipoprotein, gamma globulin, alpha-1 glycoprotein [A-1AG] and hemoglobin) also bind ligands. The binding is nearly always quickly reversible and only rarely is a strong covalent bond formed.[39] Albumin usually binds to acidic drugs such as phenytoin, phenobarbital, digoxin, aspirin, diazepam, and warfarin. Basic drugs can also bind to albumin but usually prefer other proteins, such as gamma globulin, lipoprotein, and A-1AG. A-1AG binds to alprenolol, dipyramidole, imipramine, lidocaine, prilocaine, alfentanil, sufentanil, propranolol, and quinidine.

Factors that affect the degree of plasma protein binding to drugs include the amount of protein available, the affinity constant of the drug for the proteins, the number of binding sites available, the effects of disease, and the presence of inhibitory compounds.[3,45,46] The **amount** of total protein (TP), globulin, and, in some cases, albumin concentrations is reduced at birth. TP reaches concentrations close to the adult at 1 year.[3,47] Adult albumin values are reached at about 26 weeks,[48] although it may be longer in some small-for-gestational-age (SGA) premature infants.[49] A-1AG and gamma globulin are also significantly reduced at birth.[45,50,51]

Binding is also determined by the binding **affinity** that the particular protein has for the drug. It has been suggested that the affinity of neonatal albumin is reduced.[2,51] The decreased binding of albumin to acidic and other drugs is therefore most likely due to decreased affinity[2,40,52] but may also be due to interference by globulins.[53] Kurz et al.[53] proposed four mechanisms for the decreased binding to albumin and globulins seen in the neonate: (1) displacement of drugs by bilirubin; (2) different binding properties of cord and adult albumin; (3) different properties of the globulins, although this was inconclusive; and (4) interaction of albumin with globulins in the newborn. Binding to neonatal albumin, particularly, seems to be susceptible to interference by endogenous substances.[54] The affinity that albumin has for bilirubin is

reduced at birth also.[55,56] True adult values are felt to be reached at 5 months.[56] The general consensus in the literature is that albumin-drug binding is diminished in the neonate, but whether it is due to a decreased affinity or for other reasons is not clear. Adult binding capacity for albumin has been reported to be attained at around 2 to 3 years of age[2]; it varies, however, with the drug in question. For phenytoin, it is said to be reached at 2 to 3 months,[40] and for salicylate at 10 to 12 months.[52]

The globulin fraction, in general, is lower in the neonate and probably accounts for the lower binding seen for certain drugs (but not for salicylate). It is not definite that the affinity of neonatal globulins is reduced.[53] The reduced binding of the globulin A-1AG to basic drugs in the newborn on the basis of a lower glycoprotein concentration and not a reduced affinity supports this.[57] Bupivicaine, sufentanil, and alfentanil binding may be affected as a consequence.

Effect of Displacement on Drug Distribution

It seems evident that the developing infant has reduced drug-protein binding and that this may be reduced even further by displacement. However, certain criteria need to be fulfilled, in vivo, before the displacement is significant. First, for there to be a significant shift of displaced drug from plasma to periphery, there must originally have been a relatively high amount of drug in the plasma. This translates into plasma protein binding rates of 90% to 95%,[39] and clinically important displacement is probably limited to drugs that are bound more than 80% to 90%.[40,58] Second, the drug must be free to bind to the receptor in the target organ, which may not be the case if there is a high degree of nonspecific protein binding in the tissues.[39] This is illustrated by the use of digoxin, in which the neonatal myocardium accumulates the drug to a higher degree than in the adult, but the vast majority of this drug is bound nonspecifically to tissue proteins.[4] Therefore, the Vd may potentially increase with displacement as more drug is free to go into the tissues. Endogenous substances, such as free fatty acids (FFA) and bilirubin among others, may cause this displacement of the bound drug.

Protein Binding Interactions and Bilirubin Displacement

Due to the higher concentrations of competitive substances, such as free fatty acids (FFA)[46,52,59–61] in the plasma of the younger patient, it is more likely that displacement interactions will occur. The clinical consequences of this on displacement are not clear.[1,39] In one report, reduced binding of salicylic acid, dicoumarol, and phenytoin to albumin was shown to occur at high FFA levels,[62] and, in another report, an increase in the free phenytoin level coincided with increasing FFA in the neonate.[63] Further evidence is needed to quantify this displacement for various drugs.

Bilirubin can displace xenobiotics from albumin as well and consequently affect their distribution.[1–3,51] The lower binding in the neonate of phenobarbital, theophylline, salicylate, phenytoin, and propranolol may be secondary to competition for sites by bilirubin, among other substances.[3,6,63–65] The reverse, however, is also true, and drugs may compete for the same bilirubin-binding site on albumin, resulting in bilirubin displacement and the potential for kernicterus.[65] Ninety-nine percent of the unconjugated bilirubin anion is bound to plasma albumin, and it is harmless in this form.[66,67] Normally, albumin is probably always present in the plasma in molar excess of bilirubin, and a certain number of vacant binding sites are always present. Unbound, unconjugated bilirubin in high concentrations is believed to be the toxin. Plasma to tissue transfer of bilirubin is reversible but may be irreversible in acidotic tissues[65] (Fig. 48-1).

Bilirubin diffusion into tissues is dependent on the plasma concentration of the unconjugated form, whereas the back-transport is dictated by the presence of vacant sites on albumin. Some sulfonamides and other drugs bind to the same site as bilirubin on albumin and thus decrease reserve albumin, which, in effect, "displaces" bilirubin into tissue.[68] This does not imply that the bilirubin molecule is physically ousted from its albumin site by the drug. The drug merely occupies the vacant sites and pushes the bilirubin equilibrium in the direction of higher tissue concentrations. Brodersen[65] outlined a few rules to determine the "displacing" potential of a drug: (1) Drugs that are given in low doses (hormones, digoxin, potent diuretics) are not dangerous because they do not occupy a significant fraction of the reserve albumin; (2) cationic drugs and most electroneutral substances (aminoglycosides, antihistamines, general anesthetics, and benzodiazepines) are not bound to the bilirubin-binding site; (3) sulfonamides show various effects, sulfadiazine being the weakest competitor and probably safe at usual doses; (4) several analgesics and antiinflammatory drugs are potent competitors; (5) x-ray contrast media for choliangiography have the highest potential to cause displacement because they are given in high doses and occupy the reserve albumin very efficiently. A list of drugs that may displace bilirubin has been reported.[69] Salicylate, ceftriaxone, moxalactam, cefoperazone, and even diazepam have been implicated in the neonate to a greater or lesser degree.[65,70,71] Cefotaxime and ceftazidime are 26% and 10% protein-bound, respectively, and do not significantly reduce reserve albumin concentrations.[72]

Little is known about the influence of disease on drug-protein binding other than hyperbilirubinemia in neonates. Renal and liver diseases, which decrease binding in adults, are not so common in pediatrics.[39] The phenomenon probably does occur, though, resulting in an increase in the free fraction and subsequent distribution into tissues, and this, most likely, is caused by endogenous

inhibitors of the binding. Decreased albumin seems to be of lesser importance as a cause of reduced binding. At the same time, there may be lack of binding sites as a result of hypoalbuminemia because children with kwashiorkor show decreased binding of salicylates, warfarin, and thiopental.[73]

The Effect of Development on Drug Metabolism

Drug Biotransformation: Enzyme Systems

Metabolism is the body's strategy of defense to render xenobiotics more polar so that they are suitable for rapid excretion. *Clearance* is a kinetic term describing drug elimination from the body and is defined as the volume of blood cleared of drug per unit time. Hepatic clearance or metabolism is not synonymous with detoxification, as active metabolites and active and reactive intermediates may be formed (e.g., codeine to morphine).[74] The microsomal enzymes of the liver are responsible for biotransformation of the majority of drugs, and they are located in the smooth endoplasmic reticulum (SER) of the hepatocyte.[75] They are also present, along with other enzyme systems, in the plasma, kidney, lung, and gut. Nonmicrosomal enzymes in liver mitochondria and cytosol also metabolize drugs. Biotransformation of drugs is classified as phases 1 and 2. Phase 1 reactions are oxidation, reduction, and hydrolysis. Phase 2 covers conjugation reactions. The microsomal enzymes catalyze most of the oxidations and all of the glucuronide conjugations. Reduction and hydrolysis are catalyzed by both nonmicrosomal and microsomal enzymes. The remainder of the conjugation reactions, other than glucuronidation, are catalyzed by nonmicrosomal enzymes. The microsomal enzymes include cytochrome P450 (P450), uridine diphosphate glucuronosyltransferase (UDP-GT), and epoxide hydrolase.[76] Oxidations performed by P450 include (1) side-chain oxidation (phenobarbital, phenytoin, lidocaine), (2) aromatic hydroxylation (steroid hormones), (3) dealkylation (morphine, meperidine, diazepam, lidocaine, theophylline, cefotaxime), (4) hydroxylation, (5) deamination, and (6) desulfura-

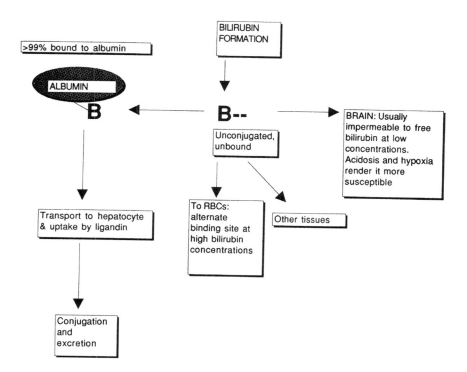

Figure 48-1. Binding of bilirubin to albumin and distribution to tissues.

tion. Oxidation reactions may produce toxic intermediates (epoxides, etc.) that are subsequently hydrolysed by epoxide hydrolase, the activity of which is low at birth in animals, reaching adult levels within 1 month.[76] Some reduction reactions are performed by microsomal enzymes, as are some hydrolysis reactions (splitting of esters and amides). Finally, the microsomal enzyme UDP-GT catalyzes phase 2 glucuronidation. The same enzymes that catalyze the metabolism of drugs also catalyze that of endogenous fatty acids, bile acids, and steroid hormones.[2]

Induction and Inhibition of Microsomal Enzymes

When assessing the maturity of drug metabolism in the newborn infant and child, several factors should be considered, including enzyme induction. Enzyme inducers increase the synthesis of enzyme systems, of SER, and of the hepatic uptake protein, ligandin. A drug may induce its own metabolism (e.g., carbamazepine) or that of other drugs (e.g., phenobarbital induces that of warfarin). Thus, exposure to inducers postnatally can have an effect on the level of enzyme activity in the neonate as well as the child and thus on one's ability to metabolize drugs.[2,3,77] Despite controversy in the literature regarding prenatal induction due to the presence of maternal inhibitory substances,[40,54,78–80] it may be significant in the fetus during late gestation.[76] P450 and UDP-GT enzymes are inducible,[75] unlike nonmicrosomal enzymes. Enzyme induction is manifested in the newborn as an increased metabolism of other drugs. Neonates who were exposed to phenobarbital during pregnancy were noted to have reduced bilirubin concentrations[81] as well as a decrease in the half-life of diazepam.[3,82,83] Postnatally, phenobarbital therapy is known to enhance the glucuronidation pathway, a phenomenon that is exploited in the treatment of hyperbilirubinemia. In the same vein, phenobarbital exposure increases the elimination of phenytoin and salicylamide in the infant.[77,84–86] On the other hand, certain drugs (cimetidine, erythromycin, etc.) may inhibit P450 activity, resulting in increased serum drug concentrations (SDCs).

The possibility of previous exposure to inducing agents should always be considered when planning a therapeutic schedule in the newborn and child, as usual doses may be ineffective, secondary to increased clearance.[3] One should start at recommended doses, but if the SDCs or responses are inadequate at steady state, the possibility of induction may offer an explanation. Similarly, drug doses should be decreased if enzyme inhibitors are added to the regimen.

Developmental Aspects of Metabolism

The rate of development of the microsomal enzyme system may vary widely between individuals and in the same individual for different drug substrates.[54] As already noted, exposure to inducing agents may be of paramount importance in determining the child's metabolic rate. In general, there is a reduced capacity to dispose of drugs in the first 15 days after birth unless there is exposure to inducers.[2] After the first 2 weeks of life, a dramatic increase in metabolism can occur, with a period of enhanced metabolism for many drugs.[40] For some, such as theophylline[87] and quinidine,[88] this can last up to 12 years. Adult rates can be reached anywhere from the fifth day of life (e.g., salicylamide[54]) to after puberty (e.g., theophylline[87]), depending on the xenobiotic and the enzyme systems that metabolize it.

Phase One Reactions
Oxidation, Reduction, Hydrolysis

Ligandin or Y protein is present in hepatocytes and secures organic acids within the cell so that they can be metabolized.[89] Its level is low in the fetus and newborn but matures during the first 5 to 10 days of life. The lack thereof may play a role in "physiologic jaundice."[73,90] Whether it contributes to the lower hepatic clearance of certain xenobiotics in the newborn period is not clear.[1,76]

In the liver, the SER contains the microsomal P450 enzymes responsible for phase 1 catalysis, and this reportedly is present as early as 6 weeks of fetal age in human hepatocytes.[54] In vivo evidence suggests that P450 enzyme oxidative activity is low at birth.[91] The system then develops quite rapidly after birth, reaching a maximum at various ages according to the drug and pathway.[54] The concomitant exposure to inducers, increased bilirubin levels, and disappearance rates of endogenous inhibitors, such as progesterone, may all play a role in determining the final P450 enzymatic activity.[3] In general, oxidation (hydroxylation, demethylation, and oxidation) appears to be the most deficient phase 1 reaction at birth. Reduction is more efficient, and many hydrolytic reactions approach adult rates.[92] Again, among the P450 oxidative reactions, there is much variation. In the newborn, reduced hydroxylation rates have been reported for phenobarbital, phenytoin, mepivacaine, lidocaine, and prilocaine.[2,93] Dealkylation appears to be less impaired at birth as regards mepivacaine, diazepam, and lidocaine,[3] but the contrary is true for theophylline, where it is the most deficient step.[94,95] Desacetylation of cefotaxime to its active metabolite, desacetylcefotaxime, is also decreased in the neonate, effectively doubling the half-life seen in adults.[96] Maturation rates of P450 vary for different drugs and between individuals and are probably related to different P450 subclasses and their substrate specificity.[40] The apparent half-lives for phenobarbital[97] and phenytoin[98] are prolonged (100–500 hours) in the neonate but may be shorter (40–300 hours), implicating pre- and postnatal autoinduction.[97,99–102] During the first 15 to 30 days, the clearance of phenobarbital increases steadily, and half-lives of 30 to 100 hours may be found at 3 to 4 weeks.[2] For many drugs, including phenobarbital,[103–106] a period of enhanced clearance is usually evident from 2 to 3 months up to 2 to 3 years of age, after which it gradually decreases and reaches adult levels after puberty.[2,40] Theophylline clearance is depressed also in the newborn[95,107] and in early infancy and appears to reach adult levels at 6 months of age.[108,109] Children from 1 to 9 years have a faster clearance than the adult,[110–112] with average half-lives of 3 to 4 hours and 6 to 10 hours, respectively. These variations in clearance reflect the changing dosage requirements for theophylline with age. After birth, the rate of enzyme maturation seems to be quicker with phenytoin and phenobarbital than with the methylxanthines. Body clearance for phenytoin actually surpasses adult values by age 2 weeks,[40,113] whereas theophylline clearance is still deficient at 2 to 3 months.[108,109] The clearance of propofol also appears to be increased in children compared with adults, and larger maintenance doses may be required.[43] This latter drug is not recommended for use in children less than 2 years of age.

Differences may also arise between adults and children in their order of preference for the phase 1 pathway. In step one of its metabolism, phenobarbital was found to be hydroxylated in the same proportion in the newborn as in the adult, but the phase 2 step of glucuronidation was deficient in the former.[100] On the other hand, the hydroxylation of phenytoin may be depressed at birth.[3] The rate of diazepam metabolism is lower in the premature than in the full-term infant, with hydroxylation and conjugation being more limited than demethylation.[114] For theophylline, N-demethylation, which is the phase 1 pathway in the adult, is deficient in the newborn.[115] Instead, the neonate methylates it (phase 2) to produce the active metabolite, caffeine.

Other Phase 1 Reactions

Some phase 1 reactions are not catalyzed by microsomal enzymes. Most of these occur in the liver but may also occur elsewhere, such as in the gut and blood. Dehydrogenation of alcohol by alcohol dehydrogenase (ADH) is a nonmicrosomal activity that was studied in humans.[116] Liver ADH was detected in 2-month-old fetuses, but the activity was no more than 2% to 4% that of the adult. Adult activity is reached around 5 years,[116] although there is considerable variation in the activity of ADH between adults. Certain elixirs may have a high alcohol content (e.g., phenobarbital), and these should be avoided, if possible, in the neonate.

Catalysis of hydrolysis by a group of nonspecific esterases can occur in blood, liver, and tissues.[75] They cleave esters and amide bonds in aspirin, succinylcholine, procaine, procainamide, and meperidine. Infants less than 6 months of age have less than half the adult level of esterases. The clearance of anesthetics by esterases may be prolonged in the newborn, but there is no evidence that this is clinically significant.[93] To date, there is no documentation of decreased clearance by esterases of the neuromuscular blockers (NMBs), succinylcholine and mivacuronium, in infants.[117] Vecuronium clearance is decreased in the infant, but this NMB is not metabolized by esterases. Instead, it is mostly excreted unchanged in the bile and urine. On the other hand, infants clear atracurium, which is only partially degraded by esterases, faster than the older child and adult. Various blood esterases reach adult levels by approximately 10 to 12 months of age.[47,52] An important exception is glucuronidase. This esterase is located in the gut and is responsible for deconjugation of drugs and bilirubin excreted into the bile, thus promoting their reabsorption.[76] Kendall et al.[118] noted the activity of glucuronidase to be 7 times that of the adult in the first 4 days after birth. This promotes enterohepatic cycling,[54] prolonging the action of drugs, such as indomethacin, and it may contribute to the hyperbilirubinemia seen in the neonate.

Phase Two Reactions
Glucuronidation

Substances that undergo conjugation become more polar and thus are easily excreted by the kidney.[76] The conjugation reactions include glucuronidation, acetylation, sulfation, and methylation, and conjugation with glutathione and other amino acids. Of these, **glucuronidation** is the most important because of its versatility with respect to multiple substrates, the large quantities formed in a variety of tissues, and the generally inactivating function of the reaction. UDP-GT microsomal enzymes catalyze glucuronidation, while nonmicrosomal enzymes catalyze remaining conjugations.[76] At birth, the ability to glucuronidate drugs is low. The classic example of decreased glucuronidation in the newborn is the excretion of bilirubin. Significantly prolonged half-lives have been reported for bilirubin in infants up to 30 days old, compared with children 4 months to 2 years of age.[54] It must be remembered, however, that decreased glucuronidation is not the only factor that figures in the elimination of bilirubin, because hepatic uptake and secretion into the bile are also involved. The capacity to glucuronidate increases rapidly after birth,[119] and 1-month- to 3-year-olds can adequately glucuronidate some substrates.[1] For other drugs (e.g., acetaminophen), however, adult activity may not be reached till age 12 years.[120] There may be considerable variation, depending on exposure to inducers, the substrate involved, and other variables. Children compensate for the decreased glucuronidation of acetaminophen[121] and morphine by increasing the rate of sulfation, and the overall half-life remains unchanged compared

with that of the adult. Thus, there seems to be considerable variation in the rate at which glucuronidation reaches adult values. This depends on the UDP-GT enzyme, the substrates, the presence of inducers, and the individual. Drugs that the adult customarily glucuronidates are morphine, benzodiazepines, acetaminophen, salicylamide, chloramphenicol, phenobarbital, and phenytoin.[1,40,74] As a corollary, evidence exists that morphine-6-glucuronide is an active metabolite.[122]

Other Conjugation Reactions

The remainder of the conjugation reactions are not catalyzed by the microsomal system. In the newborn, sulfation is more efficient than that seen in adults,[120,123] providing an alternative for the deficiency in glucuronidation.[121] **Methylation** by catechol-O-methyltransferase inactivates the endogenous transmitters, epinephrine, norepinephrine, and histamine. In the neonate, theophylline is **preferentially methylated** to caffeine, as the ability to N-demethylate it, as in the adult, is reduced.[4] Conjugation with **glutathione** to form a mercapturate derivative is not very important, but it does contribute to the inactivation of toxic intermediate epoxides mentioned earlier. One exploits this pathway in acetaminophen poisonings by using thiols (e.g., N-acetyl-cysteine) to increase glutathione conjugation with the toxic metabolite, a quinone. Aromatic carboxylic acids, such as salicylic acid, may be inactivated by conjugation with **glycine,** and this process appears deficient at birth.[39,124] **Acetylation** involves conjugation, with acetyl coenzyme A as the donor, and several N-acetyl transferases. These enzymes appear to represent multiple genes because genetic polymorphism (slow or fast acetylation by different individuals) is exhibited only to some substrates, such as isoniazid, hydralazine, and sulfas. Monomorphic acetylation, purportedly, is more prominent in newborn infants than in older children.[76]

Overall, glucuronidation is the most important phase 2 reaction and is catalyzed by microsomal enzymes, unlike the other conjugation reactions. It is depressed at birth and reaches maturity at 1 month to 3 years, depending on the substrate, but may take longer for drugs such as acetaminophen. Glucuronidation reaction rates will increase if there is exposure to inducers. The neonate's ability to sulfate drugs surpasses that of the adult, and the methylation and acetylation pathways are also well developed. In conclusion, most hepatic biotransformation enzymes do not reach adult levels until after birth,[76] but a few are more active prenatally (glutathione transferase, some UDP-GT) and postnatally (sulfation, glucuronidase) than in adults.

The Effect of Development on Renal Excretion

Drug metabolism and renal excretion cooperate in an effort to rid the body of the foreign material as soon as possible. These two processes develop at different rates in the first few months, and drug therapy needs to be modified during this period. Renal excretion depends on glomerular filtration, tubular reabsorption, and tubular secretion as well as renal plasma flow and the extent of drug protein binding.[125,126] In the newborn, all aspects of renal function are reduced.[127,128] In this section, we will discuss the developmental aspects of renal function.

Ontogeny of Renal Function
Glomerular Filtration Rate and Excretion of Drugs

The two factors that mainly condition the development of renal function are gestational age (GA) and renal plasma flow (RPF).[2] RPF is reduced in the neonate, secondary to a decreased cardiac output and an increased peripheral vascular resistance. At birth, RPF is 12 ml/min and increases to 140 ml/min at 1 year of age.[129,130] The glomerular filtration rate (GFR) is also reduced at birth, and its development is age-related, being directly so to postconceptual age (PCA).[128,131,132] However, prior to 34 weeks' gestation, there is no such direct relationship with GA, and the GFR is constantly low at 0.45 ml/min[131] (Fig. 48-2). After 34 weeks PCA, there is a rapid increase in function.[133,134] At birth, the full-term infant has a GFR of about 2 to 4 ml/min,[131] and there is a marked increase to 8 to 20 ml/min after 2 to 3 days. In contrast, the premature infant has a much lower GFR of 1 ml/min at birth and only increases 2 to 3 ml/min over the same period.[128,134,135] Therefore, this rapid improvement, seen in the first week of life in the full-term infant, is not evident in the premature neonate. In the full-term newborn, this increase in the first week postnatally is most likely secondary to an increased cardiac output, decreased peripheral and renal vascular resistances, and greater surface area for filtration.[1,2] Adult values for GFR are reached at age 2.5 to 5.0 months in normal infants[129] but may take at least 9 months in very-low-birth-weight babies.[132] These trends in developing renal function have a great impact on drug therapy. The aminoglycosides are excreted almost entirely by GFR, and their urinary excretion is closely related to the maturation of GFR.[136–138] Not surprisingly, renal clearance for aminoglycosides has been found to correlate with PCA,[139,140] as does the elimination half-life.[139,141–145] Gentamicin half-lives in the range of 8 hours for babies less than 34 weeks PCA, 6.5 hours for 35 to 37 weeks, and 5 hours for term infants over 37 weeks have been reported.[143,145] Therefore, the dosage interval should be increased to every 18 hours in premature infants less than 34 weeks of age and every 12 hours in the neonate greater than 34 weeks of age. Most of the literature on aminoglycosides is concerned with the neonate, and information is sparse on the older infant and child. It is recommended that serum concentrations and plasma creatinine (as a measure of GFR) be monitored to appropriately adjust therapy.

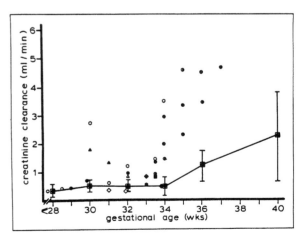

Figure 48-2. Increase in creatinine clearance with GA (gestational + postnatal ages). Infants studied at birth were grouped for GA and are represented by mean values ± 1SD connected by the solid line. Infants studied during extrauterine life are represented by a mass plot of data with GA, in which studies from one infant at different ages are indicated by the same symbol. (From BS Arant. Developmental patterns of renal functional maturation compared in the human neonate. *J Pediatr* 92(5):705–712, 1978. With permission.)

Tubular Function and Excretion of Drugs

Renal tubular function is another important factor governing renal excretion. Certain substances appear to be limited by a transport maximum (Tm), and so measurement of the Tm of these substances has been used as an index of tubular function: the Tm of glucose (TmG) as a measurement of reabsorption and the Tm of para-amino-hippurate (TmPAH) as a measurement of secretion.[146] Tubular secretion is depressed at birth and seems to mature more slowly than GFR after birth. Using PAH, West et al.[129] found a tenfold increase in tubular secretion in the first year of life, going on to reach adult levels at 7.5 months of age. This is similar to the data of Gladtke and Heimann.[147] The depressed function is probably due to decreased blood flow to peritubular regions, immaturity of cellular energy supply processes,[130] and the small mass and size of the tubular cells.[2] The development of tubular secretion may be further complicated by the phenomenon of substrate stimulation, whereby a substrate stimulates its own or another's secretion into the tubules. This has been noted in animals[148–152] and probably occurs in humans.[153,154] The penicillins and phenobarbital have been shown to stimulate tubular secretion. The tubule's capacity to reabsorb also seems limited in the newborn. However, it may be because glucose transport, which is a measure of it, appears to be a function of proximal sodium reabsorption[155]; that is, when the fraction of Na^+ reabsorbed is large, the ratio of TmG-GFR—a more accurate measure of reabsorption—is large and vice versa. Although it is not clear if the TmG-GFR is reduced in the neonate as a result either of a decreased intrinsic capacity of the tubule or in consort with an associated reduction in sodium reabsorption,[156–158] Arant's work implies that, generally, in infants of less than 34 weeks' gestation, the reduced tubular reabsorption of glucose is indeed a reflection of decreased tubular transport capacity[131] (see Fig. 48-2).

For renal excretion, many drugs rely on the organic anion or cation transport systems involved in tubular secretion. The penicillins are actively secreted via the PAH pathway and their elimination half-lives vary inversely with gestational and postnatal age. The elimination half-life for the penicillins may vary considerably but generally hover around 1 to 2 hours by 2 weeks' postnatal age.[159–161] Ampicillin clearance is reduced at birth but increases rapidly during the first week of life, the increased clearance being parallel to that of PAH.[162] Axline et al.[163] found that the serum half-life declined rapidly during the first 2 weeks of postnatal life, that the change was less marked from 2 to 4 weeks, and that there was no further decline beyond 1 month of age. This decrease in half-life for ampicillin and other penicillins may actually be a result of substrate stimulation, as mentioned earlier. Schwartz et al.[154] reported a case in which they were unable to maintain dicloxacillin levels in a neonate once parenteral penicillin was started, and it may be that penicillin stimulated the secretion of dicloxacillin. There are other reports supporting this belief.[148–150,153] The diuretic furosemide is both filtered and secreted into the tubule and thus can reach its site of action in the tubules. Only the free drug can be secreted, however, and the high protein binding of the drug may render it less available for this purpose. The general practice of administering albumin before furosemide to promote a diuresis is of interest, as one may speculate that it may in fact reduce the amount secreted into the tubule and thus the amount reaching the receptor.[164] In addition, reabsorption of drugs will also be affected by urinary pH, where a decreased pH would favor the reabsorption of acidic drugs and vice versa.

Pharmacodynamics

Use of Diuretics in the Developing Patient

There are many differences between the mature and immature kidney: In the neonate, the GFR is lower, and the effective tubular reabsorption and secretion are also lower. The fractional tubular reabsorption of sodium appears to be the same in the adult as in the neonate during nondiuresis[146]; it is reduced, however, in a proximal diuresis.[157] Therefore, the neonate loses more sodium than does the adult with an osmotic load. Because the absolute amount being filtered is small, a distal diuresis might be less effective in the neonate than in the adult.[146] The neonate cannot excrete a sodium load and becomes fluid overloaded and edematous. In this situation, the adult increases the GFR and decreases proximal and distal reabsorption to get rid of extra sodium and water. The neonate, likewise, increases the GFR and decreases proximal reabsorption of sodium but, unlike the adult, appears to increase distal reabsorption.[146,165,166] It is felt that this is the major defect in the young patient's ability to handle a sodium load. Regarding a water load, the neonate's response is impaired because of the low GFR, in spite of the fact that she can dilute her urine to 50 mosm/liter,[167–169] as can the adult. Adult capacity to excrete a water load is reached by 1 month of age. On the other hand, the newborn's inability to recycle urea to create and maintain a medullary osmotic gradient means that he cannot concentrate the urine maximally during water deprivation. The adult can concentrate the urine up to 1400 mosm/liter, whereas the newborn can only manage to do so up to 600 to 700 mosm/liter.[167,170–173] Other factors that may result in a decreased response in the infant to diuretics include a reduced carbonic anhydrase activity, decreased Na/K ATPase, lack of substrate delivery to the distal nephron, hyperaldosteronism, and decreased levels and/or response to ADH.[146,174] Surprisingly though, both the loop diuretics and the thiazides, especially the former, are quite effective in the newborn.

Use of Catacholamines in the Developing Patient

The neonate may respond to catacholamine inotropic agents differently than the mature patient in both cardiovascular and renal terms. The physiologic aspects responsible for the myocardial pharmacodynamics peculiar to the neonate are several. Even though the sensitivity of myocardial adrenergic receptors is well developed at birth, receptor innervation by the sympathetic nervous system (SNS) is not complete.[175] This, in addition to decreased neural stores of norepinephrine (NE) would indicate decreased **inotropy** and a decreased response to the indirect NE-releasing effects of dopamine. On the other hand, there is decreased NE uptake in neonatal myocardium, resulting in increased sensitivity to exogenous NE and probably to the direct actions of dopamine, which is metabolized to NE, and to dobutamine, which has direct beta-1 activity. This latter effect opposes the decreased inotropy caused by an immature SNS. The immaturity of the SNS, however, weighs more heavily, and overall there is a decrease in inotropy that improves with age.[175] Furthermore, the neonatal myocardium is less compliant, curtailing the patient's ability to increase stroke volume and thus cardiac output. In spite of these limitations, the neonate probably demonstrates inotropy, albeit somewhat diminished, when placed on dopamine.[175]

Qualitatively, the response differs as well. Seri et al.[176] noted that the increase in dopamine-induced BP was not accompanied by an increase in heart rate in **preterm neonates**, suggesting the order of sensitivity to be different from that of the adult: Alpha-adrenergic (vasoconstriction) and dopamine receptors appear more sensitive than beta-adrenergic receptors (heart rate). In fact, heart rate (HR) did not change in any group in this study. Urine output (UO) and natriuresis were maximized on 2 μg/kg/min dopamine in the first day of life, provided BP was normal.[176] Increasing the dose to 4 μg/kg/min further increased BP and GFR, but UO and natriuresis remained similar. Such findings demonstrate independent tubular effects of dopamine: inhibition of Na/K ATPase along the nephron and of Na/H exchange proximally as well as a urea washout phenomenon due to enhanced medullary blood flow. It was also noted in this study that the preterm neonate has immature cerebral bloodflow (CBF) autoregulation, and thus CBF may be sensitive to changes in systemic BP induced by dopamine.[176] This is of concern in regard to the etiology of intraventricular hemorrhage. In summary, Seri et al. suggest that the hypotensive and/or oliguric preterm infant be started at 2 μg/kg/min dopamine, as the preterm appears (1) to have an enhanced pressor response, (2) to be responsive to the renal effects at low doses, and (3) to be sensitive to dopamine-induced BP changes as autoregulation of CBF is impaired. They also showed that preterms have a reduced dopamine clearance and may require lower doses to produce similar SDCs.

In contrast, the sick **term** baby may tolerate much higher doses (up to 20 μg/kg/min), if necessary, without adversely affecting UO or HR.[177] Outwater et al.[178] showed a similar tolerance to high dopamine doses in six infants following repair of cardiac defects. Dobutamine may also be used in neonates as an inotrope, but in hypotensive babies, dopamine was more effective at increasing mean arterial pressure (MAP).[179]

In **older children** (1.5–15.0 yr), cardiac index (CI) seems to be the most sensitive parameter in response to catacholamines, with BP next, and HR being the most resistant to change.[180] Renal effects are also seen at lower doses. Girardin found no increase in HR or BP at 2.5 or 5.0 μg/kg/min, whereas CO, GFR, and urinary Na excretion increased at 5 but not 2 μg/kg/min. Finally, Berg et al.[181] studied the pharmacodynamics of dobutamine in children 2 months to 14 years of age and summarized the findings as follows: (1) There is a long linear dose-response curve—as the dose is increased, the response increases in proportion, although this proportionate rise will vary a lot between subjects; (2) a threshold concentration exists, and there is a wide variation between patients with respect to its value (one may get a response with a dose as low as 0.5 μg/kg/min dobutamine in some patients); and (3) the threshold differs for different parameters, with CI being more sensitive than BP or HR.

Use of Other Drugs in the Developing Patient

Both pharmacokinetic and pharmacodynamic reasons may be responsible for the increased risk of respiratory depression (RD) seen in infants less than 3 months of age who are receiving fentanyl and morphine.[182,183] Morphine clearance is decreased in the neonate and may contribute to this phenomenon; however, 1-month-old infants have increased morphine clearance and are still at greater risk of depression.[184] Pharmacodynamic considerations probably account for this and would include immature blood-brain barrier, decreased CNS myelinization (not mature until 18 months after birth),[93] increased CBF, altered protein binding, and differences in respiratory control mechanisms. Extremely prolonged RD can occur in newborns after fentanyl anesthesia, and serum drug concentrations must be lower in the neonate before extubation can be achieved.[185] Preliminary studies suggest that at 3 to 6 months, healthy infants have risks of RD comparable to that of the adult. Experience with sufentanil is limited in the neonate. A recent study reports its safety.[186] In contrast to neonates, older children may be less sensitive in this regard, as the apnea associated with propofol use in these patients is less than that seen in adults.[43]

References

1. Besunder JB, Reed MD, Blumer JL. Principles of drug 1 biodisposition in the neonate. Part 1. *Clin Pharmacokinet* 14:199–216, 1988.
2. Morselli PL, Franco-Morselli R, Bossi L. Clinical pharmacokinetics in newborns and infants. Age-related differences and therapeutic implications. *Clin Pharmacokinet* 5:485–527, 1980.
3. Morselli PL. Clinical pharmacokinetics in neonates. *Clin Pharmacokinet* 1:81–98, 1976.
4. Milsap RL, Szefler SJ. Special pharmacokinetic considerations in children. In WE Evans, Schentag JJ, Jusko WJ (eds): *Applied Pharmacokinetics* (2nd ed). Spokane: Applied Therapeutics, 1986. Pp 294–330.
5. Heimann G. Enteral absorption and bioavailability in children in relation to age. *Eur J Clin Pharmacol* 18:43–50, 1980.
6. Huang NN, High RH. Comparison of serum levels following the administration of oral and parenteral preparations of penicillin to infants and children of various age groups. *J Pediatr* 42:657–668, 1953.
7. O'Connor WJ et al. Serum concentrations of sodium nafcillin in infants during the perinatal period. *Antimicrob Agents Chemother* 5:220–222, 1965.
8. Silverio J, Poole JW. Serum concentrations of ampicillin in newborn infants after oral administration. *Pediatrics* 51:578–580, 1973.
9. Wallin A, Jalling B, Boreus LO. Plasma concentrations of phenobarbital in the neonate during prophylaxis for neonatal hyperbilirubinemia. *J Pediatr* 85:392–398, 1974.
10. Jalling B et al. Plasma concentrations of diphenylhydantoin in young infants. *Pharmacol Clin* 2:200–202, 1970.
11. Levy G et al. Pharmacokinetics of acetaminophen in the human neonate: Formation of acetaminophen glucuronide and sulfate in relation to plasma bilirubin concentrations and d-glucaric acid excretion. *Pediatrics* 55:818–825, 1975.
12. Jusko WJ et al. Riboflavin absorption and excretion in the neonate. *Pediatrics* 45:945–949, 1970.
13. Cavell B. Gastric emptying in preterm infants. *Acta Paediatr Scand* 68:725–730, 1979.
14. Siegel M, Lebenthal E, Krantz B. Effect of caloric density on gastric emptying in premature infants. *J Pediatr* 104:118–122, 1984.
15. Gupta M, Brans YW. Gastric retention in neonates. *Pediatrics* 62:26–29, 1978.
16. Friesen RH, Lockhart CH. Oral transmucosal fentanyl citrate for preanesthetic medication of pediatric day surgery patients with and without droperidol as a prophylactic anti-emetic. *Anesthesiology* 76:46–51, 1992.
17. Fisher AP, Fung C, Hanna M. Absorption of buccal morphine. A comparison with slow-release morphine sulphate. *Anesthesia* 43:552–553, 1988.
18. Bell MDD et al. Buccal morphine—A new route for analgesia? *Lancet* 1:71–73, 1985.
19. Daya MR et al. Recurrent seizures following mucosal application of TAC. *Ann Emerg Med* 17:646–648, 1988.
20. Winter ME, Tozer TN. Phenytoin. In Evans WE, Schentag JJ, Jusko WJ (eds): *Applied Pharmacokinetics.* (2nd ed). Spokane: Applied Therapeutics, 1986. Pp 493–539.
21. Matsukura M et al. Bioavailability of phenobarbital by rectal administration. *Pediatr Pharmacol* 1:259, 1981.
22. Roberts RJ. Anticonvulsants. In Roberts RJ (ed): *Drug Therapy in Infants: Pharmacological Principles and Clinical Experiences.* Philadelphia: Saunders, 1984. Pp 94–118.
23. Cote CJ. Sedation for the pediatric patient. *Pediatr Clin North Am* 41:31–57, 1994.
24. Hernandez A et al. Pharmacodynamics of H3-digoxin in infants. *Pediatrics* 44:418–428, 1969.
25. Roberts RJ. Antimicrobial agents. In Roberts RJ (ed): *Drug Therapy in Infants: Pharmacologic Principles and Clinical Experience.* Philadelphia: Saunders, 1984. Pp 39–93.
26. Ritchie JM, Greene NM. Local anesthetics. In Gilman A et al (eds): *The Pharmacological Basis of Therapeutics* (8th ed). New York: Pergamon, 1990. Pp 311–331.
27. Littrell RA. Epidural analgesia. *Am J Hosp Pharm* 48:2460–2474, 1991.
28. Pediatric Acute Pain Service. Guidelines for postoperative analgesia in pediatric patients. Boston: Massachusetts General Hospital. Unpublished data, 1994.
29. Lester RS. Topical formulary for the pediatrician. *Pediatr Clin North Am* 30:749–765, 1983.
30. Wester RC et al. Percutaneous absorption of testosterone in the newborn rhesus monkey: Comparison to the adult. *Pediatr Res* 11:737–739, 1977.
31. Nachman RL, Esterly NB. Increased skin permeability in preterm infants. *J Pediatr* 79:628–632, 1971.
32. Weatherstone KB, Rasmussen LB, Erenberg A. Safety and efficacy of a topical anesthetic for neonatal circumcision. *Pediatrics* 92:710–714, 1993.
33. Clotz MA, Nahata MC. Clinical uses of fentanyl, sufentanil and alfentanil. *Clin Pharm* 10:581–593, 1991.
34. de Boer AG et al. Rectal drug administration: Clinical pharmacokinetic considerations. *Clin Pharmacokinet* 7:285–311, 1982.
35. Knudsen FU. Plasma-diazepam in infants after rectal administration in solution and by suppository. *Acta Paediatr Scand* 66:563–567, 1977.
36. Knudsen FU. Effective short term diazepam prophylaxis in febrile convulsions. *J Pediatr* 106:487–490, 1985.
37. Knudsen FU. Recurrence risk after febrile seizure and effect of short-term diazepam prophylaxis. *Arch Dis Child* 60:1045–1049, 1985.
38. Vadja FJ, Symington GR, Bladin PF. Rectal valproate in intractable status epilepticus. *Lancet* 1:359–360, 1977.
39. Boreus LO. Distribution. In Boreus LO (ed): *Principles of Pediatric Pharmacology.* New York: Churchill Livingstone, 1982. Pp 46–74.
40. Roberts RJ. Pharmacologic principles in therapeutics in infants. In Roberts RJ (ed): *Drug Therapy in Infants: Pharmacologic Principles and Clinical Experience.* Philadelphia: Saunders, 1984. Pp 3–12.
41. Friis-Hansen B. Body water compartments in children: Changes during growth and related changes in body composition. *Pediatrics* 28:169–181, 1961.
42. Friis-Hansen B. Body composition during growth: In vivo measurements and biochemical data correlated to differential anatomical growth. *Pediatrics* 47:264–274, 1971.
43. Larijani GE et al. Clinical pharmacology of propofol: An intravenous anesthetic agent. *Drug Intel Clin Pharm* 23:743–749, 1989.
44. Cockshott ID. The pharmacokinetics of propofol in the ICU patient. *J Drug Dev* 4(Suppl 3):29–36, 1991.
45. Piafsky KM. Disease-induced changes in the plasma binding of basic drugs. *Clin Pharmacokinet* 5:246–262, 1980.
46. Rane A, Wilson JT. Clinical pharmacokinetics in infants and children. *Clin Pharmacokinet* 1:2–24, 1976.
47. Echobion DJ, Stephens DS. Perinatal development of human blood esterases. *Clin Pharmacol Ther* 14:41–47, 1973.
48. Gitlin D, Boesman M. Serum alpha fetoprotein, albumin and gamma G-globulin in the human conceptus. *J Clin Invest* 45:1826–1838, 1966.
49. Hyvarinen M et al. Influence of gestational age on serum levels of alpha-1 fetoprotein, IgG globulin and albumin in newborn infants. *J Pediatr* 82:430–437, 1973.
50. Wood M, Wood AJJ. Changes in plasma drug binding and alpha 1-

acid glycoprotein in mother and newborn infant. *Clin Pharmacol Ther* 29:522–526, 1981.

51. Kurz H, Mauser-Ganshorn A, Stickel HH. Differences in the binding of drugs to plasma proteins from newborn and adult man. Part 1. *Eur J Clin Pharmacol* 11:463–467, 1977.

52. Windorfer A, Kuenzer W, Urbanek R. The influence of age on the activity of acetylsalicylic acid-esterase and protein-salicylate binding. *Eur J Clin Pharmacol* 7:227–231, 1971.

53. Kurz H, Michels H, Stickel HH. Differences in the binding of drugs to plasma proteins from newborn and adult man. Part 2. *Eur J Clin Pharmacol* 11:469–472, 1977.

54. Yaffe SJ, Juchau MR. Perinatal pharmacology. *Annu Rev Pharmacol* 14:219–238, 1974.

55. Ebbeson F, Nyboe J. Postnatal changes in the ability of plasma albumin to bind albumin. *Acta Paediatr Scand* 72:665–670, 1983.

56. Kapitulnik J et al. Increase in bilirubin-binding affinity of serum with age of infant. *J Pediatr* 86:442–445, 1975.

57. Piafsky KM, Mpamugo L. Dependence of neonatal drug binding on alpha 1-acid glycoprotein concentrations. *Clin Pharmacol Ther* 29:272, 1981.

58. Sjoqvist F, Borga O, Orme MLE. Fundamentals of clinical pharmacology. In Speight TM (ed): *Avery's Drug Treatment* (3rd ed). Auckland: ADIS Press, 1987. Pp 1–64.

59. Krasner J, Giacoia GP, Yaffe SJ. Drug-protein binding in the newborn infant. *Ann NY Acad Sci* 226:101–114, 1973.

60. Freedman Z et al. Cord blood fatty acid composition in infants and in their mothers during the third trimester. *J Pediatr* 92:461–466, 1978.

61. Thiessen H, Jacobsen J, Brodersen R. Displacement of albumin-bound bilirubin by fatty acids. *Acta Paediatr Scand* 61: 285–288, 1972.

62. Rudman D, Bixler TJ, DelRio AE. Effect of free fatty acids on binding of drugs by bovine serum albumin, by human serum albumin and by rabbit serum. *J Pharmacol Exp Ther* 176:261–272, 1971.

63. Fredholm BB, Rane A, Persson B. Diphenylhydantoin binding to proteins in plasma and its dependence on free fatty acid and bilirubin concentration in dogs and newborn infants. *Pediatr Res* 9:26–30, 1975.

64. Ehrnebo M et al. Age differences in drug binding by plasma proteins: Studies on human foetuses, neonates and adults. *Eur J Clin Pharmacol* 3:189–193, 1971.

65. Brodersen R. Bilirubin transport in the newborn infant, reviewed with relation to kernicterus. *J Pediatr* 96:349–356, 1980.

66. Cashore WJ. Bilirubin metabolism and toxicity in the newborn. In Polin RA, Fox WW (eds): *Fetal and Neonatal Physiology*. Philadelphia: Saunders, 1992. Pp 1160–1164.

67. Diamond I, Schmid R. Experimental bilirubin encephalopathy. The mode of entry of bilirubin-14C into the central nervous system. *J Clin Invest* 45:678, 1966.

68. Silverman WA et al. Difference in mortality rate and incidence of kernicterus among premature infants allotted to two prophylactic antibacterial regimens. *Pediatrics* 18:614, 1956.

69. Brodersen R. Free bilirubin in blood plasma of the newborn: Effects of albumin, fatty acids, pH, displacing drugs and phototherapy. In Stern L, Oh W, Friis-Hansen B (eds): *Intensive Care in the Newborn. II*. New York: Mason, 1978.

70. Stutman HR, Parker KM, Markj MI. Potential of moxalactam and other new antimicrobial agents for bilirubin-albumin displacement in neonates. *Pediatrics* 75:294–297, 1985.

71. Drew JH, Kitchen WH. The effect of maternally administered drugs on bilirubin concentrations in the newborn infant. *J Pediatr* 89: 657–661, 1976.

72. Steele RW, Kearns GL. Antimicrobial therapy for pediatrics. *Pediatr Clin North Am* 36:1321–1349, 1989.

73. Buchanan N. Drug-protein binding and protein energy malnutrition. *South Africa Med J* 52:733–737, 1977.

74. Chemtob S. Basic pharmacologic principles. In Polin RA, Fox WW (eds): *Fetal and Neonatal Physiology*. Philadelphia: Saunders, 1992. Pp 107–119.

75. Benet LZ, Mitchell JR, Sheiner LB. Pharmacokinetics: The dynamics of drug absorption, distribution and elimination. In Gilman A et al (eds): *The Pharmacological Basis of Therapeutics* (8th ed). New York: Pergamon, 1990. Pp 3–32.

76. Gregus Z, Klaasen CD. Hepatic disposition of xenobiotics during prenatal and early postnatal development. In Polin RA, Fox WW (eds): *Fetal and Neonatal Physiology*. Philadelphia: Saunders, 1992. Pp 1103–1122.

77. Yaffe SJ et al. Enhancement of glucuronide-conjugating capacity in a hyperbilirubinemic infant due to apparent enzyme induction by phenobarbital. *N Engl J Med* 275:1461–1466, 1966.

78. Wilson JT. Alteration of normal development of drug metabolism by injection of growth hormone. *Nature* 225:861–863, 1970.

79. Juchao MR, Pedersen MG. Drug biotransformation in the human fetal adrenal gland. *Life Sci* 12:193–204, 1973.

80. Soyka LF, Long RJ. In vitro inhibition of drug metabolism by metabolites of progesterone. *J Pharmacol Exp Ther* 182:320–321, 1972.

81. Trolle D. Phenobarbitone and neonatal icterus. *Lancet* 1:251–252, 1968.

82. Sereni F et al. Induction of drug metabolizing enzyme activities in the human fetus and in the newborn infant. *Enzyme* 15:318–329, 1973.

83. Mandelli M et al. Placental transfer of diazepam and its disposition in the newborn. *Clin Pharmacol Ther* 17:564–572, 1975.

84. Reynolds JW, Mirkin BL. Urinary corticosteroid and diphenylhydantoin metabolite patterns in neonates exposed to anticonvulsant drugs in utero. *Clin Pharmacol Ther* 14:891–897, 1973.

85. Horning MG et al. Detection of 5-(3,4-dihydroxy-1,5-cyclohexadien-1-yl)-5-diphenylhydantoin as a major metabolite of 5,5-diphenylhydantoin in the newborn human. *Anal Lett* 4:537–545, 1971.

86. Rane A. Urinary excretion of diphenylhydantoin metabolites in newborn infants. *J Pediatr* 85:543–545, 1974.

87. Hendeles L, Weinberger M. A "state of the art" review. *Pharmacotherapy* 3:2–44, 1983.

88. Szefler SJ et al. Rapid elimination of quinidine in pediatric patients. *Pediatrics* 70:370–375, 1982.

89. Levi AJ, Gatmaitan Z, Arias IM. Deficiency of hepatic organic anion-binding protein as a possible cause of non-haemolytic unconjugated hyperbilirubinaemia in the newborn. *Lancet* 2:139–140, 1969.

90. Levi AJ, Gatmaitan Z, Arias IM. Deficiency of hepatic amino binding protein, impaired organic anion uptake by liver and "physiological" jaundice in newborn monkeys. *N Engl J Med* 283:1136–1139, 1970.

91. Nitowsky HM, Matz L, Berzofsky JA. Studies on oxidative drug metabolism in the full-term newborn infant. *J Pediatr* 69:1139–1149, 1966.

92. Done AK. Developmental pharmacology. *Clin Pharmacol Ther* 5:432–479, 1964.

93. Yaster M, Maxwell LG. Pediatric regional anesthesia. *Anesthesiology* 70:324–338, 1989.

94. Aranda V et al. Pharmacokinetic aspects of theophylline in premature newborns. *N Engl J Med* 295:413–416, 1976.

95. Bory C et al. Metabolism of theophylline to caffeine in premature newborn infants. *J Pediatr* 94:988–993, 1979.

96. Crooks J et al. Pharmacokinetics of cefotaxime and desacetyl-cefotaxime in neonates. *J Antimicrob Chemother* 14(Suppl B):97–101, 1984.

97. Boreus LO, Jalling B, Wallin A. Plasma concentrations of phenobarbital in mother and child after combined prenatal and postnatal administration for prophylaxis of hyperbilirubinemia. *J Pediatr* 93:695–698, 1978.

98. Loughnan PM et al. Pharmacokinetic observations of phenytoin disposition in the newborn and young infant. *Arch Dis Child* 52:302–309, 1977.

99. Boreus LO, Jalling B, Kallberg N. Clinical pharmacology of phenobarbital in the neonatal period. In Morselli PL, Garattini S, Sereni F (eds): *Basic and Therapeutic Aspects of Perinatal Pharmacology*. New York: Raven, 1975. Pp 331–340.

100. Boreus LO, Jalling B, Kallberg N. Phenobarbital metabolism in

adults and in newborn infants. *Acta Paediatr Scand* 67:193–200, 1978.

101. Pitlick W, Painter M, Pippenger C. Phenobarbital pharmacokinetics in neonates. *Clin Pharmacol Ther* 23:346–350, 1978.

102. Painter MJ et al. Phenobarbital and diphenylhydantoin levels in neonates with seizures. *J Pediatr* 92:315–319, 1978.

103. Heimann G, Gladtke F. Pharmacokinetics of phenobarbital in childhood. *Eur J Clin Pharmacol* 12:305–310, 1977.

104. Jalling B. Plasma and cerebrospinal fluid concentrations of phenobarbital in infants given single doses. *Dev Med Child Neurol* 16:785–793, 1976.

105. Rossi LN, Nino LM, Principi N. Correlation between age and plasma level/dosage ratio for phenobarbital in infants and children. *Acta Paediatr Scand* 68:431–434, 1979.

106. Rane A et al. Plasma disappearance of transplacentally transferred diphenylhydantoin in the newborn studied by mass fragmentography. *Clin Pharmacol Ther* 15:39–45, 1974.

107. Giacoia G et al. Theophylline pharmacokinetics in premature infants with apnea. *J Pediatr* 89:829–832, 1976.

108. Nassif EG et al. Theophylline disposition in infancy. *J Pediatr* 98:158–161, 1981.

109. Rosen JP et al. Theophylline pharmacokinetics in the young infant. *Pediatrics* 64:248–251, 1979.

110. Hendeles L, Weinberger M, Bighley L. Disposition of theophylline after a single intravenous infusion of aminophylline. *Am Rev Respir Dis* 118:97–103, 1978.

111. Jusko WJ et al. Enhanced biotransformation of theophylline in marijuana and tobacco smokers. *Clin Pharmacol Ther* 24:405–410, 1978.

112. Wyatt R, Weinberger M, Hendeles L. Oral theophylline dosage for the management of chronic asthma. *J Pediatr* 92:125–130, 1978.

113. Bourgeois BFD, Dodson WE. Phenytoin elimination in newborns. *Neurology* 33:173–178, 1983.

114. Mandelli M, Tognoni G, Garattini S. Clinical pharmacokinetics of diazepam. *Clin Pharmacokinet* 3:72, 1978.

115. Bonati M et al. Theophylline metabolism during the first month of life and development. *Pediatr Res* 15:304–308, 1981.

116. Pikkarainen PH, Raiha NCR. Development of alcohol dehydrogenase activity in the human liver. *Pediatr Res* 1:165–168, 1967.

117. Gronert BJ, Brandom BW. Neuromuscular blocking drugs in infants and children. *Pediatr Clin North Am* 41:73–91, 1994.

118. Kendall SR, Thaler MM, Erickson RP. Intestinal development of lysosomal and microsomal beta-glucuronidase and bilirubin uridine diphosphoglucuronyl transferase in normal and jaundiced rats. *J Pediatr* 82:1013–1019, 1973.

119. Weiss CF, Glazko J, Weston JK. Chloramphenicol in the newborn infant. *N Engl J Med* 262:787–794, 1960.

120. Miller RP, Roberts RJ, Fischer LJ. Acetaminophen elimination kinetics in neonates, children and adults. *Clin Pharmacol Ther* 19:284–294, 1976.

121. Alam SN, Roberts RJ, Fischer LJ. Age-related differences in salicylamide and acetaminophen conjugation in man. *J Pediatr* 90:130–135, 1977.

122. Laizure SC. Consideration in morphine therapy. *Am J Hosp Pharm* 51:2042–2043, 1994.

123. Howie D, Adriaenssens PI, Prescott LF. Paracetamol metabolism following overdosage: Application of performance liquid chromatography. *J Pharm Pharmacol* 29:235–237, 1977.

124. Levy G, Garrettson LK. Kinetics of salicylate elimination by newborn infants of mothers who ingested aspirin before delivery. *Pediatrics* 53:201–210, 1974.

125. Whelton A. Antibiotic pharmacokinetics and clinical application in renal insufficiency. *Med Clin North Am* 66:267–281, 1982.

126. Bowman RH. Renal secretion of [35-S] furosemide and its depression by albumin binding. *Am J Physiol* 229:93, 1975.

127. Barnett HI et al. Influence of postnatal age on kidney function of premature infants. *Proc Soc Exp Biol Med* 69:55–67, 1948.

128. Leake RD, Trygstad CW. Glomerular filtration rate during the period of adaptation to extrauterine life. *Pediatr Res* 11:959, 1977.

129. West JR, Smith HW, Chassis H. Glomerular filtration rate, effective renal blood flow and maximal tubular excretory capacity in infancy. *J Pediatr* 32:10–18, 1948.

130. Calcagno PL, Rubin MI. Renal extraction of para amino hippurate in infants and children. *J Clin Invest* 42:1632–1639, 1963.

131. Arant BS Jr. Developmental patterns of renal functional maturation compared in the human neonate. *J Pediatr* 92:705–712, 1978.

132. Vanpee M et al. Renal function in very low birth weight infants: Normal maturity reached during early childhood. *J Pediatr* 121:784–788, 1992.

133. Siegel SR, Oh W. Renal function as a marker of human fetal maturation. *Acta Paediatr Scand* 65:481–485, 1976.

134. Leake RD, Trygstad CW, Oh W. Inulin clearance in the newborn infant: Relationship to gestational and postnatal age. *Pediatr Res* 10:759–762, 1976.

135. Guignard JP et al. Glomerular filtration rate in the first three weeks of life. *J Pediatr* 87:268–272, 1975.

136. McCracken GH, West NR, Horton LJ. Urinary excretion of gentamicin in the neonatal period. *J Infect Dis* 123:257–262, 1971.

137. Kafetzis DA et al. Pharmacokinetics of amikacin in infants and pre-school children. *Acta Paediatr Scand* 68:419–422, 1979.

138. Khan AJ et al. Amikacin pharmacokinetics in the therapy of childhood urinary tract infection. *Pediatrics* 58:873–876, 1976.

139. Landers S et al. Gentamicin disposition and effect on development of renal function in the very low birth weight infant. *Dev Pharmacol Ther* 7:285–302, 1984.

140. Kildoo C et al. Developmental pattern of gentamicin kinetics in very low birth weight (VLBW) sick infants. *Dev Pharmacol Ther* 7:345–356, 1984.

141. Arbeter AM et al. Tobramycin sulfate elimination in premature infants. *J Pediatr* 103:131–135, 1983.

142. Granati B et al. Clinical pharmacology of netilmicin in preterm and term newborn infants. *J Pediatr* 106:664–669, 1985.

143. Kasik JW et al. Postconceptual age and gentamicin elimination half life. *J Pediatr* 106:502–505, 1985.

144. Nahata MC et al. Tobramycin kinetics in newborn infants. *J Pediatr* 103:136–138, 1983.

145. Szefler SJ et al. Relationship of gentamicin serum concentrations to gestational age in preterm and term neonates. *J Pediatr* 97:312–315, 1980.

146. Loggie JMH, Kleinman LI, VanMaanen EF. Renal function and diuretic therapy in infants and children. Part 1. *J Pediatr* 86:485–496, 1975.

147. Gladtke E, Heimann G. The rate of development of elimination functions in kidney and liver of young infants. In Morselli PL, Garattini S, Sereni F (eds): *Basic and Therapeutic Aspects of Perinatal Pharmacology*. New York: Raven, 1975. Pp 393–403.

148. Hirsch GH, Hook JB. Maturation of renal organic acid transport: Substrate stimulation by penicillin. *Science* 165:909–910, 1969.

149. Hirsch GH, Hook JB. Stimulation of renal organic acid transport and protein synthesis by penicillin. *J Pharmacol Exp Ther* 174:152–158, 1970.

150. Hook JB, Hewitt WR. Development of mechanisms for drug excretion. *Am J Med* 62:497–506, 1977.

151. Bond JT, Bailie MD, Hook JB. Maturation of renal organic acid transport *in vivo*: Substrate stimulation by penicillin. *J Pharmacol Exp Ther* 199:25–31, 1976.

152. Rennick B, Hamilton B, Evans R. Development of renal tubular transports of TEA and PAH in the puppy and piglet. *Am J Physiol* 201:743–746, 1961.

153. Kaplan JM et al. Pharmacological studies in neonates given large doses of ampicillin. *J Pediatr* 84:571–577, 1974.

154. Schwartz GJ, Hegyi T, Spitzer A. Subtherapeutic dicloxacillin levels in a neonate: Possible mechanisms. *J Pediatr* 89:310–312, 1976.

155. Kurtzman NA et al. Relationship of sodium reabsorption and glomerular filtration rate to renal glucose reabsorption. *J Clin Invest* 51:127, 1972.

156. Baker JT, Kleinman LI. Glucose reabsorption in the newborn dog kidney. *Proc Soc Exp Biol Med* 142:716, 1973.
157. Baker JT, Kleinman LI. Renal glucose and sodium excretion in the newborn dog. *Pediatr Res* 7:412, 1973.
158. Baker JT, Kleinman LI. Relationship between glucose and sodium excretion in the newborn dog. *J Physiol* 243:45, 1974.
159. McCracken GH Jr et al. Clinical pharmacology of penicillin in newborn infants. *J Pediatr* 82:692–698, 1973.
160. Sarff LD et al. Clinical pharmacology of methicillin in neonates. *J Pediatr* 90:1005, 1977.
161. Nelson JD, Shelton S, Kusmiesz H. Clinical pharmacology of ticarcillin in the newborn infant: Relation to age, gestational age and weight. *J Pediatr* 87:474–479, 1975.
162. Boreus LO. Renal excretion. In Boreus LO (ed): *Principles of Pediatric Pharmacology.* New York: Churchill Livingstone, 1982. Pp 115–134.
163. Axline SG, Yaffe SJ, Simon HJ. Clinical pharmacology of antimicrobials in premature infants. II. Ampicillin, methicillin, oxacillin, neomycin and colistin. *Pediatrics* 39:97–107, 1967.
164. Bowman RH. Renal secretion of [35-S] furosemide and its depression by albumin binding. *Am J Physiol* 229:93, 1975.
165. Kleinman LI, Hsieh NN. Renal tubular response of the newborn dog to a sodium load. *Pediatr Res* 8:456, 1974.
166. Aperia A et al. Renal response to an oral sodium load in newborn fullterm infants. *Acta Paediatr Scand* 61:670, 1972.
167. Linshaw MA. Concentration and dilution of urine. In Polin RA, Fox WW (eds): *Fetal and Neonatal Physiology.* Philadelphia: Saunders, 1992. Pp 1239–1257.
168. Barnett HL et al. Renal water excretion in premature infants. *J Clin Invest* 31:1069, 1952.
169. McCance RA, Naylor NSB, Widdowson EM. The response of infants to a large dose of water. *Arch Dis Child* 29:104, 1954.
170. Dicker SE. Renal function in the newborn mammal. In Dicker SE (ed): *Mechanisms of Urine Concentration and Dilution in Mammals.* Baltimore: William & Wilkins, 1970. Pp 133.
171. Trimble ME. Renal response to solute loading in infant rats: Relation to anatomical development. *Am J Physiol* 219:1089, 1970.
172. Sakai F, Endov H. Postnatal development of urea concentration in the newborn rabbit's kidney. *Jpn J Pharmacol* 21:677, 1971.
173. Stanier MW. Development of intra-renal solute gradients in foetal and post-natal life. *Pflugers Arch* 336:263, 1972.
174. Loggie JMH, Kleinman MD, Van Maanen EF. Renal function and diuretic therapy in infants and children. Part 2. *J Pediatr* 86:657–669, 1975.
175. Bhatt-Mehta V, Nahata MC. Dopamine and dobutamine in pediatric therapy. *Pharmacotherapy* 9:303–314, 1989.
176. Seri I et al. Effects of low-dose dopamine infusion on cardiovascular and renal functions, cerebral blood flow and plasma catacholamine levels in sick preterm neonates. *Pediatr Res* 34:742–729, 1993.
177. Perez CA et al. Effect of high-dose dopamine on urine output in newborn infants. *Crit Care Med* 14:1045–1049, 1986.
178. Outwater KM et al. Renal and hemodynamic effects of dopamine in infants following cardiac surgery. *J Clin Anesth* 2:253–257, 1990.
179. Klarr JM et al. Randomized, blind trial of dopamine versus dobutamine for treatment of hypotension in preterm infants with respiratory distress syndrome. *J Pediatr* 125:117–122, 1994.
180. Girardin E et al. Effect of low dose dopamine on hemodynamic and renal function in children. *Pediatr Res* 26:200–203, 1989.
181. Berg RA, Donnerstein RL, Padbury JF. Dobutamine infusions in stable, critically ill children: Pharmacokinetics and hemodynamic actions. *Crit Care Med* 21:678–686, 1993.
182. Berde CB. Pediatric postoperative pain management. *Pediatr Clin North Am* 36:921–938, 1989.
183. Johnson KL et al. Fentanyl pharmacokinetics in the pediatric population. *Anesthesiology* 61:A441, 1984.
184. Lynn AM, Slattery JT. Morphine pharmacokinetics in early infancy. *Anesthesiology* 66:136–139, 1987.
185. Koehntop DE et al. Pharmacokinetics of fentanyl in neonates. *Anesth Analg* 65:227–232, 1986.
186. Seguin JH, Erenberg A, Leff RD. Safety and efficacy of sufentanil therapy in the ventilated infant. *Neonat Net* 13:37–40, 1994.

John H. Arnold

Charles B. Berde

⟨49⟩ Sedation and Pain Control

The goals of sedation in the intensive care unit (ICU) include (1) analgesia for painful diseases and procedures, (2) compliance with controlled ventilation and routine intensive care, and (3) amnesia for the period of sedation. The ideal agent would not have hemodynamic or pulmonary side effects and not be associated with the production or accumulation of toxic metabolites. It would also have a short duration of action and a high therapeutic index. The wide variety of medications and combinations of agents that have been employed suggests that no single agent meets this ideal.[1-5]

Concepts regarding pain perception and treatment in the neonate have been controversial,[6] and it is likely that postoperative pain is undertreated in children of all ages.[7] It is now broadly accepted that analgesia in the neonatal and pediatric populations has important psychological and physiologic impact.[8,9] However, there is not a large published experience with sedation for the pediatric population.[10] The use of opioid and non-opioid agents in the neonatal and pediatric intensive care settings has, therefore, been extrapolated largely from experience in adults[11-13] with little regard for the important physiologic and pharmacologic considerations in pediatric patients.

The following review highlights the mechanisms of action, pharmacokinetics, and pharmacodynamics of most sedating agents used in the neonatal and pediatric critical care setting and concludes with a discussion of the important side effects associated with sedation and strategies for avoiding these complications.

Opioids

The combination of an opioid with a benzodiazepine was the most common sedation regimen in a survey of adult ICUs,[4] and opioids are the most commonly used primary agents.[1-3] The virtues of opioids include minimal effects on myocardial performance, ablation of pulmonary vascular response to nociceptive stimuli, and preservation of hypoxic pulmonary vasoconstriction.[14-16] Furthermore, there is some evidence that infants with documented pulmonary artery hypertension and right-to-left shunting have improved outcomes with the use of fentanyl for sedation.[17] These features are desirable for sedating critically ill infants with systemic and pulmonary hemodynamic instability. The pharmacokinetic data for the family of opioids in adults are presented in summary form in Table 49-1; the available neonatal and pediatric pharmacokinetic data are analyzed in the following sections.

Morphine

Morphine is the most widely used opioid and is the standard with which new opioids are compared. Morphine produces dose-related analgesia, sedation, respiratory depression, and euphoria and may also produce nausea, diaphoresis, dry mouth, and pruritus, which is most pronounced on the face. Unlike the non-opioid analgesics (i.e., nonsteroidal antiinflammatory agents), morphine relieves visceral as well as somatic pain. Clinical experience suggests that administration of morphine prior to an anticipated nociceptive stimulus results in much more effective analgesia than when administered after the nociceptive stimulus has been applied. Morphine is well absorbed from intramuscular (IM) and subcutaneous injection sites.

Peak analgesic effect after intravenous (IV) administration occurs at 20 minutes, reflecting delayed penetration of the blood-brain barrier. The relatively high pKa, high degree of ionization at physiologic pH, and the relatively low lipid solubility account for this delayed central effect. Cerebral spinal fluid (CSF) concentrations peak 15 to 30 minutes after administration and decrease more slowly than plasma levels. Acidosis decreases the volume of distribution and prolongs the CNS half-life by more than 50%.[18] The lowest plasma concentration to provide effective analgesia intraoperatively is approximately 65 ng/ml and does not appear to vary with age.[19] Morphine undergoes extensive hepatic and extrahepatic glucuronidation, and metabolites are excreted principally in the urine. Prolonged respiratory depression has been observed in patients with renal failure who are receiving morphine.[20] This has been attributed to accumulation of morphine-6-glucuronide, a morphine metabolite previously thought to be inactive.[21-23]

Morphine is frequently used for postoperative analgesia and is the most commonly used opioid in the neonatal intensive care setting.[24] Morphine administered by continuous infusion appears to be superior to IV bolus or IM administration for the relief of postoperative pain and for the preservation of ventilatory drive in adults.[25] Morphine infusions in the pediatric population have been shown to be safe in postcardiac surgical patients at rates of 10 to 30 μg/kg/hr with effective analgesia and minimal effects on ventilation.[26] However, infants have demonstrated a wide variability in the clearance of morphine during the first 6 weeks of life.[27] Lynn and Slattery[28] demonstrated that infants less than 7 days of age have significantly lower clearance and greater elimination half-lives than older infants and tend to have a smaller volume of distribution. Furthermore, there is a report of two newborns sedated with a continuous morphine infusion who developed generalized seizures with documented high plasma morphine concentrations.[27]

The use of morphine in infants less than 2 months of age must be undertaken with recognition of the pharmacokinetic variability in this population (Table 49-2). In our hospital, nonintubated infants under 2 months of age are given morphine with great caution and in a setting that permits close observation and rapid intervention.

Morphine has cardiovascular effects that occasionally limit its usefulness in critically ill patients. Morphine stimulates the release

Table 49-1. Opioid dosage and pharmacokinetics (adult data)

	Relative dose	Vd (liter/kg)	t1/2β	Clearance (ml/kg/min)
Morphine	0.1 mg	3.2	114 min	14.7
Meperidine	1.0 mg	3.8	222 min	15.1
Methadone	0.1 mg	—	15 hr	—
Fentanyl	1–5 μg	4.1	202 min	11.6
Sufentanil	0.2–1.0 μg	1.7	156 min	12.7
Alfentanil	5–25 μg	0.9	84 min	6.4

Vd, volume of distribution; t, half-life time.
Data from Stoelting (P 76)[69] and Goodman et al. (P 519).[178]

Table 49-2. Morphine pharmacokinetics

Age	Vd (liter/kg)	t1/2β (hrs)	Clearance (ml/kg/min)
0–7 d	3.4	6.8	6.3
2 wk–2 mo	5.2	3.9	23.8
1–17 yr	3.1	2.2	23.4
Adults	3.2	2.0	14.7

Data from Lynn and Slattery,[28] Stanski et al.,[206] and Dahlstrom et al.[19]

of significant amounts of histamine and inhibits compensatory sympathetic nervous system responses. Like all potent opioids, morphine also induces central parasympathetic stimulation and may also directly depress the sinoatrial node. In supine, normovolemic patients, morphine causes little change in hemodynamics. Rapid administration of IV morphine to hypovolemic or upright patients, however, may provoke significant hypotension. Naloxone does not inhibit morphine-induced histamine release. Direct myocardial depression is not produced by morphine, even in large doses. However, the combination of morphine or any other opioid and potent volatile anesthetic agents, nitrous oxide, or benzodiazepines may produce cardiovascular depression in critically ill patients, which is not seen when these agents are administered alone.[29–31]

In the pediatric population, morphine is generally well tolerated by ventilated patients, provided they are not severely hypovolemic. In the spontaneously breathing patient, morphine can be administered safely by judicious dosing and recognition that the peak analgesic effect coincides with peak respiratory depressant effect.

Meperidine

Meperidine is a synthetic opioid of the phenylpiperidine class and is structurally similar to atropine, accounting for its mild vagolytic effect. Meperidine has approximately one tenth the analgesic potency of morphine, with a clinical duration of action of 2 to 4 hours after IM administration. Despite an early suggestion that meperidine may cause less respiratory depression than equianalgesic doses of morphine in the neonatal population,[32] it is not commonly used in the intensive care setting. Furthermore, experience in adults suggests that meperidine may, in fact, produce **more** respiratory depression than other opioid agonists.[33]

Normeperidine is the principal meperidine metabolite, has an elimination half-life of 15 to 40 hours, and appears to accumulate in patients with impaired renal function. Normeperidine is epileptogenic and may produce myoclonus and seizures during prolonged administration of meperidine.[34]

Meperidine has a vagolytic action not shared by the other potent opioids, and tachycardia rather than bradycardia is frequently seen. In addition, meperidine, unlike other commonly used opioids, is a myocardial depressant in high doses and is therefore relatively contraindicated in patients with hemodynamic instability. Given the potential cardiovascular and neurologic side effects, meperidine has limited usefulness in the management of critically ill patients.

Methadone

Methadone has undergone a recent revival owing to its potent analgesic effects, minimal hemodynamic side effects, and pro-

longed and predictable elimination half-life. Absorption after oral administration is reliable and produces serum levels approximately 50% to 70% of those seen after IV administration.

Methadone is roughly equipotent to morphine following a single IV dose. Metabolism occurs in the liver, with no active metabolites known. The elimination half-life is approximately 35 hours following IV administration in adults, and postoperative analgesia lasts as long as 24 hours following large intraoperative doses (20 mg IV). In adults, a direct correlation between age and elimination half-life, as well as a high degree of interindividual variability, has been noted.[35] In the only study available in the pediatric population, a correlation between age and pharmacokinetic parameters was not found.[36] The mean elimination half-life was 19.2 hours in this group of children and adolescents.

In children as well as adults, the duration of analgesia depends in part on the loading dose. If standard analgesic doses (e.g., 0.1 mg/kg) are used, analgesic duration is typically 3 to 4 hours until a steady state is achieved, generally after three doses. Thereafter, analgesia may be maintained for 6 to 12 hours between doses.

Because of the high degree of interindividual variability in clearance and duration of action, careful titration to clinical effect is the safest mode of administration. In equianalgesic doses, methadone has a side-effect profile similar to morphine, except that the sedative and euphoric properties of methadone may be less pronounced than those of morphine.

Fentanyl

Fentanyl is a synthetic phenylpiperidine with approximately 100 times the analgesic potency of morphine. The pKa of fentanyl is significantly lower than morphine, and its high lipid solubility provides a rapid onset of action, as well as a short duration of effect via rapid redistribution. Fentanyl is widely regarded as a short-acting agent, and this is true when used in small dosages, which are rapidly redistributed to peripheral compartments. The phenomenon of redistribution can be quantified by calculation of a redistribution half-life or t1/2α (Table 49-3) and is an important consideration when administering relatively lipid-soluble agents (fentanyl, alfentanil, midazolam, barbiturates). When used in larger doses (15–20 μg/kg) or over prolonged periods, fentanyl is, in fact, a long-acting agent by virtue of its relatively long elimination half-life (see Tables 49-1 and 49-3).

A second peak in plasma fentanyl concentration has been reported by many authors following IV bolus administration,[37–39] and this may explain the delayed respiratory depression seen after

Table 49-3. Fentanyl pharmacokinetics

	Vd (liter/kg)	t1/2α (min)	t1/2β (min)	Clearance (ml/kg/min)
0–7 d	4.7	—	234	19.5
7 d–3 mo	8.3	—	250	28.9
3–12 mo	2.8	3.0	105	27.4
1–5 yr	3.1	10.0	244	11.5
5–12 yr	1.9	3.8	208	7.1
12–41 yr	2.9	6.3	175	13.7

Data derived from McClain and Hug,[38] Koehntop et al.,[42] Baskoff and Stevenson,[207] Singleton et al.,[208] Johnson et al.,[209] Koren et al.,[210] and Gauntlett et al.,[211] with all patients undergoing abdominal procedures excluded.

intraoperative use of fentanyl in adults.[40] This same phenomenon has been described in neonates, and release of sequestered fentanyl from skeletal muscle or lung has been proposed to explain this observation. Maximal analgesic effects are seen at plasma concentrations greater than 25 to 30 ng/ml, and respiratory depression may be produced with plasma levels above 1 to 2 ng/ml.

Metabolism of fentanyl occurs almost exclusively in the liver, with very little unchanged drug excreted in the urine.[38] Clearance is therefore profoundly affected by hepatic blood flow,[41] which may be significantly altered during intraabdominal procedures.[42,43] Halothane has been shown to alter fentanyl pharmacokinetics,[44] presumably through changes in regional splanchnic blood flow.[45] In the neonatal population, the functional maturity of the cytochrome P450 pathways may change significantly in the first few weeks of life.[46] These factors may explain the wide pharmacokinetic variability seen in infants (see Table 49-3).

Calculated steady-state volumes of distribution may be larger in infants due to a greater percentage of body lipid or to age-related changes in plasma protein binding. Increased clearance rates may reflect either increased hepatic extraction or increased hepatic blood flow in infants.[47] Elimination half-life appears to be prolonged in infants less than 3 months of age, an important factor during repetitive dosing of fentanyl.

Fentanyl is widely used in the intensive care setting because of its limited hemodynamic effects and intermediate duration of action. Fentanyl as a sole anesthetic in doses of 30 to 50 μg/kg produces minimal hemodynamic change, even in critically ill premature infants,[14,48,49] and may have beneficial effects in patients with pulmonary hypertension.[15,17] Even in such large doses, fentanyl does not release histamine. Bradycardia is more commonly seen with fentanyl anesthesia than with morphine at equipotent doses.

Fentanyl at a dose of 1 to 5 μg/kg/hr by continuous infusion is reported to be a safe and effective sedation regimen in newborns,[9] and significant bradycardia does not occur in this dose range. We have noted, however, a high rate of apparent tolerance and subsequent evidence of opioid withdrawal in newborns who have been sedated with large doses of fentanyl (20–30 μg/kg/hr) for prolonged periods.[50] Sufentanil is a structural analogue of fentanyl that is significantly more potent, has a small volume of distribution relative to fentanyl, and an elimination half-life that is slightly shorter than fentanyl. The elimination half-life is significantly prolonged in neonates and infants,[51] however, and sufentanil offers no distinct advantage over fentanyl in the critical care setting.

Alfentanil

Alfentanil is the newest fentanyl analogue, with one fifth to one tenth the potency and approximately one third the duration of action of fentanyl. Alfentanil has a very low pKa, with roughly 90% of the drug in the nonionized form at physiologic pH. The high degree of lipid solubility explains its rapid redistribution and short duration of action. The redistribution half-life of alfentanil is comparable to thiopental and fentanyl, but unlike those compounds, there is not a cumulative effect with prolonged administration.

Alfentanil is metabolized in the liver via pathways identical to those described for sufentanil, and no active metabolites have been identified. The elimination half-life is significantly prolonged in patients with hepatic dysfunction,[52] and the plasma free fraction also appears to be increased in these patients. These effects may account for the exaggerated and prolonged drug action seen in these patients.

The volume of distribution is small relative to fentanyl because of extensive protein binding, and the elimination half-life is significantly shorter than any of the currently available opioids (see Table 49-1). A high degree of interpatient variability has been seen in all pharmacokinetic studies of alfentanil, however.[53]

A pharmacokinetic study in children confirmed this variability in the pediatric population and noted that there appears to be a trend toward more rapid clearance in patients less than 1 year of age.[54] This finding has been confirmed[55] and may be attributed to both increased hepatic blood flow and increased hepatic microsomal activity in this age group (Table 49-4). There are no data available for infants less than 2 months of age. As alfentanil undergoes hepatic biotransformation by the same pathways as sufentanil, it is likely that there is similar prolongation of alfentanil elimination in infants less than 2 months of age. The significantly smaller Vd in children than in adults is likely due to age-related changes in body composition rather than differences in protein binding.[56]

The pharmacologic and pharmacodynamic effects of alfentanil are equivalent, implying that a gradient across the blood-brain barrier and drug sequestration in the CNS are not important, even during prolonged alfentanil administration. The extensive hepatic biotransformation and the absence of cumulative drug effects[57] make this a potentially useful drug in the intensive care setting. Like fentanyl and sufentanil, alfentanil may produce bradycardia when administered in large bolus doses. However, several studies in the adult literature document the hemodynamic stability, effective analgesia, and potent sedation offered by alfentanil in the intensive care setting.[58,59]

After a loading dose of alfentanil (15–25 μg/kg over 60 seconds), an infusion rate of 0.4 to 2.5 μg/kg/min appears to produce adequate sedation for ventilation without bradycardia or hypotension.[60] Supplementation with benzodiazepines appears to improve hemodynamic control and provide additional sedation while ensuring amnesia. Prolonged awakening and significant respiratory depression have not been reported despite infusion periods as long as 49 days, although there have been reports of unexplained prolongation of alfentanil elimination in patients without hepatic dysfunction.[58,61] Interestingly, even patients treated for periods longer than 14 days did not appear to develop tolerance or dependence.[60]

There is limited published experience with alfentanil for sedation in children. In a pediatric intensive care setting, where sedation is required for periods of hours, days, or weeks, it is usually inappropriate to use an agent as short-acting as alfentanil. It may have use when intensive analgesia is required for brief painful procedures, such as dressing changes, lumbar puncture, or bone marrow aspiration.

Benzodiazepines

The benzodiazepines have a variety of desirable clinical effects, which include hypnosis, anxiolysis, anticonvulsant activity, antero-

Table 49-4. Alfentanil pharmacokinetics

Age	Vd (liter/kg)	t1/2α (min)	t1/2β (min)	Clearance (ml/kg/min)
2–12 mo	0.6	12.6	76.2	8.4
1–14 yr	0.4	12.4	84.0	7.7
Adults	1.0	9.4	93.7	7.6

Data from Goresky et al.[54] and Bovill et al.[212]

grade amnesia, and muscle relaxation. The amnestic properties of the benzodiazepines may well be affected by the anxiety level of the patient prior to administration,[62] and the administration of benzodiazepines in the presence of a painful stimulus may produce hyperalgesia and agitation.[63] These problems are generally not seen when benzodiazepines are combined with opioids.

Diazepam

Diazepam has been the most widely used drug in this class and is the standard with which new benzodiazepines are compared. Diazepam is not water-soluble and must be dissolved in an organic solvent for parenteral use. IV administration and IM administration are limited by pain on injection due to the organic diluent. A less irritating lipid emulsion preparation of diazepam for IV use is now available.

The high degree of lipid solubility explains rapid distribution to the CNS and rapid onset of action. The drug is extensively protein bound, and volume of distribution may be greatly increased in patients with hypoalbuminemia. Metabolism occurs principally in the liver, with the production of an active metabolite, desmethyldiazepam, via oxidative pathways. Prolonged sedation following administration of diazepam has been attributed to enterohepatic recirculation of diazepam and to the accumulation of desmethyldiazepam.[64] The elimination half-life of diazepam is 21 to 37 hours, and desmethyldiazepam has an elimination half-life of 48 to 96 hours. These half-lives may be prolonged up to fivefold in patients with hepatic dysfunction. Obesity and aging further contribute to prolonged elimination by increasing the volume of distribution.

Diazepam does not typically produce significant respiratory depression in doses less than 0.2 mg/kg. However, there have been reports of apnea in this dose range,[65] and in larger doses there are clear effects on the carbon dioxide response curve.[66] It is well known that the combination of modest doses of diazepam with other respiratory depressants (e.g., alcohol, opiates, barbiturates) may produce profound respiratory depression, occasionally requiring airway intervention.

Diazepam was widely used as a primary sedating agent in the 1970s, but because of its long elimination half-life and the production of active metabolites, its use has been greatly reduced. Significant drug accumulation following prolonged administration makes this agent less desirable in the intensive care setting.[67]

Lorazepam

Lorazepam is 5 to 10 times more potent than diazepam and produces profound and prolonged anterograde amnesia. Oral administration results in reliable absorption, with maximal plasma concentrations in 2 to 4 hours. In doses of 0.05 mg/kg (maximum 4 mg), therapeutic levels may persist for 24 to 48 hours, with anterograde amnesia for up to 6 hours. Although lorazepam is water-insoluble, when combined with an organic solvent it is suitable for IM or IV injection, with much less tissue irritation than diazepam.[68] Lorazepam is glucuronidated by hepatic and extrahepatic conjugation to form pharmacologically inactive metabolites. The elimination half-life is 10 to 20 hours, but clinical effects may be prolonged due to pharmacodynamic differences from the other benzodiazepines. The metabolism of lorazepam is less likely to be affected by age or alteration in hepatic function than is that of diazepam. The cardiovascular and respiratory effects of lorazepam are very similar to those of diazepam. Lorazepam should be used judiciously for sedation in the intensive care setting because of prolonged effects on mental status and respiratory drive.

Midazolam

Midazolam is a shorter acting benzodiazepine that has become popular for sedation for brief procedures in adults and children. Midazolam is a water-soluble, fused imidazole ring with a pKa of 6.15 that is available in aqueous solution as the hydrochloride salt. At pH less than 4, the ring structure is open, which accounts for the hydrophilic properties of the parenteral preparation, and is buffered to a pH of 3.5. At physiologic pH, the ring is closed, and the compound becomes highly lipophilic.[69] Consequently, the incidence of thrombophlebitis and veno-irritation on injection is significantly lower than with other IV benzodiazepines (10% versus up to 39%)[70,71] and approaches the incidence found after injection of normal saline.[72]

Midazolam is hydroxylated via hepatic microsomal oxidation with the formation of one principal metabolite, 1-hydroxymidazolam. Glucuronidation of the 1-hydroxy, 4-hydroxy, and 1,4-dihydroxy metabolites occurs, and the conjugates are excreted in the urine. Unconjugated forms of the 1-hydroxy and 4-hydroxy metabolites are detectable and have some pharmacologic activity, though they are much less potent than the parent compound.[73]

After IV administration, midazolam has a very rapid onset owing to its high lipophilic properties and a short duration because of its rapid redistribution and high rate of clearance. There are limited pharmacokinetic data available, but most studies report significant interindividual variability in clearance rate and elimination half-life (Table 49-5). Midazolam is rapidly absorbed from the GI tract but undergoes extensive first-pass metabolism in the liver, producing wide variability in response to oral administration. Rectal administration requires 20 to 30 minutes to achieve adequate sedation, and the quality of sedation is inconsistent.[74] Intranasal administration of 0.2 mg/kg produces reliable sedation 5 to 10 minutes after administration.[75] Marked obesity increases the volume of distribution and prolongs the elimination half-life. Therefore, single doses should be based on total body weight, while continuous infusions should be calculated using ideal body weight.[76] Duration of effect is not altered significantly by renal failure.[77]

Table 49-5. Benzodiazepine dosage and pharmacokinetics (adult data)

	Relative dose (mg/kg)	t1/2α (min)	t1/2β (hr)	Vd (liter/kg)	Clearance (ml/kg/min)
Diazepam	0.30—0.50	30–60	21–37	1.0–1.5	0.2–0.5
Lorazepam	0.05	—	10–20	0.8–1.3	0.7–1.0
Midazolam	0.15–0.30	6–15	1–4	1.0–1.5	6–8

Data from C Prys-Roberts, CC Hug Jr (eds). *Pharmacokinetics of Anesthesia.* Oxford: Blackwell Scientific, 1984, Pp 157–186, and Stoelting (Pp 117–133).[69]

Midazolam has become very popular in the operating room and ICU because of its hemodynamic stability, rapid onset, and relative lack of accumulation when compared with other benzodiazepines. In addition, midazolam is a potent amnestic agent, producing reliable, dose-related, anterograde amnesia.

In adults, midazolam produces hemodynamic changes similar to thiopental when used as an anesthetic induction agent, with a greater decrease in BP and increase in heart rate than seen with diazepam.[72] Midazolam does reduce tidal volume in healthy volunteers[78] and reduces the ventilatory responsiveness to carbon dioxide.[79] Respiratory depression is clearly dose-related, and transient apnea may occur following rapid administration of large doses (>0.15 mg/kg), particularly in the presence of opioids.[80] Midazolam is said to be 2 to 3 times as potent as diazepam, based on demonstrated receptor affinity.[72,81] However, there is tremendous interindividual variation in clinical response,[72,82] and there are reports of respiratory arrest following administration of small doses to otherwise healthy patients.

Administration of midazolam by continuous infusion has been reported in adults requiring prolonged ventilation[83-85] and following coronary bypass surgery.[86] Midazolam infusion produced complete amnesia with hemodynamic stability but in all reports required an opioid supplement to provide analgesia. The imidazole ring structure, similar to that of etomidate, has raised concerns regarding adrenal axis suppression. Several studies, however, have documented the normal response of the adrenal axis during prolonged infusions.[83,85,87]

There are a number of reports of prolonged awakening following cessation of infusion, suggesting drug accumulation in critically ill patients with impaired hepatic function or reduced splanchnic perfusion.[85,86,88] In one study of adult patients receiving midazolam by continuous infusion, prolonged awakening was associated with high serum levels of 1-hydroxy-midazolam-glucuronide in a patient with impaired renal function.[89] Furthermore, pharmacokinetic variables were highly variable and not correlated with renal function or age.

There is limited published experience with midazolam in the pediatric population. Midazolam is an unreliable induction agent for anesthesia in premedicated pediatric patients in doses as high as 0.6 mg/kg,[90] and doses as high as 0.3 to 0.5 mg/kg are required for reliable sedation.[91] Pharmacokinetic studies in children reveal a wide range in clearance rate (6.7–11.2 ml/min/kg),[88] which is significantly greater than the range previously reported for adults (see Table 49-5). Likewise, elimination half-life was found to be shorter (1.4 hours) than the range found in adults.

Midazolam has been administered by continuous infusion without supplemental opioids to provide sedation for ventilation in pediatric patients.[92] The infusion rate varied from 0.1 to 1.2 μg/kg/min and produced reliable sedation. Tolerance and prolonged sedation were not noted in this small series despite continuous administration for up to 8 days. An acute withdrawal syndrome, characterized by confusion, hallucinations, and seizures, has been described in children requiring prolonged sedation with large doses of midazolam.[93–95]

In summary, midazolam is a potent hypnotic and amnestic agent with minimal hemodynamic effects. Although elimination may be unreliable in critically ill patients with altered renal and hepatic function, it is much more predictable than other benzodiazepines in this setting. By using incremental dosing and careful titration to clinical effect, midazolam is a valuable addition to the armamentarium of the ICU.

Flumazenil (Ro 15-1788)

Flumazenil (Ro 15-1788) is a specific benzodiazepine receptor antagonist that has been shown to rapidly reverse sedation and amnesia produced by the benzodiazepines.[96,97] There has been a report of an acute anxiety reaction to the administration of flumazenil,[96] but later studies have shown that careful titration of dosage to the appropriate clinical endpoint does not produce such effects.[97,98] Administration of flumazenil in incremental doses of 0.01 mg/kg produces prompt reversal of benzodiazepine-induced sedation without significantly increasing circulating stress hormones or producing clinically evident anxiety or dysphoria.[98] The relatively short elimination half-life of flumazenil (0.7–1.8 hours) may allow recurrence of sedation when large doses of long-acting benzodiazepines are antagonized.[99]

There has been limited experience with flumazenil in the ICU after prolonged benzodiazepine infusion. Niv and colleagues[63] reported that administration of flumazenil in incremental doses to adults sedated with midazolam by infusion for as long as 14 days produced no untoward hemodynamic or respiratory effects. They did not report on the incidence of anxiety reactions following this therapy. Recurrence of sedation within 1 hour of flumazenil administration has been described in patients sedated with large doses of midazolam, and these patients were successfully managed with a continuous infusion of flumazenil.[100] There is no published experience with flumazenil in the pediatric population.

Barbiturates

The barbiturates are all derivatives of the cyclic compound barbituric acid. Substitutions at the 2 and 5 carbon positions impart varying degrees of hypnotic, sedative, and anticonvulsant activity. The rapid onset and prompt recovery are explained by the high degree of lipid solubility and rapid redistribution to peripheral sites. The oxybarbiturates (methohexital, pentobarbital) are metabolized only by the liver, whereas the thiobarbiturates (thiopental) are metabolized in extrahepatic sites as well. Essentially, no unchanged drug is excreted in the urine, and elimination from the body depends primarily on hepatic oxidation.

The clearance rate of thiopental in pediatric patients is approximately twice as great as in adults (6.6 vs. 3.1 ml/kg/min), accounting for a greatly reduced elimination half-life (6 vs. 12 hours).[101] There do not appear to be differences in volumes of distribution or degree of protein binding between pediatric and adult patients.

The barbiturates have limited use in the ICU because of their prolonged elimination and cumulative effects. Thiopental and methohexital are frequently used for induction of anesthesia and are very effective for use during endotracheal intubation. Thiopental and pentobarbital have been commonly used for the acute and chronic management of head injury and intracranial hypertension, but recovery of consciousness may take up to 4 days after prolonged use.[102] Furthermore, head-trauma patients treated with high-dose barbiturates may have an increased incidence of sepsis and pulmonary complications,[103] and outcome is not altered in most instances.

Phencyclidines

Ketamine

Ketamine is a dissociative anesthetic that has been used as an induction agent for anesthesia, an analgesic for conscious sedation, a premedicant, and a sedative for critically ill patients. There is a broad range of experience with this agent, as well as a host of opinions regarding its usefulness in the anesthetic armamentarium.[104]

Ketamine is chemically related to phencyclidine, is water soluble as the hydrochloride salt, and exists in two enantiomeric forms, which differ in their anesthetic potency and possibly in the incidence of emergence reactions.[105,106] Only the racemic mixture containing equal amounts of the (+) and (−) enantiomers is commercially available. Ketamine produces reliable serum levels when administered intravenously (within 1 minute) or intramuscularly (within 5 minutes). The pKa of ketamine is 7.5, and its high lipid solubility explains its very rapid onset. Ketamine is rapidly redistributed, with awakening occurring in 10 to 15 minutes. The redistribution half-life is approximately 5 minutes, and the elimination half-life is 130 minutes.[107] Similar pharmacokinetic parameters have been demonstrated in children.[108] Extensive hepatic biotransformation necessitates higher doses when administered orally or rectally. The most important metabolite is norketamine, which has approximately one third the anesthetic potency of ketamine, and elevated norketamine concentrations appear to explain the prolonged clinical effects noted after oral administration. Norketamine is hydroxylated, conjugated, and excreted in the urine. Renal dysfunction does not prolong the clinical effects of ketamine.

Tolerance and hepatic enzyme induction has been demonstrated during chronic administration. Analgesia and anesthesia appear to be related to CNS action of the parent compound, although pharmacodynamic effects appear to outlast predicted CNS concentrations.[109] Cross-tolerance with opiates has been demonstrated in two animal species,[110,111] but convincing evidence in humans is lacking. Elucidation of the precise CNS site of action of ketamine is currently inconclusive, despite suggestions that ketamine may interfere with excitatory transmission via N-methyl-aspartate receptors,[112] which may represent a subgroup of opiate receptors.

The anesthetic effects of ketamine have been attributed to electrophysiologic dissociation between the thalamoneocortical and limbic systems. The clinical effects at anesthetic plasma concentrations include catalepsy, nystagmus, hypertonicity, and nonpurposeful movements.

Ketamine is a potent stimulator of the cardiovascular system, presumably via central sympathetic effects, as well as inhibition of catecholamine reuptake.[113] Heart rate, mean arterial pressure, and systemic vascular resistance all increase. Pulmonary vascular resistance does not appear to be altered in infants with or without preexisting pulmonary hypertension.[114] In an isolated heart preparation, ketamine has been shown to inhibit contractile function.[115] Without compensatory sympathetic stimulation, therefore, ketamine may produce hypotension. For critically ill patients with moderate hypovolemia, however, low doses of ketamine (e.g., 1–2 mg/kg) are safer than barbiturates as rapid induction agents prior to tracheal intubation.

There are a number of animal studies that demonstrate a significant increase in cerebral blood flow and intracranial pressure following ketamine administration.[116] Hypocapnia has been shown to limit this response in animals[117] and in newborns.[118] In patients with altered intracranial compliance, however, ketamine should be avoided. Ketamine produces dose-related respiratory depression and shifts the carbon dioxide response curve to the right.[119] The bronchodilating properties of ketamine are well known and are likely the result of increased levels of endogenous catecholamines. Ketamine is as effective as halothane in preventing bronchoconstriction in dogs[120] and has been used with success in the therapy

of life-threatening bronchospasm.[120,121] Oral and tracheal secretions are increased by ketamine, but this may be ameliorated by co-administration of an anti-sialagogue, such as glycopyrrolate or atropine.

Emergence reactions have been commonly reported in patients receiving ketamine and appear more commonly in females greater than 16 years of age after rapid administration of a large dose.[122] Emergence phenomena include visual, auditory, and proprioceptive hallucinations, as well as delirium, and may occur up to 24 hours after administration. Long-term changes in personality or behavior have not been seen in adults[123] or children[124] anesthetized with ketamine, as compared with other agents. Benzodiazepines are effective in preventing these phenomena, with some data suggesting that midazolam is more potent in this regard than diazepam.[125,126]

In the pediatric population, ketamine has been most frequently used for patients undergoing repetitive radiotherapy[127] and burn-dressing changes. In these patients, significant tolerance to the anesthetic effects of ketamine with chronic use has been described.[128] Although ventilation and airway reflexes are usually preserved with small doses, this cannot be assumed in patients at risk for aspiration of gastric contents and an unprotected airway. Ketamine is less useful as a sedative for bronchoscopy because it does not reliably suppress airway reflexes and increases tracheobronchial secretions.

There has been some experience with ketamine in the intensive care setting as sedation for ventilation. In adults, when administered as a continuous infusion, ketamine and midazolam produced less hemodynamic instability than fentanyl and midazolam.[129]

Chloral Hydrate

Chloral hydrate is a sedative and hypnotic, with CNS effects similar to the barbiturates. This drug is soluble in both water and oil and is unstable when exposed to light or air. The mechanism and site of action are unknown. Chloral hydrate is rapidly absorbed following oral or rectal administration, producing sedation within 30 minutes and lasting for 4 to 8 hours.[130] Chloral hydrate is rapidly metabolized in the liver, with the formation of large quantities of an active metabolite, trichloroethanol. The plasma half-life of chloral hydrate is only several minutes; trichlorethanol is primarily responsible for the prolonged clinical effect seen after administration of chloral hydrate. Trichlorethanol has a plasma half-life of 8 to 11 hours and is oxidized and conjugated to inactive metabolites.[131]

Chloral hydrate is a useful short-term hypnotic, with tolerance and dependence developing during chronic administration. Prolonged administration may produce protracted depression of mental status and confusion that may resemble an organic neurologic syndrome. Sedation is reliable, although paradoxical excitement, delirium, and paranoia may occur. These paradoxical effects are seen less frequently than with the barbiturates and are uncommon in children. Chloral hydrate has no analgesic properties, and in the presence of pain may produce excitement or delirium. Clinical experience suggests that chloral hydrate demonstrates cross-tolerance with the benzodiazepines and opioids and may be valuable in suppressing symptoms of opioid withdrawal.

Chloral hydrate has been commonly used in the sedation of ventilated infants with chronic lung disease.[24] The dose for sedation is 25 to 75 mg/kg, with a maximum single dose of 1 g and a maximum daily dose of 2 g. At doses of 50 mg/kg, chloral hydrate does not alter the carbon dioxide response curves of healthy full-term infants.[132] However, in infants with preexisting hypoxemia, chloral hydrate in standard sedating doses may produce significant respiratory depression and should be used with caution in any patient with compromised respiratory function.[133] Chloral hydrate is a potent inhibitor of myocardial contractility, shortens the refractory period, and sensitizes the myocardium to catecholamines, accounting for potentially fatal ventricular arrhythmias.[134] There is a narrow therapeutic index with cardiac arrhythmias and death described with doses of 100 to 150 mg/kg.[131] Significant drug accumulation may occur in patients with renal or hepatic dysfunction. Toxic levels of trichloroethanol have been documented in premature infants sedated with modest doses of chloral hydrate for as little as 3 days.[135] Chloral hydrate is very irritating to mucosal surfaces, and repeated administration may cause gastritis or irritation of the rectum. Recent concern has been raised about the carcinogenic potential of chloral hydrate metabolites,[136] although at present there is no evidence that chloral hydrate is carcinogenic in humans.

Propofol

Propofol is an IV agent structurally unrelated to the barbiturate, steroid, or imidazole compounds currently available. It has been evaluated primarily as an anesthetic induction agent. The pharmacologic and clinical data regarding propofol have been reviewed in detail.[137] In animals, propofol produces unconsciousness as rapidly as thiopental, with a slightly longer duration of action. The currently available preparation, a 1% emulsion with soy bean oil, glycerol, and egg phosphatide, does not release histamine, has no effect on bronchomotor tone, and produces profound and reversible EEG depression. Unlike thiopental, propofol does not appear to have anticonvulsant properties. Induction with propofol produces a decrease in mean arterial pressure greater than that seen with thiopental or methohexital, attributable to a decrease in systemic vascular resistance. This agent should, therefore, be used cautiously in patients with compromised cardiac function or decreased intravascular volume. Propofol produces respiratory depression comparable to that seen with thiopental, and this effect appears to be potentiated by opioids. A decrease in cerebral blood flow and an increase in cerebral vascular resistance have been attributed to propofol. Cerebral perfusion pressure has also been shown to be significantly decreased, however, and propofol should be used with caution in patients with altered intracranial compliance.

Propofol is primarily excreted in the urine, with a small amount appearing in the feces. However, studies in patients with liver and renal disease have not shown significant prolongation of elimination half-lives. Awakening occurs 4 to 8 minutes after a standard anesthetic induction dose (1.5–3.0 mg/kg), and the elimination half-life is between 30 and 90 minutes in adults. There is some evidence that elimination half-lives may be shorter in children, but these data are only preliminary.[138] The incidence of pain on injection of propofol has been reported as high as 58%[139] and may be an important limitation for conscious sedation or induction in the pediatric population. This side effect has been greatly decreased by coadministration with lidocaine.[127,140]

There has been limited experience with propofol in the intensive care setting, and the drug is not currently approved for pediatric use. When administered by continuous infusion, propofol did not appear to affect the adrenocortical axis over an 8-hour period of administration.[141] In a study of ten mechanically ventilated adult patients who received propofol by bolus followed by continuous infusion, significant decreases in mean arterial pressure were observed and necessitated alteration of the infusion rate in three patients.[141] Propofol has been shown to produce shorter recovery times and more rapid return to spontaneous ventilation in adults sedated for ventilation, when compared with midazolam.[142] Satisfactory sedation was reported in 91% of patients, but the authors emphasized the absence of analgesic properties. In addition to significant hypotension, propofol has been shown to produce green-colored urine, attributable to the accumulation of urinary phenols.[143] It should be noted that despite enthusiastic use in the United Kingdom,[141,144] there have been reports of unusual movement disorders following propofol administration[145,146] and a recent letter from the manufacturer cautions against prolonged use in children.[147]

Volatile Agents

The use of volatile agents in the intensive care setting offers a reliable route of administration, a dependable mode of excretion, and limited accumulation of active or toxic metabolites.

Nitrous oxide in oxygen (Entonox) has been a popular method of postoperative sedation in Great Britain for many years and produces reliable sedation, adequate analgesia, and rapid awakening on discontinuation. Bone marrow depression with megaloblastic changes has been well described,[148] and nitrous oxide has been shown to interfere with vitamin B_{12} metabolism after as brief an exposure as 12 to 24 hours.[149]

Halothane[150–153] has been widely reported in the treatment of status asthmaticus. The high solubility and extensive in vivo metabolism of halothane, however, make it less attractive for long-term administration.

Isoflurane, a widely-utilized fluorinated volatile agent, undergoes limited metabolism, and has a relatively low blood-gas partition coefficient of 1.4.[154,155] Of the volatile agents currently available, isoflurane appears the best suited for long-term use in the critical care setting.[156] Isoflurane has been successfully used in the management of status asthmaticus, and there are anecdotal reports that describe the use of isoflurane in the ICU for as long as 150 hours.[157,158]

Beechey and colleagues[158] reported the "routine use of isoflurane as a sedative agent for postoperative cardiac surgical patients." The authors described the use of 0.5% to 1.0% isoflurane in ventilated patients for approximately 6 to 10 hours prior to planned extubation. They reported "minimal disturbances" of cardiovascular, renal, or hematologic parameters, with exposure times as long as 150 hours. Liver function tests exhibited "limited elevations," with return to baseline by 1 week. They also reported rapid awakening on discontinuation, a feature consistent with the low solubility and limited metabolism of isoflurane. Kong and colleagues[159] compared isoflurane in subanesthetic concentrations (0.1%–0.6%) with midazolam infusion (0.01–0.2 mg/kg/hr) for prolonged sedation for ventilation in 60 adults. The study was limited to 24 hours, and the authors reported greater cooperation, less confusion, and more rapid awakening in patients sedated with isoflurane.

The effects of lengthy exposure to potent volatile anesthetics are unknown. Tolerance has been demonstrated after prolonged exposure of rats to nitrous oxide but not to isoflurane.[160] Tolerance to the analgesic effect of nitrous oxide has also been reported in humans.[161,162] There are animal data suggesting that prolonged exposure to subanesthetic concentrations of halothane but not enflurane or isoflurane produces hepatomegaly and hepatitis.[163] All of the volatile agents contain inorganic fluoride, and fluoride-induced nephrotoxicity, characterized by renal tubular dysfunction, may occur with plasma fluoride levels in excess of 50 μmol. Renal dysfunction is most common after enflurane administration, and a decrease in urine concentrating ability has been noted following 9.6 MAC hours of enflurane anesthesia.[164] Obesity,[165] untreated diabetes,[166] and isoniazid administration[167] appear to increase plasma fluoride concentrations in patients receiving fluorinated volatile anesthetics. A report describes a patient who received approximately 40 MAC hours of isoflurane with a maximum plasma fluoride concentration of 93 μmol/liter, well above the level associated with nephrotoxicity.[168]

Despite the conceptual appeal of sedation with potent volatile agents, there is limited experience regarding the potential for hepatic or renal toxicity during prolonged exposures. For the moment, the use of isoflurane in the intensive care setting can be regarded only as an interesting possibility requiring further study. Special attention must be given to considerations of scavenging and breathing circuit design, potentially cumbersome problems in the ICU.

Side Effects

Respiratory Depression

All opioids produce dose-related respiratory depression characterized by decreased ventilatory responses to, and the subjective distress produced by, hypoxemia and hypercarbia. The carbon dioxide response curve is displaced to the right, and resting pCO_2 rises. Clinically, the respiratory rate decreases, with an incomplete compensatory increase in tidal volume. Although the opioid-induced shift in the carbon dioxide response curve is well known, it is not as widely appreciated that standard doses of morphine (e.g., 0.1 mg/kg) nearly abolish ventilatory responses to hypoxemia. In patients with airway obstruction or atelectasis following surgery, blunting of hypoxic drive can lead to dangerous hypoventilation.

It has long been believed that infants and children are more prone to respiratory depression following administration of opioids than adults, and it has been speculated that immaturity of the blood-brain barrier explains this unusual sensitivity.[32] However, rigorous study of newborn pharmacodynamic responses to opioids have not been performed, and data from older infants suggest fentanyl-induced apnea is less common than in adults at similar plasma concentrations (Fig. 49-1).[169]

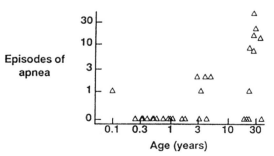

Figure 49-1. The number of episodes of apnea (defined as breath-to-breath interval exceeding 10 seconds in infants and children and 20 seconds in adults) is plotted against age. The incidence of apnea as well as the number of episodes increased with age. (From RE Hertzka et al. Fentanyl-induced ventilatory depression: Effects of age. *Anesthesiology* 70:213–218, 1989. With permission.)

At equi-sedating doses, benzodiazepines produce less respiratory depression than opioids. The respiratory depression of benzodiazepines is extremely variable; it may be exaggerated in patients with chronic pulmonary disease. When combined with opioids, the benzodiazepines may produce life-threatening respiratory depression,[170,171] and this combination should be administered only in settings in which cardiorespiratory monitoring is available. Respiratory depression from benzodiazepines is reversed by flumazenil, a specific benzodiazepine antagonist, but not by naloxone.

Chest Wall Rigidity

Chest wall rigidity is a well-described complication of opioid administration in adults and has been reported during use of all opioids.[172] In a careful electromyographic (EMG) study of rigidity during alfentanil induction, EMG activity was significantly increased in the muscles of the abdomen, chest, and extremities to a similar degree.[173] Simultaneous EEG recordings revealed no corresponding cortical activity, eliminating seizures as a possible etiology. Rigidity on induction of anesthesia has been avoided by pretreatment with a "subrelaxant" dose of pancuronium (0.01–0.02 mg/kg)[174] and by slow IV infusion of opioid.[175,176] There are few data available regarding fentanyl-induced rigidity in pediatric patients,[177] although clinical practice suggests a similar pattern.

Tolerance and Dependence

Tolerance occurs when there is a reduction in physiologic response to a drug with repeated administration.[178] The rate of development of tolerance to the analgesic effects of opioids is extremely variable. In adult cancer patients, stable doses of opioids generally produce effective analgesia for long periods.[179] Extensive experience with other chronic pain syndromes has shown that most patients treated with opioids for extended periods can be maintained on a stable dose.[180] However, in the absence of nociceptive stimulation, there is evidence that tolerance may occur much more rapidly.[181] There are also abundant animal data[182–185] and some human experience,[50,186] suggesting that tolerance is much more likely during continuous as opposed to intermittent opioid administration. These considerations are important when selecting the appropriate regimen for long-term sedation.

Acute tolerance to opioids developing over hours to days has been observed in intensive care settings in both infants and adults.[50,186] Tolerance has also been described during therapeutic use of the benzodiazepines,[187] as well as during repetitive use of ketamine.[128]

Dependence is the requirement for continued drug administration to prevent withdrawal symptoms, including agitation, dysphoria, tachycardia, tachypnea, piloerection, nasal congestion, temperature instability, and feeding intolerance. Tolerance and dependence have been described in neonatal and pediatric patients during therapeutic use of opioids.[50,188,189]

The development of physical dependence is quite variable, and withdrawal symptoms have been observed following periods of administration as short as 5 days (Figs. 49-2 and 49-3).[50] It is to be emphasized that fear of precipitation of the abstinence syndrome should not inhibit appropriate administration of opioids, because withdrawal symptoms can be eliminated by gradually tapering opioid dosage over 5 to 7 days. Dependence is also seen during therapeutic use of benzodiazepines[93,94,187,190–195] and may necessitate gradual dosage reduction during long-term usage.

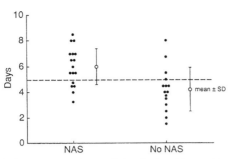

Figure 49-2. In neonates receiving fentanyl by continuous infusion, a total fentanyl dose of 1.6 mg/kg was a useful threshold in separating infants who manifested the neonatal abstinence syndrome (NAS).[50]

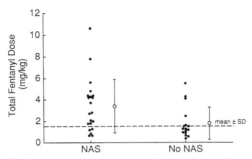

Figure 49-3. In neonates receiving fentanyl by continuous infusion, an infusion duration of 5 days was a useful threshold in separating infants who manifested the neonatal abstinence syndrome (NAS).[50]

Dependence is a set of physiologic responses that should be distinguished from addiction, which is a behavioral syndrome of compulsive drug seeking. Addiction is extremely rare in patients of all ages who are receiving opioids or benzodiazepines for pain or sedation. Addiction is not caused by administration of opioids to treat pain, and fear of addiction should not inhibit appropriate administration for acute pain and sedation in neonatal and pediatric intensive care.

Pulmonary Effects

All anesthetic agents have been shown to decrease functional residual capacity, with a resulting decrease in measured pulmonary compliance.[196-198] In addition, opioids may decrease airway diameter, adversely affecting airway resistance.[199] There is much debate about the effect of histamine release on bronchial smooth muscle and whether histamine-releasing agents such as morphine are contraindicated in patients with reactive airway disease. Although morphine has clearly been shown to release significant amounts of histamine in some patients, when compared with fentanyl,[200] precipitation of bronchospasm has not been reported after the administration of morphine. In fact, IV morphine has frequently been employed in patients with severe asthma requiring mechanical ventilation.[201] There is also evidence that morphine may in fact inhibit bronchoconstriction and mucous hypersecretion in patients with reactive airway disease.[202,203]

Gastrointestinal Effects

All opioids delay gastric emptying, decrease intestinal motility, produce nausea via direct stimulation of the chemoreceptor trigger zone, and induce an increase in common bile duct pressure. Impaired absorption of enteral nutrients is obviously undesirable, and opiate-induced ileus may increase the risk of regurgitation and aspiration of gastric contents. Spasm of the sphincter of Oddi may be antagonized by atropine or glucagon.[5,204] All opioids may produce some degree of nausea by action at brain stem sites. This effect is idiosyncratic and not clearly dose-dependent. In particular, nausea appears to be suppressed by very large doses of opioids.[205]

Summary

The goals of sedation in the critical care setting include the provision of adequate analgesia and amnesia without compromising hemodynamic stability. Opioids, alone and in combination with benzodiazepines, have become the mainstays of sedation in intensive care. Continuous infusion of agents with a short duration of action and lack of accumulation is the logical approach to the sedation of critically ill patients with cardiovascular instability. Tolerance and dependence are important complications of this strategy, and further data are necessary to elucidate the precise mechanisms involved and to develop more effective agents and modes of administration. Incremental titration to a desired clinical effect is critical when administering sedating agents in the ICU. By understanding the important pharmacokinetic and pharmacodynamic differences between infants, children, and adults, the clinician can avoid drug accumulation, the production of toxic metabolites, and untoward side effects that may add to overall morbidity in the critically ill population.

References

1. Merriman HM. The techniques used to sedate ventilated patients. A survey of methods used in 34 ICUs in Great Britain. *Intensive Care Med* 7:217–224, 1981.
2. Gast PH, Fisher A, Sear JW. Intensive care sedation now (letter). *Lancet* 2:863–864, 1984.
3. Miller Jones CM, Williams JH. Sedation for ventilation. A retrospective study of fifty patients. *Anaesthesia* 35:1104–1106, 1980.
4. Bion JF, Ledingham IM. Sedation in intensive care—A postal survey (letter). *Intensive Care Med* 13:215–216, 1987.
5. Aitkenhead AR. Analgesia and sedation in intensive care. *Br J Anaesth* 63:196–206, 1989.
6. American Academy of Pediatrics, Committee on Fetus and Newborn, Committee on Drugs, Section on Anesthesiology, Section on Surgery. Neonatal anesthesia. *Pediatrics* 80:446, 1987.
7. Schechter NL, Allen DA, Hanson K. Status of pediatric pain control: A comparison of hospital analgesic usage in children and adults. *Pediatrics* 77:11–15, 1986.
8. Anand KJ, Hickey PR. Pain and its effects in the human neonate and fetus. *N Engl J Med* 317:1321–1329, 1987.
9. Truog RD, Anand KJ. Management of pain in the postoperative neonate. *Clin Perinatol* 16:61–78, 1989.
10. Chernow B. *The Pharmacologic Approach to the Critically Ill Patient.* Baltimore: Williams & Wilkins, 1988. P 880.
11. Oh TE, Duncan AW. Sedation in the seriously ill. *Med J Aust* 152:540–545, 1990.
12. Matuschak GM, Rinaldo JE. Organ interactions in the adult respiratory distress syndrome during sepsis. Role of the liver in host defense. *Chest* 94:400–406, 1988.

13. Crippen DW. The role of sedation in the ICU patient with pain and agitation. *Crit Care Clin* 6:369–392, 1990.

14. Hickey PR et al. Pulmonary and systemic hemodynamic responses to fentanyl in infants. *Anesth Analg* 64:483–486, 1985.

15. Hickey PR et al. Blunting of stress responses in the pulmonary circulation of infants by fentanyl. *Anesth Analg* 64:1137–1142, 1985.

16. Bjertnaes L, Hauge A, Kriz M. Hypoxia-induced pulmonary vasoconstriction: Effects of fentanyl following different routes of administration. *Acta Anaesthesiol Scand* 24:53–57, 1980.

17. Vacanti JP et al. The pulmonary hemodynamic response to perioperative anesthesia in the treatment of high-risk infants with congenital diaphragmatic hernia. *J Pediatr Surg* 19:672–679, 1984.

18. Finck AD et al. Pharmacokinetics of morphine: Effects of hypercarbia on serum and brain morphine concentrations in the dog. *Anesthesiology* 47:407–410, 1977.

19. Dahlstrom B et al. Morphine kinetics in children. *Clin Pharmacol Ther* 26:354–365, 1979.

20. Hasselstrom J et al. Long lasting respiratory depression induced by morphine-6-glucuronide. *Br J Clin Pharmacol* 27:515–518, 1989.

21. Pasternak GW et al. Morphine-6-glucuronide, a potent mu agonist. *Life Sci* 41:2845–2849, 1987.

22. Osborne RJ, Joel SP, Slevin ML. Morphine intoxication in renal failure: The role of morphine-6-glucuronide. *Br Med J [Clin Res]* 292:1548–1549, 1986.

23. Sear JW et al. Studies on morphine disposition: Influence of renal failure on the kinetics of morphine and its metabolites. *Br J Anaesth* 62:28–32, 1989.

24. Franck LS. A national survey of the assessment and treatment of pain and agitation in the neonatal intensive care unit. *J Obstet Gynecol Neonatal Nurs* 16:387–393, 1987.

25. Rutter PC, Murphy F, Dudley HA. Morphine: Controlled trial of different methods of administration for postoperative pain relief. *Br Med J* 280:12–13, 1980.

26. Lynn AM, Opheim KE, Tyler DC. Morphine infusion after pediatric cardiac surgery. *Crit Care Med* 12:863–866, 1984.

27. Koren G et al. Postoperative morphine infusion in newborn infants: Assessment of disposition characteristics and safety. *J Pediatr* 107:963–967, 1985.

28. Lynn AM, Slattery JT. Morphine pharmacokinetics in early infancy. *Anesthesiology* 66:136–139, 1987.

29. Stoelting RK, Gibbs PS. Hemodynamic effects of morphine and morphine-nitrous oxide in valvular heart disease and coronary artery disease. *Anesthesiology* 38:45–52, 1973.

30. Stanley TH et al. Cardiovascular effects of diazepam and droperidol during morphine anesthesia. *Anesthesiology* 44:255–258, 1976.

31. Burtin P et al. Hypotension with midazolam and fentanyl in the newborn. *Lancet* 337:1545–1546, 1991.

32. Way WL, Costley EC, Way EL. Respiratory sensitivity of the newborn infant to meperidine and morphine. *Clin Pharmacol Ther* 6:454–461, 1965.

33. Foldes FF, Tarda TAG. Comparative studies with narcotics and narcotic antagonists in man. *Acta Anaesthesiol Scand* 9:121–138, 1965.

34. Armstrong PJ, Bersten A. Normeperidine toxicity. *Anesth Analg* 65:536–538, 1986.

35. Gourlay GK, Wilson PR, Glynn CJ. Pharmacodynamics and pharmacokinetics of methadone during the perioperative period. *Anesthesiology* 57:458–467, 1982.

36. Berde CB et al. Pharmacokinetics of methadone in children and adolescents in the peri-operative period. *Anesthesiology* 67:A519, 1987.

37. McQuay HJ et al. Plasma fentanyl concentrations and clinical observations during and after operation. *Br J Anaesth* 51:543–550, 1979.

38. McClain DA, Hug CC Jr. Intravenous fentanyl kinetics. *Clin Pharmacol Ther* 28:106–114, 1980.

39. Stoeckel H et al. Plasma fentanyl concentrations and the occurrence of respiratory depression in volunteers. *Br J Anaesth* 54:1087–1095, 1982.

40. Becker LD et al. Biphasic respiratory depression after fentanyldroperidol or fentanyl alone used to supplement nitrous oxide anesthesia. *Anesthesiology* 44:291–296, 1976.

41. Mather LE. Clinical pharmacokinetics of fentanyl and its newer derivatives. *Clin Pharmacokinet* 8:422–446, 1983.

42. Koehntop DE et al. Pharmacokinetics of fentanyl in neonates. *Anesth Analg* 65:227–232, 1986.

43. Masey SA et al. Effect of abdominal distension on central and regional hemodynamics in neonatal lambs. *Pediatr Res* 19:1244–1249, 1985.

44. Borel JD et al. The influence of halothane on fentanyl pharmacokinetics. *Anesthesiology* 57:A239, 1982.

45. Gelman S, Fowler KC, Smith LR. Liver circulation and function during isoflurane and halothane anesthesia. *Anesthesiology* 61: 726–730, 1984.

46. Mannering GJ. Drug metabolism in the newborn. *Fed Proc* 44:2302–2308, 1985.

47. Singleton MA, Rosen JI, Fisher DM. Plasma concentrations of fentanyl in infants, children and adults. *Can J Anaesth* 34:152–155, 1987.

48. Robinson S, Gregory GA. Fentanyl-air-oxygen anesthesia for ligation of patent ductus arteriosus in preterm infants. *Anesth Analg* 60:331–334, 1981.

49. Yaster M. The dose response of fentanyl in neonatal anesthesia. *Anesthesiology* 66:433–435, 1987.

50. Arnold JH et al. Tolerance and dependence in neonates sedated with fentanyl during extracorporeal membrane oxygenation. *Anesthesiology* 73:1136–1140, 1990.

51. Greeley WJ, de Bruijn NP. Changes in sufentanil pharmacokinetics within the neonatal period. *Anesth Analg* 67:86–90, 1988.

52. Ferrier C et al. Alfentanil pharmacokinetics in patients with cirrhosis. *Anesthesiology* 62:480–484, 1985.

53. Maitre PO et al. Population pharmacokinetics of alfentanil: The average dose-plasma concentration relationship and interindividual variability in patients. *Anesthesiology* 66:3–12, 1987.

54. Goresky GV et al. The pharmacokinetics of alfentanil in children. *Anesthesiology* 67:654–659, 1987.

55. Roure P et al. Pharmacokinetics of alfentanil in children undergoing surgery. *Br J Anaesth* 59:1437–1440, 1987.

56. Meistelman C et al. A comparison of alfentanil pharmacokinetics in children and adults. *Anesthesiology* 66:13–16, 1987.

57. Ausems ME, Hug CC Jr, de Lange S. Variable rate infusion of alfentanil as a supplement to nitrous oxide anesthesia for general surgery. *Anesth Analg* 62:982–986, 1983.

58. Yate PM et al. Comparison of infusions of alfentanil or pethidine for sedation of ventilated patients on the ITU. *Br J Anaesth* 58:1091–1099, 1986.

59. Yate PM, Thomas D, Sebel PS. Alfentanil infusion for sedation and analgesia in intensive care (letter). *Lancet* 2:396–397, 1984.

60. Cohen AT, Kelly DR. Assessment of alfentanil by intravenous infusion as long-term sedation in intensive care. *Anaesthesia* 42:545–548, 1987.

61. McDonnell TE et al. Nonuniformity of alfentanil pharmacokinetics in healthy adults. *Anesthesiology* 57:A236, 1982.

62. Desai N, Taylor Davies A, Barnett DB. The effects of diazepam and oxprenolol on short term memory in individuals of high and low state anxiety. *Br J Clin Pharmacol* 15:197–202, 1983.

63. Niv D et al. Analgesic and hyperalgesic effects of midazolam: Dependence on route of administration. *Anesth Analg* 67:1169–1173, 1988.

64. Klejin Evander et al. Pharmacokinetics of diazepam in dogs, mice and humans. *Acta Pharmacol Toxicol (Copenh)* 3:109–127, 1971.

65. Braunstein MC. Apnea with maintenance of consciousness, following intravenous diazepam. *Anesth Analg* 58:52–53, 1979.

66. Gross JB, Smith L, Smith TC. Time course of ventilatory response to carbon dioxide after intravenous diazepam: *Anesthesiology* 57:18–21, 1982.

67. Korttila K, Mattila MJ, Linnoila M. Prolonged recovery after diazepam sedation: The influence of food, charcoal ingestion and injection

rate on the effects of intravenous diazepam. *Br J Anaesth* 48:333–340, 1976.

68. Hegarty JE, Dundee JW. Sequelae after the intravenous injection of three benzodiazepines—diazepam, lorazepam, and flunitrazepam. *Br Med J* 2:1384–1385, 1977.

69. Stoelting RK. *Pharmacology and Physiology in Anesthetic Practice.* Philadelphia: Lippincott, 1987. P 125.

70. Pakkanen A, Kanto J. Midazolam compared with thiopentone as an induction agent. *Acta Anaesthesiol Scand* 26:143–146, 1982.

71. Korttila K, Aromaa U. Venous complications after intravenous injection of diazepam, flunitrazepam, thiopentone, and etomidate. *Acta Anaesthesiol Scand* 24:227–230, 1980.

72. Reves JG et al. Midazolam: Pharmacology and uses. *Anesthesiology* 62:310–324, 1985.

73. Ziegler WH et al. Comparison of the effects of intravenously administered midazolam, triazolam and their hydroxy metabolites. *Br J Clin Pharmacol* 16:63S–69S, 1983.

74. Saint-Maurice C et al. Premedication with rectal midazolam. Effective dose in pediatric anesthesia. *Ann Fr Anaesth Reanim* 3:181–184, 1984.

75. Wilton NC et al. Preanesthetic sedation of preschool children using intranasal midazolam. *Anesthesiology* 69:972–975, 1988.

76. Greenblatt DJ et al. Effect of age, gender, and obesity on midazolam kinetics. *Anesthesiology* 61:27–35, 1984.

77. Vinik HR et al. The pharmacokinetics of midazolam in chronic renal failure patients. *Anesthesiology* 59:390–394, 1983.

78. Forster A et al. Ventilatory effects of various doses of IV midazolam assessed by a noninvasive method in healthy volunteers. *Anesthesiology* 57:A480, 1982.

79. Forster A et al. Respiratory depression by midazolam and diazepam. *Anesthesiology* 53:494–497, 1980.

80. Kanto J, Sjovall S, Vuori A. Effect of different kinds of premedication on the induction properties of midazolam. *Br J Anaesth* 54:507–511, 1982.

81. Stoelting RK. *Pharmacology and Physiology in Anesthetic Practice.* Philadelphia: Lippincott, 1987. P 125.

82. Dirksen MS, Vree TB, Driessen JJ. Clinical pharmacokinetics of long-term infusion of midazolam in critically ill patients—Preliminary results. *Anaesth Intensive Care* 15:440–444, 1987.

83. Shapiro JM et al. Midazolam infusion for sedation in the intensive care unit: Effect on adrenal function. *Anesthesiology* 64:394–398, 1986.

84. Michalk S et al. Long-term midazolam infusion for basal sedation in intensive care: A clinical and pharmacokinetic study. *Anesthesiology* 65:A66, 1986.

85. Geller E et al. Midazolam infusion and benzodiazepine antagonist for sedation in ICU—A preliminary report. *Anesthesiology* 65:A65, 1986.

86. Westphal LM et al. Use of midazolam infusion for sedation following cardiac surgery. *Anesthesiology* 67:257–262, 1987.

87. Booker PD, Beechey A, Lloyd Thomas AR. Sedation of children requiring artificial ventilation using an infusion of midazolam. *Br J Anaesth* 58:1104–1108, 1986.

88. Byatt CM et al. Accumulation of midazolam after repeated dosage in patients receiving mechanical ventilation in an intensive care unit. *Br Med J [Clin Res]* 289:799–800, 1984.

89. Oldenhof H et al. Clinical pharmacokinetics of midazolam in intensive care patients, a wide interpatient variability. *Clin Pharmacol Ther* 43:263–269, 1988.

90. Salonen M et al. Midazolam as an induction agent in children: A pharmacokinetic and clinical study. *Anesth Analg* 66:625–628, 1987.

91. Lam TK, Ng WK, Chan YS. Use of midazolam in children (letter). *Lancet* 2:565, 1988.

92. Silvasi DL, Rosen DA, Rosen KR. Continuous intravenous midazolam infusion for sedation in the pediatric intensive care unit. *Anesth Analg* 67:286–288, 1988.

93. Sury MR et al. Acute benzodiazepine withdrawal syndrome after midazolam infusions in children (letter). *Crit Care Med* 17:301–302, 1989.

94. Mets B, Horsell A, Linton DM. Midazolam-induced benzodiazepine withdrawal syndrome. *Anaesthesia* 46:28–29, 1991.

95. Bergman I et al. Reversible neurologic abnormalities associated with prolonged intravenous midazolam and fentanyl administration. *J Pediatr* 119:644–649, 1991.

96. Ricou B et al. Clinical evaluation of a specific benzodiazepine antagonist (RO 15-1788). Studies in elderly patients after regional anaesthesia under benzodiazepine sedation. *Br J Anaesth* 58:1005–1011, 1986.

97. Ghoneim MM, Dembo JB, Block RI. Time course of antagonism of sedative and amnesic effects of diazepam by flumazenil. *Anesthesiology* 70:899–904, 1989.

98. White PF et al. Benzodiazepine antagonism does not provoke a stress response. *Anesthesiology* 70:636–639, 1989.

99. Klotz U et al. Pharmacodynamic interaction between midazolam and a specific benzodiazepine antagonist in humans. *J Clin Pharmacol* 25:400–406, 1985.

100. Bodenham A, Park GR. Reversal of prolonged sedation using flumazenil in critically ill patients. *Anaesthesia* 44:603–605, 1989.

101. Sorbo S, Hudson RJ, Loomis JC. The pharmacokinetics of thiopental in pediatric surgical patients. *Anesthesiology* 61:666–670, 1984.

102. Stanski DR et al. Pharmacokinetics of high-dose thiopental used in cerebral resuscitation. *Anesthesiology* 53:169–171, 1980.

103. Ward JD et al. Failure of prophylactic barbiturate coma in the treatment of severe head injury. *J Neurosurg* 62:383–388, 1985.

104. Reich DL, Silvay G. Ketamine: An update on the first twenty-five years of clinical experience. *Can J Anaesth* 36:186–197, 1989.

105. White PF et al. Comparative pharmacology of the ketamine isomers. Studies in volunteers. *Br J Anaesth* 57:197–203, 1985.

106. White PF et al. Pharmacology of ketamine isomers in surgical patients. *Anesthesiology* 52:231–239, 1980.

107. Domino EF et al. Ketamine kinetics in unmedicated and diazepam-premedicated subjects. *Clin Pharmacol Ther* 36:645–653, 1984.

108. Grant IS et al. Ketamine disposition in children and adults. *Br J Anaesth* 55:1107–1111, 1983.

109. Clements JA, Nimmo WS. Pharmacokinetics and analgesic effect of ketamine in man. *Br J Anaesth* 53:27–30, 1981.

110. Winters WD et al. Ketamine- and morphine-induced analgesia and catalepsy. I. Tolerance, cross-tolerance, potentiation, residual morphine levels and naloxone action in the rat. *J Pharmacol Exp Ther* 244:51–57, 1988.

111. Finck AD, Samaniego E, Ngai SH. Morphine tolerance decreases the analgesic effects of ketamine in mice. *Anesthesiology* 68:397–400, 1988.

112. Thomson AM, West DC, Lodge D. An N-methylaspartate receptor-mediated synapse in rat cerebral cortex: A site of action of ketamine. *Nature* 313:479–481, 1985.

113. Lundy PM et al. Differential effects of ketamine isomers on neuronal and extraneuronal catecholamine uptake mechanisms. *Anesthesiology* 64:359–363, 1986.

114. Hickey PR et al. Pulmonary and systemic hemodynamic responses to ketamine in infants with normal and elevated pulmonary vascular resistance. *Anesthesiology* 62:287–293, 1985.

115. Saegusa K et al. Pharmacologic analysis of ketamine-induced cardiac actions in isolated, blood-perfused canine atria. *J Cardiovasc Pharmacol* 8:414–419, 1986.

116. Michenfelder JD. *Anesthesia and the Brain.* New York: Churchill Livingstone, 1988. P 125.

117. Pfenninger E, Dick W, Ahnefeld FW. The influence of ketamine on both normal and raised intracranial pressure of artificially ventilated animals. *Eur J Anaesthesiol* 2:297–307, 1985.

118. Friesen RH et al. Changes in anterior fontanel pressure in preterm neonates receiving isoflurane, halothane, fentanyl, or ketamine. *Anesth Analg* 66:431–434, 1987.

119. Bourke DL, Malit LA, Smith TC. Respiratory interactions of ketamine and morphine. *Anesthesiology* 66:153–156, 1987.

120. Hirshman CA et al. Ketamine block of bronchospasm in experimental canine asthma. *Br J Anaesth* 51:713–718, 1979.

121. Rock MJ et al. Use of ketamine in asthmatic children to treat respira-

tory failure refractory to conventional therapy. *Crit Care Med* 14:514–516, 1986.

122. White PF, Way WL, Trevor AJ. Ketamine—its pharmacology and therapeutic uses. *Anesthesiology* 56:119–136, 1982.

123. Moretti RJ et al. Comparison of ketamine and thiopental in healthy volunteers: Effects on mental status, mood, and personality. *Anesth Analg* 63:1087–1096, 1984.

124. Modvig KM, Nielsen SF. Psychological changes in children after anaesthesia: A comparison between halothane and ketamine. *Acta Anaesthesiol Scand* 21:541–544, 1977.

125. Cartwright PD, Pingel SM. Midazolam and diazepam in ketamine anaesthesia. *Anaesthesia* 39:439–442, 1984.

126. Toft P, Romer U. Comparison of midazolam and diazepam to supplement total intravenous anaesthesia with ketamine for endoscopy. *Can J Anaesth* 34:466–469, 1987.

127. Bennett JA, Bullimore JA. The use of ketamine hydrochloride anaesthesia for radiotherapy in young children. *Br J Anaesth* 45:197–201, 1973.

128. Byer DE, Gould AB Jr. Development of tolerance to ketamine in an infant undergoing repeated anesthesia. *Anesthesiology* 54:255–256, 1981.

129. Adams HA et al. Sedation and ventilation during ventilation treatment: A comparison of two regimens. *Anaesthetist* 37:268–276, 1988.

130. Reynolds JEF (ed). *The Extra Pharmacopoeia.* London: Pharmaceutical Press, 1977.

131. Graham SR et al. Overdose with chloral hydrate: A pharmacological and therapeutic review. *Med J Aust* 149:686–688, 1988.

132. Lees MH et al. Chloral hydrate and the carbon dioxide chemoreceptor response: A study of puppies and infants. *Pediatrics* 70:447–450, 1982.

133. Mallol J, Sly PD. Effect of chloral hydrate on arterial oxygen saturation in wheezy infants. *Pediatr Pulmonol* 5:96–99, 1988.

134. Marshall AJ. Cardiac arrhythmias caused by chloral hydrate. *Br Med J* 2:994, 1977.

135. Hartley S, Franck LS, Lundergan F. Maintenance sedation of agitated infants in the neonatal intensive care unit with chloral hydrate: New concerns. *J Perinatol* 9:162–164, 1989.

136. Smith MT. Chloral hydrate warning. *Science* 250:359, 1990.

137. Sebel PS, Lowdon JD. Propofol: A new intravenous anesthetic. *Anesthesiology* 71:260–277, 1989.

138. Valtonen M et al. Propofol as an induction agent in children: Pain on injection and pharmacokinetics. *Acta Anaesthesiol Scand* 33:152–155, 1989.

139. Valanne J, Korttila K. Comparison of methohexitone and propofol ('Diprivan') for induction of enflurane anaesthesia in outpatients. *Postgrad Med J* 61:138–143, 1985.

140. Brooker J, Hull CJ, Stafford M. Effect of lignocaine on pain caused by propofol injection (letter). *Anaesthesia* 40:91–92, 1985.

141. Newman LH et al. Propofol infusion for sedation in intensive care. *Anaesthesia* 42:929–937, 1987.

142. Grounds RM et al. Propofol infusion for sedation in the intensive care unit: Preliminary report. *Br Med J [Clin Res]* 294:397–400, 1987.

143. Bodenham A, Culank LS, Park GR. Propofol infusion and green urine (letter). *Lancet* 2:740, 1987.

144. Harris CE et al. Propofol for long-term sedation in the intensive care unit. A comparison with papaveretum and midazolam. *Anaesthesia* 45:366–372, 1990.

145. Borgeat A, Wilder-Smith O. Acute choreoathetoid reaction to propofol (letter). *Anaesthesia* 46:797, 1991.

146. Imray JM, Hay A. Withdrawal syndrome after propofol (letter). *Anaesthesia* 46:704, 1991.

147. Rodgers EM. Diprivan intensive care sedation in children. *Br J Anaesth* 67:505, 1991.

148. Lassen HCA. Treatment of severe tetanus: Severe bone marrow depression after prolonged nitrous oxide anaesthesia. *Lancet* 1:527–530, 1956.

149. Amess JA et al. Megaloblastic haemopoiesis in patients receiving nitrous oxide. *Lancet* 2:339–342, 1978.

150. Colaco CM, Crago RR, Weisbert A. Halothane for status asthmaticus in the intensive care unit—A case report. *Can Anaesth Soc J* 25:329–330, 1978.

151. Raine JM et al. Near-fatal bronchospasm after oral nadolol in a young asthmatic and response to ventilation with halothane. *Br Med J [Clin Res]* 282:548–549, 1981.

152. ORourke PP, Crone RK. Halothane in status asthmaticus. *Crit Care Med* 10:341–343, 1982.

153. Schwartz SH. Treatment of status asthmaticus with halothane. *JAMA* 251:2688–2689, 1984.

154. Holaday DA et al. Resistance of isoflurane to biotransformation in man. *Anesthesiology* 43:325–332, 1975.

155. Eger EI II. Isoflurane: A review. *Anesthesiology* 55:559–576, 1981.

156. Carpenter RL et al. The extent of metabolism of inhaled anesthetics in humans. *Anesthesiology* 65:201–205, 1986.

157. Bierman MI et al. Prolonged isoflurane anesthesia in status asthmaticus. *Crit Care Med* 14:832–833, 1986.

158. Beechey AP et al. Sedation with isoflurane (letter). *Anaesthesia* 43:419–420, 1988.

159. Kong KL, Willatts SM, Prys Roberts C. Isoflurane compared with midazolam for sedation in the intensive care unit. *Br Med J* 298:1277–1280, 1989.

160. Smith RA Tolerance to and dependence on inhalational anesthetics. *Anesthesiology* 50:505–509, 1979.

161. Kripke BJ, Hechtman HB. Nitrous oxide for pentazocine addiction and for intractable pain: Report of case. *Anesth Analg* 51:520–527, 1972.

162. Whitwam JG et al. Pain during continuous nitrous oxide administration. *Br J Anaesth* 48:425–429, 1976.

163. Plummer JL et al. Effects of chronic inhalation of halothane, enflurane or isoflurane in rats. *Br J Anaesth* 58:517–523, 1986.

164. Mazze RI, Calverley RK, Smith NT. Inorganic fluoride nephrotoxicity: Prolonged enflurane and halothane anesthesia in volunteers. *Anesthesiology* 46:265–271, 1977.

165. Strube PJ, Hulands GH, Halsey MJ. Serum fluoride levels in morbidly obese patients: Enflurane compared with isoflurane anaesthesia. *Anaesthesia* 42:685–689, 1987.

166. Pantuck EJ, Pantuck CB, Conney AH. Effect of streptozotocin-induced diabetes in the rat on the metabolism of fluorinated volatile anesthetics. *Anesthesiology* 66:24–28, 1987.

167. Gauntlett IS et al. Metabolism of isoflurane in patients receiving isoniazid. *Anesth Analg* 69:245–249, 1989.

168. Willatts SM et al. Isoflurane compared with midazolam in the intensive care unit (letter). *Br Med J* 299:389, 1989.

169. Hertzka RE et al. Fentanyl-induced ventilatory depression: Effects of age. *Anesthesiology* 70:213–218, 1989.

170. Bailey PL et al. Frequent hypoxemia and apnea after sedation with midazolam and fentanyl. *Anesthesiology* 73:826–830, 1990.

171. Yaster M et al. Midazolam-fentanyl intravenous sedation in children: Case report of respiratory arrest. *Pediatrics* 86:463–467, 1990.

172. Bovill JG, Sebel PS, Stanley TH. Opioid analgesics in anesthesia: With special reference to their use in cardiovascular anesthesia. *Anesthesiology* 61:731–755, 1984.

173. Benthuysen JL et al. Physiology of alfentanil-induced rigidity. *Anesthesiology* 64:440–446, 1986.

174. Bailey PL et al. Anesthetic induction with fentanyl. *Anesth Analg* 64:48–53, 1985.

175. Comstock MK et al. Rigidity and hypercarbia associated with high dose fentanyl induction of anesthesia (letter). *Anesth Analg* 60:362–363, 1981.

176. Freye E, Hartung E, Buhl R. Lung compliance in man is impaired by the rapid injection of alfentanil. *Anaesthesist* 35:543–546, 1986.

177. Marty J, Desmonts JM. Effects of fentanyl on respiratory pressure-volume relationship in supine anesthetized children. *Acta Anaesthesiol Scand* 25:293–296, 1981.

178. Gilman AG, Goodman LS, Gilman A (eds). *The Pharmacologic Basis of Therapeutics.* New York: MacMillan, 1980. P 505.

179. Portenoy RK, Foley KM. Chronic use of opioid analgesics in non-malignant pain: Report of 38 cases. *Pain* 25:171–186, 1986.

180. Taub A. Opioid analgesics in the treatment of chronic intractable pain of non-neoplastic origin. In Kitahata L, Collins J (eds): *Narcotic Analgesics in Anesthesiology*. Baltimore: Williams & Wilkins, 1982.

181. Colpaert FC et al. The effects of prior fentanyl administration and of pain on fentanyl analgesia: Tolerance to and enhancement of narcotic analgesia. *J Pharmacol Exp Ther* 213:418–424, 1980.

182. Hovav E, Weinstock M. Temporal factors influencing the development of acute tolerance to opiates. *J Pharmacol Exp Ther* 242:251–256, 1987.

183. Cheney DL, Goldstein A. Tolerance to opioid narcotics: Time course and reversibility of physical dependence in mice. *Nature* 232:477–478, 1971.

184. Dewey WL. Various factors which affect the rate of development of tolerance and physical dependence to abused drugs. *NIDA Res Monogr* 54:39–49, 1984.

185. Cochin J, Mushlin BE. Effect of agonist-antagonist interaction on the development of tolerance and dependence. *Ann NY Acad Sci* 281:244–251, 1976.

186. Shafer A et al. Use of a fentanyl infusion in the intensive care unit: Tolerance to its anesthetic effects. *Anesthesiology* 59:245–248, 1983.

187. Miller NS, Gold MS. Abuse, addiction, tolerance, and dependence to benzodiazepines in medical and nonmedical populations. *Am J Drug Alcohol Abuse* 17:27–37, 1991.

188. Hasday JD, Weintraub M. Propoxyphene in children with iatrogenic morphine dependence. *Am J Dis Child* 137:745–748, 1983.

189. Miser AW et al. Narcotic withdrawal syndrome in young adults after the therapeutic use of opiates. *Am J Dis Child* 140:603–604, 1986.

190. Boisse NR et al. Tolerance and physical dependence to a short-acting benzodiazepine, midazolam. *J Pharmacol Exp Ther* 252:1125–1133, 1990.

191. Lopez F et al. Chronic administration of benzodiazepines—V. Rapid onset of behavioral and neurochemical alterations after discontinuation of alprazolam. *Neuropharmacology* 29:237–241, 1990.

192. Edwards JG, Cantopher T, Olivieri S. Benzodiazepine dependence and the problems of withdrawal. *Postgrad Med J* 66(Suppl 2):S27–S35, 1990.

193. Rickels K et al. Long-term therapeutic use of benzodiazepines. I. Effects of abrupt discontinuation. *Arch Gen Psychiatry* 47:899–907, 1990.

194. Lader M, Morton S. Benzodiazepine withdrawal syndrome. *Br J Psychiatry* 158:435–436, 1991.

195. Greenblatt DJ, Shader RI. Dependence, tolerance, and addiction to benzodiazepines: Clinical and pharmacokinetic considerations. *Drug Metab Rev* 8:13–28, 1978.

196. Don HF et al. The effects of anesthesia and 100 percent oxygen on the functional residual capacity of the lungs. *Anesthesiology* 32:521–529, 1970.

197. Westbrook PR et al. Effects of anesthesia and muscle paralysis on respiratory mechanics in normal man. *J Appl Physiol* 34:81–86, 1973.

198. Kallos T, Wyche MQ, Garman JK. The effects of Innovar on functional residual capacity and total chest compliance in man. *Anesthesiology* 39:558–561, 1973.

199. Yasuda I et al. Tracheal constriction by morphine and by fentanyl in man. *Anesthesiology* 49:117–119, 1978.

200. Rosow CE et al. Histamine release during morphine and fentanyl anesthesia. *Anesthesiology* 56:93–96, 1982.

201. Soleymani Y et al. Management of life-threatening asthma in children. A preliminary study of the use of morphine in respiratory failure. *Am J Dis Child* 123:533–540, 1972.

202. Eschenbacher WL et al. Morphine sulfate inhibits bronchoconstriction in subjects with mild asthma whose responses are inhibited by atropine. *Am Rev Respir Dis* 130:363–367, 1984.

203. Rogers DF, Barnes PJ. Opioid inhibition of neurally mediated mucus secretion in human bronchi. *Lancet* 1:930–932, 1989.

204. Jones RM, Fiddian Green R, Knight PR. Narcotic-induced choledochoduodenal sphincter spasm reversed by glucagon. *Anesth Analg* 59:946–947, 1980.

205. Blancquaert JP, Lefebvre RA, Willems JL. Emetic and antiemetic effects of opioids in the dog. *Eur J Pharmacol* 128:143–150, 1986.

206. Stanski DR, Paalzow L, Edlund PO. Morphine pharmacokinetics: GLC assay versus radioimmunoassay. *J Pharm Sci* 71:314–317, 1982.

207. Baskoff JD, Stevenson RL. Fentanyl pharmacokinetics in children with heart disease. *Anesthesiology* 55:A194, 1981.

208. Singleton MA, Rosen JI, Fisher DM. Pharmacokinetics of fentanyl for infants and adults. *Anesthesiology* 61:A440, 1984.

209. Johnson KL et al. Fentanyl pharmacokinetics in the pediatric population. *Anesthesiology* 61:A441, 1984.

210. Koren G et al. Pediatric fentanyl dosing based on pharmacokinetics during cardiac surgery. *Anesth Analg* 63:577–582, 1984.

211. Gauntlett IS et al. Pharmacokinetics of fentanyl in neonatal humans and lambs: Effects of age. *Anesthesiology* 69:683–687, 1988.

212. Bovill JG et al. The pharmacokinetics of alfentanil (R39209): A new opioid analgesic. *Anesthesiology* 57:439–443, 1982.

Nishan Goudsouzian

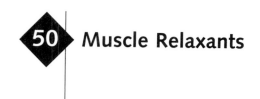

50 Muscle Relaxants

Neuromuscular Transmission

Anatomically, the neuromuscular junction is divided into three components: the neural element, which is the terminal part of the axon; the synaptic gap; and the muscular part with its specialized receptors (Fig. 50-1). As they reach the myoneural junction, the motor nerve endings lose their myelin but retain their cover of Schwann cells and are filled with mitochondria. They end as complex multibranching structures arranged in complicated arrays in a tiny area of the muscle surface forming the myoneural junction.

The nerve synthesizes acetylcholine by enzymatic esterification (choline acetyltransferase) of choline by acetate, the acetyl group being transferred from acetylcoenzyme A:

choline + acetylcoenzyme A → acetylcholine + coenzyme A.

The synthesized acetylcholine molecules are stored in small uniformly sized packages known as vesicles. The diameter of each vesicle is about 650 nm. In the resting state, small quantities of acetylcholine are continuously released, creating a miniature endplate potential. On stimulation of the nerve, the Ca^{++} traverses and enters the presynaptic area, causing the vesicles to fuse with the presynaptic membrane and release their contents of acetylcholine into the cleft separating the nerve from the muscle.

The gap between the presynaptic terminal and the cell body of the neurons is known as the synaptic cleft. The synaptic cleft has an average width of 20 nm and is in continuity with the extracellular fluid.[1,2] To exert their action, muscle relaxants have to reach the synaptic cleft. They act mainly at the site of the nicotinic receptors of the muscular side on the neuromuscular junction.

The motor endplate is the chemosensitive, highly folded area of the muscle membrane located opposite the motor nerve terminal. The postsynaptic receptors for the cholinergic transmitter are located primarily at the crests of the junctional folds as part of the integral membrane protein.[3] The receptors are in the form of discrete rings (8–9 nm in diameter) with a central pit, looking like a donut. They protrude for about 5 nm into the extracellular space and about 2 nm intracellularly. Each of these rings is made up of five polypeptide rosette types of unit: alpha (of which there are two), beta, gamma, and delta (Fig. 50-2). The two identical alpha units are the site of competition between cholinergic agonists (acetylcholine) and antagonists (nondepolarizing muscle relaxants). When both alpha units are occupied by an agonist, the protein molecule undergoes conformational changes to form a channel for ions to flow.

A nerve impulse releases 200 to 500 quanta of acetylcholine, each containing about 5000 acetylcholine molecules. Within microseconds, a portion of this released acetylcholine binds to the receptors on the postsynaptic membrane, changing their conformational shape and inducing the opening of discrete ion channels. Each quantum of acetylcholine is capable of generating about 1500 open channels in the postsynaptic membrane to cause an endplate current of about 4 nA and a potential of -80 mV. A single channel is usually open for 1 ms. Within that interval, about 10,000 ions, mainly Na^+ and K^+ and to a lesser extent Ca^{++}, cross the membrane. With the opening of the ion channels, an endplate potential is created that triggers a wave of depolarization and hence causes the muscle to contract. This depolarization signal is several

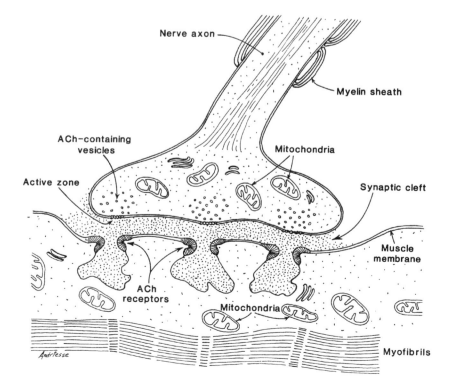

Figure 50-1. A diagramatic representation of the neuromuscular junction.

Figure 50-2.   A schematic of the postsynaptic acetylcholine receptor.

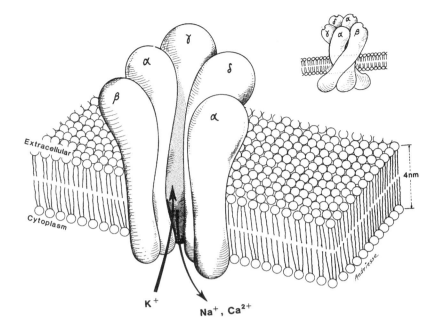

times greater than the threshold for muscle stimulation, providing a margin of safety in neuromuscular transmission.

The depolarization wave is of a very short duration. This is because acetylcholine is hydrolyzed almost immediately by the cholinesterases present at junctional folds to its components, acetyl and choline. The choline molecule is reuptaken by the nerve terminal to resynthesize acetylcholine (Fig. 50-3).

Evaluation of Neuromuscular Transmission

There are two principal methods for evaluating neuromuscular transmission: clinically and/or by a monitor. The principle of the neuromuscular monitor is straightforward. A nerve is stimulated and the resultant contraction of its motor branch evaluated. The ulnar nerve is most commonly used in this determination, with the force of contraction of the adductor of the thumb being measured. This system is the closest one can get to the single muscle nerve preparation.[4]

Several frequencies of stimuli can be used (Fig. 50-4):

1. Single twitches (0.1 cycles/sec or 6 cycles/min). In the presence of a muscle relaxant, the amplitude of the twitch stimulus is diminished. A simple comparison of these values and the control twitch response gives a percentage change. It is estimated that at least 70% of the receptors need to be blocked to obtain a depression of the twitch response.[5] If the neuromuscular blockade is deep, no response is detected. Because the diaphragm recovers faster from the effect of a relaxant than do the peripheral muscles, it is possible to have some diaphragmatic action (e.g., hiccup) in the absence of a twitch response.

2. Tetanic stimuli (50 cycles/sec for 5 seconds). It takes a greater degree of neuromuscular blockade to abolish completely a tetanic response than a twitch response. With nondepolarizing relaxants during tetanic stimulation, a characteristic fade is detected (i.e., the evoked response is stronger at the beginning of stimulation than at the end). This most probably results from progressive

Figure 50-3.   The acetylcholine cycle.

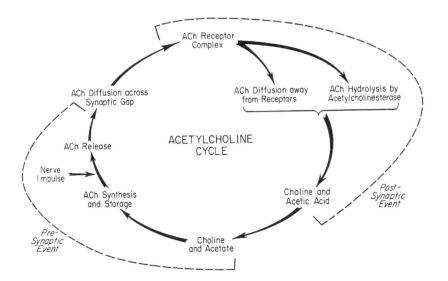

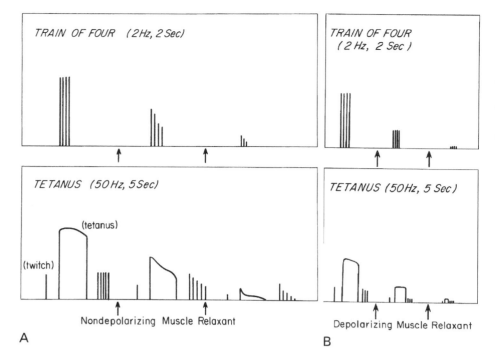

Figure 50-4. Representation of twitch, train-of-four, and tetanic responses of the thumb to stimuli applied to the ulnar nerve. With nondepolarizing block, fade **(A)** is noted during train-of-four and tetanic stimulation, and posttetanic facilitation is seen in the twitch response following the tetanus. During depolarizing block **(B),** the amplitude of tetanus is diminished but is sustained.

depletion of acetylcholine stores as the stimuli continues. Fade is not seen during normal transmission, primarily because of the presence of a large safety factor at the junction. During competitive block, however, this safety factor is diminished, and a larger number of acetylcholine molecules are required to overcome the block. The force of contraction is thus less near the end of stimulation than at the beginning (see Fig. 50-4a). During nondepolarizing block, the amplitude is diminished but no fade is seen (see Fig. 50-4b).

3. Posttetanic facilitation. If during competitive blockade a second stimulus is given after the termination of a tetanic one, the posttetanic response will be higher than the pretetanic one. The main reason is that after tetanic stimulation, the production of acetylcholine still continues; hence, if another stimulus is applied at this period, the twitch response is increased. In normal situations and during nondepolarizing block, no significant posttetanic facilitation is seen.

4. Train-of-four stimulation (2 cycles/sec for 2 seconds, 4 stimuli). Train-of-four stimulation is more versatile than either single or tetanic stimulation. Its advantage over single twitch is that a numerical value can be obtained in the absence of a control response. By comparing the fourth response with the first one, a ratio can be obtained. The advantage of train-of-four over tetanic stimulation is that it can be repeated and is not as painful. It has been noted that if the train-of-four value is more than 70%, the respiratory mechanics of an individual are near normal.[6]

Clinical Evaluation of Neuromuscular Blockade

In the absence of a neuromuscular monitor (twitch monitor), a reasonable evaluation of neuromuscular function can be obtained by observing a spontaneously moving patient. Obviously, not all signs will be present in a single patient. In a spontaneously breathing infant, a reasonable guess can be obtained by watching the respiration. If during spontaneous respiration the intercostals are not contracting, the clinician might suspect an inadequate recovery, because the diaphragm recovers before the intercostal muscles.

Retractions at the suprasternal and at the supraclavicular areas are also indications of insufficient recovery. Feeling the tone of abdominal muscles is informative, especially during coughing.

In a tracheally intubated patient, a negative inspiratory force more than 25 cm H_2O is a clear indication of adequate reversal. A crying vital capacity of more than 15 ml/kg is another such sign.[7] In a moving child, an adequate evaluation can be made by observing the movement of the upper and lower limbs.[8] The ability of the patient to lift up and maintain the elevation of the arms or legs also gives a clear indication of the absence of the neuromuscular blockade. This latter determination must, however, remain secondary to the evaluation of the adequacy of respiration. Of prime concern should be the patient's ability to maintain oxygenation and carbon dioxide excretion.

Neuromuscular Blocking Agents

Muscle relaxants act by two different methods. The first is by prolonged depolarization, and the prototype of this group is succinylcholine. All of the other clinically used relaxants act by competitive mechanisms at the receptors of the myoneural junction. This group of drugs is also known as nondepolarizing muscle relaxants. The doses clinically used for these agents are listed in Table 50-1.

Succinylcholine

Succinylcholine is the muscle relaxant with the fastest onset and the shortest duration of action. In contrast to other muscle relaxants that act by competitive inhibition, succinylcholine acts by depolarization. Its initial effect is similar to that of acetylcholine (i.e., depolarization), but because it is not hydrolyzed by the true tissue cholinesterases present at the myoneural junction, the depolarization persists until the drug diffuses out of the myoneural junction to be hydrolyzed by plasma nonspecific cholinesterase (pseudocholinesterase).

The onset of relaxation with succinylcholine is extremely fast;

Table 50-1. Clinical initial doses of relaxants in children

Succinylcholine	1.0–2.0 mg/kg IV 3–4 mg/kg IM
Mivacurium	0.2–3.0 mg/kg IV
Atracurium	0.4–0.6 mg/kg IV
Vecuronium	0.1 mg/kg IV
Rocuronium	0.6 mg/kg IV
Doxacurium	0.05 mg/kg IV
Pipecuronium	0.08 mg/kg IV
Pancuronium	0.1 mg/kg IV
Metubine	0.3 mg/kg IV
Tubocurarine	0.6 mg/kg IV

evidence of paralysis can be detected within one circulation time, and full paralysis can be obtained in less than a minute.[9] The usual recommended dose in children is 1.5 to 2.0 mg/kg. Because of their larger extracellular volume, infants require a higher amount, 2 to 3 mg/kg.[10] The neuromuscular blockade from these effective doses will usually last 5 to 10 minutes. Succinylcholine's fast onset of action makes this drug invaluable in situations in which rapid control of the airway is desirable. It is essential in these situations that a qualified person be present to manage the airway, either to ventilate by face mask or endotracheal intubation, because the patient will be apneic during neuromuscular paralysis.

Another advantage of succinylcholine is that in a dire emergency it can be given intramuscularly. Here, the amount is 2 to 3 times the intravenous (IV) dose, and as long as tissue perfusion is present, its effects can be detected within minutes.[11]

Succinylcholine has several **side effects;** they are relatively minor, but they must not be ignored.[12]

Arrythmias

Arrythmias are more commonly seen in children than in adults and are usually benign in nature and self-limiting. They can vary from a few premature atrial or ventricular contraction to a series of bigeminy for a few minutes. Sinus arrest has also been reported but usually occurs after a second dose of the drug. These cardiac manifestations can be prevented by the prior administration of IV atropine 0.01 mg/kg.

Fasciculations

Succinylcholine causes contraction of all of the muscles before relaxing. It is more manifest in children older than 4 years, but it can be seen in its milder form in smaller children; it is not observed in infants. These fasciculations can cause a rise of intragastric pressure in susceptible children. Mild hyperkalemia can also occur after the administration of succinylcholine, but it is marked in severely burned patients, the victims of extensive trauma, and in patients with paralysis or muscular dystrophies.

Malignant Hyperthermia

Succinylcholine is one of the rare agents that can trigger malignant hyperthermia, which is an acute hypermetabolic state that leads to hypercarbia, acidosis, and tachycardia, and if not actively treated can be fatal. Dantrolene is the specific treatment for malignant hyperthermia.

Mild myoglobinemia and myoglobinuria are frequently associ-

ated with succinylcholine in children,[13] although the clinical importance of this side effect is unknown. Interestingly, myoglobinuria is not seen after puberty.

A rise of intraocular pressure due to prolonged contraction of extraocular muscles may also occur with succinylcholine. This side effect is significant in patients with open-eye injury.

Recently, the Federal Drug Administration issued a warning stating that succinylcholine should not be used for routine, elective pediatric surgery and that nondepolarizing agents are effective for routine use. This was based on the observation that unexpected major complications such as malignant hyperthermia or cardiac arrest had occurred in susceptible individuals or in children with myopathies. The mortality rate in these patients was 55%. However, succinylcholine may be used in situations when the rapid establishment of an airway is critical, such as in severe laryngospasm, or for rapid intubation in an emergency.[14]

Mivacurium

Mivacurium is a short-acting relaxant. An intubating dose of mivacurium 0.25 mg/kg induces complete paralysis in about 1.5 minutes in children. The complete paralysis lasts for about 8 minutes and full recovery occurs in about 20 minutes.[15] Therefore, the duration of action of this drug is in between succinylcholine and intermediate acting drugs. Despite its short duration, its onset is similar to that of intermediate-acting relaxants. A side effect of mivacurium is histamine release, especially at larger doses. At 0.3 mg/kg, a flush can be seen that fades within 5 to 10 minutes. This flush is usually not accompanied by adverse cardiovascular signs or symptoms in children.

Intermediate-Acting Relaxants

The intermediate-acting relaxants—atracurium, vecuronium, and rocuronium—are relatively new. Similar to the long-acting ones, they are nondepolarizing and act by competitive binding of the alpha receptors at the myoneural junction. Their main advantage is the relative absence of side effects.

Atracurium is an imidazoline derivative and has a unique process of elimination. In plasma and extracellular fluid, it undergoes alkaline hydrolysis (Hoffman elimination), which is not dependent on hepatic or renal function.[16] Similarly, the dose of the drug (mg/kg) is not affected by the age of the individual.[17] The dose used for endotracheal intubation is 0.4 to 0.6 mg/kg. Larger doses can cause temporary flushing of the skin at the neck and upper chest, presumably from histamine release. This might be accompanied by a slight diminution of BP, which usually goes unnoticed because of its short duration and the antagonistic effect of endotracheal intubation. These side effects can be avoided if the drug is given slowly (60 seconds) intravenously. The absence of major side effects and its predictable mode of elimination has made this compound the frequent choice in patients with single- or multiple-organ failure; it is also used frequently by continuous infusion when prolonged periods of relaxation are required. To achieve such levels in humans is very difficult and should probably not be of clinical concern unless the drug is to be given continuously for days in patients with hepatorenal failures, as laudanosine, one of atracurium's metabolites, under normal conditions is metabolized by the liver and the kidneys.

Vecuronium is virtually free from cardiovascular side effects. Its usual recommended dose for tracheal intubation is 0.1 mg/kg, and this dose in children will provide complete neuromuscular paralysis for 20 minutes, and in another 20 minutes, the effect of the drug is dissipated. Vecuronium is mostly metabolized by the liver and excreted in the bile.[18] Because of this mode of elimination, the effect of vecuronium is cumulative (i.e., with repeated doses a lesser amount of the drug is required). Also, because of its route of metabolism, the duration of action of vecuronium is prolonged in neonates.[19]

Rocuronium is the newest of the intermediate-acting nondepolarizing muscle relaxants. Its main advantage is its rapid onset of action, fastest of all non-depolarizing relaxants, but slower than succinylcholine.[20] The usual recommended dose, 0.6 mg/kg, causes complete paralysis in about 1.2 minutes in children. The duration of action of such a dose is comparable to that of atracurium and vecuronium. Rocuronium is mainly metabolized by the liver and excreted by the kidney.

Long-Acting Relaxants

Presently, there are five long-acting relaxants available. They are tubocurarine, metubine pancuronium, doxacurium, and pipecuronium.[21] Of these, the most popular for use in infants and children has been pancuronium, because frequently, tachycardia (a side effect of the drug) may improve cardiac output. The usual dose of pancuronium is 0.1 mg/kg, which provides complete paralysis for 1 hour. Thereafter, another 40 to 60 minutes are required for complete recovery. The comparable doses of tubocurarine and metubine are 0.5 mg/kg and 0.25 mg/kg, respectively. Tubocurarine and, to a lesser degree, metubine cause histamine release with some possibility of decrease in BP. All of these three drugs are metabolized and excreted by the kidneys, but with tubocurarine there is an alternate hepatic route of metabolism. Pancuronium in combination with fentanyl (or sufentanyl) is frequently used in small infants during cardiac surgery and in the postoperative period. Here, the tachycardic properties of pancuronium are used to good effect in counteracting the bradycardia induced by fentanyl, and its relaxant properties counteract the respiratory muscle stiffness caused by fentanyl.[22] Two long-acting relaxants have become available, doxacurium and pipecuronium; they are both nondepolarizing agents. Their main advantage is the absence of side effects. They do not cause cardiovascular perturbations. In children, the recommended intubating dose of doxacurium is 0.05 mg/kg and of pipecuronium is 0.08 mg/kg.[23]

Antagonism of Neuromuscular Blocking Agents

In an intensive care setting, reversal of action of relaxants is infrequently needed, because most patients are allowed to recover spontaneously. If the need arises, however, for a rapid recovery, such as for evaluating the clinical neurological status, a reversal agent can be given. The most commonly used reversal agents (neostigmine and edrophonium) are cholinesterase inhibitors for the nicotinic receptors at the myoneural junction. Following their administration, the amount of acetylcholine at the receptor site is increased, which competitively displaces the relaxants from the myoneural junction. Because these drugs have vagomimetic effects that can cause alarming bradycardia, they are always preceded by an anticholinergic agent such as atropine or glycopyrrolate. Several combinations of these reversal agents can be given, but the standard has been atropine 0.02 mg/kg and neostigmine 0.06 mg/kg. Within minutes after their administration, improvement of the neuromuscular function can be seen if its weakness was in fact due to the effect of relaxant (Fig. 50-5).

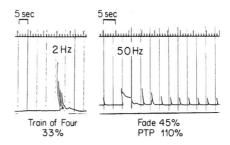

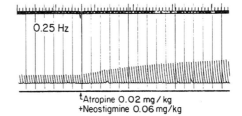

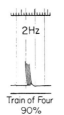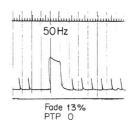

Figure 50-5. Pattern of reversal of 5-day-old 2.9-kg baby. Note the fade in train-of-four and the fade of tetanus before the reversal. The amplitude of the recording was increased during the initial train-of-four recording. PTP, posttetanic potentiation; Hz, cycle/sec.

Specific Conditions

Burns

The slight hyperkalemia seen in response to the administration of succinylcholine in normal individuals is exaggerated in the burn patient; the more extensive the burn, the more likely is the hyperkalemic response and the possibility of cardiac arrest. The exaggerated hyperkalemic response is probably due to the development of new acetylcholine receptors along the surface of the muscle membrane in the post-burn phase.[24] These new receptors may also be responsible for the resistance to nondepolarizing muscle relaxants seen in burned patients.

Although no case of cardiac arrest has been reported in the first few days following a burn, the use at that time of succinylcholine is avoided because of the ever-present possibility of hyperkalemic response. If the requirement of muscle relaxant is for a short duration, such as for an intubation, atracurium 0.6 mg/kg, vecuronium 0.12 mg/kg, or rocuronium 0.9 mg/kg can provide satisfactory relaxation in the first few days after a burn. If the burn is extensive (more than 40%) and more than 5 days have passed, however, these doses should be increased by a factor of 2 to 3.[24] For prolonged paralysis, these patients need and tolerate larger doses of nondepolarizing relaxants. As long as renal function is present, patients excrete relaxants effectively, and if the need arises, the effect of the nondepolarizing relaxant can be antagonized by the usual dose of reversal agents.[25]

Extensive Injuries

Patients with extensive nerve and muscle injuries, as well as those who have been immobilized for a long time, develop extrajunctional receptors that can predispose to a hyperkalemic response to succinylcholine. Again, this drug should be avoided whenever possible. However, if the need is immediate, such as in response to respiratory arrest or in a case of acute airway obstruction due to laryngospasm, succinylcholine use can be justified because it is the fastest acting relaxant available.

Malignant Hyperthermia

Succinylcholine is the most likely of all relaxants to be responsible for triggering of the malignant hyperthermia syndrome. Malignant hyperthermia is a hypermetabolic syndrome with a very acute onset. During one of these episodes, a marked increase in the metabolic activity of the skeletal muscles leads to increased carbon dioxide production and acidosis. The patient usually manifests with tachycardia, hypercarbia, and metabolic acidosis with a consequent hyperventilation. This is followed by a rapidly developing hyperthermia. The carbon dioxide production is increased so markedly that ventilation cannot catch up with it. The result is marked carbon dioxide retention, which is one of the pathognomonic features of this syndrome.

Of the drugs that are known to trigger malignant hyperthermia, the foremost is succinylcholine; this is followed by the halogenated anesthetic inhalational agents. Nondepolarizing muscle relaxants can be used safely.[26] The specific treatment of malignant hyperthermia is IV dantrolene, which is started at a dose of 3 mg/kg IV and continued until all the symptoms subside (see Malignant Hyperthermia by Ryan, this volume).

Progressive Muscular Dystrophy

Duchenne-type muscular dystrophy is the one most susceptible to untoward effects of succinylcholine. In these patients, succinylcholine causes rhabdomyolosis, as evidenced by myoglobinurea, increased creatine kinase (CK), hyperkalemia, and occasionally metabolic acidosis. Patients with myocardial involvement may develop tachycardia, ventricular fibrillation, and even cardiac arrest. Because of their prominent cardiac and muscular effects, succinylcholine should be avoided, but nondepolarizing muscle relaxants can be used safely.[27]

Myotonia

Because the effect of succinylcholine is similar to acetylcholine but of longer duration, in myotonic patients, it induces an exaggerated myotonic response causing respiratory and jaw muscle rigidity, leading to anoxia and inability to relax jaw muscles. Occasionally, increased myotonia has been seen following neostigmine, presumably from the stimulating effect of acetylcholine.

Asthma

In an asthmatic patient, it is important to realize that more critical than the choice of relaxant is the stimulation of the trachea by the insertion of an endotracheal tube during light planes of anesthesia, inducing an asthmatic attack.[28] This is especially important in an asthmatic patient who is asymptomatic or mildly symptomatic who will require endotracheal intubation and ventilation for another condition. In such patients, the pulmonary reflexes can be ob-tunded in several ways. The afferent part of the reflex can be blocked by the prior spraying of the vocal cords and the trachea with a local anesthetic, such as lidocaine 1% to 2%. The central part of the reflex can be blocked or attenuated by administering general anesthesia or strong sedation, the efferent part by the administration of antiasthmatic medication. In the patient who is in status asthmaticus and respiratory failure, this factor is probably of little significance because these patients are maximally broncho-constricted, but blocking the reflex may be an additional factor in breaking the vicious circle.

Of the relaxants available, tubocurarine and atracurium are mild histamine releasers. This designation alone should not preclude their usage in asthmatic patients, because there is no direct evidence of these drugs inducing asthmatic episodes. Further, the histamine-releasing potential of these drugs can be attenuated or abolished by slow IV administration (60–90 seconds).

Seizures

During a seizure, the amount of oxygen and energy substrate consumed by the brain may be markedly increased. This increase in oxygen consumption may exceed the body's capacity to increase delivery of oxygen and nutrition by increasing cerebral blood flow. In this event, portions of the brain may become ischemic and sustain permanent damage. Therefore, it is essential to control seizures to ensure adequate oxygenation. This is usually achieved by antiseizure medications. In refractory cases, muscle relaxants and positive pressure ventilation may be required. Because muscle relaxants act peripherally, they have no specific effect on the brain. By masking the motor response, they may block the clinical sign that is used to judge the effectiveness of the anticonvulsant medications. Although any of the nondepolarizing muscle relaxants can be used, atracurium would probably be the most convenient because of its noncumulative properties when administered via continuous infusion. The predictable pattern of recovery, evidence of returning neuromuscular function within 15 minutes of the infusion's discontinuation, can be detected regardless of how long the infusion has been running or how much drug can be delivered.[29,30] Atracurium infusion, however, should not be continued for more than a few days, because one of the metabolites is laudanosine, which in itself is a convulsant in animals at very high concentrations.

Neonates

For a long time, pancuronium was the relaxant most frequently used in neonatal ICUs to achieve neuromuscular paralysis as an adjunct in the management of severe pulmonary disorders such as hyaline membrane disease and persistent pulmonary hypertension of the newborn. Neuromuscular relaxation may aid in optimizing ventilation when the infant requires a respirator. In addition, the peak transpulmonary pressures are diminished, resulting in a decrease in the incidence of pneumotharaces.[31]

Vecuronium has become more popular in ICUs because it does not have cardiovascular effects. It is usually given by a continuous infusion (0.06–0.14 μg/kg/hr after an initial 0.1-mg/kg dose).[32,33] Although most of vecuronium is excreted in the bile, in an infant, a proportionally larger dose is excreted by the kidneys. Therefore, its effects are prolonged in this group of patients, especially in infants with renal failure.[34]

The frequent use of muscle relaxants in extremely vulnerable patients has led clinicians to attribute (sometimes unjustifiably) several complications to these drugs. These have included hypotension in an infant with borderline blood volume, joint contractures that might have been overcome with appropriate physiotherapy, and "gasless abdomen" on abdominal roentgenograms. The latter is probably due to evacuation of abdominal gases from the intestine in the absence of swallowing.[35] The increase in heart rate and BP and the rise of plasma epinephrine and norepinephrine levels associated with the administration of pancuronium in neonates have aroused the concern that pancuronium is a contributing factor in the occurrence of intracerebral hemorrhage or myocardial dysfunction. It should be noted, however, that the hemodynamic changes are less pronounced during tracheal intubation in infants on pancuronium than in those in whom neuromuscular paralysis has not been induced.[31]

In recent years, case reports have appeared that implicate neuromuscular blocking agents as a cause of residual weakness after discontinuation of the drug in adults.[36–38] The condition appears to be one in which acute generalized myopathy becomes apparent as neuromuscular blockade recovers. It appears that most episodes of myopathy are caused by some adverse interaction between neuromuscular blocking agents, especially pancuronium and vecuronium (which have a steroidal structure) and corticosteroids. Experimentally, the administration of steroids combined with surgical denervation causes greater muscle atrophy than either intervention alone. The atrophy reversed over several weeks when innervation of the muscle was restored.[39] Thus, it behooves us to titrate muscle relaxants carefully by monitoring the extent of the blockade both clinically and with the use of a peripheral nerve stimulator.

References

1. Goudsouzian NG, Standaert FG. The infant and the myoneural junction. *Anesth Analg* 65:1208–1217, 1986.
2. Adams PR. Acetylcholine receptor kinetics. *J Membr Biol* 58:161–174, 1981.
3. Standaert FG. Basic physiology and pharmacology of the neuromuscular junction. In Miller RD (ed): *Anesthesia*. New York: Churchill Livingstone, 1986. Pp 835–871.
4. Ali HH, Savarese JJ. Monitoring of neuromuscular function. *Anesthesiology* 45:216–249, 1976.
5. Waud BE, Waud DR. The relation between the response to "train-of-four" stimulation and receptor occlusions during competitive neuromuscular blockade. *Anesthesiology* 37:413–416, 1972.
6. Ali HH et al. The effect of tubocurarine on indirectly elicited train-of-four muscle response and respiratory measurement in humans. *Br J Anaesth* 47:570–574, 1975.
7. Shimada Y et al. Crying vital capacity and maximal inspiratory pressure as clinical indicators of readiness of weaning of infants less than a year of age. *Anesthesiology* 51:456–459, 1979.
8. Mason LD, Betts EK. Leg lift and maximum respiratory force, clinical signs of neuromuscular blockade reversal in neonates and infants. *Anesthesiology* 52:441–442, 1980.
9. Cunliff M, Lucero VM, McLeod ME. Neuromuscular blockade for rapid tracheal intubation in children: Comparison of succinylcholine and pancuronium. *Can Anaesth Soc J* 33:760–764, 1986.
10. Meakin G et al. Dose response curves for suxamethonium in neonates, infants and children. *Br J Anaesth* 62:655–658, 1989.
11. Liu LMP et al. Dose response to intramuscular succinylcholine in children. *Anesthesiology* 55:599–603, 1981.
12. Goudsouzian NG. Muscle relaxants in children. In Coté CJ et al. (eds): *A Practice of Anesthesia for Infants and Children*. Philadelphia: Saunders, 1992. Pp 151–170.
13. Laurence AS. Biochemical change following suxamethonium. Serum myoglobin, potassium and creatinine kinase, changes before commencement of surgery. *Anaesthesia* 40:854–859, 1985.
14. Kent RS. Revised label regarding use of succinylcholine in children and adolescents. *Anesthesiology* 80:242–245, 1994.
15. Goudsouzian NG et al. Neuromuscular and cardiovascular effects of mivacurium in children. *Anesthesiology* 70:237–242, 1989.
16. Miller RD. Pharmacokinetics of atracurium and other non-depolarizing neuromuscular blocking agents in normal patients and those with renal or hepatic dysfunction. *Br J Anaesth* 58:11S–13S, 1986.
17. Goudsouzian NG. Atracurium in infants and children. *Br J Anaesth* 58:23S–28S, 1986.
18. Lebreault G et al. Pharmacokinetics and pharmacodynamics of vecuronium in patients with cholestasis. *Br J Anaesth* 58:983–987, 1986.
19. Meretoja O. Is vecuronium a long-acting neuromuscular blocking agent in neonates and infants? *Br J Anaesth* 62:184–187, 1989.
20. Magorian T, Flannery KB, Miller RD. Comparison of rocuronium, succinylcholine and vecuronium for rapid sequence induction of anesthesia in adult patients. *Anesthesiology* 79:913–918, 1993.
21. Goudsouzian NG et al. Comparison of equipotent doses of non-depolarizing muscle relaxants in children. *Anesth Analg* 60:862–866, 1982.
22. Hickey P, Hansen DD. Fentanyl and sufentanil oxygen pancuronium anesthesia for cardiac surgery in infants. *Anesth Analg* 63:117–122, 1984.
23. Goudsouzian NC et al. Neuromuscular and cardiovascular effects of doxacurium in children anaesthetized with halothane. *Br J Anaesth* 62:263–268, 1989.
24. Goldhill DR, Martyn JAJ. Succinylcholine induced hyperkalemia. In Azar I (ed): *Muscle Relaxants*. Place: Marcel Dekker, 1987. P 93.
25. Martyn J, Goldhill DR, Goudsouzian N. Clinical pharmacology of muscle relaxants in patients with burns. *J Clin Pharmacol* 26:680–685, 1986.
26. Gronert GA. Malignant hyperthermia. *Anesthesiology* 53:395–423, 1980.
27. Sethna NV, Rockoff MA, Worthen M. Anesthesia related complications in children with Duchenne muscular dystrophy. *Anesthesiology* 68:462–465, 1988.
28. Murray J. Anesthesia for thoracic surgery. In Gregory GA (ed): *Pediatric Anesthesia*. New York: Churchill Davidson, 1983. P 669.
29. Delgado-Escueta AV et al. Management of status epilepticus. *N Engl J Med* 306:1337–1339, 1982.
30. Goudsouzian NG et al. Continuous infusion of atracurium in children. *Anesthesiology* 64:171–175, 1986.
31. Greenough A et al. Pancuronium prevents pneumothoraces in ventilated premature babies who actively expire against positive pressure inflation. *Lancet* 1:8367, 1984.
32. Fitzpatrick KTJ et al. Continuous vecuronium infusion for prolonged muscle relaxation in children. *Can J Anaesth* 38:168–174, 1991.
33. Eldadah MK, Newth CJL. Vecuronium by continuous infusion for neuromuscular blockage in infants and children. *Crit Care Med* 17:989–992, 1989.
34. Haynes SR, Morton NS. Prolonged neuromuscular blockade with vecuronium in a neonate with renal failure. *Anaesthesia* 45:743–745, 1990.
35. Dillard RG, Crowe JE, Sumner T. Pancuronium and abnormal roentgenograms. *Am J Dis Child* 134:821–827, 1980.
36. Hansen-Flaschen J, Cowen J, Raps EC. Neuromuscular blockade in the intensive care unit more than we bargained for. *Am Rev Respir Dis* 147:234–236, 1993.
37. Griffen D et al. Acute myopathy during treatment of status asthmaticus with corticosteroids and steroidal muscle relaxants. *Chest* 102:510–514, 1992.
38. Segredo V et al. Persistent paralysis in critically ill patients after long-term administration of vecuronium. *N Engl J Med* 327:524–528, 1992.
39. Massa R et al. Loss and renewal of thick myofilaments in glucocorticoid treated rat soleus after denervation and renervation. *Muscle Nerve* 15:1290–1298, 1992.

Angela Anderson
Michael Shannon

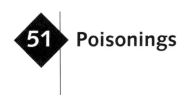

51 ◆ Poisonings

Epidemiology

While poisonings generally account for only 5% to 10% of intensive care unit (ICU) admissions in both pediatric and adult series[1,2] up to 64% of pediatric poisonings require admission to pediatric intensive care units (PICUs) as a part of initial management.

Although intoxications occur through several potential routes of exposure (Table 51-1), they most commonly are a result of ingestion, which accounts for 75% to 80% of all intoxications.[3] Other important routes of toxic exposure that may lead to life-threatening illness include dermal, inhalation, and envenomation (by toxic reptiles, arachnids, and marine life).

The age distribution for ingestions in the pediatric population is distinctly bimodal, with most ingestions occurring in toddlers 1 to 3 years of age and the remainder in adolescents. Each peak, however, provides different implications for etiology and management. In the toddler, ingestions are most commonly of a single agent and are accidental. With a carefully obtained history, the toxin is usually identifiable. In contrast, poisonings in adolescents are typically multiple and intentional. In these cases, the ingested toxin is often unknown.[3–6]

Adjunctive Measures in the Diagnosis of Poisonings

Toxic Screen Analysis

In the approach to suspected intoxications, one of the most important laboratory tests is the analysis of biologic specimens for toxic substances, commonly known as the toxic screen. The toxic screen is considered the most important adjunct to the clinical history in the diagnosis of toxic exposures.[7,8]

Many biologic specimens can be used for toxic screen analysis, including blood, urine, vomitus, hair, sweat, saliva, skin, nails, and meconium. However, the proper biologic specimen to test after a suspected intoxication generally depends on the suspected toxin.

Typically, some combination of serum, urine, and gastric contents is sent for drug analysis. The use of gastric contents for toxic screen analysis is rarely useful because this fluid is technically difficult to analyze and uncommonly yields more information than the combined analysis of urine and serum. Toxic screen analysis of serum is most useful when quantitative drug concentrations are desired, particularly for those toxins in which some correlation exists between serum concentration and clinical effect. Also, quantitative drug concentrations are often necessary because they dictate intervention strategies for many intoxications (e.g., aspirin, acetaminophen).

Analysis of urine also offers advantages. Although the information obtained is generally qualitative, quantitative urine concentrations of drug can occasionally be correlated with serum concentration (e.g., ethanol). Also, because urinary excretion is the major elimination pathway for most drug metabolites, urine often identifies the presence of drugs that may not be detected in serum analysis (e.g., cocaine).

In toxic screen analysis, biologic specimens are subjected to a battery of tests. These include thin-layer chromatography (TLC), enzyme-multiplied immunologic testing (EMIT), high-performance liquid chromatography (HPLC), gas chromatography (GC), and gas chromatography/mass spectrometry (GC/MS). Each test has its own sensitivity and specificity for the detection of toxic substances. GC/MS, for example, because it performs an analysis of chemical structure, is considered the standard against which all other diagnostic tests are measured.[9]

Comprehensive drug analyses employ all of the aforementioned analytic techniques on each specimen. Such toxic screens are able to detect more than 100 drugs, including many that are used in the therapeutic setting (e.g., diphenhydramine). These panels are usually performed by off-site commercial toxicology laboratories. Many hospitals, however, are capable of performing an on-site toxic screen. These screening panels use only one to three analytic tests in an attempt to reduce the cost and technical proficiency required to perform these tests. On-site toxic screens typically seek only agents that have been most consistently identified in toxic exposures[8] (Table 51-2).

When the diagnosis and management of drug intoxication revolves around the toxic screen result, the physician must know whether the suspected drug is detectable by the methods being used. For example, toxic screens rarely seek the presence of iron, lead, arsenic, lithium, cyanide, and other toxic substances (Table 51-3). Also, because specimen analysis by several different laboratories may be ultimately necessary to establish the diagnosis of intoxication, it is always advisable to obtain extra whole blood and urine samples at the time of initial patient evaluation.

Table 51-1. Distribution of route of exposure for human poisonings

	All cases:		Fatalities	
Route	No.	(%)	No.	(%)
Ingestion	944,603	(77.5)	310	(75.2)
Dermal	83,912	(6.9)	4	(0.9)
Ophthalmic	72,180	(5.9)	0	(0.0)
Inhalation	64,190	(5.3)	60	(14.6)
Bites and stings	42,026	(3.4)	2	(0.5)
Parenteral	3,452	(0.3)	22	(5.3)
Other/unknown	7,882	(0.6)	14	(3.4)

From TL Litovitz et al. 1988 annual report of the American Association of Poison Control Centers National Data Collection System. *Am J Emerg Med* 7:495–545, 1989. With permission.

Table 51-2. Drugs commonly identified in drug screen analysis

Ethanol	Barbiturates
Benzodiazepines	Tricyclic antidepressants
Aspirin	Cocaine
Acetaminophen	Opiates

Table 51-3. Drugs typically not detected in drug screen analysis

Beta-blockers

Calcium channel blockers

Pesticides

Hydrocarbons

Metals and minerals

Camphor

Table 51-4. Commonly used cathartics

	Child	*Adolescent*
Magnesium sulfate	25 mg/kg	25 g
Magnesium citrate	4 ml/kg	300 ml
Sorbitol, 70%	2 ml/kg	50–150 ml

From MW Shannon et al. Cathartics and laxatives—Do they still have a place in the management of the poisoned patient? *Med Toxicol* 1:247, 1986. With permission.

Use of the Regional Poison Center

Regional poison control centers (RPCCs) have been established nationally for the purpose of providing information and a central site for data collection on poison exposures. These poison centers are designed to serve both the general population as well as the health professional. All RPCCs provide 24-hour access to trained poison specialists and clinical toxicologists. Additionally, as a data collection source, the RPCC gathers a base of epidemiologic data through which experience with intoxications can be collected.

The national network of RPCCs now assures that the physician managing a critically ill, poisoned patient has access to a clinical toxicologist who can provide current recommendations for therapy as well as appropriate references. RPCC resources are also potentially useful in the identification of unknown medications and unlabeled household products.

Therapeutic Modalities in the Treatment of the Poisoned Patient

Activated Charcoal

The cornerstone of management in toxic ingestions is the administration of activated charcoal. Prepared by the controlled pyrolysis of wood, followed by its treatment with steam, acids, oxygen, and carbon dioxide, activated charcoal is a fine, granular black powder with extensive interstices. Activated charcoal preparations have a surface area of approximately 1000 m²/g. (In an adult, one dose of activated charcoal would contain the absorptive area of ten football fields.) By adsorbing drugs that are in the GI lumen and expelling them in the feces, activated charcoal significantly increases toxin elimination.[10]

Although activated charcoal has been used in treating toxic ingestions for decades, its role has expanded.[11,12] This comes as a result of findings indicating that the efficacy of activated charcoal far surpasses that of gastric emptying procedures (gastric lavage, ipecac-induced emesis) in decreasing the absorption of ingested toxins. GI absorption of drug may be reduced by as much as 85% with the timely administration of activated charcoal. These data have led to recent trends to administer activated charcoal alone after toxic ingestions, without prior gastric emptying.

The administration of activated charcoal may delay GI transit time. Because of this recognized effect, coupled with the ability of many drugs to slow gut motility, the coadministration of a cathartic with activated charcoal is recommended to facilitate expulsion of the drug-charcoal complex.[13] Commonly used cathartics are listed in Table 51-4.

Multiple-Dose Activated Charcoal

The administration of repetitive doses of activated charcoal has become an important technique to further enhance the elimina-

Table 51-5. Mechanisms of action of multiple-dose activated charcoal

Reducing the absorption of poorly absorbed drugs
    Sustained-release tablets
    Drugs with anticholinergic activity
    Drugs with erratic absorption

Interruption of enterohepatic circulation
    Tricyclic antidepressants
    Digitoxin
    Thyroid hormone
    Valproic acid
    Phenothiazines
    Diazepam
    Carbamezepine

Gastrointestinal dialysis
    Phenobarbital
    Aspirin
    Theophylline
    Meprobamate

tion of many drugs. At least three mechanisms exist by which multiple-dose activated charcoal (MDAC) has been shown to abbreviate the duration of clinical toxicity after drug intoxications (Table 51-5).[11,14-19]

Poorly Absorbed Drugs

Administration of MDAC is effective in the pre-absorptive phase of drug ingestion by adsorbing drugs that are slowly absorbed, particularly in overdose. These include sustained-release preparations (whose peak absorption may be delayed to 17–24 hours after overdose) and drugs with slow and erratic absorption (e.g., phenytoin, whose peak absorption may not be attained for 3–5 days after overdose). Finally, many medications possess among their actions nonspecific anticholingergic activity. Included among these agents are the tricyclic antidepressants, phenothiazines, antihistamines, and antispasmodics. Because anticholingergic activity is associated with reduction in GI transit time and a prolonged systemic drug absorption, MDAC increases the opportunity for drug adsorption.

Interruption of Enterohepatic Circulation

For most drugs, hepatic metabolism is initiated by phase I (synthetic) or phase II (conjugation) alteration of the parent substance. For several drugs (tricyclic antidepressants, diazepam, meperidine, glutethimide), the metabolites retain much of the pharmacologic activity of the parent drug and, in some cases, have a longer elimination half-life or greater toxicity (e.g., meperidine, diazepam, glutethimide). The fate of these pharmacologically active metabolites is typically secretion into the bile. Once a part of biliary fluid, these metabolites are secreted into the proximal duodenum. However, they may be reabsorbed along with the bile salts in the distal ileum. Such enterohepatic circulation leads to prolonged drug elimination and, occasionally, a cyclic course in the clinical manifestations of toxicity. The administration of MDAC interrupts enterohepatic circulation by providing a constant source of charcoal to the gut lumen for adsorption of metabolite as it is secreted (see Table 51-5).[15]

Gastrointestinal Dialysis

MDAC also enhances the elimination of certain drugs through a mechanism known as GI dialysis. This theorized mechanism of enhanced postabsorptive clearance is based on the observation that the elimination of phenobarbital and theophylline is enhanced by MDAC, even if these drugs are administered intravenously.[16,17,20,21] Because neither drug has significant enterohepatic circulation, another mechanism of enhancing drug elimination must exist. In the GI dialysis model, activated charcoal in the GI lumen is thought to create a drug "sink." In response, certain drugs will demonstrate enhanced diffusion across the GI mucosa from the splanchnic circulation into the gut lumen. Once there, drug is adsorbed to activated charcoal and expelled.

Other drugs appear to be eliminated through GI dialysis, particularly aspirin and mepbrobamate.[22] Interestingly, these drugs share two pharmacokinetic features: They have a small apparent volume of distribution (<0.8 liter/kg) and are poorly bound to circulating plasma proteins. These characteristics may therefore be the prerequisites needed for GI dialysis to occur. If true, any drug with these properties might be capable of enhanced elimination with MDAC.[23,24]

The recommended dose of activated charcoal is 1 g/kg. Theoretically, this dose is administered regardless of body weight. Because large doses of activated charcoal may lead to nausea and vomiting, however, adolescents and adults receive a maximum dose of 50 to 60 g. The advent of "super-activated" charcoal preparations, which have 3 to 4 times the binding surface area of conventionally activated charcoals, may permit the administration of smaller doses of activated charcoal without a compromise in efficacy.[25]

MDAC may be administered by using several dosing regimens. The most commonly used schedule is 1 g/kg every 4 hours. In patients with significant nausea and vomiting, MDAC is better tolerated if smaller doses are administered more frequently. Therefore, an alternative schedule is 0.5 g/kg every 2 hours. Continuous nasogastric infusion of activated charcoal in a dose of 0.25 to 0.5 g/kg/hr has also been successfully employed.[26]

Dosing of cathartics with MDAC must be individualized based on the substance(s) ingested and the appearance of charcoal stools. MDAC should be administered cautiously in the absence of bowel sounds.

Naloxone

Continuous Naloxone Infusion

Naloxone is a competitive antagonist of the opiate receptor that is highly effective in reversing the clinical manifestations of opioid overdose. Naloxone also has a large margin of safety; single doses as large as 20 mg in children and 50 mg in adults have been administered without adverse effect.[27] However, naloxone has a brief clinical duration of action (approximately 30–90 minutes), which often requires that it be administered repeatedly to sustain reversal of the manifestations of opioid intoxication. This brief

duration of action of naloxone also requires that victims of opioid overdose who receive naloxone be monitored closely and continuously for the reappearance of severe CNS depression.

An alternative to the frequent administration of naloxone is continuous naloxone infusion. Although a list of potential indications for the continuous infusion of naloxone are found in Table 51-6, the primary purpose for continuous naloxone infusion is to prevent the need for repetitive dosing with naloxone to maintain the desired effect (e.g., severe opiate overdose).[28]

Several dosing schedules have been proposed for continuous naloxone infusion.[29–32] The most accurate dosing schedule, however, is an empiric one determined by recording the quantity of naloxone that must be administered over one hour to achieve a desired level of consciousness. That same dose is subsequently adminstered as a continuous hourly intravenous (IV) infusion. Weaning from a continuous naloxone infusion is based on the indications that led to its use, although weaning should be attempted at 6- to 8-hour intervals. In tapering naloxone infusion, the dose should be decreased by 25% to 35%, followed by a period of observation for signs of recurrent opiate intoxication. In the absence of these, weaning of naloxone can continue. If evidence of opiate toxicity reappears, naloxone infusion should be resumed at the former dose after a repeat bolus.

Naloxone Infusion in Non-Opiate Overdose

Naloxone may also have beneficial effect in the reversal of toxicity by several drugs that are not true opiates. Included here are the synthetic opioids and imidazoline compounds.

Many drugs with opiate properties do not possess the opium nucleus. The most common members of this synthetic opioid class are fentanyl and its derivatives. Other opioids, however, may be included in this category (pentazocine, propoxyphene). Because of the structural dissimilarity of these agents to opiates, overdoses may require larger single doses of naloxone (up to 8–10 mg) to achieve reversal of clinical toxicity.

The antihypertensive agent clonidine has its primary action as a central alpha-2 adrenergic agonist. Clonidine, however, also possesses opiate agonist activity; this forms the basis for its use as a methadone adjunct or alternative in drug treatment programs. In overdose, clonidine, like opiates, leads to coma, miosis, and respiratory depression. Dramatic clinical improvement in patients with clonidine overdose has been reported after administration of naloxone.[33–37]

Clonidine is a member of a class of compounds known as imidazolines.[38] Other drugs in this class include the nasal decongestant oxymetazoline and the optic solution tetrahydrozyline. In overdose, these agents also lead to coma, miosis, and respiratory depression. Administration of naloxone may reverse much of these toxic manifestations.

Table 51-6. Indications for continuous naloxone infusion

Requirement for repeat bolus therapy
Requirement of a large initial bolus dose
Ingestion of a large amount of opiate
Ingestion of a long-acting opiate
Decreased opiate metabolism (e.g., hepatic dysfunction)

From M Tenenbein. Pediatric toxicology: Current controversies and recent advances. *Curr Probl Pediatr* 16:145, 1986. With permission.

Intoxications by other drugs, including ethanol and the benzodiazepines, may be partially reversed by administration of naloxone. This beneficial effect, however, appears to be the result of naloxone-induced stimulation of cortisol and catecholamine secretion.

Antidotal Therapies

Advances in clinical toxicology have led to the discovery of specific therapies for the treatment of toxic exposures. Table 51-7 provides a partial list of specific therapeutic agents. Several of these agents will be discussed in more detail.

Common Serious Poisonings

Cyclic Antidepressant Overdose
Clinical Presentation
The clinical features of cyclic antidepressant (CA) overdose result from their effects on the cardiovascular, respiratory, autonomic, and central nervous systems. Antidepressants possess quinidine-like membrane stabilizing effects that precipitate conduction and rhythm abnormalities. Cardiac dysrhythmias are often aggravated by concomitant hypoxemia or acidosis. These agents also cause direct myocardial depression and peripheral vasodilitation. Hypotension is therefore a common manifestation of toxicity.[39,40] However, hypertension may occur in the initial phase of intoxication as a consequence of antidepressant-induced blockade of norepinephrine reuptake. Tachycardia is a nearly universal finding after significant overdose.

The most common CNS complications of CA overdose are agitation, lethargy, seizures, and coma. Ophthalmoplegia and absent brain stem reflexes may be present after severe overdose.[41] Neuromuscular manifestations may range from myoclonus to diffuse rigidity to generalized convulsions.[41,42]

CNS depression and seizures may lead to respiratory compromise as a result of aspiration. Pulmonary edema is also recognized as a complication of severe CA overdose.[43]

The spectrum of toxic manifestations is similar for most of the CAs. However, trazodone, amoxapine, and maprotiline, which are nontricyclic antidepressants, have uniquely different toxicities. Trazadone has significantly less cardiotoxicity and neurotoxicity than the other CAs. Amoxapine is less cardiotoxic than other antidepressants but is a potent analeptic and well known for its ability to precipitate intractable seizures. The toxicity of maprotiline most resembles that of tricyclic antedepressants (TCAs), although prolonged coma (greater than 24 hours) is a characteristic of severe maprotiline overdose.

Assessment
Serum Cyclic Antidepressant Concentrations
Because of their large volume of distribution, antidepressants are widely dispersed in tissues; therefore, there is typically poor correlation between serum antidepressant concentrations and clinical presentation. However, patients with combined (parent drug and demethylated metabolite) antidepressant levels greater than 1000 ng/ml are at greatest risk for serious complications (e.g., seizures, coma, dysrhythmias, respiratory depression). Serum concentrations greater than 4000 ng/ml are usually fatal.

Electrocardiogram
Sinus tachycardia is common after antidepressant overdose but is rarely clinically important. Conduction disturbances may include

Table 51-7. Selected antidotes and special therapies

Poison	Antidote	Dosage
Acetaminophen	N-acetylcysteine (Mucomyst)	140 mg/kg PO initial dose, then 70 mg/kg PO q4h for 17 doses
Anticholinergics	Physostigmine (Antilirium)	Adult: 2.0 mg IV Child: 0.5 mg IV
Carbon monoxide	100% oxygen	Consider hyperbaric administration
Cholinesterase inhibiting agents (organophosphates, carbamates)	Atropine	Adult: 1–2 mg IV Child: 0.05 mg/kg IV
	Pralidoxime (2-PAM)	25–50 mg/kg IV up to 2 g IV q6h or infusion of 0.5 g/hr
Cyanide	Amyl nitrite Sodium nitrite	Inhale pearls 30 sec/min Adult: 10 ml of 3% solution IV over 3 min Child: 0.33 ml/kg
	Na thiosulfate	Adult: 50ml of 25% solution IV over 10 min Child: 1.65 ml/kg IV
Isoniazid	Pyridoxine	1 g IV per 1 g isoniazid ingested. If unknown, 2–5 g IV
Lead	EDTA	50–75 mg/kg/24 hr IM or IV. Consider the addition of BAL for lead > 70 μg/dl
Mercury arsenic	Dimercaprol (BAL)	3–5 mg/kg IM q4–12h
Methanol ethylene glycol	Ethanol	600 mg/kg IV or PO initial dose, then 110 mg/kg/hr IV or 450 mg/kg q4h PO. Maintain blood level at 100 mg/dl.
Methemoglobinemia	Methylene blue	0.2 ml/kg IV of 1% solution over 5 min

Use should be in consultation with poison control center.

abnormalities in P-R or Q-T intervals, although widening of the QRS complex is most characteristic.[40,44] These conduction abnormalities are associated with the appearance of ventricular or supraventricular tachyarrythmias.

A QRS duration of 0.10 seconds or longer has been correlated with an increased risk for the development of seizures.[45] QRS durations greater than or equal to 0.16 seconds are associated with an increased risk of ventricular arrhythmias.[45] A QRS duration of less than 0.10 seconds, however, may not exclude the patient from the risk of having these events.[46]

Data suggest that a right axis deviation of 130 degrees to 270 degrees in the terminal 40-ms frontal plane QRS axis is a sensitive indicator of significant CA intoxication.[47]

Blood Gas Determinations
Metabolic acidosis is the most common acid-base disturbance seen with CA ingestions and may occur with or without the presence of hypotension.[41]

Urine Analysis
Rhabdomyolysis and myoglobinuria may result from prolonged seizure activity.

Management
Decontamination
Anticholinergic activity of CAs decreases the rate of gastric emptying. Gastric lavage, therefore, may be effective up to 12 hours postingestion.

Elimination Enhancement
Multiple doses of activated charcoal appear to enhance the elimination of CAs.[48,49] Hemodialysis and hemoperfusion are of no proven value in the treatment of antidepressant toxicity.

Supportive Care
Maintenence of normal electrolytes and continuous electrocardiographic monitoring are essential in the management of antidepressant overdoses. Patients should be monitored in a critical care setting until a normal level of consciousness and a normal ECG have been maintained for approximately 24 hours.[50]

Hypotension. Trendelenburg positioning and prudent fluid administration are the primary therapeutic interventions for antidepressant-induced hypotension. Hypotension is often refractory to these measures, however, and the addition of vasopressor support may be necessary. Norepinephrine appears to be more effective than dopamine in reversing antidepressant-induced hypotension.[51]

Dysrhythmias. Ventricular dysryhthmias are typically treated with lidocaine, although phenytoin is suggested as an equally effective agent.[40,52]

Procainamide, disopyramide, and quinidine have membrane-stabilizing effects similar to those of the CAs and are contraindicated in the treatment of antidepressant-induced dysrhythmias. Prophylactic administration of antiarrhythmics is not advocated.

Normalization of the QRS interval and termination of ventricular tachyarrythmias have been accomplished with the administration of sodium bicarbonate and/or hyperventilation.[53-56] This effect appears to result from serum alkalinization as well as an increase in extracellular sodium concentration.[57] Therefore, the serum pH should be maintained between 7.40 and 7.50.

The use of physostigmine is not recommended for the treatment of CA overdoses because it may induce asystole and precipitate seizures.[40,58]

Seizures. Seizures are treated with a benzodiazepine followed by phenytoin. Seizure activity may persist after amoxapine overdoses despite conventional therapy. In these instances, the use of thiopental and skeletal muscle paralysis may be indicated.

Beta-Adrenergic Antagonist Poisoning
Clinical Presentation
Beta-blocker intoxication is characterized by cardiovascular and neurologic abnormalities. The spectrum of cardiovascular compromise after beta-blocker overdose is dependant on three factors: (1) the cardioselectivity of the preparation, (2) the presence or absence of intrinsic sympathomimetic activity (ISA) in the preparation, and (3) the membrane-stabilizing activity (MSA) of the medication. Beta-1 blockade results in a slowing of the sinus rate and a decrease in contractility. Selective beta-1 antagonists are less likely to cause bronchospasm and hypoglycemia than are nonselective beta-blockers. In high doses, however, all beta-blockers become nonselective in their properties[59] (Table 51-8).

Table 51-8. Beta-adrenergic antagonists

Generic name	Brand name	Relative B-1 selective	ISA	MSA	Lipid solubility	Peak effect (hr)	Elim. t1/2 (hr)	Route of elimination
Acebutolol	Sectral	+	+	+	Moderate	?	6–9	Liver
Alprenolol	Aptin, Betatin, Betacard	0	+ +	+	High	1–3	2–3	Liver
Atenolol	Tenormin	+ +	0	0	Low	2–4	6–9	Kidney
Metoprolol	Lopressor, Betablock	+ +	0	+/−	Moderate	1–2	3–4	Liver
Nadolol	Corgard	0	0	0	Low	3–4	20–24	Kidney
Oxprenolol	Trasicor	0	+ +	+	Moderate	1–2	1–2	Liver
Pindolol	Visken	0	+ + +	+	Moderate	1.25	3–4	Kidney
Practolol	Eraldin	+	+ +	0	Low	3	5–10	Kidney
Propranolol	Inderal, Avlocardin	0	0	0	High	1.0–1.5	3–5	Liver
Sotalol	Betacordone, Sotocor	0	0	0	Low	2–3	5–12	Kidney
Timolol	Blocadren	0	+/−	0	Moderate	1–2	4–5	Liver and kidney

ISA is a property of certain beta-blockers, that leads to simultaneous beta-1 stimulation and blockade.[60] These agents generally do not cause significant bradycardia and hypotension and may actually precipitate tachycardia and hypertension.

MSA is a "quinidine-like" effect that impairs conduction and thereby causes electrocardiographic changes similar to those seen with CA intoxication (prolonged QRS interval and AV block).

The neurologic consequences of beta-blocker intoxication include hallucinations, delirium, respiratory depression, coma, and seizures. The potential of beta-blockers to cause CNS derangements is dependent on their degree of lipid solubility and the MSA of the particular medication.[61] Those beta-blockers that are highly lipid-soluble, such as propranolol, are more likely to produce CNS effects.

Assessment
Serum Concentrations
Serum concentrations of these agents may confirm toxicity but are of little use in the management or prognosis of beta-blocker intoxication.

Electrocardiographic Changes
Bradycardia, tachycardia, S-T segment elevation (secondary to myocardial ischemia), and AV block are common ECG abnormalities. Peaked T waves have been observed with severe propranolol poisoning.[62]

Glucose
Hypoglycemia is rare in adults but may occur in children and diabetics with significant beta-blocker intoxication. Disturbances in glucose homeostasis are thought to be a consequence of inhibition of the beta-2–mediated glycogenolysis that occurs in response to hypoglycemia.[59,63]

Management
Decontamination
Gastric lavage is recommended for beta-blocker ingestions occuring within 4 hours of presentation, followed by the administration of activated charcoal with cathartic. MDAC may enhance the elimination of beta-blockers and/or their pharmacologically active metabolites.[63]

Elimination Enhancement
Most beta-blocking agents have a large volume of distribution and a high degree of protein binding. Consequently, extracorporeal elimination is generally considered ineffective. However, the pharmacokinetic properties of atenolol, nadolol, practolol, and sotolol are such that hemoperfusion or hemodialysis may be of some utility, although literature supporting this theory is sparse.

Pharmacologic Therapies
Atropine. Atropine may be used to decrease vagal tone and increase heart rate, although it is frequently ineffective in severe overdoses. Doses as high as 0.04 mg/kg or 3 mg total may be necessary.

Isoproterenol. Isoproterenol is a nonselective beta agonist with both chronotropic and inotropic properties. It may be used to reverse bradycardia and/or AV block. Doses up to 200 µg/min may be necessary to achieve the desired effect.[64] The addition of an alpha-adrenergic agonist may be necessary to prevent isoproterenol-induced vasodilatation and hypotension.[65]

Glucagon. Many case reports have identified glucagon as effective therapy for beta-blocker–induced hypotension and bradycar-dia.[63,64,66] Glucagon has both inotropic and chronotropic properties that are mediated by myocardial glucagon receptors, which activate adenyl cyclase. The toxicity of glucagon is limited to nausea, vomiting, and decreased GI motility.

The initial dose of glucagon is 50 to 150 µg/kg (5–10 mg for adults) intravenously over 1 minute. This is followed by a continuous infusion of 70 µg/kg/hr (1–5 mg/hr for adults).[22] The diluent for lyophylized glucagon contains phenol, a potential toxin when administered in the doses required for continuous infusion; glucagon should therefore be reconstituted in normal saline or sterile water.

Supportive Care
Seizures. Benzodiazepines are the drugs of choice for beta-blocker–induced seizures. Thiopental and muscle relaxants may be necessary for refractory seizures.

Bronchospasm. Aminophylline, tertbutaline, and isoproterenol are generally effective for beta-blocker–induced bronchospasm. Aminophylline should be used with caution because it lowers the seizure threshold.

Hypotension. Dopamine, norepinephrine, and/or glucagon may also be used to treat hypotension. Hypotension refractory to pharmacologic therapies may respond to the placement of an intraaortic balloon pump.[67]

Cocaine Poisoning
The most common routes of cocaine abuse are intranasal and inhalational. Cocaine smoking is associated with a more rapid onset of symptoms due to its rapid absorption. Less commonly, cocaine is injected. Finally, cocaine may be ingested, in an attempt either to smuggle it or to escape prosecution for drug possession.

The purity of street cocaine varies widely. A list of common adulterants is found in Table 51-9. Epidemiologic data also indicate that up to 95% of those who abuse cocaine simultaneously use another psychoactive agent, usually ethanol, marijuana, a benzodiazepine, or heroin. These co-exposures may confuse the clinical picture of suspected cocaine intoxication.[68]

Clinical Presentation
Cocaine stimulates the release of endogenous catecholamines and prevents their reuptake by the presynaptic neuron. Therefore, sympathetic nervous system activation mediates the primary manifestations of cocaine overdose, which are neurologic and cardiovas-

Table 51-9. Common adulterants of cocaine street samples

Sugars	Mannitol, lactose, glucose, inositol, maltose, sucrose
Inert substances	Magnesium silicate (talc), flour, cornstarch
Local anesthetics	Procaine, lidocaine, tetracaine, benzocaine
Stimulants	Theophylline, strychnine, ergotamine methylphenidate, caffeine, amphetamine
Hallucinogens	Phencyclidine, marijuana, hashish, lysergic acid diethylamide (LSD)
Depressants	Alcohol, methapyrilene
Miscellaneous	Quinine, magnesium sulfate, thiamine, tyramine, sodium bicarbonate, salicylamide

From M Shannon. The clinical toxicity of cocaine adulterants. *Ann Emerg Med* 17:1243–1247, 1988. With permission.

cular. Pulmonary, GI, and musculoskeletal disturbances are also part of the spectrum of cocaine toxicity.

Central Nervous System
Increased stimulation of dopaminergic neurons is thought to be responsible for the euphoria associated with cocaine use.[69] Marked CNS sympathetic discharge also results in agitation, mydriasis, hyperpyrexia, diaphoresis, and seizures.

Cocaine-induced seizures may be generalized or partial motor.[70] Intracerebral hemorrhage may also occur.[71]

Cardiovascular
Cocaine-induced chest pain is multifactorial. True cardiac pain may result from myocardial ischemia. Ischemic heart disease is thought to be caused by a combination of coronary artery vasospasm, increased cardiac afterload, increased oxygen consumption, and/or coronary artery thrombosis secondary to enhanced platelet aggregation. These myocardial effects make cardiac dysrhythmias common in cocaine overdoses. Chronic cocaine abuse may lead to the formation of myocardial contraction bands (clumps of myocardial sarcomeres). These bands serve as a potential nidus of reentrant dysrhythmias.[72,73]

Pulmonary
Pulmonary consequences of cocaine intoxication include pneumomediastinum, pneumothorax, or pneumopericardium, all of which may be associated with chest pain. These phenomena most characteristically occur after cocaine smoking.[74] Chronic cocaine smoking leads to a reduced capacity for gas exchange, with little or no impairment of ventilatory function.[69]

Gastrointestinal
Localized vasoconstriction and smooth muscle contraction may cause GI ischemia. This may be manifested by abdominal cramping, or diarrhea, which may be bloody. Intestinal gangrene has also been described.[69] GI manifestations have been described with both the inhalational and oral routes of cocaine abuse.[69]

Assessment
Serum Concentrations
Serum cocaine concentrations are of little utility, in part because cocaine metabolism continues in vitro, such that its concentrations are markedly reduced by the time the laboratory begins its measurement. In addition, serum cocaine concentrations do not correlate well with clinical signs.

Cocaine is excreted in the urine as benzoylecgonine, which may be detected in the urine as early as 1 hour and as late as 72 hours postexposure. In patients with chronic, high-level abuse, cocaine may be recovered in the urine up to 10 days postexposure.

Electrocardiograms
Monitor for evidence of dysrhythmias and myocardial ischemia.

Musculoskeletal
Both skeletal and cardiac muscle enzymes may be elevated with cocaine intoxication. Malignant hyperthermia and/or a variant of neuroleptic malignant syndrome have been described in victims of cocaine intoxication. Manifestations include hyperthermia, altered mental status, muscular ridgidity, and rhabdomyolsis.[75]

Urinary Analysis
Urine should be monitored for evidence of myoglobinuria and acute tubular necrosis.

Radiography
Abdominal radiographs may identify up to 50% of cocaine ingestions, particularly in body packers.[76]

Management
Decontamination
Lavage and ipecac are generally not warranted for cocaine intoxication (because ingestion is uncommon) unless toxic coingestions are suspected. In cocaine ingestions, decontamination methods, if too rigorous, may break cocaine packages, increasing the risk of severe intoxication. Activated charcoal with cathartic should be administered after cocaine ingestion and should be continued until cocaine packages are passed.

Supportive Therapy
Seizures. Benzodiazepines, phenytoin, and phenobarbital are effective agents for seizure management. If seizures are refractory to these anticonvulsants, the use of thiopental and muscle relaxants may be indicated.

Hypertension. Nifedipine, phentolamine, nitroprusside, esmolol, and labetolol are potentially effective for the treatment of hypertension.[69,77]

Dysrhythmias. Ventricular dysrythmias are typically treated with lidocaine.

Hyperthermia. Severe hyperthemia is treated with cooling blankets and ice baths. Dantrolene sodium has been recommended for patients with signs of malignant hyperthermia and neuroleptic malignant syndrome.

Agitation. Benzodiazepines and/or haloperidol may be administered to control agitation. Phenothiazines should be used with extreme caution because they are known to lower the seizure threshold and may precipitate neuroleptic malignant syndrome.

Digoxin Poisoning
Clinical Presentation
While cardiac arrhythmias are the most common clinical manifestations of digoxin overdose, GI manifestations may include nausea, vomiting, and diarrhea. Neurologic manifestations may include visual symptoms (scotoma, blurred vision, photophobia, transient blindness) or neurobehavioral abnormalities (confusion, hallucinations, and delirium).

Any cardiac dysrhythmia may occur after digoxin intoxication. Although the dysrhythmias most classic for digoxin intoxication are atrial tachycardias with concomitant AV block, premature ventricular extrasystoles may also occur and are usually multifocal. Patients without preexisting cardiac disease, however, have a high degree of tolerance to digoxin toxicity; sinus bradycardia and first- or second-degree AV nodal block are usually their only cardiac manifestations.

Other physical findings in digoxin toxicity are nonspecific. Tachypnea may be noted because digoxin has direct effects on the CNS, causing hyperventilation.[78]

Assessment
Serum Concentrations
Because digoxin has a prolonged distribution phase, concentrations that are initially elevated after overdose may fall dramatically over 1 to 4 hours.[79] As a result, serum concentrations obtained before 4 hours are of little utility. Even after tissue distribution is complete, the correlation between serum concentration and clinical toxicity may be poor.

Potassium

Because digoxin acts by inhibiting transcellular sodium-potassium exchange, increases in serum potassium are common and directly reflect the degree of digoxin intoxication.

Magnesium, Calcium, Sodium, Phosphorus, and Potassium

Imbalances in these electrolytes can enhance digoxin toxicity.

Management
Decontamination

Lavage is recommended for ingestions that have occured within 4 hours of presentation.

Elimination Enhancement

MDAC may enhance the elimination of digoxin (and digitoxin).[80] Because of the large volume of distribution of digoxin, hemodialysis is ineffective for removing digoxin, but it may be indicated for severe hyperkalemia. Anecdotal data suggest a role for hemoperfusion in massive digoxin overdose.[81]

Supportive Therapy

Dysrhythmias. Phenytoin may increase the threshold for ventricular fibrillation and improve conduction through the AV node. Phenytoin is therefore frequently recommended as the drug of choice for ventricular arrhythmias. Lidocaine may also be used. Premature ventricular contractions and ventricular tachydcardia have been treated successfully with propranolol. Bradycardia may be treated with atropine or a pacemaker if necessary.

Hyperkalemia. Hyperkalemia should be treated with glucose, insulin, bicarbonate, and kayexalate. Dialysis may be indicated if hyperkalemia does not respond to these methods.

Hypokalemia. Correct hypokalemia slowly. Nonglucose-containing solutions should be used to administer potassium because glucose may promote intracellular potassium shifts.

Antidotes

Digoxin-specific antibody fragments (Fab fragments) have been developed to treat digoxin toxicity. Fab fragments have a greater affinity for digoxin than does the Na^+-K^+-ATPase receptor. The resulting antibody-digoxin complex is inactive and renally excreted.[82] Indications for the use of Fab fragments are (1) life-threatening dysrhythmias that are unresponsive to conventional therapy and (2) digitalis-induced hyperkalemia (>5 mEq/liter) with concurrent signs of severe digitalis toxicity.[83,84]

Dosing: 40 mg (one vial) of Fab fragments will bind 0.6 mg of digitalis. If the amount of digitalis ingested is known, the following formula may be used to determine the dose of Fab fragments:

$$\text{Fab dose (no. of vials)} = \frac{\text{amount digitalis ingested (mg)} \times F^a}{0.6 \text{ mg/vial}}$$

where F^a (bioavailability factor) is 0.8 for digoxin tablets; 1.0 for digoxin elixir, capsules, or digitoxin.

If the serum concentration of digitalis is known,

$$\begin{aligned}&\text{Fab dose (no. of vials)}\\&= \frac{[\text{digoxin conc. (ng/ml)} \times V_d^b \times \text{patients wt. (kg)}]/1000}{0.6 \text{ mg/vial}}\end{aligned}$$

where V_d^b (volume of distribution) is 5.6 liter/kg for digoxin and 0.56 liter/kg for digitoxin.[83]

If the amount ingested is not known, the serum concentration is not yet available, and the patient has cardiovascular instability,

$$\begin{aligned}\text{Fab dose (no. of vials)} = \;&20 \text{ vials (800 mg) if}\\&> 30 \text{ kg, or } 10 \text{ vials (400 mg) if}\\&< 30 \text{ kg}\end{aligned}$$

The digoxin antibodies should be infused over 15 to 30 minutes, although bolus doses may be given if cardiac arrest appears to be imminent or has occured.[82]

Monitoring during Fab administration: As digoxin is removed from the Na^+-K^+-ATPase receptor and normal Na^+/K^+ exchange is restored, hypokalemia may theoretically ensue.[83] Therefore, serum potassium levels should be monitored closely after the administration of Fab fragments.

Conventional methods for detecting serum digoxin concentrations will measure both bound and free digoxin concentrations, resulting in misleading digoxin concentrations.[84,85] Therefore, digoxin concentrations are of no value after the administration of digoxin antibodies.

Iron Poisoning
Clinical Presentation

The toxic dosage of elemental iron is greater than 60 mg/kg, and 180 mg/kg may be lethal. The clinical manifestations of acute iron poisoning have been divided into four stages. Stage I appears within 6 hours of ingestion, when direct gastric irritation causes vomiting, abdominal pain, and diarrhea. This phase is rarely fatal, although severe hemorrhagic gastritis may occur. CNS effects may also be seen in this phase after severe poisonings, with lethargy, coma, and seizures. Finally, hypotension may occur as a result of the vasodilatory effects of free iron, ferritin, and released histamine and serotonin.[76,86-88]

Stage II, a quiescent period, begins approximately 6 hours postingestion. In this phase, GI and CNS symptoms may subside. This period usually lasts less than 24 hours but may extend up to 48 hours.[88]

Stage III begins approximately 12 to 48 hours after severe intoxication. Abnormalities may include (1) gastrointestinal (hematemesis, melena, GI perforation); (2) CNS (lethargy, coma, seizures); (3) cardiovascular (hypotension, pulmonary edema); and (4) liver/kidney (hepatorenal failure, coagulopathy, and hypoglycemia). Because of iron redistribution into the tissues, serum iron levels may be normal during this phase.[88]

Stage IV is characterized by the development of gastric and pyloric strictures secondary to the corrosive effects of iron. This occurs 2 to 5 weeks after ingestion.

Assessment
Serum Iron and Total Iron Binding Capacity (TIBC)

Serum iron levels peak approximately 4 to 6 hours postingestion and decline rapidly thereafter as iron is redistributed into the tissues.[87] Because of this redistribution phase, serum iron levels may not correlate with the clinical manifestations of iron poisoning.

Serum iron levels of 300 to 400 μg/dl indicate mild poisoning, 400 to 500 μg/dl indicate moderate poisoning, and greater than 500 μg/dl suggest severe iron poisoning. The cellular toxicity of iron occurs when serum iron levels exceed the TIBC. Serial iron levels should be obtained because large ingestions typically lead to bezoar formation and cause prolonged absorption of iron.

White Blood Cell Count

A WBC greater than 15,000/μL suggests that the serum iron level in that patient will be greater than 300 μg/dl.[89] A WBC less than 15,000/μL, however, does **not** exclude the diagnosis of iron intoxication.[89]

Serum Glucose

Patients with an initial serum glucose greater than 150 mg/dl may also have a significant likelihood of a serum iron greater than 300 μg/dl. A serum glucose less than 150 mg/dl, however, does not rule out the possibility of iron poisoning.[89]

Hepatic Function

Mild-to-moderate elevations in SGPT, prolongation of the prothrombin times, and increases in total iron binding capacity reflect iron-induced hepatic damage.

Blood pH

Metabolic acidosis can occur secondary to hypoperfusion and/or the production of hydrogen ions by the oxidation of iron from the ferrous to the ferric state.[90]

Hematocrit

Increases in capillary permeability may lead to hemoconcentration, while blood loss from hemorrhagic gastritis may lead to anemia.[88]

Abdominal Radiographs

Abdominal radiographs typically demonstrate the presence of radiopaque iron preparations. The absence of a positive film may be misleading because up to 70% of patients with iron poisoning may have negative x-rays.[91]

Desferoxamine Challenge Test

Desferoxamine is a known iron chelator. The desferoxamine chelation test is used to help evaluate the need for iron chelation. An intramuscular 25- to 50-mg/kg (maximum 1-g) dose of desferoxamine is administered. Urine is then collected and visually inspected for the presence of an orange to reddish brown color (vin rose), which indicates the presence of an iron-desferoxamine complex (ferrioxamine) and the need for continued chelation therapy.

Management

Decontamination

Gastric lavage should be performed for all significant ingestions (> 60 mg/kg of elemental iron) occurring within 6 hours of presentation and in any patient with a positive abdominal radiograph. A 5% sodium bicarbonate solution is administered for lavage to create nonabsorbable ferric carbonate. Because of the possibility of bezoar formations, lavage may be indicated later than 6 hours postingestion if serum iron levels continue to rise. Positive abdominal radiographs should be repeated following lavage to ensure proper decontamination. Activated charcoal does not bind iron salts and therefore is not recommended.

Whole bowel irrigation has been recommended for patients in whom gastric lavage has been unsuccessful at evacuating iron tablets. This is accomplished by infusing a polyethylene glycol electrolyte lavage solution (PEG-ELS), such as Golytely or Colyte, via nasogastric tube. The infusion rate is 2 liter/hr for adults and 500 ml/hr for children.[92]

If gastric lavage and/or whole bowel irrigation are unsuccessful in expelling significant amounts of iron, gastrotomy is a potential recourse.[93]

Elimination Enhancement

Because of the wide tissue distribution of iron, hemodialysis and hemoperfusion are ineffective.

Antidotes

Desferoxamine appears to protect the body from the harmful effects of excess free iron by (1) trapping free iron in the extracellular space, (2) enhancing urinary iron excretion, and (3) binding free iron in the cytoplasm so that it cannot interfere with mitochondrial membranes.[87]

The dose of desferoxamine for iron chelation is 15 mg/kg/hr. This dose is continued until serum iron levels fall below the TIBC or below 300 μg/dl. In severe ingestions, higher infusion rates of desferoxamine may be required.[87] Hypotension is the major reported side effect of desferoxamine infusion, although it rarely occurs at infusion rates less than 45 mg/kg/hr.[86] If hypotension occurs, vigorous fluid resuscitation should be attempted before decreasing the dose of desferoxamine.

Serum iron levels should be monitored during chelation therapy. However, iron levels that are measured by colorimetric assays may be falsely low in the presence of desferoxamine.[88]

Supportive Care

Vasopressors and aggressive fluid resuscitation are indicated to maintain an adequate BP.

Theophylline Poisoning

Clinical Presentation

Theophylline poisoning may occur as a consequence of excessive theophylline ingestion or IV administration. The most common clinical manifestations of theophylline intoxication are vomiting, tachycardia, and CNS excitation.[94] Abdominal pain, diarrhea, headache, altered mental status, seizures, and dysrhythmias are also seen. Although these manifestations generally correlate with peak serum theophylline concentrations, this correlation depends on whether the intoxication is a result of an acute or a chronic overdose. In patients with chronic overdoses, correlations tend to be less accurate (see section on Serum Concentrations).

Tachycardia is seen in almost 100% of patients with serum theophylline concentrations above 20 mg/dl. Central stimulation may cause tachypnea.[95] Hypertension is usually seen initially, although hypotension can be observed in very large overdoses. A widened pulse pressure is characteristic of theophylline intoxication.

Neuromuscular effects of theophylline intoxication include generalized or focal seizures, tremor, myoclonus, and agitation.[96]

Assessment

Serum Concentrations

Because of the potential for prolonged absorption of theophylline in overdose, especially with sustained-release preparations, serial theophylline concentrations should be obtained until a plateau has been reached.[97,98] It has also been shown that theophylline absorption may intermittently stop and restart without additional dosing.[97] Hence, if the patient does not appear to respond to therapy or worsens despite therapy, theophylline levels should be repeated, even if a plateau has previously been observed.[97]

Serum theophylline concentrations may predict life-threatening events (seizures and serious cardiac dysrhythmias) in patients with acute theophylline intoxication. However, there does not appear to be a correlation between theophylline levels and the incidence of life-threatening events after chronic theophylline intoxication.[99,100] In general, patients who ingest single toxic amounts of theophylline do not have a significantly high incidence of seizures and severe dysrhythmias until serum levels exceed 100 μg/ml. In contrast, patients with chronic theophylline poisoning develop life-threatening events across a wide range of theophylline levels, with seizures occurring at levels as low as 25 µg/ml and cardiac dysrhythmias occurring at levels as low as 40 µg/ml.[99,100]

Potassium

Hypokalemia is common, particularly after acute theophylline ingestions, when it is seen in up to 95% of patients. Hypokalemia appears to be a consequence of an intracellular shift of potassium that results from a theophylline-induced elevation of catecholamines, insulin, and glucose, as well as a respiratory alkalosis.[101–104]

Glucose, Calcium, Phosphorus, and Magnesium

Hyperglycemia, hypercalcemia, hypophosphatemia, and hypomagnasemia may be observed.[101–106]

White Blood Cell Count

Leukocytosis may occur secondary to catecholamine release and resultant WBC demargination.

Acid-Base Disturbances

Central medullary stimulation may cause a respiratory alkalosis. Metabolic acidosis has also been described and is attributed to lactic acid production from increased glycolysis and unmet increases in oxygen demand.[104]

Electrocardiogram

The most common ECG findings are tachyarrhythmias. Ventricular and supraventricular arrhythmias occur with equal frequency.

Management

Decontamination

Lavage is typically recommended for theophylline ingestions that have occured within 4 hours of presentation. If ingestion of a sustained-release preparation is suspected, lavage may be effective up to 6 to 8 hours postingestion. If serum theophylline levels continue to rise despite decontamination and elimination enhancement, endoscopy may be indicated to evaluate the possible presence of a bezoar.

Elimination Enhancement

Charcoal and cathartic should be given q2–4h until clinical evidence of intoxication has ceased. MDAC is also effective after IV theophylline overdosage (see section, Multiple-Dose Activated Charcoal). If vomiting precludes the administration of charcoal, more frequent administration of smaller amounts or a continuous infusion of charcoal should be considered. Antiemetics such as IV metaclopramide or droperidol may also be effective.

Hemoperfusion can increase theophylline elimination by five-fold.[107] Indications for hemoperfusion in the pediatric population include (1) a theophylline concentration greater than 100 µg/ml after acute intoxication, (2) a theophylline concentration greater than 50 to 60 µg/ml for patients who are chronically poisoned with theophylline, (3) hepatic insufficiency, (4) hemodynamic instability, (5) theophylline-induced seizures, and (6) a theophylline elimination half-life of greater than or equal to 24 hours. Hemodialysis may also be used but is inferior to hemoperfusion and is no better than MDAC. Peritoneal dialysis is inefficient and not recommended for treatment of severe theophylline intoxication.[108]

Supportive Therapy

Cardiovascular Support. Propranolol and verapamil have been used successfully to treat both supraventricular and ventricular arrhythmias. Propranolol may also reverse hypotension by blocking the vasodilator properties of theophylline.[108] Because of the risk of bronchospasm, propranolol should be used cautiously, particularly in patients with a history of reactive airways disease.

Seizures. Seizures may be refractory to the usual anticonvulsant regimens. Because seizures appear to involve disturbances in GABA-containing neurons, phenobarbital, a known GABA agonist, may be a superior anticonvulsant. Hemoperfusion should be performed if seizures are intractable.[107]

Electrolyte Abnormalities. Hypokalemia should be treated cautiously because total body potassium may be unaffected after intoxication, and potassium levels may rise spontaneously as theophylline levels decrease. Hypercalcemia, hyperglycemia, hypomagnasemia, and hypophosphatemia rarely require therapy.

Salicylate Poisoning

Clinical Presentation

A toxic ingestion of salicylate (ASA) is defined as the ingestion of greater than 150 mg/kg. The clinical picture of ASA poisoning includes GI, metabolic, CNS, pulmonary, and hematologic abnormalities. The features that are seen most frequently in significant overdoses include tinnitus, nausea, vomiting, agitation, and hyperventilation.

Clinical Manifestations

Cardiovascular

Tachycardia may be noted in up to 70% of patients with ASA intoxication.[109]

Pulmonary

Noncardiogenic pulmonary edema has been described and may be complicated by overzealous attempts at fluid diuresis.[110,111]

Neurologic

Agitation, asterixis, hallucinations, lethargy, seizures, and coma may be present. Fundoscopic examination may reveal papilledema from cerebral edema.

Skin

Petechiae may be seen and most commonly appear on the eyelids, face, and neck.

Assessment

Serum Concentration

The Done nomogram has been used to relate serum ASA concentrations to the severity of poisoning. It is only useful, however, in interpreting blood samples drawn 6 hours or more after an acute ASA ingestion. Peak ASA concentrations are usually reached approximately 6 hours postingestion, although formation of concretions and/or ingestion of enteric-coated preparations may delay peak absorption for up to 24 hours. Therefore, serial serum measurements should be obtained until a plateau has been observed.

Arterial Blood Gases

Because direct stimulation of the medulla leads to hyperventilation, and uncoupling of oxidative phosphorylation produces metabolic acidosis, respiratory alkalosis typically coexists with metabolic acidosis.

Sodium

Hyponatremia is occasionally seen and may be a consequence of the syndrome of inappropriate antidiuretic hormone secretion.

Potassium

Hypokalemia results from increased urinary potassium excretion and from intracellular movement of potassium ions during respiratory alkalosis. It may worsen during treatment with urinary alkalinization.

Glucose

Glucose usually decreases in children secondary to increased metabolic rate. In adults, hyperglycemia is more commonly seen. CNS glucose levels may be decreased despite normal serum glucose levels.

Calcium

Hypocalcemia may occur and may worsen with treatment with urinary alkalinization.

Renal Functions

Papillary necrosis, interstitial nephritis, rhabdomyolysis, and acute renal failure have been described following ASA overdose.

Coagulation Profile

ASAs inhibit the synthesis of Vitamin K–dependent and –independent factors. Platelet aggregation is also impaired and may be manifested in prolonged bleeding times.

Liver Function Studies

Chemical hepatitis is seen more commonly in children than in adults and is usually mild and reversible.

Management

Decontamination

Lavage is recommended up to 4 to 6 hours postingestion. If the presence of bezoars or the ingestion of enteric-coated preparations is suspected, lavage may be indicated much later than 4 hours postingestion. Subsequently, activated charcoal and cathartic are administered every 4 to 6 hours.

Elimination Enhancement

Urinary ASA excretion is enhanced in urine, with a pH of 7.5 or greater. Urine alkalinization is therefore warranted for serum ASA concentrations greater than 35 mg/dl. Because pulmonary and cerebral edema are potential complications of ASA intoxication, fluids should be administered cautiously. Hemodialysis is recommended for ASA levels greater than 100 mg/dl in acute ingestions and for levels greater than 60 to 80 in chronic intoxications. Seizures suggest a poor prognosis and are an indication for hemodialysis.

Supportive Therapy

Vitamin K may be beneficial in reversing prolonged prothrombin times.

Acetaminophen

Although one of the most common serious ingestions worldwide, acetaminophen requires only brief mention. In doses of 150 mg/kg or greater, acetaminophen results in a clinical picture of nausea and vomiting, followed by progressive hepatotoxicity (appearing approximately 24 hours after ingestion), which may lead to complications including coagulopathy, hyperammonemia, and the hepatorenal syndrome.[112] In survivors, the period of hepatic dysfunction is extraordinarily brief, resolving by 7 to 9 days postingestion; by 30 days postingestion, the liver is histologically normal.

Acetaminophen has limited importance in the critical care setting for several reasons. First, despite its morbidity, acetaminophen is associated with a low overall mortality (2%–5% based on large series). This low mortality is because acetaminophen does not typically lead to any acute, life-threatening events (although the hepatotoxicity, like that from any disease process, may lead to metabolic derangements that require ICU support). Also, the hepatic injury of acetaminophen intoxication is a gradual process. Thus, the clinician has ample opportunity to monitor for metabolic dysfunction, making it possible to anticipate complications. Finally, acetaminophen intoxication has a highly effective treatment in N-acetylcysteine (Mucomyst).[113–115] When initiated within 24 hours of ingestion, Mucomyst substantially reduces the risk of fulminant hepatic failure to as low as 1% to 2%. Mucomyst appears to be ineffective if initiated more than 24 hours after acetaminophen intoxication. Mucomyst therapy does not require the ICU setting for its administration.

References

1. Stern TA et al. Complications after overdose with tricyclic antidepressants. *Crit Care Med* 13:672–674, 1985.
2. Fazen LE, Lovejoy FH Jr, Crone RK. Acute poisoning in a children's hospital—A 2 year experience. *Pediatrics* 77:144–151, 1986.
3. Litovitz TL et al. 1988 annual report of the American Association of Poison Control Centers National Data Collection System. *Am J Emerg Med* 7:495–545, 1989.
4. Centers for Disease Control. Unintentional poisoning mortality—United States, 1980–1986. *MMWR* 38:153–157, 1989.
5. Dean B, Krenzelok EP. Adolescent poisoning: A comparison of accidental and intentional exposures. *Vet Hum Tox* 30:579–582, 1988.
6. Centers for Disease Control. Update: Childhood poisonings—United States. *MMWR* 34:117–118, 1985.
7. Helper B, Sutheimer C, Sunshine P. Role of the toxicology laboratory in suspected ingestions. *Pediatr Clin North Am* 33:245–255, 1986.
8. Brett AS. Implications of discordance between clinical impression and toxicology analysis in drug overdose. *Arch Intern Med* 148:437–441, 1988.
9. Council on Scientific Affairs. Scientific issues in drug testing. *JAMA* 257:3110–3114, 1987.
10. Neuvonene PJ, Olkkola KT. Oral activated charcoal in the treatment of intoxications. *Med Toxicol* 3:33–58, 1988.
11. Katona BG, Siegel EG, Cluxton RJ. The new black magic: Activated charcoal and new therapeutic uses. *J Emerg Med* 5:9–18, 1987.
12. Watson WA. Factors influencing the clinical efficacy of activated charcoal. *Drug Intell Clin Pharm* 21:160–166, 1987.
13. Shannon M, Fish SS, Lovejoy FH Jr. Cathartics and laxatives—Do they still have a place in the management of the poisoned patient? *Med Toxicol* 1:247, 1986.
14. Neuvonen PJ, Olkkola KT. Oral activated charcoal in the treatment of intoxications—Role of single and repeated doses. *Med Toxicol* 3:33–58, 1988.
15. Derlet RW, Albertson TE. Activated charcoal—Past, present and future. *West J Med* 145:493–496, 1986.
16. Pond SM. Role of repeated oral doses of activated charcoal in clinical toxicology. *Med Tox* 1:3–11, 1986.
17. Pond SM et al. Randomized study of the treatment of phenobarbital overdose with repeated doses of activated charcoal. *JAMA* 251:3104–3108, 1984.
18. Jones J et al. Repetitive doses of activated charcoal in the treatment of poisoning. *Am J Emerg Med* 5:305–310, 1987.
19. Park GD et al. Expanded role of charcoal therapy in the poisoned and overdosed patient. *Arch Intern Med* 146:969–973, 1986.
20. Berg MJ et al. Acceleration of the body clearance of phenobarbital by oral activated charcoal. *N Engl J Med* 307:642–644, 1982.
21. Shannon M, Amitai Y, Lovejoy FH Jr. Multiple dose activated char-

coal for theophylline poisoning in young infants. *Pediatrics* 80: 368–370, 1987.

22. Hillman RJ, Prescott LF. Treatment of salicylate poisoning with repeated oral charcoal. *Br Med J* 291:1472, 1985.

23. Mofenson HC et al. Gastrointestinal dialysis with activated charcoal and cathartic in the treatment of adolescent intoxications. *Clin Pediatr* 24:678–684, 1985.

24. Levy G. Gastrointestinal clearance of drugs with activated charcoal. *N Engl J Med* 307:676–679, 1982.

25. Krenzelok EP, Heller MB. Effectiveness of commercially available aqueous activated charcoal products. *Ann Emerg Med* 16:1340–1343, 1987.

26. Olnay BL, Reed MD, Blumer JL. Continuous nasogastric administration of activated charcoal for the treatment of theophylline intoxication. *Pediatr Pharmacol* 5:241–245, 1986.

27. Handal KA, Schauben JL, Salamone FR. Naloxone. *Ann Emerg Med* 12:438–445, 1983.

28. Tenenbein M. Pediatric toxicology: Current controversies and recent advances. *Curr Probl Pediatr* 16:213–214, 1986.

29. Goldfrank L et al. A dosing nomogram for continuous infusion intravenous naloxone. *Ann Emerg Med* 15:566–570, 1986.

30. Mofenson HC, Caraccio TR. Continuous infusion of intravenous naloxone. *Ann Emerg Med* 16:600, 1987.

31. Romac DR. Safety of prolonged, high-dose infusion of naloxone hydrochloride for severe methadone overdose. *Clin Pharm* 5: 251–254, 1986.

32. Tenenbein M. Continous naloxone infusion for opiate poisoning in infancy. *J Pediatr* 105:645–648, 1984.

33. Tenenbein M. Naloxone in clonidine toxicity. *Am J Dis Child* 138:1084, 1984.

34. Niemann JT, Getzug T, Murphy W. Reversal of clonidine toxicity by naloxone. *Ann Emerg Med* 15:1229–1231, 1986.

35. Farsang C et al. Reversal by naloxone of the antihypertensive action of clonidine: Involvement of the sympathetic nervous system. *Circulation* 69:461–467, 1984.

36. North DS et al. Naloxone administration in clonidine overdosage. *Ann Emerg Med* 10:397, 1981.

37. Kulig K et al. Naloxone for treatment of clonidine overdose. *JAMA* 247:1697, 1982.

38. Jensen P et al. Hemodynamic effects following ingestion of an imidazoline-containing product. *Pediatr Emerg Care* 5:110–112, 1989.

39. Frommer DA et al. Tricyclic antidepressant overdose. *JAMA* 257(4):42, 1987.

40. Pentel PR, Benowitz NL. Tricyclic antidepressant poisoning—Management of arrhythmias. *Med Toxicol* 1:101–121, 1986.

41. Crome P. Poisoning due to tricyclic antidepressant overdosage—Clinical presentation and treatment. *Med Toxicol* 1:261–285, 1986.

42. Braden NJ, Jackson JE, Walson PD. Tricyclic antidepressant overdose. *Pediatr Clin North Am* 33:2, 1986.

43. Shannon MW, Lovejoy FH Jr. Pulmonary consequences of severe antidepressant overdose. *J Toxicol Clin Toxicol* 25:443–461, 1987.

44. Ware MR. Tricyclic antipressant overdose: Pharmacology and treatment. *South Med J* 80:111, 1987.

45. Boehnert MT, Lovejoy FH. Value of the QRS duration versus the serum drug level in predicting seizures and ventricular arrhythmias after an acute overdose of tricyclic antidepressants. *N Engl J Med* 313:474–479, 1985.

46. Foulke GE, Albertson TE. QRS interval in tricyclic antidepressant overdosage: Inaccuracy as a toxicity indicator in emergency settings. *Ann Emerg Med* 6:160–163, 1987.

47. Wolfe TR, Caravati EM, Rollins DE. Terminal 40-ms frontal plane QRS axis as a marker for tricyclic antidepressant overdose. *Ann Emerg Med* 18:348–351, 1989.

48. Swartz CM, Sherman A. The treatment of tricyclic antidepressant overdose with repeated charcoal. *J Clin Psychopharmacol* 4:336–340, 1984.

49. Hedges JR et al. Correlation of initial amitriptyline concentration

50. Goldberg RJ, Capone RJ. Cardiac complications following tricyclic antidepressant overdose—Issues for monitoring policy. *JAMA* 254:1772–1775, 1985.

51. Teba L et al. Beneficial effect of norepinephrine in the treatment of circulatory shock caused by triclyclic antidepressant overdose. *Am J Emerg Med* 6:566–568, 1988.

52. Mayron R, Ruiz E. Phenytoin: Does it reverse tricyclic antidepressant-induced cardiac conduction abnormalities? *Ann Emerg Med* 15: 33–37, 1986.

53. Brown TCK et al. The use of sodium bicarbonate in the treatment of tricyclic antidepressant-induced arrhythmias. *Anaesth Intensive Care* 1:203–209, 1973.

54. Sasyniuk BI, Jhamandas V, Valois M. Experimental amitriptyline intoxication: Treatment of cardiac toxicity with sodium bicarbonate. *Ann Emerg Med* 15:97–104, 1986.

55. Nattel S, Mittleman M. Treatment of ventricular tachyarrhythmias resulting from amitriptyline toxicity in dogs. *J Pharmacol Exp Ther* 231:2, 1984.

56. Bessen HA, Niemann JT. Improvement of cardiac conduction after hyperventilation in tricyclic antidepressant overdose. *Clin Toxicol* 23:537–546, 1986.

57. Levitt MA et al. Amitriptyline plasma protein binding: Effect of plasma pH and relevance to clinical overdose. *Am J Emerg Med* 4:121–125, 1986.

58. Pentel P, Peterson CD. Asystole complicating physostigmine treatment of tricyclic antidepressant overdose. *Ann Emerg Med* 9:73–75, 1980.

59. Lewis RV, McDevitt DG. Adverse reactions and interactions with B-adrenoceptor blocking drugs. *Med Toxicol* 1:343–361, 1986.

60. Heath A. B-adrenoceptor blocker toxicity: Clinical features and therapy. *Am J Emerg Med* 2:518–525, 1984.

61. Mofenson HC, Caraccio TR, Schauben J. Poisoning by antidysrhythmic drugs. *Pediatr Clin North Am* 33:3, 1986.

62. Gwinup GR. Propranolol toxicity presenting with early repolarization, ST segment elevation, and peaked T waves on the ECG. *Ann Emerg Med* 17:103–106, 1988.

63. Critchley JAJH, Ungar A. The management of acute poisoning due to B-adrenoceptor antagonists. *Med Toxicol* 4:32–45, 1989.

64. Agura ED, Wexler LF, Witzburg RA. Massive propanolol overdose. Successful treatment with high dose isoproterenol and glucagon. *Am J Med* 180:755–757, 1986.

65. Dymowski JJ, Turnbull T. Glucagon and beta-blocker poisoning. *Ann Emerg Med* 15:183–184, 1986.

66. Zaloga GP et al. Glucagon reversal of hypotension in a case of anaphylactoid shock. *Ann Intern Med* 105:1, 1986.

67. Lane AS, Woodward AC, Goldman MR. Massive propranolol overdose poorly responsive to pharmacologic therapy: Use of the intra-aortic balloon pump. *Ann Emerg Med* 16:103–105, 1987.

68. Shannon M. The clinical toxicity of cocaine adulterants. *Ann Emerg Med* 17:1243–1247, 1988.

69. Buchanan JF. Cocaine intoxication: A review of the presentation and treatment of medical complications. *Hosp Physician* 29:24–28, 1988.

70. Mody CK et al. Neurologic complications of cocaine abuse. *Neurology* 38:1189–1193, 1988.

71. Lehman LB. Intracerebral hemorrhage after intranasal cocaine use. *Hosp Physician* 21:69–70, 1987.

72. Tazelarr HD et al. Cocaine and the heart. *Hum Pathol* 18:195–199, 1987.

73. Karch SB, Billingham ME. The pathology and etiology of cocaine-induced heart disease. *Arch Pathol Lab Med* 112:225–230, 1988.

74. Luque MA et al. Pneumomediastinum, pneumothorax and subcutaneous emphysema after alternate cocaine inhalation and marijuana smoking. *Pediatr Emerg Care* 3:107–109, 1987.

75. Kosten T, Kleber H. Rapid death during cocaine abuse: A variant

of the neuroleptic malignant syndrome? *Am J Drug Alcohol Abuse* 14(3):335–346, 1988.

76. McCarron MM, Wood JD. The cocaine "body packer" syndrome. Diagnosis and management. *JAMA* 250:1417–1420, 1983.
77. Gay GR, Loper KA. The use of labetalol in the management of cocaine crisis. *Ann Emerg Med* 17:282–283, 1988.
78. Bigger JT. Digitalis toxicity. *J Clin Pharmacol* 25:514–521, 1985.
79. Lewander WJ et al. Acute pediatric digoxin ingestion—A ten year experience. *Am J Dis Child* 140:770–773, 1988.
80. Lalonde RL et al. Acceleration of digoxin clearance by activated charcoal. *Clin Pharmacol Ther* 37:367–371, 1985.
81. Mathieu D et al. Massive digitoxin intoxication treatment by Amberlite XAD-4 resin hemoperfusion. *J Toxicol Clin Toxicol* 19:931–950, 1982.
82. Fazio A. Fab fragments in the treatment of digoxin overdose: Pediatric considerations. *South Med J* 80:1553–1556, 1987.
83. Stolshek BS, Osterhout SK, Dunham G. The role of digoxin-specific antibodies in the treatment of digitalis poisoning. *Med Toxicol* 3:167–171, 1988.
84. Martiny SS, Phelps SJ, Massey K. Treatment of severe digitalis intoxication with digoxin-specific antibody fragments: A clinical review. *Am J Emerg Med* 4(4):364–368, 1986.
85. Lemon M et al. Concentrations of free serum digoxin after treatment with antibody fragments. *Br Med J* 295:1520–1521, 1987.
86. Lovejoy FH. Chelation therapy in iron poisoning. *J Toxicol Clin Toxicol* 19:871–874, 1982.
87. Proudfoot AT, Simpson D, Dyson EH. Management of acute iron poisoning. *Med Tox* 1:83–100, 1986.
88. Robotham JL, Lietman PS. Acute iron poisoning. *Am J Dis Child* 134:875–879, 1980.
89. Lacouture PG et al. Emergency assessment of severity in iron overdose by clinical and laboratory methods. *J Pediatr* 99:89–91, 1981.
90. Vernon DD, Banner W, Dean JM. Hemodynamic effects of experimental iron poisoning. *Ann Emerg Med* 18:863–866, 1989.
91. James JA. Acute iron poisoning: Assessment of severity and prognosis. *J Pediatr* 77:117–119, 1970.
92. Tenenbein M. Whole bowel irrigation in iron poisoning. *J Pediatr* 111:142–145, 1987.
93. Foxford R, Goldfrank L. Gastrotomy—A surgical approach to iron overdose. *Ann Emerg Med* 14:127–130, 1985.
94. Baker MD. Theophylline toxicity in children. *J Pediatr* 109:538–542, 1986.
95. Albert S. Aminophylline toxicity. *Pediatr Clin North Am* 34:61–73, 1987.
96. Paloucek FP, Rodvold KA. Evaluation of theophylline overdoses and toxicities. *Ann Emerg Med* 17:53–62, 1988.

97. Rogers RJ et al. Inconsistent absorption from a sustained-released theophylline preparation during continous therapy in asthmatic children. *J Pediatr* 106:496–501, 1985.
98. Haltom JR, Szefler SJ. Theophylline absorption in young asthmatic children receiving sustained-release formulations. *J Pediatr* 107:805–810, 1985.
99. Shannon M, Lovejoy FH. Life-threatening events after theophylline intoxication: A prospective analysis of 144 cases. *Ann Emerg Med* 18:166, 1989.
100. Aitken ML, Martin TR. Life-threatening theophylline toxicity is not predictable by serum levels. *Chest* 91:10–14, 1987.
101. D'Angio R, Sabatelli F. Management considerations in treating metabolic abnormalities associated with theophylline overdose. *Arch Intern Med* 147:1837–1838, 1987.
102. Bertino JS, Walker JW. Reassessment of theophylline toxicity—Serum concentrations, clinical course, and treatment. *Arch Intern Med* 147:757–760, 1987.
103. Hall KW et al. Metabolic abnormalities associated with intentional theophylline overdose. *Ann Intern Med* 101:457–462, 1984.
104. Sawyer WT et al. Hypokalemia, hyperglycemia, and acidosis after intentional theophylline overdose. *Am J Emerg Med* 3:408–411, 1985.
105. Kearney TE et al. Theophylline toxicity and the beta-adrenergic system. *Ann Intern Med* 102:766–769, 1985.
106. McPherson ML et al. Theophylline-induced hypercalcemia. *Ann Intern Med* 105:52–54, 1986.
107. Park GD et al. Use of hemoperfusion for treatment of theophylline intoxication. *Am J Med* 74:961–966, 1983.
108. Gaudreault P, Guay J. Theophylline poisoning—Pharmacological considerations and clinical management. *Med Toxicol* 1:169–191, 1986.
109. Thisted B et al. Acute salicylate self-poisoning in 177 consecutive patients treated in ICU. *Acta Anaesthesiol Scand* 31:312–316, 1987.
110. Fisher CJ, Albertson TE, Foulke GE. Salicylate-induced pulmonary edema: Clinical characteristics in children. *Am J Emerg Med* 3:33–37, 1985.
111. Maron MB. Effect of high doses of aspirin on pulmonary hemodynamics and lung water. *Am J Physiol* 248:225–231, 1985.
112. Rumack BH. Acetaminophen overdose in children and adolescents. *Pediatr Clin North Am* 33:691, 1986.
113. Smilkstein MJ et al. Efficacy of oral N-acetylcyteine in the treatment of acetaminophen overdose—Analysis of the National Multicenter Study (1976 to 1985). *N Engl J Med* 319:1557–1562, 1988.
114. Riggs BS et al. Acute acetaminophen overdose during pregnancy. *Obstet Gynecol* 74:247, 1989.
115. Flanagan RJ. The role of acetylcysteine in clinical toxicology. *Med Toxicol* 2:93–104, 1987.

James W. Ziegler　◆ **51.1**　**Infant Botulism**

Botulism is a disease caused by a heat-labile toxin produced by four families of anaerobic, spore-forming rods grouped together and called *Clostridium botulinum* (CB). Only organisms of groups I and II cause human disease, usually by production of toxins type A or B.[1] The spore form of this organism, representing a dormant state, is ubiquitous and found in soil and dust and often on clothes, shoes, and other household items.[2] When exposed to appropriate conditions, including anaerobiosis, a neutral pH, adequate nutrients, and the absence of competing microorganisms, these spores germinate and the resultant bacteria replicate and produce toxin.

The toxin produced by CB is one of the most potent toxins known. On gaining access to the human circulation, it travels to any peripheral synaptic connection (it cannot cross the blood-brain barrier[3]) where acetylcholine (Ach) acts as the neurotransmitter.

There, the toxin binds irreversibly to the presynaptic membrane, blocking the release of Ach into the synaptic cleft. Thus, neurotransmission of autonomic ganglia, parasympathetic nerve endings, Ach-releasing sympathetic nerve endings, and neuromuscular junctions is inhibited. This inhibition accounts for the characteristic symptomatology of botulism, namely anticholinergic signs, muscle weakness, and paralysis. Because binding of toxin is irreversible, recovery depends on the formation of new synaptic connections.

Paralysis caused by neuromuscular blockade is the most life-threatening effect of botulism toxin. The progression of weakness and paralysis with botulism poisoning is very similar to that seen with the administration of sequential doses of nondepolarizing muscle relaxants, which competitively block receptors on the postsynaptic membrane (Table 51.1-1); it can best be understood utilizing the concept of margin of safety.[4] Following low-frequency stimulation, peripheral muscles will maintain normal strength and function until greater than 75% of receptors are blocked; for the diaphragm, loss of strength is first noted when 92% of receptors are blocked. Thus, there is a wide margin of safety. With increased frequency of stimulation, the margin of safety narrows. Based on this concept, one can predict that the progression of neuromuscular blockade, with both botulism and the use of muscle relaxants, involves: first, muscles used in repetitive activities such as sucking, swallowing, and maintaining head control, which require a high frequency of stimulation; second, peripheral muscles; and last, the diaphragm. Resolution of muscle weakness occurs in the reverse order.[5]

It is important to realize that when near the threshold for muscle dysfunction, events that additionally stress the neuromuscular junction can rapidly result in decompensation. Flexion of the neck during the performance of a lumbar puncture, with further obstruction of the airway, has been reported to precipitate respiratory arrest in this instance.[5]

History

Cases of paralytic disease following the consumption of a common, contaminated food source date back to the days of the Roman Empire. The cause, however, was not discovered until 1895 when Von Ermenger investigated an outbreak affecting 24 musicians and established that their disease was caused by a substance produced by an anaerobic bacterium.[6] In 1919, following several deaths from botulism, most of which were associated with the ingestion of canned foods, California established a Botulism Commission. This commission was key in advancing knowledge about botulism. It was discovered that spores were ubiquitous, primarily in topsoil, and harmless when ingested. Only consumption of preformed toxin resulted in disease.[7] Strict standards were set and an educational campaign begun, and in subsequent years only about ten outbreaks of food-borne botulism occurred annually, usually associated with faulty home canning techniques. From 1899 to 1973, more than 1800 cases of botulism were reported to the Centers for Disease Control (CDC)[8]; none of these occurred

Table 51.1-1. Clinical progression of botulism poisoning versus competitive blockade by nondepolarizing muscle relaxants

Infant botulism	Competitive blockade
Constipation, tachycardia	Blurred vision, tachycardia
↓	↓
Loss of head control*	Loss of head lift*
Difficulty feeding*	Weakness in jaw muscles
Weak cry*	Decreased hand grip (sustained)*
Depressed gag reflex*	Bulbar weakness
↓	↓
Peripheral motor weakness	Peripheral motor weakness
↓	↓
Diaphragmatic weakness	Diaphragmatic weakness

*Repetitive muscle activity
From C L'Hommedieu, RA Polin. Progression of clinical signs in severe infant botulism. *Clin Pediatr* 20:90–95, 1981. With permission.

in infants. It was thought that, perhaps because of their restricted diets, young infants were spared exposure.

Then, in 1976 two cases of botulism were reported in infants less than 4 months of age who had no identifiable exposure to preformed toxin.[9] These infants had evidence of intestinal colonization by CB with in vivo production of toxin; it seemed that, unlike adults, these infants' GI tracts were permissive to the growth of CB and to the production of toxin.[10] Since these initial two cases, several hundred cases of botulism in infants have been reported across the United States.

Types of Botulism

We now recognize three distinct types of botulism (food-borne, wound, infant), although the signs and symptoms of the three overlap. Classic, food-borne disease occurs when food is contaminated by CB spores and processed under anaerobic conditions, allowing the spores to germinate and produce toxin; the preformed toxin is then ingested. Symptoms usually develop within 36 hours of ingesting the contaminated food, although the disease can sometimes progress to complete paralysis over hours.

Wound botulism is rare.[11] It occurs when a deep, dirty wound, usually of an extremity, is contaminated by CB spores, which then germinate under local anaerobic conditions and release toxin directly into the bloodstream. Prodromal GI symptoms are often not encountered prior to the onset of muscular weakness.

Infant botulism, as noted, was first described in 1976 in California. It is now the most common form of botulism in the United States, with greater than 50% of cases occurring in California, Utah, and Pennsylvania. Because CB spores are ubiquitous and exposure universal, and because ingestion of spores is harmless in the adult, multiple factions must interact to influence disease activity in the infant.

Disease frequency is highest in areas with high spore counts in the soil, presumably accounting for localized geographic "hotbeds" of disease. An excellent example of this is the Philadelphia experience, in which 44 cases of infant botulism were reported over a 7-year period in a ring of counties surrounding Philadelphia[12] (Table 51.1-2). It is interesting that only one case occurred in Philadelphia proper, and no cases occurred in the counties surrounding the ring of disease.

Case studies have demonstrated that the same type of organism and toxin isolated from an affected individual is often present around that individual's home.[12] A history of nearby construction stirring up dirt or of unusually dusty conditions predating the onset of symptoms is commonly noted.[13] Often, the father's occupation is one that brings him into contact with soil on a daily basis and, if so, spores can frequently be found on workclothes and/or shoes.[12] In 1979, in California, three cases of infant botulism were traced back to contaminated honey containing spores of CB.[14] At that time, sampling of honey specimens around the state of California revealed that about 30% carried spores of CB. Presently, despite attempted educational campaigns, approximately 10% of causes of infant botulism still result from honey ingestion. **Honey should never be fed to any child less than 1 year old.**

What makes certain infants susceptible is unclear, but a certain patient profile can be developed based on reported cases. Most infants are less than 6 months old, Caucasian, and from intact two-parent families.[12,13] Breast feeding is a definite risk factor,[12,15] and in a majority of patients, the first solid food has been introduced into the diet within the 4 weeks preceding the onset of illness. Experimental studies in mice have revealed that the intestinal

Table 51.1-2. Characteristics of forty-four infants with botulism

	No.	%
Past history and family history		
Male	23	52
White race	44	100
Term gestation	44	100
Previously healthy	44	100
Purely or predominately breast-fed	44	100
Immunizations appropriate for age	34/35	97
Two-parent family	44	100
Homemaker mother	42	95
Father's occupation includes daily contact with soil	22/43	51
History of illness and physical findings		
Constipation	42	95
Weakness	44	100
Temperature $\geq$ 38.3°C at hospitalization	6	14
Decreased spontaneous movement	36	82
Hypotonia	42	95
Facial diparesis or ptosis	37	84
Diminished gag or sucking reflex	40	91
Decreased deep tendon reflexes	25	57
Absent deep tendon reflexes	3	7
Decreased tearing or salivation	8	18
Flushed or robust appearance	8	18

Reproduced by permission of *Pediatrics* 75:935, 1985. From SS Long et al. Clinical, laboratory, and environmental features of infant botulism in southeastern Pennsylvania.

bacterial flora play the major role in inhibiting growth and toxin production by CB.[16,17] It is hypothesized that in breast-fed babies, the introduction of foods other than breast milk into the diet disrupts the enteric flora, allowing overgrowth of CB. The relative immunocompetence of the very small infant may also influence disease activity.

Clinical Presentation

Clinically, there is a broad spectrum of disease presentations[13] (Table 51.1-3). The most common initial symptom is constipation, sometimes associated with other anticholinergic signs, including decreased salivation, urinary retention, and tachycardia. Within

Table 51.1-3. Clinical spectrum of infant botulism

Asymptomatic carrier of organism $\pm$ toxin

Mild involvement
  Failure to thrive
  Poor feeding
  Mild hypotonia
  Outpatient treatment

Classic disease (subacute prodrome 4–5 days from onset to hospitalization)
  Constipation
  Hyptonia
  Poor feeding
  Respiratory distress

Rapidly progressive form (brief, few hours, to absent prodrome)
  Sudden infant death

Reproduced by permission of *Pediatrics* 66:936, 1980. From JA Thompson et al. Infant botulism: Clinical spectrum and epidemiology.

days to weeks, muscle weakness develops, first of the facial and oropharyngeal muscles resulting in poor suck, weak cry, and loss of the gag reflex. Inability to handle secretions and prominent head lag are manifest, followed by weakness of peripheral skeletal muscles and finally the diaphragm. By the time of presentation to the hospital, most patients have evidence of bulbar dysfunction and generalized weakness[15] (Table 51.1-4). Deep tendon reflexes, which are usually intact on admission, are lost over time.[18] Sluggish pupils, the inability to fix and follow, and ptosis are common accompanying symptoms. Throughout the progression of symptoms, the patient remains alert, with an intact mental status.

Muscle weakness reaches a plateau and then remains there for a variable period, usually 10 to 20 days, followed by gradual recovery in reverse order of the presentation. Complete recovery takes several months.

Some patients have more mild symptoms, consisting of only constipation or failure to thrive with hypotonia; these cases are diagnosed and managed as outpatients. Although CB is not a normal inhibitant of the human GI tract, in one series of patients, 10% of case controls were found to have positive stool assays for CB organisms and/or toxin, proving that asymptomatic carriage does occur.[13]

Some early series of patients with infant botulism revealed cases that progressed extremely rapidly, with fulminant respiratory failure developing within hours of the initial onset of weakness. This prompted investigators to question whether botulism might be a cause of sudden infant death syndrome (SIDS). The overlapping age distribution of these two diseases lends further support to this theory. To examine this association, a study was done with 211 patients dying of SIDS in California and Washington; approximately 5% of these patients had CB organisms or toxin isolated from their stools postmortem.[19] It is interesting that all of these patients had been bottle-fed, suggesting that breast-feeding, although permissive to botulism in general, might be protective against severe disease.[20] A later study disputed this point.[21]

Diagnosis

When confronted with a hypotonic infant, the differential diagnosis is extensive (Table 51.1-5). The diagnosis of botulism should be suspected in any infant with muscle weakness preceded or accompanied by constipation. Usual laboratory tests, including lumbar

Table 51.1-4. Complications of forty-four infants with botulism

	No.	%
Respiratory failure	39	89
Failure of oral feeding	41	93
Otitis media	13	30
Pneumonia	11	25
Syndrome of inappropriate secretion of antidiuretic hormone	8	18
Adult respiratory distress syndrome	2	5
Autonomic instability	5	11
Convulsion	1	2
Death	1	2

Reproduced by permission of *Pediatrics* 75:928, 1985. From SS Long. Epidemiologic study of infant botulism in Pennsylvania: Report of the infant botulism study group.

Table 51.1-5. Abbreviated differential diagnosis of the hypotonic infant

Systemic
  Sepsis meningitis
  Encephalitis
  Encephalopathy
  Electrolyte abnormalities
  Metabolic disease
  Intoxication
  Hypothyroidism

Spinal cord and neuromuscular
  Poliomyelitis
  Spinal cord trauma
  Werdnig-Hoffman disease
  Guillain-Barré syndrome
  Familial dysautonomia
  Tick paralysis
  Myasthenia gravis
  Muscular dystrophy
  Myopathy
  Infant botulism

puncture, blood studies, metabolic screens, and head CT scan, are normal. Nerve conduction studies are also normal, but EMG lends supportive evidence with a characteristic pattern showing incremental response to rapid stimulation, with brief, small amplitude, overly abundant action potentials, a so-called BSAP pattern.[18,22] Repeat EMGs should be considered if the first is negative and clinical suspicion remains high. Although not diagnostic, the finding of a BSAP pattern on EMG in a patient with an appropriate history is strongly suggestive of infant botulism.

The diagnosis of infant botulism is confirmed by isolating CB organisms from stool or CB toxin from stool or, on rare occasions, from blood. CB can be grown from stool by using anaerobic procedures with special enrichment techniques. The toxin is identified from a sterile filtrate of stool by using a mouse toxin neutralization test and is typed by using specific antitoxins. Isolation of organism and toxin is performed by some state laboratories and also by the CDC. Stool remains positive for organisms and toxin for prolonged periods, even after the infant is well on the way to recovery[2,22]; thus, the diagnosis can be confirmed after the episode of acute illness.

Treatment

Treatment of infant botulism is primarily supportive, with attention focused on two organ systems: respiratory and GI. Throughout the course of illness, close monitoring with anticipation of complications is essential. Because clinical decompensation can occur suddenly, access to a pediatric intensive care unit (PICU) is crucial.

The most critical component of therapy is maintenance of the airway and assurance of adequate gas exchange. Respiratory failure, which occurs in over 50% of hospitalized patients, is multifactorial. Pooling of secretions, poor gag reflex, and inability to maintain airway patency may necessitate placement of an artificial airway. Aspiration pneumonia is a constant threat and can cause rapid deterioration. Diaphragmatic paralysis may necessitate mechanical ventilation to assure adequate gas exchange.

In patients requiring installation of mechanical ventilation, recurrent atelectasis and nosocomial pneumonia are always potential complications. Once intubated, patients usually require airway support for 10 to 20 days.[12,13,23] Extubation is attempted when diaphragmatic function returns and protective reflexes, including a good cough, are present. We usually use a maximum negative inspiratory force of less than -25 cm H_2O and an expiratory volume of greater than 10 to 15 ml/kg as signs of adequate ventilatory function. It is important to remember that the return of diaphragmatic function always precedes the return of protective airway reflexes.

Because of the inability to suck and swallow, along with constipation and relative atony of the bowel, enteral feedings are problematic. In severe cases, hyperalimentation may be necessary. Bolus feeds are poorly tolerated,[23] but continuous nasogastric feedings, starting at low volumes and gradually increasing, are usually successful. Slightly less than calculated maintenance calories is a reasonable caloric goal. The inability to feed orally usually remains long after the need for artificial airway support has passed and can last for several months. With demonstration of an adequate gag reflex and reasonable head control, oral feeds can be slowly reinitiated.

Antibiotics are commonly employed on admission, as sepsis is one of the most commonly entertained initial diagnoses. Two points with regard to antibiotics are that (1) aminoglycosides should not be used, as they can potentiate the effect of the botulism toxin at the neuromuscular junction[24]; and (2) antibiotics do not alter the course of the disease, nor do they hasten elimination of organisms and toxin from the GI tract.[18] Theoretically, antibiotics might have detrimental effects, including alteration of the enteric bacterial microecology, allowing CB overgrowth. Also, on killing organisms, large amounts of toxin might be liberated.

Autonomic dysfunction is an integral part of this disease. Constipation and urinary retention may require therapy. Fluctuations in heart rate, BP, and skin color, although at times alarming, generally require no therapy.

Botulism antitoxin, which is derived from horse serum, is indicated in food-borne disease, whereby toxin is ingested and then absorbed into the bloodstream[25] in an all-or-none fashion. In infants, where there is colonization of the GI tract with CB organisms and continued production and absorption of toxin in small amounts into the circulation, antitoxin would not be expected to influence the disease progression. Antitoxin has been used in two instances[18]: In one case, it did not appear to alter the disease, and in the other, its administration resulted in anaphylaxis.

Agents that act at the neuromuscular junction to increase the release of Ach from nerve terminals have been tried with variable results. The use of guanidine hydrochloride in adults had no demonstrable beneficial effects[26] in food-borne disease.

Prognosis

With early recognition, vigilant observation, and prompt institution of therapy, prognosis remains excellent, with full recovery the rule. Recovery occurs despite persistence of toxin in the patient's GI tract. Why and how the infant develops tolerance to the toxin are not understood; possibilities include local intestinal neutralization by antitoxin or local or systemic antibody production.

References

1. Long SS. Botulism in infancy. *Pediatr Infect Dis* 3:266–271, 1984.
2. Long SS et al. Clinical, laboratory, and environmental features of infant botulism in southeastern Pennsylvania. *Pediatrics* 75:935–941, 1985.

3. Brown LW. Infant botulism. *Adv Pediatr* 28:141–157, 1981.

4. Paton WDW, Waud DR. The margin of safety of neuromuscular transmission. *J Physiol* 191:595, 1967.

5. L'Hommedieu C, Polin RA. Progression of clinical signs in severe infant botulism. *Clin Pediatr* 20:90–95, 1981.

6. Van Ermenger E. A new anaerobic bacillus and its relation to botulism (a reprint). *Rev Infect Dis* 1:1701, 1979.

7. Geiger JC, Dickson EC, Meyer KF. The epidemiology of botulism. Public Health Bull 127:1–119, 1927.

8. Center for Disease Control. *Botulism in the United States, 1899–1977. Handbook for Epidemiologists, Clinicians, and Laboratory Workers.* Atlanta, 1979.

9. Pickett J et al. Syndrome of botulism in infancy: Clinical and electro-physiologic study. *N Engl J Med* 295:770–771, 1976.

10. Midura TF, Arnon SS. Infant botulism identification of clostriduim botulinum and its toxin in feces. *Lancet* 2:934–936, 1976.

11. Merson MH, Sowell VR. Epidemiologic, clinical and laboratory aspects of wound botulism. *N Engl J Med* 289:1005, 1973.

12. Long SS. Epidemiologic study of infant botulism in Pennsylvania: Report of the infant botulism study group. *Pediatrics* 75:928–934, 1985.

13. Thompson JA et al. Infant botulism: Clinical spectrum and epidemiology. *Pediatrics* 66:936–942, 1980.

14. Arnon SS et al. Honey and other environmental risk factors for infant botulism. *J Pediatr* 94:331–336, 1979.

15. Long SS et al. Clinical laboratory and environmental features of infant botulism in south eastern Pennsylvania. *Pediatrics* 75:935–941, 1985.

16. Burr DH, Sugiyama H. Susceptibility to enteric botulism colonization of antibiotic treated adult mice. *Infect Immun* 36:103, 1982.

17. Well GL, Sugiyama H, Bland SE. Resistance of mice with limited intestinal flu to entire colonization by clostridium botulinum. *J Infect Dis* 146:791–796, 1982.

18. Johnson RO, Clay SA, Arnon SS. Diagnosis and management of infant botulism. *Am J Dis Child* 133:586–593, 1979.

19. Arnon SS et al. Intestinal infection and toxin production by clostridium botulinum as one cause of sudden infant death syndrome. *Lancet* 1:1273–1277, 1978.

20. Arnon SS et al. Protective role of human milk against sudden death from infant botulism. *J Pediatr* 100:568–573, 1982.

21. Spika JS, Shaffer N, Hargrett-Bean N. Risk factors for infant botulism in the United States. *Am J Dis Child* 143:828–832, 1989.

22. Arnon SS, Midura TF, Clay SA. Infant botulism: Epidemiological, clinical, and laboratory aspects. *JAMA* 237:1946–1951, 1977.

23. Schreiner MS, Field E, Ruddy R. Infant botulism: A review of 12 years' experience at the Children's Hospital of Philadelphia. *Pediatrics* 87:159–165, 1991.

24. L'Hommedieu C et al. Potentiation of neuromuscular weakness in infant botulism by aminoglycosides. *J Pediatrics* 95:1065–1070, 1979.

25. Merson MH et al. Current trends in botulism in the United States. *JAMA* 229:1305–1308, 1974.

26. Kaplan JE et al. Botulism: Type A and treatment with quanindine. *Ann Neurol* 6:69–71, 1979.

XI ◆ Surgically Related Conditions

I. David Todres

◆52 Postanesthesia Recovery

The pediatric intensivist, along with the surgical team, plays a vital role in caring for the postoperative patient once the patient is transferred from the operating room to the intensive care unit (ICU). As a result, the intensivist's care covers a period when the child is emerging from the anesthetic process that was induced to perform the necessary surgery. This chapter reviews the effects of the anesthetic gases and other agents on the body's organ systems and the physiologic responses. One of the hallmarks of safe postoperative care is anticipation of potential problems in the recovery phase. Commonly occurring problems will be discussed with regard to their significance and expeditious management.

Recovery from anesthesia begins in the operating room the moment the surgical procedure is completed and anesthesia is discontinued. Thus, the first phase of anesthetic recovery is monitored in the operating room. This phase is followed by a second phase when the child is transported from the operating room to a designated environment for postoperative care. The third phase occurs either in a postanesthesia care unit (PACU) or pediatric intensive care unit (PICU), depending on the needs of the patient following surgery. The PICU is usually reserved for patients undergoing complex major surgery in whom postoperative care requires sophisticated monitoring and the skills of the personnel in an ICU. On occasion, admission is required for patients undergoing less complex surgery but in whom an adverse event necessitates their postoperative course to be followed in an ICU.

Recovery from Anesthesia

Anesthetic practice commonly employs a combination of (1) inhalation anesthetics, (2) muscle relaxants, and (3) intravenous (IV) hypnotics and opioids. The effects of these agents may be synergistic. Each group is discussed separately.

Recovery from Inhalational Anesthesia

The inhalation agents employed in children are nitrous oxide, halothane, enflurane, and isoflurane. Recovery from the effects of these gases to a state of wakefulness depends on (1) rate of alveolar ventilation, and hence the degree of reduction in alveolar concentration of the gas; (2) the anesthetic gas solubility (i.e., the blood/gas solubility coefficient); and (3) the cardiac output. Recovery from anesthesia is referred to as MAC-awake, with MAC-awake being defined as the alveolar concentration of a volatile anesthetic at which eye opening to a verbal command occurs during emergence from anesthesia in 50% of patients.[1] This level is approximately 60% of MAC, with MAC defined as the minimum alveolar concentration of the inhalation agent necessary to abolish purposeful movements in 50% of patients. Halothane has a higher solubility than enflurane and isoflurane. Despite the differences in anesthetic solubility, however, the recovery from these three agents was found to be similar in one study.[2] By contrast, in another study, in adults the shortest wake-up time was observed with halothane. A longer wake-up time was noted with enflurane, reflecting a greater anesthetic concentration between MAC and MAC-awake. Isoflurane was intermediate between halothane and enflurane in their

wake-up times.[3] Nitrous oxide is eliminated rapidly. MAC-awake is generally reached in a few minutes. At MAC-awake, patients are able to protect and maintain a clear airway spontaneously and continuously. Spontaneous eye opening in children is a good indication of the child's ability to maintain and exhibit airway protective reflexes.

Recovery from Muscle Relaxants

Reversal of neuromuscular blockade in the child is indicated by (1) wide opening of the child's eyes, (2) forceful coughing, and (3) ability to flex and elevate the lower limbs. Evidence of paradoxical ventilation is a signal that residual neuromuscular blockade may be contributing to compromised respiratory effort and reflects inadequate reversal of the neuromuscular blockade. Reversal may be effected by spontaneous weaning of the actions of the neuromuscular blocking agent or administration of the antidote to the agent, namely neostigmine. At times, depending on the nature of the surgery, the patient is returned to the ICU undergoing mechanical ventilation via an endotracheal tube (or tracheostomy) with active neuromuscular blockade in effect so that mechanical ventilation is facilitated. The effects of the blockade are then allowed to wear off spontaneously at a time that is considered appropriate to the postoperative management. Testing with a peripheral nerve stimulator is an important step in evaluating the presence of residual neuromuscular blockade. In neuromuscular blockade testing with the peripheral nerve stimulator, a train-of-four impulse is administered and the ratio of the fourth twitch height to the first twitch height is noted (see Muscle Relaxants, by Goudsouzian, this volume). If the percentage is more than 75%, it is likely that spontaneous respiration will be adequate.[4] One makes this presumption, although muscular effort of the diaphragm is not specifically assessed. Because the diaphragm is more resistant to nondepolarizing muscle agents than skeletal muscles in adults and children, however, peripheral nerve stimulation of the ulna nerve provides a practical assessment of recovery from the effects of neuromuscular blockade.[5]

An inspiratory force greater than -20 cm H_2O suggests that the child will be able to sustain adequate spontaneous respiratory movements and indicates adequate recovery from neuromuscular blockade. Incomplete recovery is potentially dangerous, as it may cause airway obstruction and diminished ventilation, leading to hypoxemia, hypercarbia, and acidosis. Also, the ability to cough effectively and eliminate secretions is diminished. It can be particularly dangerous in the presence of residual inhalation anesthesia or IV opioids.

Should there be inadequate return of functioning motor power, particularly of the diaphragm and intercostals, and should blockade monitor testing reveal residual neuromuscular blockade, an antidote (neostigmine, also known as prostigmin) to the neuromuscular blocking agent is administered. Atropine or glycopyrolate is administered before or with the neostigmine to counteract undesirable cholinergic side effects (bradycardia, increased secretions). In some cases, neuromuscular blockade may be continued into the postoperative recovery phase, should mechanical ventilation be required.

Recovery from Hypnotics and Opioids

Awakening from IV narcotics and hypnotics is extremely variable in children. These agents are cleared by redistribution, followed by slower elimination via hepatic metabolism and renal excretion. Active metabolites of these agents, such as diazepam metabolites, may prolong the anesthesia during the recovery phase. These agents depress the ventilatory response to carbon dioxide and may also depress the hypoxic drive. There is synergistic depression of respiratory and cardiovascular reflexes, when IV opioids and hypnotics are combined with inhalation agents. This is particularly noted with combinations of opioids and benzodiazepines (e.g., fentanyl and midazolam). The administration of ketamine and droperidol are often associated with prolongation of recovery time.

Recovery of Respiratory Reflexes

Recovery of the child's respiratory reflexes (i.e., responses to carbon dioxide and oxygen) is an important process in recovery from anesthesia. The reduction in response to carbon dioxide is a dose-related response. At MAC levels of 0.6 to 1.0, airway and lung function are generally adequate. However, patients with obstructive lung disease (e.g., bronchopulmonary dysplasia) may become hypercarbic. The magnitude of alveolar ventilation is also a function of the intensity of surgical stimulation. If the patient perceives pain, there is a much greater stimulus to respiration. After major surgical procedures (thoracic and abdominal), however, pain may interfere with the depth of ventilation, resulting in hypoventilation, with its potential dangers of hypoxemia and hypercarbia.

The recovery phase is critical from the point of view of adequate oxygenation to the tissues, especially brain and myocardium, and this is a time when the child is particularly liable to develop hypoxemia. There are many possible reasons for this: upper airway obstruction, central hypoventilation, and ventilation/perfusion imbalance from the atelectasis that may accompany prolonged surgical procedures. In addition, tidal volumes may be inadequate because severe pain limits ventilatory excursions or because of restrictions imposed by orthopedic casts and tight dressings. Peripheral chemoreceptors govern the hypoxic drive, and their response is blunted by inhalational anesthetic agents. For example, as little as 0.1% of alveolar concentration of halothane blunts this response, and the drive is completely abolished at 1.1% halothane.[6]

Following major surgery, the patient experiences some degree of hypoxemia, which is readily corrected by the administration of supplemental oxygen. Therefore, the patient should be closely monitored in the early recovery phase with pulse oximetry to ensure adequate oxygen saturation and given appropriate inspired concentrations of supplemental oxygen to correct the hypoxemia. A study of postoperative hypoxemia in adults concluded that its etiology is based on the interaction of two factors: (1) a gas exchange abnormality (i.e., ventilation/perfusion mismatching) induced during anesthesia that may persist for hours or days in the postoperative phase, and (2) an abnormality of control of breathing that is evident by episodic obstructive apnea rather than a sustained decrease in the respiratory rate. This may last for several days and nights following the surgery.[7] Because metabolic rate and oxygen consumption in the infant is approximately twice that of the adult, the infant cannot deal very effectively with developing hypoxemia, and for a similar reason, hypercapnia develops twice as fast as it does in the adult. The infant may therefore readily develop both metabolic and respiratory acidosis.

The effects of environmental temperature are important for the young child or infant. Should this be outside the thermoneutral range, cold stress is readily produced in the child or, conversely, heat stress, placing additional metabolic demands on the child. Hypothermia, especially in the infant, may lead to respiratory depression, hypoxemia, and acidosis.

Structural immaturity of the infant's and small child's chest wall is an important limitation in the young child's ability to deal with stress in the postoperative phase.[8] The chest wall is extremely compliant and provides very poor stability for the respiratory demands of the infant in the postoperative phase. Thus, with increased airway resistance (airway obstruction) or atelectasis (reduced lung compliance), the infant exhibits marked retractions and paradoxical movement of the chest wall. In the first 2 years of life, there is a tendency for the small airways to close, leading to increased intrapulmonary shunting. The infant's rib cage is not as well designed for respiratory efforts as it is later in life. The ribs are short and horizontally placed, and the normal bucket handle motion of the chest wall is reduced. Thus, the infant relies primarily on the movements of the diaphragm, and these are seriously compromised if there is marked abdominal distension. The respiratory muscles of the infant have a low percentage of type 1 muscle fibers, the slow-twitch and high-oxidative type, which fatigue rapidly when the respiratory load is increased.[9] Fatigue then leads to underventilation, hypoxemia, and hypercarbia. In some cases, the surgical procedure may be complicated by phrenic nerve palsy and compromise diaphragmatic function. In this situation, prolonged respiratory support may be required.[10]

The respiratory reserve of the child may already be compromised preoperatively by an underlying medical condition that may make the child susceptible to postoperative respiratory failure. Children with kyphoscoliosis, cystic fibrosis, and congenital heart lesions are particularly liable to experience postoperative respiratory compromise; respiratory support (i.e., mechanical ventilation) becomes an important part of postoperative anesthesia care. Anticipating these problems is important in ensuring safe recovery from the surgical procedure.

An important consideration in the young child is the size of the airways. The tracheal diameter in the newborn is approximately one third that of the adult, and the bronchioles are half the diameter of those in the adult. Obstruction readily occurs from blood and mucus. In children, relatively small decreases in airway diameter are associated with large increases in airway resistance, compared with those in the adult.

Transport to the Pediatric Intensive Care Unit

Transport to the PICU is a critical phase during which the infant or child should be closely monitored. Monitoring of the child is carried out to ensure maintenance of a clear airway, and adequacy of ventilation, oxygenation, and perfusion. Adequacy of ventilation is determined by clinical observation of bilateral chest movements and oxygenation by monitoring oxygen saturation using pulse oximetry. In many situations it is prudent to transfer the child with an endotracheal tube in place and artificially ventilated. The tube must be meticulously fastened in place so that accidental extubation does not occur enroute to the ICU. Its patency must be assured, and thus, portable suctioning equipment should accompany the patient. Assessing adequacy of perfusion includes continuous monitoring of heart rate and BP for the complex major surgical procedures. BP monitoring is carried out via an intraarterial catheter that is transduced to an oscilloscope machine for constant visual monitoring. The patient's perfusion may need to be supported with vasopressor drugs. These agents must be maintained for the transit phase and their infusion carefully calibrated with the use of battery-powered infusion pumps. In situations in which the child is taken from the operating room to the ICU and is not intubated, equipment for tracheal intubation should be available (i.e., endotracheal tube, laryngoscope, face mask, Ambu-bag with oxygen source, and medications that may be required to facilitate intubation).

Arrival in the Intensive Care Unit

On arrival in the ICU, the child is assessed for patency of airway, and adequacy of ventilation and perfusion. Mental status, heart rate, BP, respiratory rate, and temperature are recorded and oxygen administered according to the child's needs. Following attention to these immediate concerns, the anesthesiologist then provides a report of the anesthetic events to the nurses and physicians who will be directly attending to the child in the ICU, while directives from the surgical team regarding possible problems to be anticipated in the initial recovery phase are emphasized. The anesthesiologist informs the ICU team of the patient's medical history, the anesthetic procedure performed, the agents employed, antibiotics administered, analgesics given for postoperative pain control, any known allergies, the operative procedure, fluid replacement and fluid/blood loss, and any intraoperative complications that may have occurred. The ICU team must be familiar with possible problems that may occur in this recovery phase so that they may be anticipated and expeditiously treated.

Recovery Problems

Postoperative Pain

Control of pain in the early hours following surgery is crucial both from the point of view of the harm that pain may cause physically, as well as its emotional impact. Untreated pain exacerbates any emergence delirium that might occur. Pain may lead to tachycardia, hypertension, nausea, vomiting, and increasing anxiety in the child.[11–14] Also, pain may lead to hypertension and agitation, causing bleeding from the wounds. An assessment of pain should be made as to its severity and location. In preparing the child for surgery, according to the developmental age, the experience of anticipated pain postoperatively should be explained, with assurance that there will be efforts to control it. Explanation can go a long way toward reducing the feelings of helplessness and anxiety that the child may experience through fear of the unknown. In an effort to optimize pain control it should be remembered that **postoperative anxiety or agitation in the child may be due to underlying hypoxemia and/or underventilation** and may not necessarily reflect pain. In many cases, analgesia provided intraoperatively continues into the recovery phase. Another method of providing postoperative analgesia consists of local infiltration of the surgical wound with long-acting anesthetics, such as bupivacaine. Locally infiltrating with anesthetic (e.g., intercostal nerve blocks for pain from thoracotomy) and regional blocks and caudal and epidural analgesia may have been performed at either the beginning or the conclusion of surgery and used to assist in postoperative pain control. Caudal and epidural routes may be used on a single-injection basis, providing long-acting analgesia (e.g., bupivacaine,

for approximately 6–10 hours). In appropriate cases, an epidural catheter placed at the commencement of the surgical procedure or at its conclusion provides a route for the continuous administration of long-acting local analgesic agents.

For moderate and severe pain, IV opioids (e.g., morphine or fentanyl) are administered. These agents are most effective when given intravenously. The dose should be titrated to effect as a continuous IV infusion using a calibrated infusion pump. This method avoids the peaks and troughs of narcosis associated with intermittent doses. With opioid administration, the patient should be closely monitored for signs of possible overdose. For example, with an overdose of morphine, one might anticipate a depression in ventilation, and this is particularly liable to occur in the infant in the first 2 months of life, when the elimination half-life of the drug is much more prolonged than it is in the adult. If the patient is mechanically ventilated, one has more latitude with increasing doses of morphine or alternative opioids and analgesics. Any compromise in hepatic or renal function may prolong the effect of the opioid, and this must be taken into account in titrating the dose of the drugs. The tendency is for pain in children during the recovery phase to be undertreated rather than overtreated. This approach stems from the notion of the child experiencing pain less than the adult and also inappropriate fears of addiction from the use of opioids. With proper administration of these agents and vigilance by medical and nursing staff, one should be able to provide optimal pain relief without undesired complications. Should respiratory depression occur, however, it is essential that ventilation is immediately augmented. This is readily accomplished with a face mask-and-bag device with supplemental oxygen, and if necessary, opioid antagonists are administered, namely, naloxone (0.01–0.1 mg/kg).

The experience of pain is exaggerated by the fear of a frightening, unfamiliar environment (i.e., the PICU and large numbers of "strangers" descending on the child). The presence of parents and a familiar and favorite personal object belonging to the child can help make this phase of recovery more comforting and secure.

Anxiety and Agitation

Following surgery and emergence from anesthesia, the child may exhibit extreme restlessness and agitation. The child's behavior may reflect an emergent delirium from inhalational anesthesia that is compromised by the response to awakening from anesthesia in an unfamiliar environment. There appears to be a higher incidence of emergence delirium when enflurane is employed.[15] It is imperative, however, that one first investigates for serious signs of physiologic abnormality before concluding that the anxiety is based on the child's emotional reaction. Hypoxemia and hypercarbia secondary to airway obstruction or ventilation/perfusion imbalance may present with agitation in the child. Hypoxemia postoperatively may be due to the effects of the inhalational agents if inadequately reversed, and also to airway obstruction from secretions or from the tongue and soft palate partially or totally occluding the airway with the child supine and not yet fully recovered from anesthesia. In the anesthetized state, as with unconsciousness from other states, the muscle tone is depressed, and in the supine position, a clear airway may not be spontaneously maintained. Hypoxemia may be due to obstruction of the endotracheal tube from mucus or blood or misplacement of the endotracheal tube from its original intratracheal position, either proximally out of the airway or distally into a mainstream bronchus, leading to ventilation of only one lung. One should consider the site of the surgical procedure as a possible underlying cause of the problem. For example, if thoracic surgery is performed, postoperative hypoxemia may be due to the development of a tension pneumothorax. Other causes of anxiety and agitation may be hypotension leading to inadequate perfusion, which may be due to hypovolemia or depressed cardiac contractility. Metabolic disturbances, such as hypoglycemia and hyponatremia, and increased intracranial pressure may cause agitation in the child. In some cases, the effects of the drugs (e.g., ketamine) carry over into the recovery phase and can produce excitatory effects. Agitation and anxiety can also be due to untreated or undertreated pain. Not infrequently, the cause of the pain is remote from the major operative site and thus may be overlooked; the child may experience discomfort from a nasogastric tube, Foley catheter, or a chest tube.

Nausea and Vomiting

Nausea and vomiting are common problems in postoperative recovery from anesthesia. Generally, the nausea and vomiting are unpleasant experiences and recollections for the child and appear to be more common than in adult postoperative recovery. They can be life-threatening, however, if the airway is unprotected in the partially anesthetized child and pulmonary aspiration should occur. Thus, patients who are at potential risk for vomiting, if they are not intubated, should have their reflexes intact and be maintained in the lateral position to reduce the risk of aspiration. If there is concern about airway protection and the patient is not fully awake, it may be prudent to have the child remain intubated until the child's airway reflexes (i.e., ability to perform laryngeal closure and cough effectively) are intact once again.

The use of opioids such as morphine may be associated with an increased incidence of vomiting. The opioid stimulates the chemoreceptor trigger zone in the brain, leading to vomiting. This incidence may be reduced if continuous infusions are used, as lower doses of the agent are then required. Patients with a history of increased tendency to motion sickness are more liable to vomit. To control nausea and vomiting and the potential danger to young infants because of the loss of fluids and electrolytes, various agents have been employed with mixed success. Droperidol was found to be effective in doses of 75 to 100 μg/kg.[16,17] At these doses, no extrapyramidal reactions were noted. Other groups have reported the effectiveness of droperidol at much lower doses (10–30 μg/kg) and have documented higher incidences of extrapyramidal symptoms with higher doses.[18,19] Metoclopromide in a dose of 0.15 mg/kg may be effective in reducing gastric motility and controlling vomiting.[20] Ondansetron is a recently developed antiemetic that appears to be well tolerated in children (0.15 mg/kg IV) and not associated with cardiovascular compromise.[21,22] It has no sedative effect as compared with droperidol, which may produce prolonged sedation.[23]

Unresponsiveness or Delayed Emergence

Following the surgical procedure, the time of the child's awakening is anticipated based on the anesthetic procedure. Should the child not awaken at the anticipated time, however, there may be some underlying problem that requires investigation. In considering possible causes, it is necessary to address factors relating to the anesthetic procedure and its postoperative effects, the child's underlying medical/surgical condition prior to surgery, and complications arising out of the surgery performed. Conditions that are life-threatening need to be to considered first. Causes of unresponsiveness include (1) hypoxemia; (2) hypercarbia (CO_2 narcosis is a CNS depressant); (3) hypovolemia, leading to inadequate cerebral perfusion; (4) hypothermia; (5) residual anesthetic (inhalational, opioid, and sedative); (6) residual neuromuscular blockade; (7) increased intracranial pressure (e.g., due to an intracranial hemorrhage); (8) hypoglycemia; (9) electrolyte imbalance (hyponatremia); and (10) postictal state.

Respiratory Insufficiency

Respiratory insufficiency arising in the respiratory system is due to (1) airway obstruction, (2) apnea, and (3) respiratory failure. The child may present with anxiety and agitation, wheezing, stridor, tachypnea, retractions, apnea, tachycardia, bradycardia, hypertension, arrhythmias, seizures, or cardiac arrest.

Airway Obstruction

Upper airway obstruction may be the result of (1) posterior displacement of the tongue and soft palate and inability to cough up secretions as a result of depressed level of consciousness from residual anesthetic, (2) effects of edema or hemorrhage in the nasopharynx following a surgical procedure, (3) subglottic edema following tracheal intubation (i.e., postintubation croup, and (4) laryngospasm following the emergence from anesthesia. Postextubation laryngospasm may lead to serious hypoxemia if not relieved. Generally, the application of positive-pressure ventilation with oxygen via a face mask-and-bag device will relieve the laryngospasm and hypoxemia. Occasionally, the use of IV succinylcholine is required to break severe laryngospasm associated with oxygen desaturation that is unresponsive to positive pressure and face-mask bagging.

Intubation croup or subglottic edema has been associated with a number of factors, namely, traumatic intubation, too large an endotracheal tube, coughing on the tube, changes in the position of the patient during surgery, prolonged duration of intubation, and surgery performed on the head and neck. Children less than 4 years of age seem to be more susceptible to croup,[24] but it is very unusual postoperatively in the first few months of life.[25] Postintubation croup usually occurs within 30 to 60 minutes of extubation and is reflected in increasing inspiratory stridor and chest wall retractions. The airway obstruction may progress to the point of severely compromising the child and requiring urgent therapeutic maneuvers. Rigid bronchoscopy in some infants produces swelling of the subglottic area of the trachea.

The child may initially respond to the inhalation of racemic epinephrine (2.25% solution). Steroid administration (e.g., dexamethasone [0.3–0.5 mg/kg]) may be beneficial in reducing the edema. Its effect, however, may not be seen for a few hours. Occasionally, reintubation may be required. An alternative is continuous positive airway pressure via nasal prongs. This maneuver stabilizes the upper airway, preventing dynamic airway collapse associated with markedly increased intrathoracic airway pressures. Should reintubation be required, the endotracheal tube should be one size smaller in diameter than the one used in the first instance. With surgery of the nasopharynx and the neck, there is the potential for postoperative obstruction of the airway. In selected cases, it is appropriate to leave the nasotracheal or orotracheal tube in place until the child is fully awake and the danger period for airway obstruction has passed. If significant edema is anticipated, the endotracheal tube ensures a clear airway, should significant hemorrhage occur at the operative site. The child may require 24 to 48 hours postoperative intubation.

Apnea

Postoperative apnea is a potential problem in infants of low birth weight who are subsequently undergoing surgery. Infants who have a history of preterm delivery accompanied by episodes of recurrent apnea, which may or may not be associated with bradycardia, seem to revert to this behavior when stressed by anesthesia and surgery. These attacks are more common during the rapid eye movement (REM) phase of sleep. Apnea may be central, obstructive, or mixed in origin.[26] Maturation of the respiratory control of respiration in the infant is related to postconceptional age rather than to postnatal age.[27,28] Generally, preterm infants less than 46 weeks postconceptional age are at risk.[29] Postoperative apnea, however, has been demonstrated in preterm infants 55 weeks postconception, including those who do not have a history of preoperative sleep apnea.[30] A recent combined analysis study determined that apnea was strongly and inversely related to gestational age and postconceptional age. In addition, anemia was a significant risk factor.[31] Apnea spells may occur up to about 12 hours postoperatively, and thus the child should be monitored for this possibility for 12 to 24 hours following surgery.[30]

Postoperative sleep apnea in these preterm infants following surgery varies from minimal apneic spells requiring nothing more than stimulation to more severe spells requiring medical therapy in the form of theophylline or caffeine administration.[32,33] On rare occasions, the infant may not respond to medical therapy and will require mechanical ventilation. There are many other causes for apnea, and these must be excluded; these include hypothermia, metabolic imbalance such as hypoglycemia, drug effects from opioids such as morphine, and sepsis. Having excluded these possibilities, one can probably assume that the underlying cause is the child's immature respiratory control mechanism that has been reactivated under the stress of surgery and anesthesia.

Some children develop obstructive sleep apnea associated with upper airway obstruction from enlarged tonsils and adenoids. In addition, these children may develop pulmonary hypertension. Though the surgery should correct the underlying condition, one may still see evidence of chronic obstructive sleep apnea post-surgery and postanesthesia. Children with macroglossia or micrognathia (e.g., Pierré Robin, Treacher Collins syndromes) are at risk for upper airway obstruction.

Respiratory Failure

Respiratory failure may occur early in the postoperative period. This may be due to airway obstruction, pulmonary aspiration of gastric contents, pneumothorax, atelectasis, and hypoventilation due to the residual effects of anesthesia or neuromuscular blocking drugs. Signs of respiratory failure are evident in increased or weakening respiratory effort, lethargy, and effects on the cardiovascular system, leading to bradycardia, hypotension, and poor peripheral perfusion. The result is hypoxemia and acidosis, which further aggravates the child's cardiopulmonary status. The appearance of any of these signs of respiratory distress requires a full evaluation of the child, including a chest x-ray and blood gases to assess the severity of the respiratory compromise. A well-conceived plan to treat the underlying respiratory failure should be performed while assessing the underlying cause of the compromise. One should have a high index of suspicion for the development of respiratory failure in those children coming to surgery with existing compromise of their cardiopulmonary function; for example, the child

with kyphoscoliosis undergoing spinal surgery may readily develop respiratory failure, should the child not be able to adequately cough up secretions. Atelectasis rapidly develops, leading to hypoxemia, which can then progress to a life-threatening state. In addition, the use of opioids in these children should be titrated carefully to avoid precipitating respiratory failure. Careful preoperative evaluation of such children allows one to plan the postoperative care safely.

Inadequate Perfusion and Hypotension

Inadequate peripheral perfusion is the result of inadequate cardiac output to meet the child's metabolic needs. The most common cause in children of a reduced cardiac output is hypovolemia as a result of blood loss or inadequate correction of the child's hydration status. It is important to appreciate that hypotension is a late sign in children with hypovolemia. Children tend to compensate extremely well for intravascular volume deficits, and inadequate perfusion should be recognized before hypotension develops. If the child is hypotensive, at least 30 ml/kg of fluid infusion is required to correct the blood volume deficit. Hypotension may follow administration of opioids if the child is hypovolemic, and especially if placed in an orthostatic position. Large doses of opioids are well tolerated cardiovascularly, provided the child is euvolemic; note, however, that with large doses of opioids, respiratory depression is likely, and therefore ventilation will need to be assisted. In evaluating hypovolemic situations leading to hypoperfusion and possibly hypotension, one must also consider conditions that interfere with the venous return (e.g., tension pneumothorax, pericardial tamponade, and compression of the inferior vena cava). When poor perfusion is considered to be due primarily to inadequate myocardial contractility, administration of inotropic agents such as dopamine or dobutamine is recommended. Other causes of inadequate cardiac output are particularly seen in children undergoing repair of congenital heart disease defects.

Hypertension

Postoperative hypertension is seen less commonly. First, one must assess that measurements are not spurious (e.g., use of an inappropriately small BP cuff). Other factors that may lead to hypertension are hypervolemia, pain, distended bladder, hypercarbia, and drugs such as epinephrine and ketamine.

Tachycardia and Bradycardia

Should tachycardia occur, one must consider the underlying reason for the child to respond in this manner. Tachycardia reflects the body's attempt to compensate and maintain an adequate cardiac output in the presence of hypovolemia or heart failure, hypoxemia, hypercarbia, fever, response to reflex stimuli such as pain, or to drugs such as epinephrine and atropine.

Bradycardia in the recovery phase should make one suspect the possibility of underlying hypoxemia. It may be a vagal response to stimuli, such as passage of a nasogastric tube. Drugs may induce bradycardia (e.g., high doses of opioids [morphine and fentanyl]). Prostigmine (neostigmine), which is used to reverse the effects of nondepolarizing neuromuscular blocking agents, may also produce profound bradycardia, hence the need to administer atropine or glycopyrolate with it. In neurosurgical patients, the occurrence of bradycardia may reflect increased intracranial pressure and a warning sign that requires urgent intervention to relieve the increased pressure.

Body Temperature Alterations

The patient's body temperature should be recorded on the return to the ICU. Generally speaking, the child's temperature is restored to near normal prior to leaving the operating room environment, but in transport from the operating room to the ICU, the core temperature may drop and the child arrive in the ICU hypothermic. This may lead to serious decompensation, as the cold stress may adversely affect hemodynamic and respiratory stability. The younger the infant, the more vulnerable to cold stress.[34] The infant responds to cold stress through either shivering or nonshivering thermogenesis (oxidation of brown fat). The child may be compromised due to its inability to respond to the stress that increases the demand for oxygen delivery to the cell. Oxygen should be administered to assist the child with increased demand in oxygen consumption. Alternatively, heat stress may also compromise cardiopulmonary function. Although this is less likely to happen, the technology employed to provide a neutral thermal environment for the child may malfunction and cause overheating. Hyperthermia may be due to bacterial sepsis, dehydration, and pyrogenic reaction to the infusion of fluid and blood. Hyperthermia may reflect the development of the malignant hyperthermia syndrome.

Oliguria

Oliguria is defined as a urine output of less than 1 ml/kg/hr. Before assuming that the patient is truly oliguric, it is advisable to insert a Foley catheter to exclude urinary retention. Should a Foley catheter already be in place, its patency should be checked. Urine output is thus a valuable indicator of the adequacy of the cardiac output. Oliguria may be due to acute tubular necrosis, usually the result of preoperative or intraoperative renal ischemia. Oliguria may occur with intraoperative manipulation of the kidney or the aorta. In assessing the patient with oliguria, one must look for a possible cause of inadequate perfusion by assessing the state of the child's intravascular volume and cardiac contractility.

Seizures

The child may exhibit seizures in the recovery phase. There may be a history of seizure disorder, and inadequate anticonvulsant therapy may be at fault. One should consider hypoxemia or metabolic imbalance, such as hypoglycemia or hyponatremia, as a possible cause. It is essential that a clear and secure airway is established and adequate ventilation and oxygenation ensured while investigating the underlying cause.

Psychological Implications

The administration of a general anesthetic to the child places the child in a state of loss of control, which can destroy the basic trust necessary between the child and the caretaker.[35] With elective surgery, there should be an opportunity for explanation of what is to be anticipated, and this information will depend on the child's developmental age. Included in this explanation is the use of monitoring devices and possible pain and discomfort that may follow the surgical procedure. Pain control techniques, such as patient-controlled analgesia (PCA), are very effective in children, placing them in control while providing more effective manage-

ment of their pain. The younger the child, the more the psychosocial stress produced as a result of the surgical procedure. In this situation, increased contact and presence of family and the health care team is required in dealing with the psychosocial issues.

Recovery from the psychological trauma is more complex when the child has to undergo an emergency operation. In this situation, there is a sudden onset of a crisis in which time does not allow for adequate psychological preparation for the child. The parents are frequently separated from their child and often much less participatory in the process. They tend to assume a more complaint role with the physicians and nurses. The child waking up in the ICU may suddenly find an endotracheal tube, nasogastric tube, or Foley catheter in place. In addition, multiple invasive procedures in a frightening, alarm-sounding environment overwhelms the child, who feels utterly helpless. Under these conditions, it is difficult for physicians and nurses to engender the trust required for a nurturing doctor-patient relationship. However, every effort should be made to help the child cope as best as possible with this phase of management. Bringing the parents to the child's bedside as soon as it is feasible, and reassurance and gentleness in dealing with the child as treatment proceeds will assist the child at this difficult time.

References

1. Stoelting RK, Longnecker DE, Eger EI II. Minimum alveolar concentration in man on awakening from methoxyflurane, halothane, ether, and fluronene anesthesia: MAC awake. *Anesthesiology* 33:5, 1970.
2. Fisher DM et al. Comparison of enflurane, halothane, and isoflurane for diagnostic and therapeutic procedures in children with malignancies. *Anesthesiology* 63:647, 1985.
3. Gaumann DM, Mustaki J-P, Tassongi E. MAC-awake of isoflurane, enflurane and halothane evaluated by slow and fast alveolar washout. *Br J Anaesth* 68:81, 1992.
4. Ali HH, Kitz RJ. Evaluation of recovery from nondepolarizing neuromuscular block using a digital neuromuscular transmission analyzer—Preliminary report. *Anesth Analg* 52:740, 1973.
5. Laycock JRD et al. The potency of pancuronium at the adductor pollicis and diaphragm in infants and children. *Anesthesiology* 68:908, 1988.
6. Knill RL, Gelb AW. Ventilatory responses to hypoxia and hypercapnia during halothane sedation and anesthesia in man. *Anesthesiology* 49:244, 1978.
7. Jones JG, Sepsford DF, Wheatley RG. Post-operative hypoxemia, mechanisms and time course. *Anesthesia* 45:566, 1990.
8. Muller NL, Bryan AC. Chest wall mechanics and respiratory muscles in infants. *Pediatr Clin North Am* 26:503, 1979.
9. Keens TG et al. Developmental pattern of muscle fiber types in human ventilatory muscles. *J Appl Physiol* 44:909, 1978.
10. Lynn AM et al. Diaphragmatic paralysis after pediatric cardiac surgery: A retrospective analysis of 34 cases. *Crit Care Med* 11:280, 1983.
11. Anderson R, Krogh K. Pain as a major cause of post operative nausea. *Can Anaesth Soc J* 24:366, 1976.
12. Berde CB. Pediatric post operative pain management. *Pediatr Clin North Am* 36:921, 1989.
13. Kehlet H. Surgical stress: The role of pain and analgesia. *Br J Anaesth* 63:189, 1989.
14. Mitchell RWD, Smith G. Control of acute post operative pain. *Br J Anaesth* 63:147, 1989.
15. Steward DJ. A trial of enflurane for paediatric outpatient anaesthesia. *Can Anaesth Soc J* 24:603, 1977.
16. Abramowitz MD et al. Antiemetic effectiveness of intraoperatively administered droperidol in pediatric strabismic outpatient surgery. Preliminary report of a controlled study. *J Pediatr Ophthalmol Strabismus* 18:22, 1981.

17. Abramowitz MD et al. The antiemetic effect of droperidol following strabismus surgery in children. *Anesthesiology* 59:579, 1983.

18. Dupre LJ, Stieglita P. Extrapyramidal syndromes after premedication with droperidol in children. *Br J Anaesth* 52:831, 1980.

19. Patton CM. Rapid induction of acute dyskinesia by droperidol. *Anesthesiology* 43:126, 1975.

20. Ferrari LR, Donlon JV. Metoclopramide reduces the incidence and severity of vomiting after tonsillectomy in children. *Anesth Analg* 75:351, 1992.

21. Rose JB et al. Ondansetron reduces the incidence and severity of post strabismus repair vomiting in children. *Anesth Analg* 79:486, 1994.

22. Rose JB, McCloskey JJ. Rapid intravenous administration of ondansetron or metoclopramide is not associated with cardiovascular compromise in children. *Pediatr Anesthesia* 5:121, 1995.

23. Lin DM, Furst SR, Rodarte A. A double-blind comparison of metoclopramide and droperidol for prevention of emesis following strabismus surgery. *Anesthesiology* 76:357, 1992.

24. Koka BV et al. Post intubation croup in children. *Anesth Analg* 56:501, 1977.

25. DiCarlo JV, Sanders AI, Sweeney MF. Airway complications of endotracheal intubation in pediatric patients: Effect of endotracheal tube fit. *Anesthesiology* 69:A775, 1988.

26. Rigatto H. Apnea. In Thibeault DW, Gregory GA (eds). *Neonatal Pulmonary Care.* Norwalk, CT: Appleton-Century-Crofts, 1986. Pp 641–653.

27. Rigatto H, Brady JP, de La Torre Verduzco R. Chemoreceptor reflexes in preterm infants. I. The effect of gestational and postnatal age on the ventilatory response to inhalation of 100 percent and 15 percent oxygen. *Pediatrics* 55:604, 1975.

28. Thatch BT. Sleep apnea in infancy and childhood. *Med Clin North Am* 69:1289, 1985.

29. Liu LMP et al. Life-threatening apnea in infants recovering from anesthesia. *Anesthesiology* 59:506, 1983.

30. Kurth CD et al. Post operative apnea in preterm infants. *Anesthesiology* 66:483, 1987.

31. Coté CJ et al. Postoperative apnea in former preterm infants after inguinal herniorrhaphy. *Anesthesiology* 82:809, 1995.

32. Aranda JV, Trumen T. Methylxanthines in apnea of prematurity. *Clin Perinatol* 6:87, 1979.

33. Welborn LG et al. The use of caffeine in the control of post-anesthetic apnea in former premature infants. *Anesthesiology* 68:796, 1988.

34. Heim T. Homeothermy and its metabolic cost. In Davis JS, Dobbing J (eds): *Scientific Foundations of Paediatrics* (2nd ed). London: Heinemann, 1981. Pp 91–128.

35. Hersh SP. Psychological implications of operations in children. In Welch KJ et al. (eds): *Pediatric Surgery.* Chicago: Year Book, 1986. Pp 125–128.

Daniel P. Ryan

53 Management of Postoperative Patients

The invasion of the body by the hands of the surgeon sets in motion a number of events that lead to profound metabolic changes within the human organism. As a species, we have adapted many responses to trauma that have been recognized for many years but still remain somewhat mysterious in their etiology and interrelationships. The care of surgical patients in the early postoperative period has improved and changed a great deal in the recent past, along with the establishment of long-term "recovery rooms," now called intensive care units (ICUs). This chapter covers the physiologic responses to injury and surgery, along with their implications to the practical care of patients. In addition, aspects of nutrition and pain control are discussed. Finally, a few specific examples of postoperative patients are presented to highlight the special aspects of critical care related to the type of operation involved.

Pathophysiology

Much of the information concerning the human response to injury (including surgery) began to be accumulated in the early part of the twentieth century.[1] The pattern of response is always the same and can be separated into four somewhat distinct phases. The duration of each phase is dependent on many factors, including the type of injury, the presence of infection or other complications, the status of the patient prior to surgery, provision of nutritional support at critical times, and, finally, physical activity to help return the patient to full function. There is little information available on the specific differences between growing children and adults concerning these phases, but the general scheme of responses is the same.

From the moment of injury or the making of an incision, the body's neurohormonal environment is radically altered.[2,3] Pain, local inflammatory mediators, and tissue destruction initiate the acute changes of the "stress response." This is more than the catecholamine surge felt when faced with life-threatening danger and includes alterations of nearly all of the normal homeostatic mechanisms. The net result is a loss of body cell mass; sodium and fluid retention; "capillary leak" locally at the injury site and, to a lesser degree, systemically; metabolic shifts in energy supply; and often the onset of acute starvation. At the present time, the various effects of stress, trauma, hemorrhage, starvation, and sepsis have only been evaluated individually in the laboratory. Applying the laboratory findings may have little relevance to the clinical situation, however, because many of the factors coexist in the usual patient, and the patient has been influenced by the administration of intravenous (IV) fluids, electrolytes, glucose, and other medications, including pain medications, antibiotics, anesthetics, and so on. In spite of many types of intervention, we have not yet been able to alter the basic pattern of the response.

Acute-Phase Response

The initial injury causes the acute-phase response, a group of changes characterized by the appearance of new proteins in the blood. The response is thought to help limit the extent and magnitude of the injury and promote wound healing. The response is the same, regardless of the initiating event, and is seen in nearly all mammals.[4,5] The systemic changes include mobilization of amino acids from peripheral tissues to provide energy and substrate for hepatic protein synthesis, but a net nitrogen loss from the body results. The hepatic acute-phase proteins include fibrinogen, C-reactive protein, serum amyloid A protein, ceruloplasmin, haptoglobin, alpha-2-macroglobulin, alpha-1-glycoprotein, and complement components. Serum trace metals are altered as well. Zinc and iron levels are depressed, but copper is increased due to a higher level of ceruloplasmin.

Mediators of the Acute-Phase Response

Research has implicated a number of mediators that initiate and modulate the acute-phase response, including interleukin-1 (IL-1) and -6 (IL-6), tumor necrosis factor (TNF), colony stimulating factor, platelet-derived growth factor, interferon, and the lipid mediators of the prostaglandin system.[4–6] Macrophages that are activated at the site of injury or infection initiate the tissue response by releasing interleukins and TNF, and these factors in turn have a critical role in the overall response. The nervous system, with its endogenous opiates and modulation of catecholamine release and cortisol production, has a central role in the overall response.

Catecholamines

The interplay of the multiple mediators that have been described has not been fully solved.[4–7] The overall response is the net result of modulation in both a positive and negative manner simultaneously by many different agents. The earliest hormones involved are the catecholamines from the sympathetic nervous system. Epinephrine from the adrenal medulla and norepinephrine released from peripheral nerve terminals are responsible for the adrenergic receptor activation at the end tissues and organs. The cardiovascular system is a primary target and results in a modulation of vasomotor tone in the arterial resistance and venous capacitance vessels, along with chronotropic and inotropic changes in the heart. The net result is to conserve intravascular volume through (1) a reduction in renal blood flow from vasoconstriction, (2) activation of the renin-angiotensin-aldosterone system by beta-adrenergic release of renin from the juxtaglomerular apparatus, and (3) direct action on the brain to release arginine vasopressin. Perfusion of vital areas is augmented by the increased cardiac output caused by the direct action on the heart.

Along with the effects on the cardiovascular system, the catecholamines exert direct changes to the metabolism. These are primarily the result of beta-adrenergic activation of receptors. Hyperglycemia results from the net inhibition of insulin release and stimulation of glycogenolysis in tissues. Lipolysis and increases in plasma free fatty acids are also seen.

Adrenal Cortex

Cortisol and other glucocorticoids are essential to surviving surgical stress. The production and release of cortisol is the result of a series of interactions within the hypothalamic-pituitary-adrenal axis. Hypotension and shock release ACTH through the baroreceptor mechanism. Angiotensin II production and antidiuretic hormone secretion in response to hypovolemia stimulate ACTH release. Neurologic mechanisms are also involved because neural blockade and opioid analgesics can blunt the cortisol response to certain types of surgery.[8] Other modulators exist in the endogenous opioid peptides that inhibit both ACTH and corticotropin releasing factor (CRF) release and TNF, IL-1, and endotoxin, which increase ACTH release. The feedback mechanisms for the control of cortisol production are partially overridden in severe stress states.

Cortisol acts on tissues by controlling the rate of cellular protein synthesis,[2,9] acting predominantly in a regulatory fashion to either augment or suppress cellular processes mediated by other hormones or factors. Cortisol augments the sympathetic nervous system by stimulating increases in the synthesis of catecholamines and by increasing the number and sensitivity of adrenergic receptors. High levels of cortisol inhibit the production of beta-endorphin, countering vasodilation. Cortisol promotes catabolism through the induction of hepatic enzymes involved in gluconeogenesis and amino acid metabolism through facilitation of lipolysis and through its permissive effects on the metabolic actions of catecholamines and glucagon. The antiinflammatory properties of cortisol are related to its inhibitory effect on neutrophil lysosomal enzyme release, on phospholipase in the eicosanoid synthetic pathway, on the production of TNF, and on the production of IL-1.

Endogenous Opioid Peptides

In recent years, the role of endogenous opioid peptides within the brain and peripheral tissues has been investigated. The peptides act collectively at multiple opiate receptors. Three classes of opioid peptides have been described. The brain, hypothalamus, pituitary gland, and adrenal medulla are the major sites of synthesis and storage of the endogenous opioid peptides. The targets of the opioid's hormonal actions are not yet fully known; however, opioid receptors are present in the brain, spinal cord, and peripheral sites. The biologic actions of the endogenous opioid peptides include the modulation of behavior, inhibition of pain reception, and modulation of ventilatory drive, heart rate, vasomotor tone, temperature, metabolism, and immunity. Reports of the use of naloxone, an opiate antagonist, to reverse the hypotension of endotoxic shock[10] led to the investigation of the role of endorphins in the pathophysiology of shock.

The mechanisms that regulate the release of the endogenous opiates are similar and probably closely related to those involved in the regulation of the hypothalamic-pituitary-adrenal axis and the sympathetic nervous system.[11] Stress induces the release of both ACTH and beta-endorphin in the pituitary gland. Feedback inhibition of glucocorticoids inhibits CRF release and subsequent formation of proopimelanocortin.[12] Release of enkephalins from the adrenal medulla appears to be controlled by the sympathetic nervous system because enkephalins are released in conjunction with catecholamines.

It appears that the endogenous opiates are involved in the cardiovascular effects of hemorrhagic, septic, neurogenic, cardiogenic, and anaphylactic shock states. In addition, opiate receptor agonists diminish the stress response to surgical operations.[13] High levels of beta-endorphin have been found in models of hemorrhagic and endotoxic shock, human sepsis, and human surgical stress. The mechanisms involved with the effects of naloxone in shock states probably occur at several levels. The effects on the blood vessels are probably dependent on the presence of endogenous catecholamines. Cardiac actions of naloxone may occur through the prevention of the release of myocardial depressant factor. Unfortunately, the clinical use of naloxone to treat cardiovascular shock has not been shown to be of any significant benefit.[14,15]

Local Mediators
Prostaglandins

Local tissue trauma or the surgical wound contributes to the changes within the organism we recognize as the stress response. Tissue macrophages synthesize and release TNF, IL-1, and eicosanoids such as the leukotrienes. Local injury to the vascular endothelium and platelets within the wound release other eicosanoids, such as prostacyclin and thromboxane. The eicosanoids act locally and participate in a wide range of physiologic processes and act as mediators in inflammation, platelet function, fever, vascular smooth muscle contraction, and the immune system. The role of the eicosanoids in shock and trauma has been implicated but incompletely understood. They have important roles in the autoregulation of the regional microcirculation, renal function, and platelet-vascular interactions.[16] PGI_2 is a potent endogenous vasodilator and may be responsible for both the early and late falls in BP during endotoxin exposure. Thromboxane A_2 induces severe local vasoconstriction, increases pulmonary vascular resistance, and promotes platelet aggregation, leading to thrombogenesis. It also increases the permeability of both cellular and lysosomal membranes. The leukotrienes are potent vasoconstrictors, bronchoconstrictors, myocardial depressants, and chemotactic factors for leukocytes and macrophages.[17] The leukotrienes cause fluid leakage across the capillary endothelial membrane of virtually all vascular beds. PGE_2 has an inhibitory effect on cellular and humoral immunity and is involved in the mediation of fever and muscle catabolism.

The actions of the eicosanoids are not all deleterious to the host, and some actions are protective. The prostacyclins and prostaglandins of the E and F series counteract the thromboxane and noradrenergic-induced vasoconstriction.[16] They also counter intravascular thrombosis, stabilize membranes, possess end-organ cytoprotective effects, sensitize afferent nerve endings to mechanisms causing pain, and play an important role in the preservation of renal function in states of low perfusion.

Multiple factors regulate or initiate the synthesis of the eicosanoids. Hypoxia, ischemia, and acidosis all result in the production of eicosanoids. Complement components are potent stimulators for the release of prostacyclin and the thromboxanes.[18] Bradykinin initiates prostaglandin biosynthesis through the activation of complement and Hagemann factor. The effects of endotoxin, TNF, and IL-1 have indirectly been shown to occur through activation of the arachidonic acid synthetic pathway. Corticosteroids inhibit the production of all eicosanoids through multiple pathways, and substrate availability also appears to be an important factor in eicosanoid production. The clinical modulation of the eicosanoid pathway has not yet been found to be useful, but many areas of investigation are being followed.

Tumor Necrosis Factor

TNF is a polypeptide product of activated macrophages and has been found to be an important mediator in infection and inflammation. TNF has been implicated in the pathogenesis of septic shock and as part of the stress response in the hyperdynamic state seen following major surgery, trauma, burn injury, and tissue necrosis. The administration of endotoxin has been shown to result in a large increase in the circulating levels of TNF,[19] and the direct infusion of TNF reproduces most of the toxic effects of endotoxin, including hypotension, metabolic acidosis, hemoconcentration, pulmonary inflammation, ischemic and hemorrhagic necrosis of the GI tract, and acute tubular necrosis.[20,21]

TNF possesses multiple biologic actions that can account for many of the pathophysiologic conditions present in sepsis, various forms of shock, and the acute response to injury. TNF can exacerbate tissue injury, cause direct toxicity to the vascular endothelium, elaborate eicosanoids, and generate oxygen free radicals. TNF activates polymorphonuclear leukocytes and promotes the elaboration and potentiates the actions of other inflammatory mediators, such as IL-1. Systemic metabolic alterations may be a direct action of TNF-induced decreases in lipoprotein lipase activity and increases in plasma insulin, glucagon, epinephrine, and cortisol levels. The metabolic alterations leading to cachexia of chronic disease may be due to TNF.

Interleukin-1

IL-1 is another polypeptide produced by the mononuclear phagocyte system and acts as a primary mediator of the acute-phase response to infection and injury.[22] The biologic actions of IL-1 may also account for many of the physiologic changes observed during the stress response. Some of these responses, such as the activation of the immune system, induction of fever, and alteration of trace metal distribution, may have beneficial effects on host survival, whereas the precipitation of hypotension, intravascular coagulation, and excessive catabolism may be detrimental. IL-1 has direct effects on the CNS and induces fever at the level of the hypothalamus by activating phospholipases, resulting in increased levels of PGE_2. This finding partly explains the antipyretic activity of the cyclooxygenase inhibitors.

The hepatic production of acute-phase proteins such as C-reactive protein, fibrinogen, haptoglobin, and serum amyloid A protein is also mediated through the direct effects of IL-1 within the CNS. IL-1 also stimulates the secretion of prolactin, luteinizing hormone, thyrotropin releasing factor, and CRF. IL-1 is involved in protein catabolism by inducing proteolysis of skeletal muscle through the enhanced production of PGE_2, which activates lysosomal proteases.[23]

IL-1 production is influenced by cortisol similar to other components of the stress response. IL-1 increases ACTH and glucocorticoid production, and glucocorticoids inhibit monocyte production of IL-1. Production of IL-1 is enhanced along with TNF and other cytokines by the neuropeptide substance P and substance K, which are released in response to trauma and inflammation.[24] An amplification system appears to exist because circulating intermediaries in infection and inflammation, such as antigen-antibody complexes, complement components, lymphokines, TNF, and arachidonic acid metabolites, also promote IL-1 synthesis. The biologic actions have beneficial roles in the response to infection and sepsis. When the same effects occur as a result of noninfectious causes of inflammation and tissue injury, however, a deleterious situation may result, with profound hypotension, fever, or excessive catabolism.

Interleukin-6

IL-6 has multiple biologic functions.[25] One role seems to be mediating many of the hepatic aspects of the acute-phase response. It does not promote inflammation but in fact decreases TNF production. IL-6 causes an increase in the synthesis of the acute-phase proteins listed previously and a decrease in serum albumin. It acts with TNF and IL-1 to mediate many of the effects seen with either TNF or IL-1 infusions.[4,5,25,26]

Coagulation Factors

The initial life-saving response to injury is the activation of the blood clotting system to stop the loss of intravascular volume and provide the framework within the wound to begin the healing process. The elements involved with platelet activation, intrinsic

and extrinsic clotting cascades, and the cross-activation of the kinin system are beyond the scope of this chapter but are nonetheless important. The systems listed previously are turned on by tissue trauma and pain and are also activated by the events set into motion by the blood clotting systems. The fibrin matrix produced by the clotting blood is eventually removed and replaced by fibroblasts and collagen to heal the wound. The local activation of macrophages, polymorphonuclear leukocytes, and monocytes by the tissue trauma starts the release of the mediators essential to the healing process, which also have a systemic effect.

The Overall Clinical Response

The Acute Phase

Once the hemorrhage has stopped and if the organism has survived, a shift of body fluids from the extracellular space to the intravascular compartment follows rather quickly. The kidneys are influenced by hypovolemia, aldosterone, antidiuretic hormone, and atrial natriuretic factor to conserve intravascular volume by restricting sodium loss and increasing free water reabsorption. The systemic capillary endothelium becomes more permeable, as a result of the inflammatory mediators, to increase the flow of fluid from the extravascular to the intravascular space.

In the clinical situation, when the patient is receiving IV fluids for resuscitation, large volumes of crystalloid are needed to replace the lost intravascular volume.[27] Roughly three times the lost blood volume must be given as crystalloid to maintain the intravascular volume because of the capillary permeability described earlier. The total body edema that follows volume resuscitation of the surgical patient is a common finding. If systemic infection is present, the degree of capillary leak is exaggerated even further. Patients who have suffered major body burns exhibit the most extreme situation of total body edema formation following resuscitation, because the burn wound, even though it is a local injury, has affected the systemic capillary endothelium in the organism's attempt to replace the volume of fluid lost in the area of direct injury.

The effects of the initial injury on stimulating the body to conserve sodium and water persist for 24 to 72 hours, even if the patient's intravascular volume has been restored by IV blood or crystalloid. The clinical changes are seen with diminished urine output and minimal sodium excretion in the urine.[1,2] Free water is conserved more efficiently than sodium, and a mild dilutional hyponatremia is the result. Usually, between 24 and 72 hours after the injury or surgery, the capillary leak stops, and a diuresis usually begins shortly thereafter. The changes triggered in the metabolism of the body persist much longer.

At the time of injury or surgery, a period of acute starvation often begins. The secretion of large amounts of catecholamines, glucocorticoids, and glucagon, along with TNF, IL-1, IL-6, and other mediators, causes a systemic change in cellular fuel utilization. Hyperglycemia is the net result of the hormonal changes. High blood sugars are due to increased endogenous glucose production, high insulin levels, and insulin resistance of tissues. Fat stores are hydrolyzed as the primary energy source. Skeletal muscle proteins are broken down to provide amino acids for hepatic protein synthesis, and large amounts of alanine are supplied for gluconeogenesis.

The Catabolic Phase

The catabolic phase after surgery is also perhaps related to the immobility of the postoperative patient. Certainly, motion and muscular contractions are the best stimuli to replace the lost muscle mass in the recovery phase following injury, but postoperative pain, along with the real need for physical and psychological rest, inhibits mobility. Pain relief does not in itself prevent the systemic changes of the catabolic response.

The catabolic state persists until wounds are healed or sepsis has been drained and cured. An interesting aspect of the systemic protein breakdown is that wounds heal during this catabolic phase and develop full tensile strength even at a time when visible muscle wasting is present. The rare patient who develops a wound dehiscence almost never does so because of biologic tissue factors, and usually a technical problem or infection can be identified as the cause. A notable exception is seen in the patients on high-dose glucocorticoids for various reasons, because these agents directly affect the quality of healing.

Nutritional Considerations

Many attempts have been made to modify the metabolic response to injury.[28-30] The advent of total parenteral nutrition (TPN) has provided a means to give "high-quality" carbohydrate, lipid, and protein intake, even during periods of complete starvation following surgery.[31-34] The benefit of TPN in surgical patients has been difficult to measure, except in certain defined disease states, such as Crohn's disease, multiple intestinal fistulae, or inflammatory bowel disease when total bowel rest is necessary to quiet the intestine. In the pediatric population, the care of surgical infants has been greatly improved by the use of IV nutrition over the long term, but the catabolic phase is still present in spite of delivery of what would seem to be adequate substrates for the body.

The catabolic phase of injury persists for variable lengths of time, depending on the type of surgery, the presence of infection, and the ability to have a clean, closed wound. The patients at the extreme are those with large body surface burns who may not be able to have closed wounds for many weeks and have a tremendous metabolic effect of the burn wound itself. The calculated energy requirements of these patients have been carefully worked out from past experiences with large numbers of burn patients, and formulas have been published to calculate the metabolic needs by the size of the patients and the amount of body surface area burned.

Some of the problems produced by IV nutrition have been correlated with excess provision of the various components of the solutions, including overall calories. Investigators have been directly measuring resting energy expenditure and total energy expenditure in various patients and have found a very wide variation in energy needs, even among patients with isolated head injuries.[35] Interestingly, patients with isolated head injuries sometimes have the highest energy expenditure, probably related to a large amount of uncontrolled muscular contractions during posturing.[36] One must actually measure the energy requirements in a patient and tailor the nutrition, either enteral or parenteral, in a rational manner to the patient's needs. Commercially produced "metabolic carts" are available to perform the measurements in a systematic manner at the bedside.[37]

The most striking feature of the catabolic phase is the breakdown of skeletal muscle and the negative nitrogen balance produced. The loss of nitrogen continues for a variable time following surgery, usually less than a week in uncomplicated cases. The infusion of various, defined enteral or parenteral nutritional formulations has not been able to show a significant alteration in the loss of body protein mass.[38-40] The nitrogen loss can be slowed but not stopped

in the early period, although stores of body fat can be replenished with vigorous nutritional supplementation.[41]

The clinical effect of the use of TPN following surgery is difficult to quantify.[42-44] Considering the large costs and potential problems from its use, including acidosis, hyperglycemia, protein overload, fatty liver, metabolic complications, and so on,[45,46] one must rationally consider its use on an individual basis. In the routine postoperative surgical patients who will be able to resume an enteral diet in 3 to 7 days, the use of TPN has not been shown to have any significant effect in reducing morbidity or mortality. Even in adult patients who are severely malnourished or have sepsis following trauma or surgery, the benefits are not clear.[47-50]

In children, however, one must perhaps consider the potential benefits of providing the nutritional substrates needed to maintain growth.[51,52] The metabolic environment within the injured child will not permit these nutrients to be used until the acute catabolic phase of the illness has resolved, so this argument is not sound. In infants, who are growing rapidly one cannot argue with instituting aggressive nutritional support after the first 36 to 72 hours following surgery, when the acute injury phase should have resolved. The benefits in older children are questionable unless a prolonged period of starvation is anticipated. No studies have documented a clinical benefit of TPN when used for less than a week or so.

Recovery and Anabolic Phase

As the catabolic phase ends, the patients gradually "look better" and certainly feel better. They are more active and more interested in their surroundings and personal appearance. Metabolically, the nitrogen loss slows and stops. A gradual nitrogen gain is seen and usually continues after the patient is discharged. The elevated hormone levels return to normal, and the high metabolic rate of the catabolic phase returns to normal. During the anabolic phase, the muscle protein that has been lost is gradually replaced, and this is aided by active and passive mobility. The patients often say they are weak, tire out easily, and need more sleep than normal, often including an afternoon nap. The duration of the anabolic phase is related to the severity and duration of the catabolic phase and usually lasts 2 to 5 times longer. After the body's protein has been replenished, it is not unusual for patients to report that they have gained extra weight as fat. This occurs even in children and represents the excess intake of calories over their expenditure as exercise due to their diminished level of activity. The extra weight is usually lost easily when full activity is resumed.

Pain Management

All patients who have undergone surgery experience pain. This seems obvious, but it is often minimized by physicians and other health care workers.[53] The incision, retraction of muscles or skeletal elements, sutures, and the need for intravenous lines, urinary catheters, chest tubes, and endotracheal tubes are all sources of discomfort to various degrees. In addition, the altered states of consciousness caused by anesthesia and other drugs, and at times sensory deprivation or overload, contribute to anxiety that can magnify the perception of discomfort. The critical care unit is familiar to all of us, but it can be a very frightening place for a patient.

We would all agree that patients with pain should be relieved of it. The perception of pain and its degree of relief by various interventions often are markedly different to patient, nurse, and physician. The training of physicians and nurses has often led to the development of attitudes about pain control that have only recently been documented and challenged.[54,55] Many physicians have a tendency to minimize a patient's level of discomfort, and at times patients are reluctant to express their pain and ask for adequate relief for a number of reasons. The nursing personnel have the most intimate contact with a patient and at times are caught among their own perceptions, what the patient says and looks like, and the physicians orders for medications. In recent years, more realistic attitudes have developed, and education of patients, physicians, and others is improving.[53,56]

Even the most premature infant can perceive pain,[11,57] and all patients in the critical care setting experience multiple noxious stimuli during their routine care. The postoperative patients have incisional and posttraumatic pain as well. Many new techniques for pain management have been initially evaluated in adults and are now available for children. The decision about which medication, the route of administration, the dose, frequency, or alternative devices or techniques must be made in a rational manner and obviously tailored to the individual patient and situation. One must also consider the overall duration of the drugs used and consider changing to other agents to prevent withdrawal symptoms when appropriate.[58]

Opiate Analgesia

The most widely used potent analgesics are of the opiate class, and much has been learned about their function and receptors in the nervous system. The various forms available have different advantages and disadvantages for each, but one must remember that in doses that are equivalent in analgesic effect, all opiates produce similar degrees of respiratory depression, sedation, nausea, and constipation. The pharmacokinetics of the opiate drugs can be variable between infants, children, and adults.[54] A similar dose of morphine in infants below 1 month of age produces a higher serum level that is eliminated more slowly than in older infants or children. Fentanyl has a higher volume of distribution in infants, but its elimination half-life is very prolonged compared with children or adults. One must take into account these differences in the critical care setting and be aware of the use of these and similar agents by the anesthesia team in the operating room. For example, repeated doses of fentanyl for maintenance of analgesia during surgery may lead to accumulation of the drug and its respiratory depressant effects, or a very large single dose may have long-lasting effects because the blood level has not fallen below the threshold level required to start breathing.

Despite all of the potential problems with opiates, they continue to be relatively safe and effective. Systems for continuous infusion of morphine postoperatively[59–61] or for patient-controlled analgesia (PCA)[62] have been used safely and effectively for children. In the PCA system, a locked, preset infusion pump delivers a continuous "background level" of medication (e.g., morphine sulfate), and a signal can be delivered to the pump to deliver a preset bolus of the drug. The sophisticated pumps now available provide information about when and how many times a bolus was requested and correlate this with the patient's subjective reports of pain relief, allowing one to increase or decrease the infusion parameters. The acceptance of the medication is much increased, and yet the overall utilization is decreased compared with intermittent bolus injections. In children, anxiety about the needle and its pain can cause some to suffer in silence instead of requesting relief; the IV systems are more well tolerated. Utilizing analog "pain scales" to assess the level of discomfort can be very useful to monitor the effectiveness of the pain management.[63–65]

Newer Options for Pain Management

In the postoperative patient, many more options for pain relief have emerged in the past few years. Placement of an epidural catheter prior to an operation for intra- and early postoperative pain control has been very successful. Depending on the operative site, an epidural injection by the caudal route is helpful for lower abdominal, genitourinary, and rectal procedures. Injections of either a long-lasting anesthetic (e.g., bupivacaine) or opiates (e.g., morphine, fentanyl, or sufentanyl) have been successful.[66–70] The use of epidural infusions is not without problems or complications.[71] For thoracic or upper abdominal surgery, intercostal nerve blocks[72] or infusion of anesthetics through an intrapleural catheter[73,74] have been effective. Using combinations of these techniques is gaining in acceptance as well.[56] For a more detailed description of analgesics and sedatives, see Sedation and Pain Control, by Arnold and Berde, this volume.

Practical Considerations for Specific Surgery

Abdominal Surgery

Intraabdominal manipulations are usually followed by a large volume of fluid lost into the so-called third space. During extensive surgery, with the intestines exposed, fluid requirements are in the range of 5 to 8 ml/kg/hr in excess of maintenance requirements. Some of this loss is seen as edema of the bowel wall, mesentery, and sometimes the retroperitoneum at the end of a long operation. The excess fluid requirements continue for a variable period following the surgery and should be anticipated and added to the postoperative maintenance IV fluids. The body requires both extra sodium and water due to the changes set into motion by the surgical trauma, as explained previously, and the syndrome of **appropriate** ADH excretion. Depending on the amounts of fluid and sodium replaced in the operating room, the volume and type of fluid required postoperatively can be estimated. The response of the patient's vital signs, urine output, and urine osmolarity or specific gravity will reflect the accuracy of the initial estimation of requirements. A very close monitoring of these parameters is necessary to prevent under- or overhydration in the early period following surgery.

The fluid shifts set into motion by the surgery continue for varying lengths of time postoperatively but in an uncomplicated case usually slow and stop within 12 to 36 hours after the operation. Clinically, the change is seen as an increasing urine output and a lowering of the urine specific gravity. At this point in time, maintenance fluid volume can be resumed to prevent overhydration and electrolyte imbalance. In complicated situations, involving massive intraabdominal inflammation or sepsis, the volume of fluids required during the diuretic phase must often be restricted severely to allow the body to return to its preoperative "dry weight" and avoid prolonging the edematous phase. Attempts to promote edema mobilization with the use of diuretic medications can be dangerous and lead to intravascular dehydration in the presence of total body fluid overload.

If adequate fluid and sodium have been provided intraoperatively, a practical method to prevent hyponatremia and hypovolemia is to provide IV fluid containing twice the maintenance level of sodium at one and a half the maintenance rate (i.e., D5 + 1/2 NS + 20 KCl/liter at 1.5 × maintenance rate calculated by body mass or surface area). The urine output, vital signs, and urine specific gravity should be checked at least every 4 hours to be certain the initial estimate is close to the body's requirements. Providing the increased fluid volume without the higher level of sodium leads to hyponatremia that can rapidly approach dangerous levels and provoke seizures. The once-feared complication of postoperative renal failure has become nearly nonexistent in the pediatric population because the need for adequate hydration has been recognized.

In patients who will have extra ongoing losses from tubes and drains, the volume of these losses must be monitored carefully and appropriate replacement fluids added to the maintenance volume to prevent hypovolemia. The best method is to directly measure the electrolyte content of the losses, but usually this is not necessary. Pediatric patients usually do not produce the large volumes of acid from the stomach that are seen in adults, so a fluid with less chloride is used for replacement of these losses. Having the nursing staff measure the output every 4 or fewer hours and replace the loss over the next 4 hours will prevent nearly all cases of bad guessing concerning how much fluid will be lost. This method is reliable over the wide range of volumes that may be produced from a functioning nasogastric tube. In children, we use D5 + 1/2NS + 10 KCl/liter to approximate stomach losses. Biliary or small intestinal drainage is best replaced with Ringer's lactate. Protein losses from ascites, pleural fluid, and lymphatic leaks can be replaced with 5% albumin or a combination of Ringer's lactate and 25% albumin.

After nearly every extensive abdominal operation, a nasogastric or gastrostomy tube is maintained to keep the stomach empty and prevent gastric distention, vomiting, and possible aspiration. Acute gastric distention in children can mimic a severe intraabdominal catastrophe. Retching after an abdominal procedure produces unnecessary discomfort, and vomiting by the patient not fully free of the effects of anesthesia and analgesic medications could lead to aspiration. Most of the tubes found on the pediatric wards were designed for feeding and not for continuous aspiration of fluid and air from the stomach. The "sump" tubes have a second lumen to provide a continuous flow of air to keep the openings of the tube from sucking in the gastric mucosa. These tubes come in many sizes, ranging from 10 to 18 Fr. (Salem sump, Anderson 10–11, Replogle tube, etc.). The smaller-diameter tubes must also be matched to the patient's stomach size in relation to the length of tubing with holes in it. For example, a Salem sump may be available in 10-Fr. size, but the holes cover a distance of nearly 3 inches. Although the diameter may be appropriate for a toddler or an infant, if the tube is placed in an infant, the tip may be at the pylorus, and the upper holes, where the sump action is created, is in the lower esophagus, thus not effectively draining the stomach. The Replogle 10-Fr. tube has only about 1 inch of holes in it and is obviously a better design for infants.

Maintaining the function of the nasogastric tubes requires diligence by the nursing and physician staffs. The sump tubes are easily checked, because if air is constantly being sucked into the sump component of the tube, it usually is working. If it is not, the tube should be disconnected from the suction and a small volume of air or liquid injected to free the tube from the stomach lining. Also, a small volume of air can be injected into the sump component of the tube to be certain it is clear. If these measures are not successful, the tube may need to be repositioned or changed.

Enteral nutrition can be started as soon as the muscular bowel function returns, as evidenced by passage of flatus and stool. The presence of bowel sounds without functional passage of gas can at times be misleading, and starting oral feedings before the patient is really ready can lead to distention, vomiting, and a generally miserable feeling that may take a few extra days to resolve. If a nasogastric tube is present, the volume and character of the fluid changes with the onset of effective peristalsis, from the bilious green produced in an ileus or obstruction to the lighter, clear yellow fluid from the stomach and oral secretions. In patients who have had a prolonged ileus or an obstruction, many will have a few days of diarrhea after the bowel begins to function.

Most patients can resume enteral feedings within a few days of the surgery. IV hyperalimentation is probably vastly overutilized in routine patients. For the reasons mentioned earlier, the body cannot utilize the large load of calories and protein in the early catabolic phase of edema formation and wound healing. Most uncomplicated patients will be resuming enteral feedings within 2 to 7 days of the operation, and the risks and expense of IV hyperalimentation have not been justified by a lowering of the morbidity and mortality in previously healthy patients.[44,48] Even with the complicating features of sepsis and preexisting malnutrition in adults, studies have not shown a clear benefit of IV nutrition in the postoperative period.

Thoracic Surgery

Noncardiac chest operations are not common in the pediatric age group. Congenital malformations, tumors, and infectious problems requiring surgical treatment cover the entire age and size ranges, from premature infants to adults. Chest surgery is, as a whole, different from abdominal or extensive orthopedic surgery in that less tissue trauma is induced as a rule. Along with decreased tissue trauma, there is less systemic response in the forms of capillary leak and fluid losses. In addition, because of the increased risk of pulmonary complications with chest surgery, the primary goal in the perioperative period is to prevent any overhydration, which will further impair pulmonary function. Early extubation is usually associated with a good outcome because a patient's vigorous cough reflex is almost always better at clearing secretions than any suctioning could ever be. Also, normal negative-pressure ventilation provided by the diaphragm and chest wall is preferable to positive pressures from the ventilator to avoid trauma to the suture lines and the lung tissue. Avoiding direct trauma to airway suture lines with endotracheal tubes and suction catheters is another important reason for early extubation.

Nearly all patients who have undergone chest surgery will have some system of chest drainage to prevent fluid and air accumulation within the pleural space. The basics of the underwater seal drain and the closed suction systems deserve some mention. The commercially available drainage systems combine all of the features of the old "three-bottle suction" apparatus described in the historical texts. The tube draining from the patient is connected to the chamber, which will collect and provide some measurement of the volume of output. This chamber is connected to a "water seal" chamber, which prevents air and fluid from being siphoned into the chest. The level of fluid in this chamber and the presence of any air bubbles coming through it can indicate the presence of an air leak in the system or from the lung. The third chamber sets the level of suction by using a column of water 5 to 30 cm high to regulate the amount of vacuum applied to the drainage tube. The entire system is closed to the environment to prevent any outside contamination that could lead to ascending infection of the pleural space. The level of suction will be dictated by the type of surgery, the reason for the drainage tube, and the preferences and past experiences of the surgeon.

Usually, chest drains are not removed until after the patient is extubated and has exhibited the absence of a large fluid leak or any air leak from the drainage tube. As a general rule, one should never clamp a chest tube, because the accumulation of air or fluid could lead to a tension process within the chest, leading to cardiovascular collapse. The type of surgery will also dictate the reasons for and goals of the chest drainage system. Evacuation of air from the pleural cavity at the time of closing the chest incision may be all that is necessary in an uncomplicated procedure that does not produce the risk for air leak from the airway or pulmonary parenchyma. In contrast, multiple tubes may be necessary to evacuate hematoma, infection, persistent air leaks, and so on.

The goals of IV fluid administration following a chest operation should be to maintain the circulatory system without giving excess fluid, which may contribute to respiratory compromise. As a general rule, maintenance fluid volumes with extra sodium are usually adequate (i.e., D5 1/2 NS + 20 KCl/liter). If no concurrent abdominal surgery is done, often the patients can begin to eat the day after surgery and regulate their own intake. Early mobilization to the upright position, either walking or at least sitting in a chair, will help prevent many of the complications of chest operations. This is one area of care that has been improved greatly with the use of continuous epidural infusions and PCA.

Conclusion

This chapter covered much of what is known about the physiologic processes involved with surgery and injuries. The goals for the future are to develop biologic modifiers that can augment the normal responses to trauma and stress, while at the same time minimizing the deleterious effects on the patient. For example, preventing the capillary leak that accompanies all trauma and surgery, minimizing or preventing the catabolic phase, and rapidly entering the anabolic phase of recovery, while at the same time providing well-healed, strong wounds, early return of function of injured areas, and rapid recovery from the pain and psychological stresses, would be the ideal we should strive to attain. Until these goals are met, some practical management strategies are included, to be evaluated within the reader's own clinical experience.

References

1. Moore FD. Homeostasis: Bodily changes in trauma and surgery. In Sabiston DC (ed): *Textbooks of Surgery* (11th ed). Philadelphia: Saunders, 1977. Pp 27–64.
2. Metuid M, Moore FD. Homeostasis and nutrition in the surgical patient: The metabolic and endocrine response to injury. In Goldsmith HS (ed): *General Surgery*. Vol. 1. Philadelphia: Harper & World, 1981.
3. Cheung AT, Chernow B. The stress responses to critical illness. *Probl Anesth* 3:165–179, 1989.
4. Ott L et al. Cytokines and metabolic dysfunction after severe head injury. *J Neurotrauma* 11:447–472, 1994.
5. Gibran NS, Heimbach DM. Mediators in thermal injury. *Semin Nephrol* 13:344–358, 1993.
6. Pomposelli JJ, Flores EA, Bistrain BR. Role of biochemical mediators in clinical nutrition and surgical metabolism. *J PEN* 12:212–218, 1988.
7. Bessey PQ et al. Combined hormonal infusions stimulate the metabolic response to injury. *Ann Surg* 200:264–281, 1984.
8. Hull, CJ. Control of pain in the perioperative period. *Br Med J* 4:341–356, 1988.
9. Hensle TW, Askanazi J. Metabolism and nutrition in the perioperative period. *J Urol* 139:229–339, 1988.
10. Holaday JW, Faden AI. Naloxone reversal of endotoxin hypotension suggests role of endorphins in shock. *Nature* 275:450, 1978.
11. Anand KJS, Carr DB. The neuroanatomy, neuropsychology, and neurochemistry of pain, stress and analgesia in newborns and children. *Pediatr Clin North Am* 36:795–818, 1989.
12. Simantore R. Glucocorticoids inhibit endorphin synthesis by pituitary cells. *Nature* 270:618, 1977.
13. Carr DB, Murphy MT. Operation, anesthesia and the endorphin system. *Int Anesthesiol Clin* 26:199, 1988.
14. DeMaria A et al. Naloxone versus placebo in treatment of septic shock. *Lancet* 1:1363, 1985.
15. Groeger JS, Carlton GC, Howland WS. Naloxone in septic shock. *Crit Care Med* 11:650, 1983.
16. Oates JA et al. Clinical implications of prostaglandin and thromboxane A2 formation. *N Engl J Med* 319:689–761, 1988.
17. Lefer AM. Leukotrienes as mediators of ischemia and shock. *Biochem Pharmacol* 35:123, 1986.
18. Flohe L, Giertz H. Endotoxins, arachodonic acid and superoxide formation. *Rev Infect Dis* 9:S553, 1987.
19. Mitchie HR et al. Detection of circulating tumor necrosis factor after endotoxin administration. *N Engl J Med* 318:1481, 1988.
20. Tracey KJ et al. Shock and tissue injury induced by recombinant human cachectin. *Science* 234:470, 1986.
21. Lundsgaard-Hansen P, Blauhut B. Markers and mediators in enterogenic infectious-toxic shock. *Curr Stud Hematol Blood Transfus* 59:163–203, 1992.
22. DeClamp M, Demling R. Posttraumatic multisystem failure. *JAMA* 260:529, 1988.
23. Baracos V et al. Stimulation of muscle degradation and prostaglandin E-2 release by leucocyte pyrogen (Interleukin-1): A mechanism for the increased degradation of muscle proteins during fever. *N Engl J Med* 305:553, 1983.
24. Desodovsky H et al. Immunoregulatory feedback between interleukin-1 and glucocorticoid hormones. *Science* 8:652, 1986.
25. Ohzato H et al. Interleukin-6 as a new indicator of inflammatory status: Detection of serum levels of interleukin-6 and C-reactive protein after surgery. *Surgery* 111:201–209, 1992.
26. Murata A et al. Serum interleukin 6, C-reactive protein and pancreatic secretory trypsin inhibitor (PSTI) as acute phase reactants after major thoracoabdominal surgery. *Immunol Invest* 19:271–278, 1990.
27. Scheinksteel CD et al. Fluid management of shock in critically-ill patients. *Med J Aust* 150:508–517, 1989.
28. Warner BW, Sax HC, Fischer JE. Tailoring nutritional support for specific tissues and organs. *Curr Surg* 45:2–6, 1988.
29. Nordenstrom J, Persson E. Energy supply during total parenteral nutrition—How much and what source? *Anesthesiol Scand* 29:95–99, 1985.
30. Wernerman J, Vinnars E. The effect of trauma and surgery on intraorgan fluxes of amino acids in man. *Clin Sci* 73:129–133, 1987.
31. Shaw JHF, Wolfe RR. An integrated analysis of glucose, fat, and protein metabolism in severely traumatized patients. *Ann Surg* 209:63–72, 1989.
32. Brennan MF, Horowitz GD. Total parenteral nutrition in the surgical patients. *Adv Surg* 17:1–36, 1984.
33. Keller U et al. Protein-sparing therapy in the postoperative period. *World J Surg* 10:12–19, 1986.
34. Burns HJG. Nutritional support in the perioperative period. *Br Med Bull* 44:357–373, 1988.
35. Robertson CS, Grossman RG. Energy expenditure in the head-injured patient. *Crit Care Med* 13:336, 1985.
36. Clifton GL et al. The metabolic response to severe head injury. *J Neurosurg* 60:687–696, 1984.
37. Cortes V, Nelson LD. Errors in estimating energy expenditure in critically ill surgical patients. *Arch Surg* 124:287–290, 1989.
38. Oki JC, Cuddy PG. Branched-chain amino acid support of stressed patients. *Drug Intell Clin Pharm* 23:399–410, 1989.
39. Baker JP et al. Randomized trial of totally parenteral nutrition in

critically ill patients: Metabolic effects of varying glucose-lipid ratios as the energy source. *Gastroenterology* 87:53–59, 1984.

40. Askanazi J et al. Influence of totally parenteral nutrition on fuel utilization in injury and sepsis. *Ann Surg* 191:40–46, 1980.

41. Streat SJ, Beddoe AH, Hill GL. Aggressive nutritional support does not prevent protein loss despite fat gain in septic intensive care patients. *J Trauma* 27:262–266, 1987.

42. Detsky AS et al. Perioperative parenteral nutrition: Meta-analysis. *Ann Intern Med* 107:195–203, 1987.

43. Doinigi R et al. Nutritional assessment and severity of illness classification system: A critical review on their clinical relevance. *World J Surg* 10:2–11, 1986.

44. Dempsey DT, Mullen JL, Buzby GP. The link between nutritional status and clinical outcome: Can nutritional intervention modify it? *Am J Clin Nutr* 47:352–356, 1988.

45. Baker AL, Rosenberg EH. Hepatic complications of total parenteral nutrition. *Am J Med* 82:489–497, 1987.

46. Whitington PF. Cholestasis associated with total parenteral nutrition in infants. *Hepatology* 5:693–696, 1985.

47. Streat SJ, Hill GL. Nutritional support in the management of critically ill patients in surgical intensive care. *World J Surg* 11:194–201, 1987.

48. Buzby GP et al. A randomized clinical trial of total parenteral nutrition in malnourished surgical patients, the rationale and impact in previous clinical trials and pilot study on protocol design. *Am J Clin Nutr* 47:357–365, 1988.

49. Lowry SF, Thompson WA. Nutrient modification of inflammatory mediator production. *New Horiz* 2:164–174, 1994.

50. Grimble RF. Nutritional antioxidants and the modulation of inflammation: Theory and practice. *New Horiz* 2:175–185, 1994.

51. Cochrin EB, Phelps SJ, Helms RA. Parenteral nutrition in pediatric patients. *Clin Pharm* 7:351–366, 1988.

52. Greene HL et al. Guidelines for the use of vitamins, trace elements, calcium, magnesium, and phosphorus in infants and children receiving total parenteral nutrition: Report of the Subcommittee on Pediatric Parenteral Nutrient Requirements from the Committee on Clinical Practice Issues of the American Society for Clinical Nutrition. *Am J Clin Nutr* 48:1324–1342, 1988.

53. Majcher TA, Means LJ. Pain management in children. *Semin Pediatr Surg* 1:55–64, 1992.

54. Eland JM. Pharmacological management of acute and chronic pediatric pain. *Issues Compr Pediatr Nurs* 11:93–111, 1988.

55. Beyer JE, Levin CR. Issue and advancement in pain control in children. *Nurs Clin North Am* 22:661–676, 1987.

56. Altimier L et al. Postoperative pain management in preverbal children: The prescription and administration of analgesics with and without caudal analgesia. *J Pediatr Nurs* 9:226–232, 1994.

57. Anand KJS, Hickey PR. Pain and its effects in the human neonate and fetus. *N Engl J Med* 317:1321–1329, 1987.

58. Tobias JD, Schleien CL, Haun SE. Methadone as treatment for iatrogenic narcotic dependency in pediatric intensive care unit patients. *Crit Care Med* 18:1292–1293, 1990.

59. Beasely SW, Tibbals J. Apically and safety of continuous morphine infusion for postoperative analgesia in the paediatric surgical ward. *Aust NZ J Surg* 57:233–237, 1987.

60. McNicol R. Postoperative analgesia in children using continuous S.C. morphine. *Br J Anaesth* 71:752–756, 1993.

61. Pounder DR, Steward DJ. Postoperative analgesia: Opioid infusions in infants and children. *Can J Anaesth* 39:969–974, 1992.

62. Rogers BM et al. Patient control analgesia in pediatric surgery. *J Pediatr Surg* 23:259–262, 1988.

63. Broome ME, Lissis PP, Smith MC. Pain interventions with children: A meta-analysis of research. *J Nurs Res* 38:154–161, 1989.

64. Yaster M, Deshpande JK. Management of pediatric pain with opioid analgesics. *J Pediatr* 113:421–429, 1988.

65. Fitzgerald M, McIntosh N. Pain and analgesia in the newborn. *Arch Dis Child* 64:441–443, 1989.

66. Benlabed M et al. Analgesia and ventilatory response to CO_2 following epidural sufentanil in children. *Anesthesiology* 67:948–951, 1987.

67. Warner MA et al. The effect of age, epinephrine, and operative site on duration of caudal analgesia in pediatric patients. *Anesth Analg* 66:995–998, 1987.

68. Krane EJ et al. Caudal morphine for postoperative analgesia in children: A comparison with caudal bupivacaine and intravenous morphine. *Anesth Analg* 66:647–653, 1987.

69. Bosenberg AT et al. Thoracic epidural analgesia via caudal route in infants. *Anesthesiology* 69:265–269, 1988.

70. Payne KA, Moore SW. Subarachnoid microcatheter anesthesia in small children. *Reg Anesth* 19:237–242, 1994.

71. Wood CE et al. Complications of continuous epidural infusions of postoperative analgesia in children. *Can J Anaesth* 41:613–620, 1994.

72. Bunting P, McGeachie JF. Intercostal nerve blockade producing analgesia after appendectomy. *Br J Anaesthesiol* 61:169–172, 1988.

73. McIlvainey WB et al. Continuous infusion of bupivacaine via intraplueral catheter for analgesia after a thoracotomy in children. *Anesthesiology* 69:261–264, 1988.

74. Tobias JD et al. Postoperative analgesia following thoracotomy in children: Intrapleural catheters. *J Pediatr Surg* 28:1466–1470, 1993.

Susan E. Briggs

54 ◆ Burns and Smoke Inhalation

Burn injuries are a leading cause of accidental death in the pediatric population and the source of incalculable morbidity. Burns are the second most common cause of death in children from birth to age 4 years and the third leading cause of death in children ages 4 to 15 years. The average age of burned children is 32 months.

Flame burns account for approximately 13% of thermal injuries, and scald burns for 85% of pediatric burn injuries. Electrical and chemical injuries account for approximately 2% of burns. The most disturbing cause of burns that has dramatically increased over the past decade is child abuse. Children are frequently abused with cigarettes as well as a variety of hot implements (grills, radiators, curling irons, flat irons, matches). As with all other types of child abuse, the location and pattern of the burn, as well as the association of other social, psychological, and physical signs of child abuse, are useful guides to the diagnosis of accidental versus nonaccidental thermal injury. Immersion burns are characterized by symmetrical anatomic region involvement, as seen in the stocking/glove distribution pattern of burn injury in which both feet or hands are uniformly burned secondary to forceful immersion of a child in hot water. Most accidental minor scald burns are characterized by a scatter distribution of thermal injury, as opposed to a burn with sharply demarcated edges, because the child will attempt to escape the burning agent unless forcibly restrained. Genital and perineal burns are suspicious areas for child abuse because these are unusual areas for accidental injury unless the child falls in a bathtub![1]

Emergency Care of Thermal Injuries

The first priority in the care of the burn at the scene of the accident is to stop the burning process. It is important to remember that clothing, especially smoldering clothing or clothing soaked with chemicals, can be the source of continued burning of the patient's skin unless the clothes are promptly removed (Fig. 54-1).

In flame burns, the extent of injury is proportional to the intensity and size of the flame burn and the duration of exposure. Extinguishing the source of the flame burn promptly is the obvious first priority of treatment. Methods of accomplishing this goal are rolling of the patient on the ground, application of a blanket or coat, use of cool water or other extinguishing liquids, and the use of gelatinous-impregnated blankets. The gel penetrates hot and burning clothing and stops the burning process by transfer of heat from the skin to the blanket. Scald burns are usually self-limiting injuries. The degree of injury is proportional to the age of the patient, anatomical location of the burn, and temperature of the scalding agent. Viscous liquids such as grease and spaghetti sauce often need to be removed mechanically to stop the burning process. In very young patients with thin skin, scald burns often produce a **deep** thermal injury. In general, scald burns in individuals under 2 years of age will have a significant proportion of third-degree burn (Fig. 54-2).

Patients sustaining chemical burns should have clothing removed as quickly as possible to stop the continued injury due to absorbed chemical agents. Copious irrigation of the affected area with water, not neutralization of the offending agent, is the key to the emergency treatment of chemical burns. Following copious irrigation of the affected area with water, the burn should be covered with clean dry sheets. In chemical burns, the concentration of the agent and the duration of exposure are the key factors in determining the extent of thermal injury. Therefore, if the patient is hemodynamically stable, copious irrigation at the scene, rather than the emergency room of the hospital, is the initial key priority.

Electrical injuries require special consideration at the scene of the accident. In electrical injuries, it is important to stop the burning process by removing the patient from the source of electrical current. Caution must be utilized so that the rescue team does not become part of the electrical circuit while attempting to free

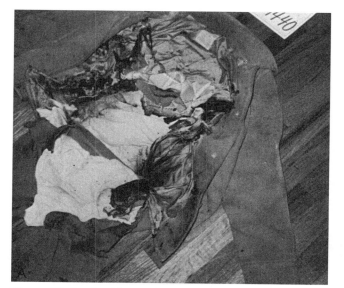

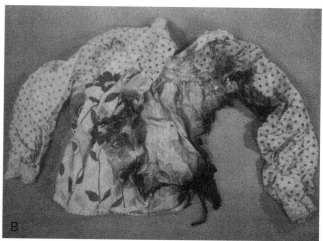

Figure 54-1. Smoldering clothes on child with thermal burns from a house fire.

Figure 54-2. Seventy percent total body surface area thermal burn in 2-month-old child suffering from scald burn.

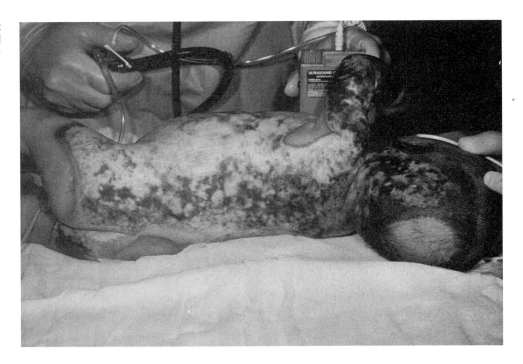

a person still in contact with a live wire. The victim must not be touched by the rescuers until the current source is either deactivated or pushed away from the patient by means of nonconducting materials such as wood.

It is important to remember that several types of injuries may occur in electrical accidents. Deep conductive electrical injuries involve extensive muscle injury, the extent of which may not be obvious at the scene. They may also involve remote areas of the body, such as the CNS and the thoracic and abdominal cavities. The presence of entrance and exit wounds should make one suspicious of deep conductive injury. Arc injuries produce limited, deep areas of coagulation damage, especially in flexion areas such as the axilla and groin. Surface thermal burns occur as a result of the flash ignition of clothing and must be treated as such with prompt stoppage of the burning process. Patients with electrical injuries often present with extensive total body surface area (TBSA) thermal burns. Associated injuries are quite common in patients with electrical burns, especially those who are thrown from the electrical source or fall from a high point. The patient must be evaluated for associated traumatic injury, especially cervical spine injury, long-bone fractures, and intrathoracic or intraabdominal injuries.[2-6]

Cooling of the thermal burn continues to be a controversial subject. Early cooling of small burns can be accomplished by application of cool water (20°C) or gelatinous-impregnated dressings to transfer heat from the wound into the dressings. Such dressings can be stored in areas where water is not readily available (e.g., airplanes). The dangers of hypothermia must be considered when cooling large burns, especially in the pediatric population. Ice packs or ice water must be used judiciously and only with small burns, as they may cause a cold injury more serious than the thermal burn or significant hypothermia with associated cardiac dysrhythmias. In general, cool solutions may reduce the pain of partial-thickness injuries with intact nerve endings but should be instituted with caution in burns greater than 20% TBSA or if the air temperature is below 50°F.

At the scene of the accident, the patient should be wrapped in clean, dry dressings. Sterile dressings are not necessary because the main goal of the dressings is to minimize contamination at the scene of the accident and to diminish the pain from exposure to the air, especially in partial-thickness burns. Application of topical agents should be avoided until the wound has been adequately debrided and evaluated as to further treatment. Oral fluids should not be given, because the patient may develop an ileus with burns greater than 15% TBSA.

The final priority at the scene is to establish whether the patient should be treated on an outpatient basis or referred to an appropriate facility for further evaluation or treatment. All burns greater than 10% to 15% of TBSA in children require fluid resuscitation and referral to a hospital facility, as do all inhalation injuries. Small burns affecting the hands, feet, face, perineum, and joint surfaces in which deep tissue involvement is suspected should also be treated as emergencies and referred to the hospital.

A brief history of the nature of the burn may prove extremely valuable in the management of the patient. Explosive burns or burns associated with motor vehicle accidents or falls should alert the physician to the possibility of associated internal injuries. A history of a fire in a closed space (e.g., a bedroom or a car with the windows up) should raise suspicion of inhalation injury. Patients with chemical and electrical burns should be sent to an appropriate facility, because damage is usually deeper than can be visualized.

Classification of Burns

Proper triage and treatment of thermal injuries require a knowledge of the pathophysiology of burn injury. Burns may be caused by heat from various sources, chemicals, electricity, and radiation. Extreme cold can also produce an injury similar to a burn. The following summarizes the major characteristics of each type of burn based on degree of skin involvement:

First degree
1. Characteristic: Cutaneous erythema
2. Pathology: Destruction of only epidermal layer of skin
3. Symptom: Pain

A first-degree burn involves only the epidermis and is characterized by cutaneous erythema and mild pain. Tissue damage is minimal, and protective functions of the skin, located in the dermis, remain intact. The chief symptom, pain, usually resolves in 48 to 72 hours. Common causes of first-degree burns are overexposure to sunlight and brief scalding by hot liquids.[2-4]

Second degree (partial thickness)
1. Characteristic: Vesicle (blister) formation (red or pink and moist)
2. Pathology: Destruction of epidermis and varying amount of dermis
3. Symptom: Painful

A second-degree burn involves injury to the entire epidermis and variable portions of the dermal layer. Vesicle (blister) formation is characteristic of second-degree burns. A superficial second-degree burn is extremely painful because large numbers of remaining viable nerve endings are exposed. Superficial second-degree burns heal in 7 to 14 days, owing to regeneration of epithelium by the epithelial cells that line the hair follicles, sweat glands, and other skin appendages deep in the dermis. A mid-level to deep second-degree burn heals spontaneously, but re-epithelialization is extremely slow. Pain is present but to a lesser degree than in more superficial burns because fewer intact nerve endings remain. Fluid losses and metabolic effects of deep dermal burns are essentially the same as those of third-degree burns.[2-4]

Third degree (full thickness)
1. Characteristic: White and dry skin (charred appearance)
2. Pathology: Total, irreversible destruction of all epithelial elements of the skin
3. Symptom: Anesthetic

A full-thickness or third-degree burn involves destruction of the entire epidermis and dermis, leaving no residual epidermal cells to repopulate. The wound will not epithelialize and can heal only by wound contraction or skin grafting.[2-4]

Resuscitation

The initial priorities in the management of the burned child are

1. establishment of an adequate airway and assessment of inhalation injury
2. calculation of burn size and initiation of fluid resuscitation
3. determination of need for escharotomy or fasciotomy

Airway Management and Assessment of Inhalation Injury

The first priority at the scene of the injury is the establishment of an adequate airway. Oxygen should be administered by face mask or endotracheal tube. Indications for intubation are the presence of massive facial swelling or inhalation injury (Fig. 54-3). Cutaneous burns of the face and neck in children may adversely affect the airway, even within a few hours. This is frequently seen

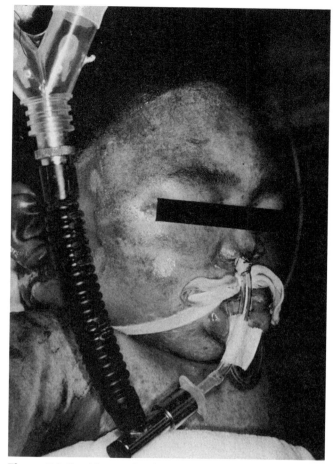

Figure 54-3. Massive facial swelling several hours after scald burn in 8-month-old child

with scald burns. Edema of the face and neck limits the victim's ability to move and open his mouth and may interfere with the clinical management of the airway. Edema of the upper airways is of concern in children because of the smaller dimension of their airways. Because resistance to flow is inversely proportional to the fourth power of the radius of the tube, decreasing the radius by half will increase resistance to flow 16 times. In an infant with a tracheal diameter of 4 mm, 1 mm of edema of the mucous membrane will increase the resistance to flow 16 times and decrease the cross-sectional area by 75%. A similar 1 mm of edema in an adult will increase resistance only 3 times and decrease the cross-sectional area by 44%.[6-8]

Pulmonary damage due to smoke inhalation and carbon monoxide intoxication is the leading cause of early death in burned children and is probably a more important determinant of survival at present than the actual size of the burn. Understanding of the distinct pathophysiology of the different types of inhalation injury has enabled the physician to better assess and treat such injuries. The hallmarks of smoke inhalation injury are hypoxia and hypercapnia. There are two distinct mechanisms of pulmonary injury following inhalation: (1) smoke toxicity and (2) carbon monoxide intoxication. Smoke toxicity is further divided into (1) direct thermal injury and (2) smoke poisoning. **Direct thermal injury** involves the inhalation of super-heated, incomplete products of combustion, such as soot and particulate matter, which cause direct mucosal damage to the tracheobronchial tree. **Smoke poisoning** results in the thermodegradation of the products of noxious gases (e.g., hydrogen cyanide). The effects of carbon monoxide intoxication are due to tissue hypoxia, and no pathologic changes are seen in the tracheobronchial tree. Carbon monoxide has a greater affinity for the hemoglobin molecule than oxygen and competes with oxygen for available hemoglobin binding sites. Increased carboxyhemoglobin levels are useful in evaluating the extent of carbon monoxide intoxication if the patient has not received oxygen during transport to the hospital. The half-life of carbon monoxide on the hemoglobin molecule is one half hour when 100% oxygen is breathed. Therefore, many patients with significant carbon monoxide intoxication on the way to the hospital will have normal carboxyhemoglobin levels if treated with oxygen.[6–8]

Clinical signs that should alert the physician to the presence of inhalation injury include

1. Upper body, especially facial burns
2. Singeing of the eyebrows and nasal hair
3. Soot in the oropharynx
4. History of impaired mentation and/or confinement in a burning environment (closed space)
5. Carbonaceous sputum (most reliable sign)

Survival from inhalation injury is dependent on the extent of pulmonary parenchymal damage. The physician's role is to prevent additional complications that further compromise the patient's pulmonary reserves. Prevention of aspiration, pulmonary edema, pneumonia and hypoxemia secondary to inadequate ventilation, mechanical ventilation, and aggressive use of bronchoscopy (flexible and rigid) to clear pulmonary secretions if needed are important adjuncts in the treatment of inhalation injuries.

Calculation of Burn Size and Initiation of Fluid Resuscitation

Calculation of the fluid requirement for resuscitation in the burned child is based on the extent of second- and third-degree burns only. First-degree burns do not involve the loss of body fluids. In children, the relative body surface area associated with the lower extremities is much less. The "rule of nines" is a useful and practical guide for determining the extent of the burn. The adult body configuration is such that anatomic regions represent 9% or a multiple of the total body surface. Tables 54-1 and 54-2 indicate the rule of nines in adults and the adjustments of percent of body surface in children according to age, respectively.[2–4]

Fluid resuscitation should be initiated with the administration of an isotonic electrolyte solution, such as lactated Ringer's (Table 54-3). The rate of fluid administration in children should be approximately 400 to 500 ml/m² of body surface area burned plus daily maintenance or a sufficient quantity of fluid to maintain the urine output at 1 ml/kg body weight/hr in infants and children. In older children, the standardized burn formulas, such as the modified Parkland formula of Table 54-3, may be utilized. The major problem with weight-related formulas is that surface area and weight relationships are not constant in the growing child.[9]

Immediately following the thermal injury, there is a rapid loss of volume from the vascular space and concomitant expansion of the interstitial space. This loss of fluid from the vascular space is rapid and maximal at 6 to 12 hours. This physiologic response is the basis of the administration of half of the calculated 24-hour fluid requirement the first 8 hours following thermal injury, one fourth the second 8 hours, and one fourth the third 8 hours. Twenty-four hours following the injury, fluid requirements decrease to a constant that remains as long as the burn wound is open. Continued controversy exists over the role of colloid replacement in acute thermal injury. Colloid is valuable, however, as an adjunct to fluid replacement in hypovolemic patients who do not respond adequately to crystalloid replacement.[2–8]

Determination of Need for Escharotomy and/or Fasciotomy

Full-thickness burns of the thorax and extremities, including digits, result in significant loss of tissue elasticity, with subsequent constriction of underlying structures. The most reliable method for

Table 54-1.   Rule of nines: Adults

Anatomic area	% body surface
Head	9
Anterior trunk	18
Posterior trunk	18
Right leg	18
Left leg	18
Perineum	1
Right arm	9
Left arm	9

Table 54-2.   Percent of body surface according to age

	Newborn (%)	3 yrs (%)	6 yrs (%)	12 + yrs (%)
Head	18	15	12	6%
Trunk	40	40	40	38
Arms	16	16	16	19
Legs	26	29	32	36

Table 54-3.   Fluid resuscitation after thermal injury during first 24 hours

Fluid	Amount	Rate	Urine output
Lactated Ringer's solution	4 ml/kg/% 2nd- and 3rd-degree burns plus maintenance	One half first 8 hr One fourth second 8 hr One fourth third 8 hr	1 ml/kg/hr (child)

measuring distal pulses in the burned extremity is with a Doppler ultrasonic flow meter. Escharotomies should be performed in the emergency room in all full-thickness circumferential burns of trunk and extremities, including the digits, regardless of the pulse status. Failure to relieve a constricting eschar of the thorax may result in life-threatening respiratory depression (Fig. 54-4). Failure to relieve a constricting eschar in the extremities may result in limb loss or permanent damage to underlying neurovascular structures. If escharotomy does not restore adequate circulation in the extremities, the possibility of compartment syndrome and need for fasciotomy should be considered.[6-8]

Secondary Priorities

Antibiotics

Prophylactic antibiotics have no proven role in pediatric burn patients and are not utilized routinely. All burns are potentially contaminated soft-tissue wounds. Tetanus toxoid (0.5 ml) should therefore be given to all burn victims. Prior immunization status is important information to obtain. Unimmunized individuals should receive 250 units of human tetanus immunoglobulin, as well as tetanus toxoid, and provisions should be made for additional tetanus boosters following discharge.[5]

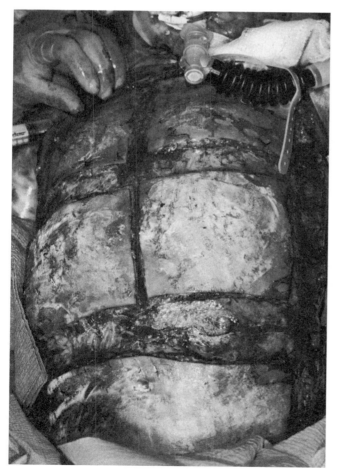

Figure 54.4. Child with 95% TBSA thermal burn requiring emergency chest escharotomies for relief of respiratory distress

Gastric Decompression

Most children with burns greater than 20% of TBSA develop a reflex paralytic ileus during the first 24 hours following thermal injury and require nasogastric tube decompression for varying periods.

Nutrition

Adequate nutrition is of utmost importance in the treatment of the burn wound because hypermetabolism, increased glucose flow, and severe protein and fat wasting are characteristic of the body's response to major trauma. Enteral feeding, either orally or via nasogastric feeding tube, is the preferred method of nutritional support if possible.

Prevention of Infection

Colonization of the nonviable and frequently necrotic burn wound eschar with bacteria and fungi presents a major risk for infection in all burned children. The sooner the burn wound is completely covered following excision of burn eschar, the less the risk of infectious complications, including death. Excision of all deep components of the burn wound, whether they be deep second-degree burns that will take more than a few weeks to heal or full-thickness third-degree burns, is the treatment of choice in all severely burned children. Early excision and grafting, as soon as the child is hemodynamically stable, remains the key to survival for children with major thermal injuries. Prior to definitive coverage of the burn wound, topical antimicrobial agents and biologic dressings are important adjuncts to treatment. The main advantages and disadvantages of current topical burn treatments are summarized in Table 54-4.

Biologic Dressings

The application of topical antimicrobial agents in all cases inhibits the rate of wound epithelialization and may cause increased metabolic rate and alterations in electrolyte concentrations. Thus, there has been a major effort to develop more effective biologic dressings to supplant the utilization of prophylactic topical antimicrobial agents.

Biologic dressings (pigskin, cadaver skin) are effective in providing temporary coverage of the burn wound when applied to fully debrided, relatively uncontaminated, burn wounds. Biologic dressings have been demonstrated to have the following advantages:

1. Adherence to wound surfaces
2. Reduction in wound colonization
3. Decrease in fluid and protein losses
4. Reduction in pain
5. Increase in rate of epithelialization over topical agents

Current uses of biologic dressings are (1) immediate coverage of second degree wounds; (2) coverage of granulating, excised wounds between autografting procedures; (3) test graft prior to autograft application, especially valuable in burned patients with limited donor sites; and (4) debridement of granulating wounds. Numerous nonbiologic synthetic substitutes, such as Biobrane and Opsite, have been developed for use in similar situations.

Table 54-4. The main advantages and disadvantages of current topical burn treatments

Silver nitrate 0.5% solution
  Antimicrobial spectrum
    Gram-positive bacteria
    Many gram-negative bacteria
  Disadvantages
    Hyponatremia (sodium leaching effect)
    Hypochloremia
    Methemoglobinemia

Mafenide (Sulfamelon)
  Antimicrobial spectrum
    Gram-positive bacteria
    Gram-negative bacteria
    Most anaerobes
  Disadvantages
    Carbonic anhydrase inhibition
    HCO_3 (urine) metabolic acidosis
    Pain on application
    Resistant organisms
    Skin allergy
  Major advantage
    Only topical agent that penetrates eschar

Silver Sulfadiazine (Silvadene)
  Antimicrobial spectrum
    Gram-positive bacteria
    Gram-negative bacteria
    Candida albicans
  Disadvantages
    Skin allergy
    Resistant organisms
    Leukopenia/thrombocytopenia (reversible)

Surgical Management of the Burn Wound

Two techniques of surgical excision, tangential excision and excision to fascia, are currently utilized in the treatment of burns. Sequential, layered, tangential excision to viable bleeding points, even to fat, is the preferred method of excision if possible and offers the best cosmetic results. Excision of burn wounds to fascia is a more rapid, technically easier, and less bloody technique and is particularly valuable in high-risk patients and in patients with thermal burns greater than 70% TBSA.

Skin Substitutes

The development of artificial skin substitutes and the use of cultured epidermal cells for coverage of the burn wound represent two methods under investigation that have the potential for providing early, permanent coverage of the burn wound, even in the severely burned child. These modalities, however, have limited applicability at this time.

Summary

Burns are a major cause of traumatic injury in children of all ages. Burns may be caused by a variety of scalding agents, chemicals, electricity, radiation, and child abuse. Regardless of the etiology of the burn, certain initial practices remain the same for all patients. The same general principles of resuscitation apply to burns as to other forms of traumatic injury. Cardiopulmonary stability must be the initial priority. Definitive care of the burn wound is a secondary priority.

References

1. Friedman S, Morse C. Child abuse: A five year follow-up of early case findings in the emergency department. *Pediatrics* 54:404, 1974.
2. Artz CP, Moncrief JA. *The Treatment of Burns.* Philadelphia: Saunders, 1969.
3. Boswick JA Jr (ed). *The Art and Science of Burn Care.* Rockville, MD: Aspen, 1987.
4. Heimbach DM, Engrav LH. *Surgical Management of the Burn Wound.* New York: Raven, 1984.
5. Kemble JVH, Lamb BE. *Practical Burn Management.* London: Hodder & Stoughton, 1987.
6. Richardson JD, Polk HC Jr, Flint LM. *Trauma: Clinical Care and Physiology.* Chicago: Year Book, 1987.
7. Dineen JJ, Moncure AC, Gross PL. *MGH Textbook of Emergency Medicine* (2nd ed). Baltimore: Williams & Wilkins, 1983.
8. Briggs SE. Rationale for acute surgical approach. In Martyn JAJ (ed): *Anesthesia and Critical Care of the Burned Patient.* New York: Grune & Stratton, 1989.
9. Briggs SE. Medical issues with child victims of family violence. In Ammerman RT, Herson M (eds): *Case Studies in Family Violence.* New York: Plenum, 1991.

John Ryan

55 Malignant Hyperthermia

The intensivist who is consulted regarding a malignant hyperthermia (MH) episode usually is confronted with a diagnostic dilemma in the operating or recovery room or is faced with the late management of MH in the intensive care unit (ICU). The proper diagnosis is paramount to appropriate therapy. An intraoperative unexpected febrile response requires a checklist of causative factors (Table 55-1).

Differential Diagnosis

In the operating room, the sudden onset of high fever can be attributed to many problems. Sepsis, neurologic injury, thyroid storm, metastatic carcinoid, or pheochromocytoma all can be associated with high fever.[1,2] At our institution, from 1974 to 1979, eight patients developed intraoperative temperatures above 108°F. These patients all had sepsis or prior neurologic trauma; the acid-base status remained normal in all of these cases. Thyroid storm has not been associated with severe acid-base abnormalities in the few anecdotal reports. Examination of the neck for thyroid nodules/enlargement may be helpful in the differential diagnosis of this entity. Muscle rigidity separates malignant hyperthermia from thyroid storm. In patients presenting with metastatic carcinoid or pheochromocytoma, the initial symptoms resemble MH, but marked cardiovascular instability persists after dantrolene therapy.[2]

The hallmark of a fulminant MH episode is hypermetabolism. Increased production of carbon dioxide and extraction of oxygen are easily detectable by capnography and a lowered oxygen saturation value despite adequate or increased ventilation and delivered oxygen concentration. In current practice, most MH episodes are aborted shortly after onset due to the anesthesiologist's early recognition that a hypermetabolic episode is present. Documentation of biochemical abnormalities with simultaneous arterial and central venous blood gas analysis is important, however, to verify the presumptive diagnosis. Creatine phosphokinase (CPK) levels are usually not elevated during the acute episode but only rise 12 to 24 hours later. Potassium levels, myoglobin determination, and thyroid studies can be useful in early aborted cases in determining the correct diagnosis.

Diagnosis

Because the first systemic effect of this syndrome is increased metabolism (increased oxygen consumption and carbon dioxide production), the cardiovascular and respiratory systems respond to this increased demand by increasing their output. Therefore, **the first clinically evident signs and symptoms of this syndrome are tachycardia and tachypnea** (Table 55-2). However, an increased end-tidal carbon dioxide ($ETCO_2$) value will precede these signs and symptoms.

The patient's response to surgery under "light" anesthesia is often tachycardia. In a healthy child of 7, however, an increase from 120 to 180 beats per minute (or an increase from 70–120 beats/min in an adult) is usually a sign of pathology; not all tachycardia or tachypnea is attributable to light anesthesia (Table 55-3). It is reasonable to deepen anesthesia, but it is also essential to immediately rule in or out other mechanical factors (endobronchial intubation, hypoventilation, circuit problem, etc.) that could cause tachycardia. If these prove normal and a brief trial of deepened anesthesia fails to slow the heart rate, a simultaneous central venous and arterial blood sample should determine the presence or absence of a hypermetabolic state. In this respect the $ETCO_2$ **monitor is particularly valuable. In hypermetabolic states, the expired carbon dioxide will be high, especially during MH.** In this condition, it becomes extremely difficult to bring the $ETCO_2$ level within the normal range, even with vigorous hyperventilation. Conversely, with airway obstruction the recorded carbon dioxide levels will be elevated; once the defect has been corrected, however, $ETCO_2$ will return rapidly to its normal value with mild-to-moderate hyperventilation.

MH can also present initially as ventricular ectopy in otherwise healthy patients; this is especially common during induction of anesthesia. If there is no airway instrumentation, hypercarbia, hypoxia, or some other stimulus to explain the arrhythmia, MH becomes suspect. Electrocardiographic investigation must also be carried out, as well as serial measurements of myoglobin and CPK levels. If the ECG is normal and the CPK and myoglobin are elevated, one can make a tentative diagnosis of MH.

Table 55-1. Unexpected febrile response during anesthesia

Diagnosis	Carbon dioxide level	Identifying factors
Sepsis	Normal	Shaking chill
Neurologic injury	Normal	CNS injury
Thyroid storm	Usually normal	Nonrigid physical examination and history
Metastatic carcinoid	Elevated	Cardiovascular instability
Pheochromocytoma	Elevated	Cardiovascular instability
Malignant hyperthermia	Elevated	Frequent rigidity, hyperkalemia
Myoglobinemia	Normal	Underlying muscle disease

Table 55-2. Signs and symptoms of malignant hyperthermia

Tachycardia

Arrhythmias

Tachypnea

Metabolic acidosis

Fever

Hyperkalemia

Cyanosis

Coagulopathy

Muscle rigidity

Myoglobinuria

Table 55-3. Presentation of malignant hyperthermia

Massive rigidity

Succinylcholine-induced muscle rigidity

Full blown in operating room

Intraoperative fever alone

Episodic fever

Neurolept malignant syndrome

Heat stroke

Central core disease

King-Denborough syndrome

Management of a Malignant Hyperthermia Episode

When a full-blown episode of MH is diagnosed, **immediate aggressive therapy** is indicated. Table 55-4 outlines the standard treatment regimen. The keystone of this approach is immediate treatment with dantrolene sodium. This drug has been shown to be effective at a dose of 2.5 mg/kg intravenous (IV) without major adverse side effects. If administered early during the episode, it reverses the biochemical changes of MH and decreases cellular metabolism.[3] If its administration is delayed for more than 24 hours, it still reverses some of the clinical signs but does not affect the mortality rate. Although dantrolene is the key to successful outcome, the other ancillary measures are also very important (see Table 55-4). Active cooling, treating the associated acidosis, and correcting the electrolyte imbalance can make the difference between a borderline or complete recovery.

Dantrolene has probably been responsible for the dramatic decrease in the mortality from MH since its IV use was introduced in the United States in 1979. The drug instructions recommend an initial dose of 1.0 mg/kg IV. A small number of patients, however, do not respond to this dosage level. Because no major side effects occur after a larger dose, the author strongly suggests an initial bolus dose of 2.5 to 3.0 mg/kg IV, followed 45 minutes later by a bolus dose of 10.0 mg/kg if **all** signs and symptoms of the syndrome have not resolved. The complete cessation of tachycardia, tachypnea, all muscle rigidity, decreased urinary output, altered consciousness, blood gas abnormalities, and electrolyte disturbances should be attained. If this does not occur with initial therapy, a repeated higher dose of dantrolene should be administered, or an alternate diagnosis for the problem should be sought.

Table 55-4. Standard treatment regimen

Stop anesthesia and surgery immediately.

Hyperventilate patient with 100% oxygen.

Administer dantrolene (Dantrium) 2.5 mg/kg IV and procainamide (up to 15 mg/kg IV slowly if required for arrhythmias) as soon as possible.

Initiate cooling.

Correct acidosis.

Secure monitoring lines: ECG, temperature, Foley catheter, arterial pressure, central venous pressure.

Maintain urine output.

Monitor patient until danger of subsequent episodes is past (48–72 hours).

Administer oral or IV dantrolene for 48 to 72 hours.

Two experiences exemplify the reasons for this recommendation. A 19-year-old patient who developed MH was treated with dantrolene at a dose of 1.0 mg/kg IV. Twelve hours postoperatively all signs of MH were absent, except tachycardia (180 beats/min) and marked hypertension (240/150 mm Hg) despite aggressive treatment with nitroprusside, nitroglycerin, and hydralazine. After IV dantrolene in a dose of 3.0 mg/kg, a brief improvement of the cardiovascular aberrations followed. Subsequent to 10.0 mg/kg of dantrolene IV given in a bolus injection, dramatic return of all parameters to normal values occurred.

The second patient developed a full-blown picture of MH and 20 hours later was still unconscious, with marked left gastrocnemius muscle rigidity. He was receiving 1.0 mg/kg of dantrolene IV every 8 hours as a maintenance dose to prevent recurrence of MH; 30 minutes following IV dantrolene in a dose of 10.0 mg/kg, the patient was awake and the muscle rigidity was relieved.

In my experience, the response to dantrolene takes 6 to 20 minutes. End-expired PCO_2 begins to decrease in about 6 minutes, and monitored arterial blood gas analysis will demonstrate significant restoration toward normal within 20 minutes. If not, intensive therapy should be pursued. Ten percent of MH patients following a full-blown episode redevelop the syndrome, so-called recrudescence. This usually occurs 4 to 8 hours after the initial episode and has been noted up to 36 hours after initial therapy. Characteristically, patients "smolder" along with modified symptoms of a continuing subclinical episode of MH.

Patients with recrudescence have died of a change in muscle cellular permeability.[4] Such patients require enormous volume infusions to maintain intravascular volume. Muscles immediately take up this volume and swell dramatically. The two patients described gained 24 kg in 18 hours, and 15 kg in 36 hours, respectively.

Once the initial episode has been successfully treated, patients traditionally have been given 1.0 mg/kg of dantrolene IV every 6 hours for 24 hours, or by mouth for an additional 48 to 72 hours. There are no data to substantiate the efficacy of this therapy.

Actions of Dantrolene

Dantrolene's action has been identified as being specific for skeletal muscles.[5,6] It does not affect neuromuscular transmission or have measurable effects on the electrically excitable surface membrane. It does, however, produce muscle weakness and may potentiate nondepolarizing neuromuscular blocking agents. Indirect evidence indicates that the site of action of dantrolene sodium is

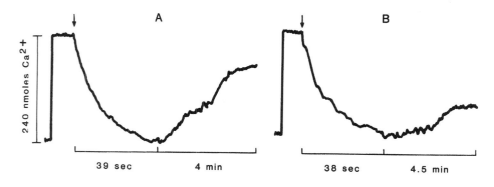

Figure 55-1. This dual spectrophotometric tracing captures the uptake and release of calcium into and from the sarcoplasmic reticulum. The tracing on the left was taken before the addition of dantrolene. The effect of dantrolene (tracing on the right) is to inhibit calcium release from the sarcoplasmic reticulum. (From WB Van Winkle. Calcium release from skeletal muscle sarcoplasmic reticulum: Site of action of dantrolene sodium? *Science* 193:1130–1131, 1976. With permission.)

within the muscle itself and is related to the caffeine-sensitive calcium stores. It is suggested that dantrolene sodium prevents the release of calcium from the sarcoplasmic reticulum or antagonizes calcium effects at the actin-myosin-troponin-tropomyosin level, or both (Fig. 55-1).[7,8] Such actions are proposed as explanations for the clinically observed skeletal muscle relaxant activity. Following are some unique properties of the drug.

1. At doses from 5 to 15 mg/kg IV it produces a significant degree of muscle relaxation.
2. In IV doses up to 15 mg/kg, it has no significant action on the cardiovascular system.
3. At IV doses up to 30 mg/kg, it does not depress respiration.
4. There is no indication of toxicity when the drug is administered intravenously on an acute basis.

Dantrolene normalizes all functions associated with muscle hypermetabolism in MH by reducing muscle rigidity and restoring normal muscle function. One important example is the rapid reduction in serum potassium, because potassium is restored to muscle cells. This helps normalize cardiac function. As cellular metabolism returns to aerobic processes and respiration normalizes, acid-base disorders are corrected. Thus, while dantrolene acts primarily on skeletal muscles, its beneficial effects are far reaching.

Incidence

MH (malignant hyperthermia, MH) is an acute, potentially fatal disorder in which skeletal muscles unexpectedly increase their metabolic rate, thereby increasing oxygen consumption above oxygen delivery, thus causing increased carbon dioxide and lactate production and greater heat production, respiratory and metabolic acidosis, muscle rigidity, sympathetic stimulation, and increased cellular permeability.

MH is a relatively rare disorder that is estimated to occur in 1 in 50,000 to 100,000 adult patients undergoing general anesthesia; in children, its incidence is reported to be 1 in 3,000 to 15,000.[9,10] This difference is more likely due to the retrospective nature of the studies and age at which most surgery is performed. MH occurs almost exclusively during or following an anesthetic procedure and is more frequently reported with halothane anesthesia, especially when succinylcholine has been utilized.[11] However, it can occur with other halogenated agents, and even in their absence.[12–14]

Although deaths from high fever were a known complication of general anesthesia, the initial descriptions of MH were not recognized as a separate entity until the syndrome was accurately characterized by Denborough and Lovell in 1960.[15] At that time, the mortality rate approached 90%. With increased awareness of the syndrome and improved symptomatic management, the mortality rate decreased to 60%. The major breakthrough in the management of this metabolic derangement, however, occurred in 1979 when the specific effectiveness of dantrolene sodium was recognized in the prevention and treatment of this syndrome.[3,16]

MH is an inherited metabolic defect best described as autosomal dominant, with reduced penetrance and variable expressivity.[17–20] Reduced penetrance implies that fewer offspring are affected than would be predicated by a totally dominant pattern. Variable expressivity implies differing susceptibility between families, with little variation within the same family. Not all patterns of inheritance fit this description, however, and consequently, it is proposed that MH is transmitted by more than one gene and more than one allele.[18–20]

Pathophysiology

Most of the investigative work on the pathophysiology of this syndrome has been performed on the pig. Swine breeders and veterinarians have long known that certain strains of pig, when exposed to stresses related to slaughter, accelerate their metabolism; the muscle from these pigs deteriorates into pale, soft, exudative pork.[21] Further observations led to the conclusion that porcine stress syndrome and MH are practically the same genetic disease.[22] Episodes of both syndromes demonstrate the same biochemical changes: fever, acidosis, cyanosis, mottling, rigidity of muscles and rhabdomyolysis, cardiac arrhythmias, and eventually shock. Consequently, some porcine pedigrees particularly susceptible to MH have been identified (e.g., Landrace, Pietrain, Poland China); these strains provide a model for the study of the human syndrome.[23] Much of our knowledge of the pathophysiology of this syndrome and the eventual identification of the specific treatment of MH are based on studies of this animal model.[24,25]

The etiologic defect responsible for MH has not been identified. Several hypotheses have been proposed. One relates to the calcium release channel of the terminal cisternae of the sarcoplasmic reticulum.[26] This channel is also termed *the ryanodine receptor* (named for the discoverer of a potent muscle toxin in the nineteenth century). Louis and Mickelson have found a greater affinity in vitro for ryanodine by human MH-susceptible sarcoplasmic reticulum than normal human sarcoplasmic reticulum.[27] This is attributed to a gene coding mutation for this calcium channel. Purification of the receptor by the same group demonstrates a similar increased affinity to ryanodine by the MH receptor in pigs.[28] Hogan et al. found human and pig receptor function to be similar.[29] This seemingly strengthens a common gene-specific etiology. Proteolytic digestion reveals a distinct difference in immunostaining of the peptides derived from the calcium release channel between MH and normal pigs. Other work demonstrates a greater sensitivity to caffeine of single calcium release channels of human MH patients compared with patients without MH (normals).[30] This mirrors the effect at the whole cell level because caffeine sensitivity has been a hallmark of MH susceptibility.

Human molecular genetic linkage studies have shown linkage between MH susceptibility and DNA markers on chromosome 19 in an area that is responsible for the activity of a hormone-sensitive lipase (Fig. 55-2); this has led to another etiologic hypothesis.[31,32] The hormone-sensitive lipase is an enzyme system that mobilizes free fatty acids (FFAs) from triglycerides. Skeletal muscle FFA metabolism is reported as abnormal in MH; the source of the elevated FFA appears to be triglycerides. The elevated FFAs are suggested as responsible for the increased calcium release and decreased sarcoplasmic reticulum calcium uptake.

The target organ in MH is skeletal muscle; the metabolic derangement is a disturbance of calcium flux from the sarcoplasmic reticulum membrane.[33–41] To understand the pathophysiologic changes that occur in skeletal muscles during an episode of MH, it is important to understand the basic physiologic changes that occur during normal contraction of skeletal muscle.[39] The nerve impulse through its action on the neuromuscular junction creates a chain of events that leads to depolarization of the muscle. The muscle action potential spreads on the surface of the muscle membrane from its center to its periphery. The action potential is transmitted to the interior of the muscle fiber by way of the T tubular system (Fig. 55-3). When it reaches the terminal sac of the sarcoplasmic reticulum, it causes a release of the calcium ion in the cytoplasm. Ionized calcium [Ca^{++}] can also be released from the sarcolemma and mitochondria. Ionized calcium bound to calmodulin initiates contraction by removing tropomyosin-troponin inhibition, which allows the actin filaments to slide across the myosin filaments, contracting the muscle fiber.[40] During relaxation, the calcium that was released during contraction is pumped back into the sarcoplasmic reticulum, sarcolemma, and the mitochondria. This restores the tropomyosin-troponin inhibition, allowing the actin and myosin filaments to separate, lengthening (relaxing) the muscle fiber. This process requires energy provided

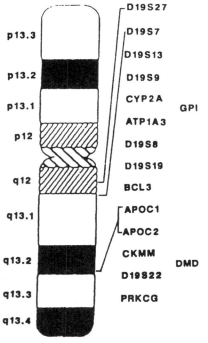

Figure 55-2. The location of MH susceptibility to DNA markers from 19q12-13.2 region of human chromosome 19, as reported by McCarthy et al.,[26] has a maximum likelihood of 450,000:1 favoring linkage of susceptibility to the cytochrome p450 (CYPZA) locus. The location of DNA marker for Duchenne muscular dystrophy is shown by (DMD). (Reprinted with permission from TV McCarthy et al. Localization of the malignant hyperthermia susceptibility locus to human chromosome 19q12-13.2. *Nature* 343:562–564, 1990. Copyright 1990, Macmillan Magazines Limited.)

Figure 55-3. The actin-myosin movement during calcium-stimulated muscle contraction. Biochemically, the relaxation phase is the energy-utilizing process, and contraction is a more passive event. It is the failure of lowering myoplasmic calcium, which occurs normally during the relaxation phase, that leads to the development of MH in a patient.

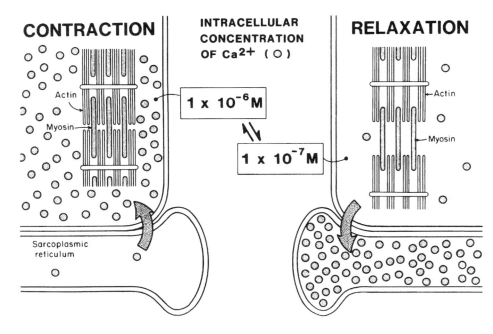

through the generation of adenosine triphosphate (ATP) within the mitochondria.

The pathogenesis of MH involves the uptake and storage of intracellular calcium. The main defect lies in the inability of the sarcoplasmic reticulum to store calcium. This is evidenced by an increase in myoplasmic free calcium.[34] At rest, the [Ca++] levels are 3 to 4 times normal. Triggering an MH episode increases the intracellular [Ca++] up to 17 times![38,41]

The elevated myoplasmic calcium level causes (1) activation of ATPase, thus accelerating the hydrolysis of ATP to adenosine diphosphate (ADP); (2) inhibition of troponin, thus permitting a biochemical contraction to occur; and (3) activation of phosphorylase kinase and glycogenolysis, with resulting production of ATP and heat. As the calcium levels further increase, calcium diffuses into a secondary storage site, the mitochondria. The [Ca++] infusion stimulates aerobic activity within this organelle as well as the sarcolemma. The ATP is rapidly diminished by this furious enzymatic activity; therefore, the supply of high energy bonds diminishes and the hypermetabolic muscles are unable to cope completely with the energy demands by means of aerobic metabolism. Consequently, the muscle resorts to anaerobic metabolism, and lactic acid accumulates. As a result of this, the metabolic rate is accelerated, causing a high rate of oxygen consumption and carbon dioxide production, as well as generation of heat. The normal circulatory response may allow heat dissipation early in this sequence, but soon, in an effort to supply the increased demands for oxygen to the muscles, peripheral vasoconstriction occurs, blood is shunted away from the skin, and the body temperature may rise dramatically.[42]

The venous blood will be markedly oxygen-desaturated because of the marked increase in the oxygen uptake of muscle cells and will have a high carbon dioxide concentration (respiratory acidosis). Due to the enhanced intracellular metabolism, lactic acidosis (metabolic acidosis) results when oxygen demands outstrip oxygen delivery. These factors have clinical importance because the earliest change in the fulminant hypermetabolic state will be mirrored on the venous side of the circulation as respiratory acidosis and markedly reduced venous oxygen values. It is therefore very helpful to obtain a central venous blood sample when seeking a diagnosis of possible MH; combined metabolic and respiratory acidosis with venous desaturation are consistent with a hypermetabolic state. ETCO₂ monitoring will serve a similar purpose and provide an early warning. Continuous measurement of ETCO₂ has enabled our pediatric anesthesia group to diagnose MH in two children.[43] The ETCO₂ is elevated prior to any clinically evident change in pulse or respirations.[44–48] The pulse oximeter may also be of value; unanticipated desaturation will occur at intermediate and lower inspired oxygen concentrations during anesthesia due to marked oxygen extraction. Both of these monitors are useful in the continued posttreatment monitoring of an MH episode.

In the ICU, placing the sensor tip of the ETCO₂ monitor 2 to 3 mm into a nares will produce a reliable trend monitor. Coupled with an oximeter, the ETCO₂ monitor represents a simple, dependable monitoring system for the post-MH episode patient.

The continued uncontrolled contraction of large groups of muscles may lead to the clinically observed muscle rigidity.[49–51] This most often occurs soon after administration of succinylcholine, but it may also be observed later. In the late stages of a full-blown MH episode, development of rigidity is attributable to the temperature rise within the muscle cell.[52] The actomyosin ATPase enzyme system ends skeletal muscle contraction. If there is an enzyme malfunction, continued contraction leads to rigidity. Our

laboratory has noted a relationship between the clinical "rigid" form of MH and the markedly lowered function of actomyosin ATPase. The presence or absence of rigidity may well be related to the level of free intracellular calcium. In animal studies, calcium concentrations that did not quite reach the threshold for muscle contraction (i.e., 1×10^6) did not result in rigidity, although the hypermetabolic aspects of the syndrome were present.[53]

Muscles are the main tissues involved in this syndrome; with a full-blown episode there may be massive swelling of the muscles, rhabdomyolysis, and clinically important leak of intracellular potassium and calcium outside the cells into the circulation. The rapid rise of potassium can result in arrhythmias that rapidly progress to cardiac arrest. However, the cardiac arrhythmias observed in this syndrome are nonspecific. Several factors contribute to their occurrence: hyperkalemia, fever, acidosis, hypoxemia, and autonomic hyperactivity. There is also the possibility that the syndrome directly affects cardiac muscle. Calcium channel blockers have produced fatal, evanescent rises in serum potassium in swine and are contraindicated in the therapy of MH.[54–56] With adequate treatment of MH with dantrolene, these electrolyte abnormalities reverse spontaneously.

If the patient survives, other complications may occur, including hemolysis, myoglobinemia, and myoglobinuria; the latter may lead to renal failure. Disseminated intravascular coagulopathy can occur; early dantrolene therapy may prevent this complication. The cause of death in this syndrome is variable and is temporally related. In the initial few hours, it is most probably due to ventricular fibrillation. Death several hours after the initial MH episode, or after a prolonged attempt at resuscitation, may be due to pulmonary edema, coagulopathy, or acid-base or electrolyte imbalance. Prior to the discovery that dantrolene was an effective treatment, recovery with supportive therapy was generally accompanied by a transient but sharp decrease in plasma potassium concentrations. This intracellular redistribution was attributed to a return of plasma pH toward normal. In the following 6 to 8 hours, a slow increase in plasma potassium usually occurred, which was extremely sensitive to IV potassium supplementation. If death occurred days after the episode, it was more likely a result of multiple organ failure, brain damage, or renal decompensation.[34]

It is interesting that the height of the fever associated with MH has no specific predictive effect on outcome.[57] The author's first MH patient had a temperature elevation greater than 43.8°C (110.8°F), with cardiac arrest and a plasma potassium level of 14.9 mmol/liter, all occurring within an 18-minute period.[58] Approximately 2 hours later, this patient was attempting to vocalize her desire to be extubated! In spite of this markedly elevated temperature, no brain damage ensued and she eventually made a complete recovery. This contrasts with the widely held view that brain damage inevitably occurs at these extreme temperature elevations.

Masseter Spasm

In the 1970s, masseter spasm following succinylcholine was recognized as a marker for the possible occurrence of MH.[59] If this tetany of the jaw muscles was appreciated by the anesthesiologist, the procedure, if elective, was usually immediately terminated. A strong correlation between succinylcholine-induced masseter spasm and MH has been described; in some patients, however, no cause was elicited.[60–62]

The inability to open the heavily sedated patient's mouth after the administration of succinylcholine is a subjective judgment. The patient can be slightly resistant or there can be active tetany.

Further succinylcholine administration does not result in paralysis of the masseter muscles. The other skeletal muscles of the body can be tetanic but more commonly respond with paralysis. The increased masseter muscle tension may last from a few minutes to half an hour. All patients can be ventilated with a face mask, despite the rigidity and the inability to open the mouth, because the chest wall is relaxed. Simple bag and mask ventilation will therefore sustain oxygenation until the masseter muscles relax.

The report that has upset this neat scenario was presented by Van der Spek et al. in 1988.[63] These authors found **routinely** increased tension in the muscles of mastication following IV administration of succinylcholine. At present, there is no physiologic explanation for this phenomenon. How can a depolarizing muscle relaxant that induces paralysis in all skeletal muscles produce increased tension in subsets of skeletal muscles at the same time? Is there an intracellular action of succinylcholine in the muscles of mastication and possibly the eye muscles that overrides the neuromuscular junctional effect of the drug? How should we now interpret masseter spasm or masseter tetany? Is it a normal phenomenon, a normal or abnormal variant, a developmental occurrence, or should we still consider increased tension as pathologic? At present, there are no definitive answers to these questions.

The relationship between succinylcholine-induced masseter spasm and a positive muscle biopsy (over half the patients studied have tested positive), however, needs to be carefully reexamined. The masseter muscles examined in one study have a predominant type I content.[64] Myoglobinemia after succinylcholine has been noted to be more frequent in childhood after halothane (40% incidence) than after thiopental (20% incidence).[65] Puberty lowers the frequency after both drugs to approximately 3%. Also, the two retrospective pediatric studies of masseter muscle rigidity following succinylcholine (as determined subjectively) was approximately 1% in patients induced with halothane; this incidence was 3% if strabismus was present.[60,66]

How should we respond to increased jaw tension after succinylcholine administration? A retrospective analysis of 68 patients recommends proceeding with the anesthetic as though the event had not occurred.[67] Previous studies recommend discontinuation of anesthesia.[60,62] Because we do not have the physiologic data to make a sound judgment based on scientific proof, caution is a

sensible refuge. After observing the patients for 15 to 20 minutes to be certain that the symptoms and signs of an MH episode do not occur, the anesthetic may be continued utilizing a nontriggering technique or halted and the surgery postponed. This decision should be made concurrently by the anesthesiologist, the surgeon, and the family. If any of the three parties is not confident with proceeding, the conservative approach (i.e., cancellation of surgery) seems appropriate. With any decision, the patient should be monitored carefully, remain in-house overnight, have a CPK level drawn at 12 and 24 hours postoperatively, have all urine samples tested for myoglobin in the first day, and have a formal neurologic examination with electromyography (EMG) to establish a baseline. The focus should be on determining the presence or absence of neuromuscular disease. As our knowledge increases, the management of patients with masseter spasm will become more rational. A recent study of three groups with varying jaw stiffness has been reported.[68] The exact relationship of physiology to this arbitrary categorization is not known.

Muscle Testing

The diagnosis of MH is primarily determined by the clinical responses. Once even a "weak" set of symptoms has been diagnosed as MH, the patient and the family are usually considered "positive" by all physicians thereafter. This may seem unjustified in some circumstances, and perhaps medically incorrect, but it is the reality of present-day medicine. It is interesting to note that in a population referred to us, 50% of family members of known MH-susceptible patients may themselves be susceptible to MH, which is consistent with the autosomal dominant mode of inheritance. This supports the need for caution when administering anesthesia to members of a family in which one person is susceptible. A metaanalysis of symptoms can give some direction regarding proclivity for susceptibility to MH, but no positive diagnosis from clinical criteria for family members is at present available.[69]

Muscle biopsy specimens have been utilized to determine the presence or absence of a consistent marker in muscle function associated with MH. One test that has gained acceptance by several laboratories is quantitation of the forces of muscle contracture following exposure of the muscle biopsy sample to halothane, caffeine, or both. If masseter spasm presents a physiologic conundrum, the present interpretation of diagnostic muscle testing is a maelstrom of confusion. In Europe, all testing follows a similar protocol.[70] Testing defined patients as positive (two tests positive), equivocal (one test positive), or negative. Approximately 15% of patients studied are "equivocal"; this diagnostic category has been questioned.[71] In North America, each laboratory and its own experience determine interpretive criteria for making the diagnosis of MH.

In an attempt to unify current methods of testing, Larach and Landis reported on 176 "normal" muscle biopsy specimens studied in 11 North American laboratories.[72] Utilizing a "common" definition of "normal," the incidence of a false-positive diagnosis in these 175 patients ranged from 10% to 70%, with a mean of 38%. This result does not examine the present unilateral criteria for diagnosis but demonstrates that standardization on this side of the Atlantic has a long way to go.

The basis for halothane, caffeine contracture testing (HCCT) is an "abnormal" response by freshly excised skeletal muscle to halothane and/or caffeine. The excised muscle is placed on stretch in a physiologic bath at 37°C. After optimal-length tension has been determined, halothane and/or caffeine are added to the bath,

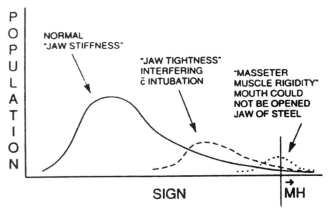

Figure 55-4. The spectrum of masseter muscle response to succinylcholine and the relationship to MH. (From R Hannallah, R Kaplan. Clinical assessment of jaw relaxation following halothane/succinylcholine in children. *Anesthesiology* 73:1189, 1992. With permission.)

the muscle is stimulated supramaximally, and the contracture amplitude is measured.[61,73] The resting membrane potential is critical in the response to caffeine.[74] A vigorous in vitro contracture of a skeletal muscle specimen to halothane, and a reduced contracture threshold to caffeine, can identify the donor as MH-susceptible (Fig. 55-5). The response to 2 mmol of caffeine and to less than 2% halothane were the only tests that unequivocally discriminated between susceptible and normal control subjects.[75] Simultaneous exposure to both halothane and caffeine, however, produces considerable overlap between normal and known MH-susceptible patients, indicating that the combined test is too sensitive (Fig. 55-6). This conclusion is controversial, depending on the laboratory involved. Any widely sensitive test to confirm an unequivocal

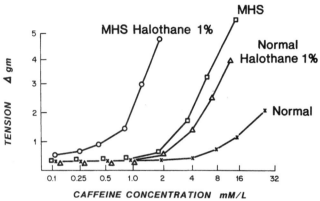

Figure 55-5. Idealized graph demonstration of the response of various classifications of patients to muscle testing by caffeine contracture. Clinically, there may be an overlap that clouds the diagnosis in an individual case.

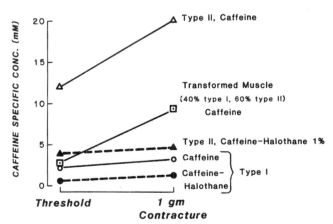

Figure 55-6. The effect of fiber type on caffeine contracture studies. Pure type I and II fever samples differ in their contracture response to caffeine and halothane-caffeine. Prolonged electrical stimulation causes type II fibers to become type I. After 3 months of low-grade stimulation, the transformed fiber content is 60/40%, as shown. The quantification of the muscle fiber type of each individual biopsy specimen is an important determinant in evaluating susceptibility to MH. (From BA Britt et al. Malignant hyperthermia: An investigation of five patients. *Can Anaesth Soc J* 20:432–467, 1973. With permission.)

diagnosis either positive or negative will have a gray zone. In MH, the problem is the clinically positive patient who tests unequivocally negative. This wide spectrum of MH susceptibility has been observed in both humans and pigs.[75] Therefore, most laboratories tend to take the conservative approach favoring the diagnosis on the positive side (false positive) because the consequences of a false-negative results are much more serious than for a false positive. It is better to treat the patient as if she is susceptible to MH, and avoid all triggering agents, than to assume the patient is negative and end with catastrophic complications. The need for immediate testing has been mitigated by the finding that cold preservation of muscle biopsy tissue for 24 hours does not affect the results.[76]

The Patient with Malignant Hyperthermia Susceptibility

Most of the time, MH occurs in situations in which it is least suspected. With a careful history, however, information can be obtained, indicating that one of the patient's relatives has had a complicated anesthetic history. There are also some disorders that have an inconstant association with MH.[77] These diseases include muscular dystrophies, and of these, the Duchenne type seems to be the one most commonly associated with MH.[33,78,79] Other associated diseases may include central core disease and neurolept malignant syndrome (see Table 55-3).[80–82] Neurolept malignant syndrome has not been described clinically in a patient who has experienced an episode of MH. Additionally, biopsy studies have presented conflicting results when attempting to relate these two syndromes.[83–86] Although patients with ptosis, squint, and skeletal deformities such as scoliosis or kyphosis have been suggested as possibly MH-susceptible, historical associations have not been successful. The reported literature and our own experience in history-taking demonstrate that the only helpful question in a medical history relates to previous difficulty or death in the family during anesthesia.[87,88] The presence of muscle cramps or an increase in muscle size with "weakness" out of proportion to apparent muscle size may also be suggestive signs and symptoms; in adults, intolerance to caffeine is often a distinctive symptom. A controlled study, however, found that a history of symptoms such as muscle cramps was similar for control and MH populations.[89] It has also been suggested that the sympathetic nervous system is abnormal in patients with MH; when utilizing norepinephrine turnover as an index of peripheral sympathetic nerve function, however, no difference was noted between age-matched controls and MH-susceptible patients.[90]

Several noninvasive tests can be performed to evaluate MH susceptibility, but none are conclusive. The most commonly used test is measurement of serum CPK, which is elevated even at rest in 60% to 70% of susceptible patients.[91] The usefulness of measuring CPK values in making the diagnosis of MH is predicated on the lack of other muscle disease that would explain the eleva-

Table 55-5. Signs and symptoms of continuing malignant hyperthermia episode

Continued hyperkalemia

Residual rigidity still present

Massive fluid requirements

Oliguria proceeding to anuria

tions; the diagnosis is also dependent on the peak CPK value. Elevation of CPK may be due to many factors and has proven useless as a screening test.[92,93] We have set an arbitrary level of tenfold increase in CPK as being diagnostic of MH in otherwise unexplainable situations. Although a useful measure if markedly elevated, a lack of CPK elevation does not exclude the diagnosis of MH. Levels of CPK above 20,000 IU in suspected patients who are biopsied have been uniformly associated with a positive diagnosis.

Another blood test that has been advocated for the detection of MH is the halothane-induced platelet ATP depletion test.[94] It appears satisfactory in the hands of the original authors but does not seem to be reproducible by other researchers.[95] A single study of calcium permeability in platelets and the effect of halothane did distinguish MH pigs from normals, utilizing a fluorescent calcium indicator dye.[96] Abnormalities in similar dye studies of pig lymphocytes and monocytes have been reported.[97,98] Conflicting data regarding the differing responses of MH porcine RBC and normals have also been published.[99,100]

Subsequent Anesthetics

Cunliffe et al. have reported that none of 1852 MH-susceptible patients developed MH when no pretreatment with dantrolene was administered.[101] The common practice is not to "routinely" use dantrolene preoperatively. This eliminates the muscle weakness and nausea frequently associated with pretreatment in adults.[102] If, however, a surgical procedure is planned in a known MH-susceptible patient, and pretreatment with dantrolene sodium is desired because of the severity of the previous episode of MH, or there is concern on the part of the patient or the anesthesiologist, dantrolene can be administered orally or intravenously.[103] The recommended oral dose is 4.8 mg/kg four times a day for 48 hours prior to anesthesia. A single IV dose of dantrolene (2.5 mg/kg) administered just prior to beginning anesthesia has been suggested as effective; this achieves a steady-state blood level of 3.6 μg/ml for approximately five and a half hours, then slowly declines.[8] Patients have been reported as "triggering" despite preoperative administration of oral or IV dantrolene.[14,104]

The IV dantrolene pretreatment does not produce any adverse cardiovascular effects and does not affect respiratory variables such as peak expiratory flow rate, vital capacity, $ETCO_2$, and respiratory rate. It is interesting that dantrolene at such doses causes peripheral muscle weakness, as evidenced by marked diminution of both twitch response and grip strength.[105] Fatigue is also a common problem for 24 to 48 hours. Consequently, common sense dictates that patients receiving dantrolene preoperatively or intraoperatively will require a smaller dose of muscle relaxant, and ambulation is preferably avoided in the first 24 hours and then performed cautiously for at least 48 hours. Such dantrolene doses in awake patients may cause dizziness or light-headedness; occasionally, nausea or difficulty in swallowing may occur during the first 24 hours of its administration.

Other measures are useful in avoiding the triggering of MH in susceptible patients.

1. Moderate to heavy premedication with tranquilizers. No phenothiazines, but barbiturates and opiates may be used, and in children, rectal methohexital is a good choice.[106]
2. A balanced anesthetic technique (nitrous oxide-oxygen, barbiturate, opioid, and any non-depolarizing muscle relaxant). Ketamine and propofol have not been reported as trigger drugs, but

desflurane and sevoflurane have been associated with the development of MH, as have all potent inhalation anesthetic drugs.[107–110]
3. Monitoring (the most important aspect of management) of all changes in heart rate should be carefully followed, and the use of an end-expired CO_2 analyzer, pulse oximeter, and a temperature monitor should be employed.
4. All local anesthetic drugs, whether amides or esters, may be used in MH-suspected or -susceptible patients.[111]
5. Immediate availability of dantrolene

Although caffeine induces contracture responses in vitro, it seems that these effects do not apply to related compounds, such as theophylline or aminophylline in vivo.[112]

The Family

Dealing with the family of the patient becomes a major challenge for the physician in the period after a possible MH episode. Most important, the family needs information and support. Frequently, the stunning effect of this complication will deter the anesthesiologist from close contact with the family, yet the psychological and legal consequences for both the family and physician of such inaction, even with a good outcome of the MH episode, can be catastrophic.[113] The intensivist can play a pivotal role in counseling family members.

The advent of genetic testing may replace muscle testing as the laboratory determinant of MH susceptibility. Until a uniform genetic test is available, it seems reasonable to document the episode by muscle biopsy at an appropriate interval after the event. It will then be necessary to determine which branch of the family is susceptible. Once these two goals have been accomplished, further testing within the family can be performed. A biopsy on other family members should be attempted only after informing them that the test is not a medical necessity—all anesthesiologists will treat the entire family as positive regardless of test results—but that this is a personal choice based on the need for peace of mind. Obtaining a muscle biopsy during incidental surgery in family members makes eminent sense. The only restriction is the withholding of dantrolene sodium and droperidol prior to excision of the muscle specimen. These two drugs have been shown to "normalize" abnormal responses of the muscle specimens in MH-susceptible individuals.[77,106]

A common practice in planning anesthesia for family members of a known MH family is to request muscle testing separately prior to the procedure. In most instances, because a balanced technique will be utilized whether the results are normal or positive, it seems easier and less expensive for the patient to have a muscle biopsy taken at the time of the planned elective operation. Obviously, the dantrolene will be available in the operating room, and the level of vigilance and awareness of the anesthesiologist will be at a peak for this patient, based on the family history.

The long-term relationship of the physician with the family of an MH survivor, continued education of the family, and easy accessibility to the physician by the family are important factors. The family needs literature; they need their questions answered. They need to know of the support group, the Malignant Hyperthermia Association of the United States. This organization maintains a hotline number (209/634-4917; ask for Index Zero), which is available 24 hours a day to physicians, for information during emergency situations and for follow-up advice and to MH families.

In summary, MH is a hypermetabolic event that can be triggered by anesthesia in genetically susceptible individuals. It has occurred in newborns and in the elderly.[114,115] With constant vigilance, it can be treated adequately with a successful outcome. If neglected, undiagnosed, or mistreated, however, MH can lead to disastrous consequences.

References

1. Bennett MH, Wainwright AP. Acute thyroid crisis on induction of anaesthesia. *Anaesthesia* 44:28–30, 1989.
2. Crowley KJ et al. Phaeochromocytoma—A presentation mimicking malignant hyperthermia. *Anaesthesia* 43:1031–1032, 1988.
3. Kolb ME, Horne ML, Martz R. Dantrolene in human malignant hyperthermia: A multicenter study. *Anesthesiology* 56:254–262, 1982.
4. Mathieu A et al. Recrudescence after survival of an initial episode of malignant hyperthermia. *Anesthesiology* 51:454–455, 1979.
5. Norwich Eaton Pharmaceuticals (Division of Norwich Eaton, Ltd). Dantrium Intravenous (Dantrolene Sodium Intravenous). Product monograph, 1979.
6. Dykes MHM. Evaluation of a muscle relaxant. Dantrolene sodium (Dantrium). *JAMA* 231:862–864, 1975.
7. Van Winkle WB. Calcium release from skeletal muscle sarcoplasmic reticulum: Site of action of dantrolene sodium? *Science* 193:1130–1131, 1976.
8. Flewellen EH et al. Dantrolene dose response in awake man. Implications for management of malignant hyperthermia. *Anesthesiology* 59:275–280, 1983.
9. Britt BA. Recent advances in malignant hyperthermia. *Anesth Analg* 51:841–849, 1972.
10. Relton JES, Britt BA, Steward DJ. Malignant hyperpyrexia. *Br J Anaesth* 45:269–275, 1973.
11. Britt BA, Kalow W. Malignant hyperthermia, a statistical review. *Can Anaesth Soc J* 17:293–315, 1970.
12. Pan TH, Wollack AR, DeMarco JA. Malignant hyperthermia associated with enflurane anesthesia. *Anesth Analg* 54:47–49, 1975.
13. Boheler J, Eger EI II. Isoflurane and malignant hyperthermia. *Anesth Analg* 61:712–713, 1982.
14. Fitzgibbons DC. Malignant hyperthermia following preoperative oral administration of dantrolene. *Anesthesiology* 54:73–75, 1981.
15. Denborough MA, Lovell RRH. Anaesthetic deaths in a family (letter). *Lancet* 2:45, 1960.
16. Harrison GG. Control of the malignant hyperpyrexic syndrome in MHS swine by dantrolene sodium. *Br J Anaesth* 47:62–65, 1975.
17. Britt BA, Locher WG, Kalow W. Hereditary aspects of malignant hyperthermia. *Can Anaesth Soc J* 16:89–98, 1969.
18. Kelstrup J et al. Malignant hyperthermia in a family: A clinical and serological investigation of 139 members. *Acta Anaesth Scand* 18:58–64, 1974.
19. Kalow W, Britt BA. Inheritance of malignant hyperthermia. In Gordon RA, Britt BA, Kalow W (eds): *International Symposium on Malignant Hyperthemia.* Springfield, IL: Charles C. Thomas, 1973. Pp. 67–76.
20. Ellis FR, Cain PA, Harriman DGF. Multifactorial inheritance of malignant hyperthermia susceptibility. In Aldrete JA, Britt BA (eds): *Second International Symposium on Malignant Hyperthermia.* New York: Grune & Stratton, 1978. Pp. 329–338.
21. Eikelenboom G, Minkema D. Prediction of pale, soft exudative muscle with a non-lethal test for the halothane-induced porcine malignant hyperthermia sundrome. *Neth J Vet Sci* 99:421–426, 1974.
22. Rutberg H et al. Metabolic changes in a case of malignant hyperthermia. *Dr J Anaesth* 55:461–467, 1983.
23. Berman MC, Kench JE. Biochemical features of malignant hyperthermia in Landrace pigs. In Gordon RA, Britt BA, Kalow W (eds): *International Symposium on Malignant Hyperthermia.* Springfield, IL: Charles C. Thomas, 1973. Pp 287–297.
24. Gronert GA, Milde JH, Theye RA. Dantrolene in procine malignant hyperthermia. *Anesthesiology* 44:488–495, 1976.
25. Gronert GA, Theye RA. Halothane-induced porcine malignant hyperthermia: Metabolic and hemodynamic changes. *Anesthesiology* 44:36–43, 1976.
26. McCarthy TV et al. Localization of the malignant hyperthermia susceptibility locus to human chromosome 19q12–13.2 *Nature* 343:562–564, 1990.
27. Louis CF, Mickelson JR. Properties of the abnormal sarcoplasmic reticulum calcium release channel of malignant hyperthermia susceptible (MHS) pigs. *J Neurol Sci* 98:507, 1990.
28. Mickelson JR, Litterer LA, Louis CF. Isolation and reconstitution of the ryanodine receptor (RyR) from malignant hyperthermia susceptible (MHS) and normal pigs. *J Neurol Sci* 98:508, 1990.
29. Hogan K, Valdivia HH, Coronado R. Ryanodine receptors of human, rabbit and pig skeletal muscle: Differential sensitivity to calcium and halothane. *J Neurol Sci* 98:137, 1990.
30. Nelson TE, Fill M, Stefani E. Malignant hyperthermia: Single Ca^{2+} release channels in human SR membranes isolated from biopsied skeletal muscle. *J Neurol Sci* 98:507, 1990.
31. McCarthy TV et al. Mapping of the gene for malignant hyperthermia susceptibility to human chromosome 19q12-13.2. *J Neurol Sci* 98:512, 1990.
32. Fletcher JE et al. Defects attributed to the Ca^{2+} release channel protein (CRCP) in malignant hyperthermia (MH) are consequences of elevated free fatty acids (FFAs) and breed differences. *J Neurol Sci* 98:508, 1990.
33. Gronert GA. Malignant hyperthermia. *Anesthesiology* 53:395–423, 1980.
34. Britt BA. Etiology and pathophysiology of malignant hyperthermia. *Fed Proc* 38:44–48, 1979.
35. Jardon OM. Physiologic stress, heat stroke, malignant hyperthermia: A perspective. *Milit Med* 147:8–14, 1982.
36. Britt BA, Kwong FHG, Endreyni L. The clinical and laboratory features of malignant hyperthermia management—A review. In Henschel EO (ed): *Malignant Hyperthermia, Current Concepts.* New York: Appleton-Century-Crofts, 1977. Pp 63–77.
37. Ohnishi ST, Taylor S, Gronert GA. Calcium-induced Ca^{2+} release from sarcoplasmic reticulum of pigs susceptible to malignant hyperthermia. *FEBS Lett* 161:103–107, 1983.
38. Lopez JR et al. Intracellular ionized calcium concentration in muscles from humans with malignant hyperthermia. *Muscle Nerve* 8:355–358, 1985.
39. Karamanian A. Muscle physiology. In Goudsouzian N, Karamanian A (eds): *Physiology for the Anesthesiologist.* Norwalk, CT: Appleton-Century-Crofts, 1984. Pp 287–299.
40. Tregear RT, Marston SB. The crossbridge theory. *Annu Rev Physiol* 41:723–736, 1979.
41. Kim DH, Sreter FA, Ohnishi ST. Kinetic studies of Ca^{2+} release from sarcoplasmic reticulum of normal and malignant hyperthermia susceptible pig muscles. *Biochim Biophys Acta* 775:320–327, 1984.
42. Muhrer ME et al. Vasoconstriction and porcine hyperpyrexia. *Science* 39:993, 1984.
43. Baudendistel I et al. End-tidal CO_2 monitoring: Its use in the diagnosis and management of malignant hyperthermia. *Anaesthesia* 39:1000–1003, 1984.
44. Lucke JN, Hall GM, Lister D. Porcine malignant hyperthermia. I: Metabolic and physiological changes. *Br J Anaesth* 48:297–304, 1976.
45. Liebenschutz F, Mai C, Pickerodt VWA. Increased carbon dioxide production in two patients with malignant hyperexia and its control by dantrolene. *Br J Anaesth* 51:899–903, 1979.
46. Rutberg H et al. Metabolic changes in a case of malignant hyperthermia. *Br J Anaesth* 55:461–467, 1983.
47. Triner L, Sherman J. Potential value of expiratory carbon dioxide measurement in patients considered to be susceptible to malignant hyperthermia. *Anesthesiology* 55:482, 1981.
48. Dunn CM, Maltry DE, Eggers GWN Jr. Value of mass spectrometry in early diagnosis of malignant hyperthermia. *Anesthesiology* 63:333, 1985.
49. Cody JR. Muscle rigidity following administration of succinylcholine. *Anesthesiology* 29:159–162, 1968.

50. Paterson IS. Generalized myotonia following suxamethonium. *Br J Anaesth* 34:340–341, 1962.

51. Inoue R et al. Generalized muscular rigidity associated with increased serum enzymes and postoperative muscular weakness induced by general anesthesia without hyperthermia. *Hiroshima J Anesth* 13: 232–235, 1977.

52. Fuchs F. Thermal inactivation of the calcium regulatory mechanism of human skeletal muscle. Actomyosin: A possible contributing factor in the rigidity of malignant hyperthermia. *Anesthesiology* 42:584–589, 1975.

53. Lopez JR et al. The effects of extracellular magnesium on muoplamic [Ca^{2+}] in malignant hyperthermia susceptible swine. *Anesthesiology* 73:109–117, 1990.

54. Saltzman LS et al. Hyperkalemia and cardiovascular collapse after verapamil and dantrolene administration in swine. *Anesth Analg* 63:473–478, 1984.

55. Harrison CG. Dantrolene-dynamics and kinetics. *Br J Anaesth* 60:279–286, 1988.

56. Rubin AS, Zablocki AD. Hyperkalemia, verapamil, and dantrolene. *Anesthesiology* 66:246–249, 1987.

57. Cabral R et al. Reversible profound depression of cerebral electrical activity in hyperthermia. *Electroencephalogr Clin Neurophysiol* 42:697–701, 1977.

58. Ryan JF, Papper EM. Malignant fever during and following anesthesia. *Anesthesiology* 32:196–201, 1970.

59. Donlon JV et al. Implications of masseter spasm after succinylcholine. *Anesthesiology* 49:298–301, 1978.

60. Schwartz L, Rockoff MA, Koka BV. Masseter spasm with anesthesia: Incidence and implications. *Anesthesiology* 61:772–775, 1984.

61. Ellis FR, Halsall PJ. Suxamethonium spasm. A differential diagnostic conundrum. *Br J Anaesth* 56:381–384, 1984.

62. Rosenberg H, Reed S. In vitro contracture tests for susceptibility to malignant hyperthermia. *Anesth Analg* 62:415–420, 1983.

63. Van der Spek AFL et al. Increased masticatory muscle stiffness during limb muscle flaccidity associated with succinylcholine administration. *Anesthesiology* 69:11–16, 1988.

64. Butler-Browne GS et al. Adult human masseter muscle fibers express myosin isozymes characteristics of development. *Muscle Nerve* 11:610–620, 1988.

65. Ryan JF, Kagen LJ, Hyman AI. Myoglobinemia after a single dose of succinylcholine. *N Engl J Med* 285:824–827, 1971.

66. Carroll JB. Increased incidence of masseter spasm in children with strabismus anesthetized with halothan and succinylcholine. *Anesthesiology* 67:559–561, 1987.

67. Littleford JA et al. Masseter muscle spasm in children: Implications of continuing the triggering anesthetic. *Anesth Analg* 72:151–160, 1991.

68. Hannala R, Kaplan R. Clinical assessment of jaw relaxation following halothane/succinylcholine in children. *Anesthesiology* 73:1189, 1992.

69. Larach MG et al. Prediction of malignant hyperthermia susceptibility by clinical signs. *Anesthesiology* 66:547–550, 1987.

70. The European Malignant Hyperpyrexia Group. A protocol for the investigation of malignant hyperpyrexia (MH) susceptibility. *Br J Anaesth* 56:1267–1269, 1984.

71. Britt BA. Comparison of the North American and European protocols for the caffeine halothane (CHC) contracture test. *J Neurol Sci* 98:522, 1990.

72. Larach MG, Landis JR. Sources of variation in false positive diagnostic rats of malignant hyperthermia using the North American protocol for caffeine halothane contracture testing. *J Neurol Sci* 98:521, 1990.

73. Britt BA et al. Malignant hyperthermia: An investigation of five patients. *Can Anaesth Soc J* 20:431–467, 1973.

74. Adnet P et al. Resting membrane potential (RMP) and in vitro caffeine test in malignant hyperthermia susceptible patients (MHS). *J Neurol Sci* 98:517, 1990.

75. Nelson TE, Flewellen EH, Gloyna DF. Spectrum of susceptibility to malignant hyperthermia—A diagnostic dilemma. *Anesth Analg* 62:545–552, 1983.

76. Kreul JF, Sufit RL, Helmer PR. Effects of cold storage on muscle biopsy contracture studies. *J Neurol Sci* 98:523, 1990.

77. Gronert GA. Controversies in malignant hyperthermia. *Anesthesiology* 59:273–274, 1983.

78. Brownell AKW et al. Malignant hyperthermia in Duchenne muscular dystrophy. *Anesthesiology* 58:180–182, 1983.

79. Miller ED Jr et al. Anesthesia-induced rhabdomyolysis in a patient with Duchenne's muscular dystrophy. *Anesthesiology* 48:146–148, 1978.

80. Frank JP et al. Central core disease and malignant hyperthermia syndrome. *Ann Neurol* 7:11–17, 1980.

81. Denborough MA, Galloway GJ, Hopkinson KC. Malignant hyperpyrexia and sudden infant death. *Lancet* 2:1068–1069, 1982.

82. Dallman JH. Neuroleptic malignant syndrome: A review. *Milit Med* 149:471–473, 1984.

83. Lopez JR, Sanchez V, Lopez MJ. Sarcoplasmic ionic calcium concentration in neuroleptic malignant syndrome. *Cell Calcium* 10: 223–233, 1989.

84. Lehmann-Horn F, Iaizzo PA, Klein W. Neuromuscular diseases and the association to malignant hyperthermia. *J Neurol Sci* 98:135, 1990.

85. Caroff SN et al. Malignant hyperthermia susceptibility in neuroleptic malignant syndrome. *Anesthesiology* 67:20–25, 1987.

86. Reyford HG et al. The in vitro exposure of muscle strips from patients with neuroleptic malignant syndrome (NMS) cannot be correlated with the clinical features. *J Neurol Sci* 98:527, 1990.

87. Ellis FR, Halsall PJ. The value of clinical predictors of MHA. *J Neurol Sci* 98:525, 1990.

88. Hackl W et al. Prediction of malignant hyperthermia susceptibility: Statistical evaluation of clinical signs. *Br J Anaesth* 64:425–429, 1990.

89. Hill J, Ryan JF; unpublished data.

90. Muldoon S et al. Sympathetic nervous system (SNS) function in malignant hyperthermia susceptible (MHS) subjects. *J Neurol Sci* 98:521, 1990.

91. Isaacs H, Barlow MG. Malignant hyperpyrexia. Further muscle studies in asymptomatic carriers identified by creatinine phosphokinase screening. *J Neurol Neurosurg Psychiatry* 36:228–243, 1973.

92. Britt BA et al. Screening of malignant hyperthermia susceptible families by creatine phosphokinase measurement and other clinical investigations. *Can Anaesth Soc J* 23:263–284, 1976.

93. Ellis FR et al. Evaluation of creatinine [sic] phosphokinase in screening patients for malignant hyperpyrexia. *Br Med J* 3:511–513, 1975.

94. Solomons CC, Masson N. Malignant hyperthermia platelet bioassay. *Anesthesiology* 60:265, 1984.

95. Giger U, Kaplan RF. Halothane-induced depletion in platelets from patients susceptible to malignant hyperthermia and from controls. *Anesthesiology* 58:347–352, 1983.

96. Maak S, Fink HS. Calcium-permeability of blood platelets in pigs with different halothane genotypes. *J Neurol Sci* 98:511, 1990.

97. Klip A et al. Halothane induces release of cytoplasmic calcium in blood mononuclear cells and muscle cells. *J Neurol Sci* 98:515, 1990.

98. O'Brien PJ, Britt BA, Kalow BI. Malignant hyperthermia: Lymphocyte Ca test for Ca-channel hypersensitivity of compensatory increase in Ca-ATPase activity. *J Neurol Sci* 98:516, 1990.

99. Ohnishi ST, Sadanaga KK. Non-invasive diagnosis of malignant hyperthermia. *J Neurol Sci* 98:515, 1990.

100. Halsall PJ. EPR measurement of membrane fluidity erythrocytes from patients tested for MH susceptibility by muscle biopsy. *J Neurol Sci* 98:516, 1990.

101. Cunliffe M, Lerman J, Britt BA. Is prophylactic dantrolene indicated for MHS patients undergoing elective surgery? *Anesth Analg* 66:S35, 1987.

102. Watson CB, Reierson N, Norfleet EA. Clinically significant muscle weakness induced by oral dantrolene sodium prophylaxis for malignant hyperthermia. *Anesthesiology* 65:312–313, 1986.

103. Flewellen EH, Nelson TE. Dantrolene dose response in malignant hyperthermia susceptible (MHS) swine: Method to obtain prophylaxis and therapeusis. *Anesthesiology* 52:303–308, 1980.

104. Ruhland G, Hinkle AI. Malignant hyperthermia after oral and intrave-

nous pretreatment with dantrolene in a patient susceptible to malignant hyperthermia. *Anesthesiology* 60:159–160, 1984.

105. Monster AW et al. Cooperative study for assessing the effects of a pharmacological agent on spasticity. *Am J Phys Med* 52:163–188, 1973.

106. Gratz DO, Reed S, Strobel GE. Chlorpromazine potentiation of halothan contractures in skeletal muscle of frog, normal and malignant hyperthermic man: Comparison with droperidol. ASA Annual Meeting Abstracts 317, 1975.

107. Dershwitz M, Sreter FA, Ryan JF. Ketamine does not trigger malignant hyperthermia in susceptible swine. *Anesth Analg* 69:501–503, 1989.

108. Gallen JS. Propofol does not trigger malignant hyperthermia. *Anesth Analg* 72:413–414, 1991.

109. Raff M, Harrison GG. The screening of propofol in MHS swine. *Anesth Analg* 68:750–751, 1989.

110. Weidel DJ, Iaizzo PA, Milde JH. Desflurane is a trigger of malignant hyperthermia in susceptible swine. *Anesthesiology* 74:508–512, 1991.

111. Dershwitz M, Ryan JF, Guralnick W. Safety of amide local anesthetics in patients susceptible to malignant hyperthermia. *J Am Dent Assoc* 118:276–280, 1989.

112. Flewellen EH, Nelson TE. Is theophylline, aminophylline, or caffeine (methylxanthines) contraindicated in malignant hyperthermia susceptible patients? *Anesth Analg* 62:115–118, 1983.

113. Gronert GA. Puzzles in malignant hyperthermia. *Anesthesiology* 54:1–2, 1981.

114. Sewall K, Flowerdew RMM, Bromberger P. Severe muscular rigidity at birth: Malignant hyperthermia syndrome. *Can Anaesth Soc J* 27:279–282, 1980.

115. Mayhew JF, Rudolph J, Tobey RE. Malignant hyperthermia in a six-month old infant: A case report. *Anesth Analg* 57:262–264, 1978.

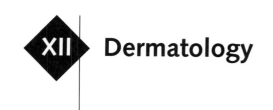

XII Dermatology

56 ◆ Dermatologic Problems

Dermatologic problems in the pediatric intensive care unit (PICU) may be conveniently divided into four groups: (1) primary skin diseases that may be life-threatening, (2) life-threatening systemic diseases with significant cutaneous involvement; (3) systemic disorders with subtle skin signs that may aid in their diagnosis, and (4) cutaneous disorders that occur as complications of bedrest or treatments administered during intensive care.[1-4]

Skin Diseases with Life-Threatening Complications

Erythema Multiforme/Toxic Epidermal Necrolysis

The term *erythema multiforme* (EM) is used to encompass a spectrum of diseases that may occur after exposure to various infectious agents, medications, or other stimuli. Most lesions are usually located acrally. A variety of morphologies may be seen, but most commonly, smooth plaques with a dusky center, commonly referred to as iris or target lesions, are present. EM minor is a benign, often recurrent disorder seen predominantly in teenagers.

In EM major, also known as Stevens-Johnson syndrome, cutaneous involvement is usually more widespread (Fig. 56-1). Mucosal involvement is always present. Ocular involvement, ranging from conjunctivitis, keratitis sicca, corneal erosions, symblepharon, and uveitis to global perforation, is present in 90% of patients. Thirty percent of patients develop pneumonia. Hemorrhagic stomatitis and erosive genital lesions may also occur.

Toxic epidermal necrolysis (TEN), also known as Lyell's syndrome, may be a separate disease but is generally regarded as the most severe and extensive form of EM (Fig. 56-2). TEN is usually caused by drug ingestion, particularly anticonvulsants, sulfa-containing antibiotics, and nonsteroidal antiinflammatory agents.[5-7] Children with HLA-B12 have a genetic predisposition

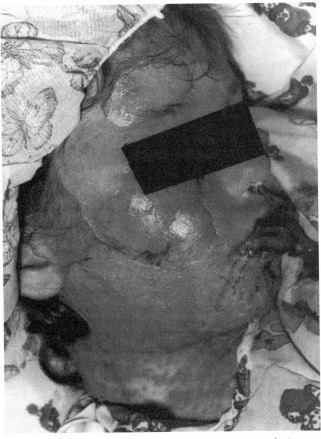

Figure 56-2. Toxic epidermal necrolysis. Note severe lesions on the face.

for TEN.[8] Patients with TEN are acutely and severely ill. Over a 2-day to 2-week period, the epidermis peels off in sheets like tissue paper, leaving oozing, raw, exposed dermis. Mucosal involvement is also generally severe, as in EM major. Gentle rubbing of the skin produces blistering, a phenomenon known as Nikolsky's sign. Severe fluid and electrolyte imbalances, sepsis, and pneumonia are common problems, just as in patients with severe thermal injury. Although the experienced physician can usually make the diagnosis of EM major or TEN clinically, a wide differential diagnosis exists (Table 56-1). A skin biopsy utilizing frozen sections will help establish the diagnosis rapidly but is not necessary in every patient.

The principles of treatment of patients with EM and TEN are (1) eliminating or treating the cause, if known; and (2) supportive care.[9] Patients should be cultured for infections and treated if an infectious trigger is likely. Patients with extensive skin sloughing may be severely dehydrated because basal metabolic rate is 2 to 3 times normal, and oral intake may be limited by pain. Nasogastric feedings with hyperalimentation are preferable to indwelling catheters, because the latter increase the risk of sepsis. Central venous catheters in particular should be avoided unless an acute episode requiring massive fluid volume over a short period exists. Foley catheters may be required for urinary retention but should be

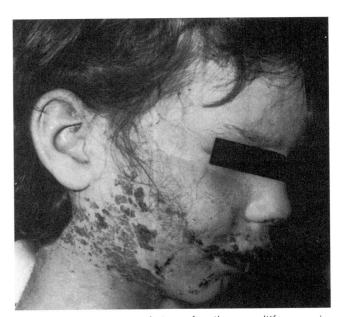

Figure 56-1. Cutaneous lesions of erythema multiforme major on the face.

Table 56-1. Differential diagnosis of toxic epidermal necrolysis.

Disease	Mucosal involvement	Nikolsky's sign	Cutaneous lesions	Etiology
Toxic epidermal necrolysis	+	+	+	Usually drug
Staphylococcal scalded skin syndrome	−	−	−	Staphylococcal toxin
Herpes gingivostomatitis	+	−	When associated with erythema multiforme	Herpes simplex
Pemphigus*	+	+	+	Autoimmune
Bechet's syndrome*	+	−	−	Autoimmune
Bullous pemphigoid*	One third of cases	−	+	Autoimmune
Erosive lichen planus	+	−	+	?

*Extremely rare in children

removed as soon as possible. Any indwelling catheters should be changed every 48 to 72 hours, and catheters should be changed every 48 to 72 hours and catheter tips cultured. Normal saline, viscous lidocaine, antibiotics, and mixtures of diphenhydramine and kaopectate all may be useful in providing symptomatic relief for the mouth. Ophthalmology consultation should be obtained whenever any eye signs or symptoms exist. Meticulous eye care, including soaks, antibiotic ointment, and lysis of synechiae several times a day, may be required.

Close observation for signs of sepsis and pneumonia are mandatory. Skin cultures should be performed on a daily basis, but positive cultures should be treated only if there are objective signs of infection. Antibiotics should be chosen on the basis of culture results if available; most infections are due to *Staphylococcus* and *Pseudomonas*. Chest x-rays should be done on a daily basis or more frequently if clinical symptoms warrant. Because patients with severe epidermal loss have difficulty with regulation of body temperature, temperature variations are common. Persistent hypo- or hyperthermia or leukopenia, however, should be presumptively treated with antibiotics.

Patients with large areas of denuded skin should be managed in a burn unit.[10] Clinicians vary in their preference for using allografts, xenografts, or bio-occlusive dressings.[10,11] Some advocate vigorous debridement in the operating room. Although some controversy remains, most recent publications stress that systemic steroids may increase morbidity and mortality and should not be used in children with EM major or TEN unless glomerulonephritis exists. A few authors recommend high-dose steroids given for 3 to 4 days if the disease is diagnosed very early.[12] Plasmapheresis, cyclosporine, and hyperbaric oxygen may be beneficial in some cases, but large prospective studies have not been performed.[13–16]

Mortality of EM major ranges from 2% to 25%; mortality of TEN may be higher than 50%. Mortality increases with percentage of surface area involved, the presence of renal involvement, neutropenia, lymphopenia, thrombocytopenia, and younger patient age. By avoiding systemic steroids and referring patients to burn centers for treatment early, mortality may be reduced to less than 20%, even for a patient with severe and extensive skin involvement. In severe cases, the skin may heal with hyper- and hypopigmentation. Permanent visual loss occurs in 10% of patients with ocular symptoms. Strictures of the respiratory tree and upper GI tract may also occur.

Erythroderma (Exfoliative Dermatitis)

Erythroderma is a term used to describe diffuse redness and scaling of the skin. Exfoliative dermatitis may occur in children with ichthyosis, psoriasis, atopic dermatitis, drug allergy, contact dermatitis, seborrheic dermatitis, an underlying malignancy, an underlying immune deficiency, acute graft versus host disease (GVH) or it can be of unknown etiology (Fig. 56-3).[17–20]

Erythroderma may be the first sign of a skin disease or may occur in a patient with a long-standing dermatologic disorder. Onset may be gradual, progressing over weeks to months, or sudden, with progression over 24 to 48 hours. Temperature instability, chills, and sepsis may occur because intact skin is required for

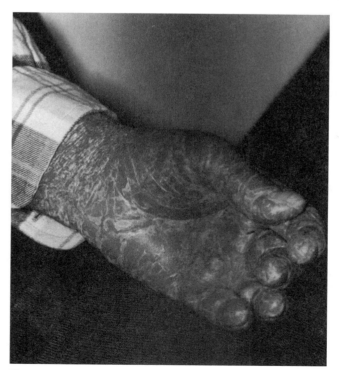

Figure 56-3. Erythroderma. Note marked scaling and a darkening (redness) of skin.

thermoregulation and serves as a barrier against infection. Massive fluid losses may occur through the skin. Leukocytosis and hypereosinophilia are commonly seen, although this varies with the underlying cause of the erythroderma.

Skin biopsy should be performed in patients with erythroderma. Biopsy may disclose a specific diagnosis; in other cases, no diagnosis can be made until the acute flare subsides. The cardiovascular, hematologic, and urologic status of the patient must be monitored. Aggressive fluid replacement, antibiotics for possible sepsis, digoxin for congestive heart failure (CHF), and rarely, dialysis may be required. If systemic or topical drug ingestion is felt to be the cause, these should be stopped. Treatment of erythroderma secondary to GVH should be discussed with a hematologist/oncologist and may include high-dose corticosteroids, antithymocyte globulin, and immunosuppressive agents. Erythroderma from atopic dermatitis, psoriasis, or seborrheic dermatitis can be treated with bland emollients and topical steroid preparations, as well as tar baths in consultation with a dermatologist. Etretinate may be considered in patients with erythrodermic psoriasis. However, because the drug is teratogenic and is stored in the body for years after it has been discontinued, this medication should only be used in males. Systemic steroids are required in patients with multisystem failure.

The prognosis for patients with erythroderma depends on the underlying disease. More than half of the patients with erythroderma secondary to atopic dermatitis or psoriasis will have episodic flares of their skin diseases and may continue to have erythroderma.[23] Patients with erythroderma from drug eruptions usually recover completely but will redevelop erythroderma if reexposed to the offending agent.

Kasabach-Merritt Syndrome

The trapping of platelets and fibrinogen within an enlarging hemangioma, resulting in consumption coagulopathy and hemolytic anemia, is known as the Kasabach-Merritt syndrome[21,22] (Fig. 56-4). This rare constellation of symptoms usually affects very young infants with large, deep hemangiomas, but patients of any age with hemangiomas of any size may be affected. The hemangioma may slowly enlarge over several weeks, but more commonly, the lesion enlarges dramatically over a period of days. The overlying skin may become shiny and woody in appearance. Ecchymoses and petechiae first develop around the hemangioma, but as the

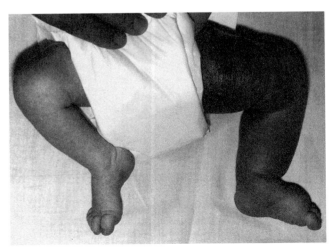

Figure 56-4. Kasabach-Merritt syndrome. Note hypertrophy of the leg and shiny, "woody" skin.

coagulopathy progresses, these become more generalized. Hematuria, GI bleeding, and/or high-output CHF may be seen. Elevated prothrombin time (PT) and partial thromboplastin time (PTT), low platelet counts, low fibrinogen levels, and elevated fibrin split products are evidence of disseminated intravascular coagulation (DIC). Hemoglobin and hematocrit are often decreased secondary to hemolytic anemia.

The vascular nature of the lesion may be difficult to appreciate if it lies deep in the dermis; radionucleotide imaging may be helpful in looking for deep visceral hemangiomas and in confirming the diagnosis in more superficial lesions.

Therapy is directed toward controlling the coagulopathy and decreasing or eliminating the lesion. Patients may require multiple transfusions of blood, platelets, and plasma. Heparin, aspirin, dipyridamole, antifibrinolytics, and ε-aminocaproic acid have all been used with some success in controlling the coagulopathy.[23] Prednisone, in dosages of 2 to 4 mg/kg/d, is the usual recommended modality of therapy, but only 50% of patients respond to this treatment. Sclerosing agents, intravascular embolization, and vascular ligation may be successful but carry a high morbidity and mortality. CHF is treated with digoxin and diuretics. Children who are not actively bleeding may be closely observed because most hemangiomas eventually resolve spontaneously and the abnormal bleeding parameters eventually correct themselves as well. Kasabach-Merritt syndrome carries a 20% to 30% mortality.

Life-Threatening Diseases with Significant Skin Involvement

Purpura Fulminans

Purpura fulminans (PF) is a rare life-threatening disease seen predominantly in children. Extensive vasculitis and thrombosis result in large ecchymotic areas, fever, hypotension, and DIC (Fig. 56-5). PF may be seen during an illness or in the convalescent period in a variety of bacterial and viral infections.[24–27] Patients develop large, symmetrical, tender, erythematous areas on the legs. These areas become purple over a period of hours. Well-demarcated areas of necrosis and gangrene may develop over the ensuing days.

Thrombocytopenia, hypofibrinogenemia, elevated PT and PTT, decreased fibrinogen levels, and increased fibrin split products are all signs of the consumption coagulopathy that usually accompanies PF. Leukocytosis, bandemia, and hemolytic anemia may also be present. Acquired deficiency of proteins C and S may occur during an episode of PF.[25]

Patients with PF who are in DIC and shock frequently develop respiratory hepatic and/or renal failure. Cardiomyopathy and GI bleeding may also occur. Compartment syndromes may develop, requiring extensive surgical debridement and/or amputation.[26] Bacterial, viral, and fungal cultures should be performed to rule out an infectious origin for PF.[27] Lesions of PF may be difficult to distinguish from necrotizing fasciitis, coumarin necrosis (which may also be associated with partial protein C deficiency), necrotizing cellulitis, and other disorders associated with purpura[28–30] or large ecchymotic plaques (Table 56-2).

Henoch-Schönlein Purpura

Henoch-Schönlein purpura (HSP) is a disease of unknown etiology in which IgA is deposited in blood vessels of the skin, kidneys, GI tract, and/or joints. The disease is primarily seen in children under the age of 10 years.

Table 56-2. Differential diagnosis of large ecchymotic plaques in the pediatric intensive care unit

	Fever	*CNS disease*	*Renal disease*
Purpura fulminans	+	–	–
Coumarin necrosis	–	–	–
Loxoscelism	+	–	+/–
Necrotizing fasciitis	+	–	–
Marantic emboli	+	+/–	+/–
Child abuse	–	–	–
	(+ with head trauma)		(+ with flank trauma)
Extravasated injection	–	–	–

+/–, often.

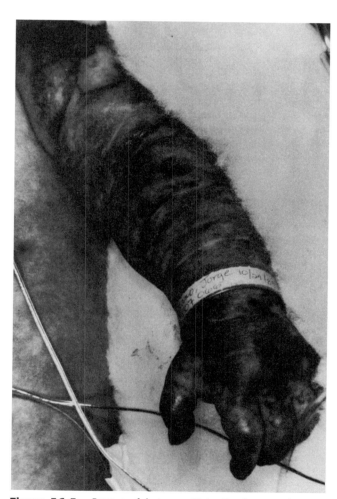

Figure 56-5. Purpura fulminans. Note the large ecchymotic areas on the arm. Extensive vasculitis and thrombosis have caused gangrene of the digits.

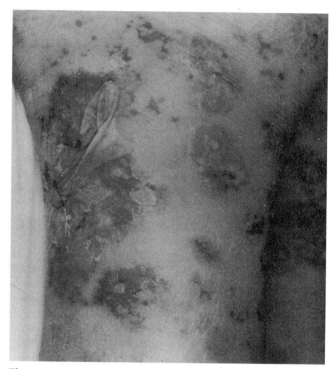

Figure 56-6. Purpuric rash of Henoch-Schönlein purpura involving the legs and buttocks.

HSP is usually a benign disorder. Patients with HSP have a characteristic symmetrical purpuric rash on the legs and buttocks (Fig. 56-6). Arthritis occurs in three fourths of the cases. Colicky abdominal pain and acute GI bleeding develop in approximately half the cases.[31] Acute abdominal pain may signal intussusception and subsequent infarction. Ten percent to 28% of patients with HSP have renal involvement ranging from microscopic hematuria to acute renal failure.[32] Mild thrombocytosis and elevation of the sedimentation rate may occur. Biopsy of affected tissues reveals vasculitis with IgA deposition in vessel walls.

Patients with multisystem involvement may require ICU management with input from surgeons, nephrologists, gastroenterologists, and dermatologists. Corticosteroids may be useful in cases with severe GI involvement. Plasmapheresis may be useful in patients with rapidly progressive renal disease. Most patients with HSP recover completely, although the disease may recur months or even years later. Three percent to 15% of children on dialysis have sustained kidney damage as a result of HSP.

Kawasaki Disease (Mucocutaneous Lymph Node Syndrome)

Kawasaki disease (KD) is a syndrome of unknown etiology primarily affecting children less than 4 years of age. Patients are febrile, irritable, and somewhat lethargic. A rash commonly begins in the perineal area and may be urticarial, morbilliform, scarlatiniform, or pustular, or may resemble erythema marginatum. Lesions usually are present for approximately a week. "Strawberry tongue" and conjunctival infection may accompany the rash. Painful erythema and edema of the palms and soles is followed approximately 2 weeks later by diffuse desquamation. During the first 1 to 2 weeks of illness, tachycardia and CHF may develop. Between days 10 and 30, life-threatening cardiac abnormalities, including CHF, arrhythmias, pericardial effusion, mitral insufficiency, or coronary artery aneurysms occur in over 20% of patients.[33,34] Aneurysms may spontaneously resolve, but death from myocardial infarction or aneurysmal rupture may occur. GI abnormalities, arthritis, and CNS abnormalities may also be seen during the acute illness.

White blood cell count is usually over 20,000 erythrocyte sedimentation rate (ESR) is high, and beginning around the second week of illness, thrombocytosis occurs. Cardiac abnormalities may be demonstrable on echo or angiography.

The diagnosis of KD is based on the fulfillment of five of six criteria, including fever, conjunctival injection, oropharyngeal changes, changes in the distal extremities, rash, and cervical adenopathy. The differential diagnosis includes scarlet fever, toxic shock syndrome (TSS), drug eruptions, and acrodynia.[35]

Intravenous (IV) gamma globulin administered during the first week of illness and high-dose aspirin given during the period of thrombocytosis significantly decrease the incidence of coronary artery abnormalities.[36,37]

Overall mortality is 0.3% to 0.5% and is highest in males less than 2 years of age. Approximately half of coronary artery aneurysms will spontaneously resolve within a year, but long-term risks of heart disease are not known.

Dermatomyositis

Dermatomyositis is an autoimmune disorder affecting multiple organ systems, particularly the musculature and skin. Immune complexes deposit around blood vessels, causing vasculitis.[38] Proximal muscle weakness develops over days to weeks. A periorbital heliotropic rash accompanied by scaly purple plaques over bony prominences (known as Gottron's papules) is pathognomonic of this disorder[39] (Fig. 56-7). Periungual telangiectasias, poikiloderma, and photosensitivity may also be seen. Acute onset of muscle weakness, dysphagia, or GI tract hemorrhage or perforation may necessitate admission to the ICU.

Muscle biopsy confirms the clinical diagnosis. Skin biopsy processed for routine histopathology and immunofluorescence help to distinguish cutaneous findings from those of other papulosqua-

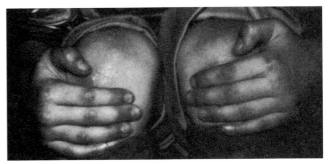

Figure 56-7. Patient with dermatomyositis, showing characteristic plaques over bony prominences of knees and hands.

mous disorders such as psoriasis and lupus. Patients have elevated CPK, lactic dehydrogenase (LDH) transaminases, aldolase, and ESR. Autoantibodies may be present. Complement levels are depressed. Patients may have either a nonprogressive course or a chronic one with intermittent acute exacerbations.

Prednisone is helpful in the majority of children with dermatomyositis, beginning at a dosage of 1 to 2 mg/kg/d. Patients who are unresponsive to higher doses of steroids or in whom complications of the disease or therapy preclude their use may be treated with plasmapheresis, cyclosporine, or other immunosuppressive agents.[40,41]

Systemic Lupus Erythematosus

Systemic lupus erythematosus (SLE) is a multisystem disease in which autoantibodies form, causing destruction of affected organs. SLE occurs most commonly in young women but may be seen in patients of either sex and may present in the first two decades of life.[42,43] Most patients have an insidious onset with acute exacerbations of their chronic disease. Cutaneous changes, arthritis, or renal symptoms may predominate. Occasional children present with an acute neurologic event, such as a seizure, sudden blindness, hemiparesis, or severe ataxia. Such an acute event may occur following sun exposure and may be accompanied by a papulosquamous rash in sun-exposed areas. When CNS and renal symptoms predominate, the differential diagnosis for SLE includes hemolytic-uremic syndrome (HUS) and thrombotic thrombocytopenic purpura (TTP)[44] (Table 56-3).

Children with lupus who require ICU management generally have multisystem disease. Antinuclear antibodies, as well as a variety of other autoantibodies, are usually present. Leukopenia, de-

Table 56-3. Differential diagnosis of palpable purpura in the pediatric intensive care unit

	Fever	*CNS disease*	*Arthritis*	*Renal disease*
Drug eruption	−/+	−	−	−/+
SLE	+	+/−	+	+/−
TTP	+	+	−	+
Sepsis	+	−/+	−	+/−
HSP	−	−	+/−	+/−
HUS	−	+	−	+

+/−, often; −/+, occasionally; SLE, systemic lupus erythematosus; TTP, thrombotic thrombocytopenia purpura; HSP, Henoch-Schönlein purpura; HUS, hemolytic-uremic syndrome.

pressed complement levels, and a false-positive VDRL are commonly seen. Skin biopsy may be helpful in establishing the diagnosis. Renal biopsy is often required to determine the type and extent of renal damage.

The mainstay of treatment of SLE is systemic steroids. Dosages should be determined in consultation with nephrologists, rheumatologists, and neurologists. Immunosuppressive agents may also be used for their steroid-sparing effects, but long-term side effects of these agents are unknown.

Five-year survival of children with SLE who do not have renal involvement is close to 100%; approximately 10% of children with SLE with renal disease succumb to their illness. Dialysis may be required in approximately 40% of children with lupus.

Rocky Mountain Spotted Fever

Envenomation by a tick harboring *Rickettsia rickettsii* causes widespread vasculitis and coagulopathy known as Rocky Mountain spotted fever (RMSF). Two thirds of the cases occur in children who are less than 15 years old; almost all cases occur between April and October.[45] Most typically, a nonpetechial rash begins on the extremities and then moves centrally (Fig. 56-8). Over the next several days, headache and fever develop. The rash becomes petechial and malaise, conjunctivitis, lymphadenopathy, myocarditis, orchitis, and CNS signs, including ataxia, coma, and seizures, may develop. Thrombocytopenia, elevated PT and PTT, and a decrease in plasma fibrinogen are signs of DIC that may occur in patients with RMSF. The diagnosis can be made by immunofluorescence of a skin biopsy or a **proteus** Ox-19 antigen agglutination test can be performed.[46] Treatment should never be delayed while awaiting laboratory confirmation of the diagnosis. The differential diagnosis of RMSF includes other causes of sepsis, SLE, drug eruptions, TTP, HSP, and HUS.

Once a diagnosis of RMSF is suspected, systemic antibiotics should be given because mortality rates are close to 0 for patients treated before the fifth day of illness. Children less than 9 years of age should receive chloramphenicol, 100 mg/kg/d; children 9 years of age or older should receive tetracycline, 30 to 40 mg/kg/d. Ventilator support, volume expanders, digoxin, and anticonvulsants may all be required. Heparin is not useful. Without antibiotic therapy, up to 70% of patients will die, but case-fatality rate is less than 3% for treated children.[47]

Hereditary Hemorrhagic Telangiectasia

Hereditary hemorrhagic telangiectasia (HHT), also known as Osler-Weber-Rendu disease, is an autosomal dominant disorder in which vascular dysplasia occurs. Arteriovenous malformations, aneurysms, and telangiectasias are responsible for the visceral and mucocutaneous hemorrhages that characterize this disorder.[48] Manifestations may begin as early as the first year of life, although most patients develop symptoms after the second decade.[49]

Children with repeated and/or unduly severe episodes of epistaxis, pulmonary atrial venous fistulas, and/or recurrent brain abscesses should be examined for the presence of telangiectasias on mucous membranes, the face, and hands. Cutaneous lesions rarely develop before age 10, however. If not seen in the child, family members should be examined and questioned for symptoms. Bleeding disorders should be ruled out by appropriate laboratory testing.

Once brisk bleeding has begun, local control measures such as direct pressure, arterial ligation, radiation, resection of the bleeding area, topical vasoconstrictors, cryosurgery, and cautery may all control bleeding. Destructive measures may cause scar tissue, potentially causing subsequent episodes to be even more severe.

One third of patients with HHT require transfusions. The severity of one bleeding episode does not predict the severity of subsequent episodes. Less than 10% of patients with HHT die of the disease or its complications.[48] Symptomatic arterial venous fistulas of the lungs, liver, and brain may develop in teenage or adult years.[49]

Skin Diseases Acquired During a Life-Threatening Illness

Drug Eruptions

Cutaneous eruptions may occur after administration of any medication, although antibiotics, anticonvulsants, and blood products are most commonly implicated[50-52] (Figs. 56-9 and 56-10). Children in the ICU often require many drugs and are thus particularly susceptible. Lesions of any morphology may be seen. Dermatologists may be helpful in determining the most likely offending

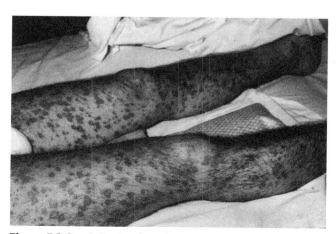

Figure 56-8. Patient with Rocky Mountain spotted fever, showing characteristic rash (nonpetechial) over legs.

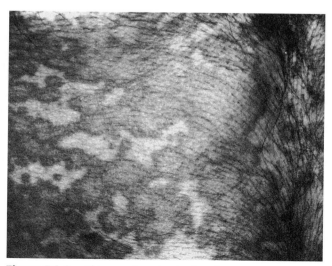

Figure 56-9. Skin eruption due to drug hypersensitivity.

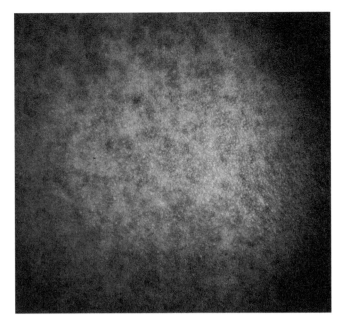

Figure 56-10. Urticarial skin eruption caused by drug hypersensitivity.

agent. For patients who develop TEN, EM major, or anaphylaxis, the offending agent must be stopped and never reintroduced. In patients with urticarial eruptions in whom no alternative treatment is available, premedication with an antihistamine may decrease the likelihood of anaphylaxis, but anaphylaxis may still occur. For patients with morbilliform drug eruptions, the medication can sometimes be continued under careful observation if there is no alternative therapy. Morbilliform eruptions rarely progress to TEN or EM major. Patients should be monitored for the development of liver and/or renal involvement.

Oral Thrush

Thrush is due to colonization and multiplication of *Candida* within the oral cavity. Children in the ICU who are debilitated by their illness are particularly prone to thrush. The patient may be asymptomatic, complain of abnormal taste sensation, or suffer a loss of appetite. White patches that bleed after being scraped are present throughout the oral cavity. Potassium hydroxide or Gram stain of the scraping reveals hyphae, pseudohyphae, and/or blastospores. Because *Candida albicans* is part of the normal oral flora, a positive culture is not diagnostic of oral thrush.[53] Treatment with oral nystatin or, in the older child, clotrimazole troches three to six times daily will temporarily eradicate signs and symptoms, but recurrence is frequent.

Contact Dermatitis

Patients in the ICU typically require external lines and monitoring devices, which are taped in place. Lubricating lotions and/or topically applied medications may also be required. These practices may result in an irritant or allergic contact dermatitis, characterized by erythema, and sometimes vesiculation, which follows the pattern of the externally applied substance. The use of hypoallergenic (satin or paper) tape and avoidance of topical preparations that contain common sensitizing agents minimize the risk of con-

tact dermatitis. Treatment involves discontinuing the offending agent combined with the use of bland lubricants and/or topical steroid preparations.

References

1. Berman RS, Silvestri DL. Dermatologic problems in the intensive care unit: Part I. *J Intensive Care Med* 1:15–28, 1986.
2. Berman RS, Silvestri DL. Dermatologic problems in the intensive care unit: Part II. *J Intensive Care Med* 1:111–118, 1986.
3. Berman RS, Silvestri DL. Dermatologic problems in the intensive care unit: Part III. *J Intensive Care Med* 1:156–170, 1986.
4. Berman RS, Silvestri DL. Dermatologic problems in the intensive care unit: Part IV. *J Intensive Care Med* 1:224–239, 1986.
5. Guillaume JC et al. The culprit drugs in 87 cases of toxic epidermal necrolysis (Lyell's syndrome). *Arch Dermatol* 123:1166–1170, 1987.
6. Jones WG et al. Drug induced toxic epidermal necrolysis in children. *J Pediatr Surg* 24:167–170, 1989.
7. Dolan PA et al. Toxic epidermal necrolysis. *J Emerg Med* 7:65–69, 1989.
8. Tadlock LM, Elias PM. Toxic epidermal necrolysis. *Curr Concepts Skin Disord* 9:15–19, 1988.
9. Halebian PH et al. Improved burn center survival of patients with toxic epidermal necrolysis managed without corticosteroids. *Ann Surg* 204:503–512, 1986.
10. Pruitt BA Jr. Burn treatment for the unburned. *JAMA* 251:2207–2208, 1987.
11. Birchall N et al. Toxic epidermal necrolysis: An approach to management using cryopreserved allograft skin. *J Am Acad Dermatol* 16: 368–372, 1987.
12. Weston WL et al. Corticosteroids for erythema multiforme? *Pediatr Dermatol* 6:229–250, 1989.
13. Kamanabroo D, Schmitz-Landgraf W, Czarnetzki BM. Plasmapheresis in severe drug-induced toxic epidermal necrolysis. *Arch Dermatol* 121:1548–1549, 1985.
14. Renfro L, Grant-Kels JM, Daman LA. Drug-induced toxic epidermal necrolysis treated with cyclosporine. *Int J Dermatol* 28:441–444, 1989.
15. Ruocco V et al. Hyperbaric oxygen treatment of toxic epidermal necrolysis. *Cutis* 38:267–271, 1986.
16. Rasmussen JE. Update on the Stevens-Johnson syndrome. *Cleve Clin J Med* 55:412–413, 1988.
17. Therstrup-Pedersen K et al. The red-man syndrome. Exfoliative dermatitis of unknown etiology: A description and follow-up of 38 patients. *J Am Acad Dermatol* 18:1307–1312, 1988.
18. Ikai K et al. Sezary-like syndrome in a 10-year-old girl with serologic evidence of human T-cell lymphotropic type 1 infection. *Arch Dermatol* 123:1351–1355, 1987.
19. Mauduit G, Claudy A. Cutaneous expression of graft-v-host disease in man. *Semin Dermatol* 7:149–155, 1988.
20. Harper JI. Cutaneous graft verses host disease. *Br Med J* 295:401–402, 1987.
21. Lel-Dessouky M et al. Kasabach-Merritt syndrome. *J Pediatr Surg* 23:109–111, 1988.
22. Loh W, Miller JH, Gomperts ED. Imaging with technetium 99m-labeled erythrocytes in evaluation of the Kasabach-Merritt syndrome. *J Pediatr* 113:856–859, 1988.
23. Larsen EC et al. Kasabach-Merritt syndrome: Therapeutic considerations. *Pediatrics* 79:971–980, 1987.
24. Chenaille PJ, Horowitz ME. Purpura fulminans, a case for heparin therapy. *Clin Pediatr* 28:95–98, 1989.
25. Powars DR et al. Purpura fulminans in meningococcemia: Association with acquired deficiencies of protein C and S. *N Engl J Med* 317:571–572, 1987.
26. Chu DZJ, Blaisdell FW. Purpura fulminans. *Am J Surg* 143:356–362, 1982.
27. Silverman RA, Rhodes AR, Dennehy PH. Disseminated intravascular coagulation and purpura fulminans in a patient with candida sepsis. *Am J Med* 80:679–684, 1986.

28. Gladson CL, Groncy P, Griffin JH. Coumarin necrosis, neonatal purpura fulminans and protein C deficiency. *Arch Dermatol* 123:1701a–1706a, 1987.

29. Marlar RA, Montogomery RR, Broekmans AW. Diagnosis and treatment of homozygous protein C deficiency. *J Pediatr* 114:528–534, 1989.

30. Umbert IJ et al. Necrotizing fasciitis: A clinical microbiologic and histophatologic study of 14 patients. *J Am Acad Dermatol* 20:774–781, 1989.

31. Saulsbury FT, Kesler RW. Thrombocytosis in Henoch-Schonlein purpura. *Clin Pediatr* 22:185–187, 1983.

32. Heng MCY. Henoch-Schonlein purpura. *Br J Dermatol* 112:235–240, 1985.

33. Barron KS, Murphy DJ Jr. Kawasaki syndrome, still a fascinating enigma. *Hosp Pract* 24:51–60, 1989.

34. Melish ME. Kawasaki syndrome (the mucocutaneous lymph node syndrome). *Pediatr Ann* 11:255–268, 1982.

35. Adler R et al. Metallic mercury vapor poisoning simulating mucocutaneous lymph node syndrome. *J Pediatr* 101:967–968, 1982.

36. Newburger JW et al. The treatment of Kawasaki disease with intravenous gamma gloubulin. *N Engl J Med* 315:341–347, 1986.

37. Nagashima M et al. High-dose gamma globulin therapy for Kawasaki disease. *J Pediatr* 110:710–712, 1987.

38. Silver RM, Maricq HR. Childhood dermatomysitis: Serial microvascular studies. *Pediatrics* 83:278–283, 1989.

39. Callen JP. Dermatomyositis and polymyositis: Continuing controversies and recent therapies. *Curr Concepts Skin Disord* Summer:18–23, 1986.

40. Dau PC, Bennington JL. Plasmapheresis in childhood dermatomyositis. *J Pediatr* 98:237–240, 1981.

41. Heckmatt J et al. Cyclosporine in juvenile dermatomyositis. *Lancet* i:1063–1066, 1989.

42. Lehman TJA et al. Systemic lupus erythematosus in the first decade of life. *Pediatrics* 83:235–239, 1989.

43. Fish AJ et al. Systemic lupus erythematosus within the first two decades of life. *Am J Med* 62:99–117, 1977.

44. Bartholomew JR, Bell WR. Thrombotic thrombocytopenic purpura. *J Intensive Care Med* 1:341–355, 1986.

45. Hemlick CG, Bernard KW, D'Angelo LJ. Rocky Mountain spotted fever: Clinical, laboratory, and epidemiological features in 262 cases. *J Infect Dis* 150:480–488, 1984.

46. Walker DH, Cain BG. A method for specific diagnosis of Rocky Mountain spotted fever on fixed paraffin-imbedded tissue by immunofluorescence. *J Infect Dis* 137:206–209, 1978.

47. Woodward TE. Rocky Mountain spotted fever: Epidemiological and early clinical signs are keys to treatment and reduce mortality. *J Infect Dis* 150:465–468, 1984.

48. Peery WH. Clinical spectrum of hereditary hemorrhagic telangiectasia (Osler-Weber-Rendu disease). *Am J Med* 82:989–997, 1987.

49. Plauchu H et al. Age-related clinical profile of hereditary hemorrhagic telangiectasia in an epidemiologically recruited population. *Am J Med Genet* 32:291–297, 1989.

50. Wintroub BU, Stern R. Cutaneous drug reactions: Pathogenesis and clinical classification. *J Am Acad Dermatol* 13:167–179, 1985.

51. Goolamali SK. Drug eruptions. *Postgrad Med J* 61:925–993, 1985.

52. Bigby M et al. Drug-induced cutaneous reactions. *JAMA* 256:3358–3363, 1986.

53. Cristlip MA, Edwards JE. Candidiasis, systemic fungal infections: Diagnosis and treatment II. *Inf Dis Clin North Am* 3:103–132, 1989.

XIII The Chronically Ill Child

Robert H. Wharton

James M. Perrin

Alice A. Curnin

Denise Lozowski

57 New Approaches to Intensive Care Unit Patients with Chronic Illness and Disability

The nature of severe chronic illness in children has changed dramatically in the past few decades. Mainly because of marked improvements in the technology of medical and surgical services and the distribution of health care, most children with severe and seemingly catastrophic illnesses currently survive rather than die.[1,2] The average life span of youngsters with cystic fibrosis has greatly improved in the past 20 years; the majority of children with acute lymphocytic leukemia achieve a remission and go on to apparent cure. New procedures correct previously fatal congenital heart lesions.

Most recent estimates suggest that between 15% and 30% of children have some chronic health condition. Of this number, about 10%, or 2% to 4% of all children, have a long-term illness likely to require daily care. Current conservative estimates are that at least 80% of children with severe long-term illnesses survive to young adulthood, although often with significant disability and potential for exacerbations that may lead to repeat hospitalizations.[3]

Improvements in technology have affected health services delivery as well. Miniaturization now makes much respiratory equipment portable, allowing ventilator-dependent youngsters to live at home rather than in hospitals. Other new technologies allowing technology-dependent children to be at home include parenteral nutrition, long-term antibiotic administration, home infusions of factor VIII for children with hemophilia, and home traction after significant trauma.[4]

In most cases, the incidence of specific diseases is stable. If more children currently survive, one may speculate that the total number of children with severe long-term illnesses will also remain unchanged over the next few decades, assuming a relatively fixed birth rate. Yet changes in the incidence of two important conditions challenge this set of assumptions. Children with bronchopulmonary dysplasia, as well as other graduates of newborn intensive care units (ICUs), now seem likely to survive, although with 1 or more years of severe respiratory distress, needing extensive home and hospital-based care. Whether the number will increase or decrease over the next decade remains a controversial question. Similarly, the increasing numbers of children with AIDS will lead to greater demands on comprehensive health care programs.

The patterns of inpatient care for children have also changed dramatically in response to the vast transfer of common acute pediatric illnesses to outpatient and home-based services and to the increasing use of day-surgery units. Recent evidence documents a marked decrease in rates of pediatric hospitalization in general, with two overlapping populations taking increasing portions of the inpatient group: poor children and children with complex long-term health conditions. (Recent estimates of the inpatients on the intensive and regular care services of the Children's service at the Massachusetts General Hospital indicate that, conservatively, 50% of all admissions are for children with preexisting chronic illness.)

These changes in the epidemiology of hospitalized children have important implications for the organization of hospital services, insofar as most pediatric beds are currently viewed as acute care beds for new cases of illness. Nowhere is this more true than in ICUs and step-down units. As we have seen, however, increasing numbers of children face long-term recuperation and rehabilitation for problems related to their chronic illness and disability. In addition, it follows that increasing numbers of families must manage the complex posthospitalization organizational and emotional requirements of their children. Therefore, much of the time spent in the ICU and intermediate units now involves careful long-term planning, collaborating with families regarding the management of care in the home, and coordinating complex services for the transition from hospital to home.[5]

Models of Care

While pediatric ICU patients have undergone significant evolution toward increased representation of chronic disease and disability and a need for heightened technological services, the general approach to children and their families has changed less. Guidelines for intervention often follow a medical model that employs specific algorithms based on deviation from statistically normal parameters of organ functioning. The focus is on the medical response to the sudden and unanticipated onset or exacerbation of serious and often life-threatening disease or injury. The goal is the total reversal of the pathological process interfering with physiologic integrity. In this medical, or more accurately, biologic model, physicians diagnose and treat diseases (i.e., the abnormalities in the structure and function of body organs and systems).[6] Children with an underlying disorder of bronchopulmonary dysplasia admitted to an ICU in respiratory distress would be treated for their pulmonary problem. If their symptoms of dyspnea could be reduced to treatable bronchospasm, this biologic reductionism would result in dramatic success. The ICU team would then comfortably utilize this model to sustain life and to prevent undesirable physical consequences of chronicity and its residual partner, disability.

The model of care that orchestrates health services to the child with chronic illness and his family, while acknowledging the importance of and overlapping with the medical model, is broader in scope. Here, professionals are more likely to accept that they are dealing with dysfunctions that are long-standing and irreversible at the physiologic level. The model recognizes that whereas organs are the targets of disease, patients suffer illnesses.[6] This "bioecologic" model addresses mutual interactions between individuals and their environment that more satisfactorily incorporate the myriad of systems that impact on the expression of illness. Now the infant with bronchopulmonary dysplasia (BPD) and respiratory distress is viewed more expansively as it is acknowledged that successful management of the infant's respiratory difficulties requires information about the child's physical environment, as well as current family or other potential emotional stresses. In addition, community resources, cultural background, and finances all are recognized as coexisting with and impacting on the health of the system.

Chronic illness in an ICU setting provides the potential for conflict between the medical and bioecologic model regarding the direction of intervention. Obviously, neither model by itself will be sufficient to treat adequately the complexities presented. On the one hand, "treatment assessed solely through the rhetoric of improvement in disease process may confound the assessment of care in the resource of illness problems."[7] The ICU faces the need to cure patients who cannot always be cured. This fragments the dynamic dialectic between biologic processes, physiologic states, and environmental situations. On the other hand, rapid, intensive, and technologically superior life-saving interventions must be available treatment modalities for all patients. The attempt to maintain the silent preexisting harmony of the bioecologic equilibrium is the motivating force for the development of new models of care, such as the bioecologic model described here for individuals and families facing chronic disease and disability.[8]

Individuals present to an ICU with or without preexisting chronic disease or disability. In the acute situation without a preexisting history, new disease may result in several alternative pathways (Fig. 57-1). First, when assuming that a person's baseline has been the total absence of illness or disability (Fig. 57-1A), a disease can be brief and resolve completely. Examples here may be uncomplicated meningitis or epiglottitis. A second scenario (Fig. 57-1B) will also be a return to previous health, but this time with a more protracted disease course, with examples being trauma or Guillain-Barré. The final possibility relates to the inability to return to baseline (Fig. 57-1C), as represented by situations such as moderate-to-severe head injury, burns, encephalitis, amputations, and spinal cord injuries. Children in this third category may leave the ICU cured of disease but with new morbidity that increases potential for exacerbations of illness due to persistent fixed disability. Individuals and families in the latter two categories will require services and interventions during their ICU course based on the bioecologic model.

Children with preexisting chronic illness who enter and survive an intensive care stay will have courses that parallel those just described (Fig. 57-2). Here, however, the baseline is shifted appreciably toward illness. In addition, after the acute illness, the individual may not be restored to her previous baseline health status. The following represent cases for each potential pathway.

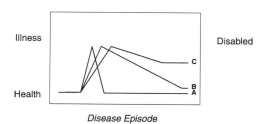

Figure 57-1. Health illness continuum: No preexisting chronic illness.

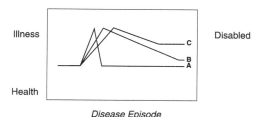

Figure 57-2. Health illness continuum: Preexisting illness.

Case 1: Acute Illness with Rapid Return to Baseline

A 5-year-old boy with spastic quadriparesis, seizure disorder, and moderate mental retardation is brought to the emergency room in status epilepticus. History on admission reveals that 2 days prior to arrival (PTA), the patient had developed cough and fever. One day PTA, he developed vomiting and lethargy. On the day of admission, he continued to vomit all of his food and medications and began to develop brief focal seizures. A generalized seizure followed after the last focal seizure, and he was brought to the emergency room (ER) having been seizing continually for 30 minutes. Past medical history (PMH) is remarkable for multiple ICU admissions for the treatment of pneumonia and status epilepticus.

In the ER, he was treated with intravenous (IV) diazepam and required intubation. When his anticonvulsant levels were found to be subtherapeutic, he received additional dilantin. A chest x-ray (CXR) revealed pneumonia. Antibiotics were begun. After seizure control was obtained, he was sent to the ICU. On reaching the ICU, he was intubated but no longer seizing. He did appear pale and thin. With vigorous hydration, antibiotics, and anticonvulsants, his condition stabilized, with a return to baseline within 24 hours.

The medical diagnosis generated by the ICU staff was status epilepticus secondary to inadequate anticonvulsant levels. They attributed the subtherapeutic levels to the vomiting brought on by the pneumonia. Their plan was to treat the child for 48 hours with IV fluids and antibiotics and discharge him home once the child could tolerate oral medication and feeds.

The family, however, felt anxious and overwhelmed. In addition to their full-time jobs and normal parenting requirements, they were responsible for this child's daily chest physiotherapy (PT), oral and gastrostomy feeds, and physical therapy exercises. Their other child and their marriage were beginning to demonstrate signs of the emotional strain caused by the caretaking responsibilities.

The team arranged a meeting with the community pediatrician. Increased nursing and therapy services were organized. Regular communication with a case manager was scheduled.

Case 2: Acute Illness with Prolonged Recovery

An 8-month-old former 850-g 27-week premature infant with bronchopulmonary dysplasia, deafness, and developmental delay was transferred from a rehabilitation hospital to the acute care hospital for gastrostomy tube placement and fundoplication. At the rehabilitation hospital, a broad-based care plan had been developed to enable this particularly disorganized, medically and developmentally fragile child to tolerate the persistent stress generated by his therapeutic needs and environment. Efforts by both staff and family had recently enabled the infant to tolerate small amounts of his feeding by mouth. Unfortunately, poor growth and frequent vomiting due to documented gastroesophageal reflux necessitated surgery.

Following uneventful surgery, he was transferred to a busy pediatric ICU. His ICU course was marked by prolonged intubation. Attempts at extubation were marked by extreme agitation with increased oxygen demands. Eight days following his surgery, he was successfully extubated. Attempts to reinstate PO feeds, however, were unsuccessful, as the infant patient refused all attempts at feeding. He would not accept a nipple in his mouth and would not suck. A neurologic consult could find no new neurologic deficits. A CT scan was unchanged.

The medical diagnosis was uncomplicated fundoplication and gastrostomy tube placement. He was seen in consult by an infant development team who found a stressed child apparently overwhelmed by his environment. He actively withdrew from physical contact, especially around his face and mouth. Their diagnosis was a child without the development of a neurologic control system that would permit the inhibition of his own exaggerated response to unregulated stimulation. The loss of a previously achieved developmental attainment highlighted the child's developmental fragility and neurologic incompetence. The recommendation was for a reinstitution of previously achieved environmental supports to enhance appropriate stimulation. Family intervention that would facilitate the child's gradual return of competence was stressed, and family support was made available. A prolonged recovery of previous skills was anticipated.

Case 3: Acute Exacerbation without Return to Baseline

A 17-year-old with Duchenne's muscular dystrophy was brought to the emergency room with a 1-day history of fever, cough, and shortness of breath. Examination revealed a severely cachectic and contracted young man in respiratory distress. ABGs demonstrated respiratory failure. CXR revealed diffuse patchy infiltrates. He was intubated, started on antibiotics, and sent to the ICU. After 48 hours of mechanical ventilation and antibiotics, his respiratory condition stabilized. Hyperalimentation was begun.

The medical history was significant for multiple admissions for pneumonia within the preceding few years. In addition to his declining respiratory status, his general medical condition had continued to deteriorate. He now demonstrated a marked cardiomyopathy, severe contractures of all four extremities, scoliosis, and inanition. He lived with his mother and 18-year-old brother, also a victim of muscular dystrophy. The three family members were exceedingly close. In addition, the two brothers maintained a special, silent symbiotic bond, with both apparently suffering when one was ill. The mother was a single parent on welfare in substandard nonhandicapped housing. The patient had not attended school in over a year.

Twelve days postadmission, he remained intubated. The ICU diagnosis was inadequate ventilation secondary to end-stage neuromuscular disease. The staff was concerned with the medical complications from prolonged endotracheal intubation. They felt the situation warranted a tracheostomy for prolonged positive-pressure ventilation. They approached the mother for consent. She refused.

A team meeting was held with representatives from the medical team, the family, and social services. It was quickly apparent that the mother was concerned that the medical intervention offered would result in her son's inability to return home, with a subsequent referral to a nursing home. She and the boy requested a second opinion from a chronic illness specialist in touch with community resources.

A second opinion recommended that the ICU team attempt to wean the patient from positive- to negative-pressure ventilation and refer **both brothers** to a local residential school specializing in individuals with respiratory complications of neuromuscular disorders. It also recommended increased attempts to provide the mother with handicapped housing so that the boys could spend weekends at home. The family consented to the plan.

These three cases illustrate that acute illness, when surrounded by precariously functioning systems, may generate a disharmony that expands symmetrically outward, like the surface rings caused when a pebble is tossed in a pond, with little apparent resistance. Therefore the effect of an apparently minor physiologic disruption of one organ system may extend to other systems quite distant from the initial site. In addition, the effects realized at these distant sites may become significantly magnified by this medical ripple effect.

In case 1, a minor pulmonary disturbance initiated a major and near fatal disturbance in the apparently unrelated neurologic system, resulting in status epilepticus. In addition, a narrow and simple explanation based on a physiologic chain of events neglected the role of the family and the community in the prevention of morbidity.

In case 2, an infant with chronic respiratory disease of infancy was transferred for a surgical procedure to diminish the morbidity generated by the GI system. The operation proceeded without apparent complications. The patient, however, faltered. Two different organ systems, again unrelated, complicated the prospect of total recovery. First, a borderline oxygen-dependent child required prolonged intubation and ventilation due to agitation and carbon dioxide retention after each attempt at extubation. Second, a recently acquired developmental achievement, the tolerance of oral feeds, was lost.

Case 3 involved a dramatic, though routine but often temporary, medical intervention (e.g., a tracheostomy), causing a potentially permanent radical alteration in a family structure. When viewed in the context of a medically indicated procedure aimed at minimizing potential complications, the tracheostomy appears to be benign. However, when understood in a larger context that would necessitate the removal of a child from his home and placement in a nursing home, the procedure can be seen in an entirely different light.

Families with Chronically Ill Children

To support families with chronically ill children effectively, health care providers must identify those who are most vulnerable, differentiating between families who have become dysfunctional and those who are stressed but coping well. This requires a clear vision of the tasks for which all families must prepare, coupled with an understanding of how the structure and coping styles of families with chronically ill children differ in ways that may promote adaptation.

While it is clear that chronic illness and disability take a toll on the child and family, a deficit or dysfunction orientation by the health care provider does not take into consideration the resilience of families. Families develop highly adaptive mechanisms for coping with the stress of chronic illness, engendering strengths in the family unit.[9] Most studies indicate the many similarities among families with and without a disabled child.[10] This may indicate a need to shift the theoretical lens through which we view families with disabled children, drawing on theories of family development such as family systems and family life cycle orientations.[2] Differences in these families may often represent adaptation and family strength rather than reflecting dysfunction or deficits.

Nevertheless, stress experienced in parenting roles is clearly higher for parents of children with a disability than for parents of healthy children, and the greatest stress is generally experienced by mothers.[11] Maternal and paternal roles may become more polarized when a child is chronically ill. The father is often primarily involved with financial concerns, while the mother tends to assume the majority of responsibility for caretaking and decision making related to medical care and education. This division of responsibility creates the clinical picture of the father on the periphery of the family unit and the mother overwhelmed with the child. When such a pattern becomes so fixed that it is unresponsive to variations in levels of family stress, long-term family dysfunction may result. With some flexibility maintained, however, this pattern may be an effective coping strategy.[12] A division of labor may be necessary to meet the multiple and long-term needs of a disabled child, with each parent developing an area of subspecialty. While this plan places great demands on the mother, it may be the most efficient method for all family members to provide support for the child and simultaneously move forward in their life as a family.

Support systems play a strong role in mediating family stress by providing both emotional support and material assistance. All families make use of both formal and informal support networks, particularly during times of crisis. When in need of aid, families with chronically ill children use supports such as community agencies no more than families with healthy children, suggesting that this population may underutilize community services.

Families coping with chronic stress related to a child's illness appear to rely heavily on an informal support network comprised of extended family, friends, or select community contacts, such as clergy. These family support networks tend to be small and highly interconnected. This pattern may have inherent stresses; however, it is consistent with the structure of many of these families in which individual members assume highly specialized roles related to the child's care. Extended family members may be incorporated into this system in a manner that can be adaptive despite the high levels of stress over time. A better understanding of how these informal networks function may shed light on the reasons why families coping with chronic illness underutilize community services. This information is critical in designing programs that are responsive to the actual needs of families.

Comprehensive Care Team

Goals

We developed a consultative service, the Comprehensive Care Team (CCT), in response to the increasing medical, psychosocial, and emotional complexity of ICU cases, such as those illustrated in Table 57-1. The goals of the CCT are to provide a hospital service to address the needs of children and families with chronic illness, to provide treatment plans for patients that address long-term as well as short-term goals, to facilitate the coordination of services and disciplines, to provide education to physicians and

Table 57-1. Comprehensive care team: Goals

Provide hospital service to address needs of children and families with chronic illness.

Provide treatment plan for patients to address short-term and long-term goals.

Facilitate the coordination of services and disciplines.

Promote education around health care issues.

Facilitate patient transfer and discharge planning.

Facilitate parent participation in decision-making process.

nurses around health care issues related to chronic illness, to support the transfer of patients out of ICUs to other medical and surgical units as well as to home or residential facilities, and to assist in maintaining open channels of communication between families and health care providers.[13]

Failure of Systems versus Systems Failure

In addressing the first goal, the team participates in the planning and management of issues related to chronic disease and disability from admission through discharge. The team helps determine the key question that assists in targeting their intervention: Did the hospitalization represent a failure of systems (i.e., physiologic failure) or a systems failure (i.e., failure of health care systems)?

An early question is whether the acute episode is consistent with the natural history of the underlying chronic disease. For example, a 9-month-old oxygen- and diuretic-dependent infant with severe BPD is hospitalized in respiratory failure. In determining the course of intervention immediately following stabilization, the ICU team needs to determine whether the respiratory compromise is initiated by a potentially reversible condition, such as pneumonia, hypochloremic metabolic alkalosis secondary to chronic diuretics, or fluid overload, or from more chronic and potentially irreversible conditions such as pulmonary hypertension and cor pulmonale.

On the other side, acknowledging the complexity of intervention required by medically fragile children, the CCT will help analyze whether a breakdown in the delivery of health care interfered with the family's ability to provide necessary and sufficient preventive care. For example, did the family not receive adequate education regarding signs and symptoms of respiratory distress; did they not have access to a primary care physician capable of providing comprehensive intervention; did they have sufficient health care services to assist in caretaking; were instructions not provided in their primary language; were instructions presented to them at a time when they were too stressed and anxious to be able to listen? What environmental factors such as insurance, finances, health care access, education, or parental support contributed to the failure? The answers to these questions are vital for developing strategies to prevent future unnecessary hospitalizations with the subsequent potential for child and family morbidity.

Longitudinal versus Acute Care

A second goal is to develop treatment plans that address the issue of short-term and long-term goals. To facilitate this effort, the team determines such factors as the projected outcome of a particular disease episode, the likely time course to resolution, the possibility of complete versus partial recovery, and the disposition following the resolution of the acute episode.[14] The CCT assists the medical team by helping to develop a picture of the longitudinal impact of the acute episode on the underlying chronic disorder and to structure interventions to assist the patients' progress toward their highest level of functioning.

For example, in the case of the child with muscular dystrophy and respiratory failure, the immediate short-term goal is treatment of the respiratory failure. The treatment provided is intubation, positive-pressure ventilation, antibiotics, hyperalimentation, pulmonary toilet, and chest physical therapy. If one proceeds solely by meeting the challenge of a succession of short-term goals, the next decision point to be faced is the question of tracheostomy versus continued intubation. For this child, a tracheostomy, given the stage of his disease and the precariousness of his home situation, while successfully managing his airway and needs for pulmonary toilet, would irrevocably limit his future possibilities for independent living and family support. By adapting a more longitudinal outlook, one can see that the goal is to treat his present and future respiratory compromise in a way that will maximize his ability to live with and achieve control over his disability.

Interdisciplinary versus Subspecialty Care

The third goal is to enlist the timely collaboration of additional health care providers, such as physical and occupational therapists, speech therapists, and social workers, and help incorporate their suggestions into the overall care plan. The CCT assists in developing interventions to mitigate the effects of acute illness on top of known disease. For instance, a primary nurse may suggest ways of modifying the environment to reduce stress for patients who have lost or have not yet attained the ability to modulate their response to their environment. The nurse then organizes developmentally appropriate patient comfort measures. The team members also reinforce the philosophy that treatment is a collaborative process between health care providers and families. Collaboration is especially important when the number of health care professionals increases, to develop a team approach to ensure coordinated intervention around mutually shared goals.

Proactive versus Reactive Intervention

Stephen Hawking, brilliant physicist, author, teacher, husband, and father, who is also mute, tetraplegic, and dependent on ventilatory support, remarks casually in the introduction to his best selling book, *A Brief History of Time*,[15] that "my disability has not been a handicap." An understanding of these and related terms are essential to all who provide care to individuals with disabilities and their families. The main terms to define are *impairment*, *disability*, and *handicap*.

The World Health Organization[16] defines *impairment* as "any loss or abnormality of physiological or anatomic structure." A *disability* is defined as "any restriction or lack of ability (due to an impairment) in performing an activity in a manner or range considered normal." Therefore, a given disability may be the result of a variety of impairments. For example, the disability of blindness may be due to corneal opacity, cataract, optic nerve damage, or cortical damage. These structural abnormalities are the impairments. A handicap is the "disadvantage encountered by an individual, resulting from an impairment or disability, that limits or prevents the fulfillment of a role that is normal for that individual." Thus, the fourth goal of the CCT is to actively promote learning and discussion of issues related to chronic disease and disability among health care workers. The team teaches precepts of long-term, holistic, family-centered care to physicians and nurses to prevent disabilities leading to handicapping conditions.

Some learning and education is on a strictly practical basis, such as identifying services required by individuals with chronic disease and disability and then targeting appropriate intervention (Fig. 57-3). Additional education serves to offer some perspective regarding where a patient is on the health/illness continuum. Specifically, ICUs can help eradicate illness, the perception— whether real or apparent—on the part of the patient that something is wrong or abnormal, that is the outcome or product of active disease. However, they cannot cure disease: the deviation from standard organ functioning. A patient with diabetes, who is in the ICU in diabetic ketoacidosis, will leave the ICU with diabetes. A patient with quadriplegia from a complete cord transection will remain quadriplegic. ICU staff will continually encounter individ-

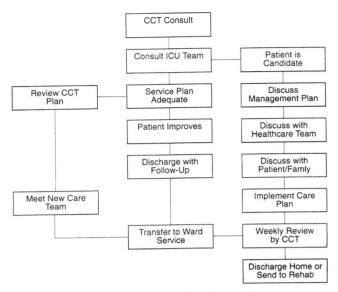

Figure 57-3. Flow chart: Comprehensive care team.

uals with these and other permanent disabilities, that is, dysfunctions that are chronic and irreversible at the physiologic level. Their disability has no bearing on the presence of medical stability.

Additional education focuses on families (parents and siblings) and intervention required to facilitate their ICU stay. When a child is a patient in an ICU, the entire family is also the patient. As an acute exacerbation of a preexisting disease disrupts the patient's function, so is it likely for the family to demonstrate signs of dysfunction early in an ICU course. Teaching in an ICU needs to focus on an understanding of the needs of this family unit as it experiences the turmoil engendered by the ICU admission.

Discharge Planning

Fifth, the CCT serves as a resource for the ICU team in the initiation of timely transfers and discharge planning. For patients admitted to the ICU for whom a continued disability is inevitable, guidelines for the determination of when the patient is medically stable and therefore ready to proceed to a next phase of intervention—whether this be transfer to an acute ward, discharge home, or discharge to a rehabilitation or chronic care facility—may often not be obvious or intuitive. The team helps to weigh the advantages of different discharge choices. Occasionally, decisions are forced to be made with less consideration of medical or nursing indicators or parameters than on the basis of a determination of allocation of scarce resources. ICUs would do well to make clearly established short- and long-term goals for patients so that determination of need for ICU beds could consistently be made by judging what is in the best interest of the patient. A patient's need to enter an ICU is clearly fairly precipitous and not subject to advanced planning. The decision on leaving an ICU should be planned and orchestrated in a manner capable of ensuring the least possible disruption.

In addition, the acute hospitalization may have significantly altered the home and community needs of the child and the family. The CCT will assist in reassessing and modifying the health care plan previously established. Even if the hospitalization has not resulted in a change in health care needs, the hospitalization will afford the team the opportunity to evaluate and modify the health care plan in effect at the time of hospitalization.

Shared Authority

Lastly, the CCT facilitates generating family-focused rather than patient-focused intervention. The CCT, cognizant of the fact that the family assumes the responsibility for daily care, coordinating multiple agencies and providers, operating and maintaining medical equipment, and remaining prepared for life-threatening emergencies, helps to develop the recognition of the central role of the family.

With this recognition comes the understanding that the moral guidelines of parental responsibility dictates that the family share in the decision-making process. For this, as was stated earlier, they need to be fully informed and their position needs complete respect and understanding. Additionally, parents of children with ill children are often accustomed to having long-standing, sharing relationships with their child's health care provider. They often negotiate health care decisions with consistent medical personnel. The occasional lack of clearly understood lines of authority in the ICU, the frequent turnover of medical personnel necessitated by the medical center delivery system, and the occasional inability to have questions answered in a consistent and unhurried manner by inconsistent and hurried personnel create unavoidable tension, anxiety, and bewilderment. The CCT's utilization of a small consistent group of providers helps to alleviate the feelings of being overwhelmed and out of control that frequently occur. The structure and intervention of the CCT more closely represents what parents have been used to outside of the ICU, and this sense of familiarity provides the comfort and reassurance that assists mutual understanding.

Physicians in roles wherein curing the patient is not the primary goal tend to operate from a broader health care base. They are generally more comfortable with methods of decision making that distribute rather than focus authority. This permits them to merge their medical intervention with that of other disciplines.

Structure

To accomplish these goals, the CCT, consisting of a physician, nurse, and social worker, each with expertise working with children and families with chronic disease and disability, was established. When consulted by the ICU team, they initially review the patient's history and the family's needs to evaluate whether the patient and family are candidates for their services. This review entails documenting services in place prior to admission, including the presence of a primary care physician, consultants, case manager, community services, and so on. They then evaluate the complexity of needs for the patient and family during the admission and consider needs relative to discharge planning, with specific attention to the community. If all services appeared in place, the CCT does not play an active role. If, however, services are required, the CCT provides a treatment plan to run in parallel to that put in place by the ICU team.

To help coordinate the two plans, a team meeting is held to discuss the CCT suggestions. The goals of the two services are defined, and individuals responsible for particular services are identified. After discussion with the family, the plan is implemented. Review of the long-term goals is the responsibility of the CCT and occurs at regular intervals, at least weekly. Once a plan is initiated, the CCT helps coordinate the plan whether the patient is transferred to home, a rehabilitation or chronic care facility, or a less acute ward. They function as the consistent thread in this sometimes patchwork quilt of care.

Treatment Plan

Case 1 illustrates how a failure of organ systems results in exacerbation of illness with erroneous blame placed on the parents' presumed faulty delivery of health care. In that case, a child who was felt to develop "too many pneumonias" was admitted in status epilepticus and discovered to have subtherapeutic anticonvulsant levels. What developed was the parents' and ICU staff's assuming adversarial positions, with each finding fault with the other. A family that had assumed responsibility for daily care, coordinating multiple agencies and providers, operating and maintaining medical equipment, and attempting to cope with life-threatening emergencies now found themselves considered to be part of the problem.

The remedy was remarkably simple. The primary care physician who had been closely involved with the child and the family since the child's birth was able to share with the ICU the extent of the family's involvement and caretaking capabilities, while also demonstrating to the parents the desire of the ICU staff to participate in the overall care and planning for the child. In addition, the social worker shared with the ICU an explanation for their perception that family dysfunction had contributed to the child's medical compromise.

Accordingly, the plans developed by the ICU were done in a collaborative fashion, taking into consideration the current framework of the family, looking to see what services could be provided to the child and family at discharge that fit all of their needs and goals. The overall focus changed from what can be done to "cure the patient" to what will enable the patient to achieve a return to the preexisting level and to prevent this disease episode from changing the baseline service needs of the patient and family and therefore furthering the degree of disability.

In case 2, the dilemma that confronts staff regards patients such as infants with BPD or head injury who cannot live without intensive care but are forced to struggle in the environment where that care is offered. It is possible that the environmental measures employed to reduce stress as well as possibly early attention to nonnutritive sucking and the judicious referral to a speech pathologist/feeding team may have reduced ventilator time and prevented the loss of recently achieved oral motor gains.

For many ICU patients, medical decisions are black and white. Decisions often fall within a gray zone, however, where several paths may be available for a particular situation. In case 3, the ICU team, appropriately concerned about the risks of prolonged intubation, suggested a tracheostomy. The mother, however, realized that she could never bring her child home again if he had a tracheostomy, due to the probable need for nocturnal positive-pressure ventilation. The mother also knew that there were no beds for ventilator-dependent children in her state, except in acute care settings. The CCT was able to suggest an alternative that provided appropriate therapy for the entire family and was acceptable to the ICU team that was primarily responsible for the patient's care.

Conclusion

The change in patients being cared for in pediatric ICUs presents a challenge to health care professionals. The dichotomy of approaches generated by health care teams with potentially contradictory goals may seem to provide more of an atmosphere for conflict than cohesion. The recognition of a commonality of purpose by all team members, however, frequently leads to resolutions that minimize morbidity and maximize the preservation of physiologic, emotional, and psychosocial functioning.

References

1. Perrin JM, Shayne MW, Bloom SR. *Home and Community Care for Chronically Ill Children.* New York: Oxford University Press, 1993.
2. Burr CK. Impact on the family of a chronically ill child. In Hobbs N, Perrin JM (eds): *Issues in the Care of Children with Chronic Illnesses.* San Francisco: Jossey-Bass, 1985.
3. Gortmaker S, Sappenfield W. Chronic childhood disorders: Prevalence and impact. *Pediatr Clin North Am* 31:3–18, 1984.
4. Office of Technology Assistance (OTA), U.S. Congress. Technology-dependent children: Hospital vs home care. Washington, DC: OTA, May, 1987.
5. American Academy of Pediatrics. Committee on Children with Disabilities: Transition of severely disabled children from hospital or chronic care facility of the community. *Pediatrics* 78:531, 1986.
6. Eisenberg L, Kleinman A. Clinical social science. In Eisenberg L, Kleinman A (eds): *The Relevance of Social Science for Medicine.* London: D. Reidel, 1981. P 13.
7. Kleinman A. *The Illness Narratives.* New York: Basic Books, 1988. P 6.
8. Engel G. The need for a new medical model: A challenge for biomedicine. *Science* 196:1246–1248, 1977.
9. Palfrey JS et al. Patterns of response in families of chronically disabled children; an assessment in five metropolitan school districts. *Am J Orthopsychiatry* 59:1, 1989.
10. Kazak A. Families with disabled children: Stress and social networks in three samples. *J Abnorm Child Psychol* 15:1, 1987.
11. Cummings, ST. The impact of the child's deficiency on the father; a study of families of mentally retarded and of chronically ill children. *Am J Orthopsychiatry* 46:2, 1976.
12. Kazak AE, Marvin RS. Differences, difficulties and adaptation: Stress and social networks in families with a handicapped child. *Fam Relations* Jan. 1984.
13. Carlson RW, Devich L, Frank R. Development of a comprehensive care team for the hopelessly ill on a University Hospital medical service. *JAMA* 259:3, 1988.
14. Gilkerson L, Gorski P, Panitz P. Hospital based intervention for preterm infants and their families. In Meisels SJ, Shonkoff JP (eds): *Handbook of Early Intervention.* Cambridge: Cambridge University Press, 1990. Pp 445–469.
15. Hawking SW. *A Brief History of Time.* Toronto: Bantam, 1988. P vii.
16. World Health Organization. International classification of impairments, disabilities, and handicaps: A manual of classification relating to the consequences of disease. Geneva: WHO, 1980.

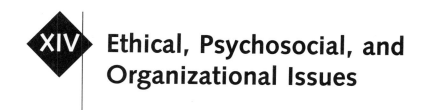

XIV Ethical, Psychosocial, and Organizational Issues

Ruth Purtilo
I. David Todres

58 ▸ Ethical Aspects of Pediatric Intensive Care

The nurturance of children, their well-being and vitality, are heralded as signs of a healthy community. The plight of children victimized by neglect, poverty, illness, and other slings and arrows of misfortune or cruelty often elicits deep sympathy, horror, and pity. For the last 25 years, the critical care medical environment has provided an additional crucial site for discussion about children: how they should be treated, what their role is in the family and larger community, and what we can reasonably expect from them. Nowhere are the ethical issues of this discussion more deeply felt and vigorously debated than in the focused environment of the pediatric intensive care unit (PICU).

The purpose of this chapter is to present basic ethical principles that can be used as guideposts in the PICU when the child, her family, caregivers, and others must maneuver through the sometimes tortuous paths of ethical deliberation. Some emerging institutional mechanisms for the resolution of such issues also are presented.

The scope of ethical issues in the PICU includes almost all that apply to critical care for any age group.[1] Still, there is reason for caution about a wholesale appeal to ethics discussions and literature not specifically focused to the pediatric context. For example, in many situations, the issue that would face an adult patient is more complicated for a young person who has never been legally competent to give consent **and** whose legal and moral status intrinsically is linked to the parent-child relationship. These and other "facts of life" about children narrow dramatically the number of analogies that easily can be drawn from positions taken regarding ethical issues in adult critical care medicine. Another challenge arises because media emphasis is on critical care for **newborns**: Baby Doe, Baby Faye, Baby M, and Baby K are just a few of the "cases" introduced into the professional and public consciousness in recent years. While their situations can help to provide important guidelines for pediatric intensive care situations, discussions skewed to the uniqueness of newborn life-and-death decisions also may lead to inaccurate or unhelpful conclusions when the issue is older children.

Ethical Principles and Practical Applications

Not Harming (The Principle of Nonmaleficence)

Medical professionals long have adopted as a basic moral principle: "First do no harm to the patient (Primum non nocere)." In modern interpretations of this general principle, a continuum of activity is inferred that includes not inflicting evil or harm, preventing it, and removing it.[2] Beauchamp and Childress limit the principle to the first activity, namely, not directly inflicting harm, on the basis that the **legal duty** is most easily interpreted in this limited fashion.[3] For example, the crucial distinction between allowing a patient to die and directly causing death is more easily understood in terms of nonmaleficence in the narrow definition.

Within the everyday practice of pediatric intensive care, the principle has many applications. Harm induced by long periods of isolation from family and loved ones, sleep deprivation, invasive interventions and restraints, and by pain and suffering associated with these conditions should be recognized as such and kept to the barest minimum possible. Many health professionals also experience a moral obligation to prevent and remove harm whenever possible. For example, in a presentation entitled, "Ethical Decision-making in the Face of Pain and Suffering in Treatment and Non-treatment of Children," Brodeur[4] highlighted several ethical obligations associated with pain in young patients that readers will recognize, among them the following:

1. Pain . . . must be properly relieved and to the extent possible prophylactically treated.
2. Better means to understand the "subjective" experience of pain in children from neonates to the age of "articulation" need to be developed.
3. Families must be educated and involved in pain management issues/techniques.
4. When the patient is dying, pain management therapies must provide as much pain relief as possible so that the patient may die comfortably, taking care not to overstep the fine line between such management and killing.

Because the PICU involves many procedures that directly cause pain or other kinds of harm, the balance of benefits to harms becomes a key criterion by which to judge whether the harmful act is ethically permissible. The ethical principle of "beneficence" described acts designed to bring about positive good or benefit to the patient.

Doing What Benefits the Patient (The Principle of Beneficence)

Health professionals can affect dramatically the well-being of a patient. Benefitting the patient is a professional duty. Of course, as the saying goes, "The devil lies in the details." For instance, some have treated preservation of life as the absolute good and death as an absolute harm to be prevented. But experience in the PICU shows that conflict arises in practice when the presumption to save life (a good) requires interventions that also are perceived by some members of the unit as creating undue suffering. In the history of health care, "doing everything possible" was usually consistent with doing what was best for the patient. The duty of beneficence required doing everything possible. Today's technological successes, a paradigm example of which is the ICU, have made available so many interventions that different questions arise: Should we be starting this procedure on this child? or Shouldn't we really be talking with the family about stopping our interventions? More discussion regarding these vital life-and-death questions is resumed later in this chapter.

Opportunities to express beneficence are by no means limited to life-and-death situations in the PICU. For instance, family support of the child is crucial. An increasing literature on the importance of acknowledging the complex interactions of family systems, of providing respite to families, and of education for family members about their child's condition are contextual considerations not directly related to the medical intervention of the patient but that substantially do affect her quality of life in the PICU.[5]

Even peer support in this high-stress setting can yield positive results for the patient. Rushton,[6] addressing caregiver suffering in the critical care setting, observes,

Nurses describe intense emotions in response to their clinical encounters. Many describe feelings of compassion toward their patients and the plight they must endure . . . In contrast, prolonged, unrecognized suffering [of the caregivers themselves] may be detrimental. Many critical care nurses experience a variety of conflicts as they carry out their care-giving roles.

Beneficence requires that everyone be working together for the well-being of the child. The fact that children are not simply "little adults" sometimes is forgotten, but the heritage they share with the adults who mold their existence sometimes also is neglected. The child's age, home environment, and religious and cultural heritage will influence her responses.

Truthtelling (The Principle of Veracity)

Veracity has long been treated as a principle that leads to the well-being of everyone involved.[7] Current thinking is that accurate information disclosed in a caring and supportive setting usually enables a patient to exercise more control over his life as well as experience the comfort of being able to address serious issues raised by the situation. Harm that ensues from "telling the truth" usually is a result of poor timing, or lack of sensitivity regarding the way the information was shared, or the fact that it became a precursor to abandonment.

Understandably, most ethics debates on this issue focus on terminally ill children. Pediatricians and parents may not be in agreement about this, though the majority seems in agreement with Bartholome's conclusion that "children do not need to be shielded or protected from the truth. Furthermore, such efforts actually make things more difficult because they cut children off from the people who can help them understand and deal with what they are experiencing."[8] He suggests that truthfulness with children involves much more than verbally providing information. Giving them the "facts" only about their condition is inadequate and can be dangerous. He suggests the following guidelines:

1. Be aware of what you are doing. Children pay more attention to what grown-ups do than to what they say.
2. Be sure that you really are ready to be honest with them.
3. Let them set the agenda for the conversation.
4. Be willing to answer any and all questions, and wait patiently for the questions to come.
5. Finally, see your task as assisting them in their efforts to become aware of their own reality.

The idea of being truthful with children sometimes is confounded by the fact that parents generally have the legal responsibility to act in accordance with their child's best interests. The health care team must make every effort to work with both the family and the child. A rule of thumb is to inform the parents or guardian and to work with them to bring the child into the conversation within a supportive context of family and professionals. When the child is not in a position to participate, extra care must be taken to work with the family to assure that the child's best interests are being served.

In summary, the duty of veracity is to act truthfully and forthrightly so as to instill the patient's and family's trust. This posture and conduct will serve everyone well in the difficult decisions surrounding the child's stay in the PICU. Because trust is one form of benefit for the patient, truthtelling carried out with sensitivity can be thought of as beneficence through the conveying of honest information.

Meeting Reasonable Expectations (The Principle of Fidelity)

Fidelity means, literally, "faithfulness." Sometimes it is translated as "loyalty." To what or whom must the doctor be faithful or loyal?

The accepted ethical and legal standards of professional medical practice provide one important general guideline for what faithfulness entails. Sometimes professional groups create statements designed to describe conduct that is appropriate for a particular group. For instance, a relevant document for families whose children are in PICUs, as well as for professionals caring for such patients, is the 1994 "Guidelines on Forgoing Life-sustaining Medical Treatment," published by the American Academy of Pediatrics.[9] The document states that the physicians' and other health care givers' primary focus of loyalty must be to the patient, then delineates rights, conditions of respect, and processes that honor that loyalty.

David Smith[10] addresses the issue of faithfulness or loyalty from the standpoint of its role as an ordering principle in the Western religious traditions. Loyalty to patients can be discerned only by understanding what it means to be loyal to any other person:

Loyalty to other persons involves care for them of the best possible sort, and changing the forms of care as needs change. It means recognizing that the time comes when we can care for them no longer, only bid them Godspeed.

Loyalty, he says, requires us to think about the things that a person lives for, what makes the person tick, but:

[T]he striking thing about babies . . . is that . . . they have never had a chance to care about or live for anything. They have not established a style of life or character.

The posture the health professional must assume, he concludes, is to work for the best that we imagine life will offer them in the future and be prepared to shift our focus of support as their needs change. Throughout, they can be offered respect, comfort for their body, and due process. This is the minimum of what the duty of fidelity requires.

Providing an Opportunity for the Patient's Voice to Be Heard (The Principle of Autonomy)

The patient's right to autonomy or self-determination has come to be accepted as a legitimate moral principle to be placed in the balance with health professionals' independent judgement about how to prevent harm or do good for the patient.

The doctrine of informed consent has made it very clear that a patient's right to autonomy includes a competent patient's right to refuse as well as to participate in any treatment. At the same time, the physical and emotional extremity of an ICU patient's condition creates barriers to her involvement through the recognized mechanisms of informed consent. This challenge is exacerbated when the patient is a child.

The major ethics discussion focuses on whether children should be involved formally, informally, or at all in the ongoing process of decision making. Legally, the parents or other guardian are responsible, but hardly ever does the ethical discussion end there. Obviously, one variable is the age and emotional stability and maturity of the child. Even the law makes accommodation for the possibility of "mature minors," invoking a common-law rule that allows select adolescents to give informed consent. The effort to assist all child patients "to become better decision makers by involving them in decisions to a degree appropriate to their current capacity" seems consistent with the ethical position of a patient's right to autonomy. Authors holding this developmental view of informed consent put the responsibility on the pediatrician to assess the patient's capacity for reasoning, understanding, and the degree of voluntariness experienced by the young patient.[11,12]

Sometimes a focus on autonomy and its emphasis on **individual** authority neglects to highlight the importance of keeping all members of the primary decision-making unit informed. Discussions about consent with children should always be conducted with the parents' sensitivities also in mind, and in such a way as to not disrupt strong parent-child support systems.

The Fair Allocation of Resources (The Principle of Justice)

The view that health care is a good provided in response to basic areas of human need—and as such should be made available to all who experience deprivation in those areas—provides a sound basis for the discussion of justice in health care. The guidelines for allocation of health care should be responsive to the essential nature of this good and, as far as the supply allows, assure that all receive a fair share of the good.[13] Obviously, as the supply decreases, the amount of deprivation overall will increase. Until there is dire scarcity of the good, withholding of needed interventions (i.e., appropriate critical care) should not be allowed to exist. Today's trends toward capitated health care systems and managed care has sometimes placed cost considerations ahead of considerations of need. These trends signal an introduction of new thinking about the role of justice in health care.

Traditionally, ICU physicians, nurses, and others have focused on the patient's health care needs, not the cost of the intervention, in determining what is appropriate for patients.

Most health care resources are in moderately scarce supply, but occasionally in the ICU, resources are in such short supply that dire scarcity exists. For example, at times, PICU beds are full. In addition, on a broader scale, there is an increasing shortage of health care personnel for ICUs. Burnout of physician and nursing personnel in ICU areas places limits on the availability of health care professionals to care for the critically ill.[14] In situations of dire scarcity, some persons may not be able to have a resource, not even a life-saving one. This is a terrible situation for everyone involved, and it should be treated as a tragedy.

If time, personnel, supplies, or bed space are in severely short supply in the PICU, the decision not to offer this valuable, often life-saving, resource should be based on the following guidelines of constraint:

1. Is the decision to exclude persons in need a "last resort" move?

2. Are the limits of due proportion being honored? (Is the least hurtful policy being adopted?)

3. Is the action being carried out with just intentions?

4. What of value is being saved by this necessary course of action?

The American Academy of Pediatrics Committee on Health Care Financing focused its comment on "the necessity of financing systems to maximize access to and ensure the quality of comprehensive patient care."[15] There is growing concern that inequalities which exist based on race and income are being felt most by children in the United States.[16,17] Therefore, the Academy Committee's position mandates the basic demand of the dictate of justice, namely to maximize access for all children, taking into account the differential treatment that will help assure that the quality of care remains high for each child.

In summary, six ethical principles help to guide ethical decision making in the pediatric intensive care setting. Each taken alone provides a necessary but not sufficient basis for decision making in the face of difficult ethical issues. The challenge is to balance the weight of the principles within the context of each patient's experience. The ethical act may not reflect an ideal resolution, but will meet the test of providing the greatest balance of benefits over harms for the patient and patient's loved ones.

In the next section, we apply the reasoning embodied in several of the principles as we address ethical dimensions of life-sustaining treatment.

Life-Sustaining Treatment in the Pediatric Intensive Care Unit

One of the most regularly encountered ethical problems in the PICU is the question of how far to go in providing life-sustaining interventions. As discussed earlier, decisions to forego life-sustaining treatment invoke the principle of beneficence. The health professional should do what is best for the patient. The good of continued life is weighed with another good, the relief of suffering. But when two goods are in conflict, which good should carry the greater weight? In today's health care environment, the principle of patient autonomy also is invoked to help answer this perplexing question. Most ethicists and clinicians would argue that the duty of nonmaleficence requires that the patient's death not be directly induced to decrease suffering. However, many recent examples of children whose lives hung in the balance have highlighted that there is a fine line between allowing a patient to die comfortably and inducing death.

The need for some more specific guides for conduct that remain true to the spirit of the principles, but give more direction for actual decisions, becomes readily apparent when the clinician, parents, children, and others are involved in life-and-death situations.

Ethically Permitted Conduct

The traditional duties of health care providers, such as beneficence and fidelity, have been thought of as ethically mandated (prescribed) conduct, while nonmalificence points to conduct that is prohibited (proscribed). With the rise in the number of possible life-prolonging interventions, however, a third area of consideration, ethical permissibility, has been introduced into analysis of ethical issues to provide breadth to the range of decisions that can be justified. Ethically permissible conduct is not activity that falls outside of the traditional duties. Rather, it provides a sphere of conduct that best approaches honoring the duties in the complex situation that faces the clinician and patient or family.

For instance, with a patient who needs permanent ventilatory support, the time may come when clinicians, families, or others will reconsider whether the treatment is providing any benefit to the patient. Patients can be maintained for days or even months or years on mechanical ventilation. Almost no one would want to return to a time when such interventions were not available. However, the initial enthusiastic response to the use of such machines has been tempered by cautions. Reiser reflects,[18]

In the debate about what should happen to Karen Quinlan, the respirator became a symbol of both the advanced technology of modern health care and the ambivalence toward it that many were coming to feel. Once turned on, the respirator seemed autonomous, its power to save life matched by its power to torment life.

And so the ventilator, initially welcomed as a means of enhancing the possibilities for a healthier life, has also become a powerful symbol of ambivalence for health professionals and patients alike. Two ethical components of good medicine are called into question: cost-effectiveness and, more importantly, the quality of life that this intervention creates for the patient and patient's family.[19] If the ventilator can reverse the underlying pathology, thereby acting solely as a bridge, almost everyone would describe the intervention as ethically mandatory. If from the patient's point of view the ventilator improves the quality of the individual's life, that too would be judged mandatory. If, however, the treatment only adds burdens to the patient without reversing the illness or improving quality of life, discontinuing the treatment may be permitted but neither prescribed nor prohibited, as long as certain other conditions are present.[1]

Withdrawing the ventilator should be accompanied by sedation on the principle that promoting comfort for the dying child becomes the primary goal of medical management.[20] Sedatives and analgesics should be titrated to **adequately** meet these needs, although the effect may hasten death through respiratory depression. This side effect of the drug should not be confused (as sometimes happens) with active euthanasia. At times, a decision to withdraw mechanical ventilation is made when the patient is pharmacologically paralyzed (e.g., pancuronium). At this time, withdrawal is seen by some as inappropriate until the muscle relaxant effects have been reversed so that death ensues as a result of the patient's respiratory failure and not the muscle relaxant. Some clinicians see reversal of muscle relaxants as "illogical," as the withdrawal of the respirator will inevitably lead to the death of the child. However, the paralyzing drugs are not promoting the "comfort" of the child in the way sedatives and analgesics do. Although patients receiving neuromuscular blocking agents are also receiving sedatives and/or opioids, it may be impossible to predict whether the paralyzed patient is comfortable and receiving adequate amounts of sedatives/opioids.[20,21] It is interesting to note that in a survey, a number of physicians and nurses erroneously believed pancuronium had analgesic and anxiolytic properties.[22]

Another example is the question of artificial administration of nutrition and hydration.[23–26] Traditionally, food and water for the patient have not been viewed as "medical treatment." However, today it is possible to provide nutrition and hydration when the patient is unable to do so naturally, and in forms (TPN, IV) not interpreted by the public as food and water per se. Because of the real symbolic and even religious significance of food and water, some view the provision of nutrition and hydration as always necessary, in spite of the method of administration. Painful sensations of hunger and thirst are concerns and should always be taken into account no matter what else is acknowledged. Some consider the fact that sometimes nutrition and hydration are artificially maintained and therefore, in those cases, perceive them as medical treatment. The courts in some states recently have supported this view, treating them as no different from other forms of medical

intervention. Thus, under certain circumstances, it is legally and ethically permissible to withhold artificial means of nutrition and hydration.[26]

Ordinary and Extraordinary Means

The key to understanding the notion of ordinary and extraordinary treatment is that **any intervention may become extraordinary.** The following statement, used by an ethics committee in the United States, provides a concise summary of the notion[27]:

Ordinary treatments are mandatory from a moral point of view; extraordinary treatments are optional or contrary to the patient's best interests. Distinguishing one from the other requires the use of two tests. First, does continued use of the intervention offer any reasonable hope of benefit to the patient? Second, if it does offer any reasonable hope of benefit, do the benefits offered significantly outweigh the burdens caused by the treatment?

To illustrate the utility of the ordinary-extraordinary notion in a life-support situation, consider the case of a 4-year-old patient who suffers a near-drowning episode and requires mechanical ventilation and other life-support measures in the PICU. The ordinary-extraordinary distinction would require consideration of the following questions, viewing the patient not only as a bundle of symptoms but also as a person undergoing an ordeal:

1. First, what can medicine do to cure the patient?
2. Taking the larger picture of the patient's life, and not just the idea that "he is breathing," can the ventilatory support be judged as providing any help at all?
3. What burdens are being incurred in order to realize the benefits?
4. How great are the burdens in relationship to the benefits (are the burdens grossly **disproportionate** to the positive ends that are realized by insisting on continued ventilatory support)?
5. If there is no hope of benefit, or if the burdens greatly outweigh the benefits, how can the process of withdrawal be accomplished in the most humane way possible?

The primary contribution of the ordinary-extraordinary distinction is that it helps to place the intervention squarely within the context of the patient's life and values, and to move thinking toward consideration of what the realistic (and therefore morally justifiable) limits of medicine are.

Futility

Medical futility is another technical way of talking about the fact that sometimes there is no reasonable hope of benefitting that patient **as a person,** even though a specific medical intervention might have a positive physiologic effect in maintaining life. More recently, the thinking has been that the concept of futility applies only to those interventions that have no known positive physiologic effect. The ethical tension arises when the doctor believes there may be some physiologic benefit, but the patient is not served well by the intervention. (In this regard it is identical to the first criterion of determining extraordinary treatment, namely, that it has no hope of benefitting the person.) In such cases, the patient's wishes to limit intervention justifiably would be honored, even though death would follow. Truog et al. state that "the notion of futility generally fails to provide an ethically coherent ground for limiting life-sustaining treatment, except in circumstances in which narrowly defined physiologic futility can be plausibly involved."[28]

The idea of medical futility carries the debate further because it gives the doctor permission to withhold or stop measures that under different circumstances would be indicated and beneficial, **and to make this decision without seeking the patient's (or family's) input and consent.** In the United States, where the competent patient's right not only to refuse treatment but also to participate in determining limits of life-saving intervention, is deeply etched into the public mind, the idea of futility seems to be shifting the sole locus of authority back to the physician. While such a return to medical paternalism surely would be met with resistance, the idea is being met with interest by both professional and laypeople because of the fear that the physician may feel compelled to continue interventions beyond the limits of benefit. In the PICU context, the physician's considered judgment that something is medically futile may save a small patient from being sustained indefinitely on machines, with little quality of life.

The futility debate has emerged in a health care setting in which the availability of interventions themselves is experienced by practitioners as ethical mandates to use them, a situation that has been called the "technological imperative."[29] The professional's perception that availability entails a moral claim is compounded when patients and their families believe that "the machine will help when the professional can't."[30] Because it is very difficult for parents to let go of the hope that their child may survive and thrive, the situation is especially common in PICUs. To complicate the situation further, each of a severely ill child's signs and symptoms may present one at a time, so that each individual intervention may seem to fall within usual and customary practices and procedures of medicine. The situation can be summarized accordingly:

At some time, almost all . . . professionals today are drawn into artful "spot-welding" attempts to mend the damage as each problem appears to spring from the very seam of the previous one, even as the dignity of the *person* continues to crumble under the activity. Clearly the perplexity is exacerbated because, as each new complication arises, the incentive to proceed assumes the power of a moral claim.[31]

Weijer and Elliott state that "futility can be used as an ethical trump card to deny demands for treatment made under the authority of patient autonomy." In addition ". . . to do what is best for patients and avoid treatment that is extravagantly expensive, futility offers the comforting advantage of pushing financial considerations to the side."[32]

Ethical Decision-Making Mechanisms and the Pediatric Intensive Care Unit

We have emphasized that the patient's well-being or "best interests" is the standard by which ethical decision making should be measured. In this section, we present some mechanisms that have been developed to help assure that the patient's best interests are realized.

Anyone who works in the PICU setting knows how stressful life-and-death decisions are for the family. Parents are often in a state of shock, angry, or feeling so guilty and depressed that they are unable to think clearly. They may make overly hasty decisions that are inappropriate or be paralyzed in their thinking and unable to arrive at a reasoned judgment. Parents as decision-makers for their child should exhibit the following guidelines[33]:

1. Commitment to the child's best interests
2. Adequate knowledge and information concerning diagnosis, treatment options, and prognosis
3. Emotional stability
4. Ability to make reasoned judgments

The staff, too, sometimes feels overwhelmed with the enormity of the consequences of its decisions and burdened by the tragedy and sorrow of the situations. In spite of these extreme circumstances, thoughtful and compassionate decision making is the norm. Consultation among professionals is—or should be—an ongoing part of the decision making. Not only physicians but also nurses, social workers, and other team members are necessary sources of information, perspective, and sharing of the burdens when so much is at stake in a decision. For the most part, families and the health professionals' team working together are able to agree on a course of action that appears to support the highest ideals and values of good health care. At the same time, conflicts sometimes arise, and then professionals must accept the burden of accountability for what happens to a young patient.

Fleischman et al. reported on the care of gravely ill children following a meeting of pediatricians and other professionals addressing this issue and seeking a principled approach.[34] The needs and interests of the child were seen as the central focus and involving the child to a degree consistent with developmental maturity. Benefits and burdens need to be carefully weighed with regard to the child's best interests and with the parents as natural guardians for their children, having great latitude in making decisions for them. It was explained that parental decisions were not absolute, and professionals needed to maintain an independent obligation to protect the child's best interests.

Two resources available to health professionals, patients, and families in complex situations are ethics consultations and ethics committees. These resources should not be a substitute for exhaustive and compassionate efforts to work out an acceptable resolution with the patient, family, and loved ones. As a "last resort" measure, the courts may be required to adjudicate.

Ethics Consultations

Ethics consultations are available at major health centers. When there is an ethics consultation service, the ethics consultant is a resource person who can help to conduct an in-depth analysis of the conflicting moral obligations, rights, responsibilities, and other ethical considerations that have bearing on the situation. Such a person can also provide reassurance that the pertinent ethical considerations have been taken into account and help to reason about the moral compromises inherent in alternative courses of action.[35]

Ethics consultants provide expert advice at the request of health professionals. To our knowledge, no consultation services have involved consults initiated by minors, though in some environments family members may initiate a consultation on behalf of a child's problem. The family may be invited by the clinician to the meeting between the ethics consultant and health professionals. The ethics consultant is similar to other consultants in providing expert advice, but differs from the clinical consultant insofar as the ethicist processes the ethical content of a decision but is not involved in the actual implementation of the decision itself. In the end, the physician, working with patient, family, and the other health professionals makes a final judgment about the course of action.[36]

Ethics Committees

Ethics committees are a widely established mechanism for assisting health professionals, families, and patients in complex decisions. Ethics committees originally were recommended by the New Jersey Supreme Court in the aftermath of the Karen Quinlan case. This court suggested a "prognosis committee" that would help clinicians assess appropriate levels of interventions in ethically charged situations, such as Ms. Quinlan's.[37] The ethics committee brings with it the advantage of having several members, each with their unique expertise and perspective.

Ethics committees as a mechanism in the neonatal and pediatric care settings became familiar to many through the so-called Baby Doe Case in 1982. Baby Doe, an infant with Down syndrome and an intestinal obstruction, became the focus of nationwide attention when surgery was withheld at the parents' request, and Baby Doe died. Along with the long public and professional reflection on what happened to this child was the Department of Health and Human Services' strong recommendation that health care institutions establish Infant Bioethics Review Committees. These committees are designed to assess ethical implications of complex clinical decisions involving newborns.[38] As a result, many pediatrics units also have established similar committees.[39]

Ethics committees may serve one or more purposes: advice on cases prospectively, retrospective review of one or more groups of similar cases, the development and review of ethics policy regarding standards of care, and education of health personnel, to name some. Committees vary in their composition but often include primary physicians, consultants in specific areas, nurses, social workers, ethicists, lawyers, theologians, and representatives of the community.[40]

The Courts

Concern over malpractice litigation may be an overriding factor in the decision to withdraw life-sustaining therapy, such as mechanical ventilation. In a survey study by Asch et al., one in five physicians considered potential legal ramifications in their therapy of the patient, although courts have upheld decisions to withdraw therapy when the decision is appropriate and made in good faith.[41] Glantz has stated, "Almost everything else physicians do (or do not do) puts them at greater risk of legal liability than withdrawing or withholding treatment in appropriate cases."[42] Some physicians appear confused regarding legal requirements on their care of the critically ill. According to Clarke, this confusion arises because there are competing legal standards co-existing (i.e., federal and state standards).[43] Clark further states there is "an emerging state legal standard that is flexible and subjective and allows quality of life analysis because it is based on parental authority. This standard conflicts with the federal standard."[43] There is a legal presumption that the parents' decisions are reasonable. However, this can be challenged if indicated.

The courts have become a mechanism for helping to arbitrate in decisions wherein the child's best interests appear not to be the focus of a parent's or guardian's decision. Sometimes, an ethics committee will recommend to the hospital or administration that they pursue judicial guidance through the vehicle of the courts or work with state child protection agencies.

The courts sometimes have been seen as eager to become involved in health care decisions. We have found them to be reluctant to do so, for good reason: They are often without the appropriate facts and background to make a considered decision; there is almost always a press of time; and these decisions fall to them on top of their other workload. Today, educational courses for probate and other judges are being offered through the National Judicial College and other organizations.

When a judge does become involved, the responsibility of the physician is to provide the courts with as much accurate data as possible and to utilize all team members who have relevant perspectives. Family members should not be completely neglected in these situations, though the impetus for involving the courts is often that parents are uninvolved or appear not to have the child's best interests in mind.

One situation in which the courts not infrequently are resorted to is when the family is Jehovah's Witnesses and blood transfusions are required for the treatment of their critically ill child. The courts usually recognize the Jehovah's Witness's right to refuse blood transfusions based on the principle of autonomy and self-determination. In addition, this right is supported by the right to religious freedom. In the case of the child, however, the principle of autonomy cannot be applied, because the child does not yet have the necessary decision-making capacity. Parents, then, cannot apply their religious principles to their child's care when there is a risk of morbidity or death from failure to administer the necessary blood transfusions. In this situation, the courts have deemed that state interests on behalf of the child outweigh the rights of the parents. Should this problem be anticipated, it is best to deal with the issue at that time and proceed through the appropriate local process for the protection of the child.

Just as ethical principles often need further interpretation in actual situations, so do areas of judicial intervention. The health professional usually is the crucial link to the judicial system and can help to clarify the situation in ways that will facilitate appropriate interpretation of judicial guidelines.

Policy Issues

Today, with increasing costs, a plethora of high technology options, the saving of low-birth-weight newborns, and society's concern about the humaneness of some of our interventions, health care providers must be both public educators and active participants in the policy process. This goes well beyond the traditional notion of the health professional's role. Furthermore, it further stresses the energies of health professionals in the PICU, many of whom are already working at near maximum capacity. However, in an economy and societal mind set where the best interests of children sometimes appear to be compromised, health professionals as a group must find ways to impact legislation. Two ways in which the health professional can foster ethically supportable policies include:

The encouragement of studies distinguishing groups of patients for whom the utility of PICU support is highly beneficial from those for whom it is only questionable. Many such studies are available today, however, that are valuable in assessing populations, and more data are needed to assist us in making decisions for the individual patient. These findings can help to assist in supporting beneficial practices and culling out unnecessary expenditures.

The support of research designed to refine present mechanisms of intervention. A difficulty is that in the case of children, research studies must be limited by the inability of a child to give informed consent. Children correctly are deemed to need added protection. The prime consideration in any research with children should be that it is not against the interests of the individual child. Developmental issues compound informed consent problems all patients/subjects face.[44,45]

Involvement in policy comes from the desire to help foster a high quality of life for patients, as well as to not allow cost to be used as an excuse to provide poorer care to some groups that are less valued to society. The ethical criteria governing the clinician's judgment about becoming involved in policy should always be the patient's medical need, human responses to those needs, and the promise of technical responsiveness to the intervention. Research about and involvement in policies can further refine the criteria for cost-effective uses of PICU interventions.

References

1. Todres ID. Ethical dilemmas in critical care medicine. *Probl Anesthesiol* 3:337–345, 1989.
2. Frankena W. *Ethics* (2nd ed). Englewood Cliffs, NJ: Prentice Hall, 1973.
3. Beauchamp T, Childress J. Nonmaleficence. In *Principles of Biomedical Ethics* (4th ed). New York: Oxford University Press, 1994.
4. Brodeur D. Ethical decision making in the face of pain and suffering in treatment and non-treatment of children. Presented at conference "Ethics Committees and the Young: Families, Hospitals and the Courts Trying to Do the Right Thing." American Society of Law, Medicine, and Ethics, St. Louis, MO, May 1994.
5. Nelson JL. Taking families seriously. *Hastings Cent Rep* 22:6–12, 1992.
6. Rushton CH. Ethical issues in critical care: Caregiver suffering in critical care nursing. *Heart Lung* 21:303–306, 1992.
7. Beauchamp T, Childress J. Veracity. In *Principles of Biomedical Ethics* (4th ed). New York: Oxford University Press, 1994.
8. Bartholome W. Care of the dying child: The demands of ethics. *Second Opinion* 18:25–39, 1993.
9. Committee on Bioethics. Guidelines on foregoing life sustaining medical treatment. *Pediatrics* 93:532–536, 1994.
10. Smith D. Our religious traditions and the treatment of infants. In Murray TH, Caplan A (eds): *Which Babies Shall Live?* Clifton, NJ: Humana Press, 1985.
11. King N, Cross A. Children as decision makers: Guidelines for pediatricians. *J Pediatr* 115:10–16, 1989.
12. Fost N. Parents as decision makers for children. *Primary Care* 13:285–293, 1986.
13. Daniels N. Health care needs and distributive justice. *Philos Public Affairs* 10:146–152, 1981.
14. Orlowski JP, Gulledge AD. Critical care stress and burnout. *Crit Care Clin* 2:173, 1986.
15. Committee on Child Health Care Financing, American Academy of Pediatrics. Principles of child health care financing. *Pediatrics* 91:506–507, 1993.
16. Elders JL. Portrait of inequality. *J Health Care Underserved* 4:153–162, 1993.
17. Marquis MS, Long S. Caring for the uninsured and underinsured. *JAMA* 268:3473–3477, 1992.
18. Reiser SJ, Anbar M (eds). *The Machine at the Bedside: Strategies for using Technology in Patient Care.* Cambridge: Cambridge University Press, 1984.
19. Purtilo RB. Ethical issues in the treatment of chronic ventilator-dependent patients. *Arch Physical Med Rehabil* 67:718–721, 1986.
20. Truog RD, Arnold JH, Rockoff MA. Sedation before ventilator withdrawal: Medical and ethical considerations. *J Clin Ethics* 2:127–129, 1991.
21. Faber-Langendown K. The clinical management of dying patients receiving mechanical ventilation. A survey of physician practice. *Chest* 106:880–888, 1994.
22. Loper KA et al. Paralyzed with pain: The need for education. *Pain* 37:315–316, 1989.
23. Paris JJ. When burdens of feeding outweigh benefits. *Hastings Cent Rep* 13:17, 1983.
24. Annas GH. Fashion and freedom: When artificial feeding should be withdrawn. *Am J Public Health* 75:685, 1985.
25. Curran WJ. Defining appropriate medical care. Providing nutrients and hydration for the dying. *N Engl J Med* 313:940, 1985.
26. American Medical Association. Statement of the council on ethical and judicial affairs. March 15, 1986.
27. Ethics Committee Statement. St. Joseph Hospital, Omaha, NE, 1993.
28. Truog RD, Brett AS, Frader J. The problem with futility. *N Engl J Med* 326:1560–1564, 1992.
29. Barger-Lux MJ, Heaney R. For better or worse: The technological imperative in health care. *Soc Sci Med* 22:1313–1320, 1986.
30. Purtilo R, Sorrel J. The ethical dilemmas of a rural physician. *Hastings Cent Rep* 16:24–31, 1986.
31. Purtilo R, O'Donohue WJ. Resources for medical decision-making in situations of high uncertainty. *Nebr Med J* 70:277–280, 1992.
32. Weijer C, Elliott C. Pulling the plug on futility. *Br Med J* 310:683–684, 1995.
33. Childress JF. Protecting handicapped newborns. In Milunsky A, Annas GH (eds): *Genetics and the Law. III.* New York: Plenum, 1985.
34. Fleischman AR et al. Caring for gravely ill children. *Pediatrics* 94:433–439, 1994.
35. Purtilo R. Ethics consultations in the hospital. *N Engl J Med* 311:983–986, 1984.
36. Purtilo R. On the concept of consultation. In Fletcher J, Quist N, Jonsen A (eds): *Ethics Consultation in Health Care.* Ann Arbor, MI: Health Administration Press, 1989.
37. Re: Quinlan; Supreme Court, State of New Jersey. 70 NJ 10, 355A, 2d 647, 669. 1976.
38. 49 *Federal Register* 1662, 1984.
39. Fost N. Infant care review committees in the aftermath of baby Doe. In Caplan A, Blank L, Merrick J (eds): *Compelled Compassion.* New York: Humana, 1992.
40. American Hospital Association. Guidelines: Hospital committees on biomedical ethics. Chicago: American Hospital Association, 1984.
41. Asch DA, Hansen-Flaschen T, Lanken PN. Decisions to limit or continue life-sustaining treatment by critical care physicians in the United States: Conflicts between physicians' practices and patients' wishes. *Am J Respir Crit Care Med* 151:288–292, 1995.
42. Glantz LH. Withholding and withdrawing treatment: The role of the criminal law. *Law Med Health Care* 15:231–241, 1987.
43. Clarke FI. Intensive care treatment decisions: The roots of our confusion. *Pediatrics* 94:98–101, 1994.
44. Nicholson RH (ed). *Medical Research with Children: Ethics, Law, and Practice.* Oxford: Oxford University Press, 1986.
45. Susman EJ, Dorn LD, Fletcher JC. Participation in biomedical research: The consent process as viewed by children, adolescents, young adults, and physicians. *J Pediatr* 121:547–552, 1992.

I. David Todres

Morris Earle, Jr.

Michael S. Jellinek

59 ▶ Communicating with Families in the Pediatric Intensive Care Unit

Robert Tuttle Morris wrote, "It is the human touch after all that counts for most in our relationship with our patients."[1] Intensive care units (ICUs) apply advanced technology with increasing numbers of diagnostic tests and therapeutic procedures with increasing subspecialization. This setting, however, contributes to a less personal environment where communication skills have become neglected, leading to a feeling of dissatisfaction with communication between the doctor, patient, and family.[2] This chapter reviews communication in the pediatric ICU (PICU), including observations of what families prefer and ways to improve our dialogue with them and in turn our ability to care for their children. We emphasize communication with the parents because the child is often too ill or too young to participate. However, the child should be included whenever this is possible.

How good a job do we do at communicating with families in the PICU? In a recent study at our institution, most parents reported being well satisfied with the care their child received; however, many identified problems with communicating.[3] Problems cited included delays in communication, insufficient updates on change in status or tests needed, lack of understanding about visiting policy and why restrictions existed, conflicting information from different members of the medical team, lack of clarity about who was in charge, physicians who seemed abrupt or insensitive, and bad news given by a junior physician at the bedside. Parents reported that the physician usually identified herself and answered all questions; however, the doctor did not sit down half the time, and all details of what the doctor said were not always understood. Parents were most worried about whether their child was in pain, would the child die, what the child would remember, and how the family would pay for everything.

Families recommended in our study that doctors should identify themselves, avoid conflicting information, limit the number of spokespersons, tell the truth, avoid serious discussion in front of the child, explain procedures ahead of time, speak to both parents at once if possible, present an organized and coherent plan, explain the role of different consultants, and that physicians need to communicate with each other! Other requests that parents made included unlimited visitation (requested by 67% of families); reduction of noise, lights, and alarms; increased number of nurses, a coffee pot, and free parking.

Others have reported similar shortcomings in the communication process between the physician and the family of the critically ill child. To correct these deficiencies, we need to understand the parents' reactions to their child's critical illness, their coping mechanisms, the importance of establishing mutual trust, and the role of empathy in giving bad news to the families.

The Family's Experience in the Pediatric Intensive Care Unit

The ICU admission of a child may represent a major loss of health and risk of death. Reactions seen in families include shock, denial, panic, protest, anger, mourning, and readjustment. Guilt is common. Parents may feel they have failed to protect the child, even when the cause of illness is beyond their control. Dealing with

Table 59-1. Parents' coping mechanisms

Focusing on the positives; hope

Support from family, friends, chaplains

Distancing (minimizing significance)

Religious faith

Preoccupation with medical details

Hostility or anger

dramatic changes in the child's condition from life-threatening to stable and suddenly back to life-threatening, often over a short period of hours, is a frightening and agonizing experience for the parents. Constant uncertainty has the effect of producing irritability and depression. Parents of children hospitalized in a PICU have reported that the most stressful aspects were seeing their child in pain, seeing the child frightened and sad, and the inability of the child to communicate with them.[4] Parents cope with their child's illness in various ways[5–11] (Table 59-1).

Coping Mechanisms

A feeling of helplessness leads parents to secure the support of close family and friends. Parents may receive support from hospital personnel (i.e., physicians, nurses, social workers, chaplains). A trusted family physician can be a valuable resource for information regarding the child and provide an important bridge between the family and the ICU staff.

To cope with their child's illness, parents need to have a sense of hope. Supporting a hopeful and positive attitude plays an important role in helping the family through the crises that often surface over each 24 hours. Other parents may try to cope by distancing themselves from the child as a way of minimizing the significance of their experience. Many parents focus on medical details as a means of coping, such as closely monitoring blood gases, oxygen saturations, and other test results. The intensive care crisis may lead to anger on the part of the parents. Guilt, blame (sometimes deserved!), and hostility toward the ICU team are ways of coping with the illness (Table 59-2). Some parents are anxious

Table 59-2. Differential diagnoses of parental hostility

Loss of control; helplessness

Guilt from failure to protect child from illness or injury

Communication difficulties between the family and the ICU team
    Getting mixed messages from different health care team members
    Insufficient relationships to the physician in charge of the child's care

Reemergence of unresolved past medical experiences (usually related to loss)

Parents with psychiatric or personality disorders

Table 59-3. Parents' needs

To receive accurate information frequently

To have an identifiable physician in charge

To be with the child

To maintain parenting role

To know the health care team cares for their child as a person

---

to talk about their feelings and others are not. Even if parents appear to be coping well, after 2 to 3 weeks in the ICU, decompensation is common. Regular ICU team meetings with the family and other additional supports are important when the ICU stay is prolonged.

Understanding parents' needs when their child is ill will assist the physician in responding appropriately, and in this way enhance communication (Table 59-3). Surveys of parents in the pediatric critical care setting identify the need for receiving honest, accurate information, frequently updated. They need to know that the health care team cares for their child as a person. Many parents express a strong need to be with their child at this time so that they can continue their parenting role. The health care team should facilitate the parents' need to have some "control" over the situation by allowing them caring responsibilities that complement the medical and nursing care. Sharp et al. studied parents' preferences when bad medical news was communicated to them.[12] The preferences were for physicians to (1) show caring, (2) allow the parents to talk, and (3) allow parents to show their own feelings. Families also wanted to meet other families with similar experiences, and when this occurred, the response was very positive; however, this occurred infrequently.

Cunningham and Sloper studied parents of Down's syndrome children and found that parents wanted to hear bad news right away—given in a realistic, sympathetic, and, if possible, positive manner.[13] They wanted to be given the bad news together, in a private setting, and to be able to be alone together afterward. They also indicated that they could only absorb the most basic information at the time of diagnosis. Quine and Pahl found that parents wanted to be given full information about the child's condition in a sympathetic and caring approach by the physician.[14] Parents expressed dissatisfaction when physicians exhibited a high degree of control of the interaction.

Harrison[15] described principles of family-centered neonatal care, many of which could be applied with positive effect to the PICU. Harrison noted the need for open and honest communication between parents and professionals on medical and ethical issues. This communication should make available to parents the same facts and uncertainties that are known by the professionals. The need to alleviate pain in intensive care was stressed. Harrison stated that professionals should acknowledge that overtreatment may be harmful or inhumane and that laws and treatment policies should be based on compassion.[15]

The Physician-Parent Relationship

When physicians are trained in intensive care, the technical and physiologic aspects may be all-consuming and overwhelming so that little time is left over for interaction with the patient's family. However, a relationship with the family that is not given short shrift is essential to providing good care. This relationship must

rest on a foundation that balances both empathy and professional judgment. Emotional detachment from the critically ill child and parent impedes good communication and is perceived as cold and inhumane. On the other hand, "overinvolvement" with the family can be emotionally draining and impair the physician's judgment. In addition, it consumes a great deal of the physician's time and energy that may be required for other tasks. The physician needs to seek a reasonable balance. Multiple brief visits are helpful and reassuring to parents. With longer visits, parents should be apprised of approximately how much time the physician has available. This should rarely exceed 30 to 45 minutes, as any extension beyond this time period is usually unproductive.

The First Communication

The first encounter between physician and family during their child's illness is crucial to developing a relationship that will make the parents feel supported. Communication should be carried out in a quiet area if possible and in an unhurried manner. The physician should sit with the family, preferably at a distance from which he is able to physically reach out to them. **Listening to** and **hearing** parental concerns is important. The family will feel relieved if their concerns are addressed. If their needs and concerns are not met, however, frustration results. Parents may be consumed with anxiety and guilt over the child's life-threatening state. The encounter may have periods of silence that may make the physician uncomfortable. The tendency then is for the physician to fill in these quiet and uneasy moments with facts and data concerning the child. Anxiety often makes it difficult for the parents to integrate information presented by the physician. What is comprehensible to the physician may be confusing to the parents. Much of what the physician says may be heard selectively or missed completely, leaving the parents confused, anxious, and frustrated. The physician should be as clear as possible and repeat important information a number of times to ensure all is understood. A few focused words will work better at getting one's message across rather than a barrage of overwhelming information.

The communication process should not be rushed. A hasty meeting in a corridor, with the physician glancing at his watch and about to sprint off, sends a signal to the parents that there is not enough time for questions. This can lead to frustration and anger on the part of the parent. Richard Asher spoke of unhurriedness as an important quality that helps the doctor deal well with people. He stated, "To give a patient the impression you could spare him an hour and yet to make him satisfied with five minutes is an invaluable gift and of much more use than spending half an hour with him during every minute of which he is made to feel he is encroaching on your time."[16]

Providing Understandable Information

Information should be presented in clearly understood words and phrases. Care should be taken to avoid technical hospital language or a patronizing tone. Asking the parents what they already understand about their child's illness provides a basis from which to proceed. Information concerning prognosis is best given and best heard when the parents request it. Predictions made may have a degree of uncertainty, and thus the physician should acknowledge this fact. If the physician makes a prediction with absolute certainty and is proved wrong, it will undermine the family's confidence. Parents should be encouraged to ask questions; frequently, however, physicians may not address their concerns and thus go unquestioned. This may be perceived as the parents fully comprehending the situation. Concerns on the part of the parents may not be raised because they do not wish to be seen as complaining and questioning the authority of the physician. Parents need to be given "permission" to ask the most simple and basic of questions. An adjunct to communication which may be helpful is drawings to explain anatomic or physiologic problems. People from different cultures may have a different understanding of their child's problems and approach to these. Some families may not understand English well. Interpreters should assist in these situations.

Establishing Trust

Establishing trust is the basis of successful communication. The intensivist builds this trust by displaying competence and control of the crisis and through repeated encounters, even if brief, in which honesty and sensitivity to the child's needs are presented. Parents cannot build relationships with every member of a large health care team—a common situation in the PICU! It is easiest for families if they can identify one physician who has the main role in communicating with them.[17] This may not always be possible, in which case the physician needs to pass this responsibility on to another **identifiable** colleague who will support a consistent plan of management. Each physician involved should explain their role and make it clear who is in charge.

Parents and the Health Care Team

Families want to be involved in the care of their child. If the child is seriously ill, the family's involvement empowers them with some degree of control over the crisis. The parents can often be very helpful because they are the ones who know their child better than anyone else. Their involvement also helps the health care team see the child as a person and not as an "interesting case" of dysfunctional organs. The parents' participation makes it easier for them to pass through the experience of their child's critical illness and the grief that may accompany it. The process is much more difficult if they are just passive bystanders.

The parents' participation and presence at the bedside a great deal of the time expose them to more interaction with the health care team, especially the nursing staff. Family dynamics and concerns expressed with the nursing staff provide important information to the intensivist and enhance his ability to communicate effectively with the family. The primary nurse often develops a very intense relationship with the family, and this can have very positive effects. At times, however, the primary nurse relationship may be an overinvolved one with the family, leading to loss of objectivity in the patient's management. The social worker is also a valuable member of the team who can provide insights into the psychosocial aspects of the family. Often, information shared with the social worker never comes to the attention of the physician or nurse.[18]

Physicians need to recognize the stress imposed on themselves by working in an ICU. The need to work closely with tense, grieving families may engender "dark" feelings regarding their own fallibility, sense of loss, frustration, limited control, and unmet expectations. These feelings should be anticipated but if unrecognized, may lead to anger, depression, and detachment.[19]

Dealing with a difficult parent may lead to the physician's aversion of that parent and abandonment at a time when the family most needs help and support.[20] Early identification of the "problem

parent" is vital so that appropriate support (e.g., social worker or psychiatrist) can assist both the parents and the health care team. Team meetings of the health care team provide a mutually supportive environment and help especially to buffer the potentially destructive efforts of the hostile parent. See Psychiatric Aspects of Pediatric Intensive Care by Jellinek, Herzog, and Todres, this volume.

When a Child Dies

An especially difficult communication situation for the intensivist occurs when the parents have to be informed of the death of their child. For the parent, death is the hardest loss of all—the ultimate unalterable loss. Parents are always unprepared for this, even when death is preceded by a period of chronic illness. They understandably expect their children to outlive them. Circumstances surrounding the death are an important consideration (e.g., a fatal crash caused by a drunken driver, a death after a prolonged illness, a suicide, AIDS). Each produces a different grief reaction.

The intensivist should find a private space where she can sit with the parents, ensured that there will be no interruptions. Sitting close to the parents so that she can reach out to touch them in a comforting manner will help bridge the emotional distance between physician and parent. She needs to inform them of their child's death sympathetically, but coming right out with the news and leaving the details until later. This may take the form of, "There is nothing I can say to take away your pain; we did the best we know how; your child has died." Allow pauses and time for the parents to express sorrow and grief through crying and sobbing. The best communication may be thoughtful silence and a tender touch. The parents are numbed by the news. They stop listening and hearing. They are asking themselves if this is really happening. There is disbelief. It must be a mistake. It is usually necessary to repeat oneself, for example, "I don't think I have made myself clear. Let me know what you think." Eventually, they have to face the truth—their loved one is dead. It is important to ensure that both parents are included and that the intensivist recognize the feelings of the quieter, less emotionally reacting parent.[21]

Acknowledgment of the parents' "feeling terrible" and the physician's acknowledgment of how terrible she feels that the life of their child could not be saved is an important first step in the parents' dealing with this tragic loss. Provision should be made for the parents to have a supportive person who can continue to be with them once the intensivist takes leave. The intensivist may be the last person with the child before he dies and becomes important to the family as a link to the final chapter. If the parents have developed a special relationship with a nurse/physician, they would have wanted her to be there at the time. Unfortunately, with the necessary changes in on-call routines, this may not always be possible.

Parents are sometimes "protected" from the dying or dead child because the sight of a body may be perceived as too traumatic a burden for the parents. In this situation, it is best if parents are given the choice, instead of an automatic screening off of the body from their view. That the parents need to be with their dead child and not be too rapidly whisked away is an important consideration.

This situation might arise following a motor vehicle accident; the ICU team may not have been able to step away from the patient to meet with the distraught family. With prolonged resuscitation, it would be helpful to have a member of the ICU team talk to the parents while the resuscitative efforts are ongoing, so that the parents are not left unsupported at this time. A progress report should be delivered in a caring, lucid, and sensitive manner, indicating that every effort is being made to save the life of their desperately injured child.

In an effort to calm or comfort the grieved parent, the nurse/physician may prescribe a sedative. This should not be a reflex response to a parent's agonizing grief. Some parents have stated that it only numbs them and puts off the inevitable—that they need to feel those feelings. One writer, describing his wife's death, says that grief has to be. "Take a valium. Relax. Try and sleep"—advice, he states, that would have trivialized his wife's memory and diminished him.[22]

Reactions of parents to the way in which the news of the death of their child was given—handled by either health professionals or police—was studied through a questionnaire answered by 150 bereaved parents of children, the majority of whom died of motor vehicle accidents. The study revealed that almost twice as many reported the interviews as sympathetically and reasonably handled than as badly handled or offensive.[23] The police were rated as more sympathetic than nurses or doctors. The survey demonstrated a serious need to improve the approach to informing parents of their child's death. Interviews reported as sympathetically handled were unhurried and conducted in private; the parents felt respected, and the informant had an understanding and caring attitude. Also, the parents had time to ask questions, with the interviewer checking that they understood the news. These parents had a designated person from whom they could subsequently ask for help or information about the death. The parents whose questions remained unanswered or evaded felt that a cover-up had occurred; some even suggested that litigation seemed their only recourse to obtain information.

After a child has died, it is helpful to the family if the physician maintains some contact with them. This can take the form of follow-up telephone calls at approximately 6, 12, and 24 months. Many physicians are reluctant to do this. However, we have found that parents appreciate the expression of continued interest and concern. This can help to screen for depression in the parents. Depression on the part of the family seriously affects their daily lives and the lives of any other children in the family. The follow-up call can also help provide closure for the physician following an intense relationship that may have terminated suddenly (Table 59-4).

When an autopsy has been performed, parents appreciate being called about the results. Preliminary results may be communicated after a few weeks following the death. More complete details, if necessary, may be provided at a later date, with a meeting between the physician and family.

Educational Approaches

Much progress in the communication process can be achieved through educational approaches, that is, recognizing communication training as part of the physician's practice in intensive care medicine. Approaches include (1) group discussion, (2) role models and mentors, and (3) follow-up of discharged patients and families.

In preparing the physician for dealing with death and dying, it is probably best to introduce a course in the clinical years of training as medical students. Black et al. identify the following elements in such a structural, comprehensive educational program.[24]

To identify the dying patient's needs and wishes

To understand the family's needs

To recognize the phases of normal grief and mourning

To be aware of cultural and religious aspects with regard to death

To appreciate the roles of other people, such as chaplains, in caring for the patient and family

To clear away the barriers erected around the subject (i.e., removal of the taboos about death)

To make the student appreciate her own death, thus contributing to her emotional development

To appreciate the need to relieve the physical and emotional distress of the dying patient

To consider ethical issues such as euthanasia, organ transplantation, and so on

The courses should be enhanced with formal lectures and discussions, interactions with patients and families, videotape illustrations, actors portraying patients and family members, and students participating in role playing. Helpful physician dos and don'ts are listed in Table 59-5.[25]

In conclusion, we need to recognize that human understanding, compassion, and sensitivity are equal partners with technical knowledge, and that all are necessary in the healing process and

Table 59-4. Questions for follow-up call to the family after a child's death

An opening general remark such as, "How are you doing?"

How are things going for you since your child (identify by name) died?

Have you been able to resume your usual routines?

How is your family coping?

How has the child's death affected your relationship with your spouse?

How are your other children (if any) reacting?

How are you sleeping and eating?

Have you returned to work?

Are you able to concentrate?

Can I do anything to help? (Provide information regarding support groups for bereaved parents.)

Table 59-5. Physician dos and don'ts

Dos
  Listen; encourage questions.
  Use clear, jargon-free language.
  Ask what parents have been told.
  Be honest.
  Identify role of each physician.
  Have repeated meetings with parents, even if brief.
  Consider family's needs, stresses, and coping mechanisms.
Don'ts
  Do not rush.
  Do not be too certain with predictions—admit uncertainty.
  Do not overwhelm with facts.
  Do not abandon the family in extremely difficult situations.

in the fulfillment in physicians dedicated to this work. As Francis W. Peabody said in the early part of this century, "for the secret of the care of the patient is in caring for the patient, . . . the treatment of disease may be entirely impersonal; the care of the patient must be entirely personal. . . ."[26]

References

1. Morris RT. *Doctors versus Folks.* Garden City, NJ: Doubleday, 1915.
2. Simpson M et al. Doctor-patient communication. The Toronto consensus statement. *Br Med J* 303:1385, 1991.
3. Earle M, Penn J, Todres ID. Improving communication with families in the pediatric intensive care unit. *Crit Care Med* 23:A195, 1995.
4. Miles MG et al. The pediatric intensive care unit environment as a source of stress for parents. *Matern Child Nurs J* 18:199, 1989.
5. Carnevale FA. A description of stresses and coping strategies among parents of critically ill children—A preliminary study. *Intensive Care Nurs* 6:4, 1990.
6. Fiser DH, Stanford G, Dorman D. Devices for parental stress reduction on a pediatric ICU. *Crit Care Med* 10:504, 1989.
7. Kasper J, Nyamalki A. Parent of children in the pediatric intensive care unit: What are their needs? *Heart Lung* 17:574, 1988.
8. Kirshbaum MS. Needs of parents of critically ill children. *Dimens Crit Care Nurs* 9:344, 1990.
9. LaMontagne L, Panlak R. Stress and coping of parents of children on a pediatric intensive care unit. *Heart Lung* 19:416, 1990.
10. Rothstein P. Psychological stresses in families of children in a pediatric intensive care unit. *Pediatr Clin North Am* 27:613, 1980.
11. Waller D et al. Coping with poor prognosis in the pediatric intensive care unit. *Am J Dis Child* 133:121, 1979.
12. Sharp MC, Strauss RR, Lock SC. Communicating medical bad news: Parents' experiences and preferences. *J Pediatr* 121:539, 1992.
13. Cunningham CC, Sloper T. Parents of Down's syndrome babies: Their earlier needs. *Child Care Health Dev* 3:325, 1977.
14. Quine L, Pahl J. First diagnosis of severe mental handicap: Characteristics of unsatisfactory encounters between doctors and parents. *Soc Sci Med* 22:53, 1981.
15. Harrison H. The principles of family-centered neonatal care. *Pediatrics* 92:643, 1993.
16. Asher R. Talk, tact, and treatment. In *Talking Sense.* London: Pitman Medical, 1972. P 117.
17. Jellinek MS et al. Facing tragic decisions with parents in the neonatal intensive care unit: Clinical perspectives. *Pediatrics* 89:119, 1992.
18. Jellinek MS et al. Coping with the truly difficult patient. *Contemp Pediatr* 8:19, 1991.
19. Jellinek MS et al. Pediatric intensive care training: Confronting the dark side. *Crit Care Med* 21:775, 1993.
20. Beresin EV. The difficult parent. In Jellinek MS, Herzog DB (eds): *Massachusetts General Hospital. Psychiatric Aspects of General Hospital Pediatrics.* Chicago: Year Book, 1990.
21. Grollman EA. *In Sickness and in Health. How to Cope When Your Loved One is Ill.* Boston: Beacon, 1987.
22. Potts M. Grief has to be. *Lancet* 343:279, 1994.
23. Finlay I, Dallimore D. Your child is dead. *Br Med J* 302:1524, 1991.
24. Black D, Hardoff D, Nelki J. Educating medical students about death and dying. *Arch Dis Child* 64:750, 1989.
25. Todres ID, Earle M, Jellinek MS. Enhancing communication: The physician and family in the pediatric intensive care unit. *Pediatr Clin North Am* 41:1395, 1994.
26. Peabody FW. *The Care of the Patient.* Boston: Harvard University Press, 1927.

Michael S. Jellinek
David Herzog
I. David Todres

60 ▶ Psychiatric Aspects of Pediatric Intensive Care

The child admitted to the pediatric intensive care unit (PICU) because of a catastrophic illness or suffering severe trauma enters a frightening environment and situation. The sudden changes in the body accompanied by immobilization and pain have psychological consequences. In this situation, special understanding of the child's and family's experience is essential, and appropriate support services need to be an integral part of management (Table 60-1).

Developmental Issues

The conscious child in an ICU usually becomes sullen and preoccupied with his physical condition. The child attempts to deal with feeling a loss of control, feeling unprotected, and at times being in excruciating pain. The child's reactions to the intensive care setting should be considered within a developmental context. The very young child will be frightened and frantically searching for a familiar face, especially a parent. He may wonder if he is being punished for having done or thought an angry or "bad" action. The school-age child will have serious fears of further impending catastrophic illness and may have a great deal of difficulty tolerating the physical restrictions often required in the intensive care setting. The child may need to have limb restraints and have his head stabilized to prevent movement and possible dislodgement of an endotracheal tube. The adolescent with a catastrophic illness is very concerned about autonomy and physical appearance. Although these classic developmental issues are well known in children facing stress or disease, the PICU environment and the stress of serious life-threatening situations often lead to regression; thus, an adolescent may at times behave like a much younger child as a solution to being overwhelmed by the pain, crisis, and setting. The role of parents includes tolerating the regressive behavior and encouraging age-appropriate behavior as soon as the child is able to.

The child in the ICU will experience marked anxiety and panic associated with the diminished sense of control in this frightening environment. Children are confused about their whereabouts in the unfamiliar surroundings and are very concerned, asking, "What is happening to me? Where am I?" They will require clear (jargon-free) and direct explanations of what is ongoing and what one plans to do, so that the child will have a sense of control and develop a sense of trust in what the clinician and nurse are required to do.

With appropriate explanation, children can comprehend the nature of their disorder and also appreciate the need for the procedures and technological equipment required for their care at this critical time. Underlying this cognitive explanation is a need to develop a trusting alliance between the physician, nurse, and child. Such trust stems from understanding the child's emotional state, respecting to the extent possible the child's wishes and privacy, easing the child's pain, and, of course, having the endorsement of parents. If at all possible, one should try to prepare the child for special procedures or maneuvers to enhance control and minimize alarm generated by sudden, unexpected events. When discussing the illness, the child should be given the opportunity to ask questions.

Of course, if the child is intubated, such verbal discussion cannot take place. However, all attempts should be made with the aid of the family to understand the child's concerns through responses such as nodding the head, blinking eyes, and tapping fingers or toes. The older child may be in a position to write down any concerns or questions.

Trust

Development of trust is crucial to the well-being of the child's experience in the PICU. The presence of a consistent physician and nurse cannot be overemphasized. It is also crucial that the medical team provide support in terms of a hopeful outcome in order to help sustain the child. Trust depends on consistency, age-appropriate communication, and empathetic care.

The child in the PICU has been removed from the familiar and secure environment of home, family, and other support systems to a new and frightening environment. In this new setting, the child should feel secure in the thought that there are people who will protect her and care for her. She needs to know that this resource and support is at hand. To cope, the child needs this security. The role of parents is key. In the crisis atmosphere of the PICU, it is important to remember that the presence of the parents is the primary support of the child. Any means to enhance the parent's role or create a more familiar environment, such as a "security" blanket, a favorite toy, or photographs, are helpful to reduce the child's anxiety. Parents should have open visitation and free access to their child in the PICU, for the sake of both the child and the parent. The presence of the parents in the PICU and the consistent contact between the parents and an identifiable physician and nurse promote a feeling of trust in the child for those primary caretakers.

The child's pain should not be minimized. Children with acute pain and the fear of impending pain should be treated, comforted, and reassured. Pain will increase anxiety, and increased anxiety

Table 60-1. Indications for child psychiatry consultation in pediatric intensive care unit settings

Psychiatric evaluation (after suicide attempt)

Mental status examination (delirium, depression)

Suicide assessment

Death of a parent (i.e., in the same motor vehicle accident)

Parental discord (especially regarding medical treatment)

Psychiatric illness in parents

Rigid denial in parents (usually blocking medical decision making)

Discord among medical team

Evaluation of psychiatric issues and major medical decisions (termination of life supports)

Team/team or team/parent communication breakdown

leads to increased perception of pain. Pain can be minimized through prevention and recognition of the settings in which this occurs and the appropriate use of local anesthesia and gentleness in the performance of the necessary procedures. One should always be aware of the "whole" child, and in this regard, it is important that one recognizes where the child is perceiving pain so that one does not accidentally "lean" on an acutely sensitive area. Pain management should be available through integrated consultation by pediatrics, anesthesia, neurology, and child psychiatry.

Parents

The ICU experience can be very difficult for the parents of the critically ill child. Parents not infrequently experience guilt about their child's state, and this feeling can be particularly disabling to them. In a family that, prior to the illness, was already experiencing severe stress, the additional stress of the critically ill child's hospitalization may be overwhelming. Parents are in a state of shock and confusion when their child is admitted and frequently feel anxious and helpless about providing their child's necessary care. The parents' guilt and shock are compounded by sleep deprivation. Very early on, the parents cannot comprehend the gravity of the reality of the circumstances, and often the whole situation feels unreal to them. Parents may need information repeated several times before they can begin to comprehend the nature of their child's illness. They may require time to have their questions answered and should feel supported in this regard. Often, the parents blame themselves for the nature of the illness (i.e., the child in an automobile accident in which the parent was the driver). At times, a diagnosis cannot be made, and there is uncertainty, causing the parents to experience frustration, anxiety, and guilt. They may have difficulty trusting the staff and may be concerned about the quality of the care that their child receives. The sight of their critically ill child, especially in a trauma case in which there is physical disfigurement, may be difficult for them to tolerate, and the addition of monitors and machines around their child combine to produce an overwhelming situation for them. Children who receive pancuronium or other muscle relaxants will lie inert and limp while receiving mechanical ventilation and other forms of support. The parents who see their child at this time may be emotionally distraught because effects of the medication convey a sense of lifelessness.

Involving parents in the care of their child should be encouraged and supported. In this way, they are allowed a sense of usefulness. Families need to express their feelings about the hospitalization and receive the necessary emotional assistance. Often, organizing a meeting with the social service team can be immensely helpful in understanding the family dynamics at this time, in addition to direct communication with the physician and nursing staff.

One aspect of the care of the critically ill child that is sometimes forgotten or overlooked is the child's siblings, who may now receive much less attention or support because of the parent's total commitment to the hospitalized child. Siblings need special consideration at this time, and attention should be given to their concerns about the critically ill child. They may develop distorted concepts of the situation that require clarification.

Meetings between the primary care health team, social services, and the family can clarify misunderstandings and provide the necessary support for the family. There are ways to support the family that will improve their coping skills and help them to deal with the situation. Communication is substantively improved when the one physician and nurse, designated as primary caretak-

ers for the child, are the ones to relate to the family. The family is then able to seek out an identifiable person for ongoing discussions. When this is not done and the family deals with multiple nurses and physicians, the parents receive inconsistent information regarding their child; in this situation, it is not uncommon that the parents will seek out those who will give the answers they wish to hear. With changing attending staff, it is imperative that the responsibilities are then appropriately passed on to another identifiable individual. Team meetings to discuss family dynamics and concerns should be held on a regular basis, as well as in response to a crisis.

The parents will frequently neglect their own special needs while caring for their child in the PICU because of exclusively focusing their energies on this child. They may find it difficult to leave the hospital or the child's bedside and should be reassured of their child's adaptation to the hospitalization. Such support can permit them to have respite schedules that will help to sustain them through their child's illness, as well as to support each other and other members of the family.

Parents may be informed of a child's poor prognosis and be unable to accept it. This form of denial is to be understood in the context of a child's illness and should be respected. The health care team can work effectively with them as they pass through this phase and accept the realities of the gravity of the situation. Parents go through reactive phases of shock, distortion, denial, and anger prior to the acceptance of the poor prognosis. The physician should confront the parent's denial when it is considered to be pathologic, that is, extreme and persisting longer than a few days, or when it prevents implementation of necessary medical interventions. For further detailed discussion of the issues relating to communication between the physician and the family of the critically ill child, see Communicating with Families in the Pediatric Intensive Care Unit by Todres, Earle, and Jellinek, this volume.

Common Psychiatric Issues

Intensive Care Unit Syndrome

The ICU syndrome is a reaction noted in children treated in ICUs and occurs primarily between the ages of 18 months and 6 years. The symptoms present as a transient psychotic state or delirium or are characterized by a state of depression, confusion, disorientation, hallucinations, and paranoid delusions. Some children will become withdrawn, refuse to speak, or in some cases, behave passively. Other children with the ICU syndrome may become deeply agitated and hostile. A number of factors contribute to this development of the syndrome, and thus recognition of this is essential to prevent the problem.

Children who are critically ill will frequently require multiple procedures and examinations around the clock, leading to constant overstimulation and sleep and sensory deprivation. Understandably, if the procedure is necessary, one cannot avoid the stimulus that accompanies the procedure. However, the presence of parents and the contact with familiar objects such as toys, along with reducing the intensity of light and noise, will help to facilitate sleep and will lessen the likelihood of this syndrome's developing. It is important that one anticipate this possibility so that if early signs are noted, it may be possible to intervene in ways that are helpful to the child psychologically without compromising his physical care. In this regard, increased visitations by the family should be promoted, and, if at all possible, the child should be moved from one part of the PICU to another where the intensity of light and sound may be less devastating.

The child's anxiety level may interfere with physiologic status (i.e., respiratory function, pain control, or necessary care, e.g., dressing changes). Anxiolytics such as short-acting benzodiazepines (e.g., midazolam 0.05 mg/kg IV titrated to effect) are often appropriate. One needs to be aware of the potential for respiratory depression, especially when opioids are also administered. Haloperidol has been effectively used when the patient does not respond satisfactorily to other anxiolytics. This drug can be repeated in 20 to 30 minutes if no effect is noted. Haloperidol can assist in control of the very agitated child.

Delirium

Delirium is a transient derangement of cerebral function, with acute global impairment of cognition and attention accompanied by disturbances of the sleep-wake cycle and changes in psychomotor activity.[1] It is common in very ill children and can be life-threatening. Clinical symptoms of delirium include the rapid development of the following: (1) reduced attention or inability to attend to external stimuli, (2) disorganized thinking (rambling, irrelevant, or incoherent speech), (3) reduced level of consciousness, (4) disorientation, (5) perceptual disturbance (evidence of hallucinations, marked distortions), (6) sleep-wake disturbance, (7) increased or decreased psychosomotor activity, and (8) memory impairment. Symptoms develop acutely and tend to wax and wane, being most obvious at night. Early signs are restlessness, drowsiness, insomnia, and nightmares.

Treatment is directed at both the cause and the symptoms. Psychiatric interventions frequently include orienting the patient to time, place, and person; decreasing the patient's sensory input (e.g., dim lighting, elimination of unnecessary noise) and increasing the patient's contact with staff and family; and administering psychotropic medication to the patient to decrease agitation, limit disruption of care, and prevent injury to self or others. A short course (2 to 3 days) of agents such as lorazepam (Ativan), 0.01 to 0.05 mg/kg intramusculary (IM), orally, sublingually, or intravenously (IV) every 6 hours is often recommended. For adolescents haloperidol (Haldol), initially 0.05 to 0.2 mg/kg IM, IV, or orally prescribed as needed, is useful to decrease agitation and can be repeated if needed and then 0.01 to 0.2 mg/kg every 6 hours IV, IM, or orally.[2] Antipsychotics (i.e., haloperidol, chlorpromazine) are useful if hallucinations or delusions are present, whereas anxiolytics (i.e., lorazepam, diazepam) assist in reducing anxiety and agitation in the absence of psychotic symptoms.

Suicide

Children and adolescents whose suicide attempt is sufficiently serious to warrant admission to the PICU are a serious challenge. Some young children will initiate a debate among the staff—Was this an accident or intentional? Frequently, the admitting history will suggest an accident, but like most "accidents" there may be family stresses or parental discord that increased the risk or lowered the level of supervision. Older children evoke confusion, sadness, and anger. The suicidal behavior makes no sense or is seen as irrational. Because staff work long hours and use expensive resources, they may come to resent rather than empathize with the suicidal patient. If rooted in depression, such children carry a high risk for recurrent depression and future, serious suicide attempts.

Overwhelming Tragedies

Some circumstances in the PICU are so tragic that they overwhelm even an experienced staff. For example, fires or motor vehicle accidents may result in the death of one or more family members, or there may be other tragic facts to tell an injured child. Violence, dashed hopes, or unexpected tragedy after long struggles may be just too much to bear.

Munchausen by Proxy

Munchausen by proxy is a syndrome in which the parent, usually the mother, falsifies illness in her child so that the child is perceived as medically ill and receives evaluation and treatment.[1-3] (Baron Munchausen is the fictional author of a German book of travels filled with tall tales.) The fabrication of the child's history and symptoms commonly yields emotional benefits for the parent.[3,4] The parental behavior is often long-standing before it is recognized and, as a result, there is commonly a history of numerous extensive workups. Parents may provide inaccurate information, alter the child's intake of medicine or food, tamper with specimens to produce false reports, obstruct hospital observations, or actively cause harm in the child. Common presenting complaints are bleeding, seizures, GI pain, diarrhea, and malnutrition.

The diagnosis should be considered when the symptoms are recurrent, seemingly intractable to treatment, and documentation of etiology is elusive.[5-7] The triad of Munchausen by proxy includes abuse of the child, deception of the physician, and passivity of the child toward the parent-perpetrator's deeds.[8] Examples include a 3-year-old child with recurrent coma in which the etiology was administration of chloral hydrate; a 2-month-old with anorexia, dehydration, and hypernatremia who was administered salt; a 4-year-old with recurrent bacterial skin and soft tissue infections who was administered injected oral and fecal matter; a 5-year-old with neurologic degenerative disease presenting for her fifth major workup with weakness and failure to thrive, who was routinely starved while calorie intake was falsified.

Clinical documentation of the means by which the illness is fabricated is difficult and may require surreptitious 24-hour video monitoring of the patient and mother, searching the mother's personal belongings, and possibly enforced separation of the mother and child.[9] All such interventions must have the whole-hearted support of the staff involved and be cleared by the senior medical, psychiatric, and hospital ethical and legal staff. Once it has been documented that the mother is making the child ill, the mother needs to be confronted and appropriate social service and legal intervention undertaken.

Munchausen by proxy is associated with long-term psychological morbidity as well as physical risk to its victims. Morbidity and mortality are exceptionally high, especially considering that the child is basically healthy. Waller reported that 5 of 23 children admitted died, and Rosenberg's review noted ten deaths in 117 cases.[10,11]

Difficult Families

Deciding that a family is difficult should be the last option after considering the overall circumstances—the communication effort of the team and the expected, wide variety of reactions as parents face uncertainty and stress. Despite the best, high-quality efforts of team members, however, some families maintain a rigid, defensive stance that impairs communication and leads to distrust. Often, these families have endured one or more tragedies before the current PICU admission; not uncommonly, they have had to cope with severe chronic disease or mental illness, and perceived the concomitant medical care as suspect rather than sincere and expert. Parents may (1) use denial in such a rigid manner as to block needed decision-making, (2) become overly dependent on the PICU staff and be so suffocating and intrusive that the staff falls into a pattern of avoidance, (3) "split" the staff by taking bits of data to many different team members as an attempt to confirm their distrust of the team, (4) become aloof and feels entitled to deal with their sense of powerlessness, or (5) be clinically depressed and in need of formal psychiatric evaluation. All of these reactions are the parents' solution to the problem of being overwhelmed by the circumstances they face. Thus the insecurity, sense of guilt, and duration of the crisis all increase the likelihood of "difficult" devaluing behavior.

Staff Stress

Although often not the identified reason for a consultation, stress on the PICU staff is a source of ongoing concern.[12] As noted earlier, a stressed staff may communicate in a more rigid or inflexible manner among themselves or with families. Although all members of the PICU team are subject to a variety of stresses and symptoms, typically attendings face the wish to control what is often uncontrollable. They have much at stake in being "perfect" and "winning" against morbidity and death. Attendings are also often stressed by competing demands of research, clinical care, and family. Fellows and residents are working long hours at the edge of their competency. Desperate not to make a mistake, they forget that errors are inevitable. Some children and families elicit strong feelings of attachment so that loss and depression may be evident after a family learns a child has died. Nurses are both somewhat protected by their years of experience and simultaneously vulnerable in their intense commitment to a family, day after day, creating an attachment that supports a child's recovery and causes true heartbreak when a child dies. Although not the focus of a child and adolescent psychiatrist's or unit chief's role, awareness of staff anger, anxiety, guilt, loneliness, and depression are all part of PICU life.

Post–Pediatric Intensive Care Unit Psychiatric Needs

Selected circumstances in the PICU should result in psychiatric follow-up, namely, after an interim consultation or the death of a child, as well as ongoing availability for post-PICU behavioral difficulties. For example, some children will suffer difficulties in school for many weeks as part of a postconcussion syndrome.

Others will have nightmares, startle reactions, anxiety, and social avoidance if the PICU experience was integrated as a trauma. The child may reexperience PICU anxieties at the sound of a monitor (during a TV show), or the sight of an ambulance serves as a trigger to PICU-related fears. These follow-up services are more likely if there is a good working relationship among the staff, referring physician, and psychiatric consultant.

Conclusion

The PICU is a hard-working setting at the edge of medical knowledge, with a child's life hanging in the balance. It is a pressured, stressful, passionate, and exciting environment that elicits a wide range of caring and painful emotions. For the children, these complex emotions are embedded in a developmental context, physical pain, uncertainty, and medical conditions that impact their mental status. Families are facing desperate circumstances, often feeling unreasonably guilty, not able to contribute to their child's care, and powerless. These issues are a key priority for the attending leadership and psychiatric consultant.

References

1. Stoddard FS, Wilens TE. Delirium. In Jellinek MJ, Herzog DB (eds): *Massachusetts General Hospital Handbook: Psychiatric Aspects of General Hospital Pediatrics.* Chicago: Yearbook, 1990. Pp 254–259.
2. Heidigenstein E, Gerrity S. Psychotropics as adjuvant analgesics. In Schecter NL, Berde CB, Yeaster M (eds): *Pain in Infants, Children, and Adolescents.* Baltimore: Williams & Wilkins, 1993. Pp 193–197.
3. Meadow R. Munchausen syndrome by proxy—The hinterland of child abuse. *Lancet* 2:343, 1977.
4. Meadow R. Management of Munchausen syndrome by proxy. *Arch Dis Child* 60:344, 1985.
5. Rosenberg DA. Munchausen syndrome by proxy. In Reece RM (ed): *Child Abuse: Medical Diagnosis and Management.* Philadelphia: Lea & Febiger, 1994.
6. Krener PKG, Wasserman AC. Diagnostic dilemmas in pediatric consultation. *Child Adolesc Psychol Clin North Am* 3:485, 1994.
7. Schreier HA, Libow JS. Munchausen by proxy syndrome: A modern pediatric challenge. *J Pediatr* 125(Suppl):110, 1994.
8. Sigal M, Gelkoph M, Meadow RS. Munchausen by proxy syndrome: The triad of abuse, self abuse and deception. *Compr Psychiatry* 30:527, 1989.
9. Sugar J. Munchausen syndrome by proxy. In Jellinek MJ, Herzog DB (eds): *Massachusetts General Hospital Handbook: Psychiatric Aspects of General Hospital Pediatrics.* Chicago: Yearbook, 1990. Pp 198–201.
10. Waller D. Obstacles to the treatment of Munchausen by proxy syndrome. *J Am Acad Child Psychiatry* 22:80, 1983.
11. Rosenberg DA. Web of deceit: A literature review of Munchausen syndrome by proxy. *Child Abuse Negl* 11:547, 1987.
12. Jellinek MS et al. Pediatric intensive care training: Confronting the dark side. *Crit Care Med* 21:775, 1993.

Brahm Goldstein

Ellen R. Feldman

Kenneth R. Scheublin

61 **Child Abuse and Neglect**

Reports of child abuse and neglect are increasing at an alarming rate. In 1977, approximately 500,000 to one million cases of child abuse and neglect occurred in the United States.[1] By 1986, over 1.5 million children were abused and neglected annually.[2] Child abuse is the single leading cause of death in children between 1 month and 1 year of age and accounts for 2000 to 5000 deaths during childhood each year.[3–5] It is the only leading cause of childhood mortality that has increased over the past 30 years.[6] Approximately 20,000 cases of child abuse and neglect annually result in "serious injuries,"[7] and many of these will eventually be cared for in an intensive care unit (ICU). Thus, it is extremely important for pediatric critical care physicians, nurses, and social workers to be aware of this problem. The recognition of child abuse and neglect as a cause of serious injury in infants and children is vital for proper care of the victims, appropriate counseling for their families, and prevention of repeat occurrences.

Pathophysiology

Head injury is the most common admitting diagnosis in cases of child abuse admitted to the pediatric intensive care unit (PICU).[8,8a] Subdural hematoma, subarachnoid hemorrhage, intracerebral hemorrhage, skull fracture, and diffuse cerebral edema are the most common clinical entities observed. Pathologic examination in cases of severe nonaccidental head trauma reveals gliding contusions in smaller children, diffuse white matter injury in older children, tearing of bridging veins, and acute subdural, parasagittal, and subarachnoid hemorrhage.[9,10]

Subdural hematomas associated with severe child abuse and neglect and head injury were described by Caffey,[11,12] who coined the terms *shaken baby syndrome* and *whiplash shaken infant syndrome.* Caffey proposed that the pathophysiologic mechanism responsible for injury was a whiplash-type motion of the head, resulting in tearing of the bridging veins secondary to acceleration-deceleration forces.

Studies by Duhaime and others[9,13,14] have revealed information concerning the biomechanical mechanisms they suggest may be responsible for head injuries seen in the shaken baby syndrome. Rather than a whiplash-type motion of the head, resulting in tearing of the bridging veins, as proposed by Caffey,[12] Duhaime et al.[13] reviewed autopsy findings of 13 fatal cases of shaken baby syndrome and found signs of blunt impact to the head in all. In a biomechanical model of a 1-month-old infant, shaking alone could not produce the accelerational forces necessary to cause injury. When the model was shaken and then impacted against a padded or unpadded surface, however, the forces necessary to produce subdural hematomas and brain parenchymal injury were present. Bruce[15,16] has used the term *shaken impact syndrome* to describe these findings.

Alexander et al.[17] suggested that the etiologic mechanism may be either shaking alone or shaking with impact. In addition, asphyxial injuries may occur,[18] with or without related trauma. Due to the number of potential mechanisms of abuse, including important legal issues, the authors prefer the terms *inflicted head injury* or *inflicted cerebral trauma* to describe this clinical syndrome.[19,20]

Distinguishing between accidental causes of head injury and inflicted head injury should not be difficult if a thorough history,

physical examination, and appropriate laboratory and radiologic tests are obtained.[21–23] Billmire and Myers[24] reviewed 84 infants less than 1 year of age who were admitted to the hospital with head injury. Sixty-four percent of all head injuries, excluding uncomplicated skull fractures, and 95% of serious intracranial injuries resulted from child abuse. Other studies have confirmed that falls from short distances are extremely unlikely to produce serious injury.[25,26] Therefore, the occurrence of intracranial injury in the absence of a history of significant accidental trauma, such as a motor vehicle accident, warrants immediate investigation for child abuse. The presence of severe neurologic injury in an infant or toddler without a history of significant trauma should be considered due to child abuse until proven otherwise.

Retinal hemorrhages on ophthalmologic examination (Fig. 61-1) are associated with severe child abuse.[3,10,11,14,20,27–37] There is good evidence that retinal hemorrhages do not occur with minor head injuries, even those that may result in skull fracture.[24] Retinal hemorrhages may rarely occur as a result of prolonged and vigorous cardiopulmonary resuscitation.[37] Other causes of retinal hemorrhages include hematologic abnormalities, CNS vascular malformations, infections, high-altitude mountain climbing, normal deliveries of newborns, and a complication of general anesthesia or pneumoencephalography.[37] The proposed pathophysiologic mechanism in the development of retinal hemorrhages is concussion to the head resulting in disruption of retinal blood vessels, most commonly between the internal limiting membrane and the ganglion cell layer, as well as in the nerve fiber layer of the retina.[36]

Clinical Presentation

Admitting Diagnosis

Victims of severe child abuse are often admitted to the PICU under a multitude of diagnoses, such as head trauma, coma, sei-

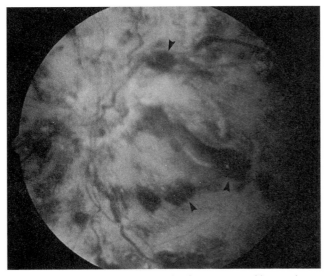

Figure 61-1. Retinal photograph of severe retinal hemorrhages *(arrowheads)* in a 4-month-old victim of shaken impact syndrome.

zures, status asthmaticus, or near-miss sudden infant death syndrome (SIDS).[8,19] It is not until a detailed history, thorough physical examination, and appropriate diagnostic tests are obtained that the underlying diagnosis of child abuse is suspected. Even so, the diagnosis of child abuse and neglect may be difficult, delayed, or even overlooked in the critically ill child. This may be due to a clinical picture confused by concurrent coma, shock, or cardiopulmonary arrest.

Few reports in the medical literature describe severe cases of child abuse and neglect admitted to the PICU.[8,38,39] The most frequent admitting diagnosis in cases admitted to the PICU is head trauma.[8] Lavaud et al.[38] described 22 cases of battered children admitted to a multiservice PICU over a 12-year period. All patients were less than 2.5 years of age. Fifty-nine percent had evidence of cranial trauma. Hauser et al.[39] and Goldstein et al.[8] similarly reported head trauma as the leading admitting diagnosis in children admitted to an ICU. Table 61-1 lists the most common admitting diagnoses in cases of severe child abuse admitted to a PICU.

History

Most victims of severe child abuse are under 1 year of age and often less than 6 months of age. The initial history may be of a minor fall or injury, seizure, respiratory arrest, or no reported predisposing event.[8,13,15,16,39,40] One case encountered by the authors involved a 4-month-old infant who was transferred to the PICU after arriving in the pediatric emergency department apneic and pulseless. The initial diagnosis was near-miss SIDS. The parents maintained the child had been well and was found lifeless after a nap. After initial resuscitation, the infant was noted to have a bulging anterior fontanelle and multiple retinal hemorrhages. A CT scan of the head revealed intracranial hemorrhages, a posterior intrahemispheric subdural hemorrhage, and massive cerebral edema (see Fig. 61-1). Multiple old rib fractures were noted on chest radiograph. Despite being confronted with these findings, the parents continued to deny any history of trauma. They asked if changing the infant's diaper too vigorously could have resulted in the infant's injuries. In a case such as this, in which the history is inconsistent with the severity of injuries, the medical team must be alert to the underlying diagnosis of child abuse.

The spectrum of child abuse and neglect has changed radically over the past 25 years.[41] The proportion of severe injuries that occurs has increased significantly.[41] The classic description of the malnourished child with multiple musculoskeletal injuries inflicted at different times by a depressed mother has changed. In our experience, as well as that of others,[41–43] there is often a history of a sudden, impulsive, and violent act on the part of the caretaker, resulting in severe injury to the child. There may be ongoing psychosocial or family problems that do not involve the child directly. Sudden acts of anger or rage are vented on the child in physical terms, resulting in violent shaking or physically striking the child with an object or by hand. This is often precipitated around the child's crying, feeding, or toilet training.[42] Cases of severe abuse involve an increasing number of single-parent families. Usually, the perpetrator in these cases is a live-in or babysitting boyfriend.[3,8] In a review of 17 cases of severe abuse resulting in admission to the Massachusetts General Hospital PICU, the perpetrator was the maternal boyfriend in two instances and the babysitter in two others.[8] Subsequent studies have confirmed this observation.[44] Table 61-2 lists the developmental pattern of predominant perpetrators and weapons used in child homicide victims.[6]

Current investigators postulate that the child is initially injured by the caretaker, loses consciousness, and is put down to rest in the hope that he will recover.[15] As a result of intracranial trauma with resultant increased intracranial pressure (ICP), coma, seizures, or respiratory arrest ensue, and only at this point is emergency medical assistance obtained. As in the case described previously, on arrival to the emergency room, the only history is of apnea or seizures and not of inflicted trauma. The diagnosis of abuse or neglect may not be considered until a complete history is obtained that proves inconsistent with the severity of the physical findings.

Head Injury

CNS damage occurs in approximately 20% of physically abused children.[27] The presence of severe neurologic injury in a child less than 1 year of age without a history of significant accidental trauma should be considered due to child abuse until proven otherwise. Infants rarely sustain nonaccidental head trauma sufficient to result in severe neurologic injury.[15,24,25,35] Minor falls may result in dramatic linear skull fractures, but rarely in significant neurologic damage.[25,43]

The anterior fontanelle may be full or tense, depending on the severity of injuries and the presence of hemorrhage. Likewise, the cranial sutures may be split. The classic clinical syndrome of pupillary dilation, bradycardia, hypertension, and decerebrate posturing may signify increased ICP. ICP, however, may be abnor-

Table 61-1. Admitting diagnoses of child abuse or neglect patients admitted to the pediatric intensive care unit

Head injury

Seizures

Burns

Multiple trauma (including gunshot wounds)

Strangulation

Overdose/ingestion

Near-drowning

Meningitis

Diabetic coma

Malnutrition

Near-miss SIDS

Table 61-2. Developmental pattern of predominant perpetrators and weapons used in child homicide victims

Age group	Predominant perpetrator	Predominant weapons
Neonates	Mother	Suffocation/drowning
Infants	Parent/acquaintance	Bodily force
Preschoolers	Parent/acquaintance	Bodily force
Adolescents	Acquaintance/stranger	Guns/knives/cars

From B Ewigman, C Kivlahan. Child maltreatment fatalities. *Pediatr Ann* 18:476, 1989. With permission.

mally elevated in the absence of these signs. The ophthalmologic examination is a vital part of the assessment of nonaccidental head injury. Presence of edema around the optic nerve and loss of venous pulsations are signs of increased ICP, although false-negative findings occur. More importantly, the presence of retinal hemorrhages are strongly associated with child abuse.[8,19,24,30-35] Retinal hemorrhages occur in 50% to 100% of abused infants and rarely occur as a result of accidental injury in children.[15,24,35]

Burns

One third to one half of all burns sustained by young children are due to passive neglect or intentional injury.[27,45,46] As with other forms of child abuse, a discrepancy between the history and the physical findings should warn the physician of the high likelihood of inflicted injury. There is an increased incidence of inflicted burns in children of single-parent families and in those with a previous history of abuse and neglect, prior ingestion, failure to thrive, or old burns.[46] Specific patterns of burns, such as stocking or glovelike distribution on the feet and hands; burns involving the buttocks, genitalia, and face; sparing of flexor surfaces; mirror-image burns; or more than two burn sites may be pathognomonic of nonaccidental injury.

Other Types of Injury

Many signs and symptoms classically associated with less severe forms of child abuse and neglect, such as bruises, internal injuries, long-bone fractures, failure to thrive, and poor hygiene,[3,11,27-29,47-51] are not seen as frequently in victims of abuse admitted to the PICU. Bony injuries, however, such as posterior rib fractures, spiral fractures, and multiple fractures of different ages, either alone or in combination with head injury, may still be observed.[52,53]

Clinical findings of intraabdominal trauma from abuse are indistinguishable from those due to accidental trauma.[27] Intraoperative findings may provide clues to the mechanism of injury. Accidental injuries resulting from motor vehicle accidents produce compressing forces that cause injuries to the antimesentery border. In contrast, the decelerating force from a punch results in a tear of the mesentery or intestine at the site of ligamental support. Rupture or injury of the duodenum, proximal jejunum, mesentery, pancreas, spleen, liver, or retroperitoneum are types of intraabdominal injuries that may occur from child abuse.[27]

Skin lesions characteristic of abuse include lacerations and bruises in various stages of healing; specific patterns seen with whipping injuries from belts or cords; posterior lesions; "finger" bruises such as grab marks, encirclement bruises, and choke marks; and bilateral bruises. Dating the injury may be possible, based on the patterns of discoloration (Table 61-3).

Suffocation[54-58] and Munchausen syndrome by proxy[57-61] are other forms of child abuse that may require admission to the PICU. Suffocation may present as SIDS, apnea, or seizures.[18,21-23] There may be petechial hemorrhages around the face and head. The mother is most often the perpetrator. Previous episodes of apnea, cyanosis, seizures, or a history of unexpected death or SIDS in an elder sibling are clues to the diagnosis. Munchausen syndrome by proxy may present as seizures, apnea, or a multitude of other signs and symptoms. Recurrent suffocation or the administration of drugs or toxic substances by the caretaker are patterns of abuse frequently observed in this syndrome.

Risk factors associated with child abuse and neglect found in children admitted to the PICU are listed in Table 61-4.[8,19] These are similar to risk factors reported in the medical literature.[29,45]

Table 61-3. Relationship between color and age of contusions

Color	Age
Reddish-blue or purple	Immediate/<1 d
Blue-purple	1–5 d
Green	5–7 d
Yellow	7–10 d
Brown	10–14 d
Resolution	2–4 wk

From M Yaster, JA Hallen. Multiple trauma in the pediatric patient. In Rogers MC (ed): *Textbook of Pediatric Care.* Baltimore: Williams & Wilkins, 1987. P 1312. Copyright © 1987 by Williams & Wilkins Co., Baltimore. With permission.

Table 61-4. Risk factors associated with child abuse and neglect in children admitted to a pediatric intensive care unit

Inconsistent history/physical examination (i.e., the history does not adequately explain the severity and/or nature of the physical injuries)

Retinal hemorrhages

Parental risk factors
    Alcohol or drug abuse
    Previous social service intervention within the family
    History of child abuse

Data from Goldstein et al.[8,19]

When compared with an age and admitting diagnosis matched control group, further analysis found the combination of parental risk factors and either retinal hemorrhage or an inconsistent history/physical examination to be 100% predictive of underlying child abuse.[8,19]

Diagnostic and Laboratory Evaluation

Skull radiographs, CT scan, and MRI are useful diagnostic imaging techniques for delineating the location of skull and brain injury in cases of nonaccidental head trauma. Skull radiographs may reveal linear or depressed fractures. In cases in which the fracture line crosses the area of the middle meningeal artery, an epidural hematoma should always be suspected in the patient with an abnormal neurologic examination. Dramatic linear skull fractures may occur with relatively minor falls but only rarely result in significant neurologic dysfunction.[43]

All infants and children with suspected intracranial injury due to inflicted trauma must undergo cranial CT scan and/or MRI.[62] The CT scan is the most readily available method of detecting underlying brain injury in cases of nonaccidental head trauma. Radiologic studies have demonstrated that the most common CT finding in victims of abuse is a parafalcine subdural hematoma in the parietal or occipital region (Fig. 61-2).[63] The presence of a subdural hematoma in the posterior interhemispheric region in the absence of a history of significant accidental trauma is considered pathognomonic of severe child abuse.[16]

MRI provides exquisite resolution of brain anatomy (Fig. 61-3). MRI has been used to detect hemorrhage when the CT scan is nonrevealing.[15,62] MRI shows chronic subdural hematomas as proteinaceous collections with variable high signal intensity (T1-weighted images [T1WI]) when CT scan may fail to differentiate old collections of blood products from cerebral spinal fluid (CSF)

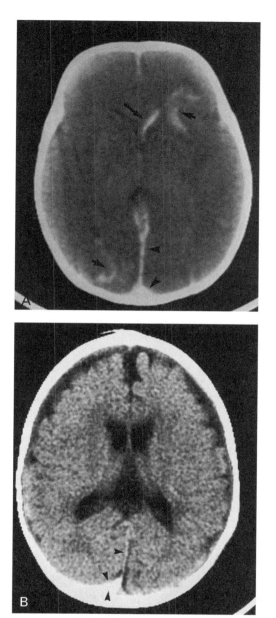

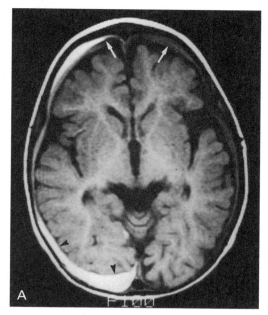

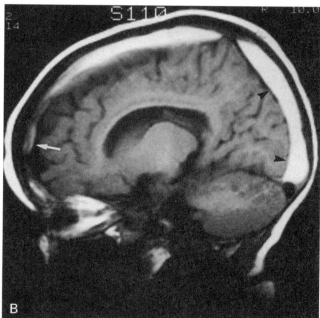

Figure 61-2. CT findings in nonaccidental head injury. Parts **A** and **B** are from different patients. **(A)** Head CT scan demonstrating subarachnoid hemorrhage, intraparenchymal hemorrhage *(small arrows)*, cerebral edema with diminished ventricular size, intraventricular hemorrhage *(large arrow)*, and posterior interhemispheric subdural hematoma *(arrowheads)* in a 4-month-old victim of child abuse. **(B)** Axial CT scan showing small right parafalcine-parietal occipital subdural hematoma in a 9-month-old infant following nonaccidental head injury.

Figure 61-3. MRI studies in shaken impact syndrome (same patient as in Fig. 61-2B). **(A)** Axial T1 (TR/TE = 600/20 msec)-weighted image demonstrates bilateral extraaxial fluid collections not demonstrated well on CT scan. The right side is hyperintense on T1 sequence *(arrowheads)*, and they both follow the calvarial topology. The hyperintensity is due to high methemoglobin concentration and is seen in subacute and chronic subdural hematomas. There is a neomembrane *(white arrows)* more prominent on the right side. The neomembrane having extensive collagen content with a few mobile protons is hypointense on both T1- and T2-weighted images. **(B)** Sagittal T1-weighted image shows high signal intensity methemoglobin in subdural hematomas over the frontal *(white arrow)*, parietal, and occipital *(arrowheads)* lobes.

or other fluid-filled spaces. MRI reveals late changes that occur after trauma as subacute cortical hemorrhagic contusions seen as cortical ribbons of high signal intensity methemoglobin.[15] Methemoglobin is formed approximately 3 days after clot formation as oxidation of deoxyhemoglobin to methemoglobin occurs. Methemoglobin initially appears intracellularly as an area of hypointensity. Approximately 1 week after bleeding, methemoglobin then appears as a high-intensity (T1WI) extracellular signal on MRI. MRI may detect altered regions of tissue water such as occur in areas of infarction

and edema. Thus, MRI is useful in detecting traumatic hematomas of varying age, as well as brain ischemia or edema.[15,62]

Laboratory investigation should include a complete blood count, platelet count, and coagulation profile to rule out underlying bleeding disorders. Urine and serum is sent for toxicology screen to evaluate for poisoning, either accidental or nonaccidental. Electrolytes, blood glucose, and renal and liver function tests should be evaluated to rule out other causes of coma, such as renal failure, hepatic encephalopathy, or Reye's syndrome. Although severe physical abuse is not frequently associated with sexual abuse, a thorough examination and appropriate cultures for venereal disease should be obtained.

Photographic documentation of significant physical findings, such as bruises, lacerations, or burns, is an important part of the evaluation for child abuse and may be crucial in a court of law.[64] Medical or forensic photographers from the hospital or police department should be consulted when available. If these professionals are unavailable, then high-quality photographs may be taken by following published guidelines.[64]

Thorough postmortem radiologic evaluation along with selected histologic studies may impact on the investigation and prosecution of cases of fatal child abuse.[51,65] Figure 61-4 demonstrates the metaphyseal injury not appreciated by routine skeletal survey but clearly demonstrated with high-contrast radiography.

Management

Pediatric Intensive Care Unit Management

The medical management of the severely abused child is no different than that of other critically ill or injured children. Immediate attention must be focused on providing the ABCs of resuscitation — airway, breathing, and circulation. In the case of intracranial injury, given current therapy and knowledge, nothing can be done about the primary neuronal injury already suffered. Therapy must be focused at preventing further secondary injury to the brain as a result of hypoxemia, hypotension, and increased ICP. Because the cerebral circulation may lose the ability to normally autoregulate following traumatic injury,[66] tracheal intubation, hyperventilation, and fluid resuscitation should be initiated when clinically indicated. If the patient presents in status epilepticus, therapy aimed

at controlling the seizures must be instituted. In the severely burned child, initial therapy must be focused around restoring fluid losses and maintaining an adequate circulation.

Once the initial evaluation and resuscitation are accomplished, further evaluation, including a detailed physical examination and diagnostic tests such as CT scan, MRI, and skull, neck, and long-bone radiographs, may be obtained. In patients with an abnormal neurologic examination, serial neurologic evaluations, including the Glasgow Coma Scale and its modification for infants,[67,68] are crucial for optimal care, because the neurologic picture may change rapidly in the presence of an enlarging subdural or intraparenchymal hemorrhage. If necessary, the patient is taken to the operating room for craniotomy, laparotomy, or burn care.

Further specific therapies are discussed in detail in the chapters Cardiopulmonary Resuscitation (by Todres, O'Malley, and Kleinman), Head Trauma (by Swearingen), Status Epilepticus (by Krishnamoorthy), and Burns and Smoke Inhalation (by Briggs).

Psychosocial Assessment and Medicolegal Aspects of Severe Child Abuse

Once the patient has been stabilized and transferred to the PICU, a detailed history may be obtained. It is not until this point that the underlying diagnosis of child abuse or neglect may surface. The psychosocial assessment and reporting of child abuse and neglect are a critical component to the overall care of the child admitted with unexplained or suspicious injuries. A thorough social assessment will help determine whether there is reasonable cause to believe that the child has suffered from abuse or neglect. The more information gathered from a number of sources and perspectives, the greater the likelihood an appropriate determination will be made. A multidisciplinary approach toward obtaining a thorough history and dealing with the family must be followed. This includes an evaluation by the physician, nurse, and clinical social worker.

The importance of the psychosocial assessment and the willingness to document and report suspected cases of abuse and neglect are underscored by the fact that every state has mandated verbal

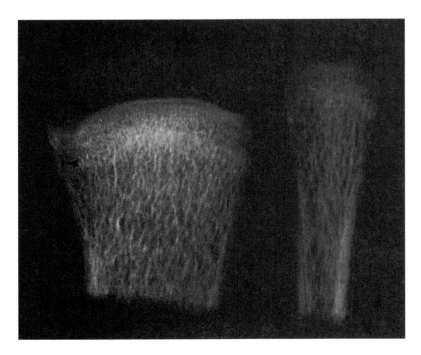

Figure 61-4. High-contrast radiograph obtained postmortem in an 11-week-old victim of shaken infant syndrome shows a metaphyseal injury *(arrowhead)* not appreciated on routine skeletal survey. (Courtesy Dr. Paul K. Kleinman, Department of Radiology, University of Massachusetts Medical School, Worcester, MA.)

and written reporting procedures. Hospital professionals must, by law, report to social service agencies and/or police departments whenever abuse or neglect is suspected.[69] The district attorney's office, in most states, needs to be notified in the event of serious physical abuse, sexual abuse, or death. Immunity from any civil or criminal action by reason of such report is offered to all mandated reporters. Nonmandated reporters may file anonymously.

These laws are particularly important to staff in a pediatric intensive care setting because they remove the burden of investigating and substantiating suspected cases of child abuse or neglect from hospital personnel to a social service agency with representatives trained and legally authorized to make professional evaluations and decisions in these areas. As a result, the hospital staff can focus their attention on the medical management of the acutely ill child.

When it has been determined that there is reasonable cause to believe that child abuse or neglect has taken place, the health care team's primary responsibility is to intervene and protect the child.[70] Whether to hospitalize a child at risk while the investigation for child abuse or neglect is conducted is usually not debated when the child's needs require admission to an ICU. The acuity of the medical problem supersedes resistance on the part of the family or caretaker, and permission for treatment is usually granted. In the rare instance when a parent or guardian threatens to remove the child from the hospital against medical advice, an emergency court order may be obtained, authorizing the hospital to hold the child in custody until a hearing can be held regarding the child's care and protection. The process for obtaining such emergency measures varies by state and institution but is generally obtained by the hospital lawyer.

A growing number of hospitals have established interdisciplinary child abuse teams knowledgeable about clinical and legal issues pertaining to child abuse and neglect, as well as institutional and state policies.[71] The role of these teams is to consult with the primary caretakers to define the diagnosis, management, and treatment needs of suspected causes of abuse and neglect. The disciplines involved may vary from one institution to another but usually include an attorney, a nurse practitioner, a pediatrician, and a social worker, who often serves as the team coordinator.

Multiagency child death review teams exist at the state and/or local level in more than 40 states.[72] The Maternal and Child Health Bureau has recommended implementation of child death review teams in all 50 states, with formation of a national team to provide leadership. The primary goal of these teams is to prevent childhood fatalities, but they also serve to identify fatalities related to child abuse and/or neglect. The effectiveness and clinical relevance of these programs have been clearly demonstrated.[73]

Repeat abuse occurs in more than 20% of all children and often leads to permanent injury or death.[27,74] Psychological help for the child and family members is important. County and state child protective services and the courts will decide on a safe environment for the child. Occasionally, the child may return to the home. Placement of the child in a safe environment outside the home may occur as a result of medical, social, and legal investigation and assessment. Close follow-up care, both medically and socially, are important components of the child's long-term management.

Outcome

Outcome from severe cases of child abuse and neglect is related to the patient's underlying diagnosis and severity of injury. In terms of survival, child abuse is the leading cause of death in children less than 1 year of age. Mortality in severe cases of abuse ranges from 22% to 36%.[8,13,19,38,39] Outcome of out-of-hospital pediatric cardiopulmonary arrests, regardless of etiology, remains grave, with mortality ranging from 71% to 93%.[75–77]

The immediate and delayed outcome in cases of head injury from child abuse is worse than any other type of head injury in childhood.[15,19] Seizures, developmental delay, motor disabilities, visual impairment, or disfigurement and contracture deformities secondary to burns are some of the more common sequelae in survivors of severe child abuse and neglect. Table 61-5 lists the neurologic sequelae found in survivors of severe child abuse and neglect admitted to the Massachusetts General Hospital PICU between 1986 and 1989.

Very little information is available concerning social service intervention and legal actions taken in cases of severe child abuse and neglect.[38,47,78–80] Kempe et al.[47] reported legal action in only 33% of abuse cases. Lavaud et al.[38] reported social service intervention or legal action in 45% of cases; seven cases resulted in foster care or adoption, and three cases led to legal proceedings. Successful social service and legal interventions following severe child abuse and neglect are a result of thorough documentation of the patient's history and physical examination (including quotes from caretakers and photographs of bruises, burns, and retinal hemorrhages), prompt consultation with the clinical social worker, and obtaining appropriate radiographic and histologic evidence of abuse. Ultimately, the willingness of physicians and nursing staff will determine the success of social service and legal actions. Previous studies have found physicians reluctant or remiss in reporting child abuse and neglect.[81,82] PICU personnel are increasingly required to identify victims of severe child abuse and neglect and institute appropriate treatment for both patients and their families.

The most effective means of dealing with child abuse and neglect is prevention. Increased awareness of the scope of the problem and improved educational and social programs are required if we are to prevent children from becoming victims of abuse and neglect.

Summary

Child abuse and neglect may be an unidentified, underlying diagnosis in some of the most common causes for admission to the PICU, such as accidental trauma, falls, seizures, apnea, drowning, burns, and near-miss SIDS. Subdural hematoma, a history inconsistent with the physical examination, or retinal hemorrhages should alert the physician to the presence of underlying abuse or neglect. Thorough documentation of history, physical findings, radiographic studies, and specialized postmortem evaluations are invaluable in substantiating cases of abuse and neglect and will likely result in appropriate social service or legal intervention. A

Table 61-5. Neurologic sequelae in survivors of severe child abuse

Seizures
Hemiparesis
Neurodevelopmental deficit (mild to severe)
Cortical blindness/retinal injury
Persistent vegetative state

history inconsistent with the physical signs and symptoms should prompt physicians to immediately consider a diagnosis of child abuse and neglect in any child admitted to the PICU. Prevention is the final answer to the growing problem of child abuse and neglect.

Acknowledgment

The authors wish to thank Peggy Hamblin, Mai Britt, and Leena M. Ketonen, MD, for their assistance in the preparation of this manuscript.

References

1. Robert Wood Johnson Foundation. *Special Report—Child Abuse.* Princeton, NJ, 1977. P 9.
2. Sedlak AJ. *Study of National Incidence and Prevalence of Child Abuse and Neglect: Final Report.* Rockville, MD: Westat, 1987.
3. Heins M. The "battered child syndrome." *JAMA* 251:3295, 1984.
4. National Center on Child Abuse and Neglect. Executive summary: National study of the incidence and severity of child abuse and neglect. Washington DC: Government Printing Office, 1981 (DHHS publication No.[OHDS]81-30329).
5. Waller RI, Baker SP, Szocka, A. Childhood injury deaths: National analysis and geographic variations. *Am J Public Health* 79:310, 1989.
6. Ewigman B, Kivlahan C. Child maltreatment fatalities. *Pediatr Ann* 18:476, 1989.
7. Krugman RD. Advances and retreats in the protection of children. *N Engl J Med* 320:531, 1989.
8. Goldstein B et al. Child abuse and neglect in the pediatric intensive care unit: Clinical presentation and predictive risk factors. *Ped Crit Care Colloquium* 137, 1989[abstract].
8a. Goldstein B et al. Presentation and risk factors of child abuse and neglect in critically ill children. *Clin Intensive Care* 2:266–269, 1991.
9. Thibault LE, Genarelli TA. Biomechanics of diffuse brain injury. In Proceedings of the Fourth Experimental Safety Vehicle Conference. New York, American Association of Automotive Engineers, 1985.
10. Calder IM, Hill I, Scholtz CL. Primary brain trauma in non-accidental injury. *J Clin Pathol* 37:1095, 1984.
11. Caffey J. On the theory and practice of shaking infants. *Am J Dis Child* 124:161, 1972.
12. Caffey J. The whiplash shaken infant syndrome: Manual shaking by the extremities with whiplash-induced intracranial and intraocular bleedings, linked with permanent brain damage and mental retardation. *Pediatrics* 54:396, 1974.
13. Duhaime AC et al. The shaken baby syndrome: A clinical, pathological, and biomechanical study. *J Neurosurg* 66:409, 1987.
14. Genarelli TA, Thibault LE. Biomechanics of head injury. In Wilkins RH, Rengachary SS (eds): *Neurosurgery.* New York: McGraw-Hill, 1985. P 1531.
15. Bruce DA, Zimmerman RA. Shaken impact syndrome. *Pediatr Ann* 18:482, 1989.
16. Bruce DA. The shaken and impacted baby. *Child Abuse Negl* 4:13, 1988.
17. Alexander R et al. Incidence of impact trauma with cranial injuries ascribed to shaking. *Am J Dis Child* 144:724, 1990.
18. Reece RM. Fatal child abuse and sudden infant death syndrome. In Reece RM (ed): *Child Abuse.* Philadelphia: Lea & Febiger, 1994. P 107.
19. Goldstein B et al. Inflicted versus nonaccidental head injury in critically injured children. *Crit Care Med* 21:1328–1332, 1993.
20. Committee on Child Abuse and Neglect. Shaken baby syndrome: Inflicted cerebral trauma. *Pediatrics* 92:872, 1993.
21. Reece RM. Fatal child abuse and sudden infant death syndrome: A critical diagnostic decision. *Pediatrics* 91:423, 1993.
22. Committee on Child Abuse and Neglect. Distinguishing sudden infant death syndrome from child abuse fatalities. *Pediatrics* 94:124, 1994.
23. Committee on Child Abuse and Neglect and Committee on Community Health Services. Investigation and review of unexpected infant and child deaths. *Pediatrics* 92:734, 1993.
24. Billmire ME, Meyers PA. Serious head injury in infants: Accidents or abuse. *Pediatrics* 75:340, 1985.
25. Lyons TJ, Oates RK. Falling out of bed: A relatively benign occurrence. *Pediatrics* 92:125, 1993.
26. Rivara FP et al. Population-based study of fall injuries in children and adolescents resulting in hospitalization or death. *Pediatrics* 92:61, 1993.
27. Kottmeier PK. The battered child. *Pediatr Ann* 16:343, 1987.
28. Reece RM, Grodin MA. Recognition of nonaccidental injury. *Pediatr Clin North Am* 32:41, 1985.
29. Yaster M, Hallen JA. Multiple trauma in the pediatric patient. In Rogers MC (ed): *Textbook of Pediatric Care.* Baltimore: Williams & Wilkins, 1987. P 1312.
30. Eisenbery AB. Retinal hemorrhage in the battered child. *Child Brain* 5:40, 1979.
31. Gilkes MJ. Fundi of battered babies. *Lancet* 2:468, 1967.
32. Kiffney GT. The eye of the "battered child." *Arch Ophthalmol* 72:231, 1964.
33. Freindly DS. Ocular manifestations of child abuse. *Trans Am Acad Ophthalmol Otolaryngol* 75:318, 1971.
34. Kanter RK. Retinal hemorrhage after cardiopulmonary resuscitation or child abuse. *J Pediatr* 108:430, 1986.
35. Rivera FP, Kamitsuka MD, Quan L. Injuries to children younger than one year of age. *Pediatrics* 81:93, 1988.
36. Rao N et al. Autopsy findings in the eyes of fourteen fatally abused children. *Forensic Sci Int* 39:293, 1988.
37. Kramer K, Goldstein B. Retinal hemorrhages following cardiopulmonary resuscitation. *Clin Pediatr* 32:366–368, 1993.
38. Lavaud J, Villey B, Cloup M. Serious cases of battered children: Experience of a multi-service pediatric intensive care department. *Child Abuse Negl* 6:231, 1982.
39. Hauser GJ, Kanda M, Holbrook PR. Child abuse and neglect: Serious cases admitted to the intensive care unit (abstract). *Pediatr Crit Care Colloq* April:81, 1988.
40. Ludwig S, Warman M. Shaken baby syndrome: A review of 20 cases. *Ann Emerg Med* 13:104, 1984.
41. Bergman A, Larson R, Mueller B. Changing spectrum of serious child abuse. *Pediatrics* 77:113, 1986.
42. Kessler DB, New MI. Emerging trends in child abuse and neglect. *Pediatr Ann* 18:471, 1989.
43. Harrwood-Nash DC. Craniocerebral trauma in children. *Curr Probl Diagn Radiol* 3:1, 1973.
44. Starling SP, Holden JR, Jenny C. Abusive head trauma: The relationship of perpetrators to their victims. *Pediatrics* 95:259, 1995.
45. Ayoub C, Pfiefer D. Burns as a manifestation of child abuse and neglect. *Am J Dis Child* 133:910, 1979.
46. Rosenberg NM, Marino D. Frequency of suspected abuse/neglect in burn patients. *Pediatr Emerg Care* 5:219, 1989.
47. Kempe CH et al. The battered child syndrome. *JAMA* 181:17, 1962.
48. Pascoe JM et al. Patterns of skin injury in non-accidental and accidental injury. *Pediatrics* 64:245, 1979.
49. Fontana VJ. The diagnosis of the maltreatment syndrome in children. *Pediatrics* 51:780, 1973.
50. Caffey J. Multiple fractures in the long bones of infants suffering from chronic subdural hematoma. *AJR* 56:163, 1946.
51. Kleinman PK, Marks SC, Blackbourne B. The metaphyseal lesion in abused infants. *AJR* 146:895, 1986.
52. Thomas SA et al. Long-bone fractures in young children: Distinguishing accidental injuries from child abuse. *Pediatrics* 88:471, 1991.
53. Gahagan S, Rimsza ME. Child abuse or osteogenesis imperfecta: How can we tell? *Pediatrics* 88:987, 1991.
54. Meadow R. Suffocation, recurrent apnea, and sudden infant death. *J Pediatr* 17:351, 1990.
55. Berger D. Child abuse simulating "near-miss" sudden infant death syndrome. *J Pediatr* 95:554, 1979.

56. Minford AMB. Child abuse presenting as apparent "near-miss" sudden infant death syndrome. *Br Med J* 282:521, 1981.

57. Meadow R. Munchausen syndrome by proxy. *Arch Dis Child* 52:92, 1982.

58. Meadow R. Fictitious epilepsy. *Lancet* 2:25, 1984.

59. Rosen CL et al. Two siblings with recurrent cardiorespiratory arrest: Munchausen syndrome by proxy or child abuse? *Pediatrics* 71:715, 1983.

60. Peters JM. Criminal prosecution of child abuse: Recent trends. *Pediatr Ann* 18:505, 1989.

61. Mitchell I et al. Apnea and factitious illness (Munchausen syndrome) by proxy. *Pediatrics* 92:810, 1993.

62. American Academy of Pediatrics, Section on Radiology. Diagnostic imaging of child abuse. *Pediatrics* 87:262, 1991.

63. Zimmerman RA et al. Computerized tomography of craniocerebral injury in the abused child. *Radiology* 130:687, 1979.

64. Ricci LR. Photographing the physically abused child. *Am J Dis Child* 145:275, 1991.

65. Kleinman PK et al. Radiologic contributions to the investigation and prosecution of cases of fatal infant abuse. *N Engl J Med* 320:507, 1989.

66. Enevoldser EM, Jensen FT. Autoregulation and CO_2 responses of cerebral blood flow in patients with acute severe head injury. *J Neurosurg* 48:689, 1978.

67. Jennett B et al. Prognosis of patients with severe head injury. *Neurosurgery* 4:283, 1979.

68. Raimondi AJ, Hirschauer J. Head injury in the infant and toddler. *Child Brain* 11:12, 1984.

69. Ballou M. Child physical abuse and crisis. *Topics Acute Care Trauma Rehabil* 2:1, 1987.

70. Litwack K, Sloan M. Physical assessment of abuse. *Topics Acute Care Trauma Rehabil* 2:10, 1987.

71. Singer B, Bourne R. Working with child abuse in a medical setting: The interweaving of law and social work. *Topics Acute Care Trauma Rehabil* 2:17, 1987.

72. Recommendations of the Child Fatality Review Advisory Group, Maternal and Child Health Bureau, USDHHS, 1993.

73. Durfee MJ, Gellert GA, Tilton-Durfee D. Origins and clinical relevance of child death review teams. *JAMA* 267:3172, 1992.

74. Alexander R et al. Serial abuse in children who are shaken. *Am J Dis Child* 144:58–60, 1990.

75. Ludwig S, Kettrick RG, Parker M. Pediatric cardiopulmonary resuscitation: A review of 130 cases. *Emerg Care* 23:71, 1984.

76. Eisenberg M, Bergner L, Hallstrom A. Epidemiology of cardiac arrest and resuscitation in children. *Ann Emerg Med* 12:672, 1983.

77. O'Rourke P. Out-of-hospital cardiac arrest in pediatric patients: Outcome. *Crit Care Med* 12:283, 1984.

78. Isaacs JL. The law and the abused and neglected child. *Pediatrics* 51:783, 1973.

79. Peters JM. Criminal prosecution of child abuse: Recent trends. *Pediatr Ann* 18:505, 1989.

80. Krugman R. Commentary on criminal prosecution in cases of child abuse. *Pediatr Ann* 18:513, 1989.

81. Mindlin RL. Child abuse and neglect: The role of the pediatrician and the Academy. *Pediatrics* 54:393, 1974.

82. Saulsbury FT, Campbell RE. Evaluation of child abuse reporting by physicians. *Am J Dis Child* 139:393, 1985.

I. David Todres

John H. Fugate

Grace T. Clancy

E. Marsha Elixson

62 ▸ The Pediatric Intensive Care Unit: Organization and Management

The success of the pediatric intensive care unit (PICU) will depend greatly on the organizational skills of the staff managing the unit. One could liken it to the performance of an orchestra, wherein the players need to perform in harmony under the leadership of a conductor. Two of the largest sections of this "orchestra" are the medical and nursing personnel. Knaus et al. demonstrated that the success in the PICU depends to a large extent on the cooperation between medicine and nursing staff.[1] Fleischman et al. aptly recognized the child as the central focus of the treatment plan, with collaborative decision making among patient, parents, and professionals.[2]

The Intensive Care Unit

A statement of Guidelines and Levels of Care for PICUs was issued in 1993 by the Committee on Hospital Care and the Pediatric Section of Critical Care Medicine.[3] In addition, much may be learned from the experience in managing adult ICUs.[4] The intensive care environment for critically ill children is a development that has followed adult and neonatal ICUs. The setting provides a physical environment in which the expertise of medicine, nursing, and other support systems are brought to the bedside of the critically ill child to optimize the potential for the child's recovery. The majority of admissions to the PICU are young children, especially under 1 year of age, requiring individuals caring for them to have the specialized technical skills. Concentrating high technological devices (e.g., monitors and mechanical ventilators) with the skilled personnel providing 24-hour-a-day medical and nursing care in a designated area allows for optimal surveillance and management of the child. There is great variation in the size of the units and also in the use of intensive care by children. There is a seasonal variation, with the highest need in winter. Most statistics on bed need, however, do not take this variation in demand into account. Provision must be made for this in terms of bed space **and** medical/nursing support.[5] Proximity or ready access to the laboratory for urgent biochemical evaluations for moment-to-moment control of the critically ill child is essential to the vital functioning of the unit.

The intensive care setting should be designed in such a way that organization is maximized. One aspect of responding to patient needs is recognition that family needs are crucial to the well-being of the child. The ICU should provide adequate space for family waiting and consulting rooms to provide a setting for family and staff to meet under optimal conditions. Conveying information to families in corridors outside the ICU in a hurried manner does not engender a trust relationship that is vital in our role as intensivists.

In providing total care for the child and the family unit in the ICU, many factors come into play. External forces include regulatory agencies defining the requirements of the ICU, and internal forces activate these defined expectations. Crucial to optimizing outcome for the **child and family** is the need to coordinate care efforts in a positive manner through good communication and planning for care, from admission to discharge from the ICU. Although ICU designs will vary and attention to the environment is important, the patient, family, health care team, and support systems are primary considerations.

In a study of the structure and organization of ICUs in the United States, Pollack et al. found substantial diversity.[6] Seventy-nine point six percent of the pediatric ICUs had full-time medical directors, and a pediatric intensivist was available to 73.7% of the units. Physician coverage for 24 hr/d, dedicated only to the PICU, was present in 48.5% of hospitals. Other ICUs providing care for children were present in 30.2% of the hospitals. The average mortality rate was 3% to 5%.

Medical Personnel

Director

Organization of a PICU, with its multidisciplinary input required for the care of the critically ill child, necessitates an individual with overall responsibility for the coordination of care and for the smooth running of the unit. Traditionally, this role is assumed by the medical director of the ICU. This position requires experience in intensive care in order to have the capacity to understand the needs of the unit from the point of view of the patient, family, and staff. It is important that the leader of the unit supports, guides, and motivates the medical and nursing staffs in their respective roles.[7] The director should be responsive to the concerns of all staff and support services while giving strong direction to the unit. Effective leadership requires credibility as a skilled intensivist with a strong presence in the unit.[8] The director should meet regularly with the nurse manager of the unit to coordinate ongoing activities and review issues that require their mutual attention. The director needs to coordinate the activities of the unit—not in isolation but as part of a system of the institution. This requires collaboration with chiefs of services that impact on the ICU and other administration offices that oversee hospital management.[9] The director should meet with consultants and support staff of the ICU to evaluate progress and problems.

Much of the smooth running of the ICU will depend on well-defined protocols established by the director of the unit in collaboration with his colleagues. When the protocols are clear to the staff (both those working full time in the unit **and** those who consult), many of the "problems" that are identified with pediatric intensive care can be eliminated. It is essential that additional stresses from confusion and lack of organization and direction be avoided.

The medical director should lead a team that regularly oversees the workings and policies of the unit and implements changes in policy. Representation on this team should include primarily ICU attendings, pediatric surgeons, nursing staff, ICU fellows (if such program exists), and the chief resident in pediatrics. This core group should also attend to quality improvement issues. Depending on the agenda of the meeting, specific consultants and other members of the health care team are invited to participate (i.e., social service, respiratory therapy, biomedical engineering, infectious disease control, etc.). The medical director should also oversee staff education in the ICU, either personally or by designating a responsible individual. The director should work closely with hospital administration to ensure there is a sound system of budget management of the ICU—no small matter in today's economic times! The medical director should have a designated associate who would ably take on the responsibilities of administrating the ICU in the absence of the director.

Intensivists

The intensivists should work closely with each other to provide continuity of care for the child and family so that there is a consistency of medical management and philosophy when the "baton of responsibility" is passed from one attending to the next. Major differences in the philosophy of medical management leave the medical and nursing staff as well as families confused. When ICU management is prolonged (i.e., weeks to months), it is advisable that the family deal primarily with a single intensivist to cope more effectively with protracted and fluctuating changes in their child's condition. Parents are under great stress when dealing with the life-threatening crisis affecting their child and cannot effectively develop the necessary relationship with an attending physician to cope with these problems if they have to relate to multiple physicians. An identifiable intensivist must be in a position to assume the leadership responsibilities when the director is absent.

Fellows

The medical team may include fellows who are engaged in a formal training program. The fellow's role at the bedside should be clearly defined. Her training is crucial to the future of intensive care practice and therefore she needs to have much of the primary responsibility for the care of the critically ill child. For the unit to run smoothly, it is essential that there is a close working relationship between the intensivist and the fellow to assist in dealing with any difficult issues and provide the teaching and experience required for this purpose. The fellow's responsibilities include both clinical and research and also preparation for future administrative duties that are required of an ICU attending. Training to be an intensivist is an exhilarating experience but also has its dark side. This needs to be appreciated so that the fellow is given the motivation and support necessary to cope with this aspect of her training.[10]

Consultants

In the operation of the ICU, there are frequently multiple consultant teams called on to provide diagnostic and therapeutic care of the critically ill child. They should be readily accessible. These teams of physicians must be aware of the protocols of the unit, and it should be clear who has the primary medical responsibility for the patient and when this changes. The consultant teams must work closely with the primary physician/nurse team. Failure to communicate with the appropriate individuals leads to disjointed care and potentially suboptimal care. Once many teams are involved, the primary intensivist must ensure a smooth coordination of the total care of the child so that the input of the many consultants' selective view of "parts" of the child is integrated into a whole. This dilemma is beautifully illustrated in the following poem.

The Blind Men and the Elephant
　It was six men of Indostan
　To learning much inclined,
　Who went to see the elephant

(Though all of them were blind),
That each by observation
Might satisfy his mind.

The First approached the elephant,
And, happening to fall
Against his broad and sturdy side,
At once began to bawl:
"God bless me! but the elephant
Is nothing but a wall!"

The Second, feeling of the tusk,
Cried: "Ho! what have we here
So very round and smooth and sharp?
To me 'tis mighty clear
This wonder of an elephant
Is very like a spear!"

The Third approached the animal,
And, happening to take
The squirming trunk within his hands,
Thus boldly up and spake:
"I see," quoth he, "the elephant
Is very like a snake!"

The Fourth reached out his eager hand,
And felt about the knee:
"What most this wondrous beast is like
Is mighty plain," quoth he;
"Tis clear enough the elephant
Is very like a tree."

The Fifth, who chanced to touch the ear,
Said: "E'en the blindest man
Can tell what this resembles most;
Deny the fact who can,
This marvel of an elephant
Is very like a fan!"

The Sixth no sooner had begun
About the beast to grope,
Than, seizing on the swinging tail
That fell within his scope,
"I see," quoth he, "the elephant
Is very like a rope!"

And so these men of Indostan
Disputed loud and long,
Each in his own opinion
Exceeding stiff and strong,
Though each was partly in the right,
And all were in the wrong!

So, oft in theologic wars
The disputants, I ween,
Rail on in utter ignorance
Of what each other mean,
And prate about an elephant
Not one of them has seen!
　John Godfrey Saxe

Residents

In academic training centers, residents rotate through the ICU for limited periods, which are based on the American Board of Pediatrics requirements for residency training programs. Guidelines on levels of care for PICUs supported by the Academy of Pediatrics strongly recommend a physician in-house at the senior resident level (i.e., the third year of training) or above in pediatrics or anesthesiology.[3] It is essential that supervision and support be carefully adjusted to the level of experience and ability of the individual resident. The resident should be made to feel a full member of the ICU team. Too often, the resident is overlooked in the decision making and treatment of the child. Teaching at the bedside and didactic conferences should provide the resident with a core curriculum of basic intensive care, especially with a view to stabilizing the critically ill patient for transport to a tertiary ICU.

Students

The student's active participation in patient care will depend on the nature and severity of the child's illness and should be carefully supported and guided by the intensivist at the bedside. The student, by being exposed to this area of medical care, is encouraged to develop an interest in it so that he may have the opportunity to consider a future career in intensive care medicine.[11] Too often, exposure to intensive care comes late, at a stage when the student may well have channeled his thoughts along another specialty track. If this experience is one in which the student is devalued or caused to feel worthless, it should not be surprising that he would turn away from such practice in the future.

Nursing Personnel

Nursing roles have changed over the years, and as Knaus et al. demonstrated, the interaction and coordination of the medical and nursing staff affect the outcome more than the technological equipment or advanced treatments.[1]

Nurse Manager/Head Nurse

The nurse/manager or senior nurse in the unit has evolved into a managerial role rather than one with bedside responsibilities. In some units, the nurse/manager may be expected to take on the larger organizational and administrative role moving her away from the bedside. It should be emphasized that the unit's organization and management is most effective when there is a designated identifiable nurse/manager with experience in the care of critically ill children and who has a heightened sensitivity of technological advances at the bedside, ensuring the very best nursing care while providing for psychological support of the staff required under these stressful conditions. The nurse/manager is a valuable member of the ICU team and should work in concert with the medical director and other interdisciplinary team members. Regular meetings held to deal with specific issues as they arise enhance the smooth, well-coordinated, organized unit that deals with its problems and solves them in a constructive manner.

Advanced Practice Nurse

The advanced practice nurse role has evolved for a specialized nurse, including the clinical nurse specialist and the acute care nurse practitioner, in the PICU. The advanced nurse practitioner, utilizing a holistic approach, is able to integrate education, research, management, consultation, and teaching within this clinical role. The Advanced Nurse Practitioner collaborates with the nurse at the bedside, physicians, and other health care team members to analyze individual patient and family needs and design interventions to meet those needs.[12] The advanced nurse practitioner is helpful in providing a perspective on the critically ill child that incorporates the importance of the primary nursing role and the progress of the child in terms of potential discharge, so

that the discharge is not a sudden, unanticipated, uncoordinated event.

Primary Nurse

The nurse is the primary caretaker at the bedside, working closely with the physician team, and is able to provide much of the compassion and care required in the child's critical illness. The nurse's close collaboration with the family makes him a surrogate for the child. Much is shared between the nurse and the family that is not brought to the attention of the physician. The nurse's input regarding the family dynamics provides valuable information for the intensive care team so that the care given to the child is optimized.

The nurse's bedside care findings and evaluations are incorporated into the physician's management plans on initial daily rounds and "plan for the day." Because the plan for the day for the critically ill child frequently changes, it needs to be constantly reevaluated. It is essential that the physician and nurse team work in harmony with the family to arrive at the appropriate treatment options.

The stressful demands of intensive care on the nursing profession has led to a phenomenon of burnout. Stress is increased on those nurses working with too large a number of critically ill children; fears of committing errors in judgment and management add to the stress. A vicious cycle is set in motion, leading to increased stress and further burnout. It is important to recognize the limits of any one individual working many hours with critically ill children and their families. Prolonged hours on duty at the bedside may lead to exhaustion, frustration, and burnout. It is essential that the medical director of the unit and the nurse/manager identify the nurse-patient ratio needs constantly so that optimal care is provided on a 24-hour basis. This requires that the administration of the hospital recognize the vital importance of supporting this need. Because of fluctuating census, often seasonally related, and thus nursing acuity needs, a system must exist that can draw on a pool of nursing expertise to deal with these periods of increased activity.

Support Personnel

There are numerous support services required in the ICU. Social service will play an important role in advising and supporting the family during this difficult period. Social service will often come to know a great deal about a family, their wishes, history, concerns, and expectations. This knowledge is invaluable to the physician/nurse team, and when incorporated into the care of the child can be most helpful. Once again, this requires cooperative and sensitive communication among all the team members, consultants, and the primary physician/nurse.

Recognizing social service concerns requires that appropriate attention and time be given to this aspect, despite the overwhelming needs to focus on the medical problems. Regular team meetings should be scheduled between the physician, nurse, and social service personnel to coordinate the care and approach to the child so that when there is a family meeting, there is a well-organized and integrated approach to care.

In addition, there are important laboratory, respiratory therapy, and radiologic services, among others, that are required. It is essential that these services are integrated into the overall care of the child, and that the individuals who represent these services are made to feel a part of the overall care plan and are valued for their knowledge and expertise beyond their technical abilities. This gives these individuals a sense of connecting their technological expertise to the human aspect of the care of the child and thus enhances and enriches their own feelings of value and worth to the unit.

Quality Assurance

Quality assurance and improvement is a necessary part of intensive care administration. This includes evaluation of patient care, cost-effectiveness, and staffing operations. The National Joint Practice Commission formulated a model for collaborative practice agreement between nurses and physicians. The model emphasized five essential factors: (1) communication, (2) competence, (3) accountability, (4) trust, and (5) administrative support.[13] The Joint-Commission for the Accreditation of Healthcare Organizations (JCAHO) currently requires evidence of monitoring of quality to address the issues of standards of care. Thus, it has become established practice to develop a quality assurance survey in ICUs to optimize and maximize outcome. The purpose of this venture is to identify issues in pediatric intensive care administration that need to be changed to improve outcome, and to recommend solutions and evaluate these solutions as to their impact on patient care. Committees given this responsibility are multidisciplinary and should include physician and nursing leadership in the unit and representatives from the residents and fellows, as well as head nurses and clinical nurse specialists. In addition, there should be representatives from pharmacy, biomedical engineering, and clinical administration.

Outcome Analysis

Pollack et al. studied the impact of quality-of-care factors in PICU mortality. Sixteen units were studied, representing 5415 admissions and 248 deaths. Analysis of risk-adjusted mortality indicated that the hospital teaching status and presence of a pediatric intensivist were significantly associated with a patient's chance of survival. A post hoc analysis indicated that the higher severity–adjusted mortality in teaching hospitals may be explained by the presence of residents caring for ICU patients.[14]

The development of illness severity scores has evolved to predict the outcome for critically ill patients and thus assist in decision making, for example, administering appropriate intensive care and avoiding useless therapy. Thus, it might be seen to aid in addressing resource allocation needs. Examples of such illness severity scores are, for adults, the Acute Physiology and Chronic Health Evaluation (APACHE I, II, and III) and the Therapeutic Intervention Scoring System (TISS) and, for pediatrics, the Physiology Stability Index (PSI) and the Pediatric Risk of Mortality (PRISM).[15–18] Most often, these scores have been designed to estimate the probability of hospital mortality. Although these scoring systems are highly specific (i.e., prediction of survival), they are not very sensitive, that is, prediction of death is less accurate, making it difficult to identify the individual child who will die. Severity scoring systems, while helpful in predicting outcome in comparable populations of patients, are blunt instruments for individual patients. In a recent study, Atkinson et al. used a modified APACHE II score (organ failure score) in adults to make predictions of individual outcomes.[19] Used prospectively, their algorithm would have indicated the futility of continued intensive care, but at the cost of 1 in 20 patients surviving with reasonable quality of life if intensive care continued. Thus, in clinical practice, the present scoring systems cannot be integrated into our decision making for the patient's management or be employed to facilitate triage decisions.

Future advances in care in the ICU may improve survival of critically ill children, and thus these scoring systems may overpredict mortality. Further development of these scoring systems, especially with regard to assessing morbidity, may prove extremely helpful in the management of ICU patients.

Admissions, Discharges, and Policy

Admissions

Admissions should be well coordinated so that the appropriate individuals who will be caring for the child are informed prior to the patient's arrival. In this way, required equipment and appropriate consultants may be arranged in advance. Failure to communicate appropriately leads to frustration, anger, and resentment, which divert attention from the primary needs of the critically ill child. When admission to the unit is difficult or impossible because of the lack of available beds, alternatives should be sought. This may entail diverting the admission of the child to an alternative intensive care area, such as a postanesthesia care unit, or if necessary, an adjacent institution where a bed is available. Under emergency conditions, to accommodate the critically ill child, this may also entail a reorganization of available space within or adjacent to the pediatric department. At these times, arrangements can be particularly stressful. It is essential that the physician director or designee (i.e., the attending on call) and the nurse manager or designee work together to establish the most effective plan of care. In this way, both medical and nursing groups **share** the responsibility and are mutually supportive.

When the demand for intensive care services exceeds the available resources, a system for distributing the available resources efficiently and equitably must be sought. A recent consensus statement on the triage of critically ill patients by the Society of Critical Care Medicine Ethics Committee was published.[20] It was recommended that patients who are not expected to benefit from intensive care (e.g., those with imminently fatal illnesses or permanent unconsciousness) should not be placed in an ICU.

Discharges

If inappropriately handled, discharges from the unit can be another instance in which further stress and strain are likely to occur with the caretakers and the family. Whenever possible, discharge from the unit should be considered as early as possible in the course of the child's illness, recognizing, of course, that critical illness is a dynamic situation with great uncertainties and unpredictable fluctuations. When discharge planning is possible early on in the illness, however, the time of discharge is carried out as an organized and well-prepared plan that is clearly understood by all and presents no surprises. The smooth discharge from the unit shows that one has considered the child's critical illness not only in the context of the ICU experience but also in the larger framework of the child's overall illness. This is important when one considers that a large number of children presenting to the ICU have an underlying chronic illness for which they are already receiving care and will continue to receive care in the future.

Policy

The policies of the ICU should be available to all in a well-documented manual. These policies need to be constantly reviewed and updated under the guidance of the multidisciplinary committee for quality assurance and protocol. Such documentation provides structure and stability to ICU functioning and is an important resource in disputes that might arise.

It should also be recognized that, as problems arise, there is a responsibility to deal with these problems and bring about resolution. Note that specific situations may be unchangeable and it is therefore necessary to come to terms with them to keep them from becoming a constant source of friction and frustration.

The importance of a well-organized and smoothly run ICU is critical to the care of the child and the family. For the intensivist, the experience can be a most rewarding one, providing a great source of satisfaction and the opportunity to be a true healer.

References

1. Knaus WA et al. An evaluation of outcome from intensive care in major medical centers. *Ann Intern Med* 104:410–418, 1986.
2. Fleischman AR et al. Caring for gravely ill children. *Pediatrics* 94:433–439, 1994.
3. Committee on Hospital Care and Pediatric Section of Critical Care Medicine. Guidelines and levels of care for pediatric intensive care units. *Pediatrics* 92:166–175, 1993.
4. Fein IA. The critical care unit. In search of management. *Crit Care Clin* 9:401–414, 1993.
5. Barry PW, Hocking MD. Pediatric use of intensive care. *Arch Dis Child* 70:391–394, 1994.
6. Pollack MM, Cuerdon TC, Getson PR. Pediatric intensive care units: Results of a national survey. *Crit Care Med* 21:607–614, 1993.
7. Owen AV. Management for doctors: Getting the best from people. *Br Med J* 310:648, 1995.
8. Zimmerman JE et al. Improving intensive care: Observations based on organizational case studies in nine intensive care units: A prospective, multicenter study. *Crit Care Med* 21:1443, 1993.
9. Simpson J. Doctors and management—Why bother? *Br Med J* 309:1505–1508, 1994.
10. Jellinek MS et al. Pediatric intensive care: Confronting the dark side. *Crit Care Med* 21:775–779, 1993.
11. Buchman T et al. Undergraduate education in critical care medicine. *Crit Care Med* 20:1595–1603, 1992.
12. Hamric AB, Spross J. *The Clinical Nurse Specialist in Theory and Practice*. New York: Grune & Stratton, 1983. Pp 40–41.
13. National Joint Practice Commission. *Guidelines for Establishing Joint or Collaborative Practice*. Chicago: The Commission, 1981.
14. Pollack MM et al. Impact of quality-of-care factors on pediatric intensive care unit mortality. *JAMA* 272:941–946, 1994.
15. Knaus WA et al. APACHE—Acute physiology and chronic health evaluation: A physiology based scoring system. *Crit Care Med* 9:591, 1981.
16. Yeh TS et al. Validation of a physiologic stability index for use in critically ill infants and children. *Pediatr Res* 18:445, 1984.
17. Pollack MM, Ruttimann UE, Getson PR. The pediatric risk of mortality (PRISM) score. *Crit Care Med* 16:1110, 1988.
18. Keene AR, Cullen DJ. Therapeutic intervention scoring system, update 1983. *Crit Care Med* 11:1–3, 1983.
19. Atkinson S et al. Identification of futility in intensive care. *Lancet* 344:1203–1206, 1994.
20. Society of Critical Care Medicine Ethics Committee. Consensus statement on the triage of critically ill patients. *JAMA* 271:1200–1203, 1994.

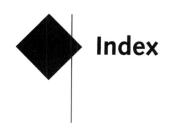

Index

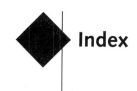

Index